Copy 2

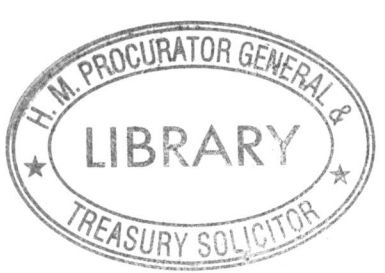

JERVIS
ON THE OFFICE AND DUTIES
OF CORONERS

AUSTRALIA
Lawbrook Co.
Sydney

CANADA and USA
Carswell
Toronto, Ontario

NEW ZEALAND
Bookers
Auckland

SINGAPORE and MALAYSIA
Sweet & Maxwell Asia
Singapore and Kuala Lumpur

JERVIS ON THE OFFICE AND DUTIES OF CORONERS

with Forms and Precedents

THIRTEENTH EDITION

by

PAUL MATTHEWS, B.C.L., LL.D.,
Solicitor-Advocate (Higher Courts: Civil), Withers LLP
H.M. Senior Coroner, The City of London
A Recorder of the County Court
Honorary Professor, King's College London

Consultant Editors

Selena Lynch
Of the Middle Temple, Barrister
H.M. Senior Coroner, South London

Michael J C Burgess, OBE
Solicitor of the Senior Courts of England and Wales (non-practising)
H.M. Assistant Coroner for Surrey, Berkshire, West Sussex, Norfolk
formerly H.M. Coroner for Surrey and of The Queen's Household, and
Hon Secretary to the Coroners' Society of England and Wales

R.N. Palmer, LL.B., M.B, B.S., F.F.F.L.M., Hon.FRC.Path.
Of the Middle Temple, Barrister
H.M. Assistant Coroner, The City of London
Formerly H.M. Senior Coroner, South London

With a Foreword by

The Rt. Hon. Lady Justice Hallett,
A Lady Justice of Appeal

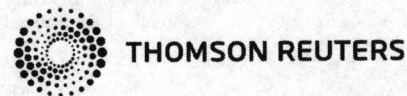

SWEET & MAXWELL   THOMSON REUTERS

First edition (1829)	By Sir John Jervis
Second edition (1854)	By W.N. Welsby
Third edition (1866)	By C.W. Lovesy
Fourth edition (1880)	By R.E. Melsheimer
Fifth edition (1888)	By R.E. Melsheimer
Sixth edition (1898)	By R.E. Melsheimer
Seventh edition (1927)	By F. Danford Thomas
Eighth edition (1946)	By W.B. Purchase
Ninth edition (1957)	By W.B. Purchase and H.W. Wollaston
Tenth edition (1986)	By Paul Matthews and J.C. Foreman
Eleventh edition (1993)	By Paul Matthews and John Foreman
Reprint (1995)	By Paul Matthews and John Foreman
Twelfth edition (2002)	By Paul Matthews
Thirteenth edition (2014)	By Paul Matthews

Published in 2014 by Thomson Reuters (Professional)
UK Limited trading as Sweet & Maxwell,
Friars House, 160 Blackfriars Road, London, SE1 8EZ
(Registered Office and address for service:
2nd floor, Aldgate High Street, London EC3N 1DL)

www.sweetandmaxwell.co.uk

Typeset by Wright and Round Ltd, Gloucestershire
Printed and bound by CPI Group (UK) Ltd, Croydon, CR0 4YY

A catalogue reference for this book is available from the British Library

ISBN 978–1–847–03114–3

FOREWORD

By The Rt Hon. Lady Justice Hallett

My experience of coroners goes back many years. As a young barrister I appeared in inquests representing the interests of the family of the deceased, and as a judge I have been asked to conduct judicial reviews of inquests at first instance and appellate level. One might imagine, therefore, that when I embarked upon the inquests into the deaths of the 52 innocent victims of the 7/7 London bombings I knew something of the system. However, I soon discovered my knowledge was very limited and my task far from straightforward. Coronial law and practice seemed to be a curious mixture of arcane history and obscure legislation, with many inquests conducted in the glare of the media spotlight.

At the time of my appointment as a deputy assistant coroner, I would have very much appreciated a new edition of *Jervis on Coroners*. The 12th edition was already 8 years old, and accompanied by a hefty cumulative supplement. At last, the new 13th edition has arrived. *Jervis* has been rewritten in the light of the significant legislative reforms proposed by *The Luce Report* and *The Shipman Inquiry*, some of which were enacted in the Coroners and Justice Act 2009 and the accompanying secondary legislation, which came into force in July 2013.

I welcome this new edition as a valuable additional resource for all those who play a part in the investigation of deaths in this country, and for judges and lawyers engaged on judicial review of coronial decisions. It is a worthy successor to the earlier editions.

Royal Courts of Justice
July 22, 2014

HEATHER HALLETT

PREFACE

"No man is an Iland, intire of it selfe; every man is a peece of the *Continent*, a part of the *maine*; if a Clod bee washed away by the *Sea*, *Europe* is the lesse, as well as if a *Promontorie* were, as well as if a *Mannor* of thy *friends* or of *thine owne* were; any mans *death* diminishes *me*, because I am involved in *Mankinde*; And therefore never send to know for whom the *bell* tolls; It tolls for *thee"*

John Donne, "Meditation XVII" from *Devotions Upon Emergent Occasions*, 1624

As the poet, lawyer and divine John Donne wrote centuries ago, the death of any member of our society is a significant event, with ramifications for the rest of us. Hence the importance of a system of death investigation. Moreover, it is all too human to want to know why people die, particularly if the cause is not a natural one. In the midst of grief, disruption and the sundering of human relationships, people seek order and explanation, knowledge of the future and, if possible, responsibility for the past, too. The coroner's inquest is the uniquely common law institution designed to provide at least some of this. For more than eight centuries an examination of the evidence, including the body of the deceased and its contents, revealed much about the medical and non-medical causes of the death, and in many cases led to punishment or compensation being awarded in criminal or civil proceedings.

In the twentieth century, however, this under-resourced and often overlooked institution was starved of national leadership and guidance and began to seem threadbare, feeble and barely fit for purpose. Numerous inquiries, some judge-led, looked long and hard into the questions of death investigation and certification, and concluded that radical solutions were called for.

Needless to say, successive governments of all political stripes have ensured that we have not had much in the way of such solutions. That we have achieved any significant reform at all is down to a number of committed reformers who doggedly chipped away at what some people might have called political pro-crastination, penny-pinching and outright obstructionism. Even after what was left of the Reform Bill had passed into law in 2009, there was a rearguard attempt to strip away from it the remaining jewel in the crown, the new national post of Chief Coroner, to be filled by a serving judge. Only a phalanx of ageing peers in the House of Lords saved the day. Glory to them and to the upper house (and not for the first time).

Notwithstanding the welcome survival of the Chief Coroner's office, coroners are still largely a local and not a national service, and different local authorities have different priorities. Some revere their coroners, or at least get on with them. Some don't. In consequence some coroners are resourced well; many, perhaps most, are not. The Chief Coroner has used his considerable "soft" power since his appointment to drive up standards and to make the service more uniform. But there is still a long way to go. It is unfortunately still something of a postcode lottery as to what kind of service you get.

I first became involved with this book some 30 years ago, and this is the fourth edition that I have edited. In the present text nothing remains of the ninth edition of 1957. The book is much longer and more complex than it was back then. This edition sees the light of day some twelve years after its predecessor, largely because of government indecision about introducing new coroner legislation. That is much too long between editions, and the next edition must be sooner rather than later. As always, suggestions for improvement are welcome.

The changes in this edition are many and important. First of all, the whole text has had to be revised, and often rewritten, in the light of the new coroner system introduced by Part I of the Coroners and Justice Act 2009, which came into force in July 2013. Secondly, four new chapters have been included for the first time: Chapter 3 on medical examiners, Chapter 4 on the territorial jurisdiction of coroners, Chapter 6 on the scope of the investigation, and Chapter 7 on information and publicity. To help make room for them, the material on death and forensic medicine from previous editions has been condensed into Appendices 5 and 6 or omitted. Coroners will almost always engage the services of expert pathologists, and the superficial medical knowledge to be gained from the medical chapters in the previous edition can nowadays be obtained from the internet. Reflecting the importance to us nowadays of the internet as a source of information, Appendix 7 gives a list of websites which may be useful to readers. Moreover, many chapters have been expanded, especially Chapter 22 on comparative death investigation law. Finally, the text has had to be revised to accommodate the effects of the ever-expanding case law, particularly the luxuriant jurisprudence of the European Court of Human Rights.

Since the last edition in 2002, two of my then consultant editors, John Burton and Bob Chambers, have died. I learned a huge amount from each. They were coroners very much of the old school, full of wisdom and humanity. I am sure that they would have approved of much of what we have achieved since. The surviving consultant editor, Michael Burgess, has now been joined by Selena Lynch and Roy Palmer. I am very grateful for all their valuable contributions, but it is right to record that, after informing me and enlightening me and sometimes arguing with me, they allowed me to finalise the text as I thought best. As before, I must therefore take full responsibility for it.

I have to thank a lot of other people too. They include Lady Justice Hallett, who despite her myriad commitments found time to contribute a Foreword; the Chief Coroner, with whom I have been fortunate to have many fruitful discussions since he was appointed; and indeed all my fellow coroners for their helpful comments and suggestions over the years. Many lawyers from other jurisdictions helped me with Chapter 22 on death investigation in other systems. They include Kai Bonitz, Jan Dalhuisen, Gordon Dawes, Daniel Feetham, Geoffrey Kertesz, John Leckey, Neil MacLean, Liana Micallef, Irini Nikolaou, Ugo Privitera, Jao Rolim, Clemens Schmölz, Roman Straka and Stefan Wenaweser. It goes without saying that none of them is at all responsible for what I have written. I have to thank the publishers,

Sweet & Maxwell and Thomson Reuters, for all their hard work and profession-alism, which is much appreciated. Lastly, I thank my wife Katie Bradford for her forbearance as once again I locked myself away for months to research and write this edition. I dedicate this edition to her.

A quotation attributed to nineteenth-century Prime Minister William Gladstone runs as follows:

"Show me the manner in which a nation or a community cares for its dead. I will measure exactly the sympathies of its people, their respect for the laws of the land and their loyalty to high ideals."

The coroner system of the English-speaking, common-law world is one way in which we care for our dead, and indeed learn from them. As an old Venetian proverb puts it: "*I morti verze i oci ai vivi.*" (The dead open the eyes of the living). My hope is that this book will continue to assist coroners and those who work with them to carry out their duties effectively and efficiently, and to produce the beneficial results that coroners' investigations are designed to do.

The City of London   PAUL MATTHEWS
July 2014

CONTENTS

PART I

THE OFFICE OF CORONER

CONTENTS

CONTENTS

Chapter 9. Disposal of Human Remains

PART III
THE INQUEST

Chapter 10. The Inquest: Preliminaries

Chapter 11. Procedure at the Inquest: Part I

Chapter 12. Procedure at the Inquest: Part II

Chapter 13. Determination and Record of Inquest

PART IV
SPECIAL CASES

PART V
AFTER THE INQUEST

Chapter 19. Appeals

Chapter 20. Further Proceedings

PART VI

The International Dimension

Chapter 21. Coroners and Human Rights

Chapter 22. Comparative Death Inquiry Law

PART VII

Appendices

TABLE OF CASES

TABLE OF CASES

TABLE OF CASES

li

TABLE OF CASES

TABLE OF STATUTES

NOTE: Bold references indicate that the relevant statutory material has been reproduced in the text

TABLE OF STATUTORY INSTRUMENTS

TABLE OF CIVIL PROCEDURE RULES

TABLE OF PRACTICE DIRECTIONS

TABLE OF NATIONAL LEGISLATION

TABLE OF INTERNATIONAL CONVENTIONS

Part I

THE OFFICE OF CORONER

Chapter 1

GENERAL INTRODUCTION

CONTEXT

This book is about the law and practice relating to certain types of death **1–01** investigation in England and Wales. Every death occurring in our society is considered a significant event, with a number of important consequences. But before these consequences can flow, there is a need to ascertain and record a number of important facts. Who exactly has died? When, where and how did the death occur? The collection of these details for every death underpins the compilation of accurate mortality statistics and will require accurate information of the pathology causing death.

Deaths in England and Wales accordingly are required to be registered with that **1–02** information.[1] The lawful disposal[2] (or removal from the jurisdiction)[3] of the remains of the deceased will involve certification, which differs according to the means of disposal. And if the death was believed not to be "natural", there will be further issues. There may be implications for the criminal[4] or civil[5] law, or lessons for our society, for our health care or other social services, or for how we cope with emergencies.

In most common law jurisdictions, therefore, there is a specialist inquiry into **1–03** what appear to be non-natural deaths, conducted by the coroner.[6] The inquiry is intended first of all to show whether the death was natural or non-natural, and secondly to produce answers to most if not all of the questions which arise in relation to the death and its causes. Many of them raise other issues about different ways of disposing of the dead, about how many public resources should be devoted to this kind of inquiry relative to other objects of public expenditure, and about the harmonisation of standards and procedures throughout Europe and indeed internationally. This book is about the coroner and the coroner's inquiry in

---

[1] See 5–3ff et seq.
[2] See 9–13 et seq.
[3] See 9–36 et seq.
[4] See Ch.14.
[5] See Ch.20.
[6] In most civil law jurisdictions, by contrast, there is no such person, and such inquiries as there may be are conducted as part of the criminal justice system: see Ch.22. This sharply differentiates England and Wales, Northern Ireland, and the Republic of Ireland, on the one hand, and Scotland and the other Member States of the EU, on the other.

England and Wales.[7] It does not cover the rest of the United Kingdom. The coroner system in Northern Ireland is significantly different, and Scotland is a "mixed" legal system, where there are no coroners at all.[8]

EARLY HISTORY[9]

Origins

1–04   The office of coroner is a very ancient one. But no one is quite sure of its origins. There is some evidence that the office of coroner existed before 1194,[10] but it is only because of art.20 of the Articles of Eyre of that year that the office can be conclusively established. The Eyre system was the means by which Royal power (including justice) travelled the whole country in the twelfth century. The Articles of Eyre set out the matters of financial interest to the King in local affairs, almost like a "checklist" for the itinerant justices. Article 20 provided for the election of three knights and clerks by every county as "keepers of the pleas of the Crown": in Latin, *custos placitorum coronae.*

1–05   Later on, grants of the right to a coroner were made by Royal Charter to boroughs, and to local "liberties" or "franchises". The role of all these "keepers of the pleas of the Crown" was to look after the records of cases in which the Crown was interested, and therefore to have regard to the financial interests of the King.

1–06   In considering the significance of the coroner's work it must be remembered that the Crown was interested not only in the due administration of criminal justice, but also in the revenue derived from that administration. This revenue would include the forfeiture of sureties, the seizure of the possessions of felons[11] and the confiscation of deodands,[12] wrecks and treasure trove,[13] and must have

---

[7] In fact there are some small differences in the coroner system between England on the one hand and Wales on the other, but on the whole it is a single system.

[8] See 22–50—22–53.

[9] For a fuller account of the history of the office of coroner, see the Historical Introduction to the 7th edn (1927) of this work, by F.J. Waldo at pp.1–18; more recently, see Ch.10 of the Report of the Committee of Death Certification and Coroners, dated September 22, 1971, Cmnd. 4810, chaired by Mr (later Judge) Norman Brodrick QC; in this work the Committee is referred to as "the Brodrick Committee", and the report as "the Brodrick Report". Chapter 10 is reproduced verbatim in Chs 1 and 2 of Thurston's *Coronership,* 3rd edn, (1985) by Knapman and Powers. The most detailed account in modern times of the early history of coroners is R.F. Hunnisett, *The Medieval Coroner* (1961), but for more recent accounts see McKeogh, *Origins of the Coronial Jurisdiction* (1983) 6 Univ. N.S.W. L.J. 191, and the Ontario Law Commission's *Report on the Law of Coroners* (1995), Ch.2.

[10] See, e.g. *Select Coroners' Rolls* (Selden Society), Vol.9, pp.xv–xix; Holdsworth, *A History of English Law,* Vol.1, pp.82–83; *Halsbury's Law of England,* 5th edn, Vol.24 at [3], fn. 2.

[11] This was only abolished in 1870, by the Forfeiture Act of that year. As to "felon," see fn.18.

[12] "Deodand" was any instrument used to kill a person, found by the coroner's jury to have been so used, and valued by them, which was then forfeit to the Crown, supposedly to be put to "pious uses" by the king's almoner. The law of deodand was abolished in 1846, but only after many persons (such as William Huskisson, the politician, in 1830) had been run over and killed by expensive railway engines, which were then forfeit as "deodand": see, e.g. *R. v Great Western Railway Co* (1842) 3 Q.B. 333; 114 E.R. 533.

[13] See 1–31 below.

been by no means negligible for the Crown in those days. Presumably it was to ensure that the tax collecting duties of coroners were properly carried out that coroners were required to be landed gentry,[14] so that any failure on their part could be made good out of their possessions.

Coroners as judges

During the thirteenth and fourteenth centuries coroners were apparently "the **1–07** principal agents of the Crown in bringing criminals to justice".[15] In addition to the coroner's inquest into violent deaths, the coroner had certain criminal jurisdiction in connection with abjurations,[16] outlawries[17] and accusations of felony,[18] which were called appeals.[19] These latter powers were quite widely used.

Although coroners were not originally intended to act as judges, it seems **1–08** nonetheless that they did sit from time to time as judges in the county court,[20] where they heard cases of felony other than homicide. Rape, burglary and robbery have all been mentioned in old authorities as crimes of violence which came within the coroner's jurisdiction.[21] At a rather lower level of criminal jurisdiction, coroners by virtue of their office were conservators of the peace[22] (as were judges and other officials such as sheriffs). They were responsible locally for preserving the peace before the rise of what are now justices of the peace.

Up until the fifteenth, and possibly sixteenth, century the coroner was a leading **1–09** figure in the county. However, with the decline in the work of the county court (caused in part by the centralisation of justice in the King's courts), and the emergence of, first, escheators and, secondly, keepers (or justices) of the peace, there was a consequential diminution in the work of coroners.[23]

---

[14] See 2–33, and also R.F. Hunnisett, *The Medieval Coroner* (1961), pp.175–176.

[15] *Select Coroners' Rolls* (Selden Society), Vol.9, p.xxiv.

[16] See R.F. Hunnisett, *The Medieval Coroner* (1961), Ch.3. An abjuration involved a confession of felony by a person who had sought sanctuary in a church or other consecrated place, followed by an oath (on the Gospels) to leave England and never return. Unless the sanctuary was a chartered sanctuary (such as an abbey), the felon had only 40 days in which to decide whether to make an abjuration, or to stand trial. If he chose to abjure the realm, the ceremony took place at the churchyard gate, and the coroner presided. On the law of sanctuary generally, see Helmholz, *The Ius Commune in England*, 2001, Ch.1. See also Bennett, *The Pastons and Their England*, 2nd edn (1932), pp.172–175.

[17] Outlawry, the process of declaring a person an outlaw, was originally a kind of punishment involving forfeiture of property and liability to be killed with impunity. However, it developed into a means of assisting the legal process, by compelling a person to stand criminal trial or defend a civil action, or to obey a court order, on pain of being made outlaw if he refused. Outlawry was abolished in civil cases in 1879 and in criminal cases in 1938, although it was obsolete much earlier. See the 7th edn (1927) of this work, at p.251, Stephen, *Digest of the Law of Criminal Procedure* (1883), art.235, and Short and Mellor, *Practice of the Crown Office* (1890), Ch.XIII.

[18] Felony was the more serious of the two kinds of offence, felony and misdemeanour, a distinction which was abolished by the Criminal Law Act 1967. Originally the *victim* of a crime (or his family) had the responsibility of finding the felon and bringing him to justice, and this process was called appeal of felony. The coroner and his jury operated as a form of check on this system.

[19] See R.F. Hunnisett, *The Medieval Coroner* (1961), Ch.4.

[20] This is not the modern county court, a civil court dealing mostly with lower value cases, but an important local criminal and civil court in medieval times before the Royal courts acquired their dominance. See, generally, Palmer, *The County Courts of Medieval England* (1982).

[21] In fact, coroners were one of the classes of officials expressly prohibited from trying criminal cases by the Great Charter (or Magna Carta) of 1215.

[22] See 2–115 below.

[23] See Hunnisett, *The Medieval Coroner* (1961), Ch.10.

1–10   Escheators began to take over the function of the coroner with regard to appraising or valuing and taking possession of lands, chattels and deodands belonging to outlaws, abjurors, suicides or the victims of homicides. This naturally reduced the financial activities of coroners. Coroners also gave up their criminal work other than inquests, for the keepers or justices of the peace took the place of coroners in becoming primarily responsible for maintaining law and order locally. The only important duty that coroners retained was that of holding inquests into cases of violent or unnatural death.[24]

STATUS AND POSITION OF CORONERS

Status of coroners

1–11   Coronership is a public office. There is however no authority for saying that a coroner is a corporation sole.[25] Unlike, say, sheriffs, coroners have never held office directly under a Royal Commission. From 1194 until 1888 county coroners were elected by the freeholders of the county, originally at the county court, pursuant to the King's writ *de coronatore eligendo*, which commanded the sheriff to hold an election.[26]

1–12   In 1888, election by the freeholders was replaced[27] by appointment by the county council, which had long been responsible for payment of the coroner's expenses and remuneration. But this change effected an alteration only in the *electorate* for the office. Writs *de coronatore eligendo* were still issued, but were directed to the county council instead of the sheriff,[28] and a coroner appointed by the county council was in the same position as if he had been elected by the freeholders of the county.[29]

1–13   The need for the writ to issue was abolished as from 1927,[30] but without otherwise affecting the coroner's position. The provision that an appointed coroner should be in the same position as an elected one was not repealed until 1974.[31] It is submitted that this repeal made no difference to his position and that a coroner, though now appointed and paid by a local authority, continued thereafter to hold office under the Crown.[32]

---

[24] For a contemporary account of a seventeenth-century inquest, see Samuel Pepys' *Diary* for January 21, 22 and 30, and February 4 and 18, 1668; and, for a modern account of a nineteenth-century one, see Thurston, *The Clerkenwell Riot* (1967), Chs 7–12. See also Dickens, *Bleak House*, Ch.11, for a fictional one (but no doubt based on Dickens' own experience as a frequent attender of inquests as a journalist).

[25] See *Coulter v Chief Constable of Dorset* [2004] 1 W.L.R. 1425 at [10] (chief constable not corporation sole).

[26] See Dalton, *The Office and Authoritie of Sheriffs* (1623), fol.169; Hunnisett, *The Medieval Coroner* (1961), Ch.9. Borough coroners were however appointed by the borough council.

[27] By the Local Government Act 1888 s.5.

[28] Local Government Act 1888 s.5(1). See the form of the writ in Short and Mellor, *Practice of the Crown Office* (1890), p.727.

[29] Local Government Act 1888 s.5.

[30] Coroners (Amendment) Act 1926 s.2(4).

[31] Local Government Act 1972 s.272(1), Sch.30.

[32] *Resolutions at Sergeants Inn upon the statute 1 Edw. 6, c. 7*, (1555) 2 Dyer 165a, 73 E.R. 359; *R. v Grimshaw* (1874) 2 New Mag. Cases 291; 10 L.T. (O.S.) 171. The Home Office continues to take this view: Home Office Circular No. 49 of 1975.

The Coroners and Justice Act 2009 ("the 2009 Act") has now largely replaced **1–14** the earlier legislation. It declares that the office of coroner is not to be regarded as a freehold office,[33] but is otherwise silent on the question of whether the office is held under the Crown. The *Chief Coroner's Guide to the Coroners and Justice Act 2009* says that "there is some doubt as to whether coroners will any longer be able to call themselves HM Coroner", in part because by virtue of the new Act, "all coroners become creatures of statute".[34]

But it is submitted that the answer is still Yes, as the 2009 Act does not expressly **1–15** or impliedly make any change to the previous position, and coroners have been "creatures of statute" since at least 1887, if not earlier. Indeed, the position is even stronger than before, as the appointment of coroners, previously made by local authorities alone, must henceforth be approved by both a senior minister of the Crown, the Lord Chancellor, and the Chief Coroner.[35] And, as will be seen, the 2009 Act and the rules and regulations made thereunder give to the Lord Chancellor and the Chief Coroner a far more extensive control over what coroners do and how they do it than central government previously enjoyed.

Like other officers of the Crown whose origin goes back to the early days of our **1–16** legal history (such as the Lord Chancellor and justices of the peace), the coroner has other than merely judicial functions. He is another exception to Montesquieu's celebrated, if descriptively inaccurate, doctrine of the separation of powers. He acted in place of the sheriff in certain circumstances until recent times.[36]

During the history of coroners their executive functions, including their duties **1–17** to have regard to the financial interests of the Crown, became steadily less important, and their judicial functions more important. Nonetheless, the office of the coroner today continues to reflect executive as well as judicial characteristics, and this is particularly so in relation to the procedure of the coroner's court.

THE CORONER'S INQUIRY

In 2013, 506,740 deaths were registered in England and Wales, and 227,984 deaths **1–18** were reported to coroners. In that year coroners (operating under both old and new systems) opened 29,942 inquests, representing about 13.1 per cent of all deaths reported to them, and about 5.9 per cent of the number of deaths registered. In the same year they returned verdicts in 31,579 inquests. A coroner's inquest is a rare (but not unique) example of inquisitorial proceedings in England and Wales.[37]

The important distinction between an accusatorial process, such as a criminal **1–19** trial, and an inquisitorial process, such as a coroner's inquest, was stated some 30 years ago by Lord Lane CJ in the following words:

---

[33] Section 23, Sch.3 para.9.
[34] Paragraph 35.
[35] Section 23, Sch.3 para.1(3).
[36] See 2–113—2–114 below.
[37] A notorious example of inquisitorial procedure in the history of English law was the Court of Star Chamber. For a more modern example, see *R. v National Insurance Commissioner Ex p. Viscusi* [1974] 1 W.L.R. 646 at 651.

"Once again it should not be forgotten than an inquest is a fact finding exercise and not a method of apportioning guilt. The procedure and rules of evidence which are suitable for one are unsuitable for the other. In an inquest it should never be forgotten that there are no parties, there is no indictment, there is no prosecution, there is no defence, there is no trial, simply an attempt to establish facts. It is an inquisitorial process, a process of investigation quite unlike a trial where the prosecutor accuses and the accused defends, the judge holding the balance or the ring, whichever metaphor one chooses to use."[38]

1–20   A more modern statement, to the same effect, albeit in the context of inquiries more generally, is that of Sir Richard Scott VC:

"In an inquisitorial Inquiry there are no litigants. There are simply witnesses who have, or may have, knowledge of some of the matters under investigation. The witnesses have no "case" to promote. It is true that they may have an interest in protecting their reputations, and an interest in answering as cogently and comprehensively as possible allegations made against them. But they have no "case" in the adversarial sense. Similarly, there is no "case" against any witnesses. There may be damaging factual evidence given by others which disparages the witness. In these events the witness may need an opportunity to give his own evidence in refutation. But still he is not answering a case against himself in the adversarial sense. He is simply a witness giving his own evidence in circumstances in which he has a personal interest in being believed."[39]

1–21   Similarly, Lord Hutton at the opening of the *Hutton Inquiry into the Death of Dr David Kelly* on August 1, 2003, said:

"It is also important that I should emphasise that this is an Inquiry to be conducted by me—it is not a trial conducted between interested parties who have conflicting cases to advance. I do not sit to decide between conflicting cases—I sit to investigate the circumstances surrounding Dr Kelly's death. I would wish to adopt what was said by Lord Justice Scarman, as he then was, at the start of the Inquiry which he conducted in 1974 into the Red Lion Square disorders. He said:

'This Inquiry is to be conducted—and I stress it—by myself. This means that all the decisions have to be taken by me. Let me indicate now, so that there need to be no misunderstanding, what are the implications of what I have just said. First of all, it is I, and I alone, who will decide what witnesses will be

---

[38] In *R. v South London Coroner Ex p. Thompson* (1982) 126 S.J. 625, DC, cited with approval in (inter alia) *Morris v Dublin Coroner* [2000] 3 I.R. 592; *Eastern Health Board v Dublin City Coroner* [2001] IESC 96; *R. (Khan) v Secretary of State for Health* [2003] EWHC 1414 (Admin); *Re Jordan's Application* [2004] NICA 29(1), 30; *R. (Paul) v Inner West London ADC* [2007] EWCA Civ. 1259; *R. (Lewis) v Mid and North Shropshire Coroner* [2009] EWHC 661 (Admin); *R. (Wilkinson) v South Greater Manchester Coroner* [2012] EWHC 2755 (Admin); *Re C's Application* [2012] NICA 47. See also *R. v Attorney General for Northern Ireland, Ex p. Devine* [1992] 1 W.L.R. 262, HL.
[39] "Procedures at Inquiries: the duty to be fair" (1995) 111 L.Q.R. 596 at 598–599. See also *R. (IPCC) v West Mercia Police* [2007] EWHC 1035 (Admin).

called. I also decide to what matters their evidence will be directed. There is, in an Inquiry of this sort, no legal right to cross-examination—but I propose within limits to allow cross-examination to the extent that I think it helpful to the forwarding of the Inquiry but no further.'

I would also add that it will be for me to decide the order in which the witnesses will be called."

Functions

The functions of an inquest on a dead body at the present day are really to   **1–22**
determine certain facts about the deceased, the cause of death, and the circumstances surrounding both death and that cause. Lord Lane CJ once summarised this
by saying that: "The function of an inquest is to seek out and record as many of the
facts concerning the death as public interest requires".[40]

Subsequently the Court of Appeal held that: **1–23**

"An inquest is a fact-finding inquiry conducted by a coroner, with or without
a jury, to establish reliable answers to four important but limited factual
questions. The first of these relates to the identity of the deceased, the second to
the place of his death, the third to the time of death. In most cases these
questions are not hard to answer but in a minority of cases the answer may be
problematical. The fourth question, and that to which evidence and inquiry are
most often and most closely directed, relates to how the deceased came by his
death . . . It is noteworthy that the task is not to ascertain how the deceased died,
which might raise general and far-reaching issues, but "how . . . the deceased
came by his death", a more limited question directed to the means by which the
deceased came by his death".[41]

Again, in the same case,   **1–24**

"It is not the function of a coroner or his jury to determine, or appear to
determine, any question of criminal or civil liability, to apportion guilt or
attribute blame."[42]

These passages have been cited and followed in later decisions.[43] In one such case   **1–25**
the court observed:

"It is of critical importance to recognise the true purpose of an inquest. Sadly,
the public's perception of such purpose does not always match the reality, and

---

[40] *R. v South London Coroner, Ex p. Thompson* (1982) 126 S.J. 625, DC.
[41] *R. v North Humberside Coroner, Ex p. Jamieson* [1995] 1 Q.B. 1, 23–24, CA.
[42] *R. v North Humberside Coroner, Ex p. Jamieson* [1995] 1 Q.B. 1, 24.
[43] *Re Ministry of Defence's Application* [1994] N.I. 279, CA (NI); *Hay v Devon Coroner* (1997) 162 J.P. 96, CA; *R. v Birmingham and Solihull Coroner, Ex p. Benton* (1997) 162 J.P. 807; *Re Bradley's Application* Unreported August 29, 1996, HC (NI); *Re Palmer's Application* Unreported December 10, 1997, CA; *Mullholland v Coroner for St Pancras* [2003] EWHC 2612 (Admin).

those caught up in the process expect more . . . than it can, or is permitted to, deliver thereby adding to their distress."[44]

1–26   The Brodrick Committee[45] exhaustively considered the role of the coroner's inquest in modern society. The committee identified the following grounds of public interest which they believed that a coroner's inquiry should serve:

"(i)   To determine the medical cause of death[46];

(ii)   To allay rumours or suspicion[47];

(iii) To draw attention to the existence of circumstances which, if unremedied, might lead to further deaths;

(iv)   To advance medical knowledge;

(v)   To preserve the legal interests of the deceased's person's family, heirs or other interested parties."

1–27   However, hitherto it has not been the function of coroner's inquest to provide a forum for attempts to gather evidence for pending or future criminal or civil proceedings.[48] Nor has it hitherto been its purpose

"to identify individual fault on the part of those involved. On the contrary it is expressly not concerned with that question. It is much more important that it identifies any deficiencies of the system and ensures that steps are recommended to deal with those deficiencies."[49]

A suggestion[50] that the European Convention on Human Rights[51] should compel a different view, and enable inquests to determine responsibility, has not so far achieved general acceptance.[52]

1–28   Until 1977, it was the specific duty of a coroner's jury in any case where they found that the deceased had died through murder, manslaughter or infanticide, to state in the verdict the name of the person or persons considered to have committed the offence, or of being accessories before the fact.[53] In such a case, the inquisition (the formal document setting out the verdict) would have the same

---

[44] *R. v Birmingham Coroner, Ex p. Benton* (1997) 162 J.P. 807; [1997] 8 Med. L.R. 362.

[45] See fn.9, above. The grounds of public interest cited were quoted with approval by the the Divisional Court in *R. v East Sussex Coroner, ex p. Homberg* (1994) 158 JP 357, the Court of Appeal in *R. v North Humberside Coroner, ex p. Jamieson* [1995] QB 1, and the Irish Supreme Court in *Morris v Dublin City Coroner* [2000] 3 I.R. 603.

[46] cf. *R. v Southwark Coroner, Ex p. Hicks* [1987] 1 W.L.R. 1624; *R. v South Glamorgan Coroner, Ex p. Basoodeo Sujeeum* [1993] C.O.D. 366, DC.

[47] cf. *R. v Greater Manchester Coroner, Ex p. Tal* [1985] Q.B. 67 at 83.

[48] *R. v Poplar Coroner's Court, Ex p. Thomas* [1993] Q.B. 610 at 629, per Dillon LJ.

[49] *Re Clegg* (1996) 161 J.P. 521 at 530; on the last point the Court appears to have overlooked the fact that the coroner's inquest not only has no power to make recommendations to deal with any deficiencies, but is specifically prohibited from doing so: see 6–02, 12–110, 13–111ff below.

[50] Sir Stephen Sedley in *Keenan v United Kingdom* Unreported April 3, 2001, para.9.

[51] See generally Ch.21 below.

[52] Though see *R. (Amin) v Home Secretary, R. (Middleton) v West Somerset Coroner* [2002] 3 W.L.R. 505, CA, reversed by the House of Lords [2004] UKHL 10 (*Middleton*) and [2003] UKHL 51 (*Amin*); and see further 6–02, 13–103ff below.

[53] See the Coroners Act 1887 s. 4, as amended by the Coroners (Amendment) Act 1926.

effect as a bill of indictment committing the person or persons named to trial at what were originally called the Courts of Assize, and later Crown Courts.[54]

The power of the coroner's jury to commit a person for murder, manslaughter **1–29** or infanticide went back to the days when coroners were first established and before there were police forces or a fully established judicial system. It resembled—and was functionally equivalent to—that of the Grand Jury in criminal cases.[55]

The continuance of this power was widely regarded as anomalous, and it was **1–30** recommended that it be abolished, first by the Departmental Committee on Coroners chaired by Lord Wright in 1935, and second by the Brodrick Report in 1971.[56] This recommendation was finally carried into effect in 1977,[57] but only after a coroner's jury had, in June 1975, named Lord Lucan as the murderer of his children's nanny.[58] Effectively, the coroner's role in the criminal justice system has now gone, but, as we shall see,[59] there are often circumstances where both systems are called into play in relation to the same facts.[60] Moreover, English judges persist in treating coroners as if they continue to play a role in the criminal justice system.[61]

OTHER FUNCTIONS

Treasure and fires

The coroner continues to have one subsidiary function. This is to inquire into cases **1–31** of suspected treasure that is found (formerly "treasure trove").[62] This function is not only an anachronism, but is also almost useless, since the inquest's verdict that the articles in question do or do not constitute treasure, or indeed any other facts which are found, are not conclusive as against any person and an action may thereafter be brought to try any such issue.[63] The only value of the coronial inquiry is that in some cases a reward may be given on the basis of the decision.[64]

The coroner for the City of London used to have jurisdiction, by virtue of a **1–32** local Act,[65] to inquire into the cause of fires in the City of London. The jury's verdict could be one of arson against a person or persons, and then the verdict and inquisition would have the force and effect of an indictment upon which such

---

[54] See, e.g. *R. v Rogers* (1531–33) Spelm. 52 (error in Latin inquisition: inquisition quashed, accused set free).

[55] *R. v Davies*, *The Times*, March 18, 1890, per Wills J, reprinted in the 7th edn (1927) of this work, pp.254–256, the 8th edn (1946), pp.296–298, and the 9th edn (1957), pp.508–510.

[56] Cmnd. 4810; see fn.9 above.

[57] Criminal Law Act 1977 ss.56 and 65; Coroners Act 1988 s.11(6).

[58] See, e.g. Marnham, *Trail of Havoc* (1987), Ch.5.

[59] See 10–73ff below, dealing with the need to adjourn an inquest where criminal proceedings are pending.

[60] See also Wells, "Inquests, Inquiries and Indictments" (1991) 11 Leg. Stud. 71.

[61] See 12–74.

[62] Coroners Act 1988 s.30; Treasure Act 1996; Coroners and Justice Act 2009 ss.25–31 and Sch.4 (not yet in force); see Ch.16 below.

[63] See 16–52, 16–61, 20–02 below.

[64] See 16–54.

[65] City of London Fire Inquests Act 1888 (repealed).

person or persons could be tried at the Central Criminal Court. This jurisdiction has been abolished.[66]

1–33   A similar jurisdiction to inquire into the cause of non-fatal fires had been claimed by some provincial coroners prior to 1860,[67] but in that year it was held that no such jurisdiction existed.[68] If and so far as the coroner's court retained (if it ever had) jurisdiction to hold inquests on non-fatal felonies, into wrecks, and into Fish Royal[69] (which was in any case doubtful),[70] all such jurisdiction was abolished in 1887.[71]

Other inquiries

1–34   Coroners' investigations are not the only means at the present day of inquiring into the circumstances or causes of deaths. There are a number of other types of inquiry required by statute, for example where there is a civil aviation accident,[72] or an accident on board ship or involving a ship,[73] or a death of a person subject to service (i.e. military) law.[74] Moreover, a statutory framework for other ad hoc inquiries is provided by statute.[75] Additionally there are judicial inquiries, where a senior judge holds an inquiry into a certain matter, usually a disaster or *cause célèbre*, although these are often conducted in a far more adversarial manner than inquests.

1–35   As with criminal proceedings, there used often to be a conflict between the coroner system and the judicial system as to which should be held first, and as to how to avoid prejudicing the other.[76] But the matter is now regulated by statute.[77] The very fact of the existence of such statutory inquiries was evidence of the perceived inadequacies of the coroner's investigation, and, in considering possible future development and reforms of the coroner system, statutory inquiries have provided many helpful comparative features.[78]

---

[66] Criminal Law Act 1977 s.56(4). A similar jurisdiction survives in some Australian states.

[67] See the 7th edn (1927) of this work, at p.252. In the 1st edn (1829) at p.34, and 2nd edn (1854) at p.44, it was recorded that in some parts of the country coroners by custom could and did inquire into other felonies.

[68] *R. v Herford* (1860) 3 E. & E. 115; see the Coroners Act 1887 s.44.

[69] Meaning whales and sturgeons: not a common subject in modern treatises, but see *Constable's case* (1601) 5 Co. Rep. 1086; and also A. P. Herbert, *"Tinrib, Rumble and Others v The King and Queen"*, in *Uncommon Law* 7, and *Halsbury's Laws of England*, 4th edn Reissue, Vol.12(1), para.229.

[70] See Hunnisett, *The Medieval Coroner*, Ch.1; cf. Grindon, *Law of Coroners* (1850), p.19, and Wellington, *The King's Coroner* (1905), Vol.I, p.6.

[71] Coroners Act 1887 s.44.

[72] See 15–38 below.

[73] Merchant Shipping (Accident Reporting and Investigation) Regulations 2012 (SI 2012/1743) (replacing the Merchant Shipping (Accident Reporting and Investigation) Regulations 1995). For a comparison between an inquest and an inquiry under the Merchant Shipping Act 1970 s.61, see *R. v East Sussex Coroner, Ex p. Healy* [1988] 1 W.L.R. 1194, DC.

[74] Armed Forces Act 2006 s.343; Armed Forces (Service Inquiries) Regulations 2008 (SI 2008/1651).

[75] Inquiries Act 2005; see also 15–38.

[76] See e.g. Wells, "Inquests, Inquiries and Indictments" (1991) 11 Leg. Stud. 71.

[77] See 10–73ff below.

[78] For a dispute about holding a statutory inquiry where an inquest would be inadequate, see *R. (Litvinenko) v Home Secretary* [2014] EWHC 194 (Admin), DC.

RELATIONS WITH CENTRAL GOVERNMENT

Although coroners in England and Wales are appointed by local authorities,[79] albeit **1–36** with the approval of the Lord Chancellor and the Chief Coroner, they are independent judicial officers,[80] not subject to local or central government control. The Lord Chancellor had and has power (formerly with the concurrence of the Home Secretary, now with that of the Lord Chief Justice) to make rules governing the practice and procedure of coroner's inquiries,[81] and also had and now has (with the Lord Chief Justice) certain powers to remove coroners from office.[82] But in law the Ministry of Justice (formerly the Department for Constitutional Affairs, and before that the Lord Chancellor's Department) has no *operational* responsibility for coronial affairs, though it sometimes acts as if it did.

Formerly, the central government department which operated as a liaison **1–37** between coroners and government was the Home Office. Since the Home Office was also responsible for prisons, police and immigration, and many controversial inquests arise out of deaths in prison, police custody and immigration centres, coroners were formerly put in a difficult position, where they were seen—however unwittingly—as an arm of central government. But now it is the Ministry of Justice which has the strategic responsibility for coroners' affairs.[83]

Review of coroners' systems

In recent years a number of common law jurisdictions have carried out a review **1–38** of their coroners' systems, all ultimately derived from the English system. These include Ontario,[84] New Zealand[85] and the Republic of Ireland.[86] In 2001 the Home Office announced a fundamental review of the English system, chaired by a retired civil servant, which reported in 2003 (the "Luce Report"). In addition, a public judicial inquiry began in February 2001 into issues arising out of the conviction in January 2000 of Dr Harold Shipman for the murders of some of his patients. This inquiry dealt (inter alia) with death and cremation certification, including the role of the coroner, and also reported in 2003.[87] Both reports recommended a national coroner system, under the guidance of a Chief Coroner.

In 2004 the Home Office published a position paper on these reports. In May **1–39** 2005 the responsibility of the Home Office for coroner matters was transferred to the Department of Constitutional Affairs, subsequently renamed the Ministry of Justice. In 2006 a draft bill to reform coroner system was prepared, but was never introduced into Parliament. In 2008 a further bill was introduced, covering both

---

[79] Para. 1–13, above, and see 2–23 below.
[80] See Home Office Circular No. 31 of 1982.
[81] See Coroners and Justice Act 2009 s.43; formerly Coroners Act 1988 s.32(1).
[82] See 2–97ff below.
[83] It also has responsibility for prisons, through the National Offender Management Service.
[84] See Ontario Law Reform Commission, *Report on the Law of Coroners*, 1995.
[85] See New Zealand Law Commission, *Preliminary Paper 36,* August 1999; *Report 62,* August 2000.
[86] See Department of Justice, Equality and Law Reform, *Review of the Coroner Service,* December 7, 2000.
[87] See the website at *http://webarchive.nationalarchives.gov.uk/20090808154959/http://www.the-shipman-inquiry.org.uk/reports.asp.* The First Report (dealing with Shipman's victims) was published on July 19, 2002.

coroners and criminal law, and finally was enacted as the Coroners and Justice Act 2009. Part I of this Act was based on the earlier draft bill. Most of Part I was brought into force on July 25, 2013.

THE NEW SYSTEM

1–40   Part I of the Coroners and Justice Act 2009 provides the new legislative basis for most of the coroner system in England and Wales. A primary change relates to nomenclature. For example, the coroner has become the "senior coroner", and the deputy and assistant deputies "assistant coroners", while the coroner's *inquest* of old has become the coroner's *investigation*. The term "inquest" is still to be used, but is now restricted to the part of the investigation that involves a court hearing evidence and reaching a verdict. There are now essentially three stages: (1) pre-investigation inquiries; (2) the investigation; (3) the inquest.

1–41   However, the system is far removed from that recommended by the two reports in 2003. In particular, it is still local rather than national, on financial grounds. In addition, parts of the Act as enacted are not to take effect. Thus, the provisions dealing with a new appeals system, to replace judicial review, have been excised from the Act,[88] and the provisions for a new national coroner for treasure[89] are not to be brought into force, at least for the present, again on financial grounds. One part of the new system which has not yet been brought into force, but was planned to be in late 2014, is that relating to medical examiners.[90]

1–42   Provision was made in the Act however for a chief coroner. The incoming coalition government in 2010 tried to abolish the post before it came into force, on costs grounds. Ultimately that attempt failed, and the introduction of the office of chief coroner therefore represents the most important part of the reforms now brought into force.

1–43   An important limitation on the new coroner system is that, with the exception of the chief coroner's office, there is no new money available. Three important new statutory instruments have been made under the 2009 Act to deal with the conduct of coroners' inquiries. They deal with coroners' investigations,[91] coroners' inquests,[92] and the allowances, fees and expenses that coroners may pay, may be reimbursed, or may charge others.[93]

1–44   The transitional provisions from the old system to the new are unfortunately not as clear as they might be. There are transitional provisions in the 2009 Act relating to existing coronial *appointments*,[94] so that office-holders are "grandfathered" into the new system. But there are no transitional provisions relevant to pre-existing *inquiries* in the 2009 Act itself, even though the Act confers power to make statutory instruments exercisable so as to make transitional provisions.[95]

---

[88] Section 40 and associated provisions: repealed by the Public Bodies Act 2011 s.33. See 19–01–19–02.

[89] Sections 25 to 31. See 16–20.

[90] Sections 18 to 21. See 3–02.

[91] Coroners (Investigations) Regulations 2013 (SI 2013/1629).

[92] Coroners (Inquests) Rules 2013 (SI 2013/1616).

[93] Coroners Allowances Fees and Expenses Regulations 2013 (SI 2013/1615).

[94] Coroners and Justice Act 2009 s.177, Sch.22, Pt I; see 2–40.

[95] Coroners and Justice Act 2009 s.176(3).

Each of the statutory instruments made dealing with coroners' investigations[96] **1–45** and coroners' inquests[97] contains a transitional provision[98] that the instrument should apply to investigations or inquests not completed before July 25, 2013, *but* that any decision made before July 25, 2013 should stand. In addition, existing legislation requires that the repeal of any legislation should not affect any obligation which has already accrued under that legislation.[99]

Where an inquest under the old system was completed before July 25, 2013 **1–46** none of the provisions of the 2009 Act nor of the statutory instruments made under it can apply. The only obligations continuing into the future must have arisen under the old legislation and be continued (if at all) by the interpretation legislation dealing with the transitional effects of repeals.[100] This may cause problems in relation to, for example, requests for access to documents relating to an old inquest.[101]

Where an inquest under the old system was *not* completed before July 25, 2013, **1–47** the provisions of the statutory instruments apply to the investigation (as it becomes) as from that date, but do not affect the validity or effect of decisions already taken.[102] What is more difficult to see is how provisions in the 2009 Act itself can apply to a continuing investigation if the conditions set out in the Act for their application are never satisfied. For example, an investigation under Part I of the Act is not required unless *either* there is a body within the coroner area satisfying certain criteria,[103] *or* the Chief Coroner has given a direction.[104] Where an inquest was opened and the body released and disposed of before July 25, 2013, the first alternative condition cannot be satisfied, because the relevant section was not in force when the body was there.

One answer to this might be that the transitional provisions of the statutory **1–48** instruments made under the Act were predicated on the footing that the statutory conditions for an investigation to take place were satisfied, so the provisions in the 2009 Act must also apply. This reasoning is both clumsy and shaky. A better, though more limited, answer might be that the obligation to inquire attached under the old law,[105] and continues despite the repeal of the legislation imposing it,[106] but now subject to new procedural rules.

This is more limited because it raises, but does not resolve, the further problem **1–49** caused by the occasional specific reference to provisions of the 2009 Act. For example, where a provision is predicated on the condition that the coroner "is under a duty to investigate a death under section 1",[107] it cannot apply to a case where the inquest was opened before July 25, because in that case the coroner's

---

[96] Coroners (Investigations) Regulations 2013 (SI 2013/1629).
[97] Coroners (Inquests) Rules 2013 (SI 2013/1616).
[98] Regulation 3 in the former; r.3 in the latter.
[99] Interpretation Act 1978 s.16(1)(c).
[100] Interpretation Act 1978 s.16(1)(c).
[101] Coroners Rules 1984 r.57; cf 7–24, 18–53.
[102] Coroners (Investigations) Regulations 2013 (SI 2013/1629) reg.3; Coroners (Inquests) Rules 2013 (SI 2013/1616) r.3.
[103] Coroners and Justice Act 2009 s.1(1); see 5–01.
[104] Coroners and Justice Act 2009 s.1(5); see 5–17.
[105] Coroners Act 1988 s.8(1); see 5–17.
[106] Interpretation Act 1978 s.16(1)(c).
[107] Coroners (Investigations) Regulations 2013 (SI 2013/1629) reg.6.

duty to inquire arises under the *previous* legislation, as continued for this case by the interpretation legislation, and not under s.1 of the 2009 Act. It is to be hoped that no one challenges these provisions in the transitional period.

1–50   The statutory rules of the new system are supplemented by guidance from various sources. The Home Office previously wrote, and the Ministry of Justice now sends, circular letters and newsletters to coroners and other concerning developments in the coroner system, including new legislation. The Coroners' Society of England and Wales provides guidance to coroners. The newly appointed Chief Coroner has provided detailed guidance to coroners and local authorities on various matters relating to the new system, and also on legal matters. But it is clear that the principle that public authorities should follow principles that they have issued and not depart from them without giving clear reasons for doing so to persons affected[108] does not apply to such guidance.[108a]

HUMAN RIGHTS

1–51   Finally, an important dimension of the law of coroners' inquiries is the law of human rights. The Human Rights Act 1998 enables UK judges to measure domestic laws against an international standard, namely, the European Convention on Human Rights, 1950. The rights conferred by this convention are now, by virtue of the Act, mirrored by equivalent rights in English domestic law. Some of the provisions of this Convention impact on inquiries into death (not necessarily inquests), and have provided a legal basis upon which the law relating to coroners has been significantly developed. The subject is dealt with throughout this work where relevant, and in detail in a later chapter.[109]

---

[108] See *Gransden & Co Ltd v Secretary of State for the Environment* [1987] P. & C.R. 86. Also *R (McLeish) v North London Coroner* [2010] EWHC 3624 (Admin).
[108a] Cf. *R (McLeish) v North London Coroner* [2010] EWHC 3624 (Admin).
[109] Chapter 21 below.

Chapter 2

THE OFFICE OF CORONER

CLASSIFICATION OF CORONERS

Until 2013

Until 2013, coroners were of three kinds, namely: **2–01**

(1) coroners ex officio, i.e. persons who were coroners by virtue of their office;

(2) franchise coroners;

(3) district (formerly called "county") coroners, each of which had a deputy, and might also have one or more assistant deputies, to cover for absence or unavailability.

Coroners ex officio

Coroners ex officio included the Lord Chief Justice and all the judges of the High   **2–02**
Court.[1] Such coroners were said to have jurisdiction unlimited in England and
Wales,[2] although in modern times there was no case of such jurisdiction being
exercised. The Coroners Act 1988 contained a saving for "the jurisdiction of a
judge exercising the jurisdiction of a coroner by virtue of his office",[3] but this has
now been repealed,[4] and the only coroners who may in future exercise jurisdiction
as such are those appointed (or treated as appointed) under the Coroners and
Justice Act 2009 ("the 2009 Act").

---

[1] *Wardens and Commonalty of Sadlers' Case* (1588) 4 Co.Rep. 54b at 57b; *Barclee's Case* (1658) 2 Sid.
101; 4 Co.Inst. 73; 1 Bl.Comm. 355; Supreme Court of Judicature Act 1873 s.12; Coroners Act 1887
s.34; Senior Courts Act 1981 s.44; Coroners Act 1988 s.33(1). See also Short and Mellor, *Practice of
the Crown Office* (1890), p.4.

[2] *Barclee's Case* (1658) 2 Sid. 101; *Halsbury's Laws of England,* 4th edn reissue, Vol.9(2), para.804.

[3] Section 33(1).

[4] Coroners and Justice Act 2009 s.178, Sch.23.

Franchise coroners

2–03 By 2013 franchise coroners were almost entirely extinct. These were coroners who were not elected by the freeholders of a county, but who were appointed by a lord or other person having the right to appoint a coroner for "any town corporate, liberty, lordship, manor, university or other place".[5] The right of any person to appoint a franchise coroner was extinguished by a combination of the Coroners (Amendment) Act 1926[6] and the Local Government Act 1972,[7] save for three special cases, namely the Queen's coroner and attorney, the coroner of the Queen's Household,[8] and the coroner of the Scilly Isles.

The Queen's coroner and attorney

2–04 The office of the Queen's coroner and attorney survives, but no longer exercises any coronial function. It is said that the origins of the office may be traced back to the ancient office of Clerk to the Crown: at some time unknown it became a separate and distinct office,[9] appointed by letters patent.[10] Among his other duties, the holder took inquisitions on the bodies of all persons dying in the King's Bench Prison.[11] On the abolition of the Fleet and Marshalsea Prisons,[12] it was provided that the coroner for the City of London should hold inquests upon persons dying in the King's Bench Prison. Since then the Queen's coroner and attorney has had no place over which to exercise coronial jurisdiction.

2–05 In 1879 the Queen's coroner and attorney and the Master of the Crown Office were both transferred, with the then Crown Office of the Queen's Bench Division, to the Central Office of the Supreme Court.[13] In 1892 it was proposed to abolish the office, but apparently Lord Halsbury and Lord Coleridge CJ defeated the proposal "on account of the great antiquity of the office".[14]

2–06 In recent times the person appointed to this office has also been the Master of the Crown Office and the Registrar of Criminal Appeals.[15] As to the former office, in the first edition of this work in 1829, it was stated[16] that the Master of the Crown Office was coroner of the King's Bench, and this may be the origin of the close connection between the two offices. As to the latter, the office of Registrar of Criminal Appeals is now by statute combined with the office of Queen's coroner and attorney and Master of the Crown Office.[17] The Queen's coroner and

---

[5] See the definition of "franchise coroner" in s.43 of the Coroners Act 1887 (repealed), and the discussion in the 7th edn (1927), of this work, at 101–104.

[6] Section 4.

[7] Section 220(1).

[8] Local Government Act 1972 s.220(2).

[9] See Hunnisett, *The Medieval Coroner* (1961) p.149.

[10] *Vyntners'* case (1558) 2 Dyer 150b.

[11] Originally in Borough High Street and later in St George's Fields, Southwark. Notable prisoners included John Wilkes, Tobias Smollett, Lord Cochrane and the King of Corsica.

[12] Queen's Prison Act 1849 s.19; Prison Act 1865 s.48.

[13] Supreme Court of Judicature (Officers) Act 1879 ss.5, 6.

[14] See the 7th edn (1927), of this work, at p.102 (repeated in the 8th and 9th editions).

[15] See *Halsbury's Laws of England*, 5th edn, Vol.24 at [745].

[16] At p.4.

[17] Courts and Legal Services Act 1990 s.78(1).

attorney and Master of the Crown Office is by virtue of his appointment a Master of the Queen's Bench Division.[18]

To be qualified for the appointment, a candidate must be a barrister or solicitor of not less than 10 years' standing,[19] and the appointment is made by the Lord Chancellor, with the concurrence of the Minister for the Civil Service (usually the Prime Minister) as to salary.[20] A full-time holder of this office may not provide advocacy, litigation, conveyancing or probate services, practise (or be involved in practice) as a UK lawyer, nor act as a remunerated arbitrator or umpire.[21]

2-07

Coroner of the Queen's Household

The coroner of the Queen's Household was originally called the coroner of the verge. He had exclusive jurisdiction within a circuit of 12 miles ("the verge") around the residence of the monarch's (movable) court. Although exclusive jurisdiction was given to him in respect of deaths within the precincts of the palace or house where the King was actually resident,[22] at an early date the jurisdiction of the coroner of the verge outside those precincts and within the verge became concurrent with that of the county coroner.[23]

2-08

Then in 1887 that part of his jurisdiction was completely transferred to the relevant county or borough coroner,[24] leaving him with exclusive jurisdiction in respect of inquests[25] on persons whose bodies were lying within the limits of any of the Queen's palaces or within the limits of any other house where Her Majesty was then residing.[26] The inquests into the deaths of Diana, Princess of Wales, and Dodi Fayed led to considerable litigation concerning aspects of the office of coroner of the Queen's Household.[27] But in 2013 the office was abolished,[28] as part of the general reform of the coroner system.

2-09

Coroner for the Scilly Isles

The coroner for the Scilly Isles was formerly a franchise coroner appointed by the Prince of Wales as Duke of Cornwall. As a result of the Local Government Act 1972, which applied to the Scilly Isles only in 1978,[29] the council of the Scilly Isles obtained power to appoint its coroner in the same way as any county council,[30] and

2-10

---

[18] Senior Courts Act 1981 s.89(2).
[19] Senior Courts Act 1981 Sch.2 Pt II para.2.
[20] Supreme Court Act 1981 s.89(1).
[21] Courts and Legal Services Act 1990 s.75 Sch.11.
[22] Offences within the Court Act 1541 s.3; Coroners Act 1887 s.29(2).
[23] Inquests within Verge, etc. Act 1399 ("*Articuli super cartas*").
[24] Coroners Act 1887 s.29(4) Sch.3, repealing the Inquests within Verge, etc. Act 1300; see now Coroners Act 1988 s.29(3).
[25] And, presumably, inquiries which did not lead to inquests: Coroners Act 1988 Sch. 2 para.5.
[26] Coroners Act 1988 s.29(2). The Queen's palaces included Buckingham Palace, St James's Palace, Windsor Castle, Kensington Palace, Hampton Court Palace, and Sandringham House. The Palace of Westminster, however, was not a royal palace, and came within the jurisdiction of the Westminster coroner. The 1988 Act applied to England and Wales only (s.37(3)), and hence palaces in Scotland or elsewhere were not included.
[27] See, e.g. *Paul v Deputy Coroner of The Queen's Household* [2007] EWHC 408 (Admin).
[28] Coroners and Justice Act 2009 s.46.
[29] Local Government Act 1972 s.265(2); the Isles of Scilly Order 1978 (SI 1978/1944), Sch., inserting a new subs.(3A) into s.220 of the 1972 Act for the purposes of the Act's application to the Isles of Scilly.
[30] Local Government Act 1972 s.34(1), but subject to s.34(2).

the coroner thereafter could no longer properly be regarded as a franchise coroner.

District coroners

2–11 Except for the dwindling number of special cases previously mentioned, all coroners in 2013 were ordinary coroners, and there was no hierarchy among them. (Their deputies and assistant deputies did not hold separate offices, but were merely persons who could deputise for them in their office.) Formerly coroners were elected by the freeholders of the county or the burgesses of the borough (as the case might be). Such election was subsequently replaced by appointment by the county or borough council.[31]

2–12 Borough coroners were abolished on April 1, 1974, consequent upon the reorganisation of local government,[32] although since 1985 certain coroners had been appointed by metropolitan district or London borough councils as if they were non-metropolitan county councils.[33] The legislation in force before 1988 referred to all these remaining non-franchise coroners as "county coroners", but the Coroners Act 1988 did not, so the preferable course was to refer to them as "district" coroners.

From 2013

2–13 From 2013, the classification is completely changed. The ex officio and franchise coroners are gone, and there is a new and distinct hierarchy of coroners:

(1) the Chief Coroner;

(2) the Coroner for Treasure;

(3) senior coroners;

(4) area coroners;

(5) assistant coroners, and assistant coroners for treasure.

The Chief Coroner

2–14 For the first time, the coroner system in England and Wales has a national head, the Chief Coroner, who must be a serving judge. He is given many powers and duties under the 2009 Act, but in general terms his responsibilities include providing leadership and guidance[33a], setting standards, and developing training for coroners and their staff, directing investigations to be undertaken, monitoring certain investigations and also coroners' reports, overseeing the transfer of cases between coroners, keeping registers of lengthy investigations, and reporting to the Lord Chancellor. He may also conduct investigations and inquests himself. The 2009

---

[31] Local Government Act 1888 s.5(1). See 1–12 above.
[32] Local Government Act 1972 s.220(1).
[33] Local Government Act 1985 s.13(2); Coroners Act 1988 s.1.
[33a] See *www.judiciary.gov.uk/related-offices-and-bodies/office-chief-coroner/guidance-law-sheets/*.

Act also confers power to appoint deputy chief coroners to assist the Chief Coroner.[34]

The Coroner for Treasure

The Coroner for Treasure is a further innovation of the 2009 Act. It is a national **2–15** post, and not local or territorial. All cases of treasure in England and Wales will be reported to him, and he or his assistants will deal with any necessary investigations or inquests. However, the provisions of the 2009 Act concerning the Coroner for Treasure have not been brought into force with the remainder of Pt I, because of a lack of resources, and for the moment the provisions relating to treasure in the 1988 Act continue to apply.[35]

Senior coroners

Under the 2009 Act, pre-existing coroner "districts" have become coroner **2–16** "areas".[36] Each such area has a senior coroner.[37] The first such senior coroners were the coroners in office under the old system when the new one came into force.[38] The intention is that, through amalgamation of existing areas over time, each area will have a caseload such that the senior coroner will be a full-time appointment. Although coroner areas are based on local government districts, most of them will ultimately cover several local government districts. The functions of senior coroners may be performed by area and assistant coroners when the senior coroner is absent or unavailable, or the senior coroner consents, and hence references in the legislation to a senior coroner include references to an area or assistant coroner.[38a]

Area coroners

The area coroner is also an innovation of the 2009 Act, although in limited respects **2–17** the office resembles that of the deputy coroner under the old system. An area coroner is a coroner for a particular coroner area,[39] appointed by the local authority, and in effect takes a part of the coroner workload.[39a] The introduction of this post (which may be full- or part-time) facilitates the creation of a team of coroners for busy coroner areas. If a vacancy occurs in the office of senior coroner, the area coroner (or one of them, if there is more than one) steps in to perform that role until the vacancy is filled.[40] However, it is not clear whether an area coroner can be appointed without an order having been made by the Lord Chancellor so to require.[41]

---

[34] See 2–20.
[35] See 16–20.
[36] See 2–30, 4–01.
[37] Coroners and Justice Act 2009 s.23 Sch.3 para.1.
[38] Coroners and Justice Act 2009 s.177 Sch.22 para.3. See 2–40.
[38a] Coroners and Justice Act 2009 s.23 Sch.3 para.8.
[39] See 2–30, 4–01.
[39a] Coroners and Justice Act 2009 s.23 Sch.3 para.8; see 2–16, 2–25.
[40] See 2–24.
[41] See 2–26.

Assistant coroners, and assistant coroners for treasure

2–18 Each coroner area[42] has at least one assistant coroner, to cover for the absence or unavailability of the senior coroner, or simply to assist in the workload.[43] This post is the functional equivalent of the old deputy and assistant deputy coroners. The main difference is that assistant coroners are appointed by the local authority and not the coroner himself. Assistant coroners for treasure are designated by the Chief Coroner from among assistant coroners,[44] and fulfil similar functions in relation to the Coroner for Treasure.[45]

APPOINTMENT[46]

The Chief Coroner

2–19 There is no requirement by law to appoint a Chief Coroner, even though the statutory scheme contemplates the existence of one. The 2009 Act in fact provides that the Lord Chief Justice *may* appoint a person as the Chief Coroner,[47] for a term decided by him, but which must expire before the appointee's 70th birthday.[48] The Lord Chief Justice must consult the Lord Chancellor over both the appointment and the term.[49] To be eligible for appointment, a person must be a High Court or circuit judge, and under the age of 70.[50] Provided he remains eligible, the Chief Coroner can be reappointed at the end of a term of office.[51] Because there is no requirement for an appointment at all, there is no statutory machinery for dealing with a vacancy in the office. The Lord Chief Justice *may* appoint another person, using the same procedure.

2–20 There is provision for the appointment of one or more deputy chief coroners,[52] although the Lord Chief Justice must first consult the Lord Chancellor as to how many deputy chief coroners should be appointed, and according to which criteria of eligibility.[53] There are in fact two separate levels of eligibility for appointment. The first is the same as for the Chief Coroner (i.e. High Court or circuit judge), and the appointment process is identical to that for the Chief Coroner.[54]

2–21 The second is that a person must be a senior coroner or the Coroner for Treasure, and under the age of 70. In this case the appointment is made by the Lord Chancellor after consulting the Lord Chief Justice, but otherwise the process is the

---

[42] See 2–30, 4–01.
[43] Coroners and Justice Act 2009 s.23 Sch.3 para.8. See 2–16, 2–27.
[44] See 2–29.
[45] Coroners and Justice Act 2009 s.25 Sch.4 para.11.
[46] See the Chief Coroner's Guidance, *How to become a coroner.*
[47] Coroners and Justice Act 2009 s.35 Sch.8 para.1(1).
[48] Coroners and Justice Act 2009 s.35 Sch.8 para.1(4).
[49] Coroners and Justice Act 2009 s.35 Sch.8 para.1(3), (4).
[50] Coroners and Justice Act 2009 s.35 Sch.8 para.1(2).
[51] Coroners and Justice Act 2009 s.35 Sch.8 para.1(5).
[52] Coroners and Justice Act 2009 s.35 Sch.8 para.2(1).
[53] Coroners and Justice Act 2009 s.35 Sch.8 para.2(3).
[54] Coroners and Justice Act 2009 s.35 Sch.8 para.2(2), (4), (5), (8)).

same as for the Chief Coroner.[55] Again, because there is no *requirement* for an appointment of deputy chief coroners at all, there is no statutory machinery for dealing with a vacancy in the office. However, no deputy chief coroners have so far been appointed, and there are no current plans to appoint any.

The Coroner for Treasure

Once the relevant provision has come into force, the Lord Chancellor may appoint   2–22
a person as the Coroner for Treasure in relation to England and Wales.[56] To be
eligible, a person must be under the age of 70, and satisfy the judicial-appointment
eligibility condition[57] on a five-year basis.[58] Once again, because there is no
requirement for an appointment at all, there is no statutory machinery for dealing
with a vacancy in the office. The Lord Chancellor may appoint another person,
using the same procedure. However, as mentioned above,[59] lack of resources means
that there are no plans at present to bring the relevant provision into force.

Senior coroners

The relevant authority[60] for each coroner area,[61] after consulting other local   2–23
authorities whose areas fall within the coroner area in question,[62] must appoint a
senior coroner for that area,[63] but only with the consent of the Lord Chancellor
and the Chief Coroner.[64] The Chief Coroner has issued guidance for local
authorities on the appointment process.[65] To be eligible, a person must be under
the age of 70, and satisfy the judicial-appointment eligibility condition[66] on a five-
year basis,[67] but must not be (or within the last six months have been) a councillor[68]
for any local authority whose area falls within the coroner area in question.[69]

If a vacancy occurs in the office of senior coroner, the relevant authority must   2–24
notify the Lord Chancellor and the Chief Coroner in writing as soon as
practicable,[70] must appoint a successor within three months (extendable by the
Lord Chancellor) of the vacancy occurring,[71] and must notify the Lord Chancellor
and the Chief Coroner in writing of the appointment as soon as practicable.[72]

---

[55] Coroners and Justice Act 2009 s.35 Sch.8 para.2(2), (6)–(8).
[56] Coroners and Justice Act 2009 s.25 Sch.4 para.1.
[57] See 2–34.
[58] Coroners and Justice Act 2009 s.25 Sch.4 para.2.
[59] See 2–15.
[60] See 2–32.
[61] See 2–15, 2–30, 4–01.
[62] Coroners and Justice Act 2009 s.23 Sch.3 para.1(2).
[63] Coroners and Justice Act 2009 s.23 Sch.3 para.1(1).
[64] Coroners and Justice Act 2009 s.23 Sch.3 para.1(3).
[65] *Chief Coroner Guidance No. 6*, 24 July 2013.
[66] See 2–34.
[67] Coroners and Justice Act 2009 s.23 Sch.3 para.3.
[68] In relation to the Common Council of the City of London, the term "councillor" includes both an alderman of the City and a common councillor: Coroners and Justice Act 2009 s.23 Sch.3 para.4(2).
[69] Coroners and Justice Act 2009 s.23 Sch.3 para.4(1).
[70] Coroners and Justice Act 2009 s.23 Sch.3 para.5(2)(a).
[71] Coroners and Justice Act 2009 s.23 Sch.3 para.5(2)(b).
[72] Coroners and Justice Act 2009 s.23 Sch.3 para.5(2)(c).

During the vacancy, the area coroner (or, if there is more than one, the one nominated by the relevant authority) acts as senior coroner,[73] and is to be treated for all the public-facing purposes of the 2009 Act as being the senior coroner.[74] If there is no area coroner, the assistant coroner nominated by the relevant authority[75] acts as senior coroner,[76] and is to be similarly treated.[77]

Area coroners

2-25   The Lord Chancellor may, after consulting the Chief Coroner and every local authority whose area falls within the coroner area in question,[78] by order require the relevant authority for a coroner area to appoint one or more area coroners,[79] and the relevant authority must make the appointment or appointments,[80] but only with the consent of the Lord Chancellor and the Chief Coroner.[81] The Chief Coroner has issued guidance for local authorities on the appointment process.[82] To be eligible, a person must be under the age of 70, and satisfy the judicial-appointment eligibility condition[83] on a five-year basis,[84] but must not be (or within the last six months have been) a councillor[85] for any local authority whose area falls within the coroner area in question.[86]

2-26   The structure of the legislative provisions is simply to place an obligation on a relevant authority to make an appointment where the Lord Chancellor makes an order. None of the provisions expressly confers power on the relevant authority to appoint one or more area coroners where the Lord Chancellor has *not* made an order. The Chief Coroner's view is however that it was the Government's intention to confer such a power in the 2009 Act.[87] If a vacancy occurs in the office of area coroner, the relevant authority must notify the Lord Chancellor and the Chief Coroner in writing as soon as practicable,[88] must appoint a successor within three months (extendable by the Lord Chancellor) of the vacancy occurring,[89] and

---

[73] Coroners and Justice Act 2009 s.23 Sch.3 para.7(2).
[74] Coroners and Justice Act 2009 s.23 Sch.3 para.7(5). But he is *not* to be so treated for the purposes of paras 1–5, 7 and 9–19 of Sch.3 of the Act, dealing with appointment, qualification, vacancies and terms of office. This means (for example) that he is not automatically entitled to the salary of the senior coroner.
[75] Presumably if there is only one there is no need for a nomination, and that one acts.
[76] Coroners and Justice Act 2009 s.23 Sch.3 para.7(3).
[77] Coroners and Justice Act 2009 s.23 Sch.3 para.7(5). See fn.74 above.
[78] Coroners and Justice Act 2009 s.23 Sch.3 para.2(2).
[79] Coroners and Justice Act 2009 s.23 Sch.3 para.2(1).
[80] Coroners and Justice Act 2009 s.23 Sch.3 para.2(3).
[81] Coroners and Justice Act 2009 s.23 Sch.3 para.2(5).
[82] *Chief Coroner Guidance No. 6*, 24 July 2013, paras 38–49.
[83] See 2–34.
[84] Coroners and Justice Act 2009 s.23 Sch.3 para.3.
[85] In relation to the Common Council of the City of London, the term "councillor" includes both an alderman of the City and a common councillor: Coroners and Justice Act 2009 s.23 Sch.3 para.4(2).
[86] Coroners and Justice Act 2009 s.23 Sch.3 para.4(1).
[87] See the Chief Coroner's Guide to the Coroners and Justice Act 2009 para.21.
[88] Coroners and Justice Act 2009 s.23 Sch.3 para.5(2)(a).
[89] Coroners and Justice Act 2009 s.23 Sch.3 para.5(2)(b).

must notify the Lord Chancellor and the Chief Coroner in writing of the appointment as soon as practicable.[90]

Assistant coroners

The Lord Chancellor may, after consulting the Chief Coroner and every local authority whose area falls within the coroner area in question,[91] by order require the relevant authority for a coroner area to appoint a minimum of assistant coroners,[92] and the relevant authority must make the appointment or appointments,[93] but only with the consent of the Lord Chancellor and the Chief Coroner.[94] The Chief Coroner has issued guidance for local authorities on the appointment process.[95] To be eligible, a person must be under the age of 70, and satisfy the judicial-appointment eligibility condition[96] on a five-year basis,[97] but must not be (or within the last six months have been) a councillor[98] for any local authority whose area falls within the coroner area in question.[99] **2-27**

If a vacancy occurs in the office of assistant coroner, which causes the number of assistant coroners to fall below or further below the minimum number referred to above, the relevant authority must appoint a successor within three months (extendable by the Lord Chancellor) of the vacancy occurring.[100] There is no obligation to notify the Lord Chancellor and the Chief Coroner in writing of the appointment, but as stated above, their consent to it is required. **2-28**

Assistant coroners for treasure

Once the relevant provision has come into force, the Chief Coroner may designate one or more assistant coroners to act as assistant coroners for treasure.[101] Such persons will have already satisfied the conditions for, and been appointed as, assistant coroners.[102] Once again, because there is no requirement for an appointment at all, there is no statutory machinery for dealing with a vacancy in the office. The Chief Coroner may designate another person, using the same procedure. However, as mentioned above,[103] lack of resources means that there are **2-29**

---

[90] Coroners and Justice Act 2009 s.23 Sch.3 para.5(2)(c).
[91] Coroners and Justice Act 2009 s.23 Sch.3 para.2(2).
[92] Coroners and Justice Act 2009 s.23 Sch.3 para.2(1); see the Coroners and Justice Act 2009 (Coroner Areas and Assistant Coroners) Transitional Order 2013 (SI 2013/1625). Although s.177 Sch.22 para.1(4) requires such an order to be made at the same time as the order bringing into force the repeal of ss.1–7 of the 1988 Act, i.e. SI 2013/1869 (made July 24, 2013), in fact it was made sooner (on July 2, 2013).
[93] Coroners and Justice Act 2009 s.23 Sch.3 para.2(3).
[94] Coroners and Justice Act 2009 s.23 Sch.3 para.2(5).
[95] *Chief Coroner Guidance No. 6*, 24 July 2013, paras 39–49.
[96] See 2–34.
[97] Coroners and Justice Act 2009 s.23 Sch.3 para.3.
[98] In relation to the Common Council of the City of London, the term "councillor" includes both an alderman of the City and a common councillor: Coroners and Justice Act 2009 s.23 Sch.3 para.4(2).
[99] Coroners and Justice Act 2009 s.23 Sch.3 para.4(1).
[100] Coroners and Justice Act 2009 s.23 Sch.3 para.6(2).
[101] Coroners and Justice Act 2009 s.25 Sch.4 para.7.
[102] See 2–27.
[103] See 2–15 above.

no plans at present to bring the relevant provision into force to make an appointment of a Coroner for Treasure, nor indeed the power to designate any assistant coroners as assistant coroners for treasure.

Coroner areas

2–30 England and Wales are required to be divided into coroner areas,[104] each consisting of the area of a local authority or the combined areas of two or more local authorities,[105] as specified (and named for this purpose) in an order made by the Lord Chancellor,[106] after consulting every local authority, the Welsh Ministers, and any other person whom he thinks appropriate.[107] The order so made[108] took the coroner districts then in existence under the old system, and renamed them as coroner areas under the new.[109]

2–31   The Lord Chancellor may make orders altering coroner areas,[110] whether by changing their boundaries, combining or dividing them, or changing their names.[111] Before making such an order, the Lord Chancellor must consult local authorities and others that he considers appropriate, and the Welsh Ministers, if the coroner area is in Wales.[112] The first such order merged a number of areas.[113] Under the previous system, where such an alteration caused loss of office or salary, compensation had to be paid, treating coroners for this purpose as local government officers.[114] But the current policy is to consider making such alterations only on a vacancy arising.

"Relevant authority"

2–32 If a coroner area consists of the area of a single local authority, that authority is the relevant authority for the coroner area. If it consists of the areas of two or more local authorities, then the relevant authority is whichever one of them they agree upon, but in default of agreement the one determined by the Lord Chancellor, after consulting the Secretary of State or the Welsh Ministers, as appropriate. For these purposes, each of a county council, a "unitary" district

---

[104] Coroners and Justice Act 2009 s.22 Sch.2 para.1(1).
[105] Coroners and Justice Act 2009 s.22 Sch.2 para.1(2). This appears to mean that no order can be made which specifies as a coroner area an area which is *less* than a local government area, or *less* than the combined areas of two or more local government areas. Unfortunately the Coroners and Justice Act 2009 (Coroner Areas and Assistant Coroners) Transitional Order 2013 (SI 2013/1625) in a few instances did just that.
[106] Coroners and Justice Act 2009 s.22 Sch.2 para.1(3).
[107] Coroners and Justice Act 2009 s.22 Sch.2 para.1(4).
[108] Coroners and Justice Act 2009 (Coroner Areas and Assistant Coroners) Transitional Order 2013 (SI 2013/1625).
[109] This was required under Coroners and Justice Act 2009 s.177 Sch.22 para.1(1), (3).
[110] Coroners and Justice Act 2009 s.22 Sch.2 para.2(1). See the Chief Coroner's Guidance No.14, *Merger of Coroner Areas.*
[111] Coroners and Justice Act 2009 s.22 Sch.2 para.2(3).
[112] Coroners and Justice Act 2009 s.22 Sch.2 para.2(2).
[113] Coroners and Justice Act 2009 (Alteration of Coroner areas) Order 2013 (SI 2013/1626).
[114] Local Government Reorganisation (Compensation for Loss of Remuneration) Regulations 1995 (SI 1995/2837), as amended by the Local Government Reorganisation (Compensation for Loss of Remuneration) (Amendment) Regulations 1996 (SI 1996/660) reg.2, as from April 1, 1996. These regulations however refer to coroners under the Coroners Act 1988, rather than to coroners under the 2009 Act, and so are strictly not applicable in their present form to the latter.

council,[115] a London borough council, the Common Council of the City of London, the Council of the Isles of Scilly, and a county borough council in Wales is a local authority.[116]

Qualification for appointment

Originally, it was a necessary qualification for a coroner that he held land in fee 2–33 (exactly how much was never quite clear),[117] but this requirement has long been abolished.[118] From 1926 to 2013, coroners had to be either lawyers or medical practitioners. However, under the 2009 Act, but subject to transitional provisions,[119] all coroners must be lawyers.

The specific qualifications for each type of appointment are set out above, but 2–34 most of them depend upon the so-called "judicial-appointment eligibility condition" being satisfied on a five-year basis. A person so satisfies this condition if he has had a "relevant qualification" for "qualifying periods" totalling at least five years.[120] A qualifying period is a period during which that person both has the relevant qualification and gains experience in law,[121] by being engaged in law-related activities.[122]

A person has a relevant qualification if he is a solicitor or barrister in England and 2–35 Wales,[123] but also if he holds another qualification which has been specified by the Lord Chancellor by order in relation to a particular office or other position.[124] A person needs a practising certificate to act as a solicitor,[125] but not to be admitted as one. So once a solicitor has been appointed a coroner it is no longer necessary to hold a practising certificate, and the accounts rules do not apply.[126]

Incompatibility with coronial appointment

At common law, occupation of the office of coroner was not of itself incompatible 2–36 for some other official or professional activity[127] except perhaps being made sheriff

---

[115] That is, the district of a council comprised in an area for which there is no county council.

[116] Coroners and Justice Act 2009 s.48(1).

[117] See, e.g. 1 Bl.Comm. 336. It was said that some coroners satisfied the requirement by ownership of burial plots. See also Hunnisett, *The Medieval Coroner*, 1961, pp. 170–177.

[118] Coroners (Amendment) Act 1926 s.1(4).

[119] See 2–39 below.

[120] Tribunals, Courts and Enforcement Act 2007 s.50(1), (2). It is not enough simply to obtain the relevant qualification by transferring from the equivalent qualification in another jurisdiction which has been held already for five years.

[121] Tribunals, Courts and Enforcement Act 2007 s.50(3).

[122] Tribunals, Courts and Enforcement Act 2007 s.52(2).

[123] Tribunals, Courts and Enforcement Act 2007 s.50(4)(a), (5), but subject to s.51(5), (6) (when a person is taken for these purposes to become a solicitor or barrister) and (7) (the effect of suspension from practice during the pendency of disciplinary proceedings).

[124] Tribunals, Courts and Enforcement Act 2007 ss.50(4)(b), 51(1). By virtue of the Judicial Appointments Order 2008 (SI 2008/2995), as amended by the Judicial Appointments (Amendment) Order 2013 (SI 2013/3022) art.3, as from December 3, 2013 this includes a Fellow of the Institute of Legal Executives.

[125] Solicitors Act 1974 s.1(c).

[126] SRA Accounts Rules 2011 r.5.1(c)(i).

[127] It is not, for example, incompatible with being a justice of the peace: *Davis v Pembrokeshire Justices* (1881) 7 QBD. 513.

(or anciently, chosen verderer)[128] with which the office is said to be incompatible,[129] and in those instances in which the person appointed had agreed personally to engage himself as coroner as a full-time office and not to pursue any other vocation. But it is now provided by statute that a "coroner appointed under section 2 of the Coroners Act 1988" and "holding a full-time appointment" may not provide legal services or act as arbitrator for personal reward.[130] This prohibition does not extend to other professional services (e.g. medical).

2–37   There are currently about 99 coronerships in England and Wales, of which about 46 are full-time appointments. The remaining appointments are held for the most part by lawyers,[131] usually in private practice, and some of them also hold other official positions, either administrative or judicial.[132] In a very few cases, the same person holds more than one coronership.

2–38   However, there are certain statutory disqualifications as regards appointment to the office of coroner. The disqualification of a serving or former councillor for being appointed coroner has already been referred to.[133] There is a converse disqualification, whereby a senior coroner, area coroner or assistant coroner is disqualified for being elected or being a member of the council of a local authority whose area falls within the coroner area.[134] A senior coroner, area coroner or assistant coroner appointed under the 2009 Act, the Coroner for Treasure, and a deputy chief coroner are all disqualified by reason of office for being elected as a Member of Parliament,[135] or a Member of the Northern Ireland Assembly,[136] but not, apparently, as a Member of the National Assembly for Wales.[137]

---

[128] A verderer is a judicial officer of a forest: see *Select Pleas of the Forest* (Selden Society), Vol.13 pp.xix–xx, xxvii–1, and Hunnisett, *The Medieval Coroner* (1961), pp.146–147. The only verderers now left are those of the New Forest in Hampshire, who have certain executive and judicial functions within the New Forest, e.g. making limited kinds of by-laws and sitting in the Court of Swainmote: see the New Forest Acts 1877 to 1949. See also *Verderers of the New Forest v Young* [2003] EWHC 3252 (Admin); [2004] 16 E.G. 112, DC (local magistrates had concurrent jurisdiction with the Court of Swainmote in respect of breaches of by-laws made by verderers).

[129] See 2–92.

[130] Courts and Legal Services Act 1990 s.75 Sch.11; there is no definition of what constitutes a "full-time appointment". It is submitted that it means an appointment the holder of which is required to devote substantially the whole of his or her working day to the requirements of the office.

[131] See 2–34—2–35 above.

[132] For example deputy district judge. At least one coroner is also a recorder. The Coroners' Society were advised by counsel in 1957 that it was not unlawful for a person to be both town clerk and coroner, though it might be considered improper. Since then one person has apparently held both offices simultaneously. The Coroners' Society has taken a similar view of membership of a hospital management committee by a coroner: see its reports for 1961–1962, at p.4.

[133] See 2–23.

[134] Coroners and Justice Act 2009 s.23 Sch.3 para.11.

[135] See the House of Commons Disqualification Act 1975 s.1 Sch.1 (as amended by the 2009 Act Sch.21 para.26). Until the 2009 Act came into force there was no disqualification. It may be noted that Thomas Wakley, founder of *The Lancet*, was MP for Finsbury in London from 1835 to 1852 and also coroner for West Middlesex (including Finsbury) from 1839 to 1862.

[136] See the Northern Ireland Assembly Disqualification Act 1975 s.1 Sch.1 (as amended by the 2009 Act Sch.21 para.27).

[137] See the National Assembly for Wales (Disqualification) Order 2010 (SI 2010/2969) art.2, Sch.

Transitional provisions

In relation to the appointment of coroners, there were three aspects to the **2–39** transition from the old system to the new. The first was to transfer previously existing coronial appointments into appointments in the new system. The second was to deal with the fact that under the old system—but not the new—it was possible for a person to be qualified for coronial appointment by virtue of a medical qualification alone, and that there were a number of such persons in post. The third was to deal with subtle changes in the rules on disqualification.

As to the first aspect, a person who was the coroner for a coroner's district under **2–40** the 1988 Act, and but for the repeal of the 1988 Act would have continued in office, has since that repeal been treated as having been appointed under the 2009 Act[138] as the senior coroner for the corresponding coroner area.[139] Similarly, a person who was the deputy coroner or an assistant deputy coroner for a coroner's district under the 1988 Act, and but for the repeal of the 1988 Act would have continued in office, has since that repeal been treated as having been appointed under the 2009 Act[140] as an assistant coroner for the corresponding coroner area.[141] A person who becomes an assistant coroner under this provision, and immediately before so becoming was remunerated by salary, will continue to be entitled to such salary.[142]

As to the second aspect, the transitional provisions were designed to protect the **2–41** positions of persons who were holding coronial office when the new system came into force in 2013, but were not qualified for that office under the new rules. First, the requirements for qualification in the 2009 Act for coronial appointment do not apply at all to a person treated under the rules just discussed as automatically appointed senior coroner or assistant coroner.[143]

But, secondly, provision is also made for the case where a new coroner area is **2–42** subsequently created by the Lord Chancellor by order.[144] In such a case a person who does not meet the qualification criteria, but was treated as automatically appointed senior coroner for a coroner area that now forms part of the new area, *and* held office as such immediately before the new area was created, may become senior coroner, area coroner or assistant coroner for the new area.[145] Likewise, a person who does not meet the qualification criteria, but was treated as automatically appointed assistant coroner for a coroner area that now forms part of the new area, *and* held office as such immediately before the new area was created, may become an assistant coroner for the new area.[146]

---

[138] s.23 Sch.3 para.1(1); see 2–23 above.
[139] Coroners and Justice Act 2009 s.177 Sch.22 para.3(2).
[140] s.23 Sch.3 para.2(4); see 2–27 above.
[141] Coroners and Justice Act 2009 s.177 Sch.22 para.3(3). Note that a deputy coroner does not become an "area coroner" under the new system.
[142] Coroners and Justice Act 2009 s.177 Sch.22 para.3(4).
[143] Coroners and Justice Act 2009 s.177 Sch.22 para.3(6).
[144] Coroners and Justice Act 2009 s.22 Sch.2 para.2; see 2–31 above.
[145] Coroners and Justice Act 2009 s.177 Sch.22 para.3(9) (senior coroner, area coroner), (10) (assistant coroner).
[146] Coroners and Justice Act 2009 s.177 Sch.22 para.3(10).

2–43   As to the third aspect, the disqualification of a person for appointment as coroner because he was at that time or within the previous six months had been a member of a local authority was expressed in complex terms in the old system.[147] In the new law it is simpler.[148] The transitional provisions therefore make clear that where a person is treated as automatically appointed into the new system, the new disqualification rule does not apply.[149] Thus a person who would not be disqualified under the old system but would under the new is not prejudiced.

2–44   Similarly, where a new coroner area is subsequently created by the Lord Chancellor by order,[150] a person who was automatically transferred into an appointment in a coroner area that now forms part of the new area, *and* held office as such immediately before the new area was created, is not affected by the new disqualification rule.[151]

Scope of appointment

2–45   Under the old system, a coroner appointed in England, although named as coroner for a particular coroner's district, was nonetheless in law a coroner for the whole administrative area which included that district.[152] And a coroner appointed for a district in Wales was treated as a coroner for the whole of Wales,[153] as is a senior coroner appointed for a coroner area in Wales under the new system.[154] But, except in certain limited and specified circumstances, an English or Welsh coroner could hold inquests only within the *district* to which he had been assigned.[155]

2–46   This rule was repealed with effect from February 12, 2013,[156] and is not carried over into the new law.[157] Under the new system, a senior coroner, area coroner or assistant coroner appointed for a coroner area having jurisdiction as to a particular death may exercise coronial powers in relation to that death anywhere in England and Wales.[158]

---

[147] Coroners Act 1988 s.2(2)–(4).
[148] See 2–23 above.
[149] Coroners and Justice Act 2009 s.177 Sch.22 para.3(6).
[150] Coroners and Justice Act 2009 s.22 Sch.2 para.2; see 2–31 above.
[151] Coroners and Justice Act 2009 s.177 Sch.22 para.3(9) (senior coroner, area coroner), (10) (assistant coroner).
[152] Coroners Act 1988 s.4(5). "Administrative area" meant a metropolitan or non-metropolitan county or Greater London (s.35(1)), so a coroner for a district of Greater London or a metropolitan county was treated as a coroner for the whole of Greater London or such metropolitan county (as the case might be).
[153] Coroners Act 1988 s.4A(8).
[154] Coroners Act 1988 s.4A(8) (*not* repealed in 2013, as amended by the Coroners and Justice Act 2009 (Consequential Provisions) Order 2013 (SI 2013/1874) art.2(2),(3)).
[155] Coroners Act 1988 s.5(2).
[156] Coroners and Justice Act 2009 (Commencement No. 11) Order 2013 (SI 2013/250) art.2. See also *Chief Coroner Guidance No. 2* on the location of the inquest: a coroner should conduct an inquest outside his area only exceptionally.
[157] cf. the 2009 Act s.24; see 10–17.
[158] See 4–02.

Matters consequent on an appointment

Under the old system, it was customary for a coroner, upon being appointed, to make a declaration of office.[159] There is nothing in the new law either to require or to prohibit this. However, the Chief Coroner's intention is that it should be a term of appointment of a senior coroner[160] that he or she should take an oath or affirmation of office before the Lord Chief Justice or another senior judge,[161] and that an area or assistant coroner should take an oath before the senior coroner.[162] The Chief Coroner has provided a form of oath or affirmation for use on such occasions.[163] The question of taking possession of coroner records, documents and other information is dealt with later.[164]

2–47

TERMS OF APPOINTMENT: THE CHIEF CORONER

Appointment and functions

The appointment of the Chief Coroner and deputy chief coroners has already been dealt with.[165] The first Chief Coroner, HH Judge Peter Thornton QC, took up his post in September 2012. The institution of the office of Chief Coroner is really the cornerstone of the new coroner system. The functions of the Chief Coroner are not set out in any one place in the legislation, but they fall into several different categories, as follows:

2–48

(1) liaison between the government (both central and local) and the coroners operating the system;

(2) a role in the appointment of coroners;

(3) providing national leadership and guidance to coroners;

(4) increasing the efficiency of the coroner system.

Thus, under the first head, the Chief Coroner must provide an annual report to the Lord Chancellor on the system.[166] Under the second, he must give his approval

2–49

---

[159] The form of declaration was set out in the Coroners Rules 1984 Sch.4 Form 1. Leckey and Greer, *Coroners' Law and Practice in Northern Ireland* (1998) para.2–07, expressed a doubt as to whether the form was intra vires the rule-making power (i.e. s.32 of the 1988 Act). That power extended to making "rules regulating the practice or procedure of or *in connection with* inquests" (emphasis supplied). It may be that the words "in connection with" extended the power sufficiently to cover the procedure of appointment of a coroner who would then hold inquests, and the power to make rules was expressed (by s.32(a)) to extend to prescribing forms. But even if this were not so it did not matter, as there was no *obligation* to make a declaration, and it would still have been open to coroners to use this form of words if they wished. The same is true for the future.

[160] As to which see 2–69 ff.

[161] See *Chief Coroner Guidance No. 3*, 16 July 2013, paras 3 and 5.

[162] See *Chief Coroner Guidance No. 3*, 16 July 2013 para.7.

[163] *Chief Coroner Guidance No. 3*, 16 July 2013, Annex A.

[164] See 18-66.

[165] See 2–19—2–20.

[166] See 2–50.

to all appointments of senior coroners, area coroners and assistant coroners.[167] Under the third, he sets national standards and provides support, leadership and guidance for coroners,[168] and makes regulations about training for coroners and their staff.[169] Under the fourth, he has power to request information from coroners about investigations,[170] keeps a register of coroner investigations lasting more than 12 months,[171] and takes steps to reduce delays,[172] monitors investigations into the deaths of servicemen overseas,[173] oversees and directs transfers of cases between coroners,[174] conducts investigations and inquests himself,[175] or directs coroners[176] or requests the nomination of judges or former judges to do so,[177] and collates, monitors and publishes coroners' reports to prevent other deaths.[178]

Duties

Reports and advice to the Lord Chancellor

2–50   The Chief Coroner must give the Lord Chancellor a report for each calendar year,[179] by July 1, in the following year.[180] The Lord Chancellor must publish it and lay a copy before each House of Parliament.[181] It must cover both matters that the Chief Coroner wishes to bring to his attention[182] and matters which the Lord Chancellor has asked to be covered.[183] It must contain an assessment for the year of the consistency of standards between coroners' areas.[184] It must also contain a summary of information about investigations which are not concluded within the period of 12 months from the date on which the coroner was made aware that the body was within the coroner's area.[185]

2–51   This information includes the number and length of such investigations notified to the Chief Coroner during the year as not having been completed or discontinued within that 12-month period, the number and length of such investigations so notified during the year as having now been completed or discontinued, and the number and length of such investigations notified during a previous year but not concluded or discontinued by the end of the year for which the report is made.[185a] It also includes the reasons for the length of all those

---

[167] See 2–54.
[168] See 2–14.
[169] See 2–56.
[170] See 2–62.
[171] See 2–62.
[172] See 2–62.
[173] See 4–25.
[174] See 5–17.
[175] See 2–57.
[176] See 2–58—2–59.
[177] See 2–60—2–61.
[178] See 2–63.
[179] Coroners and Justice Act 2009 s.36(1).
[180] Coroners and Justice Act 2009 s.36(5).
[181] Coroners and Justice Act 2009 s.36(6). The first such report, covering the period of July 25, 2013 to June 30, 2014, was laid before Parliament on July 15, 2014.
[182] Coroners and Justice Act 2009 s.36(2)(a).
[183] Coroners and Justice Act 2009 s.36(2)(b).
[184] Coroners and Justice Act 2009 s.36(3).
[185] Coroners and Justice Act 2009 s.36(4)(a).
[185a] See 10–14.

investigations and the measures taken with a view to keeping them from being
unnecessarily lengthy.

The report must also contain a summary for the year of matters required to be   **2–52**
recorded in connection with an authorisation to a coroner to enter and search any
land,[186] and of matters reported by a coroner with a view to preventing other
deaths in future and the responses to such reports.[187] If requested to do so by the
Lord Chancellor, the Chief Coroner must give advice to him about particular
matters relating to the operation of the coroner system.[188]

Other duties

The Chief Coroner has a number of other duties, dealt with elsewhere. These   **2–53**
include the duty to keep a register of notifications by coroners relating to
investigations which have lasted longer than a year,[189] the duty to monitor service
death investigations,[190] and the duty to keep a record of authorisations to coroners
to enter upon and search any land.[191] The Chief Coroner also has a role in
authorising coroners to enter upon and search any land.[192]

Powers

Appointment of coroners

The Chief Coroner is necessarily involved in the appointment by relevant   **2–54**
authorities of coroners,[193] for a number of reasons. The first is that he must be
consulted by the Lord Chancellor before the Lord Chancellor makes an order
requiring the appointment of area coroners or a minimum number of assistant
coroners.[194] The second reason is that the relevant authority must give him written
notice of a senior coroner or area coroner vacancy as soon as practicable after it
arises.[195] The third reason is that that authority must give him notice of the
appointment to fill the vacancy as soon as practicable after it is filled.[196] The fourth
reason is that his consent is required for the appointment of a senior coroner, area
coroner, or assistant coroner to take effect.[197] The Chief Coroner has issued
guidance for local authorities on the appointment process.[198]

---

[186] Coroners and Justice Act 2009 s.36(4)(c). But the provisions in Sch.5 para.4 concerning such
authorisations have not so far been brought into force, so there will be nothing to report under this
head.
[187] Coroners and Justice Act 2009 s.36(4)(d).
[188] Coroners and Justice Act 2009 s.36(7).
[189] Coroners and Justice Act 2009 s.16(3). See 2–62, 10–14.
[190] Coroners and Justice Act 2009 s.17. See 4–25.
[191] Coroners and Justice Act 2009 s.32 Sch.5 para.4(3). See 7–22. But the provisions in Sch.5 para.4
concerning such authorisations have not so far been brought into force, so there will be nothing to
record under this head.
[192] Coroners and Justice Act 2009 s.32 Sch.5 para.3(1). See 7–22. But the provisions in Sch.5 para.3
concerning such authorisations have not so far been brought into force.
[193] As to which, see 2–23—2–29.
[194] Coroners and Justice Act 2009 s.23 Sch.3 para.2(2)(a). See 2–25, 2–27.
[195] Coroners and Justice Act 2009 s.23 Sch.3 para.5(2)(a). See 2–24.
[196] Coroners and Justice Act 2009 s.23 Sch.3 para.5(2)(c). See 2–24.
[197] Coroners and Justice Act 2009 s.23 Sch.3 para.2(5). See 2–23, 2–25, 2–27.
[198] *Chief Coroner Guidance No. 6*, 24 July 2013, especially at paras 9-10 (consents), and 11-14 (the Chief
Coroner's role).

2–55   However this last provision imports an implied duty on the part of the Chief Coroner to deal with the question of consent with reasonable expedition. It is not required that he take part in the selection process itself, though of course he may do so (and it may be desirable that he do so).[199] But he must make a decision as to whether to approve a particular appointment within a reasonable time. The Chief Coroner is also the person who designates one or more assistant coroners as assistant coroners for treasure.[200] Although it does not relate to coroner appointments, the Chief Coroner must be consulted before the Lord Chancellor appoints a person to be the Medical Adviser or a deputy medical adviser.[201]

Training

2–56   The Chief Coroner may make regulations about the training of coroners and their staff, with the agreement of the Lord Chancellor.[202] They may cover the kind, the amount and the frequency of training.[203] In practice the Judicial College (responsible for training the judiciary generally) is involved in the process, and organises training courses for coroners and their staff.

Power to conduct or direct investigation

2–57   The Chief Coroner may himself conduct an investigation into a person's death.[204] Where he does so, he has the same functions in relation to the body and the investigation as if he were a senior coroner in whose area the body was situated,[205] and no other coroner has any such functions.[206] In effect, his decision to conduct an investigation deprives the senior coroner who would otherwise be under a duty to investigate of all jurisdiction in relation to the matter. The legislation is then read as including a reference to the Chief Coroner exercising functions under this provision whenever there is a reference to a senior coroner.[207] This must mean that the relevant authority for that area is responsible for all costs flowing therefrom (except his salary).

2–58   Similarly, the Chief Coroner may direct the Coroner for Treasure to conduct an investigation into a person's death,[208] and the Coroner for Treasure must do so.[209] Where he does so, the Coroner for Treasure has the same functions in relation to the body and the investigation as if he were a senior coroner in whose area the body was situated,[210] and no other coroner has any such functions.[211] The legislation is then read as including a reference to the Coroner for Treasure exercising functions under this provision whenever there is a reference to a senior coroner.[212]

---

[199] See 2–23, 2–25, 2–27.
[200] Coroners and Justice Act 2009 s.25 Sch.4 para.7. See 2–29. But these provisions have not yet been brought into force.
[201] Coroners and Justice Act 2009 s.38 Sch.9 para.4(a).
[202] Coroners and Justice Act 2009 s.37(1). At the time of writing no regulations have been made.
[203] Coroners and Justice Act 2009 s.37(2).
[204] Coroners and Justice Act 2009 s.41 Sch.10 para.1(1).
[205] Coroners and Justice Act 2009 s.41 Sch.10 para.1(2)(a).
[206] Coroners and Justice Act 2009 s.41 Sch.10 para.1(2)(b).
[207] Coroners and Justice Act 2009 s.41 Sch.10 para.1(3).
[208] Coroners and Justice Act 2009 s.41 Sch.10 para.2(1).
[209] Coroners and Justice Act 2009 s.41 Sch.10 para.2(2)(a).
[210] Coroners and Justice Act 2009 s.41 Sch.10 para.2(2)(b).
[211] Coroners and Justice Act 2009 s.41 Sch.10 para.2(2)(c).
[212] Coroners and Justice Act 2009 s.41 Sch.10 para.2(3).

The Chief Coroner also has power to give a direction to investigate a death to,   **2–59**
and thereby confer jurisdiction upon, a coroner in three other cases. The first is
where a coroner has reported that he has reason to believe that the death has
occurred in or near his area in circumstances that there should be an investigation,
but in the absence of the body there is otherwise no duty on anyone to
investigate.[213] The second is where one coroner is under a duty to investigate, but
the Chief Coroner considers that a coroner in another area should do so instead.[214]
The third arises in the case of a service death on active service or analogous
circumstances where the body has been taken to Scotland, but certain conditions
are satisfied rendering it desirable that an investigation under English law take
place.[215] These cases are discussed elsewhere.

Power to request investigation

The Chief Coroner may request the Lord Chief Justice to nominate a High Court   **2–60**
or circuit judge or former Court of Appeal or High Court judge under the age of
75 years to conduct an investigation into a person's death, and the Lord Chief
Justice after consulting the Lord Chancellor[216] may do so.[217] The Chief Coroner
may also request a former senior coroner under the age of 75 years to conduct an
investigation into a person's death.[218] If the person so nominated or requested
agrees, he comes under a duty to conduct the investigation,[219] has the same
functions in relation to the body and the investigation as if he were a senior coroner
in whose area the body was situated,[220] and no other coroner has any such
functions.[221] The legislation is then read accordingly.[222]

The Chief Coroner may also notify the Lord Advocate, in the case of a service   **2–61**
death on active service or analogous circumstances where the body has been
brought to England and Wales, but the Chief Coroner thinks that it may be
appropriate for the death to be investigated under the Scottish system of fatal
accidents inquiries.[223]

Information about investigations

The Chief Coroner has various powers to obtain information about investigations   **2–62**
which are being conducted. He may at any time require information from a
coroner in relation to a particular investigation or investigations which are being
conducted by that coroner,[224] and the coroner is obliged to provide it.[225] A coroner
conducting an investigation which has not been completed or discontinued within
a year of the date that the death was reported must notify the Chief Coroner of the

---

[213] Coroners and Justice Act 2009 s.1(4). See 5–16.
[214] Coroners and Justice Act 2009 s.3. See 4–22.
[215] Coroners and Justice Act 2009 s.13. See 4–26.
[216] Coroners and Justice Act 2009 s.41 Sch.10 para.3(6).
[217] Coroners and Justice Act 2009 s.41 Sch.10 para.3(1).
[218] Coroners and Justice Act 2009 s.41 Sch.10 para.3(3).
[219] Coroners and Justice Act 2009 s.41 Sch.10 para.3(4)(a).
[220] Coroners and Justice Act 2009 s.41 Sch.10 para.3(4)(b).
[221] Coroners and Justice Act 2009 s.41 Sch.10 para.3(4)(c).
[222] Coroners and Justice Act 2009 s.41 Sch.10 para.3(5).
[223] Coroners and Justice Act 2009 s.12(5). See 4–27.
[224] Coroners (Investigations) Regulations 2013 (SI 2013/1629) reg.25(1).
[225] Coroners (Investigations) Regulations 2013 (SI 2013/1629) reg.25(2).

fact as soon as reasonably practicable and explain why it has not been completed or discontinued.[226] Where the coroner having previously notified the matter thereafter completes or discontinues the investigation he must notify the Chief Coroner of the date on which that happened, and explain any further delay.[227]

After the investigation

2–63   Where coroners make reports intended to prevent deaths in future, they must send copies to the Chief Coroner.[228] The Chief Coroner may publish the report, or a summary, as he thinks fit,[229] and may send a copy to any person whom he thinks may find it of interest.[230] Coroners must also send the Chief Coroner copies of any response they receive to such reports,[231] and he may publish such response, or a summary, as he thinks fit,[232] and may send a copy to any person whom he thinks may find it of interest.[233] If a respondent to a report makes written representations to the coroner about release or publication of the response, the coroner must pass them to the Chief Coroner, who may then consider them and decide whether there should be any restriction on release or publication.[234] The Chief Coroner also has power to require a coroner and his relevant authority to provide him with copies of any accounting records held by them.[235]

Staff

2–64   The Lord Chancellor must appoint staff to assist the Chief Coroner and any deputy chief coroner in the performance of their functions.[236] They are appointed on whatever terms the Lord Chancellor thinks appropriate.[237] The office of the Chief Coroner is located at the Royal Courts of Justice in London.[238]

Termination of office

2–65   It will be recalled that the Chief Coroner is appointed by the Lord Chief Justice after consulting the Lord Chancellor, and a deputy chief coroner is appointed either by the Lord Chief Justice or by the Lord Chancellor, in either case after involving the other.[239] The Chief Coroner or a deputy chief coroner may resign from office by giving notice in writing to the person (Lord Chancellor or Lord

---

[226] Coroners (Investigations) Regulations 2013 (SI 2013/1629) reg.26(1).
[227] Coroners (Investigations) Regulations 2013 (SI 2013/1629) reg.26(2).
[228] Coroners and Justice Act 2009 s.32 Sch.5 para.7(3); Coroners (Investigation) Regulations (SI 2013/1629) reg.28(4)(a). See 13–122 ff.
[229] Coroners (Investigation) Regulations (SI 2013/1629) reg.28(5)(a).
[230] Coroners (Investigation) Regulations (SI 2013/1629) reg.28(5)(b).
[231] Coroners (Investigation) Regulations (SI 2013/1629) reg.29(6)(a).
[232] Coroners (Investigation) Regulations (SI 2013/1629) reg.29(7)(a).
[233] Coroners (Investigation) Regulations (SI 2013/1629) reg.29(7)(b).
[234] Coroners (Investigation) Regulations (SI 2013/1629) reg.29(10).
[235] Coroners Allowances, Fees and Expenses Regulations 2013 (SI 2013/1615) reg.14(2). See 18–43.
[236] Coroners and Justice Act 2009 s.35 Sch.8 para.9(1).
[237] Coroners and Justice Act 2009 s.35 Sch.8 para.9(2).
[238] The address is: 11th floor, Thomas More Building, Royal Courts of Justice, Strand, London WC2A 2LL. Website: *http://www.judiciary.gov.uk/about-the-judiciary/office-chief-coroner*. [Accessed June 4, 2014].
[239] See 2–122ff.

Chief Justice) who made the appointment.[240] However the resignation does not take effect unless and until it is accepted, and the recipient has consulted the other office holder (Lord Chancellor or Lord Chief Justice) concerned.[241]

The Lord Chief Justice, after consulting the Lord Chancellor, may remove the **2–66** Chief Coroner or a deputy chief coroner that he appointed from office for incapacity or misbehaviour.[242] The Lord Chancellor, after consulting the Lord Chief Justice, may remove a deputy chief coroner that he appointed from office for incapacity or misbehaviour.[243]

Remuneration, allowances and expenses

The Lord Chancellor may pay the Chief Coroner remuneration or allowances, or **2–67** expenses incurred in performing his functions, in amounts which the Lord Chancellor determines.[244] For this purpose "expenses" also include costs reasonably incurred in connection with proceedings in respect of the performance of functions, costs reasonably incurred in disputing claims in such proceedings, damages or costs ordered to be paid by the Chief Coroner, and reasonable sums paid to settle such proceedings or claims.[245] There is a similar regime in relation to deputy chief coroners.[246] In practice, the Chief Coroner, being a serving judge, has his salary and pension in place already, and there is no need for the Lord Chancellor to make separate provision for them.

Power of a deputy chief coroner to act

A deputy chief coroner may perform any functions of the Chief Coroner during **2–68** a vacancy in the office of Chief Coroner, if the Chief Coroner is absent or unavailable, or otherwise with the consent of the Chief Coroner.[247] Hence references in the legislation to the Chief Coroner are to be read where appropriate as including a deputy chief coroner.[248]

---

[240] Coroners and Justice Act 2009 s.35 Sch.8 para.3(1) (Chief Coroner), (3) (deputy chief coroner).
[241] Coroners and Justice Act 2009 s.35 Sch.8 para.3(2) (Chief Coroner), (4) (deputy chief coroner).
[242] Coroners and Justice Act 2009 s.35 Sch.8 para.4(1).
[243] Coroners and Justice Act 2009 s.35 Sch.8 para.4(2).
[244] Coroners and Justice Act 2009 s.35 Sch.8 para.5.
[245] Coroners and Justice Act 2009 s.35 Sch.8 para.7.
[246] Coroners and Justice Act 2009 s.35 Sch.8 paras 6, 7.
[247] Coroners and Justice Act 2009 s.35 Sch.8 para.8(1).
[248] Coroners and Justice Act 2009 s.35 Sch.8 para.8(2).

Senior, Area and Assistant Coroners: Terms of Appointment

Contract

2–69   Because coronership is a statutory office,[249] rather than an employment, and the terms on which the appointee holds office are prescribed by statute, there is no room for any "contract of employment".[250] Hence attempts by appointing authorities to exact undertakings of a contractual nature[251] might appear to be of doubtful utility. Having selected the best candidate for appointment, it would be improper not to appoint that candidate for failing to give collateral undertakings which by law there is no obligation to give. An attempt simply to impose such terms, e.g. as a "condition of appointment", would fare no better. The appointing authority has no power unilaterally to impose any non-statutory terms, or exact any contractual consideration for the appointment.[252]

2–70   That said, an element of consensus is imported by statute law itself into the terms in two respects. The first is in relation to the amount of salary to be paid. This is dealt with below.[253] The second is in relation to terms not otherwise provided for by the statute itself. As to the latter, subject to the statutory terms, a senior coroner, area coroner or assistant coroner holds office on whatever terms are from time to time agreed by that coroner and the relevant authority for the area.[254] But such agreement does not make the term part of a contract, nor any obligation contained in the term a contractual one. Instead, it imports the agreed obligation into the statutory framework. In practice appointing authorities and coroners execute—and happily operate—documents often ineptly headed "Terms and conditions of employment", containing all kinds of matters which they have "agreed" between them.

Residence

2–71   It was formerly a requirement for county (but not borough) coroners that they should reside within the district for which they were coroners or in some place wholly or partly surrounded by such districts and not more than two miles beyond the boundary of them.[255] However, this requirement was abolished long ago.[256]

---

[249] *Re Saunders* (1744) 3 Atk. 184; 26 E.R. 908; cf. *Leconfield v Thornley* [1926] A.C.10 (Clerk of the Peace of a county).

[250] See *Chief Coroner Guidance No. 6* para.4. cf. *Roy v Kensington and Chelsea and Westminster Family Practitioner Committee* [1992] 1 A.C. 624 at 630, 649; *Leconfield v Thornley* [1926] A.C. 10 at 20, per Lord Buckmaster.

[251] e.g. to retire on being given notice, not to carry on other businesses, or (more prosaically) not to smoke on the authority's premises; see also Leckey and Greer, *Coroners' Law and Practice in Northern Ireland* (1998) para.2–06.

[252] cf. *Leconfield v Thornley* [1926] A.C. 10 at 35, per Lord Sumner.

[253] See 2–79—2–81 below.

[254] Coroners and Justice Act 2009 s.23 Sch.3 para.19. See *Chief Coroner Guidance No. 6* para.4.

[255] Coroners Act 1844 s.5.

[256] Local Government Act 1972 s.272(1) and Sch.30. The Coroner of the Queen's Household continued to have a residence requirement, but that office has itself now been abolished: see 2–09.

Availability

In each coroner area, a coroner (who may be a senior coroner, an area coroner, or   2–72
an assistant coroner) must be available "at all times" to address urgent matters
relating to an investigation into a death which must be dealt with immediately and
cannot wait until the next working day.[257] As the Chief Coroner has noted,[258] this
rule is drafted more restrictively than the previous law,[259] and requires less of the
coroner.

In practice, the on-call coroner's officer[260] is likely to be the first point of   2–73
contact, who will normally have sufficient authority from the coroner to deal with
administrative matters, and who will contact the on-call coroner for specific
instructions where judicial functions are to be exercised.[261] Before dealing with the
question of what matters are urgent, and cannot wait until the next business day,
it is first necessary to be clear what are "matters relating to an investigation". If the
matter concerned does not fall within that phrase, in law it is irrelevant how urgent
it is.[262]

The meaning of the phrase "relating to" is flexible, and depends on the statutory   2–74
context.[263] Here, "matters relating to an investigation" must mean matters
intended to assist or form part of a particular investigation. Therefore it will include
removing the body to a suitable mortuary, directing an autopsy or other
examination, whether that examination should be invasive or not, and if so how
far, and seeking statements or other information in relation to the identity of the
deceased, or how, when and where the deceased came by his or her death.

Questions of whether to permit organ removal for transplantation[264] or to   2–75
release[265] the body for a funeral however do not assist or form part of the
investigation. They are for a collateral purpose, and can only "relate to" an
investigation in the negative sense that, if the organ were removed or the body
released, it would no longer be available to the coroner for the purposes of his
investigation. But the same could be said of many coronial decisions which do not
assist or form part of the inquiry.

---

[257] Coroners (Investigations) Regulations 2013 reg.4. See 2–16 for the power of area and assistant
coroners to carry out the functions of senior coroners.
[258] *The Chief Coroner's Guide to the Coroners and Justice Act 2009*, 2nd edn (July 2013) para.46. See also
Chief Coroner, *Release of the Body for Burial or Cremation*, 1 May 2014, [21]–[31].
[259] See previously Coroners Rules 1984 r.4, which stated that "A coroner shall at all times hold himself
ready to undertake, either by himself or by his deputy or assistant deputy, any duties in connection
with inquests and post-mortem examinations." It may be noted that the Home Office suggested, in
a circular letter dated December 14, 1999 to all coroners that this required: "a *full* call-out service by
all coroners at all times", including what were called "applications for permission to remove a body
abroad" when neither inquest nor post-mortem examination was contemplated. Plainly the old rule
did no such thing. As to notices of intention to remove the body, see 9–36 below.
[260] See 2–134 below.
[261] See 2–142.
[262] As to so-called "out of England" orders, see 9–38.
[263] See, e.g. *Svenska Petroleum Exploration AB v Lithuania* [2006] EWCA Civ. 1529 [137]; *Veolia ES
Nottinghamshire Ltd v Nottingham CC* [2009] EWHC 2382 (Admin) [56].
[264] See 8–78 ff.
[265] In practice, this means deciding whether the coroner needs to retain legal possession (as to which
see 8–11). If the coroner decides that he does not, and "releases" the body, he is not responsible if
the local authority for its own reasons does not immediately allow the relatives access to the body in
its mortuary (see 8–12).

2-76   The better view is that deciding about organ removal for transplantation and release of the body are not in themselves sufficiently closely connected to *the investigation itself* to fall within the phrase "matters relating to an investigation". Going even further in the same direction, the giving of an acknowledgement relating to the removal of a body from the jurisdiction (the so-called "out of England" order)[266] where the death is not itself under investigation is not a matter "relating to an investigation" either, and also falls outside the scope of this provision.[267]

2-77   But if a matter *is* one relating to an investigation, then it is necessary to go on and consider whether it "must be dealt with immediately and cannot wait until the next business day". Most coronial work can be done within the business day, waiting its turn from one day to the next, if need be. This rule however treats certain things as taking priority over other work. So the effect ought to be proportionately small. Matters connected with the immediate investigation of a homicide (for the purposes of so-called "hot pursuit") are the obvious examples.

2-78   Where the bereaved would like the body released as soon as possible for funeral reasons, that does not make the logically *preceding* decision (e.g. as to whether and how to carry out a post-mortem examination) one which must be dealt with immediately, for the urgency relates to the release (not a matter relating to the investigation) rather than to the decision on the examination (which would be such a matter).

Salary and fees

2-79   Every senior coroner for a coroner area and every area coroner[268] is entitled to a salary,[269] in whatever amount is from time to time agreed by that coroner and the relevant authority for the area.[270] The relevant authority is responsible for paying the salary.[271] If they cannot agree on an alteration, either may refer the matter to the Lord Chancellor, who may determine the amount and the date on which it becomes payable.[272] The alteration takes effect in accordance with the determination.[273] The Lord Chancellor must have regard to the nature and extent of the coroner's functions and indeed to all the circumstances.[274] In practice, coroners' salaries are negotiated nationally by a Joint Negotiating Committee for Coroners,[275] in which both coroners and local authorities are represented, although a few coroners make their own separate arrangements.

---

[266] See 9–36 ff.
[267] See 9–41.
[268] Coroners and Justice Act 2009 s.23 Sch.3 para.15(6).
[269] Coroners and Justice Act 2009 s.23 Sch.3 para.15(1). See formerly Coroners Act 1988 s.3(1) Sch.1 para.1(1).
[270] Coroners and Justice Act 2009 s.23 Sch.3 para.15(2).
[271] Coroners and Justice Act 2009 s.23 Sch.3 para.15(5).
[272] Coroners and Justice Act 2009 s.23 Sch.3 para.15(3).
[273] Coroners and Justice Act 2009 s.23 Sch.3 para.15(3).
[274] Coroners and Justice Act 2009 s.23 Sch.3 para.15(4). See formerly Coroners Act 1988 s.3(1) and Sch.1 para.1(3).
[275] At the time of writing the latest agreed pay scale is that set out in Circular No. 51, dated April 14, 2011. Circular No. 55 of July 30, 2012 indicated that there would be no pay award for 2012.

If the Lord Chancellor fixes the rate of the salary of the coroner,[276] then it appears that, at any rate as long as the Lord Chancellor does not take into account irrelevant considerations, or fail to consider relevant ones, his decision is final and there is no appeal from it.[277] Although (unsurprisingly) there is no direct authority for saying that the exercise by the Lord Chancellor of his rate-fixing power if made in bad faith,[278] for an improper purpose,[279] or after taking into account irrelevant considerations or failing to take into account relevant ones,[280] would be struck down by the courts, it can hardly be doubted that this would be the case.[281] **2–80**

Every assistant coroner for a coroner area is entitled to fees,[282] in whatever amount is from time to time agreed by that coroner and the relevant authority for the area.[283] The relevant authority is responsible for paying the fees.[284] There is no provision for the Lord Chancellor to fix the amount of the fees in case of disagreement. **2–81**

Remedy for non-payment of salary or fees

In the nineteenth century it was held that the coroner's remedy for non-payment of his salary was to seek an order for mandamus compelling the council to perform its statutory duty and pay the sums due.[285] It was also decided that a claim for a declaration of rights by the coroner would not lie,[286] though the decision was almost certainly wrong in this respect.[287] **2–82**

But the current system of judicial review requires an initial distinction to be drawn between matters of public law and matters of private law. The two categories were originally said to be mutually exclusive, so that the judicial review procedure could only be used for matters of public law, and writ actions, whether for a money sum or for a declaration, or for some other relief could only be used for private law matters.[288] As a result, the courts have been working out the **2–83**

---

[276] See 2–79 above.
[277] See *Ex p. Driffield* (1871) L.R. 7 Q.B. 207, decided under the County Coroners Act 1860 s.4, the forerunner of para.(2) of Sch.1 to the 1988 Act.
[278] See, e.g. *Associated Provincial Picture Houses Ltd. v Wednesbury Corporation* [1948] 1 K.B. 223 at 229; *R. v Governor of Brixton Prison Ex p. Soblen* [1963] 2 Q.B. 243.
[279] See, e.g. *Congreve v Home Office* [1976] Q.B. 629 at 641.
[280] See, e.g. *Anisminic Ltd. v Foreign Compensation Commission* [1969] 2 A.C. 147 at 171, 195, 210; *Prest v Secretary of State for Wales* (1982) 266 S.J. 708, CA.
[281] See generally de Smith, Jowell and Woolf, *Judicial Review of Administrative Action*, 5th edn (1995); Wade and Forsyth, *Administrative Law*, 8th edn (2000). cf. *Re South Down Coroner's Application* [2004] NIQB 86: the High Court of Northern Ireland dismissed a judicial review claim by a part-time coroner that the remuneration of part-time coroners there constituted unlawful discrimination compared to that of full-time coroners.
[282] Coroners and Justice Act 2009 s.23 Sch.3 para.16(1). There was no similar provision under the 1988 Act.
[283] Coroners and Justice Act 2009 s.23 Sch.3 para.16(2).
[284] Coroners and Justice Act 2009 s.23 Sch.3 para.16(3).
[285] *Baxter v LCC* (1890) 63 L.T. 767.
[286] *Baxter v LCC* (1890) 63 L.T. 767.
[287] RSC Ord.XXV r.5 (as it then was; it is now CPR r.40.20), which had been made only seven years previously, in 1883, for the first time empowered the courts to make binding declarations of right "whether or not any consequential relief is or could be claimed". Doubts about the validity and extent of the new rule persisted until the decision of the Court of Appeal in *Guaranty Trust Co of New York v Hannay* [1915] 2 K.B. 536.
[288] See *O'Reilly v Mackman* [1983] 2 A.C. 237; *Cocks v Thanet DC* [1983] 2 A.C. 286.

principles which must be applied to decide whether ordinary action (called a "Pt 7 claim" by the CPR) or judicial review should be used.[289]

2–84   It is not entirely free from doubt under which category a claim by a coroner for his salary should now fall. On the one hand, the coroner is seeking proper performance of the statutory duty of a public body, i.e. the relevant authority, and local authorities have long been subject to orders of mandamus (now, a "mandatory order")[290] to compel them to perform their statutory duties, even when they consist merely of the payment of money.[291] On the other hand, it has been held that judicial review was inappropriate "for enforcing performance of ordinary obligations owed by a master to his servant".[292]

2–85   Thus, in one case, a superintendent registrar of births, marriages and deaths, appointed by the Registrar-General under statutory powers,[293] but paid by the local authority, brought a writ action for unpaid salary, withheld by the authority to reflect industrial action taken by the registrar. The House of Lords held that the claim failed, because he was unwilling to perform some of the duties of his office. But there was no suggestion that the registrar's remedy lay by way judicial review rather than by action.[294] And in another case,[295] the House of Lords held that a claim by a general medical practitioner against his family practitioner committee, for unpaid basic practice allowance, was properly brought by ordinary action rather than judicial review. The claim was for a private law right to remuneration, whether conferred by contract or by statute.[296]

2–86   It is therefore submitted that, notwithstanding previous authority to the contrary, the procedural changes arising from the revisions the rules relating to judicial review mean that the coroner's remedy for unpaid salary is nowadays by way of ordinary CPR Pt 7 claim, and not by way of judicial review.

---

[289] See, e.g. *Davy v Spelthorne BC* [1984] A.C. 262; *Wandsworth LBC v Winder* [1985] A.C. 461; *R. v East Berkshire Health Authority Ex p. Walsh* [1985] Q.B. 152; *Gillick v West Norfolk Health Authority* [1986] A.C. 112; *R. v Derbyshire CC Ex p. Noble* [1990] I.C.R. 808; *McLaren v Home Office* [1990] I.C.R. 824; *Doyle v Northumbria Probation Committee* [1991] 1 W.L.R. 1340; *Roy v Kensington and Chelsea and Westminster Family Practitioner Committee* [1992] 1 A.C. 624, HL; *Mercury Ltd v Telecommunications Director* [1996] 1 W.L.R. 48, HL; *Clark v University of Lincolnshire and Humberside* [2000] 1 W.L.R. 1988, CA; *Wandsworth LBC v A* [2001] 1 W.L.R. 1264, CA.

[290] Senior Courts Act 1981 s.29(1).

[291] See, e.g. *R. v Treasurer of Oswestry* (1848) 12 Q.B. 239 (to compel the borough treasurer to pay the expenses of a prosecution); *R. v Liverpool City Council Ex p. Coade, The Times,* October 10, 1986 (to compel local authority to discharge statutory obligation to pay teachers pursuant to their contracts of employment).

[292] *R. v BBC Ex p. Lavelle* [1983] 1 All E.R. 241 at 248, approved by the Court of Appeal in *Law v National Greyhound Racing Club* [1983] 1 W.L.R. 1302, and followed in *Evans v University of Cambridge* [2002] EWHC 1382 (Admin); *R. (Tucker) v National Crime Squad Director General* [2003] EWCA Civ. 57; *R. (Gamesa Energy UK Ltd) v The National Assembly for Wales* [2006] EWHC 2167 (Admin); *R. (Shoesmith) v Ofsted* [2010] EWHC 852 (Admin).

[293] Registration Service Act 1953; Local Government Act 1972.

[294] *Miles v Wakefield MDC* [1987] A.C. 539. The position of the registrar at that time was peculiarly analogous to that of the coroner, being paid by the local authority but acting independently of it, and indeed holding office under the Crown: see 1–11 ff above. The legal status of the registrar has since changed from independent office-holder to local authority employee, by virtue of the Statistics and Registration Service Act 2007 s.69.

[295] *Roy v Kensington and Chelsea and Westminster Family Practitioner Committee* [1992] 1 A.C. 624, HL.

[296] See also *R. v Secretary of State for Transport Ex p. Sherriff & Sons, The Independent,* January 12, 1988 (mandamus not possible to enforce private right to recovery of a debt).

Fee or remuneration not authorised by statute

Save as authorised by Act of Parliament,[297] a senior coroner, area coroner or   **2–87**
assistant coroner is not permitted to take any fee or remuneration in respect of
anything done by him in the performance of his functions.[298] So, for example,
coroners may not charge for providing an interim certificate of the fact of
death.[299]

No penalty is specifically prescribed for contravention of this prohibition, but   **2–88**
historically it was a principle of the criminal law that "all acts or omissions contrary
to the prohibitions or command of [statutes of this type] are [offences] at common
law punishable by indictment unless such method manifestly appears to be
excluded by statute".[300] Modern authority, however, turns the presumption the
other way, and it requires clear language, or a very clear inference, in a modern
statute to create a crime.[301] It is therefore submitted that breach of the prohibition
is not *of itself* an offence.

Where a gift or payment is made to a coroner to influence his behaviour in the   **2–89**
conduct of his office, both donor or payer and coroner formerly committed the
common law offence of bribery,[302] and now the statutory offences under the
Bribery Act 2010.[303] A coroner who receives a bribe has long been liable to be
punished by loss of office.[304] Furthermore, even where a coroner is not convicted
of any offence in connection with taking money or other rewards, demanding fees
to which a coroner is not entitled[305] or any other corrupt practice[306] has been held
to constitute such misbehaviour on the part of the coroner as to justify his removal
from office.[307]

Reimbursement of expenses

A coroner is of course entitled to be reimbursed the expenses which he is by law   **2–90**
authorised to incur or pay in the conduct of his office and the performance of his
duties,[308] and although in some cases he should give advance notice of them to the
relevant authority,[308a] also to be indemnified in respect of costs, damages and

---

[297] So requiring *primary* legislation to give the authority, even if the amount is quantified by *secondary* legislation. There are three main matters: the coroner's salary (2–79 above) his pension (2-110—2–111 below), and fees for copies for documents supplied (18–34 below).

[298] Coroners and Justice Act 2009 s.23 Sch.3 para.18; formerly Coroners Act 1988 s.3(2).

[299] See 8–20 below.

[300] *R. v Lennox-Wright* [1973] Crim.L.R. 529; see also *R. v Hall* [1891] 1 Q.B.747; *Rathbone v Bundock* [1962] 2 Q.B. 260.

[301] *Attorney-General Ex rel. McWhirter v Independent Broadcasting Authority* [1973] Q.B. 62, CA; *R. v Horseferry Road Justices Ex p. Independent Broadcasting Authority* [1987] Q.B. 54, DC.

[302] Co. Inst. 145, 147; 1 Hale P.C. 262; 1 Hawk. P.C. c. 67; 4 Bl.Comm. 139; Bac. Abr., *Offices and Officers* (N); *R. v Gurney* (1867) 10 Cox C.C. 550.

[303] s.1 (donor or payer); s.2 (recipient), in force July 1, 2011 (SI 2011/1418).

[304] 3 Co. Inst. 145, 147; 1 Hawk. P.C. c. 67; *R. v Harrison* (1800) 1 East P.C. 382 (coroner fined, imprisoned and removed from office for corruptly demanding money not to hold an inquest).

[305] 3 Co. Inst. 149.

[306] *R. v Coates* (cited in Dickinson's *Justices*, p.515); *R. v Harrison* (1800) 1 East P.C. 382.

[307] See 2–96 below.

[308] Coroners and Justice Act 2009 s.34 Sch.7 para.9; Coroners Allowances, Fees and Expenses Regulations 2013 (SI 2013/1615); formerly Coroners Act 1988 s.27(3). See *Forrest v Lord Chancellor* [2011] EWHC 1421 (Admin), and 18–33 ff.

[308a] Coroners Allowances, Fees and Expenses Regulations 2013, SI 2013 No.1615, reg.7; see 5–65.

expenses in relation to legal proceedings in respect of his duties.[309] Receipt of the reimbursed expenses or satisfaction of the indemnity is obviously not taking a fee or remuneration, because it is not a profit to the coroner. But even if it were, it would be within the exception for receipts authorised by Act of Parliament.

Term of office

2–91 Since coronership was formerly a freehold office,[310] there was no power at common law in the appointing council to impose conditions at the time of appointment, such as a condition of retirement from the office at a certain age, or termination of the appointment upon certain notice.[311] And although the office was held under the Crown,[312] the appointment did not terminate on the demise of the Crown.[313] In principle, therefore, a coroner once appointed was entitled to hold office for life.[314] But this was subject to a number of limitations.

2–92 First, it was said that the offices of sheriff and of verderer[315] were so inconsistent with that of coroner, that upon a coroner being appointed or elected to either office, his appointment as coroner automatically terminated.[316] Given the greatly reduced functions of all three offices in modern times, so that none of their functions now overlap, it must be doubted how far this remains true. Secondly, a coroner might resign his office by giving notice in writing to the council having power to appoint his successor, but the resignation did not take effect unless and until it was accepted by the council.[317]

2–93 Thirdly, a coroner appointed after May 1, 1927 and before April 6, 1978 (not having opted out of the pension provisions of the 1926 Act), could in some circumstances be required to vacate his office if called upon to do so.[318] Fourthly, the coroner could be removed from office in a number of ways, either by the Lord Chancellor or by a competent court.[319] Fifthly, a coroner who ceased to hold the

---

[309] Coroners and Justice Act 2009 s.34 Sch.7 para.9; Coroners Allowances, Fees and Expenses Regulations 2013 (SI 2013/1615) reg.37; formerly Coroners Act 1988 s.27A. See 18–44.

[310] *Re Saunders* (1744) 3 Atk. 184; 26 E.R. 908.

[311] cf. *Leconfield v Thornley* [1926] A.C. 10, HL (appointment of Clerk of Peace of a county).

[312] See 1–13 above. As to whether this is still so, see 1–15.

[313] *Resolutions at Sergeants Inn* (1558) 2 Dyer 165a; 73 E.R. 359; *Tombes v Ethrington* (1663) 1 Lev. 120; 83 E.R. 327; Demise of the Crown Act 1901 s.1(1).

[314] *Jervis on Coroners,* 1st edn (1829), p.53. See *Londonderry and North Tyrone Coroner's Application for Judicial Review,* July 4, 2003, HC (NI) (Weatherup J), (the Lord Chancellor's Department had sent a letter to a coroner stating that when he reached the age of 75 years his appointment would terminate automatically, but stated at the hearing that it accepted that it had no power to require the coroner to retire merely on age grounds, and confirmed that the letter did not have the effect of terminating the coroner's tenure of his office).

[315] See 2–36.

[316] Staunford P.C., c.51, fol.48b; cf. Blackstone, who says only that he "may be removed": 1 Bl.Comm. 336; and also Hunnisett, *The Medieval Coroner* (1961), pp.168–170; and see the 9th edn of this work at pp.11 and 38. For the appointment of sheriffs, see *Halsbury's Laws of England,* 4th edn reissue Vol.42, paras 1101–1110.

[317] Coroners Act 1988 s.3(3). It was no longer necessary for a writ *de coronatore exonerando* to be issued in respect of the resignation of a coroner: Coroners (Amendment) Act 1926 s.2(4) (repealed).

[318] Coroners Act 1988 Sch.1 para.2(3). If the coroner's retirement was brought about by these means, he was entitled to a statutory pension of the maximum that could be granted: 2–110 below.

[319] See 2–96 below.

legal or medical professional qualification by virtue of which he was appointed would cease also to hold the office of coroner.[320]

A senior coroner, area coroner or assistant coroner appointed under the 2009 Act is in a very different position, although for those in office under the old system and deemed appointed into the new[321] there are important transitional provisions. The office is not a freehold office,[322] and there is a statutory retirement imposed at the age of seventy years.[323] A senior coroner, area coroner or assistant coroner may resign office by giving notice to the relevant authority and having the resignation accepted.[324]   **2–94**

But such a coroner may also lose office on a merger of coroner areas,[325] or may be removed from office as described below. Finally, where a senior coroner, area coroner or assistant coroner loses his professional qualification, as where he is struck off the roll of solicitors, or is disbarred, then he ceases to be qualified to be coroner at all,[326] and he vacates office automatically.[327] It is also possible for the coroner on appointment *to agree* a term[328] that he should vacate office at some other point, e.g. when the particular case which he was appointed to conduct has come to an end.   **2–95**

Removal from office, correction or punishment

There have long been various powers, both at common law and conferred by statute, vested in the Lord Chancellor and in the High Court to remove a coroner from office, or to correct or punish him. The 2009 Act has extended the statutory powers to cover not just senior coroners, but area and assistant coroners as well.   **2–96**

Power of Lord Chancellor and Lord Chief Justice

The Lord Chancellor[329] has statutory power, with the agreement of the Lord Chief Justice (or his delegate),[330] to remove a senior coroner, area coroner or assistant coroner from office for incapacity or misbehaviour.[331] The Lord Chancellor[332] also had power at common law to remove coroners from their office for neglect of   **2–97**

---

[320] But see Thurston's *Coronership,* 3rd edn (1985) para.4.08, where the opposite view is taken.
[321] As to which see 2–40.
[322] Coroners and Justice Act 2009 s.23 Sch.3 para.9.
[323] Coroners and Justice Act 2009 s.23 Sch.3 para.10.
[324] Coroners and Justice Act 2009 s.23 Sch.3 para.12.
[325] See 2–31 above.
[326] See 2–23 above.
[327] But see Thurston's *Coronership,* 3rd edn (1985) para.4.08, where the opposite view is taken.
[328] As to which see 2–70.
[329] The Chancellor of the Duchy of Lancaster used to exercise this power in relation to Lancashire (Coroners Act 1887 s.39), but this has long been abolished: Local Government Act 1972 s.272(1).
[330] Coroners and Justice Act 2009 s.23 Sch.3 para.13(2).
[331] Coroners and Justice Act 2009 s.23 Sch.3 para.13(1), formerly Coroners Act 1988 s.3(4).
[332] Quaere whether the common law power, in relation to Lancashire, if it still exists, is exercisable by the Lord Chancellor or the Chancellor of the Duchy of Lancaster, since the repeal of s.39 of the Coroners Act 1887 by the Local Government Act 1972 clearly only affected the exercise of the *statutory* power of removal.

duty.[333] If the Lord Chancellor considered that the case for removing the coroner had been made out, he made an order accordingly.[334] This common law jurisdiction was preserved by the 1988 Act,[335] but that provision has now been repealed.

2–98   Since the 2009 Act creates the new statutory offices of senior coroner, area coroner and assistant coroner, and makes fresh provision for their removal from office, it is submitted that the common law power has gone, and only the statutory power remains. In practice, it is that power which will be exercised. The powers to remove a coroner are exercised judicially, and such exercise may in an appropriate case be subject to judicial review.[336]

2–99   In relation to the *common law* power to remove, it was formerly held that it was not necessary to give notice of the petition for removal to the coroner concerned,[337] and still less to hear him before making the order. But this approach would not be followed today.[338] Certainly, where the former statutory power was being exercised, the coroner concerned was generally given an opportunity of being heard.[339]

2–100   However, the procedure to be followed today is the judicial discipline procedure laid down in the Constitutional Reform Act 2005. The Lord Chancellor's power to remove a coroner can only be exercised after he has complied with "prescribed procedures".[340] In addition, the disciplinary powers short of removal from office that apply to other judicial holders apply also to the offices of senior coroner, area coroner and assistant coroner.[341]

2–101   "Prescribed procedures" are those prescribed by the Lord Chief Justice with the agreement of the Lord Chancellor, to be followed in the investigation and determination of allegations of judicial misconduct and in reviews by the Ombudsman.[342] They involve a complaint to the Judicial Conduct Investigation Office,[343] which is investigated in accordance with rules made by the Lord Chief

---

[333] *Re Saunders* (1744) 3 Atk. 184; 26 E.R. 908; *Ex p.Parnell* (1820) 1 J. & W. 451; 37 E.R. 439; *Ex p. Pasley* (1842) 3 Dr. & W. 34.

[334] In the case of exercise of the common law power, this involved ordering the issue of a writ *de coronatore amovendo*: *Ex p.Parnell*, above. cf. 2 Hawk. P.C. c. 9 s.12, which referred to discharge of a coroner by the writ *de coronatore exonerando* (the need for this writ where a coroner *resigns* was removed by the Coroners (Amendment) Act 1926 s.2(4)).

[335] Coroners Act 1988 s.33(2).

[336] See *Forrest v Lord Chancellor* [2011] EWHC 1421 (Admin), and Ch.19 below.

[337] *Ex p. Parnell* (1820) 1 J. & W. 45; 37 E.R. 439. In *Ex p. Pasley* (1842) 3 Dr. & W. 34, the petition was served personally on the coroner in prison. However, in *Re Saunders* (1744) 3 Atk. 184; 26 E.R. 908 the Lord Chancellor stood over a petition for removal until service had been effected at the coroner's last known place of abode.

[338] For the development of the principle *"audi alteram partem"*, see Halsbury's *Laws of England*, 4th edn reissue, Vol.1(1), paras 94–100; for the impact of the Human Rights Act 1998, see Ch.21.

[339] *Re Ward* (1861) 3 De G.F. & J. 700; 45 E.R. 1049; *Re Hull* (1882) 9 Q.B.D. 689.

[340] Constitutional Reform Act 2005 s.108. It applied to coroners (but not deputy or assistant deputy coroners) under the 1988 Act since 2006, by virtue of the Discipline of Coroners (Designation) Order 2006 (SI 2006/677), made under s.118 of the 2005 Act.

[341] Coroners and Justice Act 2009 s.23 Sch.3 para.14; Judicial Discipline (Prescribed Procedures) Regulations 2013 (SI 2013/1674) (in force October 1, 2013, replacing the Judicial Discipline (Prescribed Procedures) Regulations 2006) reg.3(b).

[342] Constitutional Reform Act 2005 s.115; Judicial Discipline (Prescribed Procedures) Regulations 2013.

[343] Judicial Discipline (Prescribed Procedures) Regulations 2013 reg.6.

Justice.[344] Investigation of a complaint normally ceases if the office-holder vacates office before a decision is made.[345]

The Lord Chief Justice has power to suspend an office-holder from office **2–102**
pending a decision on a complaint.[346] Before doing so, he must notify the office holder of the proposed suspension, the reasons for it and the time when it is proposed that it will come into effect.[347] He must also notify the office holder of the factors that will be taken into account in determining when the suspension will end,[348] and invite the office holder to make representations.[349] The office holder must make any representations within ten business days of the notification.[350] The Lord Chief Justice and the Lord Chancellor must keep the position under review, and the office-holder informed.[351]

Before making a decision[352] in relation to a case, the Lord Chancellor and the **2–103**
Lord Chief Justice (or his delegate)[353] must consider any advice provided by a person who or a body that has conducted an investigation into a complaint in accordance with the rules made by the Lord Chief Justice.[354] If the Lord Chancellor and the Lord Chief Justice having considered such advice require further investigation before making a decision, they may refer the complaint to a nominated judge, investigating judge or disciplinary panel to investigate it further.[355]

Where the advice does not recommend removal from office, but the Lord **2–104**
Chancellor and the Lord Chief Justice consider it the appropriate disciplinary action, they must constitute a disciplinary panel and refer the complaint to it.[356] In such a case the Lord Chancellor and the Lord Chief Justice must consider the advice provided by the disciplinary panel before making a decision.[357] In other cases the Lord Chancellor and the Lord Chief Justice may agree to dismiss a complaint or take other disciplinary action.[358] If the complaint is dismissed they may agree that the Lord Chief Justice should deal with the matter informally.[359] The Judicial Conduct Investigation Office must notify the final decision to various persons including the complainant and the office holder complained of.[360] The decision may be published.[361]

What amounts to incapacity or misbehaviour is a fact-sensitive question. **2–105**
Unfitness owing to age or illness was formerly stated to be grounds for removing

---

[344] Judicial Discipline (Prescribed Procedures) Regulations 2013 reg.7.
[345] Judicial Discipline (Prescribed Procedures) Regulations 2013 reg.23.
[346] Constitutional Reform Act 2005 s.108(4)(a), (6), (7).
[347] Judicial Discipline (Prescribed Procedures) Regulations 2013 reg.17(1)(a).
[348] Judicial Discipline (Prescribed Procedures) Regulations 2013 reg.17(1)(b).
[349] Judicial Discipline (Prescribed Procedures) Regulations 2013 reg.17(1)(c).
[350] Judicial Discipline (Prescribed Procedures) Regulations 2013 reg.17(2).
[351] Judicial Discipline (Prescribed Procedures) Regulations 2013 reg.17(3).
[352] Under Judicial Discipline (Prescribed Procedures) Regulations 2013 reg.15.
[353] Judicial Discipline (Prescribed Procedures) Regulations 2013 reg.20.
[354] Judicial Discipline (Prescribed Procedures) Regulations 2013 reg.12.
[355] Judicial Discipline (Prescribed Procedures) Regulations 2013 reg.13.
[356] Judicial Discipline (Prescribed Procedures) Regulations 2013 reg.14(2).
[357] Judicial Discipline (Prescribed Procedures) Regulations 2013 reg.14(4).
[358] Judicial Discipline (Prescribed Procedures) Regulations 2013 reg.15(2).
[359] Judicial Discipline (Prescribed Procedures) Regulations 2013 reg.15(3).
[360] Judicial Discipline (Prescribed Procedures) Regulations 2013 reg.16.
[361] Judicial Discipline (Prescribed Procedures) Regulations 2013 reg.18.

a coroner for inability,[362] and may satisfy the current test of "incapacity".[363] Absence, whether owing to imprisonment[364] or otherwise,[365] was also a ground of removal for inability. Bankruptcy, however, does not necessarily constitute incapacity or misbehaviour.[366] Holding an incompatible office, or being too much engaged in other business, may constitute incapacity, and also given as grounds for removal.[367]

2–106 Most of the examples of what constitutes misbehaviour in decided cases date from earlier centuries, and recent examples are rare. In some cases, absence might constitute misbehaviour.[368] Examples of misbehaviour are improper refusal to hold an inquest,[369] intoxication,[370] corruption,[371] demanding fees to which the coroner was not entitled,[372] and repeated failure to make the coroner's annual return to the Secretary of State.[373] The most recent example concerned unreasonable behaviour on the part of the coroner, stemming from a mistaken perception of his relationship with his local authority.[374]

2–107 The terms of appointment of all Northern Ireland coroners[375] warn them that the Lord Chancellor regards conviction "for an offence of dishonesty, or moral turpitude or an otherwise serious nature (including drink driving) as constituting misbehaviour". In November 2000 Lord Irvine of Lairg LC wrote to all coroners warning them that he regarded "a drink-driving conviction as an extremely serious matter, potentially amounting to misconduct".[376]

Power of the court

2–108 Formerly, a court that convicted a coroner of extortion, corruption or wilful neglect of his duty or misbehaviour in the discharge of his duty might remove him from his office, and disqualify him from acting as coroner.[377] But this statutory power was without prejudice to the jurisdiction of the High Court in relation to or over a coroner or his duties.[378] This jurisdiction permitted the High Court not merely to review any act done or any order made by a coroner,[379] but to treat any offence on the part of a coroner as contempt of court, and to visit it accordingly

---

[362] Fitz.Nat.Brev. 163 N. A coroner was removed in 1941 for insanity.

[363] See 2–97 above.

[364] See *Ex p. Parnell* (1820) 1 J. & W. 45; 37 E.R. 439; *Ex p. Pasley* (1842) 3 Dr. & W. 34.

[365] *Re Saunders* (1744) 3 Atk. 184; 26 E.R. 908. In 1903 a coroner was removed for indefinite absence. In 1941 a coroner who had absconded and could not be found was removed (he was also bankrupt).

[366] But see previous note.

[367] Fitz.Nat.Brev. 163 N; Com.Dig.Officer G. 4; 2 Co.Inst. 32; 2 Hawk. P.C. c. 9 s.12.

[368] See the cases cited in fnn.364 and 365.

[369] *Re Ward, Re Hull*, above, fn.339.

[370] *Re Ward*, above, fn.339; *Ex p.Pasley*, above, fn.364.

[371] *R. v Coates* (cited in Dickinson's Justices, 515).

[372] 3 Co.Inst. 149; cf. *R. v Harrison* (1800) 1 East P.C. 382.

[373] A coroner was removed on this ground in 1944.

[374] *Forrest v Lord Chancellor* [2011] EWHC 1421 (Admin).

[375] Unlike in England and Wales, the Lord Chancellor makes these appointments.

[376] Circular letter dated November 20, 2000.

[377] Coroners Act 1988 s.3(6). For *civil* liability to third parties, see 2–120 ff below.

[378] Coroners Act 1988 s.33(2)(b).

[379] *R. v Stanlake* (1672) 1 Mod. 82, 86 E.R. 749. See generally 19–25 ff below.

with censure or other punishment, including removal from office.[380] The court's statutory power of removal from office has been repealed.[381] Presumably, however, the common law jurisdiction of the court remains.

Restraint by injunction and declaring office vacant

A person ceasing to be a coroner (whether by removal, ceasing to be qualified, or otherwise) or indeed any other person who purports to exercise the powers of a coroner may be restrained by injunction from so acting, and the High Court also has power (if appropriate) to declare the office vacant.[382] There are old authorities supporting the proposition that, where a person who usurps the office of coroner from the true holder receives any of the profits[383] of that office, an action for money had and received will lie by the true coroner against the usurper,[384] but it would seem that the better view is that the action will not lie to recover salary payable in respect of work that the plaintiff has not performed.[385] A usurper who has acted in good faith and under an apparent right is probably entitled to deduct his necessary expenditure from the profits for which he is accountable.[386]

2–109

Pension

Councils responsible for paying a coroner's salary were given power in 1926 to grant him a non-contributory pension on his retirement in certain circumstances.[387] However, these provisions only applied to coroners who were appointed before April 6, 1978 and who did not elect in writing before July 6, 1978 that those provisions should not apply to them after that date. All other coroners (i.e. all those

2–110

---

[380] *Lord Buckhurst's Case* (1662) 1 Keb. 280 (coroner fined £100 and removed from office for keeping the inquisition in his pocket, the jury having returned a murder verdict, and failing to return it at the next gaol delivery); *R. v Wakefield* (1717) 1 Str. 69, 93 E.R. 390 (coroner imprisoned for deceiving the jury into returning a suicide verdict instead of finding that the deceased was a lunatic); *R. v Harrison* (1800) 1 East P.C. 382 (coroner fined £100 and imprisoned for six months for accepting money for not holding an inquest, although the case was not one where an inquest should have been held). See also *R. v Stukely* (1701) 12 Mos.Rep. 493; *R. v Marsh* (1703) 3 Salk. 172; 91 E.R. 759; *R. v Storey* (1748) 1 Leach C.L. 43.

[381] Coroners and Justice Act 2009 s.178 Sch.23 Pt I.

[382] Senior Courts Act 1981 s.30. The injunction is now sought by application for judicial review: see CPR rr.54.2(d), 54.3(1)(b) (formerly RSC, Ord.53 r.1(1)(b)), and 19–25 below. The present procedure was introduced in 1938 to replace information in the nature of *quo warranto*, which formerly served the same purpose. For examples, see *R. v Grimshaw* (1847) 10 Q.B. 747, 116 E.R. 284, and *R. v Diplock* (1869) L.R. 4 Q.B. 549; and, for *quo warranto* generally, Short and Mellor, *Practice of the Crown Office* (1890), Ch.VIII.

[383] But this does not include gratuities; *Boyter v Dodsworth* (1796) 6 T.R. 681.

[384] *Arris v Stukely* (1677) 2 Mod. 260; *King v Alston* (1848) 12 Q.B. 971; *Brown and Green Ltd. v Hays* (1920) 36 T.L.R. 330.

[385] *Lawlor v Alton* (1873) I.R. 8 C.L. 160; *Miles v Wakefield MDC* [1987] A.C. 539, HL.

[386] *Mayfield v Moore*, 53 Ill. 428 (1870); *Booker v Donohue*, 95 Va. 359, 28 S.E. 584 (1897); *Albright v Sandoral*, 216 U.S. 331 (1910); and see Williams, Mortimer and Sunnucks, *Executors, Administrators and Probate*, 18th edn (2000) para.8–35.

[387] See ultimately the Coroners Act 1988 s.3(1) and Sch.1 para.2 (now repealed). These provisions never applied to the coroner of the Queen's Household (see the 1988 Act Sch.2 para.1), nor, it appears, to the Queen's coroner and attorney (who has no "relevant council").

who did so elect[388] and all those appointed on or after April 6, 1978) were taken outside the ambit of these provisions by statutory instrument.[389] For the first time they became eligible to join the local government superannuation scheme, with certain modifications.[390] For the purposes of the relevant regulations, coroners are deemed to be employees of the relevant council,[391] and in practice cease to be in pensionable service at 70.[392]

2–111   This position continues, and is indeed extended, under the current legislation, which obliges a relevant authority for a coroner area to make provision for the payment of pensions to or in respect not only of senior coroners, but also of area coroners for the area.[393] There is no express pension provision for assistant coroners, but recent decisions[394] on the legislation relating to part-time workers[395] in relation to other part-time judicial officers probably mean that provision will have to be made for them in future.

Duties of coroners

2–112   The duties remaining to the coroner at the present day fall into four main areas, of which only the first two are of any significance: (1) to inquire into the death (including cause and surrounding circumstances) of certain persons; (2) to hold inquests on treasure; (3) (possibly) to take the place of the sheriff in certain limited circumstances; (4) to act as a conservator of the peace. The first and second categories will be considered at length hereafter,[396] but something may now be said briefly in relation to the third and fourth categories.

---

[388] Where a coroner held office before April 6, 1978 and then elected not to continue to be covered by the earlier provisions, his reckonable service was increased by multiplying it by five-thirds for five years' service or less, and by multiplying it by four-thirds for more than five years' service: Local Government Superannuation Regulations 1986 (SI 1986/24) reg.D1(1)(h).

[389] The Social Security (Modification of Coroners (Amendment) Act 1926) Order 1978 (SI 1978/374).

[390] Originally the Local Government Superannuation Regulations 1986 (SI 1986/24), and successively the Local Government Pension Scheme Regulations 1995 (SI 1995/1019), the Local Government Pension Scheme Regulations 1997 (SI 1997/1612), and now the Local Government Pension Scheme (Benefits, Membership and Contributions) Regulations 2007 (SI 2007/1166), the Local Government Pension Scheme (Transitional Provisions) Regulations 2008 (SI 2008/238) and the Local Government Pension Scheme (Administration) Regulations 2008 (SI 2008/239).

[391] 1986 Regulations regs B1(14), B7; 1995 Regulations regs B4, M2 Sch.B2 para.4; 1997 Regulations reg.131(2)(b), (5); Local Government Pension Scheme (Administration) Regulations 2008 (SI 2008/239) reg.9(1)(b), (2), (4).

[392] 1986 Regulations reg.B8, as amended by reg.G4 and Sch.15 Pt IV; 1995 Regulations reg.M2 Sch.M2 paras 1, 5; 1997 Regulations reg.135. Note that this does not mean that they are obliged to vacate office, merely that the pension entitlement will not increase further.

[393] Coroners and Justice Act 2009 s.23 Sch.3 para.17.

[394] *O'Brien v Ministry of Justice* [2010] UKSC 34; *O'Brien v Ministry of Justice* [2012] ICR 955, ECJ; *O'Brien v Ministry of Justice*, Case Number: 2202623/05, August 19, 2013, ET.

[395] Council Directive 97/81/EC of 15 December 1997, concerning the Framework Agreement on part-time work concluded by UNICE, CEEP and ETUC, as applied to the UK by Council Directive 98/23/EC of 7 April 1998, and transposed into UK law by the Part-time Workers (Prevention of Less Favourable Treatment) Regulations 2000 (SI 2000/1551).

[396] See Chs 5 (deaths) and 16 (treasure).

Replacement of sheriff

Under the law before 2003, when any just exception was taken to a sole sheriff,[397]   **2–113**
writs were awarded instead to all the coroners of the county jointly to perform the
sheriff's ministerial duty.[398] The coroner was in such cases in all respects considered
as the immediate officer of the court in place of the sheriff, becoming the *locum
tenens vicecomitis* and might do all lawful acts which the sheriff might have done. But
the rule did not apply if there were two (or more) sheriffs[399] and the objection of
interest applied only to one. In such a case the writ was directed to the other (or
others), and not to the coroners.[400] Nor was process awarded to the coroner in the
case of the death of the sheriff but instead to the under-sheriff, who was
empowered to act until another sheriff is appointed.[401]

However, the role of the sheriff in the enforcement of High Court writs of   **2–114**
execution was abolished in 2003,[402] and a new system of court enforcement
officers introduced. It may be considered that consequently the role of the coroner
in substituting for the sheriff has now also disappeared. Unfortunately, the
legislation does not refer to coroners at all (if only to make clear that their role has
been abolished). Moreover the new statutory scheme does not refer to the
possibility that an enforcement officer may be disqualified through interest.
Nevertheless it must be unlikely that a situation could arise where the writ could
not be directed to another such officer. For this reason, the old law relating to
coroners as a substitute for the sheriff is no longer set out here.[403]

Conservator of the peace[404]

Before the rise of justices of the peace, who as early as the fourteenth century   **2–115**
became the chief instrument for preserving the peace,[405] there were conservators
of the peace at common law. Amongst them were the judges and the most
important officials of the county, namely, the sheriffs and coroners. The main
weapon used by conservators of the peace in keeping the peace was the power to
take surety of the peace.[406] Not all conservators of the peace had identical
powers,[407] and it is a question of exactly what powers to act as conservator a

---

[397] e.g. because he is a party to or otherwise interested in an action in which he may be called upon to
execute process, i.e. enforcing a judgment by seizing goods or taking possession of land.

[398] 4 Co.Inst. 271; Dalton, *The Office and Authoritie of Sherifs* (1623), ff.41b–42b; *Wimbish v Willoughby*
(1552) 1 Plow. 73; *Cumberland v Cumberland* (1615) Hob. 85; *Weston v Coulson* (1764) 1 W.Bl. 506,
96 E.R. 292; *R. v Dolby* (1823) 2 B. & C. 104, 107 E.R. 323. The Coroners Act 1887 s.15 (repealed),
formerly entitled the coroners to the same fees or other compensation for this service as the sheriff
would have been entitled to.

[399] As in the City of London.

[400] *R. v Warrington* (1692) 1 Salk 152; 91 E.R. 141; *Letsom v Bickley* (1816) S.M. & S. 144; 105 E.R.
1004. But this apparently did not happen in *R. v Dolby*, above; cf. Dalton, *The Office and Authoritie
of Sherifs* (1623), f. 43a.

[401] Sheriffs Act 1887 s.25(1)

[402] Courts Act 2003 s.99, Sch.7.

[403] Readers are referred to earlier editions of this work, where the position was set out in more detail:
see, e.g. the 12th edn (2002) at 3–42 to 3–45.

[404] This was dealt with in greater detail in earlier editions of this work.

[405] See 1–09 above.

[406] *Entick v Carrington* (1765) 19 St.Tr. 1029 at 1059–1061; 1 Bl.Comm. 338.

[407] See 1 Bl.Comm. 338–339.

coroner actually possessed. Hawkins[408] said that he might "certainly bind any person to the peace who makes an affray in his presence."

2–116   The power of a coroner to take surety of the peace for affrays in his presence has never been expressly repealed, but it is at least obsolescent, having been largely, if not wholly, swallowed up in the wider power of a coroner to commit for contempt of court.[409] Wellington[410] took the view in 1905 that coroners still retained the conservator's power to issue warrants for the arrest of suspected felons, burglars and robbers, basing himself upon the authority of Hale,[411] but added that this was in any event best left to the justices.

2–117   It has sometimes been suggested that a coroner is a justice of the peace by virtue of his office.[412] However, when the various authorities are examined, the authorities on which they themselves rely are seen not to support the proposition stated, but the quite different proposition that a coroner is a conservator of peace by virtue of his office.[413] No useful purpose is served by treating coroners as also justices of the peace. Their functions today are quite different. It is therefore submitted that a coroner does not become one merely by virtue of his office.[414]

Privileges and immunities

Immunity from arrest

2–118   A coroner was entitled at common law to immunity from arrest on civil (but not criminal) process when engaged in the discharge of his official duties.[415] The immunity was held to extend to a deputy coroner,[416] which was consistent with the statutory provision[417] that a deputy coroner in acting as authorised should be deemed to be the coroner. Arrest on civil process is however nowadays virtually obsolete. In any event the old office of coroner has been replaced by the new statutory offices of senior coroner, area coroner and assistant coroner, and since the legislation is silent on the matter it must be doubtful whether immunity at common law can extend to these new offices.

---

[408] 2 Hawk. P.C. c. 8 s.5, 7th edn (1795), Vol.III, p.52.

[409] See 11–20 below.

[410] *The King's Coroner*, Vol.II, p.100. A similar view was taken by the learned editor of the 5th edn of this work, in 1888, p.22.

[411] 2 Hale P.C. 107; and see also the *Mirror of Justice*, c.1 s.13; Britton, Bk.1, c.2. It is unclear to what extent Hale's view was based upon the provisions of the Pursuit of Felons Act 1275 and Office of Coroner Act 1276, both of which either assume or confer powers of arrest, and both of which were repealed by the Coroners Act 1887 s.45 and Sch. 3. cf. Blackstone, who considered that the coroner might "apprehend any felon within the country without warrant" (4 Bl.Comm. 289).

[412] *Jervis on Coroners*, 4th edn (1880), p.27; Stephen, *Commentaries*, 7th edn, p.641; Umfreville, *Lex Conoratoria*, Ch.15 para.32, and Archbold, *Quarter Sessions Practice*, 6th edn, p.48.

[413] See also *Entick v Carrington* (1765) 19 St.Tr. 1029 at 1060, per Lord Camden CJ.

[414] See also the 7th edn of this work (1927), at pp.253–254 (to the same effect).

[415] *Callaghan v Twiss* (1847) 9 Ir.L.R. 422. A rare example of arrest on civil process arises under the Insolvency Act 1986 s.364.

[416] *Ex p.Middlesex Deputy Coroner* (1861) 6 H. & N. 501, 158 E.R. 207.

[417] Coroners Act 1988 s.7(4).

Ineligibility for jury service

Coroners, deputy coroners and "assistant coroners" were formerly ineligible for **2–119**
jury service,[418] but this ineligibility has now gone.[419] It is also said that coroners,
at least, are more generally exempt from serving in any office which is inconsistent
with the duties of a coroner.[420] However, it seems unlikely at the present day that
this latter point remains of any significance.

Judicial immunity

A potentially much more important privilege of the coroner is that of judicial **2–120**
immunity. As Lord Tenterden CJ put it:

> "The Court of the coroner is a Court of Record of which the coroner is the
> Judge; and it is a general rule of very great antiquity, that no action will lie
> against a Judge of Record for any matter done by him in the exercise of his
> judicial functions."[421]

More recently Laws LJ said: **2–121**

> "Certain things are beyond contention. The Coroner is a judge; and neither [the
> relevant council] nor anyone else, save a properly constituted court of appeal or
> review, has the least business interfering with his judgments or how he arrives at
> them. His independence as a judge is a matter of constitutional guarantee.
> Nothing could be more elementary."[422]

Thus no action will lie against a coroner who, in the course of his duties, **2–122**
properly turns the plaintiff out of a room where an inquest is to be held,[423] or who
defames the plaintiff during the course of his address to the jury,[424] nor indeed who
causes any harm to the plaintiff by any act within the jurisdiction of the coroner.[425]
The immunity exists even if the acts were done or the words were spoken
maliciously and without reasonable or probable cause.[426] The immunity, however,
does not extend to acts done, or words spoken while a coroner is acting in excess
of, or without, jurisdiction.[427]

---

[418] Juries Act 1974 s.1 Sch.1 Pt.I Group B.
[419] Criminal Justice Act 2003 s.321 Sch.33, as from April 5, 2004, by virtue of SI 2004/829.
[420] Roll.Abr. 632, Trial, Jurors B s.4; Fitz.Nat.Brev; *Jervis on Coroners,* 1st edn (1829), p.63; cf. *Ex p. Jefferies* (1829) 6 Bing. 195. See 2–36 above.
[421] *Garnett v Farrand* (1827) 6 B. & C. 611 at 625; 108 E.R. 576 at 581.
[422] *Forrest v Lord Chancellor* [2011] EWHC 142 (Admin).
[423] *Garnett v Farrand* (1827) 6 B. & C. 611 at 625; 108 E.R. 576 at 581.
[424] *Thomas v Churton* (1862) 2 B. & S.475; 121 E.R. 1150; *Scott v Stansfield* (1868) L.R. 3 Ex. 220.
[425] *Anderson v Gorrie* [1895] 1 Q.B. 668.
[426] ibid; *Anderson v Gorrie* [1895] 1 Q.B. 668.
[427] *Foxhall v Barnett* (1853) 2 E. & B. 928; *McC. v Mullan* [1984] 2 All E.R. 908, HL; *R. v Waltham Forest Justices Ex p.Solanke* [1986] Q.B. 479, QBD; cf. *Desmond v Riordan* [2000] 1 I.L.R.M. 502, Irish High Ct (Morris P.): coroner loses immunity only once he *knows* he is not performing a coronial function.

2–123   The justification for this immunity is that it

> "is not for the protection or benefit of a malicious or corrupt Judge, but for the benefit of the public, whose interest it is that the Judges shall be at liberty to exercise their functions with independence and without fear of consequences."[428]

2–124   Not all the acts of a coroner can be classed as judicial; some may be regarded as administrative.[429] How far a coroner is protected from civil proceedings in respects of acts done, or words spoken, in the exercise of administrative duties is not clear, for there has never been a case on the point. However, it is almost certainly the law that if the coroner acts in good faith he is immune from suit.[430] On the other hand, if he acts in bad faith or (possibly) without reasonable cause in his administrative capacity, then he may be liable for the tort of misfeasance in a public office.[431]

2–125   It should further be noted that the coroner's privilege is to be personally immune from civil liability for actions carried out by him in the course of his duties. This privilege relates to private law alone, and has nothing to do with the courts' public law powers to review coroners' decisions and inquisitions, by means of judicial review[432] and otherwise,[433] and the various powers exercisable by the courts and the Lord Chancellor and the Lord Chief Justice to discipline the coroner or remove him from office in case of various kinds of wrongdoing or default.[434]

Precedence of coroners

2–126   In England and Wales the order of precedence on official and ceremonial occasions is based on social, and not official, rank unless special precedence has been assigned by statute or otherwise.[435] No such special precedence has been assigned to coroners,[436] and therefore it is common for precedence on official and ceremonial occasions to be based on official rank.

2–127   On county occasions it is common for the coroners to be given precedence next to the sheriff because of the great antiquity of the two offices, and also the historical fact that the coroner could, in special circumstances,[437] act for the sheriff. This view has, however, been criticised.[438] Thurston[439] argued on historical grounds

---

[428] *Scott v Stansfield* (1868) L.R. 3 Ex. 220 at 223.

[429] See 2–142—2–143.

[430] *Everett v Griffiths* [1921] 1 A.C. 631; *Docker v Chief Constable of West Midlands Police* [2001] 1 A.C. 435, HL; *Karling v Purdue, The Times,* October 15, 2004, CS(OH).

[431] *Calveley v Chief Constable of Merseyside* [1989] A.C. 1228, HL; *Jones v Swansea City Council* [1990] 1 W.L.R. 1453, HL; *R. v Bowden* [1995] 4 All E.R. 505, CA; *Three Rivers DC v Bank of England* [2001] 2 All E.R. 513, HL; *Docker v Chief Constable of West Midlands Police* [2001] A.C. 435, HL; *Akenzua v Home Secretary* [2002] EWCA Civ. 1470; *Watkins v Home Secretary* [2006] UKHL 17, HL.

[432] See 19–25 ff and cf. *R. v Hallstrom Ex p. W* [1986] Q.B. 824, CA.

[433] e.g. under the Coroners Act 1988 s.13: see 19–05 below.

[434] See 2–96 ff above.

[435] See generally, Squibb, *Precedence in England and Wales* (1981).

[436] Squibb, *Precedence in England and Wales* (1981).does not even mention them; cf. pp.72–74.

[437] See 2–113—2–114 above.

[438] Waldram, *Civic Ceremonial,* 3rd edn (1979), p.38.

[439] Thurston's *Coronership,* 3rd edn (1985), paras 05.03, 05.06. But the Lord Lieutenant, not the coroners, represents the Queen in the county.

that coroners should precede justices of the peace, since the institution of the former office antedated that of the latter by at least a hundred years, and that, as representatives of the Queen, coroners should not be preceded by councillors or corporation officials.[440]

Robes for coroners

In 1905 the Coroners' Society discussed the question of whether coroners should **2–128** wear wigs and gowns in court, and there was significant disagreement on the subject.[441] More than 100 years later, there is still no officially recognised dress for coroners, even though over the years a few coroners have appeared in robes and wigs when discharging their duties in court, and a few more on civic or ceremonial occasions.[442] Judges in the higher civil courts nowadays do not wear wigs, and judges in the Supreme Court do not wear robes either. The modern practice is for coroners to preside over inquest hearings unrobed, and this is the approach advised by the Chief Coroner.[443] However, ultimately it is a matter for the coroner concerned.[444]

Despite the lack of official recognition, and indeed of modern usage, the form **2–129** and style of both wig and gown are traditionally distinct from those worn by barristers and judges: the wig is like a judge's but without the back curl, and the robe is dark blue with black velvet yoke, black lace strips on the facings, and sleeves with four pleats.[445] If a gown is worn, it is usual also to wear a wing collar and bands.

The coroner's officers and other staff[446]

It is impossible for a coroner to carry out all of his functions entirely on his own. **2–130** Generally, he receives information through, and makes his enquiries by means of, his officer or officers. Such officers deal with investigations on the coroner's behalf, and prepare cases for inquest hearings. In busy areas there will be a need for other staff too, such as personal assistants, receptionists or financial clerks. Where a part-time coroner runs a solicitor's or doctor's practice as well, the staff of that practice may (formally or informally) provide similar services to him as coroner.

A busy coroner's area will have several coroner's officers, and may be subdivided, **2–131** one officer taking responsibility for each sub-area. Until recently the need for and indeed the ubiquitous existence of such officers and staff had no statutory recognition, but the position is now different. The relevant authority for a coroner area must now secure the provision of whatever officers and other staff are needed

---

[440] cf. Squibb, *Precedence in England and Wales* (1981), pp.74–77.
[441] See Burney, *Bodies of Evidence: Medicine and the Politics of the English Inquest, 1830–1926* (Baltimore: Johns Hopkins University Press, 2000), pp.102–103.
[442] See *Chief Coroner Guidance No. 3*, 16 July 2013, paras 8–15.
[443] *Chief Coroner Guidance No. 3*, 16 July 2013 para.10.
[444] cf. *St Edmundsbury and Ipswich Diocesan Board of Finance v Clark* [1973] Ch 323, 330.
[445] Messrs Ede & Ravenscroft, Chancery Lane, London, WC2, make coroners' gowns to this traditional design.
[446] See generally the Home Office's *Coroner Service Survey*, 1998 (Research Study 181), pp.9–13, 34–35, and Home Office Circular No. 46 of 2002, and the *Report of the Coroners' Officers' Working Party*.

by the coroners for that area to carry out their functions,[447] *except* to the extent that such officers or staff are provided by a police authority.[448]

Remuneration and employment

2–132   A coroner's officer or member of staff who is also a police officer (or a civilian employed by the Police Authority) is paid by the Police Authority, and not by the coroner.[449] Those who are not police officers or civilian employees of the Police Authority are usually employed directly by the relevant authority rather than by the coroner.[450] From the coroner's point of view this is preferable, as it avoids problems with unfair dismissal and redundancy, and it may also avoid vicarious liability in tort for their actions. The downside is that the coroner does not have the same control over the officer or other member of staff.

2–133   Despite the judicial independence of the coroner, he does not possess exclusive powers over his staff, and there is no foundation in law for an assertion that staff seconded by another employer to work for a coroner remain entirely under his control. On the contrary, the employer has appropriate powers of control and direction over the staff, to be exercised consistently with the coroner's judicial independence and proper freedom of action as a judge.[451]

Duties

2–134   The coroner's officer is usually the first point of contact with the coroner system, especially out of office hours. Although legally speaking the duty to be available is cast upon the coroner,[452] in fact the coroner's officer shoulders the direct and immediate burden. He or she acts as a filter, carrying out the instructions (standard or non-standard, as the case may be) of the coroner, keeping him informed, and seeking further instructions as appropriate.

2–135   He may visit the scene or place where the body lies; alternatively he may receive a report from police attending the scene. As the coroner's representative, the officer cannot be denied access to the body, over which the coroner has exclusive jurisdiction.[453] In either event he will commonly have to make the actual arrangements for removal of the body to a mortuary or other suitable place, acting under instructions (whether standing or case-specific) from the coroner.

2–136   The duties of the coroner's officer may also include making the administrative arrangements for any post-mortem examination, searching for evidence relevant to the investigation or inquest,[454] interviewing potential witnesses and taking statements, and dealing with lawyers and others representing interested parties. If a post-mortem examination is made, he will notify the persons who have the right

---

[447] Coroners and Justice Act 2009 s.24(1)(a).
[448] Coroners and Justice Act 2009 s.24(2).
[449] Police Act 1964 s.55.
[450] The Joint Negotiating Committee for Coroners' position is that arrangements between coroners and local authorities to pay an allowance to cover office expenses (including clerical assistance) should be settled locally.
[451] *Forrest v Lord Chancellor* [2011] EWHC 142 (Admin) at [27]–[33].
[452] See 2–72 ff above.
[453] See 8–11 below.
[454] See 5–64, 10–65 below.

to be informed of this.[455] If an inquest is to be held, the coroner's officer or other members of staff, on the direction of the coroner, will notify the interested persons,[456] and will summon the witnesses[457] and the jurors (if a jury is required).[458] The officer will liaise with the press and will probably also organise the actual sitting of the court, acting as a mixture of usher and clerk of the court, and supervising the recording equipment.

Any other members of the coroner's staff, such as secretary/receptionist, **2–137** bookkeeper or clerk, will have narrower and more conventional office roles. Mortuary technicians are not normally part of the coroner's staff, but are employed by the local authority as part of their public mortuary service, or by a hospital as part of theirs.

In their relations with members of the public the coroner's staff will come into **2–138** contact with relatives of deceased persons in times of stress, and often in very difficult circumstances. The public reaction to the service rendered by the coroner system will depend largely upon the impression that is made by the first contact with it; this depends on the coroner's staff, and in particular on the coroner's officers. At the same time, the officers are not the coroner, and they must never appear to assume more than transitory responsibility for what is being done, ordered or arranged. They must report to, and receive instructions from, the coroner, though they may know from experience the likely sequence of events in certain fairly common and well-defined circumstances.

The practice by some coroners of delegating limited decision-making powers to **2–139** officers in standard cases was criticised in the *Report on the Retention of Organs at the Royal Liverpool Children's Hospital, Alder Hey*,[459] in the context of deciding whether a post-mortem examination should be carried out.[460] The Report expressed the view that "the wording of the Rules clearly lays the responsibility on the coroner personally, and not on his Officer, of taking decisions regarding the authorisation of a post-mortem examination".[461]

This statement betrayed a serious confusion of thought, as well as an error. The **2–140** question was not whether the rules made the coroner *responsible* for what is done; it was clear that they did. Instead it was whether the coroner might give the officer *authority* to take the decision *on his behalf*, in accordance with whatever criteria the coroner thought proper. Prima facie, a decision taken by the officer within that authority, and following those criteria, would be a decision *of the coroner*, for which he alone would be responsible.

Secondly, the then rules relating to directing or requesting post-mortem **2–141** examinations[462] did not (as other rules[463] did) make clear that the decision was one for the coroner personally. Accordingly, the Report was led into error in

---

[455] See 8–60 below.
[456] See 10–22 ff below.
[457] See 10–29 below.
[458] See 10–43 ff below.
[459] Inquiry ordered December 3, 1999, under the National Health Act 1977 s.2; report ordered to be published January 30, 2001.
[460] *Report*, paras 19–24.
[461] *Report* para.19.2
[462] Coroners Rules 1984 rr.5–6.
[463] Coroners Rules 1984 rr.29, 31.

concluding that the decision to order a post-mortem examination was one incapable of delegation.

2–142 In practice, of course, even if the rules permitted it, no sensible coroner would attempt to delegate any but the most straightforward cases to officers, and officers would refer all other cases to the coroner. But, if everything in the coroner's service had to be done personally by the coroner, the service would grind to a halt. This is recognised by the regulations made in 2013 under the 2009 Act, which provide variously that a coroner "may delegate administrative functions to coroner's officers and other staff",[464] and that a coroner "may delegate administrative, but not judicial functions, to coroner's officers and other support staff".[465] This requires a distinction to be made between administrative and judicial functions, neither of which terms is defined for this purpose.

2–143 A judicial act has been defined for the purposes of judicial review in the following terms:

> "the term "judicial' does not necessarily mean acts of a judge or of a legal tribunal sitting for the determination of matters of law, but for the purpose of this question an act done by competent authority, upon consideration of facts and circumstances, imposing liability and affecting the rights of others."[466]

2–144 On this basis there can be no doubt that, for example, a decision as to whether there should be a post-mortem examination in a particular case *is* a judicial act, because it affects the rights of the personal representatives and next of kin of the deceased. The Chief Coroner advises that functions delegable to coroners' staff include contacting bereaved relatives, making inquiries on the coroner's behalf,[467] and making the necessary arrangements (though not the decision itself) to conduct a post-mortem examination.[468]

2–145 There is a question whether the coroner may lawfully pre-sign blank forms for various of the decisions that he may be called upon to make, and leave them with his officer. There can be no doubt that, if the decisions are *judicial* decisions, and the purpose of the pre-signing is to enable the officer in effect to take such decisions without disturbing the coroner, then this is an unlawful delegation.

2–146 However, if the purpose of so doing is *not* to delegate decision-making, but instead is purely logistical, it is different in law. If the decision is still *in fact* made by the coroner, who directs the officer (whether over the telephone, or by email or fax, or otherwise) as to what to insert in the pre-signed form, and then to deliver it as the coroner's decision, then it is prima facie lawful. There is no delegation of the decision. The coroner has decided.

2–147 As a matter of law the coroner is entitled to leave documents in another's hands to be released as and when the coroner so authorises, and for this purpose it does

---

[464] Coroners Allowances, Fees and Expenses Regulations 2013 (SI 2013/1615) reg.3.

[465] Coroners (Investigations) Regulations 2013 (SI 2013/1629) reg.7; the misplaced comma after "functions" is unfortunately misplaced in the regulation itself.

[466] *R v Dublin Corporation* (1878) 2 LR Ir 371, 376, per May CJ, approved by Lord Atkinson in *Everett v Griffiths* [1921] 1 A.C. 631, 683.

[467] *The Chief Coroner's Guide to the Coroners and Justice Act 2009*, 2nd edn (July 2009) para.48.

[468] *Chief Coroner Guidance No. 8*, 1 August 2013 para.10.

not matter in what order the signature and the rest of the certificate are written on the document. However, depending on the circumstances, it may be unwise to adopt this course, as it is clearly the responsibility of the coroner to ensure that certificates bearing his signature say exactly what he intends, and he takes the risk that they do not.

Recruitment

In the past, the coroner's officer could have been almost anyone. In Dickens' time   **2–148**
it might have been the parish beadle.[469] In the City of London in 1950 it was the mortuary superintendent.[470] Today a coroner's officer is often an experienced serving police constable who is specially and permanently detailed for this duty. He may well have a deputy, also a police officer, who replaces him when he is ill or on holiday. The appointment of serving policemen was already fairly common when it was recommended by the Departmental Committee on Coroners, in 1935.[471]

In the past it was suggested that, in order to keep free from suspicion the making   **2–149**
of enquiries into the deaths of persons in police custody, the coroner's officer should not be a serving police officer.[472] But where the coroner's officer is a police officer or police civilian employee, this has certain advantages, such as the free passage of information and general co-operation from the regular police forces, either or both of which may be less forthcoming in other cases. Indeed, many police forces regard this liaison as of value, and coroners themselves tend to prefer police officers to civilians.

Nonetheless there is a trend towards civilianisation of coroners' officers,[473] and   **2–150**
this trend has been supported by the Home Office, in suggesting that police civilian staff, rather than police officers, be appointed as coroners' officers.[474] Other coroners' officers may have been nurses, firefighters or undertakers in a previous career. The Coroners' Officers Association was set up in November 1997, changing its name in 2011 to the Coroners' Officers and Staff Association.[475] It holds a programme of talks and social events, as well as an annual conference.

Specialist coroners

According to the statutory scheme, the only truly specialist coroners are the   **2–151**
Coroner for Treasure and assistant coroners for treasure. Their work is confined to treasure inquests, subject to any direction by the Chief Coroner to deal with a death case.[476] Subject to that, all senior coroners, area coroners and assistant coroners are qualified to deal with any kind of case, including (for so long as the

---

[469] See, e.g. his *Bleak House*, Ch.XI.
[470] *The Corporation of London* (OUP, 1950), p.160.
[471] Cmnd. 5070 para.230.
[472] See, e.g. the Broderick Report para.21.11.
[473] Organisation and Methods Branch of the Home Office, *Review of the Work and Methods of Coroners' Officers*, March 1983.
[474] Home Office Circular No. 93 of 1985.
[475] Website at *http://www.coasa.org.uk* [Accessed June 4, 2014]. At the time of writing, the Hon. Secretary is Ms Sonia Brooks, Coroners' Officers and Staff Association, PO Box 3781, Chester, CH1 9YJ, secretary@coasa.org.uk.
[476] See 2–58.

treasure provisions of the 2009 Act are not brought into force) treasure cases.[477] But there are two non-statutory specialist cadres of coroners, trained for particular types of case. These are (i) the cadre of specialist military coroners, dealing with deaths on active service,[478] and (ii) the cadre of advisory coroners for disaster victim identification ("DVI") cases, who can advise coroners dealing with inquests arising out of mass fatality disasters.[479] Non-cadre coroners remain able to deal with both types of case, but such cases may be allocated to cadre coroners by the Chief Coroner in the exercise of his powers to do so.[480]

Part-time coroners and legal practice

2–152   A part-time coroner who also carries on a professional practice would be unwise to act professionally in connection with any legal proceedings resulting from the death of a person into whose death he has conducted or may be about to conduct an investigation (including a post-mortem examination) or hold an inquest, and, indeed, the Coroners' Society recommends that a coroner should not so act.[481]

2–153   In 1995 the Solicitors Disciplinary Tribunal found a solicitor coroner to have been guilty of unbefitting conduct. He had opened and adjourned an inquest on a deceased who (unknown to him) had been employed by one of his clients. Having discovered this, the solicitor arranged for the inquest to be transferred to another coroner. This inquest was, for unconnected reasons, quashed and a further inquest held before another coroner. At *this* inquest the solicitor appeared to represent the interests of his client, the deceased's employer. The Tribunal held that "his knowledge of the matter had not been expunged by the order quashing the first inquest and he had acted in the same matter as both coroner and advocate for an interested party [*sic*]. Such behaviour was reprehensible. The conflict of interest was clear". However, as there were mitigating factors, the Tribunal merely reprimanded the solicitor and ordered him to pay a contribution towards costs.

2–154   The Law Society's *Guide to the Professional Conduct of Solicitors* formerly stated:[482]

"**Coroners**

(e) A solicitor who is a coroner or deputy or assistant deputy coroner should not appear on behalf of a client before a coroner's court for the area or district for which he or she is appointed. Nor should such a solicitor (or any

---

[477] Coroners and Justice Act 2009 (Commencement No. 15, Consequential and Transitory Provisions) Order 2013 (SI 2013/1869) art.3(b), referring to the Coroners and Justice Act 2009 s.23. See 16–21.

[478] See Chief Coroner's Guidance No. 7, *A Cadre of Coroners for Service Deaths*, and 13–78.

[479] See *UK DVI-Cadre of Advisory Coroners, Terms of Reference,* 2008, agreed between the Home Office and the Coroners' Society of England and Wales, and 17–05 et seq.

[480] See 2–59.

[481] Coroners' Society of England and Wales Recommendations on Procedure 1975 para.2. But this was not intended to prevent a solicitor coroner from acting in non-contentious probate matters for the estate of a deceased person whose death had been reported to him. Whether the Society would take the same view today is perhaps questionable.

[482] 8th edn (1999) para.15.06(e). The regulatory function is now carried on by the Solicitors Regulatory Authority, whose Handbook does not deal with the matter in the same detailed terms.

partner or employee of the solicitor) act professionally in any civil or criminal proceedings resulting from a death where the solicitor has held an inquest into the circumstances of such death. Further, since the coroner acts in a judicial capacity, such a solicitor must make arrangements for another person to carry out an inquest into the death of a person where it might be thought that some bias could arise out of his or her personal or professional connection with the deceased, or with a near relative of the deceased."

Further, it is undesirable and inconsistent with the status of the coroner as an **2–155** independent judicial officer for him to act as a professional or expert witness at an inquest before another coroner,[483] the more so in front of a jury which is aware of his judicial status.[484] It is also undesirable for a coroner to discuss with the media any aspect of current inquest proceedings.[485]

---

[483] Home Office Circular No. 31 of 1982.
[484] cf. *R. v Hoyland-Thornton* [1984] Crim. L.R. 561, CA: conviction quashed for material irregularity where jury saw as prosecuting counsel a barrister who a few days previously had sat with them as assistant recorder.
[485] *R. v Inner West London Coroner, ex p.Dallaglio* [1994] 4 All E.R. 139, CA.

Chapter 3

MEDICAL EXAMINERS

Introduction

The Shipman Inquiry[1] identified a weakness in the death certification system. **3–01**
Where a medical practitioner gave a certificate of the cause of death which showed
an entirely natural cause, the registrar of deaths would allow the death to be
registered without any further inquiry, such as a reference to the coroner. If the
body of the deceased was to be cremated, there was an additional check, by the
cremation referee, but that would at best look only at the facts of that case and not
at all the deaths being certified by a particular doctor or those occurring in a
particular locality. If the body of the deceased was to be removed from the
jurisdiction, the undertaker had to give notice to the coroner, but the coroner
would have only the certificate of the medical practitioner to go on. If the body
was to be buried, there were no further formalities at all. A burial order would be
issued by the registrar.

The Coroners and Justice Act 2009 introduces a new office, that of the medical **3–02**
examiner. This person will be a medical practitioner, employed by the local
authority, with the role of examining every death that occurs in the locality, and
referring to the coroner those deaths which ought properly to be further
investigated. However, the provisions in the 2009 Act concerned with medical
examiners have not been brought into force at the same time as those concerning
coroners.[2] It was previously anticipated that they will not be brought into force
until October 2014, at the earliest.[3] In this chapter the main features of the medical
examiner system are described, though of course many of the details will have to
wait until the regulations are made in due course.

It is anticipated that medical examiners will fulfil the following roles: **3–03**

(1) provide medical advice to attending medical practitioners where the cause
of death is apparently natural but not clear;

---

[1] See 1–38.

[2] The medical examiner system is overseen not by the Ministry of Justice, but by the Department of
Health.

[3] Letter of June 3, 2013 from Secretary of State for Health to the Chairman of the House of Commons
Health Select Committee. These provisions are the responsibility of the Department of Health, rather
than the Ministry of Justice, responsible for the rest of Pt I of the 2009 Act. But the next general
election is due in May 2015, and implementation will be delayed until after that, because of the costs
implications.

(2) carry out an independent scrutiny of the circumstances of the death to ensure that the right cases are referred to the coroner;

(3) discuss the death with relatives of the deceased so that they can raise any concerns;

(4) provide general medical advice to coroners about specific cases;

(5) confirm the medical cause of death in all cases not investigated by a coroner.

3–04   Since 2008, some seven pilot schemes have been run in coroner districts across England and Wales to see how the medical examiner system will work in practice. A detailed study in Sheffield has suggested that nationally the number of cases *reported* to coroners will actually drop by 20–25 per cent, but that the number of cases *investigated* by the coroner will rise by 15–20 per cent.

APPOINTMENT

3–05   Local authorities[4] in England and local health boards in Wales must appoint medical examiners to carry out the functions conferred on them by the 2009 Act.[5] They must appoint enough medical examiners, and make available sufficient funds and other resources, to enable those functions to be discharged in their respective areas.[6] They must also monitor the performance of the medical examiners.[7] A person is qualified for appointment as a medical examiner if he or she is and has been a registered medical practitioner throughout the previous five years,[8] and practises or has practised as such within that time.[9]

3–06   The Secretary of State for Health (for England) and the Welsh Ministers (for Wales) may make regulations providing for (a) the terms of appointment of medical examiners and for the termination of appointment,[10] and (b) remuneration, expenses, fees, compensation for termination of appointment, pensions, allowances or gratuities,[11] and (c) training.[12] Regulations are likely to provide that persons must have completed prescribed training (probably as e-learning) before they can be appointed as medical examiners.

---

[4] The original version of the Act placed this duty on Primary Care Trusts, but this was amended to local authorities by virtue of the Health and Social care Act 2012 s.54.

[5] Coroners and Justice Act 2009 s.19(1).

[6] Coroners and Justice Act 2009 s.19(2)(a). See the Report of the Mid-Staffordshire NHS Foundation Trust Public inquiry, ("the Francis Report"), February 2013, HC 947 para.14.91, recommendation 276.

[7] Coroners and Justice Act 2009 s.19(2)(b).

[8] Coroners and Justice Act 2009 s.19(3)(a). For 'registered medical practitioner', see Medical Act 1983, s.55(1) (App.1).

[9] Coroners and Justice Act 2009 s.19(3)(b).

[10] Coroners and Justice Act 2009 s.19(4)(a).

[11] Coroners and Justice Act 2009 s.19(4)(b).

[12] Coroners and Justice Act 2009 s.19(4)(c).

FUNCTIONS

The precise functions of medical examiners are to be conferred by regulations   **3–07**
made by the Secretary of State for Health (for England) and the Welsh Ministers
(for Wales),[13] which may also make provision for the procedure to be followed in
the exercise of those functions,[14] and also the exercise of those functions by
unqualified persons during periods of emergency.[15] For this purpose, a period of
emergency is a period so certified by the Secretary of State on the basis that there
is, has been or is about to be a situation actually or potentially causing a substantial
loss of life throughout all or part of England and Wales.[16] Any such certificate must
state the beginning and end of the period,[17] though the Secretary of State can issue
a fresh certificate thereafter in respect of the same situation.[18]

  In carrying out their functions, medical examiners must have regard to guidance   **3–08**
issued by the National Medical Examiner.[19] The Secretary of State may by
regulations require medical examiners to make enquiries to establish or confirm
the cause of death,[20] to confirm the cause of death stated in the attending
practitioner's certificate and to notify a registrar of such confirmation,[21] or
alternatively to refer the case to a senior coroner,[22] and other matters besides.

Independence

It is critical that medical examiners are independent in carrying out their   **3–09**
functions.[23] This may perhaps be one reason why the original legislation was
amended so that local authorities rather than Primary Care Trusts appoint medical
examiners.[24] This is underscored by a provision that no local authority or Board
which has appointed medical examiners is to have any role in relation to the way
that such examiners exercise their professional judgment as medical practitioners.[25]
Guidance for local authorities appointing medical examiners is likely to say that
appointees may be from any speciality, or none, but (if not GPs) should be or have
been of consultant grade in order to give them the necessary seniority.

Medical examiner officers

Like coroners, medical examiners will operate through officers. They must   **3–10**
obviously have suitable expertise and sufficient independence to be able to carry
out their role. They will need sufficient clinical knowledge, confidence to discuss
cases with doctors, empathy with the bereaved and good time-management skills,

---

[13] Coroners and Justice Act 2009 s.19(4)(e).
[14] Coroners and Justice Act 2009 s.19(4)(d).
[15] Coroners and Justice Act 2009 s.19(4)(f).
[16] Coroners and Justice Act 2009 s.19(7).
[17] Coroners and Justice Act 2009 s.19(8).
[18] Coroners and Justice Act 2009 s.19(9).
[19] Coroners and Justice Act 2009 s.21(9). For the National Medical Examiner, see [3.08].
[20] Coroners and Justice Act 2009 s.20(1)(e).
[21] Coroners and Justice Act 2009 s.20(1)(f)(i).
[22] Coroners and Justice Act 2009 s.20(1)(f)(ii).
[23] The Francis Report para.14.91, recommendation 275.
[24] See 3–05.
[25] Coroners and Justice Act 2009 s.19(5).

as well as the ability to administer the system, including supplying information to the medical examiners, maintaining records and making statutory notifications.

3–11   They may be based at any convenient location. Indeed, in many cases this may be with or near the coroner's officers, although it may be that in the case of large acute hospitals some officers are based there in order to ensure timely availability of paper-based records. An alternative may be where the local authority locates its public health department. Either way, it is to be hoped that this does not compromise their independence.

NATIONAL MEDICAL EXAMINER

3–12 The Secretary of State for Health may, after consulting the Welsh Ministers,[26] appoint a person as National Medical Examiner,[27] on whatever terms and conditions the Secretary of State thinks appropriate.[28] The qualification for appointment is the same as for a medical examiner.[29] The Secretary of State may determine and pay the National Medical Examiner remuneration or allowances, and sums towards expenses incurred in performing his or her functions.[30]

3–13   The National Medical Examiner has the function of issuing guidance to medical examiners, after consulting Welsh Ministers,[31] so that they carry out their functions effectively and proportionately,[32] and also has any further functions conferred by regulations made by the Secretary of State.[33] The National Medical Examiner may, after consulting Welsh Ministers,[34] amend or revoke any such guidance.[35]

---

[26] Coroners and Justice Act 2009 s.21(3).
[27] Coroners and Justice Act 2009 s.21(1).
[28] Coroners and Justice Act 2009 s.21(5).
[29] Coroners and Justice Act 2009 s.21(4). See 3–05.
[30] Coroners and Justice Act 2009 s.21(6).
[31] Coroners and Justice Act 2009 s.21(8).
[32] Coroners and Justice Act 2009 s.21(2)(a).
[33] Coroners and Justice Act 2009 s.21(2)(b).
[34] Coroners and Justice Act 2009 s.21(8).
[35] Coroners and Justice Act 2009 s.21(8).

Chapter 4

THE TERRITORIAL JURISDICTION OF CORONERS

Territorial Jurisdiction

Under the old law, the position concerning the territorial jurisdiction of coroners was complex. It is now much simpler. England and Wales are divided into coroner areas,[1] each consisting of the area of a local authority or the combined areas of two or more such authorities.[2] Each senior coroner, area coroner or assistant coroner in England is appointed for that coroner area only.[3] Exceptionally, however, coroners appointed for a coroner area in Wales are each treated as appointed for the whole of Wales.[4]   **4–01**

Once jurisdiction has arisen for a coroner in a coroner area to inquire into a death (usually because of a report of the presence in that area of a dead body fulfilling the statutory criteria)[5] it is the coroners of that area who alone have jurisdiction to act. Even if the body thereafter is moved to another area during the investigation, that coroner continues to have jurisdiction,[6] and no coroner for any other area has any function in relation to it.[7] Two questions nevertheless arise: first, what are the limits of a coroner area, and secondly, in what circumstances does a coroner have or gain jurisdiction outside his area, or not have or lose jurisdiction within it?   **4–02**

Coastal boundaries

Coroner areas are based on local government areas. The exact boundaries of coastal counties may not be easy to determine. The Local Government Act 1972 delineates very few boundaries of counties, but refers to pre-existing administrative areas.[8] Earlier statutes do the same. Where a county has ultimately been defined in   **4–03**

---

[1] Coroners and Justice Act 2009 s.22 Sch.2 para.1(1). See 2–30.

[2] Coroners and Justice Act 2009 s.22 Sch.2 para.1(1). See 2–30.

[3] Coroners and Justice Act 2009 s.22 Sch.2 paras 1(1), 2(3), (4). See 2–23, 2–25, 2–27.

[4] Coroners Act 1988 s.4A(8), not repealed by the Coroners and Justice Act 2009, but instead modified by the Coroners and Justice Act 2009 (Consequential Provisions) Order 2013 (SI 2013/1874). See 4–17.

[5] As to which see 5–01.

[6] Coroners and Justice Act 2009 s.22 Sch.2 para.4(2).

[7] Coroners and Justice Act 2009 s.22 Sch.2 para.4(3).

[8] As to modification of seaward boundaries, see Local Government Act 1972 s.71, and as to the low water mark boundary and accretions from the sea, see s.72.

terms of parishes, it is important to recall that, at common law, coastal parishes do not extend beyond the low-water mark, unless the contrary is proved.[9]

4–04   However, where the territorial extent of a county is not referred ultimately (on the seaward side) to a parish or parishes, it does not follow that, merely because the county contains parishes, whose own jurisdiction extends only to the low-water mark, the county itself only extends thus far.[10] Indeed, it is clear that ships in harbour are within the county, at least for some purposes,[11] and coroners have in recent years exercised jurisdiction over them accordingly.[12]

4–05   In determining whether an arm of the sea or a tidal river is within the territorial extent of a county, the common law view was that an arm of the sea was within the body of a county if there was land of the same or another county within such distance that the movements of a man on one shore were discernible with the natural eye from the other.[13]

4–06   Indeed Hale specifically referred to this point in the context of the jurisdiction of coroners and sheriffs:

> "That arm or branch of the sea which lies within the *fauces terrae*, where a man may reasonably discerne between shore and shore, is or may be within the body of a county, and therefore within the jurisdiction of the sheriff or coroner."[14]

4–07   However, international conventions[15] to which the United Kingdom is signatory enable territorial seas to be distinguished from "internal waters". Internal waters are those under the full sovereignty of the territorial state. The first of these conventions was given the force of law in the United Kingdom by Order in Council in 1964.[16] The convention requires a baseline (normally the low-water mark)[17] to be drawn around the coast, and this baseline divides the territorial seas of a state from the internal waters of a state.

---

[9] *R. v Musson* (1858) 8 E. & B. 900; Hunt's *Law of Boundaries and Fences*, pp.13–15; Poor Law Amendment Act 1868 s.27 (now repealed).

[10] Note the special position of the Channel Tunnel, which from the UK coast to the Channel midpoint is within the district of Dover in Kent: Channel Tunnel Act 1987 s.10(1).

[11] *R. v Soleguard* (1738) And. 231; *R. v Keyn* (1876) 2 Ex.D. 63 at 82.

[12] See 5–58 below.

[13] 4 Co. Inst. 137, 140, 141; 3 Bl.Comm. 106; 2 Hawk. P.C. c. 9 s.14; 2 East P.C. 804; *The Public Opinion* (1832) 2 Hag.Adm.Rep. 398; *R. v Forty-Nine Casks of Brandy* (1836) 3 Hag.Adm.Rep. 257; *R. v Cunningham* (1859) Bell C.C. 72; *R. v Keyn* (1876) 2 Ex.D. 63, 157, 164–168; *The Fagernes* [1927] P. 311.

[14] *De Jure Maris*, c. 4, approved in *The Goring* [1987] Q.B. 687, affirmed [1988] A.C. 831.

[15] The Convention on the Territorial Sea and the Contiguous Zone (Geneva, April 29, 1958; T.S. 3 (1965), Cmnd. 2511), now superseded by the United Nations Convention on the Law of the Sea (Montego Bay, 10 December 1982; TS 81 (1999), Cmnd. 4524).

[16] The Territorial Waters Order in Council 1964, dated September 25, 1964, as amended by SI 1998/2564. Since, as Diplock LJ put it in *Post Office v Estuary Radio Ltd* [1968] 2 Q.B. 740: "It still lies within the prerogative power of the Crown to extend its sovereignty and jurisdiction to areas of land or sea over which it has not previously claimed or exercised sovereignty or jurisdiction", it was not necessary for any Act of Parliament to "confirm" the Order for it to have legal effect. Since October 1, 1987, this Order has had effect as if made under the Territorial Sea Act 1987 s.1. See also the Territorial Sea (Limits) Order 1989 (SI 1989/482).

[17] United Nations Convention on the Law of the Sea art.5.

Thus the latter include all rivers, harbours, anchorages, bays and estuaries and **4–08** indeed all sea areas to the landward side of the baseline.[18] There is no authority on the point, but if "internal waters" for the purposes of the Conventions are under the full sovereignty of the United Kingdom, it would be desirable that all such waters in England and Wales should fall into one or other of the administrative counties, and consequently within the jurisdiction of a coroner.

Airspace

It is even more difficult to be sure how far the territorial jurisdiction of a coroner **4–09** extends to aircraft and other machines which overfly his district. On the one hand, the old common law maxim, *cujus est solum, ejus est usque ad coelum et ad inferos*, even if it was ever to be regarded as representing English law, clearly no longer does so in relation to a property-owner seeking to prevent an overflying aeroplane from entering his "airspace".[19]

On the other hand, the coroner's jurisdiction concerns the state's powers rather **4–10** than property-owners' rights, and it is relevant to recall that the preamble to the Air Navigation Act 1920[20] declared that:

> "the full and absolute sovereignty and rightful jurisdiction of His Majesty extends and has always extended, over the air superincumbent on all parts of His Majesty's dominions and the territorial waters adjacent thereto."

In principle, there is no reason why the jurisdiction of a coroner should not **4–11** extend to overflying aircraft. However, investigations into the deaths of persons killed in aeroplane accidents will normally be conducted by coroners having jurisdiction in the place where the aircraft crashes. In-flight deaths which do not involve crashes will probably not come to the attention of the coroner while the aircraft is still in the coroner area concerned, and so are unlikely to give rise to any practical reason for that coroner to assert jurisdiction.[21]

Chief Coroner's direction

In any event, it should be noted that, in the case of a death "in or near the coroner's **4–12** area", where the body is destroyed, lost or missing, there is in certain circumstances power for the Chief Coroner to direct a named coroner to assume jurisdiction and hold an inquest.[22] The predecessor of this power was exercised in cases of deaths in coastal waters, particularly to assist relatives of the deceased to obtain a certificate which would serve as evidence of death for certain purposes.[23] It might also be used, for example, where a person vanished in open countryside and was presumed

---

[18] See generally, *Halsbury's Laws of England* (5th edn), Vol.61, paras 121–131, and also *Post Office v Estuary Radio Ltd* [1968] 2 Q.B. 740, CA.
[19] cf. *Bernstein v Skyviews Ltd* [1978] Q.B. 479.
[20] Now repealed.
[21] One possibility would be in proving certain criminal offences (*e.g.* obstructing a coroner by concealing a body) where it may be necessary to show that some coroner had jurisdiction to hold an inquest: see *R. v Purcy* (1933) 149 L.T. 432 and 5–58 below.
[22] Coroners and Justice Act 2009 s.1(5), replacing Coroners Act 1988 s.15 (power of Secretary of State). See 5–16—5–17 below.
[23] See the Brodrick Report, para.13.08.

to have died after falling into a pothole or mineshaft, but no body was ever recovered, or a body was cremated before the death was reported to the coroner.

Extra-territorial prisons

4–13   Early prison legislation provided that where a local authority constructed and occupied a prison outside its own boundaries, that prison should be treated for jurisdictional purposes (including those of the coroner) as if it was *within* its boundaries.[24] This legislation applied to a number of prisons, and was deemed to apply to others, including Holloway Prison in London.[25] This jurisdiction was expressly not affected by later legislation[26] transferring the ownership of prisons to the Prison Commissioners,[27] and then to the Secretary of State,[28] with the exception of two orders.[29] Accordingly, any such extra-territorial prisons, even though no longer the property of the local authorities that constructed them, were still technically within the jurisdiction of the coroners for districts of those authorities.

4–14   However, the current legislation now provides that an investigation (and any inquest) into a death shall, subject to transfer provisions,[30] only be conducted by the coroner in whose area the body was lying when jurisdiction arose,[31] even if the inquest may be conducted outside his area.[32] The earlier legislation[33] was a consolidation Act, and consolidation is presumed not to be intended to change the law.[34] But the current legislation makes entirely fresh provision, and therefore, whatever the position under the old law, the current position is clear.

Relationship between coroner areas in England and Wales

4–15   Under the old law there was a complex relationship between a coroner for one district of an "administrative area" and the other coroner or coroners for the same administrative area. For this purpose "administrative area" was defined[35] to mean Wales, a metropolitan or non-metropolitan county in England, and Greater London (which did not include the City),[36] except that for certain purposes[37] "administrative area" did not include any part of a non-metropolitan county forming part of a coroner's district which extends into another non-metropolitan

---

[24] Prisons Act 1823, 4 Geo. IV, c. 64 s.48.

[25] 15 & 16 Vict., c. 70. Holloway Prison was built by the Corporation of the City of London.

[26] Prisons Act 1877, 40 & 41 Vict., c. 21.

[27] Prisons Act 1877 s.30, repealed and replaced by Prisons Act 1952 s.34.

[28] Prisons Act 1952 s.35, as substituted by the Prison Commissioners Dissolution Order 1963 (SI 1963/597) art.3(2) Sch.1.

[29] S.R. & O. 1919 No. 790 (Ipswich Prison); S.R. & O 1933 No. 127 (Pentonville and Wandsworth Prisons). Both orders are now spent.

[30] See 5–16—5–17.

[31] Coroners and Justice Act 2009 s.1(1), replacing Coroners Act 1988 s.5(1), itself derived from the Coroners Act 1887 s.7(1), as amended by the Coroners (Amendment) Act 1926 ss.30, 31, Schs II, III.

[32] See 2–46 and *Chief Coroner Guidance No. 2.*

[33] The Coroners Act 1988.

[34] *Atkinson v United States of America Government* [1971] A.C. 197, HL; *Maunsell v Olins* [1975] A.C. 373 at 382.

[35] By the Coroners Act 1988 s.35(1).

[36] Coroners Act 1988 s.35(1).

[37] The application of ss.4(5), 5(3), 13(2) of the 1988 Act.

county.[38] All coroners for districts in the same administrative area were, subject to certain exceptions, coroners of that area for all purposes,[39] and in some cases could hold inquests for coroners in other districts of the same administrative area. [40]

Now, the law is simpler. Each coroner area in England is entirely separate from **4–16** each other such area, and the coroners of one area have no jurisdiction over any investigations which belong to another area. At the same time, some powers which coroners may exercise in relation to their investigations may be exercised anywhere in England and Wales.

The position in Wales is exceptional. Senior, area and assistant coroners are **4–17** appointed for coroner areas, as in England. But coroners in Wales are treated as appointed for the whole of Wales,[41] and therefore can conduct investigations and hold inquests in respect of deaths whose jurisdiction would otherwise fall on the coroners of a different coroner area than their own. This gives "additional flexibility in the deployment of resources in Wales. It means that a coroner with specialist skills can temporarily act outside his or her own district without having to be appointed as a coroner in the other district."[42] However, this comes at the cost of creating the potential problem of concurrent jurisdiction.[43]

EXTRA-TERRITORIAL JURISDICTION

The jurisdiction of the coroner is normally limited to the coroner area for which **4–18** he is appointed, and (as will be seen)[44] depends upon the fact that the body of a person, whose death it is his duty to investigate, is within that area. However, there may be circumstances in which it is desirable for a coroner other than the one who originally has jurisdiction to take charge of the matter.

Assumption by request

Thus, the senior coroner for one coroner's area having a duty to conduct an **4–19** investigation may request the senior coroner for another coroner's area to conduct the investigation.[45] If the latter agrees, then he, and not the former, must conduct the investigation, as soon as practicable,[46] unless by then the Chief Coroner has given a direction as to who should conduct it,[47] and the transfer in any event is still subject to the possibility of such a direction from the Chief Coroner thereafter.[48]

---

[38] Coroners Act 1988 s.35(1B).
[39] Coroners Act 1988 ss.4(5)(a), 4A(8)(a), 35(1).
[40] Coroners Act 1988 s.5(3).
[41] See 2–45.
[42] See *Hansard*, HL 10 July 2013, col. GC114, per Lord McNally. Why this flexibility is needed (to the extent that it is needed) only in Wales and not elsewhere is not explained.
[43] On the problem of concurrent jurisdiction, see 5–116 ff.
[44] See 5–01 below.
[45] Coroners and Justice Act 2009 s.2(1).
[46] Coroners and Justice Act 2009 s.2(2); formerly Coroners Act 1988 s.14(1), though note that the old requirement that the body be lying in the district when the request is made has now gone.
[47] Coroners and Justice Act 2009 s.2(3).
[48] Coroners and Justice Act 2009 s.2(4)(a).

The senior coroner making the request must inform the Chief Coroner in writing of the request and the response from the other senior coroner.[49]

4–20   It is common for this provision to be used when a person dies abroad[50] and the body is returned to England and Wales. If the presence of the body is reported to the coroner at the point of entry, he usually transfers jurisdiction to the coroner at the place of intended disposal. However, if multiple bodies are involved in the same incident (whether the death occurs abroad or not), it usually makes sense to transfer all jurisdiction to a single coroner. In the case of an incident abroad, this will frequently be the coroner at the point of entry.[51]

4–21   This provision applies only where a coroner is under a duty to conduct an investigation into a death. Accordingly, no transfer is possible under this provision if an investigation has already been held, unless and until that investigation has been quashed by the High Court.[52] The predecessor provision[53] applied only where the body was lying in the coroner's district at the time, and where the original coroner considered that "an inquest ought to be held", which meant that it could not apply where the body had left the district,[54] or all that was envisaged was some procedure falling short of an inquest.[55]

4–22   But since 2013 those limitations have gone. In considering whether to make or accede to a request under this provision, coroners may take into account various factors. One is how far the transfer may lead to evidence for an investigation or at an inquest that would otherwise be undisputed becoming disputed, and thus leading to difficulties in the admission of documentary evidence.[56]

Assumption by direction of Chief Coroner

4–23   If the coroner requested to assume jurisdiction declines to do so, or even where no request has been made, the Chief Coroner may direct any senior coroner to conduct an investigation into a death even though otherwise it would be the duty of a different senior coroner to conduct it.[57] Where the Chief Coroner gives a direction, written notification of which must be given to the original coroner,[58] the coroner directed must conduct (or continue)[59] the investigation, as soon as practicable,[60] though the transfer so directed is still subject to the possibility of a further direction from the Chief Coroner thereafter.[61]

---

[49] Coroners and Justice Act 2009 s.2(5).
[50] See 5–87 ff below.
[51] See Home Office Circular No. 79 of 1983. This was the case in respect of those who died in the destruction of the World Trade Center on September 11, 2001: see Home Office Newsletter No. 37 (December 31, 2001) para.3.
[52] See 18–01.
[53] Coroners Act 1988 s.14.
[54] Taking the body out of England, burial out of the district, and cremation anywhere, were conclusive. There was an uncertainty when the body was *buried within the district*.
[55] e.g. consideration under s.16(3) of the 1988 Act whether to resume an inquest adjourned under s.16(1): see 10–83 ff below.
[56] *R. v Coroner for the Queen's Household Ex p. Al Fayed* Unreported July 18, 2000, Newman J, para.18. See further 12–30 ff below.
[57] Coroners and Justice Act 2009 s.3(1); see formerly Coroners Act 1988 s.14(2), (3). As to mass fatalities and disasters, see *Mass Fatalities: The Chief Coroner's Role*, 23 July 2014, and also Ch.17.
[58] Coroners and Justice Act 2009 s.3(4).
[59] Coroners and Justice Act 2009 s.3(5).
[60] Coroners and Justice Act 2009 s.3(2).
[61] Coroners and Justice Act 2009 s.3(3)(a).

Consequential provisions

Whether the transfer arises by way of agreement between two senior coroners, or **4–24** as a result of a direction of the Chief Coroner, certain consequential provisions follow. The transferring coroner must hand over to the receiving coroner all relevant evidence, documents and information, and notify of the transfer the next of kin or personal representative of the deceased, and any other interested person who has made himself known to the coroner, within five working days of the date on which the transfer was agreed, or the direction issued, unless there are exceptional circumstances.[62]

The receiving coroner's relevant authority will be responsible for all the costs **4–25** related to the transferred investigation (and any inquest) from the date of the transfer, except that in the case of a direction to transfer, the Chief Coroner may direct otherwise.[63] This means that costs already incurred up to the time of transfer remain with the transferring coroner's relevant authority.

Service deaths outside the United Kingdom

In certain circumstances the death outside the United Kingdom of a serviceman on **4–26** active service or similar activities[64] (or of a civilian accompanying servicemen and subject to service discipline),[65] whose body is brought to Scotland, or is expected to be brought to the United Kingdom, may be the subject of an investigation by a coroner from England and Wales. The Chief Coroner has put in place a scheme to ensure that a coroner experienced in service deaths deals with the case, and may wish to intervene in order to implement this.[66]

If the Secretary of State thinks that it may be appropriate for the circumstances **4–27** of the death to be investigated under the relevant Scottish legislation,[67] he may notify the Lord Advocate to that effect.[68] But if the Lord Advocate has been so notified, the body is in Scotland, no inquiry has been held or concluded under the Scottish legislation, the Lord Advocate has notified the Chief Coroner that in his view it may be appropriate for a coroner from England and Wales to conduct an investigation, and the Chief Coroner has reason to suspect that the deceased died a violent or unnatural death, or the cause of death is unknown, or the deceased died in custody or otherwise in state detention, then the Chief Coroner may direct a senior coroner to conduct an investigation into the death.[69]

The senior coroner so directed must conduct the investigation as soon as **4–28** practicable,[70] though always subject to the Chief Coroner's power to direct a transfer of the investigation to another coroner.[71] If on the other hand the body of such a person instead comes to England and Wales, and the Chief Coroner thinks

---

[62] Coroners (Investigations) Regulations, 2013 (SI 2013/1629) reg.18.
[63] Coroners (Investigations) Regulations, 2013 (SI 2013/1629) reg.19(1) (agreement), (2) (direction).
[64] Coroners and Justice Act 2009 s.12(2).
[65] Coroners and Justice Act 2009 s.12(3).
[66] See *Chief Coroner Guidance No. 7*, and also 13–78.
[67] Fatal Accidents and Sudden Deaths Inquiry (Scotland) Act 1976; see 20–50—20–53.
[68] Coroners and Justice Act 2009 s.12(4).
[69] Coroners and Justice Act 2009 s.13(1).
[70] Coroners and Justice Act 2009 s.13(2).
[71] See 4–19.

that it may be appropriate for the circumstances of the death to be investigated under the Scottish legislation, he may notify the Lord Advocate accordingly.[72]

Location of body and powers of coroner

4–29   Formerly, it would have been necessary, in the case of a transfer of jurisdiction, for the body to be moved into the district of the coroner directed to assume jurisdiction,[73] but this has not been required for many years.[74] Whether or not the body is actually moved into the area of the senior coroner assuming jurisdiction (whether he assumes jurisdiction at the request of another coroner, or by direction of the Chief Coroner), that coroner also assumes, in relation to the investigation, all the powers and duties which he would have if the body had originally been lying within his area and the death reported to him in the usual way, to the exclusion of any other senior coroner.

Extra-territorial powers

4–30   Most coronial powers are exercisable extra-territorially since 2013. One is the power to remove a body. A senior coroner responsible for conducting an investigation into a death or needing to request a post–mortem examination for the purpose of deciding whether he has a duty to conduct an investigation may order the removal of a body to any suitable place, either within his area or elsewhere.[75] But he may not order the removal of the body to a place provided by a person who has not consented to its being removed there, unless it is a place provided within his own area by a local authority.[76]

4–31   Formerly the coroner was obliged to order the return of the body after examination to a place within his district if he did not authorise its disposal,[77] but that has gone with the 2013 reforms. Other powers exercisable extra-territorially include the powers to exhume a body,[78] to require a person to supply evidence and produce documents and other things,[79] to summon witnesses[80] and jurors,[81] and to hold an inquest,[82] anywhere in England and Wales.

---

[72] Coroners and Justice Act 2009 s.12(5).
[73] Coroners (Amendment) Act 1926 ss.16–17 (repealed).
[74] Coroners Act 1988 s.14(4).
[75] Coroners and Justice Act 2009 s.15(1), (2); formerly Coroners Act 1988 s.22(1) (restricted to coroner's district and adjoining district).
[76] Coroners and Justice Act 2009 s.15(3); formerly Coroners Act 1988 s.22(2).
[77] Coroners Act 1988 s.22(4). The 1988 Act changed the law by using the word "disposal", instead of "burial" in s.24(2) of the 1926 Act: see Law Com. No. 167.
[78] See 8–03 ff.
[79] See 7–12 ff.
[80] See 10–29—10–30.
[81] See 10–43—10–48.
[82] See 10–16.

Part II

THE INVESTIGATION

Chapter 5

BEGINNING THE INVESTIGATION

BASIS OF CORONIAL JURISDICTION

A senior coroner who is made aware that the body[1] of a deceased[2] person is within **5–01** that coroner's area,[3] and has reason to suspect that *either* the deceased died a violent or unnatural death,[4] *or* the cause of death is unknown,[5] *or* the deceased died in custody or otherwise in state detention,[6] must as soon as practicable conduct an investigation into the death.[7] "Reason to suspect" is a low threshold, not amounting even to a prima facie case,[8] and the coroner is not limited to *admissible* evidence,[9] or to information which turns out to be true: it is sufficient if the coroner in good faith believes it to be true.[10] It should be noted that it is the presence of the body that matters, not where the death itself took place.[11]

Once the coroner is so made aware and has such reason, he has a duty to **5–02** investigate, save in those cases where his jurisdiction is transferred to another coroner,[12] or otherwise specifically taken away,[13] or where the coroner in question

---

[1] See 5–03 ff.

[2] As to when a body is to be regarded as "dead", see 5–14 below and Appendix 5. Coroners are often alerted informally by doctors and police that a person is gravely ill and likely to die shortly, in circumstances which would satisfy the statutory criteria. This is usually done because questions of organ transplants may thereafter arise, with a limited timescale for action: see 8–82. But a coroner acquires no jurisdiction and no power until the person concerned dies.

[3] See 2–30.

[4] See 5–70—5–97 below.

[5] See 5–80—5–82 below.

[6] See 5–83—5–86 below; Coroners Act 1988 s.8(1).

[7] Coroners and Justice Act 2009 s.1.

[8] See *R. (Canning) v Northampton Coroner* [2006] EWCA Civ. 1225 (dealing with "reasonable cause" under the 1988 Act); *R. Gracey) v Cheshire Coroner* [2008] EWHC 957 (Admin). See also *R. v Inner North London Coroner Ex p. Linnane* [1989] 1 W.L.R. 396, DC.

[9] *R. v South London Coroner Ex p. Weeks* Unreported December 6, 1996, Scott Baker J, referring to *Hussien v Chong Fook Kam* [1970] A.C. 942 at 949B.

[10] *R. v Stephenson* (1884) 13 QBD 331.

[11] It may have occurred in another coroner area, or at sea, or abroad: see 5–87—5–97 below.

[12] See 4–22 above.

[13] See 5–98 ff below.

or some other coroner has already held a valid investigation into the death (which has not been quashed)[14] and has not been ordered by the court to hold a further investigation.[15] But if the coroner is not made aware of the presence of the body within his area until after it has gone (or has been buried or cremated),[16] he has no original power to investigate the death,[17] although it may be conferred on him by agreement between coroners,[18] or the Chief Coroner may confer it on him in an appropriate case.[19]

What Amounts to a Body

5–03   Since the power of the coroner generally depends not on the fact of *death having occurred* in his area, but on his being informed of the fact that *there is a dead body* within it, it is necessary to consider first of all what amounts to a body, and how far a duty to conduct an investigation may arise without one. This may be the subject of a pre-investigation inquiry by the coroner.[20] Clearly, the complete body of a dead human being, whether newly born child or fully grown adult, falls within the term "body". But the following cases must also be considered:

     (1) the body of a fetus or of a stillborn child;

     (2) old human remains;

     (3) a partially destroyed body or a part or parts of a body;

     (4) calcined remains or ashes.

The body of a fetus or of a stillborn child

5–04   Neither a fetus (that is, a human being still *in utero*) nor a stillborn child can be the subject of an investigation, since in neither case is there any independent life[21] and therefore in neither case can there be a subsequent death.[22] For the purposes of death registration, a "stillborn" child is one which has issued forth from its mother after the 24th week of pregnancy but which did not at any time after being

---

[14] See 18–01 below.

[15] See 19–05, 19–25; as to the time for completing an investigation, see 10–14.

[16] See 9–20 ff below.

[17] R. (Touche) v Inner North London Coroner [2001] Q.B. 1206, CA; Bicknell v Birmingham and Solihull Coroner [2007] EWHC 2547 (Admin); R. (Lawrance) v West Somerset Coroner [2008] EWHC 1293 (Admin); Connah v Plymouth Hospitals NHS Trust [2010] EWHC 1727 (Admin); this was overlooked in R. v South London Coroner Ex p. Weeks Unreported December 6, 1996, Scott Baker J.

[18] See 4–19.

[19] See 4–22, 5–17.

[20] See 8–13.

[21] cf. Attorney General's Reference (No. 3 of 1994) [1998] A.C. 245; Re MB (An Adult: Medical Treatment) [1997] 2 FCR 541, 556–557.

[22] Attorney General's Reference (No. 3 of 1994) [1998] A.C. 245; Re MB (An Adult: Medical Treatment) [1997] 2 FCR 541, 556–557; Attorney General for Northern Ireland v Senior Coroner for Northern Ireland [2013] NICA 68 at [29], [30] (confirming the position in the text for England and Wales, but concluding differently for Northern Ireland on the basis of specific Northern Ireland legislation). A similar problem arises in relation to so-called "out of England orders", concerning the removal of a stillborn child from England and Wales; see 9–36.

completely expelled from its mother breathe nor show any other signs of life.[23] But a child born with signs of life (e.g. a beating heart) is nonetheless a child, and so may be the subject of an investigation in an appropriate case, even though it suffers from defects (e.g. missing organs) making it impossible for it to survive.

Because of improvements in medical technology, "viability" of a fetus may indeed now start even earlier than the 24th week. If there is any doubt as to whether or not a child achieved an existence independent of its mother before dying, the coroner should carry out a pre-investigation inquiry, treating the question of stillbirth as a preliminary issue. If an investigation is begun, but the body turns out to be that of a stillborn child, the coroner, though there can be no conclusion as to the cause of death,[24] should nonetheless transmit to the registrar of deaths a certificate setting out the facts as far as they are known. The stillbirth is then registered by the registrar in a manner similar to that of a live birth.[25] **5–05**

Old human remains

Provided they are sufficient to demonstrate a death,[26] old human remains prima facie constitute a body for the purposes of the acquisition of jurisdiction by a coroner,[27] even if they are situated in a museum.[28] The question accordingly becomes whether the further conditions referred to above[29] are satisfied. In the case of unearthed bones, or even a complete skeleton, one consideration will be whether the site from which they have been disinterred has ever been used as a burial ground, either with regular consecration or even as a "plague pit". If this is so, the coroner will probably (but not inevitably) take the view that there is no reason to suspect a death falling within the statutory criteria, and thus that he has no duty to conduct an investigation. **5–06**

On the other hand, if the site has never been used for authorised or recognised burial purposes, the first objective will be to determine whether the remains are human. If the skeleton is incomplete, the assistance of an anatomist or anthropologist may have to be sought.[30] If the remains are human, the next question will be whether there is any reason to suspect a death falling within the statutory criteria. If there is, the coroner must investigate, so far as he is able, and he will probably begin by considering their age and possible identification. Carbon-dating may assist in relation to the former. **5–07**

Whatever the strict legal position, in practice the coroner is unlikely to consider an investigation necessary in the case of a discovery of anatomical specimens, or in **5–08**

---

[23] Births and Deaths Registration Act 1953 s.41, as amended in 1992. See Home Office Circular No. 83 of 1992.

[24] Though see 13–66 below.

[25] Births and Deaths Registration Act 1926 s.5. Registration of Births and Deaths Regulations 1987 regs 31, 32.

[26] See 5–09 below.

[27] See, e.g. the case of a mummified baby found in a suitcase more than 40 years after its death: see *The Times*, November 6, 1985 (Battersea Coroner); see also the inquest on one of the victims of the "Moors murderers", found 25 years after her death: *The Daily Telegraph*, April 13, 1988.

[28] See Department of Culture, Media and Sport, *Report of the Working Group on Human Remains*, November 2003; Department of Culture, Media and Sport, *Guidance for the care of human remains in museums*, October 2005.

[29] See 5–01.

[30] Some museums (e.g. the Museum of London) employ bone experts, who can assist in this.

a case where the death must have taken place a long time ago.[31] The coroner has power to order the exhumation of the remains for examination for the purpose of his own duties or for certain criminal proceedings.[32] In other cases the licence of the Home Secretary must be obtained.[33]

Partially destroyed body or body parts

5–09   In the case of the discovery of partially destroyed bodies or parts of bodies, or pieces of tissue, there are a number of difficult problems which may be encountered, since it cannot automatically be assumed that the body to which the piece of tissue or part belongs is dead. A skull would be sufficient, for example. But a severed arm or leg is not conclusive evidence that the body from which it comes is dead. Similarly a piece of tissue may be not sufficiently vital as to demonstrate the inevitability of death.

5–10   Thus the finding of a tattooed arm, proved to be that of a particular person, which had been cut off from the body with a sharp knife, was held by an Australian court not to constitute a body for the purpose of giving jurisdiction to the coroner, since an arm may be removed from a person's body without loss of life.[34] By contrast, in one English case, portions of human lung were found in the sea at the point at which an aircraft had crashed, without any trace of the pilot being found. The person from whom the lung material had come was shown to have had the same blood group as the missing pilot. The coroner held that the lung material constituted a body and accordingly he had jurisdiction because of its presence within his area.[35] Similarly, in another case the coroner held that he had jurisdiction to hold an inquest where the lower half only of a girl's body was found in the street, and the rest was not recovered.[36] Clearly, medical evidence may be required to satisfy the coroner that it is reasonable to assume that the tissue or part of a body discovered came from a dead body.

5–11   It is also a desirable practice for the coroner who begins an investigation upon an incomplete human body to allow time for other portions to be found. If having thus adjourned and thereafter completed his investigation, he is satisfied that some other portion of the same body has been discovered, he need not hold any further inquiry in relation to that portion.[37] In some cases it may instead be desirable for

---

[31] See *The Times*, November 13, 1984, regarding the body of a man recovered from a bog after 2,500 years. And no inquiry appears to have been carried out in relation to the body of King Richard III (died 1485), dug up from a Leicester car park: see Buckley et al, "The King in the Car Park" (2013) 87 Antiquity 519, and also *R. (Plantagenet Alliance Ltd) v Secretary of State for Justice* [2013] EWHC B13 (Admin); [2013] EWHC 3164 (Admin), Haddon-Cave J.; [2014] EWHC 1586 (Admin), DC. Cl.3 of the Coroners Bill of 2007 provided that the coroner had no duty to inquire if he had reason to believe that the death took place over 50 years before.

[32] Coroners Act 1988 s.23; see 8–03 ff below.

[33] Burial Act 1857 s.25. See 8–01 below.

[34] *Re Oram Ex p. Brady* (1935) 52 N.S.W.W.N. 109. cf. *R. v Bond* (1717) 1 Str. 22, 93 E.R. 360, where an inquisition taken on an exhumed skull was ordered not to be filed, seemingly on the ground that there could not be a view of the whole body (necessary at that date to give jurisdiction).

[35] *Re Bennett*, 1965, Lincolnshire, Louth District. Strictly this may not have been justified, since the material might have been tissue discarded after an operation and simply flushed out to sea.

[36] *Re Suha Youmis Hawa*, *The Times*, November 22, 1984, Inner West London Coroner.

[37] See also 5–23 below.

the coroner to report the matter to the Chief Coroner, with a view to the latter's directing an investigation.[38]

Calcined remains or ashes

Where calcined remains and ashes are concerned, it is again necessary in the first **5-12** instance to make sure that the remains are those of a human being. Once more, this may depend on pathological and anatomical evidence, or it may be determined by consideration of the surrounding facts. The coroner should next decide whether there are sufficient remains to constitute a body, and for this purpose it is generally necessary that some vital organ should be present, as in the case of mutilated bodies.[39] The ashes remaining after the cremation of a body are highly unlikely ever to constitute such remains as a matter of fact.

If the coroner decides that the remains do constitute a body, he must next decide **5-13** whether the statutory conditions are satisfied.[40] If they are, the coroner must conduct an investigation. Even in cases where the cause of death is unascertainable, it may still be useful for a coronial investigation to be conducted, as it may set at rest rumour, suspicion or gossip by the recording of the other facts that can be established.

Deciding whether a body is dead

The coroner may also be faced with the difficult task of deciding whether a body **5-14** in his area is actually "dead", for instance when it is connected to a life support machine in an irreversible coma. The notion of death is discussed in more detail elsewhere,[41] but it appears that, once a person has suffered brain stem death which no medical treatment is able to reverse, the person is "dead" for the purposes of the coroner's acquiring jurisdiction, even whilst a machine ventilates the body.[42]

By contrast, death of the higher brain, leaving the brain stem alive, and leading **5-15** to what is known as "persistent vegetative state", does not in law amount to death.[43] The coroner has no power to "permit" the discontinuance of treatment, or the switching off of the ventilator. Either the patient is dead already, and it makes no difference, or the patient dies as a result, and it is (potentially) homicide. The only authority which can sanction such matters (unless the patient has sufficient capacity to do so)[44] is the High Court.[45]

---

[38] See 5–16 ff.

[39] See 5–09 above.

[40] See 5–01 above.

[41] See App.5 below.

[42] *Mail Newspapers v Express Newspapers* [1987] F.S.R. 90, *Airedale NHS Trust v Bland* [1993] A.C. 789, and *Re Baby A* (1992) 3 Med. L.R. 303, Fam.D. cf. Thurston, *Coronership*, 3rd edn (1985), para.10–15, which sets out both this view and the opposing one that whilst the heart beats and the blood circulates there is no "dead" body, but without expressing a preference. Of course, in practice no coroner would insist on taking possession of the body where it was still connected to a life support system.

[43] *Airedale NHS Trust v Bland*, above; Jennett, *The Vegetative State* (2002). See App.5.

[44] As to which, see *B (Consent to Treatment Capacity), Re; sub nom. B v An NHS Hospital Trust*; B (Adult: Refusal of Medical Treatment), Re [2002] EWHC 429; [2002] 2 All E.R. 449.

[45] *Airedale NHS Trust v Bland* [1993] A.C. 789, HL; *An NHS Trust v A.* [2001] Fam. 348; *942 NHS Trust v H* [2001] 2 F.L.R. 501; cf. *R. (Pretty) v DPP* [2002] 1 All E.R. 1, HL.

Jurisdiction Without a Body

Report to the Chief Coroner

5–16   If a coroner considers that the human remains or ashes within his area do not constitute a "body", for the purposes of acquiring jurisdiction, or if there was once a body but it had gone from his area by the time he was informed,[46] he should consider whether the facts should be reported to the Chief Coroner. Where the coroner has reason to believe that a death has occurred in or near his area, that the circumstances of death are such that there should be an investigation into it,[47] and that the duty to conduct an investigation into the death does not arise because of the destruction, loss or absence of the body, he may report the matter to the Chief Coroner.[48]

5–17   The Chief Coroner may then direct a coroner (not necessarily the one making the report) to conduct an investigation into the death.[49] Subject to the power of the Chief Coroner thereafter to direct another coroner to conduct it,[50] the coroner to whom the direction is given must hold an investigation as soon as practicable. The statutory predecessor of this power was considered to apply equally to cases where there was only part of a body as it did to cases where there was no body at all. Moreover it was not necessary that the coroner believe for certain that the person concerned had died, and neither was it impermissible to seek to invoke the discretion in order to establish that death *had* occurred.[51]

Conditions for power to arise

5–18   The conditions that must be satisfied for the power to arise are stringent. In the first place, the coroner must have reason to believe that the death has taken place in or near the coroner's area. The use of the word "near" was not intended to enlarge a jurisdiction or to permit "poaching" in a neighbouring district (now "area"),[52] but was intended to cover the possibility that the missing body was not exactly where it was believed to be. It would appear to cover a death by drowning off the shore, but not persons lost overboard from a ship on the high seas.[53] What is "near" is for the coroner to judge in a reasonable manner.[54]

5–19   Secondly, the coroner must have reason to believe that the circumstances of the death are such that there should be an investigation into it. It is unclear whether this means that the coroner would consider it desirable to conduct an investigation,

---

[46] *R. (Touche) v Inner North London Coroner* [2001] Q.B. 1206, CA; *Bicknell v Birmingham Coroner* [2007] EWHC 2547 (Admin).

[47] See *Bicknell v Birmingham Coroner* [2007] EWHC 2547 (Admin), paras 19-21.

[48] Coroners and Justice Act 2009 s.1(4). cf the position in Northern Ireland: *Re Howard's Application* [2011] NIQB 125.

[49] Coroners and Justice Act 2009 s.1(5); formerly Coroners Act 1988 s.15. See Purchase [1954] Crim.L.R. 46; Harvard [1954] Crim.L.R. 782.

[50] See 4–22.

[51] *R. v Home Secretary Ex p. Weatherhead* (1995) 32 B.M.L.R. 72, [1996] C.O.D. 271, May J.

[52] *Connah v Plymouth Hospitals NHS Trust* [2010] EWHC 1727 (Admin).

[53] *R. v East Sussex Coroner Ex p. Healy* [1988] 1 W.L.R. 1194, DC: death eight or nine miles offshore following diving accident not "near" for this purpose.

[54] *R. v East Sussex Coroner Ex p. Healy* [1988] 1 W.L.R. 1194, DC; *R. v South London Coroner Ex p. Driscoll* (1993) 159 J.P. 45, DC.

or that if the body were present in his area he would be legally obliged to do so.[55] Nearly all deaths in such circumstances are likely to be violent or unnatural deaths: it is very unlikely that there would be sufficient evidence to suggest that the death was due to natural causes. Therefore, if there were a body within his area, the coroner would normally be bound to conduct an investigation.

Thirdly, the coroner must have reason to believe that the duty to conduct an investigation does not arise because of the destruction, loss or absence of the body.[56] Finally, the Chief Coroner's power only arises where the coroner reports the matter to him, and it is clear that the coroner has a discretion whether or not to do so, although the exercise of this discretion is subject to judicial review in the usual way.[57]   **5–20**

Thus deaths which are, in any event, the subject of other official inquiries may not merit a report to the Chief Coroner. On the other hand a coronial investigation would be desirable if there were facts to which public attention should be drawn or if there were any suspicious circumstances attaching to the death. When the coroner considers whether or not to report the matter to the Chief Coroner, he should also take into account any desire by the relatives that an investigation should be held.   **5–21**

Deaths were sometimes reported to the Secretary of State under the old regime in order to facilitate the registration of the death.[58] Registrars were reluctant to register death in the absence of evidence of death unless an investigation had been held or the court had presumed death,[59] and, in such cases, there was unlikely to be any person other than the coroner who was qualified to give evidence to the registrar for the registration of the death. This may still be true under the new regime. In reporting the matter to the Chief Coroner the coroner should give his reasons for considering it desirable to conduct an investigation.   **5–22**

It should be noted that the Chief Coroner cannot be compelled to exercise his power to direct an investigation to be held.[60] If the Chief Coroner does exercise it, he may direct *any* coroner to conduct the investigation, not merely his informant. The coroner so directed must conduct an investigation as soon as practicable,[61] subject to the power of the Chief Coroner to direct another coroner to conduct it.[62]   **5–23**

---

[55] *Bicknell v Birmingham Coroner* [2007] EWHC 2547 (Admin) at [19]–[21].

[56] This is less stringent than formerly, under s.15 of the 1988 Act, where it was necessary to show that the body had been destroyed *or was irrecoverable*. So the fact that the body was buried elsewhere would not necessarily have satisfied this condition, but its mere absence from the area will now do so.

[57] *Bicknell v Birmingham Coroner* [2007] EWHC 2547 (Admin); *R. (Lawrance) v West Somerset Coroner* [2008] EWHC 1293 (Admin); *Connah v Plymouth Hospitals NHS Trust* [2010] EWHC 1727 (Admin). See 19–25 ff.

[58] Though there are various provisions enabling registration of a death outside England and Wales (e.g. at sea) without the intervention of a coroner: see paras 5–58—5–59 below.

[59] As to this, see now the Presumption of Death Act 2013.

[60] *R. v Home Secretary Ex p. Weatherhead* (1995) 32 B.M.L.R. 72; [1996] C.O.D. 271, May J.

[61] Coroners and Justice Act 2009 s.1(6).

[62] Coroners and Justice Act 2009 s.3. See 4–22.

Duty to Report Death

5–24   In addition to those cases in which the duty was imposed upon some particular person,[63] at common law it was the duty of every person who was about the deceased to give immediate[64] notice to the coroner or to his officer or to the appropriate officer of police, of circumstances requiring the holding of an inquest.[65] It would seem that this was also true of circumstances that should lead to inquiry but which ultimately did not necessitate an inquest.[66]

5–25   If this more general duty still exists under the new regime, it cannot be enforced by any particular legal sanction, except insofar as it is an offence to obstruct a coroner in the exercise of his duty,[67] or to do anything to frustrate or prevent an inquest. In particular it is an indictable offence at common law to bury the body of a person before the coroner had has the opportunity of holding an inquest upon it,[68] or in any way to dispose of the body (as by burning it or removing it[69]) in order to prevent inquiries being made by the coroner as to how the person died.[70]

5–26   However, there is now provision for the Lord Chancellor by regulations to require registered medical practitioners in prescribed circumstances to notify coroners of deaths of which they are aware.[71] Before making such regulations, the Lord Chancellor must consult the Secretary of State for Health and the Chief Coroner.[72] At the time of writing, none have so far been made.

---

[63] As to which see 5–51 below.

[64] This means "while the body is fresh and while it remains in the same situation as when death occurred": *R. v Clerk* (1702) 1 Salk. 377.

[65] *R. v Clerk* (1702) 1 Salk. 377.

[66] e.g. because of the Coroners Act 1988 s.19, now the Coroners and Justice Act 2009 s.4 (see 8–36—8–37 below), or because the visiting forces provisions forbade the inquest to be held: see 5–98—5–108 below.

[67] *R. v Soleguard* (1738) And. 231 (refusing access to the place where the body lay); *R. v Purcy* (1933) 149 L.T. 432 (concealing a body); *R. v Skinner* (1993) 14 Cr. App. R. (S.) 115 (concealing a body); *R. v Godward* [1998] 1 Cr. App. R. (S.) 385 (concealing a body).

[68] 2 Hawk. P.C. Ch. 9 s.23; *R. v Clerk,* above; *R. v Davis* (1942) 42 S.N.S.W.) 263.

[69] As to the removal of bodies out of England and Wales, see 9–36—9–44 below.

[70] See *R. v Price* (1884) 12 Q.B.D. 247, 248; *R. v Stephenson* (1884) 13 Q.B.D. 331; *R. v Pearson* Unreported October 13, 1954, Newcastle Assizes (Glyn-Jones J) (preventing an inquest); *R. v Hunter* [1974] Q.B. 95 (conspiracy to prevent burial); *R. v Swindell* (1981) 3 Cr.App.R.(S.) 255, CA (preventing burial); *R. v LeGrand* [1983] Crim. L.R. 626 (preventing a burial); *R. v Ake, The Times,* December 17, 1985, Teesside Crown Court (Tucker J) (preventing an inquest); *R. v Parry* (1986) 8 Cr. App. R. (S.) 470 (conspiracy to prevent burial); *R. v Blakemore* [1997] 2 Cr. App.R. (S.) 255 (act tending to pervert course of justice); *R. v Godward* [1998] 1 Cr. App. R. (S.) 385 (concealing a body); *R. v Whiteley* [2000] All E.R. (D.) 1888, CA (conspiring to prevent burial); *R. v Lang* Unreported November 22, 2001, CA (act tending to pervert the course of public justice).

[71] Coroners and Justice Act 2009 s.18(1) (not in force at the time of writing). No regulations have so far been made.

[72] Coroners and Justice Act 2009 s.18(2) (not in force at the time of writing).

CERTIFICATE OF CAUSE OF DEATH

Certification by a registered medical practitioner

Until regulations are made by the Lord Chancellor,[73] there is no obligation on a   5–27
doctor as such to report a death to the *coroner*, although doctors are encouraged to
in cases of doubt or suspicion,[74] and in practice do so.[75] However, in the case of the
death of any person who has been attended in his last illness by a registered medical
practitioner,[76] such practitioner is under the current law obliged to sign and
transmit to the registrar of birth and deaths a certificate on a form prescribed
stating, to the best of his knowledge and belief, the cause of death.[77] It makes no
difference that the death has been, or will be, reported to the coroner, or that there
will be an investigation.[78] However, the Secretary of State for Health has power to
make regulations to change the position in future,[79] once the new system of
medical examiners[80] comes into effect.

A number of points on the existing law should be noted. First, the obligation to   5–28
give a certificate is strictly an obligation to notify the *cause* of death and not the *fact*.
Thus a doctor does not certify that death has occurred,[81] only what in his opinion
was the cause, assuming that death has taken place. Secondly, arising out of the first,
there is no obligation on the doctor even to see, let alone examine the body before
issuing a certificate. The Brodrick Report recommended that the certifying doctor
should be required to inspect the body of a deceased person before issuing a
certificate,[82] but this recommendation has not so far been implemented.

Thirdly, it should be noted that the only practitioner who can be required by law   5–29
to sign a medical certificate as to the cause of death is one who has "attended" the
deceased "during his last illness". Neither expression is defined. The Select
Committee on Death Certification in 1893 pointed out that the words "during his

---

[73] See Coroners and Justice Act 2009 s.18(1) (not in force at the time of writing), and 5–26 above.

[74] *Guidance for Doctors completing Medical Certificates of Cause of Death in England and Wales*, Office for National Statistics, July 2010, para.4.

[75] For two studies on the ability of (1) hospital clinicians and (2) general practitioners to recognise reportable deaths, see (1) *Start and others*, (1993) 306 B.M.J. 1038 (see also (1993) 306 B.M.J. 1018 at 1539, 1540), (2) *Start and others*, (1995) 45 B.J.G.P. 191. Another study in 1993 suggested that 18 per cent of junior doctors would alter a cause of death to avoid involving the coroner: *Maudsley and Williams*, (1993) 15 J. Public Health. Med. 192.

[76] This term includes provisionally registered persons, i.e. the status accorded to persons for the first year after graduation. The Brodrick Report (at para.5–05) recommended that only fully registered persons should be able to certify the cause of death.

[77] Births and Deaths Registration Act 1953 s.22(1). The form of certificate is prescribed by the Registration of Births and Deaths Regulations 1987 Sch.2, Form 14 (for all persons aged more than 27 days) and 15 (for persons aged less than 28 days). Bilingual forms are prescribed for use in Wales: see the Registration of Births and Deaths (Welsh Language) Regulations 1987 Sch. 2, Forms 11 and 12 (see App.2). In practice the doctor who issues a certificate hands it to a relative of the deceased (or other "qualified informant") who will take it to the registrar to register the death. In so doing the relative or other person is acting as the agent of the medical practitioner, and fulfilling the latter's duty to transmit the certificate.

[78] See Home Office Circular, dated October 21, 1923.

[79] Coroners and Justice Act 2009 s.20 (not in force at the time of writing).

[80] See Ch.3.

[81] In practice in modern times the fact of death *having occurred* is frequently certified by health professionals who are not registered medical practitioners, such as paramedics attending the scene of an accident.

[82] At para.5–22.

last illness" had been interpreted very flexibly, and suggested that they ought to be defined as meaning "personal attendance by the person certifying upon at least two occasions, one of which should be within eight days of death". This suggestion too was never taken up.

5–30   Nonetheless, it is clear that in imposing an obligation on a medical practitioner to certify the form of death without having seen the patient after death, the law contemplates that the doctor has had a sufficient opportunity to confirm a diagnosis of a illness which causes the patient's death. Thus "attendance" must be substantial (e.g. a house call or appointment), rather than casual, and "last illness" must mean the illness which caused the death.

5–31   Accordingly, it is submitted that, where a patient is received into a hospital, he is not being attended for this purpose by any hospital doctor until he has been examined and a decision concerning his condition reached. If the patient dies before a decision has been reached, then, unless the doctor who last attended him before admission is prepared to certify, the death is likely to be a death of which the cause is unknown and of which the coroner should accordingly be informed.[83]

The condition of attendance

5–32   Although a medical practitioner cannot be *required* to give a certificate unless the condition of attendance is satisfied, the question arises whether he has *power* to do so in any other case. The Brodrick Report recommended[84] that a doctor should be permitted to certify the cause of death only if he had attended the deceased at least once during the seven days preceding death, but this recommendation too has never been implemented. The result is that a doctor may in theory certify the cause of death though he has not seen the deceased alive during his last illness, nor indeed even before death.[85] In practice, this is rare, but it does happen,[86] and leads to a so-called "legally uncertified" death.[87]

Report by the registrar of deaths

5–33   In any event, the registrar of deaths is obliged to notify the coroner of any death taking place where the deceased was seen neither during the 14 days preceding death nor at any time afterwards by a certifying medical practitioner.[88] Whilst a doctor who does not know the cause of death could give a certificate stating the cause as "unknown", he should not do so as (in this case also) the registrar will inform the coroner, and unnecessary delay will be caused.

Certification in cases to be reported to coroner

5–34   Accordingly, if the death is one which the registrar of births and deaths is likely to report to the coroner, the medical practitioner can (and should) save the relatives

---

[83] See 5–01.

[84] At para.5–12.

[85] See also App.5.

[86] e.g. where the doctor caring for the deceased is unavailable, and a partner in the same practice gives the certificate based on medical records.

[87] Gastrell and others, "An analysis of legally uncertified deaths 1979–2002" (2004) *Health Statistics Quarterly* 24.

[88] See 5–47 below.

unnecessary frustration[89] and delay by reporting the death directly to the coroner and, whether or not he issues a medical certificate, by informing the relatives that the death cannot be registered until the coroner has dealt with the case.[90] If the practitioner does issue a certificate but rings the printed statement on the face of it to the effect that he has reported the death to the coroner,[91] the registrar of births and deaths will refrain from registering the death until he has been informed by the coroner of the action taken or to be taken in regard to the death. If the coroner decides not to do anything,[92] the death can then be registered immediately from the medical certificate issued by the practitioner. This prevents delay in making funeral arrangements.

Post-mortem examinations for certification purposes

The practitioner should not himself arrange a post-mortem examination of the body (with the consent of the deceased's personal representatives or relatives)[93] unless it is clear that the coroner would have no jurisdiction and, in particular, that the death is not a death of which the cause is unknown. If, however, in the case of a natural death a post-mortem examination is made to afford him more exact and complete information as to the extent of the disease process, it is desirable that a certificate should be issued indicating that further information about the disease process causing death may become available after a post-mortem examination.   **5–35**

DEATHS ASSOCIATED WITH OPERATIONS OR ANAESTHESIA

The reporting of deaths to the coroner where the death is associated with an operation or anaesthetic is a sensitive and problematic area. It overlaps with the question whether the death can properly be regarded as violent or unnatural, discussed later.[94] Although there may be no question of negligence, the very fact of a report to a coroner is sometimes taken, by some doctors and members of the public, as a suggestion that some medical error has occurred. It is not.   **5–36**

Report by the registrar of deaths

Although there is no statutory duty upon a doctor to report such deaths to the coroner, the registrar of deaths is required to report (a) deaths which appear to have occurred during an operation before full recovery from the effect of an anaesthetic and also (b) deaths which the registrar has reason to believe to have been unnatural or to have been caused by violence or neglect.[95] The two categories will cover   **5–37**

---

[89] Especially interruption of funeral arrangements.

[90] See *Guidance for doctors completing Medical Certificates of Cause of Death in England and Wales*, Office for National Statistics, July 2010, para.4.

[91] This statement is repeated on the reverse and is called "Statement A".

[92] Issuing a so-called "Form A" to the registrar: see 8–15 below.

[93] If carried out without consent and not under any lawful authority (such as the coroner's direction), the examination probably amounts to an actionable trespass: *Clerk and Lindsell on Torts*, 18th edn (2000), para.14–45.

[94] See 5–70 ff.

[95] See 5–47 below.

most (if not all) deaths associated with operations or anaesthesia. As stated above,[96] where a death will be reported by the registrar to the coroner, it is desirable for the doctor himself to report such death.

Cause of death

5–38 In deciding whether the cause is related to an operation or anaesthesia, the doctor must ask the question: would the patient have died from this cause and at this time if the operation has not been performed or the anaesthetic administered? Another way to put the point is, did the treatment do any more than fail to save the patient's life?[97] In some cases, the answer to this question is difficult or impossible to give, since the disease from which the patient was suffering would be expected to result in death and the operation or anaesthetic may merely alter the time or mechanism of death. Where there is doubt, the doctor should err on the side of caution and make the report.

5–39 Operations and their associated anaesthetics are performed to save life, improve the quality of life or diagnose a condition, which may be treatable. All surgery and anaesthesia have known, associated, risks, and the doctor will use clinical skill to weigh the expected benefit to the patient from surgery against the likely risks. The decision will also be one involving the clinical judgments of both surgeon and anaesthetist, who use different criteria in assessing patients but who will jointly arrive at a decision as to whether or not to proceed with an operation.

5–40 Most deaths associated with surgery and anaesthesia are not due to error or negligence on the part of the medical team, but are due to the disease process in the patient or a recognised complication of the surgery or anaesthetic which could not be avoided in the necessary treatment of the patient. If a patient who is bleeding internally is operated upon to stop that bleeding but dies from haemorrhage on the operating table before the surgeon can find the source of bleeding, the death is clearly not associated with the operation or anaesthetic, even though the patient may have been in a poor condition for an anaesthetic. Clearly, in these circumstances, death would have been inevitable without the operation and any attempt to save the life is justifiable.[98]

5–41 A patient may undergo surgery in non-urgent circumstances for a non-life threatening condition, such as the removal of haemorrhoids ("piles"). Between 10 and 14 days after the operation the patient may die suddenly from a pulmonary embolus. The formation of blood clots in the deep veins of the leg after an operation is a well-recognised complication of surgery, and may occur despite measures to prevent it. Such a clot can then cause sudden death from pulmonary embolism. Death in these circumstances may not be attributable to any error or negligence in the surgery[99] but is clearly a consequence of the surgery, and death from this cause would not have occurred in the absence of surgery.[100] It must be reported. In such a case, the coroner may need to investigate, for example, whether

---

[96] See 5–34 below.
[97] *R. v Birmingham and Solihull Coroner Ex p. Benton* (1997) 162 JP 807, 8 Med. L.R. 362.
[98] cf. *R. v Birmingham and Solihull Coroner Ex p. Benton* (1997) 162 JP 807, 8 Med. L.R. 362.
[99] There may, of course, be other questions relating to pre- and post-operative care, e.g. the administration of blood-thinning agents as a prophylactic.
[100] See also 14–80 ff.

the doctors paid due regard to guidance (e.g. from the National Institute for Health and Clinical Excellence) and VTE prophylaxis.

In attempting to analyse deaths associated with anaesthesia and surgery, the **5–42** following questions may assist:

(a) Was the death due to the pre-existing disease or injury for which the surgery was being performed, and would death have occurred at the time it did without surgical intervention? Or did the operation or anaesthesia cause or contribute to the death?

(b) Was there informed consent, i.e. did the patient know of and accept the risks involved?

(c) If the cause of death was the pre-existing condition rather than the operation or anaesthesia, was there a failure to prevent the death by other means?

(d) If the operation or anaesthesia did cause or contribute to the death, was this a justified response to the pre-existing condition?[101]

(e) Was there any accident or defect in the pre-operative, operative or post-operative care, without which the death would not have occurred?

(f) If not, was the death otherwise preventable by other means? Was national and local guidance followed, and if not, why not?

Although it may seem to a medical practitioner that the death of a patient is free **5–43** from any suggestion of error, that is not the test for the coroner's involvement:[102] even where there was no error, there are still circumstances in which a coroner must be involved. Thus it may be a death of which the cause is not known.[103] Or adverse comment may be made in relation to the treatment of the deceased (even by himself).[104] Or there may be a belief in the relatives or friends of the deceased that the recent or earlier employment, occupation or experience of the deceased or some accident or other unnatural event, though it was considered trivial at the time of its occurrence, may have some bearing upon the death. In such cases, the medical practitioner should not see the coroner's investigation as a threat, but rather as an *opportunity*: there is value in an objective inquiry being set in motion at the earliest moment (although of course there are other means to carry out such inquiries today).

---

[101] Compare (1) an operation, not without risk, for cosmetic purposes; (2) an urgent, but non-life-threatening operation; (3) a "heroic" attempt to save life in emergency.

[102] See the studies on (1) hospital clinicians and (2) general practitioners' ability to recognise reportable deaths: (1) *Start and others* (1993) 306 B.M.J. 1038; (2) *Start and others* (1995) 45 B.J.G.P. 191.

[103] See 5–01 above.

[104] Raising a suspicion of neglect: see 5–74 below.

Doctor's Knowledge of Criminal Acts

5–44   Sometimes a medical practitioner, during the course of his treatment of a patient, obtains information, which reveals the actual or probable commission of a criminal act either by the patient or by another person in relation to the patient. It is clear law that the doctor, unlike the lawyer, has no right or privilege to refuse to answer questions in a court of law or otherwise to give information which he is statutorily required to give, merely by reasons that in doing so he would be breaking a professional confidence.[105] But the question here is whether a medical practitioner is under an obligation to speak at an earlier stage, in order to inform the authorities.

5–45   It has already been stated that he is normally under no specific legal duty to inform the coroner.[106] Nonetheless there are circumstances in which there is a duty to speak to the police or to some other authority.[107] One such case is where vital evidence would be lost if the authorities were not alerted in time.

5–46   Thus in one case, Avory J said:

> "It may be the moral duty of the medical man, even in cases where the patient is not dying, or not unlikely to recover, to communicate with the authorities when he sees good reason to believe that a criminal offence has been committed. However that may be, I cannot doubt that in such a case as the present, where the woman was, in the opinion of the medical man, likely to die and, therefore, evidence was likely to be lost, it was his duty, and that some one of those gentlemen [i.e. the medical practitioners who attended the woman] ought to have done it in this case."[108]

Registrar's Report to Coroner

5–47   It is the duty of the registrar of deaths to report certain deaths to the coroner.[109] These are:

    (a)   the death of any person not attended during his last illness[110] by a registered medical practitioner;[111] or

---

[105] See 7–71 below.

[106] See 5–24—5–26. But he may have professional obligations to do so.

[107] See also the BMA guidance "Confidentiality and Disclosure of Health Information", available at *http://www.bma.org.uk* [Accessed June 4, 2014].

[108] Charge to Grand Jury at Birmingham Assizes on December 1, 1914, later circulated to all coroners with the authority of the Lord Chief Justice.

[109] Registration of Births and Deaths Regulations 1987 reg.41(1). "Coroner" for this purpose includes a senior coroner, area coroner or assistant coroner, and the Chief Coroner, a judge former judge or former coroner when conducting an investigation under Sch.10 to the 2009 Act: Registration of Births and Deaths Regulations 1987 reg.2(1), as amended by SI 2013/1869. The registrar in reporting to the coroner should use Form 52: Home Office Circular No. 28 of 2003.

[110] See 5–29 above.

[111] This means a fully registered medical practitioner: Medical Act 1983 Sch.6 para.11(2).

(b) a death in respect of which the registrar is unable to obtain the delivery of a duly completed certificate of cause of death; or

(c) any death with respect to which it appears to the registrar from the certificate of cause of death that the deceased was seen by a certifying medical practitioner neither after death nor within 14 days before death; or

(d) any death the cause of which appears to be unknown;[112] or

(e) any death which the registrar has reason to believe to have been unnatural or caused by violence[113] or neglect,[114] or by abortion, or to have been attended by suspicious circumstances; or

(f) any death which appears to have occurred during an operation or before recovery from the effects of an anaesthetic;[115] or

(g) any death which appears from the contents of any medical certificate to have been due to industrial disease[116] or industrial poisoning.

The registrar is not released from his duty otherwise to report a death to the coroner merely because the coroner will be unable to hold an investigation, whether because of the visiting forces provisions,[117] or by reason of diplomatic or other immunity.[118] **5–48**

If the registrar has reason to believe that it is the duty of some other person or authority than himself to report the death to the coroner, he is obliged to satisfy himself that the death has been duly reported.[119] The registrar must refrain from registering any death which he has himself reported to the coroner, or which to his knowledge it is the duty of some other person or authority to notify the coroner, or which has been notified to the coroner until (in any of these cases) he has received a coroner's certificate after inquest held[120] or notification from the coroner that he does not intend to hold an inquest.[121] The registrar must also report to the coroner any alleged stillbirth if he has reason to believe that the child was born alive,[122] and may not register such stillbirth until he has received either a coroner's certificate after inquest, or a notification that the coroner does not intend to hold an inquest.[123] **5–49**

---

[112] This includes a statement in a medical certificate of the cause of death that the death was due to "natural causes": Home Office Circular No. 28 of 2003.

[113] This is held to include accidental bone fractures.

[114] This is held to include self-neglect, such as death through starvation because of *anorexia nervosa*.

[115] Recovery from anaesthetic is customarily measured as taking approximately 24 hours from the conclusion of the operation, but there is no legal definition.

[116] See paras 15–34—15–35.

[117] See 5–98—5–108 below.

[118] See 5–109—5–115 below.

[119] Registration of Births and Deaths Regulations 1987 reg.41(2).

[120] See 18–11 below.

[121] Registration of Births and Deaths Regulations 1987 reg.41(3) (not apparently amended in light of the bringing into force of the 2009 reforms in 2013).

[122] Registration of Births and Deaths Regulations 1987 reg.33(1).

[123] Registration of Births and Deaths Regulations 1987 reg.33(2) (not apparently amended in light of the bringing into force of the 2009 reforms in 2013).

Other Reports to Coroner

5–50   Apart from the duty of those about the deceased to give notice to the coroner,[124] a few persons have imposed upon them the duty of notifying certain deaths to the coroner or to some other person or authority. There are also more general obligations on a wider range of individuals to notify the circumstances of the death to the registrar of births and deaths.

5–51   The death of a person in legal custody in a prison,[125] detention centre[126] or young offender institution[127] must be reported forthwith by the governor or manager to the coroner. Similarly, the death of a person under sentence in service custody premises[128] must be reported by the commandant to the coroner. By contrast, where a child accommodated in a children's home dies, the death need not be reported to the coroner, but must be notified by the responsible authority as soon as possible to a variety of other persons and authorities.[129]

5–52   Since 1959,[130] there has been no specific requirement that the death of a person resident (whether voluntarily or compulsorily) in a mental hospital or other similar institution must be reported either to the coroner or to some other authority. The Brodrick Report[131] recommended that there should be an obligation to report to the coroner the death of a compulsorily detained mental patient, but this has not been implemented. However, the 2013 reforms have extended the range of deaths which engage the duty of the coroner to conduct an investigation to include those in state detention,[132] and this will cover the deaths of persons compulsorily detained on mental health grounds.

Report to Registrar

5–53   Even in cases where there is no requirement to notify the coroner of the fact or circumstances of a death, there is nonetheless a general requirement that any death which takes place in England and Wales should be reported to a registrar of births and deaths. Originally this had to be the registrar for the sub-district in which the death took place or, where a dead body was found and no information as to the place of death was available, for the sub-district in which the dead body was

---

[124] See 5–24 above.
[125] Prison Rules 1999 r.22(2).
[126] Detention Centre Rules 2001 r.36.
[127] Young Offender Institution Rules 2000 r.29(2).
[128] Service Custody and Service of Relevant Sentences Rules 2009 r.39(1)(a).
[129] Children's Homes Regulations 2001 reg.30, Sch.5; Children's Homes (Wales) Regulations 2002 reg.29 Sch.5.
[130] Mental Health Act 1959 ss.1, 149(2) and Sch.8 Pt I, repealing provisions for reporting and notifying such deaths to coroners. This followed the recommendation of the Report of the Royal Commission on the Law relating to Mental Illness and Mental Deficiency (1957 Cmnd. 169, para.169). The 1959 Act has been substantially replaced by the Mental Health Act 1983.
[131] At 12–09.
[132] See 5–85, where "deprivation of liberty" orders are also considered.

found.[133] But the report can now be made to any registrar in England and Wales.[134] The primary purpose of such report is to enable registration of the death to take place.[135]

Death in a house

Under the current law,[136] where a person dies in England and Wales in a house, it **5–54** is the duty of a "qualified informant" to give to the registrar, within five days[137] from the date of the death, information to the best of his knowledge and belief of the particulars required to be registered concerning the death, and in the presence of the registrar to sign the register.[138] For these purposes, each of the following persons is a "qualified informant":

(a) any relative of the deceased person present at the death or in attendance during his last illness;

(b) any other relative of the deceased residing or being in the sub-district where the death occurred;

(c) any person present at the death;

(d) the occupier of the house if he knew of the happening of the death;

(e) any inmate of the house who knew of the happening of the death;

(f) the person causing the disposal of the body.[139]

The duty falls first on the nearest relative in category (a). If there is none in **5–55** category (a), then on all those in category (b). If there is none in category (a) or (b), then on all those in categories (c) or (d). If there is none in category (a), (b), (c) or (d), then on all those in categories (e) or (f).[140]

Death elsewhere than in a house

Where a person dies elsewhere in England and Wales than in a house, or a body **5–56** is found and no information is available as to the place of death, a similar duty is imposed, with similar time limits,[141] upon the following persons, who are "qualified informants" for this purpose:

---

[133] Births and Deaths Registration Act 1953 ss.15, 16(3), 17(3) and 41. For reports where death takes place out of England and Wales, see 5–59 below.

[134] Births and Deaths Registration Act 1953 s.23A; Registration of Births and Deaths Regulations 1987 reg.42A (added by SI 1997/844 reg.3).

[135] Births and Deaths Registration Act 1953 s.15. For registration of deaths taking place out of England and Wales, see 5–59 below.

[136] It will change when the new provisions on medical examiners are brought into force: see Ch.3.

[137] Births and Deaths Registration Act 1953 s.18, extends the period to 14 days in cases where within five days of the death a qualified informant has sent written notice of the death together with a notice of the signing of a medical certificate of the cause of death under s.22(2) of the Act.

[138] Births and Deaths Registration Act 1953 s.16(3).

[139] Births and Deaths Registration Act 1953 s.16(2).

[140] Births and Deaths Registration Act 1953 s.16(3).

[141] Births and Deaths Registration Act 1953 ss.17(3), 18.

(a)　any relative of the deceased who has knowledge of any of the particulars required to be registered concerning the death;

(b)　any person present at the death;

(c)　any person finding or taking charge of the body;

(d)　any person causing the disposal of the body.[142]

Failure to supply required information

5–57　In case of failure to supply the required information, the registrar has power to require the attendance of a qualified informant at the registrar's office (or some other place appointed by the registrar within his sub-district) to give the necessary information and to sign the Register.[143] Failure to supply information (where that information is not otherwise given), failure to comply with a requirement of the registrar, and wilful refusal to answer questions put by the registrar are all criminal offences.[144]

OTHER REPORTS

5–58　In addition to the general duty to report deaths to the registrar of births and deaths,[145] there are special regulations dealing with deaths in ships, hovercraft and aircraft registered in the United Kingdom and deaths of persons employed in UK-registered ships, deaths in ships not registered in the United Kingdom which thereafter (but during the same voyage) call at ports in the United Kingdom, deaths of persons on or in circumstances connected with an offshore installation within the UK jurisdiction, deaths occurring outside the United Kingdom amongst members of or civilians employed in the armed forces of the Crown and their families, and deaths on board HM ships or aircraft.[146] It is true that a ship in harbour in England and Wales,[147] a ship in internal waters[148] or an aircraft overflying a coroner's district,[149] may all be within the jurisdiction of a senior coroner, but for the most part, compliance with these regulations is unlikely to lead to a coronial investigation in this country, and accordingly is not further considered from a jurisdictional point of view.

5–59　　However, compliance with these and other regulations may lead, contrary to the normal rule,[150] to registration of a death which took place out of England and

---

[142] Births and Deaths Registration Act 1953 s.17(2).

[143] Births and Deaths Registration Act 1953 s.19.

[144] Births and Deaths Registration Act 1953 s.36(a), (e).

[145] See 5–53.

[146] The Civil Aviation (Births, Deaths and Missing Persons) Regulations 1948 (SI 1948/1411) (civil aircraft); the Service Departments Registers Order 1959 (SI 1959/406) (HM forces, ships and aircraft); the Hovercraft (Births, Deaths and Missing Persons) Regulations 1972 (SI 1972/1513) (hovercraft); the Offshore Installations (Logbooks and Registration of Death) Regulations 1972 (SI 1972/1542) (offshore installations); the Merchant Shipping (Returns of Births and Deaths) Regulations 1979 (SI 1979/1577) (merchant ships). See Home Office Circular No. 42 of 1982.

[147] See 4–04.

[148] See 4–08.

[149] See 4–11.

[150] For which see 5–53.

Wales. In addition to the cases already mentioned, provision is made for the registration of deaths occurring abroad and originally registered by the British Consul or High Commission in the country of death.[151] This is a system of voluntary death registration, and deaths registered under it do not attract the same consequences[152] as deaths where registration is compulsory (i.e. those in England and Wales). But it does mean that the need for an official certificate of death (e.g. for insurance purposes) can be satisfied in some cases.[153]

Finally, there is an example of an obligation on *the coroner* to report a death he   **5–60** is aware of to someone else. Where a coroner decides to conduct an investigation into a death or directs that a post-mortem examination should be made, and the coroner believes that the deceased was under the age of 18 years, the coroner must notify the appropriate Local Safeguarding Children Board within three days of making the decision or direction.[154] This involves providing all information relating to the death of the person who was or may have been under the age of 18 years at the time of death and held by him for the purposes of his investigation.[155]

CORONER'S ENQUIRIES

Where a coroner is informed, by whatever means, of the presence of a dead body   **5–61** within his area, he has the right to possession, and must consider the circumstances.[156] As already stated, the duty to conduct an investigation arises where he has reason to suspect that certain criteria are satisfied.[157] In considering all the relevant material, the coroner is not limited to *admissible* evidence.[158] Moreover, since 25 July 2013, the coroner may make whatever enquiries seem necessary in order to decide whether the duty to conduct an investigation arises, creating a kind of preliminary stage inquiry.[159] As will be seen, this can involve the exercise of various coronial powers.[160]

Once the coroner has reason to suspect that the criteria are satisfied, the coroner   **5–62** is under a duty to conduct an investigation,[161] which may lead to an inquest in due

---

[151] Registration (Entries of Overseas Births and Deaths) Order 1982 (SI 1982/1526).

[152] See, e.g. 5–91, 18–13 below.

[153] See Home Office Circular No. 42 of 1982, which also suggests that a death certificate is needed for probate purposes. In fact, English law does not require the production of a death certificate for the grant of probate, as the applicant swears to the death, and normally the Probate Registry will seal the grant on that basis alone.

[154] Coroners (Investigation) Regulations 2013 reg.24(1).

[155] Coroners (Investigation) Regulations 2013 reg.24(2), (3).

[156] See 8–11. In 2013, 227,984 deaths were reported to coroners, about 45 per cent of the number of deaths registered that year (this proportion had been steadily rising for many years, from about 12 per cent in the 1920s, although in recent years it has flattened or even dipped slightly).

[157] See 5–01.

[158] *R. v South London Coroner Ex p. Weeks* Unreported December 6, 1996, Scott Baker J, referring to *Hussien v Chung Fook Kam* [1970] A.C. 942 at 949B; *R. (Canning) v Northampton Coroner* [2006] EWCA Civ. 1225; see also *R. (Gracey) v Cheshire Coroner* [2008] EWHC 957 (Admin).

[159] Coroners and Justice Act 2009 s.1(7)(a); *Chief Coroner's Guide to the Coroners and Justice Act 2009*, para.55.

[160] See Ch.8.

[161] Coroners and Justice Act 2009 s.1(1); formerly Coroners Act 1988 s.8(1). This assumes that an inquest has not already been held: see 18–01—18–09 below on the concept of *functus officio*.

course,[162] and the next of kin or personal representative of the deceased may require the claimant to provide an interim certificate of the fact of death.[163] However, his duty can be discharged in some cases,[164] and, indeed, in a few exceptional cases he may be prohibited from investigating at all.[165]

5–63   It is apparent from this that, if there is no reason to suspect that the person has died in circumstances satisfying the statutory criteria, the coroner has no jurisdiction and therefore neither power nor duty to interfere. It would be intolerable if the coroner had power to intrude without adequate cause upon the privacy of a family in distress and to interfere with their arrangements for a funeral.[166] Nor can the coroner acquire jurisdiction to conduct an investigation by consent,[167] or by undertaking to someone to do so.[168]

Preliminary inquiry by coroner's officer

5–64   The normal practice is for the coroner's officer to make a preliminary inquiry, especially in cases of possible unnatural deaths, to see if there are grounds for suggesting that the coroner has jurisdiction, and he will report his findings to the coroner. The coroner has various powers to obtain information compulsorily from others,[169] although in practice (and certainly at the outset, in dealing with the emergency services, hospital staff, GPs and relatives) he and his officers usually have little difficulty in obtaining the relevant information voluntarily, without the need to resort to compulsion. Where an unidentified body is the subject of the inquiry, medical evidence may assist in establishing identity.[170] In addition, the charity Missing People (formerly the National Missing Persons Helpline) may be of assistance.[171]

Exercise of coronial powers

5–65   The coroner may then, as a result of the preliminary inquiries, exercise various powers. First of all, he may order an exhumation to be carried out.[172] Second, he may direct the removal of the body to a suitable place.[173] Third, he may request that a post-mortem examination be made.[174] It must be borne in mind, however, that the coroner's jurisdiction is based on his having "reason to suspect" that the criteria are satisfied. Though there is an element of objectivity, it is not dependent solely on the actual results of his preliminary inquiries. Subject to the exceptional cases to be mentioned below,[175] it also exists if he honestly believes information

---

[162] See Chs 10, 11.
[163] Coroners (Investigations) Regulations 2013 (SI 2013/1629) reg.9; see 8–20, 10–12.
[164] See 4–22, 8–16, 8–36 below.
[165] See 5–98 ff below (visiting forces) and 5–190 ff below (state and diplomatic immunity).
[166] *R. v Price* (1884) 12 Q.B.D. 247 at 248, per Stephen J.
[167] *Re Aylmer Ex p. Bischoffheim* (1887) 20 QBD 258, 262; *R. v Social Services Secretary Ex p. Child Poverty Action Group* [1990] 2 QB 540, CA.
[168] *Connah v Plymouth Hospitals NHS Trust* [2010] EWHC 1727 (Admin).
[169] See 7–12 ff.
[170] See App.6.
[171] Tel: 020 8392 4590, Freefone 116 000; *http://www.missingpeople.org.uk* [Accessed June 5, 2014]; see Home Office Newsletter for Coroners No. 26 para.4.
[172] Coroners and Justice Act 2009 s.32, Sch 5 para.6(1), (2). See 8–03 ff.
[173] Coroners and Justice Act 2009 s.15(1)(b). See 2–135, 4–29, 8–11, 8–58.
[174] Coroners and Justice Act 2009 s.14(1)(b). See 8–39 ff.
[175] See 5–98—5–85.

which, if true, would give him jurisdiction.[176] The coroner may also seek information, or further information, from potential witnesses.[177] Unusual costs in exercising powers should be notified to the relevant authority, preferably before they are incurred.[178]

Bias, conflict of interest and similar problems

Although there may be no relevant legal disqualification,[179] there are cases in which **5–66** it would be improper for the coroner to act as such, and he should recuse himself. The coroner is a judicial officer, and should not act as such if he has some interest (personal or professional) which might (consciously or otherwise) influence his decision-making.[180] Thus, at common law, wherever there was a real danger of bias on the coroner's part, for example arising out of his personal or professional connection with the deceased or the deceased's family, he should make arrange-ments for another person to act in his place as coroner,[181] even if he himself believed that he was capable of acting impartially.[182] And if he had a pecuniary or proprietary interest in the matter, he must not act, even if there was no danger of bias.[183]

The common law test has been modified in the case of *litigation*, to comply with **5–67** art.6 of the European Convention on Human Rights. Now the court must first ascertain all the circumstances that had a bearing on the suggestion of bias, and then ask whether they would lead a fair-minded and informed observer to conclude that there was a real possibility that the tribunal was biased.[184] Strictly speaking, art.6 does not normally apply to decisions of the coroner's court, as typically they do not determine anyone's "civil rights and obligations".[185]

---

[176] *R. v Stephenson* (1884) 13 Q.B.D. 331; *Re Hull* (1882) 9 Q.B.D. 689.

[177] See 10–65.

[178] Coroners Allowances, Fees and Expenses Regulations 2013, SI 2013 No.1615 reg.7; see 18–40.

[179] See 2–36.

[180] See, e.g. *Halsbury's Laws of England*, 5th edn, Vol.61, paras 631–638. See also Stout, *Judicial Bias* [2011] JR 258; Sedley, "When should a judge not be a judge?" (2011) 23 *London Review of Books*, 9–12.

[181] *R. v Gough* [1984] A.C. 646, HL, followed in *R. v Inner West London Coroner Ex p. Perks* (1993) 157 J.P. 985, reversed on facts [1994] 4 All E.R. 139, CA; see also *R. v West Yorkshire Coroner, Eastern District Ex p. Smith, The Times,* November 6, 1982, QBD; *R. v South Yorkshire Coroner Ex p. Stringer* (1993) 158 J.P. 453, DC; *Matthews v Hunter* [1993] 2 N.Z.L.R. 683; *R. v East Sussex Coroner Ex p. Homberg* (1994) 158 J.P. 357, DC; *Re Sutherland* [1994] 2 N.Z.L.R. 242; cf. *R. v Wilson, The Times,* February 2, 1995, CA; *R. (Chaudhari) v Walthamstow Coroner's Court,* Unreported, March 26, 2002, Sedley LJ; *R. (Francis) v Southwark Coroner* [2012] EWHC 712 (Admin), permission to appeal refused [2013] EWCA Civ. 313. The question of possible bias is judged as at the time when the supervisory court considers the matter, and the facts to which the court has regard are all those in evidence of the date of the application to such court, above. For an example of the controversy that can arise, see *Re Jeremy Turner, The Independent,* January 9, 11, 1992.

[182] His successor should start all over again: cf. *R. v South London Coroner Ex p. Driscoll* (1993) 159 J.P. 45, DC.

[183] See also *R. v Bow Street Metropolitan Stipendiary Magistrate Ex p. Pinochet Ugarte (No. 2)* [2000] 1 A.C. 119, HL. The fact that the local authority which pays his salary is involved in the case does not disqualify the coroner: *R. v South Yorkshire Coroner Ex p. Stringer* (1993) 158 J.P. 453, DC.

[184] *Director General of Fair Trading v Proprietary Association of Great Britain, re Medicaments (No. 2)* [2001] 1 W.L.R. 700, CA; *Porter v Magill* [2002] 1 A.C. 357, HL; *Taylor v Lawrence* [2002] 3 W.L.R. 640, CA; cf. the test in Australia: *Johnson v Johnson* (2000) 74 A.L.J.R. 1380 at 1382; *Ebner v Official Trustee in Bankruptcy* (2000) 75 A.L.J.R. 277 at 283, 290, 294, 309–310.

[185] See 21–22 below.

Nevertheless, on a number of occasions the court has applied the modified test to a coroner's decisions or inquisitions.[186]

5–68   In one coroner's case,[187] the matter was put in this way:

"The fair-minded and informed observer is neither unduly sensitive nor suspicious yet he is not complacent. He is assumed to have taken the trouble to acquire knowledge of all relevant information before coming to a conclusion . . . [188] The fair-minded and informed observer is also expected to be aware of the law and the functions of those who play a part in its administration . . . [189] When applying the test, any Court will take account of an explanation given by the tribunal and assume that the hypothetical observer is also aware of that explanation."[190]

The court also indicated "that if there were real ground for doubt, the doubt should be resolved in favour of recusal".[191]

5–69   A coroner should raise with the interested persons at the first appropriate opportunity (e.g. a pre-inquest review) any matters which might be thought to indicate the possibility of bias, so that the interested persons may consider what, if anything, they wish to do.[192] An interested person who with knowledge of the relevant facts giving rise to an appearance of bias does not challenge a coroner's refusal to recuse himself before the inquest may be taken to have waived the objection.[193]

VIOLENT OR UNNATURAL DEATHS

Basic distinctions

5–70   The distinction between a violent or unnatural death and natural death is one of the most difficult to draw. The question will arise in the context of the coroner's deciding whether or not there is "reason to suspect that . . . the deceased died a

---

[186] *R. v East Riding and Kingston-upon-Hull Coroner Ex p. Dawson* [2001] EWHC Admin 352, [2001] A.C.D. 68, Jackson J; *R. (Pounder) v North and South Durham and Darlington Coroner (No. 2)* [2010] EWHC 328 (Admin); see also *Paul v Deputy Coroner of The Queen's Household* [2007] EWHC 408, *R. (Ahmed) v South and East Cumbria Coroner* [2009] EWHC 1653 (Admin), *Dowler v North London Coroner* [2009] EWHC 3300 (Admin), *Re Ramsbottom's Application* [2009] NIQB 55; *Re Donaldson's Application* [2010] NIQB 144; and *R. (Butler) v Black Country District Coroner* [2010] EWHC 43 (Admin).

[187] *R. (Pounder) v North and South Durham and Darlington Coroner (No. 2)* [2010] EWHC 328 (Admin) at [12].

[188] See *Helow v Secretary of State for the Home Department* [2008] 1 W.L.R. 2416 at [1]–[3].

[189] See *Lawal v Northern Spirit* [2003] UKHL 35 at [21]–[22].

[190] See *Director General of Fair Trading v Proprietary Association of Great Britain, re Medicaments (No. 2)* [2001] 1 W.L.R. 700, CA at [67].

[191] *R. (Pounder) v North and South Durham and Darlington Coroner (No. 2)* [2010] EWHC 328 (Admin) at [12], referring to *AWG Group v Morrison* [2006] EWCA (Civ) 6, [2006] 1 W.L.R. 1163 at [8]; see also *R. (Sreedharan) v Greater Manchester Coroner* [2013] EWCA Civ. 181 at [57]–[60].

[192] *R. (Shaw) v Leicester City and South Leicestershire ADC* [2013] EWHC 386 (Admin) at [102]–[105], affirmed [2014] EWCA Civ. 294.

[193] *R. (Shaw) v Leicester City and South Leicestershire ADC* [2013] EWHC 386 (Admin) at [62], [101], affirmed [2014] EWCA Civ. 294.

violent or unnatural death", and thus whether or not he has the duty to conduct an investigation,[194] and in some cases whether he has a duty to summon a jury.[195]

For present purposes the following generalisations can be made. A violent death **5–71** involves an injury of some sort. The most obvious example is that of a person deliberately killing himself or being deliberately killed by another, but if accidental occurrences such as a cut, a fall or a road accident cause death, that death too will be violent. Further, the concept of violent death also includes deaths from violence without human intervention, such as a person being struck by lightning or being killed by a wild animal.

There is no legal definition of what constitutes an unnatural death.[196] However, **5–72** from early statutes and writers it appears to have been one where there was some suspicion of foul play or other wrongdoing.[197] Hale, for example, contrasted "unnatural or violent death" with death through "fever or apoplexy or other visitation of God".[198] Thus it has been said that, "no doubt the main object of all such inquiries is to ascertain whether the death has been caused by any violence or criminal act",[199] and that there must be "a reasonable suspicion that there may have been something peculiar in the death; that it may have been due to other causes than common illness".[200] However, recently it has been made clear that at this stage there is no need to demonstrate a causative link between the wrongdoing and the death.[201]

Where death is due to an event which is itself a response to an underlying cause, **5–73** that underlying cause must be considered. If it is not in itself unnatural, for example a cancer, or a heart condition, and the response was a natural consequence of the disease (e.g. the usual and appropriate treatment, properly administered), the fact that a recognised complication of the response led to death does not make the death unnatural. So care is necessary, for example, in considering deaths of individuals within a few weeks of chemotherapy for malignant disease.[202] The treatment may have simply failed to prevent the death, or it may have contributed to it. It will often be necessary to examine the propriety of the treatment administered.

However, it is now clear that unnatural death is wider than death from unnatural **5–74** causes.[203] Thus, where neglect[204] is a cause or contributory cause of a death whose underlying cause is otherwise natural, that is an unnatural death for this purpose.[205] Moreover, the same is true "whenever a wholly unexpected death, albeit from

---

[194] See 5–01 above.
[195] See 10–34.
[196] See Pilling (1967) 7 Med. Sci. & Law 59.
[197] See, e.g. the statute *De Officio Coronatoris*, 4 Edw. 1, stat. 2; 1 East P.C. 382.
[198] 2 Hale P.C. 57.
[199] *Re Hull* (1882) 9 Q.B.D. 689 at 700.
[200] *R. v Price* (1884) 12 Q.B.D. 247 at 248; *R. v Stephenson* (1884) 13 Q.B.D. 331 at 337.
[201] *Bicknell v Birmingham and Solihull Coroner* [2007] EWHC 2547 (Admin).
[202] See NCEPOD Report, "For Better, For Worse": *http://www.ncepod.org.uk/2008sact.htm*.
[203] See App.5.
[204] Formerly "lack of care"; see 13–83 ff below.
[205] *R. v Poplar Coroner Ex p. Thomas* [1993] Q.B. 610; *R. v Avon Coroner Ex p. Smith* (1998) 162 J.P. 403; *R. (Touche) v Inner North London Coroner* [2001] Q.B. 1206, CA; *R. (Canning) v Northampton Coroner* [2006] EWCA Civ. 1225.

natural causes, results from some culpable human failure".[206] So a culpable failure to prevent death from natural causes is an unnatural death; but a non-culpable failure to do so is not.[207] Medical treatment for a non-potentially fatal condition but which causes death will continue to be unnatural,[208] but appropriate medical treatment for an otherwise fatal condition resulting in recognised complications leading to death is not. Again, death from natural disease transmitted unnaturally (e.g. deliberately[209] or by reason of work)[210] is unnatural.

Death in the elderly

5–75　　Particular difficulty may be encountered in dealing with reported deaths of elderly persons. As people age, they may develop diseases that impact on daily life, resulting in cardiovascular insufficiency, and rendering them liable to sudden collapse and therefore injury. Again, old bones may become osteoporotic, rendering them liable to break with the most trivial of injury in carrying out normal activities. The ageing brain shrinks, and vigorous head movements may lead to the tearing of small veins between the skull and the surface of the brain, leading to the development of subdural haematomas. The overweight are liable to suffer diabetes and its complications, cardiac, renal, visual and arteriosclerotic. Dementia may lead to loss of the swallowing reflex, making a choking fit more likely. Many elderly people have several co-morbidities.

5–76　　An elderly person who suffers a long bone fracture is at much greater risk of death than a younger person, whether from heart failure following blood loss from the fracture, or from pneumonia as a result of immobility following treatment. People who have suffered neurological illness (e.g. stroke) may become bedbound and immobile, rendering them more liable than the young to the development of pressure sores, which may lead to fatal sepsis.

5–77　　Where such a person dies, the coroner will have to consider carefully whether the death was "violent or unnatural", or whether it was a natural consequence of the (natural) disease process(es) suffered by the individual. If there is the suspicion of violence contributing, whether as the result of a (non-natural) accident or of the acts of a third party, the coroner must investigate. But if there is no reason so to suspect, and the death can be explained as the natural consequence of natural disease, then there is no duty to investigate.

5–78　　Ultimately, however, "unnatural" is an ordinary word of the English language which should be given its ordinary meaning.[211] Thus:

> "it is for the tribunal which decides the case to consider, not as law but as fact, whether in the whole circumstances the words of the statute do or do not as a matter of ordinary usage of the English language cover or apply to the facts

---

[206] *R. (Touche) v Inner North London Coroner* [2001] Q.B. 1206 at [43]; *R. (Canning) v Northampton Coroner* [2006] EWCA Civ. 1225.

[207] cf. *R. v Birmingham and Solihull Coroner Ex p. Benton* (1997) 162 J.P. 807, 8 Med LR 362.

[208] *R. v Birmingham and Solihull Coroner Ex p. Benton* (1997) 162 J.P. 807, 8 Med LR 362.

[209] cf. *R. v Clarence* (1888) 22 Q.B.D. 23, CCR (knowingly infecting wife with gonorrhoea not an assault).

[210] *R. v Poplar Coroner Ex p. Thomas* [1993] Q.B. 610, 627, CA; *Terry v East Sussex Coroner* [2002] Q.B. 312, CA, at [1]. See 13–44 below.

[211] *R. v Poplar Coroner Ex p. Thomas* [1993] Q.B. 610, CA.

which have been proved. If it is alleged that the tribunal has reached a wrong decision then there can be a question of law but only of a limited character. The question would normally be whether their decision was unreasonable in the sense that no tribunal acquainted with the ordinary use of language could possibly reach that decision."[212]

Accordingly, the view taken by a coroner as to whether a particular death is "unnatural" will not be interfered with by the courts, unless the decision was *Wednesbury* unreasonable.[213] **5–79**

DEATH OF WHICH THE CAUSE IS UNKNOWN

From a legal point of view, under the law in force up to July 25, 2013 a death **5–80** would not fall within this category unless it was a *sudden* death of unknown cause. In 2013 the law was changed so that the requirement that death must have been "sudden" (the meaning of which was in any event obscure)[214] was removed. But the requirement that the cause be unknown remains. For this purpose, the cause of death is unknown if (not being a violent or unnatural death) it is not positively known to be natural,[215] or if the death cannot be certified by a doctor.[216] This may be because the terminal cause of death is not known, or because the terminal cause of death is known, but not the underlying condition which is the real cause of death.

Even where there *are* medical opinions, such as where there is a dispute between **5–81** doctors with rival views, or a clinician offers a view which the family does not accept, the cause of death can in appropriate cases still be "unknown" to the coroner. His view that it is unknown can only be attacked on ordinary judicial review principles.[217]

A coroner responsible for conducting an investigation may request a post- **5–82** mortem examination of the body.[218] If this reveals the cause of death before the coroner begins holding an inquest into the death,[219] and the coroner thinks it unnecessary to continue the investigation, he must discontinue the investigation,[220] unless he has reason to suspect that the deceased died a violent or unnatural death or died in custody or otherwise in state detention.[221] So where the coroner's duty to conduct an investigation arises only from having reason to suspect that the person has died from an unknown cause, the coroner will usually request that a

---

[212] *Brutus v Cozens* [1973] A.C. 854, per Lord Reid.
[213] *R. v Poplar Coroner Ex p. Thomas* [1993] Q.B. 610, CA; see also *R. v East Sussex Coroner Ex p. Healy* [1988] 1 W.L.R. 1194, DC, and *R. v East Sussex Coroner Ex p. Homburg* (1994) 158 J.P. 57, and *R. v Birmingham and Solihull Coroner Ex p. Benton* (1997) 162 J.P. 807; *R. (Canning) v Northampton Coroner* [2006] EWCA Civ. 1225..
[214] *R. (Kasperowicz) v Plymouth Coroner* [2005] EWCA Civ. 44.
[215] *R. v Greater Manchester Coroner Ex p. Worch* [1988] QB 513, CA.
[216] *R. (Kasperowicz) v Plymouth Coroner* [2005] EWCA Civ. 44.
[217] See 19–25.
[218] Coroners and Justice Act 2009 s.14; see 8–39 ff.
[219] As to which see 10–05 ff.
[220] Coroners and Justice Act 2009 s.4(1); formerly Coroners Act 1988 s.19(1), (4); See 8–36.
[221] Coroners and Justice Act 2009 s.4(2).

post-mortem examination be carried out, and (assuming that it shows a natural death) will then be able to discontinue the investigation.[222]

DEATH IN CUSTODY OR STATE DETENTION

5–83 Formerly it was the coroner's duty is to hold an inquest if he had reasonable cause to suspect that the body within his district was that of a person who had died "in prison".[223] It represented a statutory recognition that, because of the nature of prison institutions, there was a special need for an independent investigation into deaths which occurred within their walls.[224]However, as "prison" was not defined, it was not clear whether it should bear the same narrow meaning as it did in the prison legislation,[225] or a more general interpretation as "a place where a person is restrained of his liberty",[226] or "in prison custody".[227] But express provision was made for coroners to hold inquests into the deaths of members of the armed forces dying in detention barracks or detention quarters,[228] suggesting that "prison" did not include a detention centre, youth custody centre, or community home, and neither would the duty to hold an inquest arise in the case of the death of a person detained under the provisions of the Mental Health Act 1983,[229] or in police custody or at a police station.[230]

5–84 In 1969, the Home Office nevertheless recommended that coroners should hold an inquest on the death of any person in any kind of legal custody,[231] and even though the person concerned actually died in hospital after having been held in such custody.[232] Although it was never tested, art.2 of the European Convention on Human Rights and the enactment of the Human Rights Act 1998 might have

---

[222] See 8–36 below.
[223] Coroners Act 1988 s.8(1)(c). See generally, Creighton and King, *Prisoners and the Law*, 2nd edn (2000), paras 10.105–10.167.
[224] *Re Rapier, deceased* [1988] Q.B. 26, DC; *R. v Southwark Coroner Ex p. Hicks* [1987] 1 W.L.R. 1624, DC; *R. v North Humberside Coroner Ex p. Jamison* [1995] Q.B. 1, CA.
[225] See the Prison Act 1952 ss.1, 53(1); *Nicoll v Catron* (1985) 149 J.P. 424, DC; *R. v Moss and Harte* (1986) 149 J.P. 26, CA.
[226] *Hobert and Stroud's Case* (1630) Cro. Cas. 210.
[227] See Thurston, *Coronership*, 3rd edn (1985) para.15–04, and *R. v Greater Manchester Coroner Ex p. Worch* [1988] Q.B. 513, CA.
[228] Army Act 1955 s.128(2); Air Force Act 1955 s.128(2); Naval Detention Quarters Rules 1973 r.93.
[229] cf. *R. (Wilson) v Northamptonshire Coroner*, decision on papers, July 24, 2002 (death of person detained under Mental Health Act was not death in prison or police custody so as to attract *jury requirement* under s.8(3)); renewed application withdrawn. See also *R (Antoniou) v Central & NW London NHS Foundation Trust* [2013] EWHC 3055 (Admin) (suicide of detained patient).
[230] cf. *Nicoll v Catron* (1985) 149 J.P. 424, DC. Indeed, in the case of death in the police station there was not even a specific duty to report the death to the coroner at all, although in 1980 the then Home Secretary thought that all deaths in custody *should* be reported to the coroner: House of Commons Official Report, November 11, 1980, col. 151. In practice the death was likely to be such as would be reported to him anyway.
[231] See also *R. v North Humberside Coroner Ex p. Jamieson* [1995] Q.B. 1 at 26C.
[232] Home Office Circular No. 35 of 1969. cf. *R. v Inner North London Coroner Ex p. Linnane* [1989] 1 W.L.R. 395, DC.

compelled a different reading of the statute since 2001, taking the wider view.[233] There was also a question as to whether the criteria were apt to cover the death of a non-prisoner (such as a prison officer or visitor) who happened to be in a prison at the time of death.[234] Certainly they were applied to cases going wider than the convicted prisoner serving his sentence in the prison where he died.[235]

But the old law has now gone. Since 2013 the criterion is whether the coroner **5–85** has reason to suspect that the deceased died while in custody or otherwise in state detention. A person is in state detention if he or she is compulsorily detained by a "public authority" within the meaning of the Human Rights Act 1998.[236] This will cover deaths of those compulsorily detained in prison, police stations, service detention, mental hospitals, and immigration detention centres, amongst others. It will not however cover those who, not being in custody or state detention, happen to die in any of those places. Nor will it cover the deaths of persons merely by reason that they die whilst subject to a "deprivation of liberty" order,[237] both because for this purpose "deprivation of liberty" extends more widely than cases of ordinary physical detention, to cases where the person lives in relative normality but has never sought to leave, or complained of being restrained, but would be restrained if he or she sought to do so,[238] and because the person authorised to detain the deceased may have been a private individual or company, rather than an organ or agent of the state, or other "public authority".[239]

Custody or state detention abroad

A question that was never decided under the old law was whether "prison" **5–86** included prisons outside England and Wales.[240] A similar question remains open today. Although the statute applies only in England and Wales,[241] it is presence of the body at the time of being made aware of it that gives the coroner jurisdiction, and not the place where the other statutory criteria (e.g. violent or unnatural death, death in custody or otherwise in state detention) have been satisfied.[242] It is

---

[233] See 21–05 below. cf. *R. (Wilson) v Northamptonshire Coroner*, decision on papers, July 24, 2002 (death of person detained under Mental Health Act was not death in prison or police custody so as to attract jury requirement under s.8(3)); renewed application withdrawn.

[234] *R. v Graham* (1905) 93 L.T. 371 at 374: "It is for the general protection of those who would not have protection unless there be an inquest" (per Lord Alverstone CJ). The Prison Act 1865 s.48, expressly limited the duty to hold an inquest to the case of *prisoners* dying in prison, but this provision was not repealed until 1893, and so subsisted for six years concurrently with the apparently more general obligation in the Coroners Act 1887 s.3(1) (later s.8(1) of the 1988 Act).

[235] See *R. v Surrey Coroner Ex p. Campbell* [1982] Q.B. 661, DC (unconvicted prisoner on remand); *R. v Southwark Coroner Ex p. Hicks* [1987] 1 W.L.R. 1624 at 1627, DC (convicted prisoner, sentenced to hospital order, awaiting transfer to mental hospital).

[236] Coroners and Justice Act 2009 s.48(2), referring (in part) to Human Rights Act 1998 s.6, subs.(2) of which provides that "public authority" includes "(a) a court or tribunal, and (b) any person certain of whose functions are functions of a public nature". On para.(b), see *YL v Birmingham City Council* [2008] 1 A.C. 95, HL (by a majority, a private care home was not carrying on "functions of a public nature", and therefore not a "public authority" in this sense).

[237] Mental Capacity Act 2005 ss.4A, 4B.

[238] *P v Cheshire West and Chester Council* [2014] UKSC 19 [48]–[50]. See also *RB v Brighton & Hove C.C.* [2014] EWCA Civ 561.

[239] See in particular *YL v Birmingham City Council* [2008] 1 A.C. 95, HL, and fn.238 above.

[240] Though cf. a dictum of Staughton LJ in *Re Neal* (1995) 37 B.M.L.R. 164, DC.

[241] Coroners and Justice Act 2009 s.181(1); formerly Coroners Act 1988 s.37(3).

[242] See 5–87 below.

therefore submitted that the criteria include custody and other state detention in Scotland, Northern Ireland, and indeed any other country.[243]

Deaths Outside England and Wales

Historical requirements

5–87   The primary requirement for jurisdiction has always been the presence of the body. Initially this was because no inquest could be held without a view of the body in the coroner's own jurisdiction:[244] the inquest was *super visum corporis*. The requirement for a view has long been abolished,[245] though the requirement of presence of the body in the coroner's area (with some exceptions)[246] still remains.[247] But originally a coroner had no jurisdiction to inquire into the death of a person unless, further, both the cause of death and the death itself also took place in his area.[248] In criminal cases, statutes of 1548[249] and 1728[250] extended the coroner's jurisdiction to cases where *either* the cause of death *or* the death itself took place in his area. However, neither statute had any effect in cases of accidental (non-criminal) death, where the old common law rules continued to apply.[251] Thus, if in such a case the cause of death took place in one area and the death itself in another, no coroner could have jurisdiction.

5–88   Accordingly, it was provided by the Coroners Act 1843[252] that:

> "The Coroner only within whose jurisdiction the body of a person upon whose death an inquest ought to be holden shall be lying dead shall hold the inquest, notwithstanding that the cause of death did not arise within the jurisdiction of such Coroner."[253]

This provision was considered to confer jurisdiction upon the coroner in whose area the body lay, not only where death took place in his area, but also in cases where death took place outside his area, and the only factor connecting the case with the coroner was the presence of the body.[254]

---

[243] cf. the Home Office view on the benevolent exercise of discretion to hold an inquest, 5–84.

[244] *R. v Hinde* (1844) 5 Q.B. 944; 113 E.R. 1504.

[245] Coroners Act 1980 s.1.

[246] See 5–16 ff above.

[247] Coroners and Justice Act 2009 s.1(1); formerly Coroners Act 1988 s.8(1).

[248] 2 Hale P.C. 66; Umfreville, *Lex Coronatoria*, Ch.15, paras 15–16; *R. v Great Western Railway Co* (1842) 3 Q.B. 333, 114 E.R. 533. Contrast the position in criminal law, where by the Offences against the Person Act 1861 s.9, murder or manslaughter committed abroad *by a British subject* (and whoever the victim) is within the jurisdiction of the English courts.

[249] Criminal Law Act 1548.

[250] Murder Act 1728.

[251] *R. v Great Western Railway Co* (1842) 3 Q.B. 333, 114 E.R. 533 (death within area, cause of death outside area: held, no jurisdiction).

[252] 6 & 7 Vict., c. 12.

[253] Section 1, later consolidated into the Coroners Act 1887 as s.7(1).

[254] *R. v Hinde* (1844) 5 Q.B. 944; 113 E.R. 1504, at 948, 1506, per Lord Denman CJ.

Discretion or duty where death occurred outside area

In the years up to 1982, coroners held many inquests where both cause of death **5-89** arose and death itself took place outside England and Wales.[255] These were, however, treated by both writers and coroners alike as a matter of *discretion* for the coroner as to whether to hold an inquest, and not as a matter of duty.[256] The question whether the coroner had a discretion or a duty to hold an inquest arose in an acute form in 1982, in a case where a British subject died a violent death abroad, and the body was brought back to England. The coroner in whose area the body lay declined to act, not in the purported exercise of discretion, but upon the ground of absence of all jurisdiction. On an application for judicial review of the coroner's decision, the majority of the Court of Appeal (reversing the Queen's Bench Divisional Court)[257] held that the coroner had not only power but indeed a *duty* to hold an inquest, because the body was in his area, even though both cause of death and death itself had happened outside England and Wales.[258] The 2013 reforms do not affect this position. Indeed, they confirm it.[259]

The coroner is therefore generally obliged to treat bodies lying in his area of **5-90** persons who die outside England and Wales[260] in the same way as those who die there. This mean conducting investigations and holding inquests into their deaths when the jurisdictional conditions (including that the coroner is made aware of the death)[261] are satisfied,[262] and not doing so when they are not.

There are however two matters to note. The first is that the provisions of the **5-91** Human Rights Act 1998 and the European Convention on Human Rights may not always apply to such deaths, because of the territorial scope of those instruments.[263] This may affect the *scope* of such investigations.[264] The second is that, as the deaths of persons dying outside England and Wales are not *required* to be registered in England and Wales,[265] the coroner has never had any obligation to send certain certificates to the registrar after he has dealt with the case.[266]

Acquisition of relevant extra-jurisdictional evidence

When the coroner is obliged to inquire into a death which has already been subject **5-92** to an inquiry or inquest outside England and Wales, his task may be made easier

---

[255] See *R. v West Yorkshire Coroner Ex p. Smith* [1983] Q.B. 335 at 341, DC.

[256] See the 9th edition of this work (1957), p.69; *Halsbury's Laws of England*, 4th edn, Vol.9 (original), para.1013; Thurston, *Coronership*, 3rd edn (1985) p. 39.

[257] *R. v West Yorkshire Coroner Ex p. Smith* [1983] Q.B. 335.

[258] [1983] Q.B. 335.

[259] See , e.g. Coroners and Justice Act 2009 ss.12, 13.

[260] i.e. including elsewhere in the United Kingdom: see 18–02—18–04 below.

[261] See 5–01. So if death occurs in Scotland or Northern Ireland, and a cremation certificate is issued there valid for England and Wales, it will be unnecessary to inform the relevant coroner in England and Wales, and therefore such coroner will never acquire jurisdiction.

[262] See , e.g. *R. (Sutovic) v North London Coroner* [2006] EWHC 1095 (Admin); in Northern Ireland, cf. *Re Forde's Application* [2008] NIQB 40 (where the law is slightly different). As to the appropriate conclusions to reach where criminal acts abroad are involved, see 13–56.

[263] *R. (Al Skeini) v Secretary of State for Defence* [2008] A.C. 153; *R. (Gentle) v Prime Minister* [2008] A.C. 1356; *R. (Smith) v Secretary of State for Defence* [2011] 1 AC 1; *Al-Skeini v UK* (2011) 53 EHRR 18; *Smith v Ministry of Defence* [2014] AC 52. See 21–12.

[264] See Ch.6.

[265] Although there are provisions *enabling* registration in some cases: see 5–59 above.

[266] See 18–11 below.

by obtaining reports or documents prepared in connection with that earlier inquiry or inquest. Coroners in Northern Ireland are usually happy to assist their counterparts in England and Wales.[267] The Home Office was apparently willing to approach the Scottish Crown Office for copies of the informal investigation by the Procurator Fiscal in case of a death which has occurred in Scotland,[268] and coroners may be able to secure documentary evidence relating to inquiries or inquests held in other countries.[269]

5–93   Where the deceased was a serviceman, his commanding officer will usually send to the coroner certain certificates and other useful information, including information about any service investigation that may be being or may have been held.[270] Calling witnesses from abroad to give evidence,[271] if they are willing to attend, will be very costly, and may sometimes (e.g. where United Kingdom servicemen are involved) interfere substantially with work and other matters in the foreign country. There are provisions for the admission of documentary evidence (in the form of statements or otherwise)[272] and it is submitted that this would be a suitable case for their use, in a case where the evidence is not disputed.[273]

5–94   An additional method for the coroner to seek evidence from abroad is to *ask* the judicial authorities of the relevant state to provide it in accordance with their own rules. This is done by way of a formal "letter of request". It is clear that the High Court has an inherent jurisdiction to issue a letter of request for evidence including—or even consisting solely of—the production of documents.[274] But the notion of inherent jurisdiction applies to inferior courts, such as the county court,[275] so there is no reason for it not to apply to the coroner's court.[276] Essentially the coroner, as a judicial officer in England and Wales, in the exercise of his inherent jurisdiction,[277] makes a request to the foreign court asking it to obtain and transmit to him the evidence required.[278]

5–95   Of course, unless the foreign court is bound by some treaty or convention obligation (and there is none for coroners' courts) the foreign court need not respond to the letter, positively or otherwise. But the comity of nations is a

---

[267] On the Northern Irish law, see Leckey and Greer, *Coroners' Law and Practice in Northern Ireland* (1998).

[268] Home Office Circular No. 79 of 1983, para.6. Now it would fall to the Ministry of Justice. On the relevant Scottish law, see generally, Carmichael, *Sudden Deaths and Fatal Accidents Enquiries,* 2nd edn (1993).

[269] The coroner should approach the Consular Division, Foreign and Commonwealth Office, G/99, Old Admiralty Building, London, SW1A 2PA (Tel: 020 7008 0216; Fax: 020 7008 0160): Home Office Newsletter for Coroners, No. 25, para.11 (August 22, 2002).

[270] Home Office Circular No. 16 of 1988. Service investigations are held under the Armed Forces (Service Inquiries) Regulations 2008, SI 2008 No.1651.

[271] See 10–25 ff below.

[272] See 12–30ff below.

[273] See also Home Office Circular No. 79 of 1983, para.10. If the evidence is disputed, it may not be possible to admit it (see 12–32), and the coroner is often left with virtually nothing with which to hold the inquest: cf. *R. v Coroner of the Royal Household Ex p. Al Fayed*, unreported, July 18, 2000, Newman J.

[274] *Panayiotou v Sony Music Entertainment (UK) Ltd* [1994] Ch. 142.

[275] *Langley v North West Water Authority* [1991] 1 W.L.R. 697, CA.

[276] See *R. v North Humberside Coroner Ex p. Jamieson* [1995] Q.B. 1, CA, holding that the coroner is the master of his own procedure.

[277] As to which see *Connelly v DPP* [1964] A.C. 1264 at 1301 per Lord Morris.

[278] See examples in App.3.

powerful, if sometimes rather slow, catalyst. It is important to ensure that all the usual, very formal, diplomatic language is used in the letter of request, and to have it properly translated into the official language of the court. Moreover, if this route is used, it is highly desirable that the Foreign and Commonwealth Office should be kept informed.[279]

Where a body arrives in England and Wales, the question arises as to which   **5–96**
coroner should make any necessary enquiries. Strictly it seems that the coroner at the point of entry (once having been informed of the presence of the body) should act,[280] but, except in the case of multiple deaths in a single incident,[281] it seems to be the practice for the coroner having jurisdiction at the place of intended burial or cremation to inquire,[282] and in the past the Home Office approved of this practice.[283]

If the first coroner to be informed of the presence of the body within his district   **5–97**
is that of the point of burial or cremation, then he will have original jurisdiction. Otherwise there must be a transfer of jurisdiction between the two.[284] If the jurisdictional conditions are not satisfied in respect of the body, the coroner has no jurisdiction to investigate, and cannot give any certificates in relation to the disposal of the body.[285]

DEATHS INVOLVING VISITING FORCES

Lord Chancellor's direction for investigation

If the coroner otherwise having jurisdiction to conduct an investigation into a   **5–98**
death is satisfied that the deceased person at the time of his death had a relevant association[286] with a visiting force,[287] the coroner cannot, without a direction from the Lord Chancellor, begin an investigation.[288] There is no requirement that a coroner inform the registrar of deaths of his being so satisfied, but the Registrar-General supplies a convenient form[289] for doing so. The prohibition does not

---

[279] Coroners should contact the coroners liaison officer, Emma Nicholson, at the Foreign and Commonwealth Office, King Charles Street, London, SW1A 2AH, tel. 020 7008 1500.

[280] See 5–61 above.

[281] See, e.g. *Re Canberra Aeroplane Crash, The Times*, November 24, 1984, Swindon coroner; *Re RAF Autobahn Crash, The Times*, August 17, 1985, Swindon coroner; *Re Gulf War Deaths, The Times*, May 15, 1992, Oxford coroner. See also Ch.17.

[282] See, e.g. *Re Paul Fleming, The Times*, November 2, 1983, North London coroner; *Re William Russell, The Times*, September 18–19, 1985, Western Cornwall coroner; *Re Christopher King, The Independent*, August 24, 1989, Southampton coroner; *Re Malcolm Olson, The Independent*, August 15, 1992, Mid-Hampshire coroner.

[283] Home Office Circular No. 79 of 1983, para.11.

[284] See 4–19 ff.

[285] See 9–21, 9–28.

[286] As to this term, see 5–104 ff below.

[287] As to this term, see 5–75 below.

[288] Visiting Forces Act 1952 s.7(1A).

[289] Form 90. Where such deaths are certified by a medical practitioner with the visiting forces, who is not registered with the General Medical Council, and the coroner conducts an investigation, the death is technically "legally uncertified" for registration purposes: Gastrell and others, "An analysis of legally uncertified deaths in England and Wales, 1979–2002" (2004) *Health Statistics Quarterly* 24.

extend to the coroner's preliminary inquiries designed to enable him to decide whether he has a duty to conduct an investigation, so if as part of such preliminary inquiries the coroner directs a post-mortem examination which shows a natural death, that will be the end of the matter.[290]

5–99 If an investigation into such a death has begun but not yet been completed, the coroner shall suspend it unless directed not to do so by the Lord Chancellor.[291] If an inquest is being held as part of such an investigation, the coroner must adjourn[292] the inquest and discharge the jury (if any).[293] Again there is no requirement that a coroner inform the registrar of deaths, but in practice coroners complete the usual certificate after inquest[294] as far as possible.[295] Suspension of an investigation under these provisions does not prevent its suspension under the provisions[296] so requiring because criminal proceedings have been or may be begun in respect of the death, and vice versa.[297]

5–100 In order that the Lord Chancellor may consider whether there are special circumstances justifying conducting an investigation into the death of such a person, the coroner should report the matter to the Lord Chancellor giving all available information, such as whether an inquiry is being held by the visiting force's own authorities, and including any reasons the coroner may have for thinking that an investigation would be of value.[298]

5–101 It is unlikely that the Lord Chancellor would issue a direction for conducting an investigation unless it appeared that the visiting force authorities were not proposing to hold an inquiry, or it appeared that the circumstances would prevent any such inquiry bringing to light the facts. Of course, where the visiting serviceman causes the death of someone who is not connected with a visiting force, and himself survives, these provisions do not apply.

What constitutes a visiting force

5–102 A visiting force for these purposes is any body, contingent or detachment of the forces of a country to which the visiting forces provisions apply who are at present in the United Kingdom[299] at the invitation of the UK government.[300] The visiting

---

[290] See 8–16. Registrars of deaths and the police will report deaths as usual to the coroner, and it is for the latter to decide whether the visiting forces provisions apply: Home Office Circular No. 54 of 1981, paras 7, 8.

[291] Visiting Forces Act 1952 s.7(1B).

[292] The adjournment should be without setting a date for resumption, that is, *sine die*: Home Office Circular No. 54 of 1981, para.9.

[293] Visiting Forces Act 1952 s.7(2A).

[294] Form 99 REV: see 18–11 below.

[295] Endorsing Pt 2 with words such as "Inquest adjourned under the Visiting Forces Act 1952, s. 7(2A), and not resumed".

[296] See 10–73 ff.

[297] Visiting Forces Act 1952 s.7(2B).

[298] cf. Home Office Circular No. 54 of 1981, para.2 (issued before the 2013 reforms). This may, of course, cause delay in the registration of the death, and the coroner should explain this to those involved: above, para.3.

[299] This includes UK territorial waters and any place on, under or above an installation in a designated area within the Continental Shelf Act 1964 s.1(7), or any waters within 500m of such an installation: 1952 Act ss.12(1), 12(1A) (as amended by the Criminal Justice Act 1988 s.170 and Sch.15, para.14).

[300] Visiting Forces Act 1952 s.12(1).

forces provisions apply to most of the Commonwealth countries[301] and to any other country designated for the purpose by Order in Council.[302] They have also been applied to members of certain international military headquarters.[303]

A certificate issued by or on behalf of the appropriate authority of a country,   **5–103** stating that a body, contingent or detachment of the forces of that country is, or was at the time specified in the certificate, present in the United Kingdom, is conclusive evidence of that fact.[304] Further, where it is admitted or proved that such a body, contingent or detachment was at any time present in the United Kingdom, it is assumed until the contrary is shown that it is or was so present at the invitation of the UK government.[305]

Persons associated with a visiting force

A person having a relevant association with a visiting force is defined as one falling   **5–104** into any of three categories:[306]

(1) a member of that force for the time being appointed to serve with it;[307]

(2) a member of a civilian component of that force, being someone who holds a foreign passport containing an uncancelled entry stating that he is a

---

[301] Visiting Forces Act 1952 s.1(1)(a), which contains a list, as amended from time to time. At the time of writing it is: Canada, Australia, New Zealand, South Africa, India, Pakistan, Ceylon, Ghana, Malaysia, the Republic of Cyprus, Nigeria, Sierra Leone, Tanganyika, Jamaica, Trinidad and Tobago, Uganda, Kenya, Zanzibar, Malawi, Zambia, Malta, the Gambia, Guyana, Botswana, Lesotho, Singapore, Barbados, Mauritius, Swaziland, Tonga, Fiji, the Bahamas, Bangladesh, Solomon Islands, Tuvalu. Dominica, St Lucia, Kiribati, St Vincent and the Grenadines, Papua New Guinea, Western Samoa, Nauru, Zimbabwe, the New Hebrides, Belize, Antigua and Barbuda, St Christopher and Nevis, Brunei, Maldives, Namibia, Cameroon, Mozambique.

[302] Visiting Forces Act 1952 s.1(1)(b). The following countries have been so designated: Belgium, France, the Netherlands, Norway and the United States of America (SI 1954/634), Luxembourg, Turkey, Greece, Denmark, Portugal and Italy (SI 1956/2041), the Federal Republic of Germany (SI 1961/1511), Spain (SI 1989/1329), Albania, Bulgaria, the Czech Republic, Estonia, Hungary, Latvia, Lithuania, Poland, Romania, the Slovak Republic, Slovenia and Sweden (SI 1997/1779), and Armenia, Austria, Azerbaijan, Belarus, Finland, Georgia, Kazakhstan, Kyrgyzstan, the Former Yugoslav Republic of Macedonia, Moldova, Russia, Switzerland, Turkmenistan, Ukraine and Uzbekistan (SI 1998/1268), Bosnia-Herzegovina, Croatia, Ireland, Jordan, Montenegro, Serbia and Tajikistan (SI 2008/299), Algeria (SI 2010/2970).

[303] International Headquarters and Defence Organisations Act 1964 s.1(2), Sch. para.6. The following headquarters have been designated (SI 1965/1535, as amended by SI 1987/927, SI 1994/1642, SI 1999/1735, and SI 2009/704): the Headquarters of the Supreme Allied Commander Transformation (HQ SACT); the Supreme Headquarters Allied Powers Europe (SHAPE); Maritime Component Command Headquarters Northwood (CC-MAR HQ NORTHWOOD); Commander Submarines Allied Naval Forces North (COMSUBNORTH); NATO Airborne Early Warning and Control Force (NAEW&CF); NATO Joint Electronic Warfare Core Staff (NATO JEWCS); Headquarters United Kingdom–Netherlands Amphibious Force (UKNLAF); Headquarters United Kingdom–Netherlands Landing Force (UKNLLF); the European Air Group (EAG); the Intelligence Fusion Centre (IFC); Headquarters Allied Rapid Reaction Corps (HQ ARRC).

[304] Visiting Forces Act 1952 s.16(1)(a). Any purported certificate on behalf of such appropriate authority is presumed to be such a certificate until the contrary is proved, and any authority on whose behalf such document purports to be made is presumed to be the appropriate authority until the contrary is proved: above s.16(3). A certificate under s.16(1)(a) may be procured by informing the Under Secretary of State, Home Office (C Division): Home Office Circular No. 68 of 1955, para.27.

[305] Visiting Forces Act 1952 s.16(1)(b).

[306] Visiting Forces Act 1952 s.12(2).

[307] Visiting Forces Act 1952 ss.12(2)(a) and 12(1).

member of such civilian component, and which entry is accompanied by a note of recognition given or made on behalf of the Secretary of State and not subsequently notified to the sending country as having been withdrawn;[308]

(3) a dependant (i.e. spouse or other person wholly or mainly maintained by the member[309] or in his or her custody, charge or care, and probably including a domestic servant) of a person in (1) or (2) alone, not being a United Kingdom or Colonies citizen, nor being ordinarily resident[310] in the United Kingdom.[311]

Lack of relevant association

5–105   If the deceased person himself did not have a relevant association with the visiting force, then, assuming the coroner otherwise has jurisdiction, he is bound to conduct an investigation.

Where a person has been charged with the homicide of the deceased

5–106   If, however, the coroner is satisfied that a person who is subject to the jurisdiction of the service courts of a country to which the Visiting Forces Act 1952 applies[312] has been charged before a court of that country with the homicide[313] of the deceased person, whether or not that charge has been dealt with, or is being detained by an authority of that country with a view to being so charged, he must suspend the investigation (including adjourning an inquest and discharging any jury),[314] unless the Lord Chancellor otherwise directs, and must supply a certificate stating the particulars necessary for the registration of the death so far as ascertained.[315]

---

[308] Visiting Forces Act 1952 ss.12(2)(a) and 10(1). For this purpose it is assumed until the contrary is proved that any document purporting to be a foreign passport issued to the person in question, any entry in such passport stating that the holder is a member of the civilian component, and any purported mark or note of recognition by the Secretary of State are genuine and what they purport to be: Visiting Forces Act 1952 s.10(3).

[309] For the concept of whole or main maintenance, see, e.g. *Re Coventry* [1980] Ch. 461, CA.

[310] For the concept of ordinary residence, see *R. v Barnet LBC Ex p. Shah* [1983] 2 A.C. 309, HL; *Nessa v Chief Adjudication Officer* [1999] 1 W.L.R. 1937, HL ; *Collins v Secretary of State for Work and Pensions* [2006] 1 W.L.R. 2391, CA. However, it is specifically provided that in determining whether a person is (or was at any time) ordinarily resident in the United Kingdom, no account is to be taken of any period during which he has been or intends to be present in the United Kingdom while a member of a visiting force or of a civilian component of such a force or while a dependent of such persons: s.12(3).

[311] Visiting Forces Act 1952 s.12(2)(b).

[312] See the Visiting Forces Act 1952 s.2(2): broadly this includes members of a visiting force and all other persons who are subject to the service law of the country in question and who are not also either (i) citizens of the United Kingdom or Colonies, or (ii) ordinarily resident in the United Kingdom, or (iii) only so subject by reason of being members of the country's force.

[313] By s.7(6)(as amended), this term includes:(a) murder, manslaughter or infanticide;(b) any offence under the law of the country in question which is analogous to any of the offences within paragraph (a); and(c) any offence under the law of the country in question which is analogous to the offence of encouraging or assisting suicide.

[314] Visiting Forces Act 1952 s.2(2A).

[315] Visiting Forces Act 1952 s.7(2). According to the Home Office in 1981, this adjournment too should be sine die: Home Office Circular No. 54 of 1981, para.11.

The form of certificate to the registrar is not prescribed, but the usual certificate **5–107** after inquest[316] is normally used, so far as relevant.[317] There is no need to wait for the result of any service court proceedings.[318] However, if such person is charged by the service court with an offence other than homicide, the inquest must continue, and if he is tried by an English court, the same consequences will follow as with any other English prosecution.[319]

Procedure for suspended investigation

Where an investigation has been suspended by reason of the visiting forces **5–108** provisions, the coroner must not resume it except on the direction of the Lord Chancellor.[320] As with deaths of persons having a relevant association with a visiting force,[321] the coroner should report all the facts of such cases to the Lord Chancellor, to enable him to decide whether to direct an investigation, or a resumption of one.[322] If the coroner does resume the investigation, he must resume any inquest that was adjourned because of the visiting forces rules,[323] and any such resumed inquest may be held with a jury if the coroner thinks there is sufficient cause for it to be held with one.[324]

State and Diplomatic Immunity

Immunity from suit and all legal process is accorded to a Head of State,[325] an **5–109** ambassador of a foreign country and High Commissioners of Commonwealth countries, and other diplomatic agents, and their families.[326] Administrative and technical staff of a diplomatic mission (and their families) enjoy similar privileges, except that they are not exempt from the civil and administrative jurisdiction of a receiving state in respect of acts performed outside the course of their duties.[327] The domestic staff of members of a diplomatic mission enjoy a more limited immunity.[328] Immunity also applies to a former head of state for acts done in his official capacity as head of state, except for acts amounting to international crimes

---

[316] Form 99 REV: see 18–11 below.
[317] The Home Office view was that the cause of death shown should be restricted to the medical cause and should not extend to the wider circumstances: Home Office Circular No. 54 of 1981, para.10.
[318] Home Office Circular No. 54 of 1981, para.10.
[319] See 10–75 ff below.
[320] Visiting Forces Act 1952 s.7(3).
[321] See 5–104 above.
[322] Home Office Circular No. 54 of 1981, para.2.
[323] Visiting Forces Act 1952 s.7(3A).
[324] Visiting Forces Act 1952 s.7(3B).
[325] *Mighell v Sultan of Johore* [1894] 1 Q.B. 149, CA; State Immunity Act 1978 s.20.
[326] Diplomatic Privileges Act 1964 s.2, Sch.1 arts 31, 37, para.1; *Propend Finance Pty Ltd v Sing, The Times*, May 2, 1997, CA (Australian police officer attached to the Australian High Commission in London).
[327] Diplomatic Privileges Act 1964 s.2, Sch. 1 art.37, para.2; *Re B (A Child) (Care Proceedings: Diplomatic Immunity)* [2003] Fam. 16 (interim care order could be made in respect of embassy employee).
[328] Diplomtic Privileges Act 1964 art.37 para.4.

against humanity.[329] The Commissioner of the Australian Federal Police Force has been held entitled to state immunity (as part of the Government of Australia).[330] National and other representatives on, and certain officers, employees and agents of, certain international organisations also have the like diplomatic immunity.[331]

5–110   Such immunities also bring with them inviolability for embassies,[332] the private residences of diplomatic agents,[333] premises of international organisations,[334] and residences of representatives on and personnel of those organisations.[335] Both state[336] and diplomatic[337] immunity may be waived by the state[338] concerned, even against the wishes of the individual involved,[339] for it is the privilege of the state and not of the individual. Hence it may not be waived by the individual.[340]

Coroner's powers in relation to previously immune body

5–111   Whilst it is clear that the coroner and the coroner's officer will have no right of access to premises which are accorded diplomatic inviolability,[341] the exact legal position regarding the conducting of an investigation into the death of a person who until his death was entitled to diplomatic immunity is more difficult. An earlier edition of this work, before the enactment of the Diplomatic Privileges Act 1964, stated that:

> "The effect of these diplomatic immunities and privileges is to preclude a coroner from investigating the death of a person who, if alive, would have been entitled to diplomatic immunity unless the immunity is waived."[342]

5–112   Other writers have taken the same view,[343] as indeed have coroners in practice. None of the statutory provisions conferring diplomatic privileges and immunities deals expressly with the matter. However, it is provided that when the functions of a person enjoying privileges and immunities have come to an end, those privileges and immunities should cease at the moment when the person leaves the country.[344]

---

[329] State Immunity Act 1978 s.20, read with the Diplomatic Privileges Act 1964 s.2, Sch.1 art.39(2); *R. v Bow Street Metropolitan Stipendiary Magistrate Ex p. Pinochet Ugarte (No. 3)* [2000] 1 A.C. 147, HL.

[330] *Propend Finance Pty Ltd v Sing, The Times*, May 2, 1997, CA.

[331] International Organisations Act 1968 s.1, Sch.1 arts 1, 9.

[332] Diplomatic Privileges Act 1964 s.2, Sch.1 art.22. What are "diplomatic premises" within the meaning of the Schedule is now governed by the Diplomatic and Consular Premises Act 1987. As to when premises are "used" for diplomatic purposes, see *Westminster City Council v Republic of Iran* [1986] 1 W.L.R. 979.

[333] Diplomatic Privileges Act 1964 s.2, Sch.1 art.30.

[334] International Organisations Act 1968 s.1 (and orders made thereunder) Sch.1 art.2.

[335] International Organisations Act 1968 s.1 (and orders made thereunder) Sch.1 art.9.

[336] *Duff Development Co v Government of Kelantan* [1924] A.C. 797.

[337] Diplomatic Privileges Act 1964 s.2, Sch.1 art.32.

[338] Or international organisation: *Standard Chartered Bank v International Tin Council* [1987] 1 W.L.R. 641.

[339] *R. v Kent* (1941) 28 Cr. App. R. 23.

[340] *Re P* [1998] 1 F.L.R. 624.

[341] As to "diplomatic premises", see 5–110 above.

[342] 9th edn (1957), p.22. Waiver is by the state (whose immunity it is: 5–110) and not the deceased's family.

[343] e.g. *Halsbury's Laws of England*, 5th edn reissue, Vol.24 [85], and Vol.61 [274].

[344] Diplomatic Privileges Act 1964 s.2 and Sch.1 art.39 para.2.

Further, it is provided that in case of the death of a member of the mission his family continues to enjoy the privileges and immunities until the expiry of a reasonable period in which to leave the country,[345] and, as long as the deceased was not a national of or permanently resident in this country, the moveable property of the deceased may be exported from this country.[346] It is therefore submitted that, whatever the position before 1964, these provisions impliedly extend the privileges and immunities conferred upon a person whilst alive for a reasonable period after his death, so as to enable the removal of the body from this country, and that the present practice of coroners is legally (as well as politically) justified.[347]

Consular offices

Consular offices are in a different position. The authorities of this country may not enter that part of consular premises[348] which is used[349] exclusively for the purpose of the work of the consular post except with the consent of the head of the post (or his designee) or of the head of the diplomatic mission of the state concerned, which consent may be assumed in case of fire or other disaster requiring prompt protective action.[350] Consular officers and employees are not amenable to the jurisdiction of the English judicial or administrative authorities in respect of acts performed in the exercise of consular functions.[351] Further, consular officers are not liable to arrest or detention pending trial, except in the case of a grave crime, and are not otherwise liable to any form of restriction on their personal freedom except in execution of a judicial decision of final effect.[352]

    These immunities, however, do not extend to the families of consular officers or employees. In any event, these privileges and immunities may be waived by the state concerned.[353] Overall, it therefore appears that, except insofar as a coroner's inquiries into a death lead him to investigate acts performed in the exercise of consular functions (which in the normal case seems unlikely), there is no restriction on the jurisdiction of a coroner to conduct an investigation into the death of a consular officer or employee, or a fortiori that of a member of their families.

Advice on immunity

If a coroner is in doubt whether a claim to diplomatic immunity is valid, or if, although the claim may be thought valid, he considers that there are nevertheless strong reasons for his exercising jurisdiction, he should consult the Ministry of Justice coroners unit, who, after consultation with the Foreign Office, will advise

5–113

5–114

5–115

---

[345] Diplomatic Privileges Act 1964 s.2 and Sch.1 art.39 para.3.

[346] Diplomatic Privileges Act 1964 s.2 and Sch.1 art.39, para.4.

[347] A reported example was the death in a car accident of the Third Secretary at the East German embassy, where diplomatic privilege was claimed and no inquest was held: see *The Times*, October 10, 1984.

[348] See the Consular Relations Act 1968 Sch.1 art.1(j); Diplomatic and Consular Premises Act 1987.

[349] cf. *Westminster City Council v Republic of Iran* [1986] 1 W.L.R. 979.

[350] Consular Relations Act 1968 Sch.1 art.31 para.2. Presumably this assumption is not conclusive, in that consent might be expressly refused even in such cases.

[351] Consular Relations Act 1968 Sch.1 art.43 para.1.

[352] Consular Relations Act 1968 Sch.1 art.41.

[353] Consular Relations Act 1968 Sch.1 art.45.

him.[354] In any event, the certificate of the Secretary of State as to whether a particular person is entitled to a particular privilege or immunity under any of the provisions so far discussed, is conclusive.[355] Subject to that, the courts have jurisdiction to decide whether or not a person is entitled to a diplomatic or other privilege or immunity.[356]

CONCURRENT JURISDICTION

5–116   Before the division of counties into districts (now areas), each being assigned its own coroner, in 1844,[357] there might be several coroners for a county. At common law, an inquest could be taken by one of them alone: the judicial acts of the one who first proceeded to make inquiry and completed the inquest were as valid as if all had joined.[358] Conversely, after one coroner had completed an inquest, no other coroner in the county had any jurisdiction to act in the same matter.[359]

5–117   In effect, the law was that the first coroner in a county to take jurisdiction and hold an inquest excluded all the others. As Hale CJ put it, in considering the case where a county coroner and the Admiralty coroner had concurrent jurisdiction:

> "He who first seizes the Body may take the Inquisition, and the other hath lost his Opportunity."[360]

To avoid inconvenience and unseemly squabbles, coroners used sometimes (unofficially) to divide up their county between them,[361] and it was this practice that was given statutory force in 1844.[362]

5–118   With one important exception, the structure of the current legislation[363] assumes that only the senior coroner of *one* coroner area can nowadays have jurisdiction in respect of any particular body at any one time. This is subject, of

---

[354] Home Office Circular No. 68 of 1955, para.8. (The functions of the Home Office relating to coroners have been transferred to the Ministry of Justice.) Advice can be obtained, in urgent cases, by telephoning the duty officers at the Foreign Office.

[355] Diplomatic Privileges Act 1964 s.4; Consular Relations Act 1968 s.11; International Organisations Act 1968 s.8; Statement Immunity Act 1978 s.21. Such certificates may be challenged in the courts only on the grounds that they are not genuine, or that they were issued outside the scope of the relevant statutory power, and neither their contents nor the paths at which such contents were arrived at are reviewable by the courts: *R. v Secretary of State for Foreign and Commonwealth Affairs Ex p. Trawnik*, The Times, February 21, 1986, CA; cf. *R. v Governor of Pentonville Prison Ex p. Osman (No. 2)*, The Times, December 24, 1988; [1989] C.O.D. 446; (1989) 86(7) L.S.G. 36 (certificate conclusive as to facts, but not as to law, and not exclusive). See also *Re P* [1998] 1 F.L.R. 624 (certificate that children were dependants of diplomat father).

[356] See, e.g. *R. v Lambeth Justices Ex p. Yusufu* [1985] Crim. L.R. 510, DC.

[357] Under the Coroners Act 1844 ss.5 and 19.

[358] Staunford P.C. fol.53a; 2 Hale P.C. 50; 2 Hawk. P.C. c. 9 s.45. This was presumably on the general principle that the acts of one judge of a court of record are as effectual as the acts of the whole court: 2 Hawk. P.C. c. 1 s.10.

[359] 2 Hale P.C. 59; *R. v West Yorkshire Coroner Ex p. Smith* [1982] 3 All E.R. 1098 at 1108.

[360] *Atwood's Case*, P. 27 C.2, reported in Umfreville's *Lex Coronatoria*, Vol.2, Ch.15, para.11.

[361] Umfreville's *Lex Coronatoria*, Vol.2, Ch.15, paras 47–52; Hunnisett, *The Medieval Coroner*, Ch.8.

[362] Coroners Act 1844 ss.5, 19 (repealed).

[363] Coroners and Justice Act 2009 s.1 (1); see formerly Coroners Act 1988 s.5(1).

course, to the possibility that jurisdiction may be transferred, either by agreement[364] or by direction of the Chief Coroner.[365] And within each coroner area, there is a hierarchy which means that there can be identified a particular judicial officer who deals with each case, so that it may not in fact be the senior coroner of that area, but an area or assistant coroner.[366]

However, exceptionally, there is the case of Wales. A senior coroner appointed **5-119** for a coroner area in Wales is for all purposes regarded as a coroner for the whole of Wales, and has the same jurisdiction, rights, powers and authorities throughout Wales as if he had been appointed as a senior coroner for the whole of Wales.[367] Such coroners accordingly have concurrent jurisdiction in coroner areas in Wales.

Whilst it is unlikely at the present day that any of the disputes which **5-120** characterised eighteenth-century coroners' jurisdiction and practice would break out over such a matter as which coroner was to take jurisdiction, it is nonetheless submitted that in circumstances such as these the old common law rules should still apply, and the first coroner to take jurisdiction and hold an inquest thereby excludes all other persons with a concurrent jurisdiction.[368]

REFUSAL TO HOLD AN INQUEST

There are various powers and remedies available where a coroner refuses or **5-121** neglects to conduct an investigation or hold an inquest which ought to be conducted or held.

Application to High Court

First, the Attorney-General[369] or any interested person[370] with his authority[371] **5-122** may apply[372] to the High Court,[373] and the High Court, if satisfied that the coroner is indeed refusing or neglecting to conduct an investigation or hold an inquest which ought to be conducted or held, may order an investigation to be held, whether by him or a senior coroner, area coroner or assistant coroner in the same coroner area,[374] and may also order the coroner to pay such costs of and incidental to the application as seem just.[375] For this purpose "coroner" means a coroner appointed under the Coroners Act 1988, or a senior coroner, area coroner

---

[364] See 4–19 ff.

[365] See 4–22.

[366] See 2–13.

[367] Coroners Act 1988 s.4A(8), as modified by the Coroners and Justice Act 2009 (Consequential Provisions) Order 2013 art.2(2), (3). See 2–24, 4–17.

[368] See the authorities cited in 5–116—5–117 above, and also Wellington, *The King's Coroner*, Vol.1, p.30.

[369] Or, in some cases, the Solicitor General: see 5–116—5–117 below.

[370] This includes the Crown: *Re Culley* (1833) 5 B. & Ad: 230.

[371] His authority was historically known as his *fiat*, after the Latin for "Let it be done".

[372] As to procedure, see 19–22 below.

[373] See 19–22 below.

[374] Coroners Act 1988 s.13(1), (2)(a).

[375] Coroners Act 1988 s.13(2)(b). See *Terry v East Sussex Coroner* [2002] Q.B. 312, CA. As to the principles upon which the court will order costs to be paid, see 19–70 ff below.

or assistant coroner appointed under the Coroners and Justice Act 2009.[376] It was once said that, notwithstanding the Attorney-General's consent may have been given, the permission of the court was also required for such an application to be made,[377] but this seems wrong in principle; this is not judicial review.[378]

Application for judicial review

5–123   Secondly, a person aggrieved[379] by the refusal of a coroner to hold an inquest may apply for judicial review of that decision,[380] in particular for an order quashing the decision and for a mandatory order to require an inquest to be held.[381] After the claim is issued, the matter is referred to the single judge of the Administrative Court for permission, initially on paper, but if permission is refused on paper then the application is renewable in court,[382] and (if permission is given) to either another single judge or the full court for the required orders.[383] In this case, there is a time limit for making the application of three months from the date on which the grounds arose for making it.[384] The application may include a claim for damages (assuming some loss to have been incurred by the claimant).[385]

Other matters

5–124   There are two other matters that may be mentioned. First, refusal to hold an inquest may in any event be conduct amounting to misbehaviour, justifying removal from office.[386]

5–125   Secondly, there was ancient authority for the proposition that where a coroner *refused* to hold an inquest into a "*felo de se*" or "any other sudden death",[387] it could be held instead by the justices of the peace or the justices of gaol delivery or of *oyer* and *terminer* ("hear and determine") or of the Court of King's Bench.[388] There was however no modern instance of this occurring.

5–126   Similarly, it was formerly held in cases where the coroner was actually *unable* to hold an inquest *super visum corporis* (at that time, a view of the body being necessary to give a coroner jurisdiction),[389] because the body had been buried too long[390] or

---

[376] Coroners Act 1988 s.13(4).
[377] Per Comyn J in *R. v South London Coroner Ex p. Thompson*, (1982) 126 S.J. 625, DC.
[378] See next para.
[379] This means someone with a sufficient interest: see 19–37 below.
[380] Pursuant to CPR, Pt 54: see generally Ch.19 below.
[381] See, e.g. *R. v West Yorkshire Coroner Ex p. Smith* [1983] Q.B. 335, CA; *R. (Canning) v Northampton Coroner* [2006] EWCA Civ. 1225 (coroner's decision not to hold an inquest could only be impugned on *Wednesbury* grounds).
[382] See 19–53 below.
[383] See 19–55—19–62 below.
[384] CPR r.54.5. See 19–47.
[385] CPR r.54.3(2). See 19–26.
[386] See 2–106.
[387] 2 Hale P.C. 59.
[388] 2 Hale P.C. 59; 2 Hawk. P.C. c. 9 s.29, fn.7, referring to *R. v Killinghall* (1756) 1 Burr. 17; 97 E.R. 165, where earlier authorities (such as *Stanlack's case* (1672) 1 Ventr. 181) are cited and discussed, and the position agreed (by counsel) to be an as set out in the text, but where the inquisition in question (taken before a grand jury) was held invalid because the assize judge had declined to take part in the proceedings and it was accordingly *coram non judice*.
[389] See the Coroners Act 1980 s.1.
[390] *R. v Parker* (1675) 2 Lev. 140; *Anon.* (1680) 1 Ventr. 352.

could not be found,[391] that the inquest could be taken by the justices of the peace,[392] or of assize,[393] or a commission of enquiry[394] instead. No such power of justices of the peace so to act was ever expressly abolished. Courts of assize, which for the purpose of statutory interpretation included courts of gaol delivery and of *oyer* and *terminer*,[395] were abolished in 1971,[396] and no further commissions to hold such courts could thereafter be issued. However, all references in statutes and other instruments to courts of gaol delivery and of *oyer* and *terminer* were to be construed as references to the Crown Court,[397] which in general terms thereafter had a similar jurisdiction.

Thus it might have been said that the successors of the justices of gaol delivery   **5–127**
and of *oyer* and *terminer* were the judges of the Crown Court.[398] On the other hand, the jurisdiction of "the courts created by commissions of assize" was transferred to the High Court in 1875 along with the jurisdiction of the Court of Queen's Bench[399] and continues to be exercisable by judges of the High Court today.[400] Until July 25, 2013 there might have been a question whether a judge of the High Court was entitled to conduct an inquest (in addition to any other power to do so)[401] whenever a court *refused* to hold an inquest into a "*felo de se*" or "any other sudden death" , even though none in fact ever did so.

Whatever the historical merits of these arguments, the 2013 reforms must mean   **5–128**
that all of them have now gone. Parliament cannot have intended that other, more primitive (and unfunded) systems of death investigation should exist in parallel with the new coroner system under the 2009 Act.

---

[391] *R. v Montgomery Coroner* (1616) 2 Poph. 209; 79 E.R. 1298.C. Noy 87; 74 E.R. 1053.
[392] *R. v Parker* (1675) 2 Lev. 140; *R. v Montgomery Coroner* (1616) 2 Poph. 209; 79 E.R. 1298.C. Noy 87; 74 E.R. 1053.
[393] *R. v Parker* (1675) 2 Lev. 140; *Anon.* (1680) 1 Ventr. 352.
[394] *R. v Parker* (1675) 2 Lev. 140.
[395] Interpretation Act 1889 s.13(4).
[396] Courts Act 1971 s.1(2).
[397] Courts Act 1971 Sch.8, para.2.
[398] See *R. v Crown Court at Sheffield Ex p. Brownlow* [1980] Q.B. 530 at 544; *Smalley v Crown Court at Warwick* [1985] 1 All E.R. 769 at 777.
[399] Judicature Act 1873 s.16; Supreme Court of Judicature (Consolidation) Act 1925 s.18(2)(a)(ii), (vii).
[400] Senior Courts Act 1981 s.19(1).
[401] See 2–02 above.

Chapter 6

THE SCOPE OF THE INVESTIGATION

INTRODUCTION

The scope of a coroner's investigation into a death is a matter of importance. **6–01**
Amongst other things, it governs the statements and other information which must
be sought by the coroner during the investigation, the statements which must be
read, the witnesses who must be called, and the questions which may be asked of
the witnesses who are called, at any inquest forming part of that investigation. The
question of scope must be considered first of all from the point of view of the four
statutory questions which the law asks the investigation to try to determine:[1] *who*
was the deceased, and *when*, *where* and *how* did the deceased come by his or her
death?[2] Then in addition the investigation is asked to make a finding[3] as to any
particulars required to be registered concerning the death.[4]

Subject only to the power of the coroner to *report* a matter to someone who he **6–02**
believes may have power to take action to prevent other deaths in future,[5] neither
the coroner conducting the investigation nor the jury, if there is one, may express
any opinion on any other matter.[6] Thus, "recommendations" (whether from the
coroner or the jury) as to how matters should be changed in future are no longer
permissible,[7] and no determination may be framed so as to appear to determine any
question of criminal liability by a named person, or civil liability generally.[8]

THE FOUR QUESTIONS

Who, *when*, and *where* are relatively straightforward. The identity of a person is in **6–03**
English law not a matter of precise legal formality, as it is in some legal systems,

---

[1] Coroners and Justice Act 2009 s.10(1)(a); formerly Coroners Act 1988 s.11(4)(a); see 13–01.
[2] Coroners and Justice Act 2009 s.5(1)(a), (b); formerly Coroners Act 1988 s.11(5)(b), and Coroners
Rules 1984 r.36(1)(a), (b); see 13–01.
[3] Coroners and Justice Act 2009 s.10(1)(b); formerly Coroners Act 1988 s.11(4)(b); see 13–01.
[4] Coroners and Justice Act 2009 s.5(1)(c); formerly Coroners Rules 1984 r.36(1)(c); see 13–01.
[5] Coroners and Justice Act 2009 s.32, Sch.5 para.7; formerly Coroners Rules 1984 r.43; see
13–122 ff.
[6] Coroners and Justice Act 2009 s.5(3); formerly Coroners Rules 1984 r.36(2).
[7] *R. v Shrewsbury Coroner's Court Ex p. British Parachute Association* (1987) 152 J.P. 123. cf. the Coroners
Rules 1953 rr.27, 34, which expressly conferred to power to make such recommendations, but
which was abrogated in 1980.
[8] Coroners and Justice Act 2009 s.10(2); formerly Coroners Rules 1984 r.42; see 12–112, 13–57,
13–103.

where you are registered at birth with a name which you can never change, or at least only with difficulty.[9] Instead, you are *who you and others say you are*. In English law, if you wish to change your name, you simply change it, and then provide evidence of the fact that you are known by the new name.[10] Hence the importance of the so-called "deed poll".[11] So the identity of the deceased is not a matter of scientific certainty. It is simply something that can be easily established on the available evidence. By what name (whether or not it was the original one) was this person known at the time of death? If the evidence is that the deceased was known in England at the time of death as AB, it does not matter that, at another time or in another country, he or she was known as CD. There is no need to agonise over whether AB or CD is the "legally correct" name. If necessary, the fact can be found that the deceased was AB, originally (or also) known as CD.

6–04   "When" and "where" are difficult only when there is doubt as to the moment of death. For example, if a person dies as a result of going into a river, and the body is found in a different place from where the person went in, the place of death and the time may well be uncertain. Similarly, where death occurs on a vehicle that is moving. And where a person is found dead in a fixed place, doubt as to the time of death may cause some difficulty. In such cases the evidence must at least seek to establish the parameters of the possible time and place of death. If even that is not possible, the finding will be that the body was found dead at such a place and time.

6–05   The last question ("how") is usually the most difficult. The statutory task is not to ascertain how the deceased *died*, but how the deceased *came by his or her death*. This is a more limited question, directed to the means by which the deceased came by his or her death.[12] So, before the Human Rights Act 1998[13] came into force, the word "how" in the statutory question was interpreted simply as "*by what means*" the deceased came by his or her death.[14]

6–06   The question of how the deceased *came by* his or her death is of course wider than merely finding *the medical cause* of death, and therefore the coroner should inquire into acts and omissions which are directly responsible for the death.[15] But he or she need not investigate "the underlying responsibility for every circumstance which may be said to have contributed to the death",[16] still less "every issue raised

---

[9] See e.g. the French *Code Civil* arts 60 to 61-4; *Décret* 94-32 of January 20, 1994.

[10] See *Halsbury's Laws of England*, 5th edn, Vol.88, paras 326-329.

[11] That is not an *indenture*, a deed made by a two or more persons, originally a single document executed in two places and torn into two halves, with *indentured* edges, but a deed made by a single person alone, a deed *poll*, that is, with a straight edge. See *Halsbury's Laws of England*, 5th edn, Vol. 32, para.203. It can be done with a simple statutory declaration instead.

[12] *R. v North Humberside Coroner Ex p. Jamieson* [1995] Q.B. 1, 24, CA; *Re Ministry of Defence's Application*, [1994] N.I. 279, CA (NI); *R. v Coventry Coroner Ex p. O'Reilly* (1996) 160 J.P. 749, DC. cf. *R. v West Yorkshire Coroner Ex p. Clements* (1993) 158 J.P. 17 at 22, DC (pre-HRA case).

[13] As interpreted in *R. (Middleton) v West Somerset Coroner* [2004] 2 A.C. 184. This is discussed below: 6–14 ff.

[14] *R. v North Humberside and Scunthorpe Coroner Ex p. Jamieson* [1995] Q.B. 1, 24.

[15] *R. v East Sussex Coroner Ex p. Homberg* (1994) 158 J.P. 357, DC; cf. *Re Medical Defence Union Ltd. v Sinclair* [1990] 1 Med. L.R. 359, HK.

[16] *R. v East Sussex Coroner Ex p. Homberg* (1994) 158 J.P. 357, DC.

by the claimant, however peripheral to the main issues to be determined".[17] This is a question of causation,[18] though not limited to the last link in the chain.[19]

Where a person is suffering from a natural disease or some injury caused by himself or another, and a third person (e.g. a health professional) has an opportunity to take steps to prevent death from that disease or injury, but the person dies, it may be necessary to investigate the steps taken by that third person.[20] In some cases, indeed, the coroner may have to consider and rule on the lawfulness of actions taken before the death.[21] Expert evidence, or its absence, may have a critical impact on the focus of the inquiry.[22] **6–07**

The requirement to summon a jury for some inquests[23] cannot by itself enlarge the area or scope of the investigation.[24] Similarly the coroner's ability at the end of an inquest to report matters to some person believed to have power to take action to prevent future deaths[25] has been described as "ancillary to the inquest procedure and not its mainspring"[26] and should not by itself enlarge the scope of the investigation.[27] Nevertheless, the coroner may as a matter of discretion admit evidence relevant to the issue of preventing deaths in future, even if of only marginal relevance to the circumstances of the death.[28] Indeed, in art.2 cases, he or she may be obliged to.[29] **6–08**

In any event, it is accepted that "the enquiry is almost bound to stretch wider than strictly required for the purposes of a verdict. How much wider is pre-eminently a matter for the coroner."[30] Thus the investigation may behave like a funnel,[31] looking at a wide variety of facts at the outset but becoming narrower in scope as it progresses, until it arrives at a refined conclusion. If the investigation is **6–09**

---

[17] R. (Allen) v Inner North London Coroner [2009] EWCA Civ. 623 at [33]; R. (Le Page) v Inner South London Assistant Deputy Coroner [2012] EWHC 1485 (Admin.); see also R. (Rowley) v Director of Public Prosecutions [2003] EWHC 693 at [55], and R. (Shaw) v Leicester City and South Leicestershire ADC [2014] EWCA Civ. 294.

[18] R. (Allen) v Inner North London Coroner [2009] EWCA Civ. 623 at [40] ("It is implicit in such an investigation that what is being investigated caused or may have caused or contributed to the death"). cf. R. (Duffy) v Worcestershire Deputy Coroner [2013] EWHC 1654 (Admin.) at [41].

[19] R. v Inner West London Coroner Ex p. Dallaglio [1994] 4 All ER 139, 155, 164; R. (Butler) v Black Country District Coroner [2010] EWHC 43 (Admin.) at [62]; Jones v South London Coroner [2010] EWHC 931 (Admin.) at [25]; Re Chief Constable of PSNI's Application [2010] N.I.Q.B. 66.

[20] R. v Poplar Coroner Ex p. Thomas [1993] Q.B. 610; R. (Touche) v Inner North London Coroner [2001] Q.B. 1206 at [46]; R. (Takoushis) v Inner North London Coroner [2006] 1 W.L.R. 461, CA.

[21] R. (Pounder) v Durham and Darlington Coroner [2009] EWHC 76 (Admin.).

[22] R. (Shaw) v Leicester City and South Leicestershire ADC [2014] EWCA Civ. 294.

[23] See 10–34.

[24] Re Neal (1995) 37 B.M.L.R. 164, DC.

[25] Coroners and Justice Act 2009 s.32, Sch.5 para.7; formerly Coroners Rules 1984 r.43; see Chief Coroner Guidance No. 5, 16 July 2013, and 13–122.

[26] Re Kelly (1996) 161 J.P. 417, DC.

[27] Re Clegg (1997) 161 J.P. 521, DC.

[28] R. (Sreedharan) v Greater Manchester Coroner [2013] EWCA Civ. 181 at [35]–[36]; see also R. (Lewis) v Mid and North Shropshire Coroner [2009] EWCA Civ. 1403.

[29] R. (Lewis) v Mid and North Shropshire Coroner [2009] EWCA Civ. 1403: see 6–19. below.

[30] R. v Inner West London Coroner Ex p. Dallaglio [1994] 4 All E.R. 139 at 155; R. (Cairns) v Inner West London Deputy Coroner [2011] EWHC 2890 (Admin.) at [57]–[71].

[31] See R. (Lewis) v Mid and North Shropshire Coroner [2009] EWCA Civ. 1403 at [26].

to fulfil the purpose of allaying suspicion and rumour, it will undoubtedly look at matters which turn out to have no causative contribution to the death at all.[32]

6–10   Certain things will not however fall within the scope of the investigation. The most obvious examples are events after death, such as any investigation into the death by other state agents, such as the police, or the manner in which the bereaved were informed of or treated after the death (for example by health professionals). But the coroner must be careful to ensure that there is sufficient evidence of death having occurred at or by a particular time. It has unfortunately happened that a coroner in good faith and on evidence credible at the time, has formed the view that death must have occurred by a particular time, but years later further evidence has come to light casting doubt on that conclusion, and thus on the coroner's decision to cut off his inquiry at that point, and leading to the quashing of his inquisition and the re-opening of the inquiry from the beginning.[33]

6–11   Other matters that fall outside scope include questions of policy[34] and resources. Whether a juvenile should be given a custodial sentence or not as a matter of policy is not something which a coronial investigation into the death of the juvenile should go into.[35] Similarly, questions of whether a war was lawful under international law,[36] or the political decisions as to the allocation of resources to the armed forces and as between the different branches of the services,[37] are matters for public and political debate, but unsuitable for investigation by the coroner. It is also inappropriate for the coroner to investigate whether a legal decision was correctly made, e.g. to refuse bail, resulting in the deceased being in prison, where he or she died. This is because it involves the coroner's court substituting its view for that of the original court. Plainly a jury cannot do this, and even the coroner is in no position to act as a kind of court of appeal from the original decision.

6–12   Similar facts in relation to other cases may be relevant.[38] The antecedents of the deceased and indeed of witnesses may sometimes form part of the scope of the investigation. In some cases criminal convictions of the deceased may be relevant and so admissible in evidence,[39] but in others they may be irrelevant and so inadmissible.[40] Similarly, information as to the decision of the CPS to prosecute or not to prosecute persons involved in the death may sometimes be relevant, and irrelevant at others. But even if relevant, such evidence may be so prejudicial that

[32] R. (Sreedharan) v Greater Manchester Coroner [2013] EWCA Civ. 181 at [48]; cf. the inquests into the deaths of Diana, Princess of Wales, and Dodi Fayed, where Sir Scott Baker said at the outset, on October 2, 2007: "We shall investigate matters, some of which may very well turn out to be irrelevant to the causes of the deaths because one of the purposes of an inquest is to allay suspicion and rumour". See also Ramsbottom's Application for Judicial Review [2009] NIQB 55, and Re JR 29's Application [2009] NIQB 97.
[33] Attorney General v South Yorkshire (West) Coroner [2012] EWHC 3783 (Admin.) at [13]–[21].
[34] Jordan v United Kingdom (2001) 11 BHRC 1, ECtHR at [128]; cf. A v Home Secretary [2005] 2 A.C. 68 at [29]; R. (Smith) v Oxfordshire Assistant Deputy Coroner [2011] 1 A.C. 1 at [81], [127], [131].
[35] R. (Scholes) v Home Secretary [2006] EWCA Civ. 1343.
[36] R. (Gentle) v Prime Minister [2008] UKHL 20.
[37] R. (Smith) v Oxfordshire Assistant Deputy Coroner [2011] 1 A.C. 1 at [127]; Smith v Ministry of Defence [2013] UKSC 41 at [65].
[38] R. (Sreedharan) v Greater Manchester Coroner [2013] EWCA Civ. 181 at [40]–[44].
[39] R. v Inner South London Coroner Ex p. Fields (1998) 162 J.P. 411.
[40] See R. (Stanley) v Inner North London Coroner [2003] EWHC 1180 (Admin.), Silber J.

it should not be admitted.[41] And, although it is not the purpose of inquest proceedings to establish criminal or civil liability,[42] it is proper in some cases to ask questions of a witness going to credit,[43] and so it must be proper for the coroner to seek to obtain such information before any hearing.[44]

A difficult problem of scope may be posed when the subject matter of the investigation involves highly secret information, such as where members of the security services make statements or are called to give evidence at inquests. This may affect the question of disclosure of documents and other information.[45] It may also affect the identity of the coroner and any jury concerned. So far as the coroner is concerned, it is usually possible to find a person with appropriate security clearance, and the Chef Coroner can transfer the investigation to such person.[46] But where there must be an inquest as part of the investigation,[47] and that inquest is required to be held with a jury,[48] the problem is more acute. The coroner cannot ensure that all the members of the jury are of the appropriate security clearance.[49] In such cases, it may prove to be impossible to hold the inquest at all with the required scope.[50] **6–13**

THE EFFECT OF THE HUMAN RIGHTS ACT 1998

The pre-Human Rights Act position set out above will continue to have effect in many, perhaps still most, cases investigated by coroners. But, since the 1998 Act came into force, it is now clear that, where it is necessary to avoid a breach of any rights under the European Convention on Human Rights, as made justiciable under that Act, the question of "how" does not refer merely to "*by what means*", but also to "*in what circumstances*" the deceased came by his or her death. This judicial legislation[51] is now confirmed by the express terms of the 2009 Act itself.[52] So there are two classes of case: those where art.2 of the European Convention on **6–14**

---

[41] cf. *R. (Stanley) v Inner North London Coroner* [2003] EWHC 1180 (Admin.), Silber J, where two police officers had shot and killed the deceased in alleged self-defence.

[42] *Hay v Devon Coroner* (1997) 162 J.P. 96, CA.

[43] Criminal Procedure Act 1865 ss.3–5; *R. (Sreedharan) v Greater Manchester Coroner* [2013] EWCA Civ. 181 at [35]–[36].

[44] *R. (Sreedharan) v Greater Manchester Coroner* [2013] EWCA Civ. 181.

[45] *R. (Home Secretary) v Assistant Deputy Coroner for Inner West London* [2010] EWHC 3098 (Admin.); *Secretary of State for Foreign and Commonwealth Affairs v Assistant Deputy Coroner for Inner North London* [2013] EWHC 1786 (Admin.). See also *R. (MPS) v Chairman of Azelle Rodney Inquiry* [2012] EWHC 2783 (Admin.), and *R. (Litvinenko) v Home Secretary* [2014] EWHC 194 (Admin.), DC.

[46] See 4–22.

[47] See 10–05.

[48] See 10–34.

[49] Even if it it were possible, it would breach the principle of random seletion of the jury: see 10–44.

[50] See the decision by Sir Robert Owen, sitting as coroner in the *Litvinenko* case, to ask the Government to set up a public inquiry instead of an inquest, as he had ruled that certain relevant documents were too secret to be admitted in an inquest, and that proceeding without them would inevitably render the inquest "incomplete . . . potentially misleading and/or unfair": *The Guardian*, June 5, 2013. See further *R. (Litvinenko) v Home Secretary* [2014] EWHC 194 (Admin.), DC.

[51] *R. (Middleton) v West Somerset Coroner* [2004] 2 A.C. 184.

[52] Coroners and Justice Act 2009 s.5(2); see 13–01.

Human Rights is engaged (colloquially called *Middleton* investigations) and those where it is not (colloquially called *Jamieson* investigations).[53]

6–15   Whether there is any greater difference between the two classes of case than simply the verdict (as it was formerly called) or the determination (as it is now) is a matter of some debate. In one decision of the House of Lords,[54] the majority view was that there was a clear distinction in scope in the two classes of case. On the other hand, in the most recent decision of the Supreme Court to discuss the question,[55] where nine judges sat, four took the view that there was no difference in scope, whereas two took the view that there was, with one judge expressly sitting on the fence, and two others expressing no view.[56] Yet it is hard to deny that the difference in interpreting the word "how" in the statutory question must mean that there are things potentially within the scope of the inquiry in a *Middleton* case which would not be in a *Jamieson* case.[57] And the legislature has now enshrined the distinction in meaning in primary legislation, which makes it impossible for the judges to ignore.

6–16   It is submitted that there *is* a difference in scope. *Jamieson* itself was a case of death in state custody before the Human Rights Act, where the Court of Appeal[58] held that the scope of the inquest was restricted to the means by which the deceased came by his death. This was suicide by self-suspension, and the only question was whether there was any sufficient evidence of neglect by prison staff having a causative or contributory effect. A *Middleton* inquest into the same death now would probably need to look in addition at the general regime then in operation, the reception of the deceased into the institution, the communication of information between staff, the treatment of the deceased leading up to death, the training of the staff, and the events surrounding the discovery of the deceased, amongst other things. That said, it is still not necessary for the coroner to investigate every issue raised by interested persons, even in art.2 cases.[59] The coroner must decide on the appropriate scope.

6–17   The reality today, however, is that there are at least three classes of case. There are those (a decreasing proportion) which are clearly *Jamieson* from the start.[60] There are those (a still small, but nevertheless increasing proportion) which are clearly *Middleton* from the start.[61] And there are those (a proportion increasing exponentially) which at the beginning are not clearly either. In the middle category, the coroner usually plays safe, and casts the net wider rather than

---

[53] After *R. v North Humberside Coroner Ex p. Jamieson* [1995] Q.B. 1, CA.

[54] *R. (Hurst) v North London Coroner* [2007] 2 A.C. 189.

[55] *R. (Smith) v Oxfordshire Assistant Deputy Coroner* [2011] 1 A.C. 1. See also *R. (Sreedharan) v Greater Manchester Coroner* [2013] EWCA Civ. 181 at [18(vii)].

[56] See *R. (Smith) v Oxfordshire Assistant Deputy Coroner* [2011] 1 A.C. 1 at [208] per Lord Mance. See also *R. (Shaw) v Leicester City and South Leicestershire ADC* [2013] EWHC 386 (Admin.) at [7]–[8], affirmed 11 February 2014, CA.

[57] See for example the discussion in relation to shortcomings in the regulatory system, in 6–16 below.

[58] [1995] Q.B. 1.

[59] *R. (Allen) v Inner North London Coroner* [2009] EWCA Civ. 623 at [33].

[60] e.g. *R. (Cairns) v West London Coroner* [2011] EWHC 2890 (Admin.).

[61] Some would distinguish deaths in state custody ("full" *Middleton*) from other deaths in which the state may be implicated, such as public hospital deaths ("lesser" *Middleton*), where the inquiry need be *Middleton* only in certain respects.

narrower. The funnel[62] may narrow the inquiry later, but at the outset a wider range of matters is considered. Only in the first category can the coroner safely proceed on the basis of the more restricted scope of the pre-Human Rights Act era.

In 2013 the previously existing power of the coroner to make a report to an **6–18** appropriate person to prevent future deaths under secondary legislation became a qualified *duty* under primary legislation.[63] But, if the previous power to report did not enlarge the scope of the enquiry,[64] it is difficult to see why this legislative change should by itself make any difference. The critical point is whether the Human Rights Act made a difference to scope, by making the rights conferred by the European Convention on Human Rights justiciable in domestic courts.

The Court of Appeal has said, probably obiter, that it did, in the sense that the **6–19** Strasbourg caselaw relating to art.2 required that the state's own inquiry must inter alia ascertain "any shortcomings in the operation of the regulatory system", even if they were not causative of the death.[65] The coroner's previous power, now duty, to report is the means of compliance with this requirement in England and Wales.[66] This means that, in *Middleton* cases, although the inquest is not required to investigate other non-causative matters,[67] the scope of the investigation must cover non-causative system failures, so that the coroner (and not any jury that there may be) can properly perform his or her function to make a report designed to prevent future deaths.[68]

---

[62] See 6–09.

[63] Coroners and Justice Act 2009 s.32, Sch.5 para.7; formerly Coroner Rules 1984 r.43; see 13–122.

[64] See 6–08.

[65] R. (Lewis) v Mid and North Shropshire Coroner [2009] EWCA Civ. 1403 at [11], [35]. See also R. (Duffy) v Worcestershire Deputy Coroner [2013] EWHC 1654 (Admin.) at [41].

[66] R. (Lewis) v Mid and North Shropshire Coroner [2009] EWCA Civ. 1403 at, [16], [38]. The actual decision was that it was not necessary for the *jury* (where there was one) to deal with these matters. See also R. (Middleton) v West Somerset Coroner [2004] 2 A.C. 182 at [38].

[67] R. (Allen) v Inner North London Coroner [2009] EWCA Civ. 623 at [40], referred to in Lewis at [30] as not being in conflict with it. But Lewis was held by Blake J at first instance not to involve any system failures, and the Court of Appeal did not disagree. cf R. (Le Page) v Inner South London Assistant Deputy Coroner [2012] EWHC 1485 (Admin.).

[68] See 13–122.

Chapter 7

INFORMATION AND PUBLICITY

CONTEXT

When the coroner is considering whether he has an obligation to conduct an **7–01** investigation, or when he conducts one, he acquires information about the deceased, about the death, and about other persons involved. The events of and surrounding the death may have taken place in public and be well-known, or in private and not at all publicly known, or partly one and partly the other. Questions of criminal or civil liability may perhaps have to be determined in due course (though not by the coroner). The deceased or others involved may be celebrities, or they may be unknown. The facts surrounding the death may be a matter of great interest for the media, a matter of shame for the family, a matter of national or even international catastrophe, or even all of these and more. The coroner may be obliged subsequently to hold an inquest as part of the investigation. Whatever the position, the coroner must manage the information made available by virtue of the inquiries or investigation consistently with the rights of all concerned. This chapter is intended to deal with the questions impacting on that information from the beginning, concerned with publicity, disclosure of information to interested persons, data protection, freedom of information, copyright and legal privilege.

PUBLICITY

General

The public nature of the coroner's inquiries is clearly exemplified by the obligation **7–02** to hold an inquest hearing in public.[1] And the result of any inquest must be recorded in a document.[2] But it does not follow that everything which the coroner finds out during his inquiries about the deceased or the death is or should be placed in the public domain. As has already been noted, "The function of an inquest is to seek out and record as many of the facts concerning the death *as public interest requires*."[3] But the public interest, and what it demands, is not the same as what is

---

[1] Coroners (Inquests) Rules 2013 (SI 2013/1616) r.11; see 10–16.
[2] Coroners (Inquests) Rules 2013 (SI 2013/1616) r.34, Form 2; see 13–02.
[3] *R. v South London Coroner Ex p. Thompson* (1982) 126 S.J. 625, DC, per Lord Lane CJ (emphasis supplied).

interesting to the public.[4] This means that the coroner must be careful to distinguish between information which it is proper to make public and that which it is not, and also (in respect of the former) the point in time at which it is proper to make it public.

The deceased

7–03   The deceased will have enjoyed certain civil rights during life. On death, many of these, including rights in respect of confidential information and copyright, will pass as a matter of law to his personal representatives (executors or administrators) for the benefit of his estate.[5] Other rights, such as rights in respect of defamation and data protection, will die with him, and do not pass to anyone else. But members of his family and others may have their own rights of these kinds which will of course survive the death of the deceased. The coroner however has certain duties to investigate,[6] and powers to obtain information.[7] These override the ability of the deceased and those connected with him to keep such matters to themselves. But the coroner must be careful to use and preserve the information thus obtained only for the purposes for which the powers were conferred, and not to deploy it in collateral or unrelated ways.[8]

7–04   The first question for the coroner is at what point the identity or putative identity of the deceased may or should be disclosed to third parties, such as the media. If there is an inquest in due course, the identity of the deceased will be a matter for the court to find if possible on the evidence, and indeed such evidence may be given at the opening of the inquest. But under the new coroner system, an inquest may not be opened for some time after a death has been reported.[9] Indeed, in most cases reported to coroners no inquest will ever be opened. There is no legal restriction on the coroner disclosing to third parties the apparent identity of the person whose death has been reported to him, or into which he may later decide to conduct an investigation. At the same time there is no duty on him to do so at this stage. And there may be good reasons why the coroner should *not* release the details of the deceased at this stage, for example to protect from "hatemail" or similar personal attack the family of a person who has died after medical treatment was withdrawn or a ventilator was switched off, or to reduce the risk of an opportunistic burglary.

7–05   It makes no difference if the deceased was a person under 18 years (though of course in that case the obligation of the coroner to inform the Local Safeguarding Children Board is engaged).[10] By disclosing the identity of the deceased, the coroner does not normally disclose the identity of others such as interested persons. However, the coroner may need to consider whether disclosure of the identity of

---

[4] *British Steel v Granada Television Ltd* [1981] A.C. 1096, 1168, per Lord Wilberforce.
[5] See 19–02.
[6] See 5–01, 6–01.
[7] See 7–12 ff.
[8] *Marcel v Metropolitan Police Commissioner* [1992] Ch. 225, 237; *Lonrho v Fayed (No. 4)* [1994] Q.B. 775, 788-789; *Scopelight Ltd v Chief Constable of Northumberland* [2010] Q.B. 438, CA.
[9] See 10–04, 10–05.
[10] See 5–60.

the deceased will involve or lead to the disclosure of the identity of others, whose identities ought for some other reason not to be disclosed.[11]

Interested persons

At this early stage the coroner has no duty to disclose to the media or other third parties the names or other details of interested persons[12] or those who claim to be interested persons. And, in general, it would be wrong for the coroner to do so, because no useful coronial purpose is served by so doing. But there may be circumstances where it would advance the coroner's functions if some disclosure were made. For example, the coroner might make a public appeal for a particular person to come forward to assist in the inquiry. Or it may be necessary or desirable for the coroner to do so to enable or advance enquiries properly to be made by other authorities or agencies, such as the Local Child Safeguarding Board,[13] the IPCC,[14] or the Prisons and Probation Ombudsman.[15]

7–06

Where the deceased was a child, disclosure of the identity of the deceased, particularly to the media, may lead to accidental disclosure of the details of other family members, which may include other minors such as siblings. Even where the deceased was an adult, the circumstances of the death may implicate or help to identify a child (e.g. a fire at the family home started by a child). Before an inquest is opened, the statutory power to prohibit publication of details relating to certain minors involved in court proceedings[16] does not apply. In such a case if there is a risk of harm to the child concerned, the appropriate course for the coroner to take is to invite the local authority to apply to the High Court for an order making the child a ward of court, and then for that court to make an appropriate restriction order.[17]

7–07

Other information

At the outset of the inquiry the coroner may have other information, beyond the identities of the deceased and any interested persons. This may include the address of the deceased, the wishes of the family as to disposal, and the cause of death. The addresses of the deceased or interested persons may already be known, or easily discovered from other sources. But if it is not, the coroner should be cautious about disclosing it. The home of a deceased person may become a target for vandalism or even burglary if it is known that the occupant has died. Interested persons may be targeted by those wishing to express critical views in relation to the death. The wishes of the family as to disposal of the body may be a matter of media interest. But they are, generally speaking, a private matter rather than a public one. Whether the coroner has been asked to give, or has given, a burial order or cremation certificate (or what such order or certificate contains) is not normally something

7–08

---

[11] See 6–13, 7–07.
[12] As to whom, see 8–21, 8–22.
[13] See 5–60.
[14] See 8–22, 8–62; website *http://www.ipcc.gov.uk/* [Accessed 5 June 2014].
[15] See 10–70; website *http://www.ppo.gov.uk/*[Accessed 5 June 2014].
[16] Children and Young Persons Act 1933 s.39; see 11–75.
[17] Decision of the Court of Appeal in July 1995. See also *Re LM (Reporting restriction: Coroner's inquest)* [2007] EWHC 1902 (Fam).

which needs to be dealt with in public. It will be irrelevant to any inquest that may be held, and to the acts that are to be sought and recorded.

7–09   The cause of death is more complex. It may contain very personal and otherwise confidential information about the deceased's health or lifestyle (e.g. alcohol or drug addiction, sexuality). As a general rule, this is information that without the permission of those entitled to give it ought not to be disclosed, except as part of the inquest process, or as otherwise required by law.[18] Secondly, if there is to be an inquest, it will be the function of that inquest to determine, so far as possible, the cause of death. It is not for the coroner to disclose the necessarily incomplete information so far available, and still less, on that incomplete information, at this stage to reach and publish what will inevitably be perceived as a "conclusion". That said, there may be rare cases where there is a considerable public interest in disclosing some information about the cause of death even before any inquest proceedings can begin (e.g. to allay rumour and suspicion, perhaps threatening public disorder),[19] and in such cases some disclosure relating to the cause of death may be justified.

7–10   If the coroner's preliminary inquiries do not result in an investigation,[20] or if the coroner conducts an investigation, but discontinues it,[21] the case will be closed without an inquest. The only records will be the coroner's file (probably very thin) and the certificates given in respect of (i) death registration (i.e. Form A or Form B, as appropriate),[22] and (ii) (in the case of an investigation begun but discontinued) the disposal of the body.[23] For reasons elsewhere given,[24] where no investigation was ever begun, there will be no certificates relating to the disposal of the body (i.e. burial order, cremation certificate), though there may be a so-called "out of England order".[25] None of these is a public document, and ordinarily there will be no proper basis for the coroner to disclose these to the media or the public generally. Of course what the recipients of the certificates do with them is not a matter for the coroner. And interested persons may seek disclosure of documents held by the coroner, either at the time or subsequently, even where there is no inquest.[26]

Inquest

7–11   The rules relating to contempt of court[27] do not apply to the coroner's preliminary inquiries or to an investigation before an inquest is opened. But if the coroner conducts an investigation, and does not discontinue it, an inquest will be opened and in due course held. The opening of the inquest makes the proceedings "active"

---

[18] In the case of a suspected homicide where the police have attended the post-mortem examination (see 8–61), of course they too will have and be able to make use of the information for their own purposes.

[19] cf. *R. (Coker) v Inner South London Coroner* [2006] EWHC 614 (Admin.).

[20] See 8–15—8–16.

[21] See 8–19, 8–36.

[22] See 8–15—8–17, 8–37.

[23] See 9–28, 9–38.

[24] See 9–21, 9–28.

[25] See 9–38.

[26] See 9–24 ff.

[27] See 11–89 ff.

for the purposes of contempt.[28] The inquest is an explicitly public procedure[29] forming part of the investigation.[30] The position with regard to publicity of information at the opening and the holding of the inquest is accordingly different, and is discussed later.[31]

Coroner's Powers to Obtain Information

Generally speaking, the family of the deceased, the police, hospitals and other **7–12** institutions co-operate with the coroner's inquiry, and volunteer information without being required by legal process to produce it.[32] Partly for this reason, under the law until 2013 the coroner's power to obtain information from third parties was limited, and rested mainly on (i) potential witnesses volunteering information, (ii) the duty of the police to supply all relevant material in their possession to the coroner,[33] and (iii) the power of the coroner to obtain a witness summons from the High Court (and latterly the county court) to require a witness to come to the inquest and give evidence or bring documents.[34] Now the coroner's power is significantly increased, even though in most cases he will not need to use it. There are two separate provisions of importance. The first relates to the whole period of the investigation, whether before or during any inquest. The second provision relates to the inquest itself. The effect of each provision is not limited to the coroner area for which the coroner is appointed;[35] so it extends throughout England and Wales, though not to Scotland or Northern Ireland.[36]

First, a coroner who is conducting an investigation may by notice require a **7–13** person[37] (a) to provide a written statement about anything specified in the notice, (b) to produce documents in his custody or control relating to a matter relevant to the investigation, or (c) to produce for inspection, examination or testing anything in his custody or control relating to a matter relevant to the investigation, within such period as the coroner thinks reasonable.[38] So this provision has no application where the coroner merely carries out preliminary inquiries, and never comes under an obligation to conduct an investigation.[39] However, where it does apply, the coroner can now require a potential witness (whether of fact or expert opinion) to make a statement, within a stated time, so that the coroner can take into account what that person says in deciding whether to discontinue an investigation[40] or

---

[28] See 10–09, 11–92.
[29] Coroners (Inquests) Rules 2013 (SI 2013/111; see 10–09.
[30] Coroners and Justice Act 2009 s.6; see 10–04.
[31] See 10–09 (opening), and 11–04 (holding).
[32] See 10–65.
[33] See 10–65.
[34] See e.g. *Worcestershire CC v Worcestershire Coroner* [2013] EWHC 1711, QB. This is no longer available to the coroner, since there is now the statutory notice procedure under the 2009 Act: see 7–13.
[35] Coroners and Justice Act 2009 s.32, Sch.5 para.1(7).
[36] Coroners and Justice Act 2009 s.181.
[37] This includes the Crown or an agency of the Crown, such as HMRC: see *R (HMRC) v Liverpool Coroner* [2014] EWHC 1586 (Admin.) DC.
[38] Coroners and Justice Act 2009 s.32, Sch.5 para.1(2).
[39] As to which see 8–13.
[40] As to which see 8–36.

proceed to an inquest,[41] or can consider whether to call that person as a witness at the inquest. There is no statutory requirement to pay or compensate persons for their time in complying with the notice.[42] But an expert can reasonably refuse to prepare and produce a written expert opinion from nothing without a proper fee for the work.[43] The production of an existing written report, not otherwise privileged, would normally be different.

7–14   Second, a coroner who has at least decided to hold an inquest, even if it has not yet been opened, may by notice require a person to attend at a stated time and place (a) to give evidence at the inquest, (b) to produce documents in his custody or control relating to a matter relevant to the inquest, or (c) to produce for inspection, examination or testing anything in his custody or control relating to a matter relevant to the inquest.[44] There is no requirement (as there was under the old law) in respect of (b) and (c) that the production should take place at the inquest itself,[45] or even in public. It could be to the coroner or his officer at the coroner's office. Allowances, fees and expenses are payable by the coroner for work done in connection with or for attendance at an inquest.[46] A person can be punished for disobedience to a notice to attend, even without an appropriate sum by way of conduct money being paid or tendered.[47]

7–15   For the purposes of these two provisions, "document" is not exhaustively defined, but includes information stored in an electronic form.[48] It will include paper documents, photographs, and also electronic computer files, whatever the medium on which they are stored. Non-documentary things are covered by para.(c) in each of the two provisions. A document is under a person's control if it is in his possession or if he has a right to possession of it.[49] But a person cannot be required to provide evidence or documents if he could not be required to do so in civil proceedings in England and Wales (essentially because of the law of privilege, including for this purpose public interest immunity),[50] or if this would be incompatible with an EU obligation.[51]

7–16   A person who claims to be unable to comply with such a coroner's notice, or that it is not reasonable in all the circumstances to require him to comply with it, must apply to the coroner who issued it, who may revoke or vary the notice on that ground.[52] It appears that the High Court has no power to deal with the matter at least until the coroner has made a determination on the point.[53] In deciding whether to revoke or vary a notice, the coroner must consider the public interest

---

[41] As to which see 10–04.
[42] Unlike the position for work done in preparation for attendance at an inquest: see 18–36 ff.
[43] See *Seyfang v GD Searle & Co* [1973] Q.B. 148; *Lively Ltd v City of Munich* [1977] 1 Lloyd's Rep. 418; *Brown v Bennett, The Times*, 2 November 2000.
[44] Coroners and Justice Act 2009 s.32, Sch.5 para.1(1).
[45] See 18–36.
[46] Coroners Allowances, Fees and Expenses Regulations 2013 (SI 2013/1615); see cf *Khanna v Lowell White Durrant* [1995] 1 WLR 121.
[47] See 12–04—12–05.
[48] Coroners and Justice Act 2009 s.48(1).
[49] Coroners and Justice Act 2009 s.32, Sch.5 para.1(6).
[50] Coroners and Justice Act 2009 s.32, Sch.5 para.2(2). For the law on privilege and public interest immunity, see 7–60 ff.
[51] Coroners and Justice Act 2009 s.32, Sch.5 para.2(1).
[52] Coroners and Justice Act 2009 s.32, Sch.5 para.1(4).
[53] See para.1(4): the "claim . . . *is to be determined* . . . by the . . . coroner" (emphasis supplied).

in the information sought being obtained for the purposes of the inquest or investigation, having regard to the likely importance of the information.[54]

The form of notice to be given under either of these two provisions is not **7–17** prescribed.[55] But a notice so given must indicate what the recipient must do if he wishes to apply for the notice to be revoked or varied,[56] and also explain the possible consequences of non-compliance with it.[57] These include the fact that a person who without reasonable excuse fails to comply with such a notice is liable to a fine imposed by the coroner not exceeding £1,000.[58] But they also include two other offences which may be committed in connection with information sought by coroners for an investigation.

First, it is an offence for a person to do anything intended to have the effect of **7–18** (a) distorting or altering anything produced or provided for the purposes of an investigation, or (b) preventing anything from being so produced or provided.[59] Second, it is an offence for a person intentionally to suppress, conceal, alter or destroy a document which that person knows or believes to be one which the coroner (if aware of its existence) would wish to have.[60]

However, proceedings for these two offences can be instituted only by or with **7–19** the consent of the DPP.[61] A person guilty of either offence is on summary conviction liable to a fine not exceeding level 3 on the standard scale, or to imprisonment for a term not exceeding 51 weeks, or both.[62] In each case the offence cannot be committed by doing anything authorised or required by a coroner or authorised by a specific provision[63] preserving privilege, public interest immunity, and certain defences under EU law.[64]

The effect of these statutory provisions on the coroner's pre-existing common **7–20** law powers is not made express. On the one hand, this is a new statutory system intended to take the place of a partly common law and partly statutory system that has accreted over centuries. One view would therefore be that the old powers have gone. On the other hand, implied repeal is generally only accepted where it is of necessity, and there is nothing in the new statutory powers which is inconsistent with the old common law ones. The Chief Coroner's view is that they do not alter or remove those common law powers,[65] and this is the better view. But the coroner's power to seek a witness summons from the High Court in aid of inquest proceedings has now gone, because it depended on the fact that coroners had no

---

[54] Coroners and Justice Act 2009 s.32, Sch.5 para.1(5).
[55] But see App.3 for an unofficial form.
[56] Coroners and Justice Act 2009 s.32, Sch.5 para.1(3)(b).
[57] Coroners and Justice Act 2009 s.32, Sch.5 para.1(3)(a).
[58] Coroners and Justice Act 2009 s.32, Sch.6 para.6. There is nothing to prevent the coroner who issued the notice from sitting to impose the fine, though he or she must obviously hold a hearing complying with the ECHR art.6. Any fine would be collected by the magistrates' court under the Criminal Justice Act 1988 s.67(1): see 11–100.
[59] Coroners and Justice Act 2009 s.32, Sch.6 para.7(1).
[60] Coroners and Justice Act 2009 s.32, Sch.6 para.7(2), (3).
[61] Coroners and Justice Act 2009 s.32, Sch.6 para.7(5).
[62] Coroners and Justice Act 2009 s.32, Sch.6 para.7(6).
[63] Coroners and Justice Act 2009 s.32, Sch.5 para.2.
[64] Coroners and Justice Act 2009 s.32, Sch.6 para.7(4).
[65] *Chief Coroner's Guide to the Coroners and Justice Act 2009*, 2nd edn (July 2013) para.132.

other power to issue a witness summons in relation to their proceedings,[66] and that is no longer the case.

7–21   As already stated, the coroner has the right to possession of the body whilst he makes inquiries into the death.[67] It appears that at common law the coroner or his officer is entitled as part of his inquiries to search not only the body, but also property belonging to the deceased, and even the place where the body was found, if there is reasonable cause to believe that evidence bearing on the purposes of the inquest may thus be found.[68] Similarly it appears that possession may be taken of property relevant to such purposes[69] (and, indeed, of any other property where there is no other suitable person to take charge of it, though this is not part of his duties,[70] and such property must be delivered up to the person entitled to it[71] upon demand).[72]

7–22   On the other hand it is doubtful if a coroner ever had power at common law to enter premises unless the body was there. Indeed, at common law a search warrant could not be issued in cases of murder.[73] In Australia it has been held that a coroner has no common law power to enter premises and search for evidence.[74]As recommended by the Brodrick Report[75] as long ago as 1971, the 2009 Act now therefore makes provision for the coroner, when authorised by or on behalf of the Chief Coroner, to have power of entry onto and search of land, together with power to seize certain things found there.[76] But these provisions have not been brought into force with the other provisions of the Act, and there are no plans at present to do so.

7–23   The common law offence of doing acts tending and intended to pervert the course of justice can be committed in relation to a coroner's inquest. Thus, in one case, a medical practitioner, whose patient's death was the subject of a coroner's inquiry and might also lead to civil or criminal proceedings, falsified the computerised records relating to the patient, so as to make it appear that he was not at fault in connection with the death. The Court of Appeal approved the direction of the trial judge that

> "An act has such a tendency [i.e. to pervert the course of public justice] if it gives rise to the possibility that it will mislead a tribunal concerned with public justice and might cause a miscarriage of justice. Public justice is any judicial proceedings

---

[66] See CPR r.34.4(3).

[67] See 8–11.

[68] Home Office Circular No. 68 of 1955, para.16, summarising the opinion of the Law Officers (Sir Richard Webster AG, and Robert Finlay SG) given in 1896.

[69] As to its retention, see 18–57—18–61.

[70] See 18–57—18–61.

[71] Normally the personal representatives of the deceased: see 9–02 below. In rare cases it may be the Treasury Solicitor: see 9–19 below.

[72] cf. the position once the inquest is over: see 18–53 below. See also *Settelen v Metropolitan Police Commissioner* [2004] EWHC 2171 (Ch).

[73] *Ghani v Jones* [1970] 1 Q.B. 93, CA.

[74] *Ex p. Zinc Corporation* (1969) 90 W.N. (N.S.W.) 654.

[75] See para.13–07.

[76] Coroners and Justice Act 2009 s.32, Sch.5 paras 3–5.

which might arise from the death of [the patient], including an inquest, civil or criminal proceedings."[77]

The coroner who suspects the commission of such an offence should not attempt to deal with the matter himself, but should report the matter to the police.

DISCLOSURE OF INFORMATION

General rule

The law relating to disclosure of information by the coroner to interested persons   **7–24** was completely reformed in the 2013 rules. Although many organisations who investigate deaths routinely disclose reports and other documents to the bereaved family,[78] an interested person (who may not be one of the bereaved) is also entitled to seek disclosure of documents held by the coroner *during* or *after* an investigation, pre-inquest review or inquest.[79] It therefore follows that no right to disclosure arises under these rules where the coroner carries out preliminary inquiries, but never comes under an obligation to conduct an investigation.[80] Of course, interested persons may have other rights to access information about the deceased.[81]

The general rule is that, where an interested person[82] asks[83] for disclosure of a   **7–25** document held by the coroner, the coroner (subject to certain objections)[84] must provide it (or a copy), or make it available for inspection by the applicant as soon as reasonably practicable.[85] But the rules impose no duty on the coroner to tell the interested persons what documents they hold. If an applicant is likely to make a number of requests in succession, a coroner could wait (but not unreasonably) until a bundle of documents could be disclosed together.[86] There is a fee for disclosure *after* an inquest.[87] However, the coroner may not charge a fee for any document or copy disclosed before or during an inquest.[88] Although a coroner's inquiry is inquisitorial in form, coroners can nevertheless expect assistance from interested persons where appropriate, and hence full disclosure to them helps to protect the coroner from allegations of inadequate investigation thereafter.[89]

---

[77] *R. v Sinha, The Times*, July 13, 1994, CA.
[78] For example the Prisons and Probation Ombudsman, the IPCC etc.
[79] Coroners (Inquests) Rules 2013 (SI 2013/1616) r.12; see also Coroners (Investigations) Regulations 2013 (SI 2013/1629) reg.23 ("at any time during the course of an investigation").
[80] As to which see 8–13.
[81] See eg Access to Health Records Act 1990, s.3, Data Protection Act 1998.
[82] Coroners and Justice Act 2009 s.47; see 8–21—8–22.
[83] The request may be informal: *R. (McLeish) v North London Coroner* [2010] EWHC 3624 (Admin.).
[84] Coroners (Inquests) Rules 2013 (SI 2013/1616) r.15; see 7–30.
[85] Coroners (Inquests) Rules 2013 (SI 2013/1616) r.13(1).
[86] *Chief Coroner's Guide to the Coroners and Justice Act 2009*, 2nd edn (July 2013) para.123.
[87] Coroners Allowances, Fees and Expenses Regulations 2013 (SI 2013/115) reg.12; see 18–62.
[88] Coroners (Inquests) Rules 2013 (SI 2013/1616) r.16.
[89] *R. (Shaw) v Leicester City and South Leicestershire ADC* [2014] EWCA Civ. 294.

What are documents?

7–26   For this purpose "document" means any medium in which information of any description is recorded or stored,[90] and "copy" in relation to a document means anything onto which information has been copied, directly or indirectly.[91] "Document held by the coroner" is not exhaustively defined, but is stated to include (a) any post-mortem examination report, (b) any other report provided to the coroner during the course of the investigation, (c) any available recording of any inquest hearing in public (except for any part where the public was properly excluded), and (d) any other document which the coroner considers relevant to the inquest.[92] Obviously, (c) and (d) can only exist once an inquest hearing has taken place or (in the case of (d)) is at least contemplated. Where the coroner obtains statements, whether voluntarily or by compulsion,[93] from potential witnesses (whether of fact or expert opinion), these will prima facie fall within the scope of the disclosure obligation.[94]

Restrictions

7–27   One important restriction on the right to disclosure is not expressly stated, but is clearly implied from reading the whole rule.[95] This is that a "document held by the coroner" must be a document held by the coroner in the context of the *particular* investigation in relation to which the applicant is an interested person, and not merely a document held by the coroner in the context of *any* investigation which the coroner is conducting or has ever conducted. It must also follow that the coroner has no duty to provide a translation of any document he discloses.[95a]

7–28   Another restriction, which appears more clearly from the wording of the rule[96] is that whether the coroner provides the original document or a copy, or allows inspection, is a matter for *the coroner*, and not the applicant. And it is expressly provided that the coroner may manage disclosure by disclosing an electronic copy of a document instead of a paper copy, disclosing a redacted version, or making it available for inspection at a particular time and place.[97] The Chief Coroner advises that disclosure should be by electronic means wherever possible.[98]

7–29   Although nothing is expressly said about any restrictions on use by the applicant of otherwise confidential information contained in disclosed documents, this is a

---

[90] Coroners (Inquests) Rules 2013 (SI 2013/1616) r.2(1). So it will include photographs, audio and video tapes, CDs, DVDs and computer files, whatever the medium on which they are stored.
[91] Coroners (Inquests) Rules 2013 (SI 2013/1616) r.2(1). So the copy could be of the second or subsequent generation (i.e. indirect).
[92] Coroners (Inquests) Rules 2013 (SI 2013/1616) r.13(2).
[93] See 7–12 ff.
[94] In *Jordan v United Kingdom* (2001) 11 BHRC 1 at [133], [134], [142], and in *McShane v United Kingdom*, May 28, 2002 at [122]–[123], the ECtHR criticised the lack of advance disclosure of witness statements at inquests as contributing to a failure to comply with the procedural obligation under art.2.
[95] In particular the references to "interested person" and "*the* coroner" (r.13(1)), "any post-mortem examination report" (r.13(2)(a)), "*the* investigation" (r.13(2)(b)), and "relevant to *the* inquest" (r.13(2)(d)).
[95a] Cf. *Bayer AG v Harris Pharmaceuticals Ltd* [1991] FSR 170 (civil litigation).
[96] Coroners (Inquests) Rules 2013 (SI 2013/1616) r.13(1).
[97] Coroners (Inquests) Rules 2013 (SI 2013/1616) r.14.
[98] *Chief Coroner's Guide to the Coroners and Justice Act 2009*, 2nd edn (July 2013), para.119.

case of compulsory disclosure of information by the coroner to an interested person for the purposes of advancing the investigation and defending their legitimate interests. It therefore falls within the general principle that without the consent of the discloser, the information so disclosed can only be used for those purposes and no others, any breach of this restriction amounting potentially to a contempt of court.[99] The coroner would be wise to bring this point home to the applicant by attaching a notice in suitable terms to the disclosed document or copy.[100] Disclosing such documents in confidence (e.g. to lawyers) for the inquest's purposes will not terminate the restriction.[101] Where the applicant requests disclosure of a recording of an inquest hearing, there will be less risk of the recording somehow finding its way onto the internet, or being tampered with or misused, if the coroner does not send the applicant a copy, electronically or otherwise, but simply allows (auditory) inspection at the coroner's offices.[102]

Objections

The coroner may refuse to disclose a document where (a) this is otherwise **7–30** prohibited by law,[103] (b) author's or copyright holder's consent cannot be reasonably[104] obtained, (c) the request is unreasonable,[105] (d) the document relates to actual or contemplated criminal proceedings, or (e) *the coroner*[106] considers the document irrelevant[107] to the investigation.[108]

A difficult question is raised when a statement or report is supplied to the **7–31** coroner on the basis that it is for his use only, and is not to be further disseminated

---

[99] See e.g. *Marcel v Metropolitan Police Commissioner* [1992] Ch. 225, 237; *Lonrho v Fayed (No. 4)* [1994] Q.B. 775, 788-789; *Scopelight Ltd v Chief Constable of Northumberland* [2010] Q.B. 438, CA. It was held by Kerr J in *Re Jordan's Application* Unreported September 4, 2001, HC (NI), that requiring undertakings to that effect did not infringe the ECHR.

[100] The following is suggested: "This [copy] document is supplied to you under the Coroners (Inquests) Rules 2013, rule 13, only for the purposes of advancing the investigation into the death of [name] and defending your legitimate interests in connection with that investigation, including in any court proceedings for that purpose. You must not disclose or publish it or the information in it (including on the internet or in other media) more widely than is necessary for these purposes. If you do, you may be held to be in contempt of court and liable to be punished as such, including being subjected to a fine or imprisonment. You may however show it to a lawyer for the purposes of taking advice. If you are in any doubt, you should take legal advice."

[101] cf. *Distillers Co (Biochemicals) Ltd v Times Newspapers Ltd* [1975] Q.B. 613.

[102] The problem of clandestine recordings being made at the inspection, if considered to be real, can be dealt with by providing headphones rather than loudspeakers to listen to the recording, and by supervising the applicant during the inspection.

[103] e.g. the document is subject to legal privilege or public interest immunity, and the relevant person has not consented to its deployment; see 7–68. The Chief Coroner advises that police reports to the coroner fall into this category, following *R. (Lagos) v City of London Coroner* [2013] EWHC 423 (Admin): see *Chief Coroner's Guide to the Coroners and Justice Act 2009*, 2nd edn (July 2013), para. 121.

[104] e.g. the author or copyright holder seeks significant payment for consent, or insists on other unreasonable conditions.

[105] e.g. where the applicant has access reasonably available from another source, or has not made any attempt to source elsewhere, or the request requires the coroner to carry out unreasonable searches or commit unreasonably large resources in order to locate the objects of the request.

[106] Emphasis supplied. It is the coroner who decides, subject to judicial review in an appropriate case.

[107] The Chief Coroner advises that this means something which the coroner does not intend to rely on at the inquest: *Chief Coroner's Guide to the Coroners and Justice Act 2009*, 2nd edn (July 2013), para.122.

[108] Coroners (Inquests) Rules 2013 (SI 2013/1616) r.15.

without the maker's (or someone else's) consent. This is common where the police or health and safety authorities are concerned. Those particular cases will usually fall under category (d), however, as documents relating to (contemplated) criminal proceedings. In other cases, if the statement or report was voluntary, the coroner must respect the condition. But, assuming that the witness is within England and Wales, the coroner could use the compulsory power to obtain a statement or report (even in the terms already volunteered), and the statement or report so produced could not be made subject to the same condition.

Chief Coroner's power to obtain information

7–32   The Chief Coroner may at any time require information from a coroner in relation to a particular investigation or investigations which are being conducted by that coroner,[109] and the coroner is obliged to provide it.[110] He also has powers to obtain other information more generally from the coroner.[111]

Data Protection

7–33   The data protection legislation is intended to require those who control and process personal data to do so in accordance with the so-called "data protection principles".[112] The current legislation dates from 1998 and replaces an earlier system dating back to 1984,[113] which was, however, narrower in scope. The legislation is excessively technical, and it is not easy to be sure how it affects coroners. It is certainly not designed with them in mind, and can be capricious in application. Guidance of a general nature (not specific to coroners) is available from the Information Commissioner and the data protection website.[114] Neither the Home Office nor the Ministry of Justice has provided any guidance to coroners on how the legislation affects them.[115]

Data

7–34   "Data" mostly refers to information which is *automatically* processed (e.g. by computer) or recorded for that purpose. But the term extends beyond this, in particular to information recorded as part of a structured and accessible *manual* filing system.[116] However, the term *personal* data is restricted to data relating to an

---

[109] Coroners (Investigations) Regulations 2013 (SI 2013/1629) reg.25(1).
[110] Coroners (Investigations) Regulations 2013 (SI 2013/1629) reg.25(2).
[111] See 2–62—2–63.
[112] Data Protection Act 1998 s.4(1), referring to Sch.1 Pt I.
[113] Data Protection Act 1984.
[114] *http://www.ico.org.uk* [Accessed June 5, 2104].
[115] Home Office Circular No. 35 of 2000, "Responding to Tracing and Similar Enquiries", which (despite its title) represents a limited attempt to summarise the most important provisions of the 1998 Act, though without any specific reference to the position of coroners. In 2009 a judicial working group produced *A Guide to the Data Protection Act 1998 in respect of the Responsibilities of the Judiciary,* which was issued with the agreement of the Lord Chief Justice, the Senior President of Tribunals and the Lord Chancellor.
[116] Data Protection Act 1998 s.1(1), definition of "data". As to what is meant by a "relevant filing system", see *Durant v Financial Services Authority* [2003] F.S.R. 573, CA; [2003] EWCA Civ. 1746.

identifiable *living* individual,[117] and that individual is a "data subject".[118] So coroners are not concerned with data relating to the deceased persons whose deaths they investigate. But of course they may control or process personal data relating to living persons as well (e.g. relatives, interested persons, witnesses, etc.), and the legislation applies to that. The term "sensitive personal data" means personal data concerned with the person's racial origins, political opinions, religious beliefs, trade union membership, health, sex life, criminal behaviour or criminal proceedings against him.[119]

Data are "processed" if they are obtained, recorded or held, or *any operation* is   **7–35** carried out to them.[120] So coroners are certainly involved in processing data. A "data processor" is generally any person, not being an employee of the data controller, who processes personal data on behalf of the data controller.[121] The "data controller" is normally a person who (either alone or jointly or in common with other persons) determines the purposes for which and the manner in which the personal data are to be processed.[122] The coroner will accordingly be a data controller. His staff (not being his employees) who process the data will be data processors. If the coroner or his own employees process the data, the coroner will be a data processor as well.

Notification

Unless exempt from doing so, a data controller has to notify the Information   **7–36** Commissioner and be entered in the Data Protection Register[123] before processing personal data,[124] otherwise he commits an offence.[125] However, the law was amended in 2009 to exempt "judges" from the need to notify, and the Information Commissioner has accepted since 2010 that coroners fall within the wide definition of "judge" for this purpose.[126] Hence they are exempted from the obligation to notify for all processing by a coroner or person acting on a coroner's instructions or on his behalf for the purposes of exercising judicial functions.[127] There is no definition of "judicial functions". But, since coroners do not normally act as employers of their staff, it is difficult to envisage their being controllers of personal data except in relation to living persons involved in their judicial investigations. In relation to that data, the purpose of the processing will be in order

---

[117] Data Protection Act 1998 s.1(1), definition of "personal data". The definition is to be narrowly construed, to cover information which affects the privacy of the data subject, "whether in his personal or family life, business or professional capacity", and would not include for example information recorded by a public authority merely because of a complaint made to it the data subject about the conduct of a third party: *Durant v Financial Services Authority* [2003] F.S.R. 573, CA; [2003] EWCA Civ. 1746.

[118] Data Protection Act 1998 s.1(1), definition of "personal subject".

[119] Data Protection Act 1998 s.2.

[120] Data Protection Act 1998 s.1(1), definition of "processing".

[121] Data Protection Act 1998 s.1(1), definition of "data processor".

[122] Data Protection Act 1998 s.1(1), definition of "data controller".

[123] Data Protection Act 1998 s.18.

[124] Data Protection Act 1998 s.17(1).

[125] Data Protection Act 1998 s.21(1).

[126] Data Protection (Notification and Notification Fees) Regulations 2000 (SI 2000/188) Sch. para.1, definition of "judge' (as inserted by SI 2009/1677 reg.2).

[127] Data Protection (Notification and Notification Fees) Regulations 2000 (SI 2000/188) Sch. para.6 (as inserted by SI 2009/1677 reg.2).

to exercise judicial functions. (In relation to the personal data of staff not employed by the coroner, the data controller will normally be their employer.)

The data protection principles

7-37 Although exempt from notification, the coroner in processing data must still abide by the "data protection principles".[128] A serious contravention of these principles may result in a monetary penalty.[129] The principles may be summarised as follows (though the full statutory statements contain some qualifications):[130]

(1) personal data must be processed fairly and lawfully, and one or more conditions (discussed below) must also be met;[131]

(2) personal data must be obtained only for specified and lawful purposes, and not processed incompatibly with those purposes;[132]

(3) personal data must be adequate, relevant and not excessive in relation to the processing purposes;[133]

(4) personal data must be accurate and kept up to date;[134]

(5) personal data must not be kept for longer than necessary;[135]

(6) personal data must be processed in accordance with the rights of data subjects;[136]

(7) appropriate measures must be taken against unauthorised or unlawful processing of personal data, and against loss of or damage to such data;[137]

(8) personal data must not be transferred outside the EEA unless the destination ensures adequate protection for the rights of data subjects.[138]

7-38 As regards the first principle, the coroner in processing personal data must satisfy at least one of six stated conditions.[139] Normally he will satisfy at least two of them, that is (i) that the processing is necessary for compliance with a legal obligation (not being contractual) of the coroner,[140] and (ii) that it is necessary for the administration of justice, for the exercise of functions conferred on the coroner under an enactment, or for the exercise by the coroner of functions of a public

---

[128] Data Protection Act 1998 s.4(4).
[129] Data Protection Act 1998 s.55A.
[130] Data Protection Act 1998 s.4(2) requires that the principles be interpreted in accordance with Sch.1 Pt II.
[131] Data Protection Act 1998 s.4, Sch.1 Pt I para.1.
[132] Data Protection Act 1998 s.4, Sch.1 Pt I para.2.
[133] Data Protection Act 1998 s.4, Sch.1 Pt I para.3.
[134] Data Protection Act 1998 s.4, Sch.1 Pt I para.4.
[135] Data Protection Act 1998 s.4, Sch.1 Pt I para.5.
[136] Data Protection Act 1998 s.4, Sch.1 Pt I para.6.
[137] Data Protection Act 1998 s.4, Sch.1 Pt I para.7.
[138] Data Protection Act 1998 s.4, Sch.1 Pt I para.8.
[139] Data Protection Act 1998 s.4(3). The six conditions are set out in Sch.2.
[140] Data Protection Act 1998 s.4, Sch.2 para.3.

nature in the public interest.[141] In some cases he will also satisfy a third, namely, that the processing is necessary for the purposes of legitimate interests pursued by the coroner or a third party to whom he discloses the data.[142]

In addition, if the coroner processes *sensitive* personal data, he must satisfy at least   7–39
one of 11 further conditions.[143] Where an inquest is held, the coroner will generally satisfy at least two of them, that is (i) that the processing is necessary for the purposes of or in connection with any legal proceedings,[144] and (ii) that it is necessary for the administration of justice, or for the exercise of functions conferred on the coroner under an enactment.[145] Where no inquest is held, he will usually still satisfy the second.

As regards the eighth principle, this does not apply in certain circumstances.[146]   7–40
Only two of these circumstances are likely to apply to the coroner, namely (i) that the transfer is necessary for purposes of substantial public interest,[147] and (ii) that the transfer is necessary for the purposes of or in connection with any legal proceedings.[148] But a coroner will rarely have to consider the transfer of personal data outside the EEA anyway.

Some data or processing are exempt from some of the data protection principles   7–41
in certain cases. In particular, personal data is exempt from the "non-disclosure provisions"[149] of the data protection legislation when the disclosure is required by law, or under an order of the court,[150] or where it is necessary for the purposes of or in connection with any legal proceedings.[151]

Rights of data subjects

Individuals have the right under the data protection legislation, by written request,   7–42
and on payment of a fee,[152] to require a data controller (a) to inform them whether their personal data are being processed, (b) if so, to inform them what they are, for what purposes they are being processed, and the recipients to whom they are or may be disclosed, and (c) to have a copy of them accompanied by information as to their source.[153] But the data controller does not have to respond until any further information which he may reasonably require in order to satisfy himself of the applicant's identity and the location of the information sought has been supplied.[154] There are provisions to deal with the case where the data controller cannot

---

[141] Data Protection Act 1998 s.4, Sch.2 para.5(a), (b), (d).
[142] Data Protection Act 1998 s.4, Sch.2 para.6.
[143] Data Protection Act 1998 s.4(3). The 11 conditions are set out in Sch.3.
[144] Data Protection Act 1998 s.4, Sch.3 para.6(a).
[145] Data Protection Act 1998 s.4, Sch.3 para.7(1)(a), (b).
[146] Data Protection Act 1998 s.4(3). The circumstances are set out in Sch.4.
[147] Data Protection Act 1998 s.4, Sch.4 para.4(1).
[148] Data Protection Act 1998 s.4, Sch.4 para.5(a).
[149] Data Protection Act 1998 s.27(3), (4), defines these as meaning principles 1–5, and ss.10 and 14(1)–(3) of the Act. But it includes principle 1 only to the extent that it does not require compliance with the conditions in Schs 2 and 3.
[150] Data Protection Act 1998 s.35(1).
[151] Data Protection Act 1998 s.35(2)(a).
[152] Data Protection Act 1998 s.7(2).
[153] Data Protection Act 1998 s.7(1). See *P v Wozencroft*, [2002] EWHC 1724 (Fam); [2002] 2 FLR 1118; [2002] Fam. Law 806, Fam Div.
[154] Data Protection Act 1998 s.7(3).

comply with the request without disclosing information relating to another individual.[155]

7–43   The data controller must respond to a subject access request within the "prescribed period", currently 40 days[156] from the date of the request and receipt of any further information needed.[157] Coroners should not underestimate the time and effort that may be needed to comply with these requests. They may find that their funding local authority's data protection/freedom of information department (which will generally be experienced in this area of the law) is prepared to deal with such requests on their behalf, so that coroners do not have to deal personally with them.

7–44   Data subjects also have certain rights to prevent the processing of their personal data in some cases,[158] and may obtain compensation for damage suffered by reason of any contravention of the legislation by the data controller.[159] The court may also order the correction or erasure of inaccurate personal data.[160]

FREEDOM OF INFORMATION

7–45   It is desirable to mention briefly here the more general statutory obligation imposed upon "public authorities" to disclose information held by them to the public on request.[161] This does not directly affect coroners, since (like other judges) they are not "public authorities" within the meaning of the legislation.[162] Thus coroners have no obligation to respond to requests made under the Act in relation to information which coroners hold. Nor does it affect them indirectly, since the information which coroners hold is likely to be "exempt information", either because it is reasonably accessible to the applicant by other means,[163] or because it is contained in documents held by a court or inquiry for its purposes.[164] It is also exempt information if it has been obtained in circumstances where to disclose it would amount to an actionable breach of confidence,[165] or if it is subject to a prohibition on disclosure under other laws.[166]

---

[155] Data Protection Act 1998 s.7(4)–(6). As to whether the data controller should consider it reasonable to comply with a request for disclosure of personal data even though data about another person (who has not consented) is included, see *Durant v Financial Services Authority* [2003] F.S.R. 573, CA; [2003] EWCA Civ. 1746.

[156] Data Protection (Subject Access) (Fees and Miscellaneous Provisions) Regulations 2000 (SI 2000/191).

[157] Data Protection Act 1998 s.7(8).

[158] Data Protection Act 1998 ss.10–12. See *AB v Syvret* [2013] J.R.C. 170, Royal Court of Jersey.

[159] Data Protection Act 1998 s.13.

[160] Data Protection Act 1998 s.14.

[161] Freedom of Information Act 2000 s.1.

[162] Freedom of Information Act 2000 ss.3, 4, Sch.1; but the Lord Chancellor may by order so designate them under s.5.

[163] Freedom of Information Act 2000 s.21.

[164] Freedom of Information Act 2000 s.32. See also *Galloway v Information Commissioner* [2009] 108 B.M.L.R. 50 (statements for purposes of hospital SUI investigation held exempt); *Kennedy v The Charity Commission* [2014] UKSC 20 (charity inquiry documents exempt).

[165] Freedom of Information Act 2000 s.41; see *Bluck v Information Commissioner*, Information Tribunal, September 17, 2007 (medical records of deceased not to be disclosed to deceased's mother without widower's consent).

[166] Freedom of Information Act 2000 s.44.

Furthermore, if a public authority (such as a local authority) holds information **7–46** *on behalf of* the coroner, as for example where his files are stored in its archives, that information is not "held by a public authority" for the purposes of the Act,[167] and hence the authority cannot be made to respond positively to a request in relation to it. Indeed, since the information would inevitably be confidential, the authority would owe a duty to the coroner to respond *negatively* to the request. The consequence of this is that under this legislation there is in any event no obligation on any "public authority" to disclose the existence or content of such information.[168]

Where a coroner sends a report to prevent further deaths during or after an **7–47** inquest, the coroner has no obligation to respond to a freedom of information request, and ordinarily should not do so. Whether the recipient (being a public authority) must do so will depend on the circumstances.[169] Even if it is clear that the recipient would have to disclose the report, it is not appropriate for the coroner to sidestep the procedures imposed and protections conferred by the freedom of information legislation. But, except in cases where the information in the report is confidential, it does not seem that there is anything to prevent an interested person who has a copy from disclosing it.

COPYRIGHT

Copyright is a statutory monopoly for a certain length of time on the use of certain **7–48** types of intellectual work product. The discussion that follows relates to works created on or after August 1, 1989.[170] Copyright takes the form of a property right, granted to the author of (or in some cases other copyright-holder in relation to) certain works.[171] These are original literary, dramatic, musical or artistic works,[172] sound recordings,[173] films[174] or broadcasts,[175] and the typographical arrangement of published editions.[176] Letters and other written documents are "literary" works,[177] as indeed are oral statements,[178] and photographs are "artistic" works[179] for this purpose.

---

[167] Freedom of Information Act 2000 s.3(2).

[168] Freedom of Information Act 2000 s.2.

[169] e.g. it may be exempt information under s.32(1)(c)(i) or (2)(b) (document created by a court or a person conducting an inquiry, for the purposes of proceedings or the inquiry).

[170] Works made on or after June 1, 1957 and before August 1, 1957 are governed by the Copyright Act 1956, and works made on or after July 1, 1912 and before June 1, 1957 are governed by the Copyright Act 1912.

[171] Copyright, Designs and Patents Act 1988 s.1(1).

[172] Copyright, Designs and Patents Act 1988 ss.3 (literary, musical, dramatic), 4 (artistic).

[173] Copyright, Designs and Patents Act 1988 s.5A.

[174] Copyright, Designs and Patents Act 1988 s.5B.

[175] Copyright, Designs and Patents Act 1988 s.6.

[176] Copyright, Designs and Patents Act 1988 s.8.

[177] Copyright, Designs and Patents Act 1988 s.3(1); *British Oxygen Co Ltd v Liquid Air Ltd* [1925] Ch. 383; *Tett Bros Ltd v Drake and Gorham Ltd* (1934) MacG. Cop. Cas. (1928–35) 492.

[178] Although in that case copyright does not subsist in them until they are recorded, whether in writing or otherwise: s.3(2).

[179] Copyright, Designs and Patents Act 1988 s.4(1)(a).

7–49   The author of a work is the person who creates it.[180] Even a reporter who reports the words spoken on a public occasion may be regarded as an author if he uses skill, labour and judgment in doing so.[181] This is likely to mean that when police or other agencies take the statement of a witness and reduce it to writing, they rather than the witness will be the author. The author is the first owner of the copyright,[182] with certain exceptions. Two of these are of particular interest to the coroner. First, in the case of a literary, dramatic, musical or artistic work or a film made on or after July 1, 1994 by an employee in the course of his employment the first owner is the employer, subject to any agreement to the contrary.[183]

7–50   Second, where a work is made by an officer or servant of the Crown in the course of his duties, Her Majesty is the first owner of any copyright in the work.[184] There is no authority as to whether works (such as letters, memoranda, judgments or rulings) produced by a judge or a coroner in the course of his duties fall within the scope of this provision. But it is submitted that they do. The coroner, like the judge, may not be the *servant* of the Crown, but he does *hold office* under the Crown,[185] and therefore can properly be described as an "officer" of the Crown.[186]

7–51   In the case of a literary, dramatic, musical or artistic work the normal term of copyright expires at the end of the period of 70 years from the end of the calendar year in which the author dies.[187] In the case of a sound recording the term is 50 years from the end of the year in which it was first made or (if later) published or (if not published) made available to the public.[188] For a film, the period is 70 years from the end of the year in which the last of certain persons involved in the creation of the film dies.[189] For broadcasts it is 50 years from the end of the year

---

[180] Copyright, Designs and Patents Act 1988 s.9(1). In the case of a sound recording this is the producer: s.9(2)(aa). In the case of a film, it is the producer and the principal director: s.9(2)(a). In the case of a photograph it is usually the photographer, but the person who directs how and when it is taken may be the author instead, or at least a co-author, depending on the degree of control and collaboration: *Creation Records Ltd v News Group Newspapers Ltd* [1997] EMLR 444, 450–451.

[181] *Walter v Lane* [1900] A.C. 539, HL; *Express Newspapers plc v News (UK) Ltd* [1990] 3 All E.R. 376.

[182] Copyright, Designs and Patents Act 1988 s.11(1).

[183] Copyright, Designs and Patents Act 1988 s.11(2).

[184] Copyright, Designs and Patents Act 1988 s.163(1)(b).

[185] See 1–11 ff.

[186] For a contrary argument, see Laddie, Prescott and Vitoria, *The Modern Law of Copyright and Designs*, 4th edn (2011) paras 39.46–39.47. But the argument is misconceived. In part it relies on the fact that an officer can be told by the Crown what to do, and a judge (or coroner) could not be told how to decide. But the premise is false. Even if it were true for *many* or even *most* officers, that would not prove it were true for *all*. For example many ministers, in carrying out their duties, cannot be told what to do. And in part the argument relies on the fact that in the Senior Courts Act 1981 what the Act calls "judges" and "officers" are dealt with in different parts of the Act (although many of the "officers" are in fact junior judges). But the same Act also makes clear that each High Court and Court of Appeal judge holds an "office" (e.g. s.11(1), "This section applies to the office of any judge of the [Senior Courts]"), so it does not take the argument very far.

[187] Copyright, Designs and Patents Act 1988 s.12(2). Exceptional cases are dealt with in the remaining provisions of the section.

[188] Copyright, Designs and Patents Act 1988 s.13A(2). Exceptional cases are dealt with in the remaining provisions of the section.

[189] Copyright, Designs and Patents Act 1988 s.13B(2). Exceptional cases are dealt with in the remaining provisions of the section.

it which it was made.[190] In the case of Crown copyright, however, the term a literary, dramatic, musical or artistic work is 125 years.[191]

The owner of the copyright in a work has the rights to copy the work, to issue   **7–52**
copies or rent or lend it, and to perform, show or play or communicate it, to the public, or to make an adaptation of it.[192] A person who does or authorises another to do any of these things without the copyright-owner's licence infringes the copyright.[193] From the coroner's perspective, the most significant infringing act will be to copy the work without licence. In relation to a literary, dramatic, musical or artistic work this means reproducing the work in any material form, including storing the work in any medium by electronic means.[194] It is not necessary to show the intention to infringe.[195] But it is not an infringement of copyright to reproduce the *idea* in a copyright work without copying the *form* in which it is expressed,[196] nor to produce a similarity between two works by mere coincidence.[197] Other forms of infringement include renting or lending copies of the work to the public,[198] or communicating it (including making it available electronically) to the public.[199]

From the coroner's perspective, there are two separate aspects to copyright law.   **7–53**
The first is that the coroner or his staff may create works in which copyright subsists, and the question arises whether others may so act as to infringe that copyright. The second is that the coroner or his staff may do acts which might infringe the copyright of others.

As to the first of these, one problem for the coroner is that in most cases he does   **7–54**
not employ anyone personally. Usually the Police Authority or the local authority is the employer of his staff.[200] So the copyright in letters and other documents created by his staff on his behalf may belong in law to those employers rather than to him. And the copyright in photographs made by photographers employed by the police may well belong to the police. It would therefore be sensible to have an advance agreement in place between the coroner, the employer and the employee that the copyright should belong to the coroner.[201] This will make it quicker and easier in any dispute to make clear where the ownership lies. But copyright in sound recordings made by the coroner's staff (whoever employs them) at his direction will probably belong to the coroner as the "producer".[202]

Where works are created by independent contractors, such as the pathologist, to   **7–55**
whom the coroner pays a fee for the work done, the copyright in the work will

---

[190] Copyright, Designs and Patents Act 1988 s.14.
[191] Copyright, Designs and Patents Act 1988 s.163(3)(a).
[192] Copyright, Designs and Patents Act 1988 s.16(1).
[193] Copyright, Designs and Patents Act 1988 s.16(2).
[194] Copyright, Designs and Patents Act 1988 s.17(2). This will include posting to an internet website.
[195] *Sony Music Entertainment (UK) Ltd v Easyinternetcafe Ltd* [2003] EWHC 62 (Ch).
[196] *USP plc v London General Holdings Ltd* [2006] F.S.R. 65.
[197] *Mattel Inc v Woolbro (Distributors) Ltd* [2004] FSR 12, Ch D.
[198] Copyright, Designs and Patents Act 1988 s.18A.
[199] Copyright, Designs and Patents Act 1988 s.20. Again, this will include posting to an internet website.
[200] See 2–130 ff.
[201] See 7–149.
[202] See 12–104.

belong at law to the contractor. But if expressly or impliedly the copyright was to belong to the coroner, he will probably be the equitable or beneficial owner.[203] In circumstances where (i) the work product is fact-specific, every autopsy report being different, (ii) the pathologist is forbidden by law to supply a copy of the report to any other person,[204] and so cannot re-use the work for another client, and (iii) the coroner needs to be able to enforce copyright against third parties who might otherwise wish to publish it (e.g. the media), this must be implied.[205] In homicide cases where the pathologist is also retained by the police,[206] the report may belong in equity both to the coroner and to the police. Where works are created by third parties, such as the PPO or the HSE, for their own purposes, and they are shown to the coroner for his information, the position is different. Again, the copyright will belong at law to the third party, but the coroner can have no claim to equitable or beneficial ownership.

7–56   Looking at the second aspect, the coroner may make copies of a copyright work for purely internal purposes, such as research, or for placing on files, or for forensic purposes, such as inserting in an inquest bundle to be used in court, or for external purposes such as sending to another person or authority for action or by way of report (such as the Chief Coroner). Or the coroner may disclose a copyright document by making and supplying a copy of it to a person entitled to such disclosure. All of these have the potential for infringement of copyright. But there are possible defences which the coroner may rely on in the face of any such allegation.

7–57   The first is that copyright is not infringed by anything done for the purposes of judicial proceedings.[207] Once an inquest has been opened,[208] at least, there are in existence judicial proceedings for the purposes of which a potentially infringing action may be done. Indeed, since 2013, it is clear that a coroner may exercise judicial functions even before an inquest is opened, once an investigation is under way.[209] So, for example, copying bundles containing copyright material for the purposes of a contemplated or forthcoming inquest hearing would not amount to an infringement.

7–58   The second is that doing an act specifically authorised by an Act of Parliament does not infringe copyright unless that Act so provides.[210] So the question is whether, where a coroner provides a copy of a copyright work under compulsion, for example by virtue of the disclosure rules,[211] that disclosure is "specifically authorised by an Act of Parliament". The disclosure rules made in 2013 were made under powers in the 2009 Act which did not require, but did clearly permit, that they be so made.[212] It is therefore submitted that the disclosure is "specifically

---

[203] *A & M Records Ltd v Video Collection International Ltd* [1995] EMLR 25; *Ray v Classic FM plc* [1998] F.S.R. 622; *R Griggs Group v Evans* [2005] F.S.R. 706.
[204] Coroners (Investigations) Regulations 2013 (SI 2013/1629) reg.16(2); see 8–70.
[205] See *R Griggs Group v Evans* [2005] F.S.R. 706.
[206] See 8–48, 8–52.
[207] Copyright, Designs and Patents Act 1988 s.45(1).
[208] As to which see 10–05.
[209] Coroners (Investigations) Regulations 2013 (SI 2013/1629) reg.7: "A coroner may delegate administrative, but not judicial functions".
[210] Copyright, Designs and Patents Act 1988 s.50(1).
[211] Coroners (Inquests) Rules 2013 (SI 2013/1616) rr.12–16; see 7–24 ff.
[212] Coroners and Justice Act 2009 ss.43(3)(d), 45(2)(g).

authorised" by the 2009 Act. The Act specifically authorised the making of rules which could (i.e. delegated the decision whether to) require the disclosure.

A further point is that if the coroner asks for the permission of the copyright-   **7–59** holder to copy the document to the applicant, but cannot reasonably obtain permission, the coroner may refuse to give the disclosure by copy.[213] This is not a defence to an allegation of infringement. Instead it releases the coroner from the obligation he would otherwise have to do the act which might amount to an infringement. If a third party (*e.g.* the HSE) supplies a copy of a document in which it has copyright to the coroner confidentially, on terms that it is not to be disclosed further, and declines to permit the coroner to disclose it to interested persons, the coroner may refuse to disclose it on the grounds above stated. Although he would not infringe copyright by copying it, if he did so for the purposes of judicial proceedings, or because it was specifically authorised by an Act, he might find it less likely that the third party would disclose further such material to him in the future.

PRIVILEGE

This chapter is about information that the coroner may have, and the restrictions   **7–60** upon it. A very significant restriction upon such information is the law of privilege. Privilege operates to restrict the information that may be available to the coroner, or which may be deployed, at the inquest. But it can apply even before that, during preliminary inquiries or the early stages of the investigation. For example, the coroner's power to require a person to supply information or evidence[214] is subject to the law of privilege,[215] as also is the coroner's duty to disclose relevant documents in his possession to interested persons.[216]

There are three kinds of privilege which are relevant here. First, there is the right   **7–61** of a person (usually, but not always, a witness giving evidence in court) not to answer any question tending to incriminate him or her: the privilege against self-incrimination. Secondly, there is the privilege of a person who has sought or received legal advice or assistance in certain circumstances not to be compelled to reveal what has passed between him and his lawyer, or confidential information about his litigation, and further to prevent his lawyer from so revealing either. This is called legal professional privilege. Thirdly, there is the "privilege" preventing certain types or pieces of information from being disclosed in court by reason of the harm that would or might be done to the public interest if they were so disclosed. This is not a "privilege" of the same kind as the first two, and in modern times it is usually known as public interest immunity.

---

[213] See 7–30.
[214] Coroners and Justice Act 2009 s.32, Sch.5 para.1; see 7–13,—7–14.
[215] Coroners and Justice Act 2009 s.32, Sch.5 para.2.
[216] See 7–30.

Self-incrimination

7–62   Before 1953, the rule against self-incrimination in the coroner's inquiry was the ordinary common law rule, i.e. that a person[217] "cannot be caused to answer any question that would tend to incriminate him or to expose either himself or his wife to a possible criminal prosecution nor to produce any document that might have a similar effect: the rule does not apply to the danger of a mere civil liability".[218] Since then, however, it has been expressly provided by secondary legislation that a witness at an inquest is not obliged to answer any question tending to incriminate him or her.[219] This is much narrower than the common law rule. For one thing, the statutory rule in terms only applies to witnesses at an inquest. The common law rule alone applies to questions put or information sought *before* the inquest.

7–63   The statutory rule gives no definition of what is meant by "incriminate". At common law, an incriminating question is one the answer to which would tend to expose the witness to a criminal charge, penalty or forfeiture reasonably likely to be preferred or sued for,[220] and (as already stated) the rule applied to documents as well as to oral evidence.[221] The court has to be satisfied that there is a "real and appreciable" risk of prosecution.[222] A mere possibility is insufficient.[223] But the privilege applies to steps in the chain, even when there is already evidence tending to incriminate.[224]

7–64   Since 1968 the common law privilege, in *all* legal proceedings except criminal proceedings, has by statute been stated to extend only to criminal offences under the law of any part of the United Kingdom, *but* to cover incrimination of one's spouse.[225] Exposure to a penalty remains unaffected,[226] but exposure to a forfeiture is no longer an objection (except in criminal proceedings).[227] That last point apart, it has been said that the statute merely stated the common law position.[228] A witness is not, however, privileged from answering questions merely because the answers would tend to expose him to a subsequent civil action, even at the suit of the Crown[229] (unless the proceedings are for the recovery of a penalty). Strictly speaking, the wording of the rule does not require that the criminal charge or proceedings for a penalty or forfeiture are reasonably *likely* to be instituted.[230]

---

[217] In English law, this includes a corporate body: *Triplex Safety Glass Co Ltd v Lancegaye Saftey Glass (1934) Ltd* [1939] 2 K.B. 395, CA.

[218] The 8th edn of this work (1946) at p.9; in fact the rule was slightly wider, in extending beyond criminal charges to civil penalties and forfeitures: see Cross, *Evidence,* 3rd edn (1967), pp.227–231.

[219] Coroners (Inquests) Rules 2013 r.22, replacing Coroners Rules 1984 r.22, itself replacing Coroners Rules 1953 r.18. The coroner must warn the witness when the question is asked: r.22(2); see 12–94.

[220] *R. v Boyes* (1861) 1 B. & S. 311; *Blunt v Park Lane Hotel* [1942] 2 K.B. 253.

[221] *Spokes v Grosvenor Hotel* [1897] 2 Q.B. 124.

[222] *Compagnie Noga d'Importation et d'Exportation SA v Australian and New Zealand Banking Group Ltd* [2007] EWHC 85 (Comm).

[223] *Tarasov v Nassif* Unreported February 11, 1994, CA.

[224] *Tate Access Floors Ltd v Boswell* [1991] Ch. 512, 529.

[225] Civil Evidence Act 1968 s.14(1).

[226] *Re Westinghouse Electric Corporation Uranium Contract Litigation, MDL Docket No. 235* [1978] A.C. 547, CA.

[227] Civil Evidence Act 1968 s.14(1)(a).

[228] *Rio Tinto Zinc Corpn. v Westinghouse Electric Corpn.* [1978] A.C. 547 at 636, per Lord Diplock.

[229] Witnesses Act 1806.

[230] cf. *Blunt v Park Lane Hotel* [1942] 2 K.B. 253.

Whether the privilege applies where answering questions would tend to expose   **7-65**
the witness to a professional disciplinary charge is less clear. One Court of Appeal
decision assumed (without deciding) that it did apply, but held that the effect of the
professional rules in that case (concerning accountancy) meant that any such
privilege as there might be had been waived by the professional.[231] A later Court
of Appeal decision, however, held that disciplinary proceedings under the Financial
Services Act 1986 simply did not attract the privilege.[232] Where (as is the case with
the General Medical Council Fitness to Practice Panel) the function of the
proceedings is to protect the public rather than to punish the professional,[233] and
the sanctions available relate to the ability to practise rather than to financial or
similar penalties, it is submitted that the privilege is not thereby engaged.

A different problem concerns spouses. Both the common law rule and the 1968   **7-66**
statutory restatement extended the privilege to answers tending to incriminate
spouses. However, the provision in the Coroners Rules does not. Whilst it is clear
that the common law privilege continued after 1953 to apply to all stages of the
inquiry before the inquest itself, it is a question whether the statutory rule
impliedly abrogated it for the inquest. As a matter of construction, an important
privilege of this kind should not be abrogated without express, or at least
necessarily implied,[234] provision.[235] Perhaps more importantly, the statutory power
to make rules "for regulating the practice and procedure at or in connection with
inquests"[236] probably did not extend to rules removing substantive rights of this
kind.[237] Hence it seems that the common law privilege still applies in the coroner's
court along with the Coroners Rules version.

Legal professional privilege

Next, there is legal professional privilege. This is much more than a rule of   **7-67**
evidence.[238] It is a substantive legal principle.[239] A witness need not, and the lawyer
whose client[240] he is must not, without the consent of that client, disclose or give
evidence (written or oral) of confidential communications between them made
either for the purpose of seeking, obtaining or giving legal advice ("advice

---

[231] *R. v Institute of Chartered Accountants of England and Wales Ex p Nawaz* Unreported April 25, 1997, CA; at first instance the judge had *held,* rather than assumed, that the privilege applied: [1997] PNLR 433.

[232] *Official Receiver v Stern, re Westminster Property Management Ltd* [2000] 1 W.L.R. 2230, CA.

[233] *Gupta v General Medical Council* [2002] 1 W.L.R. 1691, PC; *Raschid v General Medical Council* [2007] 1 W.L.R. 1460 at [16], CA.

[234] i.e. implication "which necessarily follows from the express provisions of the statute construed in their context": *R. v Special Commissioner Ex p. Morgan Grenfell & Co Ltd* [2002] 3 All E.R. 1 at [45], per Lord Hobhouse; see also *R. v DPP* [2000] 2 A.C. 428 at 481.

[235] *R. v Home Secretary Ex p. Simms* [2000] 2 A.C. 115, HL; *R. v Special Commissioner Ex p. Morgan Grenfell & C. Ltd* [2002] 3 All E.R. 1 at [8], [44].

[236] Coroners (Amendment) Act 1926 s.26 (now replaced by Coroners Act 1988 s.32(1)).

[237] *Re Grosvenor Hotel, London (No. 2)* [1965] 1 Ch. 1210, CA (rules of court under Supreme Court (Consolidation) Act 1925 s.99, enabling rules to be made regulating practice and procedure in court, could not abrogate public interest immunity).

[238] *R. v Derby Magistrates' Court Ex p. B* [1996] 1 A.C. 487, HL.

[239] *R v Inland Revenue Commissioners Ex p Morgan Grenfell* [2003] 1 A.C. 563 at [7]; *Three Rivers DC v Bank of England (No. 6)* [2005] 1 A.C. 610 at [26].

[240] Usually the relationship is that of professional and private client, but the same principles apply to an employed lawyer and his employer, whose full-time adviser he is: *Alfred Crompton Amusement Machines v Commissioners of Customs & Excise (No. 2)* [1974] A.C. 405, HL.

privilege"),[241] or for the purpose of pending or contemplated litigation ("litigation privilege").[242] Advice privilege covers advice to an interested person for the purposes of a coroner's inquest.[243] Litigation privilege extends to confidential communications between either the lawyer or the client and third parties, where such communications are made for the purposes of pending or contemplated litigation,[244] and also extends to reports made internally in an organisation, if (in each case) the dominant purpose of making such communication or report was for use for the purposes of such litigation.[245]

7–68   The privilege is that of the client,[246] who may waive it if he chooses,[247] and not that of the lawyer[248] or third party,[249] who may not. For this purpose "lawyer" covers not only a solicitor or barrister, but any "authorised person" in relation to rights of audience, the conduct of litigation, or conveyancing or probate services,[250] and any "licensed body" providing such services.[251]

7–69   The privilege extends even to communications which—if disclosed—would help to further the defence of an accused person.[252] But it does not extend to communications between lawyer and client whereby the client seeks advice intended to facilitate or guide the client in the commission of a crime or fraud (even if the lawyer is ignorant of the purpose for which his advice is wanted),[253] nor to documents brought into existence in the course of or in furtherance of a fraud to which the client is party.[254] It should also be noted that privilege, as with self-incrimination, applies to persons and not to information. Thus a person not within the scope of the privilege, but who is able to give evidence of the communications between a lawyer and client, may do so.[255] Legal professional privilege is not lost by the death of the client, but survives for the benefit of the estate.[256]

7–70   **Privilege between trade mark or patent agent and client.** For the sake of completeness, it should be mentioned that there is a modern privilege, analogous to that for the lawyer and client relationship, for communications passing between

---

[241] *Wheeler v Le Marchant* (1881) 17 Ch. D. 675, CA; *Balabel v Air India* [1988] Ch. 317, CA; *Visx Inc. v Nidex Co* [1999] F.S.R. 91, CA.

[242] *Wheeler v Le Marchant* (1881) 17 Ch. D. 675, 681, CA; *Lee v South West Thames Regional Health Authority* [1985] 1 W.L.R. 845; *Three Rivers DC v Bank of England (No. 6)* [2005] 1 A.C. 610 at [102].

[243] *Three Rivers DC v Bank of England (No. 6)* [2005] 1 A.C. 610 at [115]; see also at [39], [56].

[244] *Three Rivers DC v Bank of England (No. 6)* [2005] 1 A.C. 610 at [102].

[245] *Waugh v British Railways Board* [1979] A.C. 521, HL; *Re Barings plc* [1998] 1 All E.R. 673.

[246] *Calcraft v Guest* [1898] 1 Q.B. 759 at 761.

[247] *Re International Power Industries NV* [1985] B.C.L.C. 128.

[248] *Procter v Smiles* (1886) 55 L.J.Q.B. 467.

[249] *Schneider v Leigh* [1955] 2 Q.B. 195, CA.

[250] Legal Services Act 2007 s.190(1), (2).

[251] Legal Services Act 2007 s.190(3), (4).

[252] *R. v Derby Magistrates' Court Ex p. B* [1996] 1 A.C. 487, HL.

[253] *R. v Cox and Railton* (1884) 14 Q.B.D 153; *Banque Keyser Ullman SA v Skandia (UK) Insurance Co Ltd* [1986] 1 Lloyd's Rep. 336, CA; *Barclays Bank plc v Eustice* [1995] 1 W.L.R. 1238, CA.

[254] *O'Rourke v Darbishire* [1920] A.C. 581, HL.

[255] *Calcraft v Guest* [1989] 1 Q.B. 759, CA; cf. *R. v Ulljee* [1982] 1 N.Z.L.R. 561.

[256] *Bullivant v Attorney General for Victoria* [1901] A.C. 196, 206, HL. See also *Bluck v Information Commissioner*, Information Tribunal, September 17, 2007 (medical records of deceased not to be disclosed to deceased's mother without widower's consent).

a patent agent and his client, and between a trade mark agent and his client, as to matters relating to the protection of various intellectual property rights.[257]

Other professions and privilege. Other professions have from time to time 7–71 claimed, either for themselves or for their clients, a similar privilege. However, it is settled that neither priests,[258] probation officers,[259] prison officers,[260] medical practitioners,[261] accountants,[262] nor (subject to one exception) journalists,[263] have any such privilege.

The one exception for journalists is that by statute no court may require a person 7–72 to disclose, nor is any person guilty of contempt of court for refusing to disclose, the source of information contained in a publication for which he is responsible, unless it is established to the satisfaction of the court that disclosure is necessary in the interests of justice or national security for the prevention of disorder or crime.[264] The prohibition extends to production of a document, if that would disclose the source of information, and it is for the party seeking disclosure to prove on the balance of probabilities that one of the four exceptions to the prohibition applies.[265] The "interests of justice" covers the administration of justice in the course of legal proceedings in a court of law,[266] such as proceedings at an inquest before a coroner, but extends beyond this, to enabling the exercise of other legal rights.[267] "Necessary" means "really needed".[268]

It should be noted that the statutory provision has been widely construed, and 7–73 covers both the case where information has been communicated for publication but not yet published,[269] and also the case where a claim to the return of property might help to identify a journalist's source.[270] Furthermore, the scope of the provision extends wider than journalists, to *anyone* responsible for the publication. The merits in the public interest of ordering a journalist to depart from their normal standards must be clearly demonstrated,[271] and there is, of course, a human rights dimension.[272] In any event, of course, a sensible coroner will not require any

---

[257] Copyright, Designs and Patents Act 1988 ss.280, 284.

[258] *Normanshaw v Normanshaw* (1893) 69 L.T. 468; *Pais v Pais* [1971] P. 119.

[259] *McTaggart v McTaggart* [1949] P. 94 at 97.

[260] *R. v Umoh* (1987) 84 Cr. App. R. 138, CA.

[261] *Duchess of Kingston's* case (1776) 20 St. Tr. 355 at 572–576; *R. v Gibbons* (1823) 1 C. & P. 97; *Hunter v Mann* [1974] Q.B. 767, DC.

[262] *R. (Prudential Insurance plc) v Special Commissioner of Income Tax* [2013] UKSC 1. There is a limited privilege for tax advisers in the tax legislation, but that will have little or no impact on coroners' inquiries.

[263] *British Steel Corporation v Granada Television* [1981] A.C. 1096, HL; *Attorney-General v Lundin* (1982) 75 Cr.App.R. 90, DC.

[264] Contempt of Court Act 1981 s.10.

[265] *Secretary of State for Defence v Guardian Newspapers Ltd* [1985] A.C. 339, HL.

[266] *Secretary of State for Defence v Guardian Newspapers Ltd* [1985] A.C. 339, HL at 350, per Lord Diplock.

[267] *X Ltd v Morgan-Grampian (Publishers) Ltd* [1991] 1 A.C. 1, HL; *Camelot Group plc v Centaur Communications Ltd* [1998] 1 All E.R. 251, CA.

[268] *Re an Inquiry under the Companies Securities (Insider Dealing) Act 1985* [1988] A.C. 660, per Lord Griffiths.

[269] *X Ltd v Morgan-Grampian (Publishers) Ltd* [1991] 1 A.C. 1 at 40.

[270] *Secretary of State for Defence v Guardian Newspapers Ltd* [1985] A.C. 331, HL.

[271] *John v Express Newspapers* [2000] 1 W.L.R. 1931, CA.

[272] See 21–42—21–42 below.

witness (much less a professional person of this kind) to answer a question which is not strictly necessary for the purposes of the inquest.[273]

7–74   **Spouses and other confidences.** To conclude the categories of person whose evidence is not privileged, there is no privilege at any inquest for spouses as such,[274] nor for confidential communications by reason merely of such confidentiality.[275] Again, however, a coroner should be careful only to require such confidences to be broken when necessary in the interests of the inquest.

Public interest immunity

7–75   Finally, it is possible for a witness to refuse to answer questions or produce documents on the grounds that the "public interest" requires him so to do.[276] Although public interest is an imprecise concept, it should not be used so as to cover cases where disclosure of information would be merely awkward or inconvenient. Accordingly, the principle is that the

> "courts have and are entitled to exercise a power and duty to hold a balance between the public interest, as expressed by a minister, to withhold certain documents or other evidence, and the public interest in ensuring the proper administration of justice."[277]

7–76   The threshold test as to when immunity may be asserted is whether disclosure will cause "substantial harm" to the public interest.[278] Once the threshold is passed, the court must carry out a balancing exercise in each particular case, considering whether the harm to the public interest is outweighed by the public interest in the administration of justice.[279] By analogy with the law relating to disclosure in civil proceedings, it seems that a claim to immunity may be made either in respect of the answer to a particular question, or to a whole category of questions.[280]

7–77   **Scope of the immunity.** The question then arises as to the exact scope of the immunity. Because of the balancing exercise to be carried out, every case must be taken on its own merits, and the following discussion understood accordingly. Information relating to national security[281] or to the formation of government

---

[273] *Attorney-General v Mulholland* [1963] 2 Q.B. 477, CA.

[274] *Shenton v Tyler* [1939] Ch. 620, CA. The Evidence Amendment Act 1853 s.3, created a privilege for spouses now abolished by the Civil Evidence Act 1968 s.16(3), and the Police and Criminal Evidence Act 1984 s.119(2) and Sch.7 Pt V.

[275] *Science Research Council v Nassé* [1980] A.C. 1028, HL.

[276] *Marks v Beyfus* (1890) 25 Q.B.D. 494, CA; *Duncan v Cammell Laird & Co Ltd* [1942] A.C. 624, per Viscount Simon LC; *Conway v Rimmer* [1968] A.C. 910, per Lord Reid.

[277] *Conway v Rimmer* [1968] A.C. 910 at 952, per Lord Reid.

[278] *R. v Chief Constable of West Midlands Police Ex p. Wily* [1995] 1 A.C. 274, HL.

[279] *Conway v Rimmer* [1968] A.C. 910, 952; *Air Canada v Secretary of State for Trade (No. 2)* [1983] 1 All E.R. 161 at 165–166 (reversed on other grounds [1983] 2 A.C. 394); *Al Rawi v Security Service* [2011] UKSC 34.

[280] cf. *Conway v Rimmer* [1968] A.C. 910.

[281] *Asiatic Petroleum Co Ltd v Anglo-Persian Oil Co Ltd* [1916] 1 K.B. 822, CA; *Duncan v Cammell Laird & Co Ltd* [1942] A.C. 624, HL. See also *R. (Home Secretary) v Inner West London Assistant Deputy Coroner* [2010] EWHC 3098 Admin; *R (Foreign Secretary) v Inner North London Asistant Deputy Coroner* [2013] EWHC (Admin).

policy at high level[282] will usually[283] be protected from disclosure on this basis. In discovery (now disclosure)[284] cases, immunity has been obtained for internal communications between the Commissioners of Customs and Excise and their staff and third parties in order to enable the Commissioners to fulfil certain of their statutory obligations,[285] for a soldier's medical sheets prepared in the course of military service,[286] for documents relating to attempts made by a military families' association to reconcile a solider and his wife who were now engaged in divorce proceedings,[287] for documents produced by the child care service,[288] for the police public order manual[289] and for the investigating officer's report commissioned by the Police Complaints Authority following the shooting by police of the deceased.[290]

On the other hand, the Home Office was held not entitled to immunity in **7–78** respect of certain documents relating to the formulation of policy on an experimental "control unit" in its prison service,[291] the police were not entitled to assert public interest immunity in respect of witness statements obtained during an investigation into the death of a demonstrator alleged to have been struck by a police officer,[292] or in respect of documents seized in the course of an investigation,[293] or police video recordings of interviews with child witnesses,[294] the Navy were obliged to disclose the report of a naval board of inquiry into a death on station abroad,[295] and local education authorities have been required to produce records and reports.[296]

As to questions in court, and witness summonses, public interest immunity has **7–79** been accorded to information as to the identity of police and other informers for whom confidentiality is said to be essential to encourage them to come forward,[297] and also to the identity of tactical firearms officers and the like.[298] This head of

---

[282] *Burmah Oil Co Ltd v Bank of England* [1980] A.C. 1090, HL; *Air Canada v Secretary of State for Trade (No. 2)* [1983] 2 A.C. 394, HL.

[283] But not invariably: see *Air Canada v Secretary of State for Trade (No. 2)* [1983] 2 A.C. 394 at 432, per Lord Fraser, and the cases there cited.

[284] See Civil Procedure Rules 1998 Pt 31, replacing RSC Ord.24.

[285] *Alfred Crompton Amusement Machines Ltd v Customs & Excise Commissioners (No. 2)* [1974] A.C. 405, HL.

[286] *Anthony v Anthony* (1919) 35 T.L.R. 559; however, the doctor concerned was permitted to give evidence of his treatment of the soldier, which seems inconsistent.

[287] *Broome v Broome* [1955] P. 190.

[288] *Re D (Infants)* [1970] 1 W.L.R. 599, CA; *Gaskin v Liverpool City Council* [1980] 1 W.L.R. 1549, CA.

[289] *Goodwin v Chief Constable of Lancashire, The Times,* November 3, 1992, CA.

[290] *Hay v Devon Coroner* (1998) 162 J.P. 96.

[291] *Williams v Home Office* [1981] 1 All E.R. 1151.

[292] *Peach v Metropolitan Police Commissioner* [1986] Q.B. 1064, CA.

[293] *Marcel v Metropolitan Police Commissioner* [1992] Ch. 225, CA.

[294] *Nottinghamshire County Council v H* [1995] 1 F.L.R. 115; *Re M (Minors)* [1995] 1 F.L.R. 57.

[295] *Barrett v Ministry of Defence, The Times,* January 24, 1990.

[296] *Thompson v ILEA* (1977) 74 L.S. Gaz. 66; *Campbell v Tameside MBC* [1982] Q.B. 1065, CA. See also *Worcestershire CC v Worcestershire Coroner* [2013] EWHC 1711, QB.

[297] *Marks v Beyfus* (1890) 25 Q.B.D. 494; *Rogers v Home Secretary* [1973] A.C. 388, HL; *D. v NSPCC* [1978] A.C. 171, HL; *Continental Reinsurance v Pine Top Insurance* [1986] 1 Lloyd's Rep. 8, CA; *R. v Rankine* [1986] Q.B. 224, CA; *R. v Johnson (Kenneth)* [1988] 1 W.L.R. 1377, CA.

[298] *R. v Crown Prosecution Service Ex p. J, The Times,* July 8, 1999, DC; *R. v Bedfordshire Coroner Ex p. Local Sunday Newspapers Ltd* (1999) 164 J.P. 283; *R. (Bennett) v Inner South London Coroner* [2004] EWCA Civ. 1439, CA. See also *R. (Metropolitan Police Service) v Chairman of Azelle Rodney Inquiry* [2012] EWHC 2783 (Admin.).

immunity, however, does not cover journalists who refuse to disclose their sources of information.[299]

7–80 **Nature of information and not area of government.** It is the nature of the information and not the area of government to which it relates that determines whether there is immunity: in other words there can in principle be immunity for matters relating to local government or statutory bodies.[300] The claim to immunity is invariably supported by a certificate, usually of a minister, setting out the basis for the claim. However, the certificate is not conclusive, and it is for the court to decide whether the claim to immunity is valid.[301]

7–81 **Power of court to assess documents.** In order to assist the court so to decide, in disclosure cases the court has power to inspect the documents in question, in private, so that the court is able to see just how useful the documents in question are likely to prove, and the balancing exercise required between the national interest and the public interest in administration of justice can be the more easily carried out. However, before the court does inspect the documents, it must be satisfied that there is a likelihood that they will assist the claims being made by the party seeking disclosure.[302] The coroner may properly call for documents from others in order to decide on relevance and also any claims to public interest immunity, rather than have to debate the latter claims with the holders without having seen the documents in question.[303]

7–82 **Witnesses in court and the application of public interest immunity.** However, in cases where a witness in court is asked a question, or a line of questioning begins, or a witness seeks to set aside a summons, the matter is more difficult. There are after all no documents for the minister to examine before issuing a certificate that giving the evidence in question would not be in the public interest,[304] and similarly, there are no documents to be inspected privately by the court. It nevertheless appears that a ministerial certificate can be used to communicate to the court the minister's views on relevant public interest issues with the object of preventing disclosure of matters contrary to the public interest by way of oral evidence.[305] But the certificate must be sufficiently explicit to enable the court to ascertain what really is the nature of the evidence for which immunity is being claimed.[306] And the court must still retain the prerogative of examining the evidence for itself.[307]

---

[299] *British Steel Corporation v Granada Television Ltd* [1981] A.C. 1096, HL; *Attorney-General v Lundin* (1982) 75 Cr.App.R. 90, DC; cf. the Contempt of Court Act 1981 s.10, see 7–72.

[300] *Rogers v Home Secretary* [1973] A.C. 388, HL.

[301] *Conway v Rimmer* [1968] A.C. 910, HL. Formerly the certificate was conclusive: *Duncan v Cammell Laird & Co Ltd* [1942] A.C. 624, HL. See also *Sethia v Stern, The Times,* November 4, 1987, CA.

[302] *Air Canada v Secretary of State for Trade (No. 2)* [1983] 2 A.C. 394, HL. cf. *Continental Reinsurance v Pine Top Insurance* [1986] 1 Lloyd's Rep. 8, CA.

[303] *Worcestershire CC v Worcestershire Coroner* [2013] EWHC 1711, QB. See 7–13, 10–65.

[304] *Broome v Broome* [1955] P. 190.

[305] *Re Ministry of Defence's Application* [1994] N.I. 279, CA (NI).

[306] *Broome v Broome* [1955] P. 190, at 199.

[307] *Re Ministry of Defence's Application* [1994] N.I. 279, CA (NI).

It may be that the proper procedure to be followed in these cases is similar to that **7–83** now obtaining in criminal trials for certain sexual offences, where certain types of question may not be put, or if put, must be disallowed.[308] It should be noted that this species of privilege is not, like private privilege, capable of being waived by the Crown: if it applies at all, effect must be given to it.[309]

---

[308] Youth Justice and Criminal Justice Act 1999 s.41. See *Continental Reinsurance v Pine Top Insurance* [1986] 1 Lloyd's Rep. 8 at 26, CA.
[309] *Duncan v Cammell Laird & Co Ltd* [1942] A.C. 624 at 641–642; *Rogers v Home Secretary* [1973] A.C. 388, HL. cf. *Alfred Crompton Amusement Machines Ltd. v Customs & Excise Commissioners (No. 2)* [1974] A.C. 405 at 434.

Chapter 8

CORONER'S POWERS BEFORE INQUEST

REFERENCE TO CORONER

Where a death is referred to the coroner, he has ultimately three possible courses **8–01** of action:

(1) he may be satisfied after preliminary inquiries that he has no duty to conduct an investigation, and he may proceed no further;

(2) he may be satisfied that he has a duty to conduct an investigation, but on the results of a post-mortem examination discontinue it; or

(3) he may be satisfied that he has a duty to conduct an investigation, including holding an inquest, usually with, but sometimes without, a post-mortem examination.

This chapter deals with the first two of these courses of action and with that part of the third which relates to carrying out a post-mortem examination. Where homicide is suspected, however, the practice is modified, and this is dealt with later.[1]

Almost every coroner's investigation begins with the body. The coroner **8–02** therefore has a number of powers in relation to dealing with and examining the body. However, the coroner's power to inquire into deaths requiring investigation would be seriously curtailed if a coroner had no power to exhume bodies which had already been buried by the time he came to make his inquiries. So if the body has already been buried, it may well need to be exhumed first of all.

---

[1] See 14–01—14–22 below.

Exhumation

8–03   Any disinterment or other disturbance without lawful authority[2] of a body that has been buried is an offence both at common law[3] and by statute,[4] although it has been doubted whether the common law offence can survive the introduction of the statutory one for the same prohibited act.[5] Where the Secretary of State for Defence has designated[6] (a) a vessel which sank or was stranded while in military service or (b) an area containing such a vessel or an aircraft which crashed on military service, it is an offence[7] to interfere with the military remains concerned, whether by an excavation, exploration, salvage or otherwise, without the Defence Secretary's licence.[8] This will obviously cover exhumation of human remains inside or near such a vessel or aircraft. The provisions of the Act are in *addition* to other relevant statutory provisions, and not in substitution for them.[9] Unless a

---

[2] e.g. a faculty granted for the purpose of reburial in consecrated ground , or the Secretary of State for Justice's (Lord Chancellor's) licence under the Burial Act 1857 s.25. Over 1,000 licences are granted every year by the Ministry of Justice. In *R. (East London Coroner) v Secretary of State for Justice* [2009] EWHC 1974 (Admin.), the Divisional Court held that the Secretary of State's refusal to grant a licence for exhumation of a body under s.25 of the Burial Act 1857 on the basis that the family (who owned the burial rights) now opposed such grant could not be impugned as irrational or *Wednesbury* unreasonable, especially since it now appeared that a faculty would also be needed. In *R. (Rudewicz) v Secretary of State for Justice* [2013] Q.B. 410, it was held that s.25 appeared to confer an unfettered discretion on the Secretary of State, and that the general presumption of permanence applicable to the faculty jurisdiction did not apply to the licence jurisdiction under s.25. Moreover, arts 8 and 9 of the ECHR were not engaged. Accordingly a licence was not granted unlawfully to reunite the remains of a priest with those of members of his order, and to make access to the grave easier for those wishing to visit. See also *R. (Plantagenet Alliance Ltd) v Secretary of State for Justice* [2014] EWHC 1668, DC.

[3] *R. v Lynn* (1788) 2 T.R. 733; 100 E.R. 395; *R. v Sharpe* (1857) Dears. & Bell 160, 169 E.R. 959; *Foster v Dodd* (1867) L.R. 3 Q.B. 67 at 77; *R. v Jacobson* (1880) 14 Cox C.C. 522; *R. v Price* (1884) 12 Q.B.D. 247 at 252; *R. v Kenyon* (1901) 65 J.P. 730; *R. v Filer, The Times*, December 22, 1960; *The Times*, February 15, 1961; *R. v Harmsworth* [1975] Crim.L.R. 525.

[4] Burial Act 1857 s.25. The exception contained in this section for an ecclesiastical faculty only applies where the faculty is for the removal of a body from one consecrated place of burial to another. Thus it does not apply, e.g. where a body is removed in order to be reburied in unconsecrated ground, and in such a case both licence *and* faculty would be required: see, e.g. *R. v Tristram* (1899) 80 L.T. 414; *Re Talbot* [1901] P. 1. For a further exception see Crossrail Act 2008, Sch 15.

[5] *R. (Rudewicz) v Secretary of State for Justice* [2013] Q.B. 410 at [21].

[6] Under the Protection of Military Remains Act 1986.

[7] Under the Protection of Military Remains Act 1986 s.2.

[8] Under the Protection of Military Remains Act 1986 s.4.

[9] *Pace* the views of the Ministry of Defence and one coroner, who each considered that they alone had exclusive power to exhume: see *The Times*, December 6, 1994. In a case reported in *The Times*, August 31, 1995, the remains of two wartime airmen were found by aviation archaeologists who had been licensed by the Ministry of Defence to dig at an aircraft crash site. The coroner was informed, but a Ministry spokesman did not "anticipate an inquest".

faculty[10] is obtained from the Ordinary,[11] removal of a body or other human remains[12] from consecrated ground is unlawful under ecclesiastical law.[13]

Historic common law powers

There is early authority[14] for the view that a coroner had power at common law   **8–04** to disinter a body within a reasonable time after death for the purpose of holding an inquest when none had already been validly held. But it was a question whether the coroner had such power without the leave of the court to order disinterment.[15] This never arose for decision in modern times, and the common law on the subject has now been replaced by statutory provision.[16] Although it is clear that where these provisions operate there is no need for the Secretary of State's licence, it is not clear how far these new provisions take away the need for a faculty under

---

[10] The purpose for which these have been granted include the following: (i) to identify a body: *R. v Tristram* [1898] 2 Q.B. 371; (ii) to obtain papers buried with the body: *R. v Hall*, cited in *R. v Tristram* [1898] 2 Q.B. 371; (iii) for public health reasons: *Rector of St Helen's Bishopsgate v Parishioners* [1892] P. 386; (iv) to widen adjoining streets: *Re Brideford Parish* [1900] P. 314; (v) for reburial in unconsecrated ground: *Re Talbot* [1901] P. 1; *Re Crawley Green Road Cemetery* [2001] Fam. 33; (vi) for cremation: *Re Matheson* [1958] 1 W.L.R. 246; cf. *Re Dixon* [1892] P. 386; (vii) to correct earlier decision on place of burial: *Re Atkins* [1989] 1 All E.R. 14; *Re Durrington Cemetery* [2000] Fam. 33; (viii) to remove body of person buried by mistake in reserved plot: *Re St Luke's, Holbeach Hurn* [1990] 2 All E.R. 749; (ix) for other public interest reasons: *Re Horner, The Times*, July 18, 1995 (body of murder victim to be exhumed and reburied secretly elsewhere to prevent killer visiting grave); *Re Radcliffe Infirmary Burial Ground* [2011] PTSR 1508 (to enable a university to redevelop a burial ground by building a school of government there; since the remains would have been exhumed for that reason, a faculty would issue also for archeological and medical research before reburial). But there must be "strong and compelling" reasons for ordering exhumation: *Re Smith* [1994] 1 All E.R. 91, Const. Ct.; see also *Re Knight, The Times*, January 27, 1994, Const. Ct. (exhumation should be ordered only for "special reasons", and not as matter of course); *Re John Stokes, The Times*, September 9, 1995 (exhumation of *cremated* remains for scattering refused); *Re Christ Church Alsager* [1999] Fam. 142, Chancery Court of York (once a body or cremated remains has been buried in consecrated ground there should be no disturbance unless good and proper reason shown; a mistake was likely to be such; a change of mind not normally so); *Re Durrington Cemetery* [2000] Fam. 33; *Re Blagdon Cemetery* [2002] Fam. 299, Arches Ct.; *Re St Andrew's Churchyard, Alwalton* [2012] PTSR 479; cf. *Re St Mary's Churchyard, Alderley* [1994] 1 W.L.R. 1478, Const. Ct. (exhumation and reinterment of remains within churchyard); *Re Jenkins' Petition* [2013] PTSR 297 (exhumation to enable reburial at greater depth in same grave).

[11] Normally the (Church of England) Bishop of the Diocese in question, who acts through the Chancellor of the Consistory Court (who actually hears and decides applications). See generally Newsom, *Faculty Jurisdiction of the Church of England,* 2nd edn (1993); Hill, *Ecclesiastical Law,* 2nd edn (2001), Chs 6–7.

[12] Including cremation ashes: *Re Atkins* [1989] 1 All E.R. 14; *Re Crawley Green Road Cemetery* [2001] Fam. 308.

[13] *Adlam v Colthurst* (1867) L.R. 2A. & E. 30. Neither faculty nor licence is necessary where the removal is effected in accordance with certain statutory and other provisions: see Town and Country Planning (Churches, Places of Religious Worship and Burial Grounds) Regulations 1950 (SI 1950/792 as amended by SI 1996/525) Pastoral Measure 1983 s.65 Sch.6; New Towns Act 1981 s.20(7); Community Land Act 1975 Sch.4 Pt III para.11(9); Development of Rural Wales Act 1976 (c.75) s.5(1) Sch.3 para.26(6); Disused Burial Grounds (Amendment) Act 1981 s.2, Sch.; Town and Country Planning Act 1990 s.240(2); Leasehold Reform, Housing and Urban Development Act 1993 Sch.20 para.6.

[14] Britton, c. 2 s.3; Staunford P.C. 51a; Hale, *Summary,* 170; 2 Hale P.C. 58, 170; 2 Hawk. P.C., c. 9 s.23.

[15] This was a case where the coroner had already held one inquest, and might therefore have been *functus officio*, but if so it would not be the *coroner* ordering exhumation, but the *court*, whereas the court in this case made it clear that it was the coroner who was acting, albeit with the leave of the court.

[16] Coroners and Justice Act 2009 s.32 Sch.5 para.6; formerly Coroners Act 1988 s.23, and before that Coroners Act 1980 s.4.

ecclesiastical law, where the body in question lies in consecrated ground. The statutory scheme for the Secretary of State's licence was held not to take away the need for a faculty under the ecclesiastical jurisdiction,[17] but the purpose of the coronial power is very different, and often needs to be exercised urgently. It would be stultified if, whenever a body buried in consecrated ground needed to be exhumed for coronial purposes, it was necessary in addition to obtaining the coroner's order to obtain a faculty as well.

Statutory powers of exhumation

8–05   A coroner may issue a direction[18] signed by him for the exhumation of a body (i) buried *anywhere within England and Wales* when he thinks that it is necessary for the body to be examined under s.14 of the Coroners and Justice Act 2009,[19] or (ii) buried *in his coroner area* when he thinks that it is necessary for the body to be examined for the purposes of any criminal proceedings[20] either instituted or contemplated in respect of the death in question, or any other death which has taken place in circumstances connected with the death in question.[21]

8–06   Hence the crucial limitation on the coroner's power to order an exhumation is that there must be a necessity to examine the body for either of the two stated purposes. So, if the coroner is not in a position to request a s.14 examination,[22] and there are no proceedings pending or contemplated for whose purposes an examination of the body is required, the coroner has no power to order exhumation. Nor does he have any power to exhume for the purposes of reburial elsewhere, or cremation. However, it is clear, since the abolition of the requirement for the coroner to view the body before holding an inquest,[23] that the power of exhumation is not now for the purpose of founding jurisdiction, but is for the purposes of the investigation, and in particular the provision of evidence as to the cause of death and other facts which must be inquired into.

High Court powers in relation to a second investigation

8–07   If the determination or findings of an investigation are quashed by order of the High Court, it seems that the High Court itself has power at common law to order the body to be disinterred for the purpose of conducting a second investigation.[24] The Court has a discretion as to whether or not to make the order, according to the circumstances of the case.[25] However, it is more likely that the question of

---

[17] See *R. v Tristram* (1899) 80 L.T. 414; *Re Talbot* [1901] P. 1.

[18] The form is prescribed by the Coroners (Investigations) Regulations 2013 reg.22, Sch. Form 4: see App.2.

[19] Coroners and Justice Act 2009 s.32 Sch.5 para.6(2); formerly Coroners Act 1988 s.23(1)(a). As to s.14 of the 2009 Act, see 8–35.

[20] This includes proceedings in respect of an offence under the Armed Forces Act 2006 s.42, the Army Act 1955 s.70, the Air Force Act 1955 s.70, or the Naval Discipline Act 1957 s.42.

[21] Coroners and Justice Act 2009 s.32 Sch.5 para.6(3); formerly Coroners Act 1988 s.23(1)(b). In this case, if there is to be any investigation at all it is likely that the circumstances are such that the coroner will be obliged to suspend it: see 10–75—10–80 below.

[22] See 8–35.

[23] See the Coroners Act 1980 s.1 (repealed).

[24] *R. v Saunders* (1719) 1 Str. 167; 93 E.R. 452.

[25] See the cases cited in fn.14 above.

exhumation will be left to the coroner with the duty to conduct the new investigation.[26]

Procedure for exhumation

If he decides to proceed with an exhumation, the coroner issues his direction,   **8–08**
signed by him, addressed to the persons in charge of the burial ground or cemetery.
The coroner must use the prescribed form,[27] although this is drafted in a curious
way, and requires the coroner to state that the direction is so that the body may be
examined for the purposes of *either* conducting an investigation into the death *or*
discharging a coroner's function in relation to the death of the deceased. Neither
of these is what the statute actually requires for the power to apply,[28] and in some
cases neither will be correct.

It was formerly usual to carry out exhumations at night.[29] Today they are usually   **8–09**
carried out early in the morning, and with privacy, although it is convenient to
open the ground to within, say, 15 to 20 centimetres of the top of the coffin
beforehand. It is desirable to ensure by the presence of the appropriate persons that
the grave[30], the coffin[31] and the body[32] be identified. In cases where this is
required, forensic scientists will take soil and other samples, and photographers will
record the various stages of the operation. In the past, examination took place in
a makeshift mortuary at the burial ground. Nowadays the body will be removed to
a mortuary licensed for examinations.[33] The various procedures are described in
more specialist works.[34]

Procedure for reinterment

Once the body has been identified, the necessary examination made, and any other   **8–10**
matters have been dealt with, the body should normally be reinterred, pursuant to
a burial order[35] issued by the coroner. The cost of an exhumation ordered by a
coroner will be part of his expenses to be reimbursed by the local authority. As
exhumations are unusual occurrences, the local authority's schedule of permitted
fees[36] may not include them, and a coroner should arrange beforehand with his
local authority what will be reasonable and proper expenses to be reimbursed. The

---

[26] Who may then exercise the power under the Coroners and Justice Act 2009 s.32 Sch.5 para.6,
discussed above.

[27] The form is set out in the Coroners (Investigations) Regulations 2013 reg.22, Sch. Form 4: see
App.2.

[28] As to the former Sch.5 para.6(2) refers more precisely to the need for an examination under s.14, and
not merely an investigation into the death. As to the latter Sch.5 para.6(3) refers to the need for an
examination for the purposes of criminal proceedings (which are not coronial functions at all).

[29] See the 9th edn (1957) of this work, at p.76.

[30] Usually a cemetery official, who will first have checked plans and records.

[31] Usually the funeral director originally concerned.

[32] Often the funeral director rather than relatives.

[33] See 8–58.

[34] Polson and Marshall, *The Disposal of the Dead,* 3rd edn (1975); Saukko, *Knight's Forensic Pathology,* 3rd
edn (2004); Mason, *Forensic Medicine for Lawyers,* 5th edn (2008). As to forensic medicine and
pathology generally, see App.6.

[35] As to burial orders, see 9–20—9–22 above. See also *R. (Plantagenet Alliance) v Secretary of State for
Justice* Unreported 15 August 2013, Haddon-Cave J, [2014] EWHC 1668, DC.

[36] As to this, see 18–40 below.

burial authority concerned is also under a duty to record the details of the disinterment and reinterment (if any).[37]

POSSESSION AND RELEASE OF BODY

8–11   During the coroner's preliminary inquiries, and even afterwards if the circumstances are such that a coroner has a duty to conduct an investigation,[38] the coroner has a right to possession of the body of the deceased for the purposes of his coronial functions until those functions are completed or he otherwise loses jurisdiction.[39] But this is subject to (i) provision for the police to seize material for the purposes of police inquiries,[40] and (ii) provisions for earlier release. As to the latter, the old law gave the coroner a *discretion* to order the earlier release of the body.[41] The new law however *requires* the coroner to release the body for burial or cremation "as soon as reasonably practicable".[42] It is therefore not an absolute but a qualified duty, and he can issue a burial or cremation order only where he no longer needs to retain the body "for the purposes of the investigation".[43] Since he must by then have come under a duty to conduct an investigation, he cannot issue such an order in any case which he disposes of by way of preliminary inquiry.

8–12   If the coroner cannot release the body within 28 days of being made aware that it is in his area, he must notify the next of kin or personal representative of the reason for the delay.[44] A decision by the coroner whether or not to release a body will be subject to judicial review by the courts in an appropriate case.[45] So, before deciding whether to release the body and make a burial or other order, the coroner ought to give to any person he is aware of who may be affected by the decision the opportunity to comment.[46] Coroners do not have their own mortuaries, but use those of hospitals and local authorities. Accordingly, a coroner who releases a body is not responsible for a failure by the mortuary owner to give immediate access to it.

---

[37] Local Authorities' Cemeteries Order 1977 (SI 1977/204) art.11 (as substituted by SI 1986/1782).

[38] i.e. in the Coroners and Justice Act 2009 s.1(1); formerly the Coroners Act 1988 s.8(1): see 5–01 above.

[39] *R. v Bristol Coroner Ex p. Kerr* [1974] Q.B. 652. This common law right is recognised by the Coroners and Justice Act 2009 s.15 (power to order the body to be removed to a suitable place: 2–135, 8–58), and the Coroners (Investigations) Regulations 2013 (SI 2013/1629) reg.20.

[40] Police and Criminal Evidence Act 1984 s.19. This allows the police to seize things found with the body, but not the body itself, since, whether or not the body is a "thing" within s.19 (cf. *Cowan v Condon* [2000] 1 W.L.R. 254, CA), it would need clear words to abrogate the common law right of the coroner to possession of the body (cf. *R. (Rottman) v Metropolitan Police Commissioner* [2002] 2 A.C. 692, HL).

[41] *R. v Bristol Coroner Ex p. Kerr* [1974] Q.B. 652; Coroners Rules 1984 r.14; *R. v Bristol Coroner Ex p. Atkinson* Unreported May 5, 1983, Forbes J.

[42] Coroners (Investigations) Regulations 2013 reg.20(1). See Chief Coroner, *Release of the body for burial or cremation*, 1 May 2014.

[43] Coroners (Investigations) Regulations 2013 reg.21(1) (emphasis supplied); see 9–21, 9–28.

[44] Coroners (Investigations) Regulations 2013 reg.20(2).

[45] *R. v Bristol Coroner Ex p. Kerr* [1974] Q.B. 652; *R. v Bristol Coroner Ex p. Atkinson* Unreported May 5, 1983, Forbes J; 9–16, 9–17, 19–31.

[46] *R. v Bristol Coroner Ex p. Atkinson* Unreported May 5, 1983 per Forbes J. See 9–16 above.

Preliminary Inquiries

Post-mortem examination to obviate need for investigation

The coroner is entitled to make preliminary inquiries before he decides whether he   **8–13**
is under a duty to investigate. The mere fact that, for example, a person collapses
and dies suddenly does not mean that the coroner must have reason to suspect a
death of which the cause is unknown. The coroner may consider that the
circumstances point towards a natural cause of death of a certain type, even if he
cannot be sure at that stage. Under the old law the coroner had no power to direct
a post-mortem or other examination whilst he was simply deciding whether he
had jurisdiction to inquire. He could only do so once he had decided that he had.
The law is now different. As part of his preliminary inquiries, and in order to
decide *whether* he is under a duty to conduct an investigation, the coroner may
request that a post-mortem examination be made,[47] and may specify the kind of
examination to be made.[48] Merely having a post-mortem carried out does not
therefore mean that an investigation has started, though commissioning further
tests normally would.[49]

Certification of death by registered medical practitioner

On the other hand, if no medical practitioner is prepared to give a medical   **8–14**
certificate of the cause of death, the coroner *may* have reason to suspect a death of
which the cause is unknown.[50] Indeed, he may have such reason even where the
deceased's own doctor is prepared to certify the cause of death as natural.[51] Either
way, if the coroner does have such reason, he will come under a duty to conduct
an investigation.[52] However, even if the deceased was attended during his last illness
by a medical practitioner who signs or is prepared to sign a certificate as to the
cause of death,[53] the death may still come to the notice of the coroner. For
example, the death may be reported to him by the registrar of births and deaths
because the cause of death appears to be one of those which he is required so to
report.[54] Or the medical practitioner may wish to discuss the case with the coroner
before actually giving the certificate. Or the death may be reported by other
persons,[55] and the coroner only subsequently finds that a medical practitioner is
willing to give a certificate.

---

[47] Coroners and Justice Act 2009 s.14(1)(b); see formerly Coroners Act 1988 s.19(1). See 8–35.
[48] Coroners and Justice Act 2009 s.14(2). See 8–35.
[49] See the Chief Coroner's *Guide to the Coroners and Justice Act 2009*, para.79, and his amended advice
of November 22, 2013, "Preliminary Inquiries or Investigation?"
[50] *R. (Kasperowicz) v Plymouth Coroner* [2005] EWCA Civ. 44 at [8].
[51] *R. v Westminster City Coroner Ex p. Rainer, The Times*, October 26, 1968; 112 S.J. 882: 81-year-old
man collapsed and died in hospital before operation; coroner ordered post-mortem examination;
court refused to prohibit it despite family doctor's willingness to certify cause of death, because it was
impossible to say coroner had no reasonable cause.
[52] Coroners and Justice Act 2009 s.1(1), (2)(b); see 5–01.
[53] See 5–27 ff above, and also *R. v Westminster City Coroner Ex p. Rainer, The Times*, October 26, 1968;
112 S.J. 882.
[54] See 5–47 above.
[55] For example, the police, who may break into a locked home to find the body of the deceased
inside.

8–15   If, as a result of his preliminary inquiries, the coroner is satisfied that the medical practitioner was or would be entitled to sign a medical certificate of the cause of death and that he (the coroner) otherwise has no duty to conduct an investigation, he may inform the medical practitioner that he does not intend to conduct one, and he may wish also to notify his informant (if this was not the doctor). The coroner concludes the matter by notifying the registrar of births and deaths of his decision, so that the death can be registered on the certificate of the medical practitioner.[56] No official form of notification to the registrar is prescribed, but the Registrar-General supplies two forms of notification (called Form 100), usually coloured peach and pink respectively, of which that marked "Form A" (peach) is the notification of the coroner's intention not to proceed further with his inquiries.[57] A copy of the form and the report of the coroner's and his officers' inquiries should be attached to the records of the case and preserved.

8–16   If the post-mortem examination reveals a cause of death and the statutory criteria for conducting an investigation are otherwise not satisfied, the coroner will be under no duty to conduct one,[58] and his preliminary inquiries will simply terminate. If the death is one which requires to be registered,[59] he sends to the registrar of deaths a certificate (the other Form 100 referred to above, headed "Form B", but often in pink), showing the cause of death as disclosed by the post-mortem examination report. The death is then registered by the registrar in accordance with this information[60] and no investigation is conducted. Neither the coroner nor the registrar has power to edit the post-mortem examination report to make it conform to the usually accepted form of setting out the cause of death.[61]

8–17   As with the Form A procedure, a copy of the form, the report of the post-mortem examination and the report of the coroner's officer or any other inquiries should be attached to the records of the case and preserved. Both procedures ("A" and "B") are available in the preliminary inquiry phase, even where the coroner is otherwise prohibited from conducting or continuing an investigation by reason of the visiting forces provisions,[62] because the coroner never reaches the point at which he comes under a duty to conduct an investigation.

---

[56] However, the coroner does not notify the registrar if the deceased died outside England and Wales, because then there is no obligation to register the death: Births and Deaths Registration Act 1953 s.15. If the doctor did not attend the deceased during his last illness, for registration purposes he is unable to certify. But if the coroner sends a Form A to the registrar, the registrar must accept it, and the death is treated as "legally uncertified": Gastrell and others, "An analysis of legally uncertified deaths in England and Wales 1979–2002" (2004) *Health Statistics Quarterly* 24.

[57] See Home Office Circular No. 12 of 1993.

[58] Coroners and Justice Act 2009 s.1(1); see 5–01, 5–62, 6–63.

[59] So, in a case where the deceased died outside England and Wales but the body has been brought here for disposal, the coroner may still employ his procedure, but he does not notify the registrar of the result of the post-mortem examination, because the registrar need not register such a death: Home Office Circular No. 79 of 1983, and cf. Births and Deaths Registration Act 1953 s.15.

[60] Births and Deaths Registration Act 1953 s.23(3).

[61] Home Office Circular No. 100 of 1955.

[62] Visiting Forces Act 1952 s.7; See 5–98 ff above.

THE INVESTIGATION

Duty to conduct investigation

On the other hand, the coroner may find, as a result of the preliminary inquiries   **8–18**
(whether or not including a post-mortem examination), that the statutory criteria
are fulfilled, and that he or she has a duty to conduct an investigation. For example,
the post-mortem may be inconclusive, and further tests necessary.[63] The coroner
will then have to set in train all the various inquiries necessary. These include
obtaining evidence of identification and of the circumstances of the death, and
relevant documents, and commissioning reports from experts and others.[64]
However, the coroner may at any time suspend an investigation if it appears that it
would be appropriate to do so.[65] If it is so suspended, the coroner must (i) adjourn
any inquest, and (ii) provide the registrar with the particulars required to register
the death.[66] No time limit is specified, and no form has so far been provided, for
such provision.

If a post-mortem examination has already been carried out, and he still has the   **8–19**
duty to investigate, there will have to be an inquest as part of that investigation in
due course. If however no such examination has been carried out, the coroner has
power to request one as part of his or her investigation. This is significant, because
the result of such an examination may *require* the coroner to discontinue the
investigation rather than continue to an inquest hearing. In cases where art.2 of the
European Convention on Human Rights is engaged, it may be necessary to have
a post-mortem examination as part of the investigation in order to satisfy the
requirements of that article.[67]

Having begun but not yet completed an investigation, the coroner, on request   **8–20**
by the next of kin or personal representative[68] of the deceased, may (not must)
provide that person with a certificate of the fact of death.[69] This is often referred
to as an "interim" certificate, as opposed to the certificate of registration of death
obtained from the registrar when the investigation is over.[70] The coroner in issuing
any such certificate must use a prescribed form.[71] But that does not mean that the
certificate must contain only that information. The form produced by the Iris
software used by coroners also allows for the provision of other information,
including the marital status of the deceased. It is a matter for the coroner whether
the additional information is included, but if it is, the recipient of the certificate
cannot for that reason complain that the certificate is not a lawful certificate of the
fact of death.

---

[63] See the Chief Coroner's *Guide to the Coroners and Justice Act 2009*, para.79, and his amended advice
of November 22, 2013, "Preliminary Inquiries or Investigation?"
[64] See 10–65. As to the time for completing an investigation, see 10–14.
[65] Coroners and Justice Act 2009 s.11 Sch.1 para.5.
[66] Coroners (Investigations) Regulations 2013 (SI 2013/1629) reg.8. See also 18–16—18–1].
[67] *AK v Turkey*, App. no. 38418/97, November 30, 2004, ECtHR.
[68] As to these expressions see 8–29—8–33.
[69] Coroners (Investigations) Regulations 2013 (SI 2013/1629) reg.9.
[70] See 18–19.
[71] Coroners (Investigations) Regulations 2013 (SI 2013/1629) Sch. Form 1.

Interested persons

8–21   It follows from the inquisitorial nature of the coroner's functions and proceedings that there are no "parties" to an investigation, in the same way that there are to accusatorial proceedings such as a civil claim or a criminal prosecution.[72] Yet where an investigation (and any inquest that forms part of it) takes place, certain persons nevertheless have interests and rights over and above those of the general public. These are known as "interested persons". In relation to the deceased and an investigation (or inquest) into a person's death,[73] there are a number of persons who qualify as such interested persons.

8–22   These persons are:

(a) a spouse, civil partner, partner,[74] parent, child, brother, sister, grandparent, grandchild, child of a brother or sister, stepfather, stepmother, half-brother or half-sister;

(b) a personal representative;

(c) a medical examiner[75] exercising functions in relation to the death;

(d) a beneficiary under a policy of insurance issued on the deceased's life;

(e) the insurer who issued such a policy of insurance;

(f) a person who may by his own, or his employee's or agent's, act or omission have caused or contributed to the death;

(g) a representative of a trade union of which the deceased was a member at death, in a case where the death may have been caused by—

   (i) an injury received in the course of an employment; or
   (ii) a disease prescribed for the purposes of certain social security benefits;

(h) a person appointed by, or representative of, an enforcing authority;[76]

(i) a chief constable,[77] or

(j), if it concerns a serviceman, a Provost Marshal,[78]

---

[72] See 1–19—1–21..

[73] There will be different criteria in relation to a treasure inquest under the new regime, when that comes into force: Coroners and Justice Act 2009 s.47(6). See Ch.16.

[74] This does not mean business or professional partner. For this purpose, a person is the partner of a deceased person (whether of the same or different sex) if the two of them were living as partners in an enduring relationship at the time of the deceased's death: Coroners and Justice Act 2009 s.47(7); see also *R. (Platts) v South Yorkshire Coroner* [2008] EWHC 2502 (Admin).

[75] See Ch.3.

[76] "Enforcing authority" has the meaning given by the Health and Safety at Work etc. Act 1974 s.18(7): Coroners and Justice Act 2009 s.48(1).

[77] Coroners and Justice Act 2009 s.47(3).

[78] Coroners and Justice Act 2009 s.47(4).

in either case where it appears that someone may have committed a homicide offence[79] or a related offence;[80]

(k) the Independent Police Complaints Commission,[81] where the death of the deceased is or has been the subject of an investigation managed or carried out[82] by that Commission;

(l) a person appointed by a government department to attend an inquest into the death or to assist in, or provide evidence for the purposes of, an investigation into the death;

(m) any other person whom the coroner thinks has a sufficient interest.[83]

In a case where art.2 of the European Convention on Human Rights is engaged **8–23** (i.e. a death arguably through state agency or in state custody),[84] the absence of legal representation for the family at the inquest may result in a breach of that article.[85] In such cases coroners should therefore encourage the family to obtain legal advice. Subject to that, however, there is no duty upon the coroner to advise interested persons of their rights.[86] One problem for coroners is that not all families are a cohesive single entity. Sometimes different members of the family take different stances.[87] In such cases the coroner should pay close attention to the wording of the rules, which were expanded under the new law to cover expressly a wider range of relatives.[88] A person entitled to claim the status of interested person is not obliged to do so. If a person so entitled declines to claim the status, the coroner is entitled to continue on the basis that that person is not an interested person.

Coroner's decision as to sufficient interest

There is a residual category for persons whom the coroner thinks have a "sufficient **8–24** interest".[89] The words "sufficient interest" are not technical, but ordinary English

---

[79] This means murder, manslaughter, corporate manslaughter, infanticide, causing death by dangerous driving, causing death by careless or inconsiderate driving, causing death by driving whilst unlicensed, disqualified or uninsured, causing death by careless driving under the influence of drink or drugs, encouraging or assisting suicide, and causing or allowing the death of a child or vulnerable adult: Coroners and Justice Act 2009 s.48(1), referring to s.11 Sch.1 para.1(6).

[80] This means an offence involving the death of the deceased (other than a homicide offence or its service equivalent) or an offence involving another death committed in circumstances connected with the death of the deceased: Coroners and Justice Act 2009 s.48(1), referring to s.11 Sch.1 para.1(6).

[81] It is not clear why the IPCC is included in the list, but not other organisations with a similar interest in carrying out an investigation into professional actions which may have resulted in death, such as the Probation and Prisons Ombudsman, the Care Quality Commission, the Local Safeguarding Children Board and the General Medical Council.

[82] Under the Police Reform Act 2002 Sch.3 Pt 3, including as extended or applied by other statutory provision: Coroners and Justice Act 2009 s.47(5).

[83] Coroners and Justice Act 2009 s.47(1), (2)(a)-(m).

[84] See 21–15.

[85] *R. (Wright) v Home Secretary* [2001] U.K.H.R.R. 1399 at [60].

[86] *R. v Central Cleveland Coroner Ex p. Dent* (1986) 150 J.P. 251; see also *Maksimovich v Attorney General* [1985] 4 N.S.W.L.R. 318, CA (NSW); and *Re Price's Application* (1986) 15 N.I.J.B. 84, CA (NI).

[87] See, e.g. *R. v South London Coroner Ex p. Driscoll* (1993) 159 J.P. 45, DC.

[88] Coroners and Justice Act 2009 s.47(2)(a).

[89] Coroners and Justice Act 2009 s.47(2)(m).

words, and it should be left to the coroner to give them an ordinary meaning. In the phrase formerly used under the old rules, "properly interested", the word "properly" imported not only that the interest was reasonable and substantial, but that the coroner might need to be satisfied that the concern of the person involved was genuinely directed to the scope of the inquest under the rules.[90] Under those rules, the fact that all other interested persons were content that a particular person be treated as "properly interested" was irrelevant.[91]

8–25   It is for the coroner to decide who has a sufficient interest. He should be a person who has himself some personal interest in the case, not merely a person who has an interest as a representative.[92] In Northern Ireland it has been held that the coroner is entitled also to have regard to whether the person concerned has the legal capacity to intervene in an inquest.[93] It may be that public bodies with an interest in the investigation, such as the Prisons and Probation Ombudsman, Care Quality Commission, Local Safeguarding Children Board and General Medical Council have a sufficient interest for this purpose,[94] at least once the inquest is over.

8–26   A medical practitioner, dental practitioner or ophthalmic practitioner in England who is, or is a director of a corporate body which is, involved in an inquest conducted as part of an investigation under the Coroners and Justice Act 2009, as a person who is found to have caused, or contributed to, the death of the deceased, or otherwise had their conduct brought into question, has obligations in certain circumstances to make declarations of these facts to the National Health Service Commissioning Board.[95] This may make such practitioners reluctant to claim "interested person" status under category (f) (person who may by his own, or his employee's or agent's, act or omission have caused or contributed to the death), even though the awarding of such status patently does not amount to a "finding" of anything. Instead they may seek it under class (m) (any other person whom the coroner thinks has a sufficient interest).

8–27   The coroner must obviously consider carefully the basis upon which such a practitioner may properly claim to be an interested person, and must not allow a

---

[90] *R. v South London Coroner Ex p. Driscoll* (1993) 159 J.P. 45, DC (decision that deceased's sisters not properly interested quashed).

[91] cf. *R. v Secretary of State for Social Services Ex p. Child Poverty Action Group* [1990] 2 Q.B. 540, CA.

[92] cf. *R. v Inner North London Coroner Ex p. GLC and others, The Times,* April 30, 1983, Woolf J (question whether the Hackney Black People's Association was a "properly interested person" within r.20(2)(h) left unresolved, although the judge indicated that on the material before him it seemed not to be such: the coroner after hearing further argument decided that it was not); see also *Re Medical Defence Union Ltd v Sinclair* [1990] 1 Med. L.R. 359, HK; *Re People First of Ontario* (1992) 87 D.L.R. (4th) 765, CA of Ont.; *R. (Southall Black Sisters) v West Yorkshire Coroner* [2002] EWHC 1914 Admin.

[93] *Re Northern Ireland Human Rights Commission's Application* [2002] N.I. 271, CA (NI), rvsd. by the House of Lords, *The Times,* June 25, 2002, on the basis that the body concerned *had* capacity to intervene, and might do so, *if so invited by the coroner.*

[94] cf. *Cleveland County Council v F* [1995] 2 All ER 236, 241; *Att-Gen for Gibraltar v May* [1999] 1 W.L.R. 998, CA.

[95] National Health Service (Performers Lists) (England) Regulations 2013 (SI 2013/335) regs 4(5)(i), 9(2)(h), (4)(i), as amended by the Coroners and Justice Act 2009 (Commencement No. 15, Consequential and Transitory Provisions) Order 2013 (SI 2013/1869) para.4, Sch, para.5. These regulations do not apply in Wales, where the equivalent rules currently in force (the National Health Service (Performers Lists) (Wales) Regulations 2004 (SI 2004/1020), as amended) make no such provision.

claim which has been made under (m), rather than (f), in order to frustrate the purposes of the relevant practitioner standards legislation. But there may be cases where the practitioner has a sufficient interest not arising from his acts or omissions possibly causing or contributing to death, and not falling within any other category, and in such a case a claim under (m) will be properly made.

As long as the coroner's decision is not one which no reasonable coroner could **8–28** have reached, it will be upheld.[96] Thus in one case under the old rules the coroner's view was upheld that the brother of a deceased was not "properly interested", where the deceased's widow had decided neither to attend nor to be represented at the inquest.[97] In another where two victims of the same road accident were the subject of two separate inquests, the coroner's decision that the father of one victim was not properly interested in the inquest into the death of the other was upheld.[98] On the other hand, in another case where the deceased as a result of mental health issues broke up with his partner shortly before death, the coroner's decision that the ex-partner was not a properly interested person was quashed.[99] The rules of natural justice have a role to play here.[100] In an inquest held as a result of a traffic accident in which an untraced motor driver was involved, the Home Office view was that the Motor Insurers' Bureau should be treated as a properly interested person.

Next of kin and personal representatives

In addition to, or instead of, dealing with "interested persons", coroners **8–29** conducting an investigation sometimes have to deal with or notify what the coroner legislation refers to as the deceased's "next of kin" or "personal representative". Neither of these phrases is defined in the legislation. "Personal representative" is a technical legal term, meaning the person who on or after death becomes the owner (and not merely an agent) of the deceased's estate, and has the obligations to collect in and administer that estate, pay debts, and distribute the balance to those entitled either under a will or on intestacy.[101] Where that person is appointed by a will, he is called an executor. Where there is no executor, and he is appointed by the court, he is called an administrator.

The phrase "next of kin" has no current[102] technical meaning in English law, **8–30** and it is surprising that it is not defined for the purposes of the coroner legislation. In some modern specific statutory contexts, one person may nominate another to have certain rights[103] or to take certain decisions[104] in the event of that person's

---

[96] *R. v Portsmouth Coroner Ex p. Keane* (1989) 153 J.P. 658 at 661; *R. v Coroner of The Queen's Household Ex p. Al Fayed* (1999) 58 B.M.L.R. 205, Hidden J; *Allman v West Sussex Assistant Deputy Coroner* [2012] EWHC 534 (Admin.).

[97] *R. v Portsmouth Coroner Ex p. Keane* (1989) 153 J.P. 658; cf. *R. v Hammersmith Coroner Ex p. Peach* [1980] Q.B. 211, CA (brother had locus standi to bring judicial review proceedings), and *R. v South London Coroner Ex p. Driscoll* (1993) 159 J.P. 45, DC (coroner misdirected himself in holding that two sisters were not "properly interested").

[98] *R. v Coroner of The Queen's Household Ex p. Al Fayed* (1999) 58 B.M.L.R. 205, Hidden J.

[99] *R. (Platts) v South Yorkshire Coroner* [2008] EWHC 2502 (Admin.).

[100] *Annetts v McCann* (1990) 65 A.L.J.R. 167, HC (Aus.).

[101] See 8–78 ff.

[102] It had one before 1926.

[103] e.g. in relation to a pension scheme.

[104] e.g. in relation to organ transplantation: see 8–78 ff.

death. In a functional sense, this may look like an appointment as next of kin for a limited purpose. But in law it is not, and moreover there is no legal basis in the legislation for the deceased to nominate someone as his next of kin for coronial purposes. Hence it is necessary to consider the meaning of the phrase for these purposes.

8-31   At common law, "next of kin" meant the person or persons closest[105] in blood[106] to the deceased.[107] This depended on the degrees of relationship, which were ascertained by counting the number of steps between the deceased and the relative in question. If they were connected lineally, the steps were counted directly. If they were related collaterally the steps were counted through their common ancestor. Thus parents and children were first-degree relatives, whereas grand-parents and siblings were of the second degree, and uncles and aunts, nephews and nieces were of the third degree. The surviving spouse was never the next of kin at common law. The "statutory" next of kin[108] were different, not only because according to the statute they included issue of pre-deceased common law next of kin, by virtue of the principle of representation, but also because the rules of entitlement were different.[109]

8-32   Neither of these is entirely appropriate for the purposes of coroners' investiga-tions. Here, the phrase "next of kin" is used to denote a person or persons who should be informed of various stages or events in the investigation. It is always an alternative to the deceased's personal representative. Closeness to the deceased, ability to receive and act on information and smallness of number are more important for this purpose than, say, the rules of inheritance or the principle of representation, which work better for the (passive) purpose of obtaining a share of the deceased's estate. And marriage or civil partnership is closer even than blood.[110]

8-33   But, in considering blood, in the lay mind descent is more powerful than ascent, and lineals are more important than collaterals. In the context of the new coroner legislation, therefore, it is submitted that "next of kin" means the first available adult or adults with capacity in the following classes of person, to the exclusion of those who are minors or without capacity, and of those further down the list: the surviving spouse or civil partner, children, grandchildren (etc.), parents, grand-parents (etc.), siblings, uncles and aunts, nieces and nephews, cousins (etc.).[111] Where there is more than one such person in a class, the whole class is treated together as a single person.

---

[105] Next = nearest.

[106] Kin, from the anglo-saxon *cynn* = family.

[107] *Re Gray's Settlement* [1896] 2 Ch. 802; *Re Clanchy's WT* [1970] 2 All E.R. 489, CA.

[108] Under the Statutes of Distribution, 1670 and 1685; see now the Administration of Estates Act 1925 s.46.

[109] The surviving spouse could take, and children were preferred to parents, for example.

[110] cf. the definition of "interested person" in the Coroners and Justice Act 2009 s.47(2)(a), placing spouse and civil partner before blood relations.

[111] This list is very similar to the list of those entitled to obtain letters of administration to the deceased's estate, under the Non-Contentious Probate Rules 1987 r.22: see 9–08—9–09. The only difference is that here grandparents take priority over siblings, on the lineal principle.

Coroner's relationship with interested persons, next of kin and personal representatives

Coroners' inquiries often involve substantial disagreement between interested   **8–34**
persons and others as to the circumstances in which death occurred, and in serious
cases, accusations may be made of civil or criminal responsibility. The coroner must
remain neutral, and his or her conduct free from suspicion of partiality, or of pre-
judging the result of the investigation. The coroner should therefore be clear on
the necessity for any pre-inquest meetings where only some of the interested
persons are present, and correspondence and telephone calls must be conducted in
an appropriately neutral way, particularly where the coroner or coroner's officers
regularly work with the persons concerned (e.g. emergency services, pathologists,
etc.).[112] Important and contentious applications should not be dealt with on paper,
but heard instead at a pre-inquest review hearing,[113] where everyone may be
present and participate.

Post-mortem examination as part of investigation

The coroner may request a suitable practitioner to make a post-mortem examina-   **8–35**
tion of the body,[114] and may specify the kind of examination to be made.[115] So it
may be a full invasive examination, a partial invasive examination, a cross-sectional
imaging scan (either computerised tomography (CT) or magnetic resonance
imaging (MRI)),[116] with or without additional radiographic techniques such as the
injection of radio-opaque dye into the coronary vasculature to aid diagnosis of
cardiac conditions, a biopsy, or a toxicological test of blood, amongst other things.
A "suitable practitioner" for this purpose is either a registered (and licensed)
medical practitioner[117] or a practitioner of a kind designated by the Chief Coroner
as suitable to make examinations of the kind required.[118] The person making the
examination must report the result to the coroner in the form required by him as
soon as practicable.[119]

Discontinuing the investigation

If the examination reveals the cause of death before the coroner has begun holding   **8–36**
an inquest into it, *and* the coroner thinks it is not necessary to continue the
investigation, the coroner must discontinue the investigation,[120] *unless* the coroner
has reason to suspect that the deceased died a violent or unnatural death,[121] or died
in custody or otherwise in state detention.[122] Where the coroner does discontinue,

---

[112] *Brown v Norfolk Coroner* [2014] EWHC 187 (Admin.) at [43]–[44].
[113] See 10–90 ff.
[114] Coroners and Justice Act 2009 s.14(1)(a); formerly Coroners Act 1988 s.20(1).
[115] Coroners and Justice Act 2009 s.14(2).
[116] See the Chief Coroner's Guidance No. 1, on *The Use of Post-Mortem Imaging (Adults)*.
[117] Coroners and Justice Act 2009 s.14(3)(a).
[118] Coroners and Justice Act 2009 s.14(3)(b). See the *Chief Coroner's Guide to the Coroners and Justice Act 2009* at [75].
[119] Coroners and Justice Act 2009 s.14(5).
[120] Coroners and Justice Act 2009 s.4(1).
[121] Coroners and Justice Act 2009 s.4(2)(a).
[122] Coroners and Justice Act 2009 s.4(2)(b).

he must record the cause of death and notify the next of kin or personal representative, using a prescribed form.[123]

8–37   Having so discontinued, the coroner may not hold an inquest into the death,[124] and no determination or finding may be made.[125] Instead, if the death is one which requires to be registered,[126] the coroner sends to the registrar of deaths a Form B, showing the cause of death as disclosed by the post-mortem examination.[127] The death is then registered by the registrar in accordance with this information.[128] But discontinuing the investigation in this way does not prevent a fresh investigation in future if the statutory criteria are later satisfied.[129] If an interested person requests the coroner in writing to give a written explanation as to why the investigation was discontinued, he must do so as soon as practicable.[130]

When further pathologist's report required

8–38   It sometimes appears certain that the death, as ascertained by a post-mortem examination, is from a natural cause, but the pathologist desires some further time to make a toxicological, histological, bacteriological or other examination before he will be able to give the complete and precise cause of death. In such cases it is not necessary to go on with the investigation and hold an inquest. The coroner can simply await the result of the further examination, and once he has the precise cause of death, he can discontinue the investigation and send Form B to the Registrar. Obviously this procedure is inapplicable to any case in which the cause of death turns out, as the result of further inquiry, to have been violent or unnatural, or where the death was that of a person in custody or state detention, because in such cases the coroner has no power to discontinue the investigation, but must go on to hold an inquest.

Post-Mortem Examinations

8–39   If the coroner does not request an examination (a "coroner's post-mortem"),[131] then except for the rare circumstances in which the medical referee for a cremation authority may carry out or request a post-mortem,[132] it may only take place with the authority of the person lawfully in possession of the body and also the

---

[123] Coroners (Investigations) Regulations 2013 reg.17, Sch. Form 2. As to the time for completing an investigation, see 10–14.

[124] Coroners and Justice Act 2009 s.4(3)(a).

[125] Coroners and Justice Act 2009 s.4(3)(b).

[126] So, in a case where the deceased died outside England and Wales but the body has been brought here for disposal, the coroner may still employ his procedure, but he does not notify the registrar of the result of the post-mortem examination, because the registrar need not register such a death: Home Office Circular No. 79 of 1983, and cf. Births and Deaths Registration Act 1953 s.15.

[127] There is no longer a legal obligation to do this: cf. Coroners Act 1988 s.19(3) (repealed); see 18–11—18–14.

[128] Births and Deaths Registration Act 1953 s.23(3).

[129] Coroners and Justice Act 2009 s.4(3). See *Terry v East Sussex Coroner* [2002] Q.B. 312, CA.

[130] Coroners and Justice Act 2009 s.4(4).

[131] See the Human Tissue Act 2004 s.11.

[132] Cremation (England and Wales) Regulations 2008 reg.24.

"appropriate authority" required by statute.[133] (This will usually be a "clinical" or "hospital" post-mortem.) In general, a coroner is not under any positive duty to request a post-mortem examination of the body of the deceased. However, as stated above, he has power to do so, and in some cases it may be arguable that a failure to exercise that power has resulted in an insufficiency of inquiry, justifying an order requiring him to have one carried out or the quashing of a determination.[134] If, on the other hand, the coroner requests a post-mortem examination, this will override the wishes of the personal representatives or family of the deceased,[135] subject only to judicial review in an appropriate case.[136] A failure to comply with the rules relating to such examinations does not render the evidence resulting from the examination inadmissible. It will be for the coroner to decide whether to admit it.[137]

Right of interested persons in relation to post-mortem examinations

The powers of the coroner to cause a post-mortem examination to be carried out **8–40** are not exclusive of the rights of others, and in particular "interested persons".[138] So even while a coroner is in possession of a body he may, and in some cases should, permit a second post-mortem examination to be carried out at the instigation of such others.[139] These will include the deceased's family who are unhappy with the results of the first examination, and also a defendant charged with an offence in relation to the death.[140] In the past, some coroners have arranged for a second, independent examination to be made and the report kept on file (sometimes even unread by the coroner), in a case where a person was being sought in connection with a death, but had not been found by the time the body was to be disposed of.[141] In such cases, of course, the second autopsy report belongs to the coroner, and not to any future defendant (although an interested person may—subject to exceptions—be now entitled to disclosure).[142]

The Home Office urged consideration of this course in cases of possible **8–41** homicide where no one had been found or charged and the family requested the

---

[133] Human Tissue Act 2004 s.5(1), referring to ss.2, 3. As to "the person lawfully in possession of the body", see 9–01 ff above. In practice, hospital post-mortems are a tiny fraction of the number carried out. The overwhelming majority are coroners' post-mortems.

[134] See Ch.19.

[135] *R. v Greater Manchester Coroner Ex p. Worch* [1988] Q.B. 513, CA; *Re Jacobs' Application for Judicial Review* (1999) 53 B.M.L.R. 21, CA; *R. (Kasperowicz) v Plymouth Coroner* [2005] EWCA Civ. 44; cf. *Abernethy v Deitz* (1996) 39 NSWLR 701, CA of NSW (no further useful information capable of being obtained through examination); *Green v Johnstone* [1995] V.R. 176, Sup. Ct. Vic. (autopsy contrary to Aboriginal culture and religion); *Ronan v State Coroner* [2000] W.A.S.C. 260 (order that no post-mortem be performed); and cf. *Pope v State Coroner* [1998] S.A.S.C. 6526 (application for such an order dismissed).

[136] As to which see Ch.19 below.

[137] *R. (Shaw) v Leicester City and South Leicestershire ADC* [2013] EWHC 386 (Admin.) at [30], affirmed [2014] EWCA Civ. 294.

[138] As to this expression, see 8–21 ff.

[139] *R. v South London Coroner Ex p. Ridley* [1985] 1 W.L.R. 1347; *R. (McLeish) v North London Coroner* [2010] EWHC 3624 (Admin), para.36.

[140] See also 14–18 ff below.

[141] Home Office Newsletter, January 21, 1985.

[142] See 7–24 ff. The person obtaining such disclosure, even if the potential defendant, would not be under any duty to reimburse the cost of the second autopsy.

release of the body for funeral purposes.[143] But it is difficult to see how the pathologist can anticipate the needs of an unknown defence.[144] The interests of family, police, defendants and others will conflict, and the coroner's role includes balancing those competing interests. The post-mortem examiner owes no duty to the deceased's estate or family to preserve tissue removed against the possibility that it might become material evidence in future litigation.[145] Any future defendant's loss of the opportunity to obtain evidence through a second post-mortem does not render a fair trial impossible so as to justify a stay of the proceedings.[146] In any event, if a defendant who has been unable to obtain a second autopsy is convicted of the homicide of the deceased, it is impossible to know whether the lack of a second autopsy made any difference to the jury. The coroner cannot be expected to second-guess the future course of events, and must accordingly be entitled to release the body without first causing a second post-mortem to be made for the benefit of a future defendant.

8–42　　In the past it has been argued that the coroners have no power to authorise a second post-mortem examination and accordingly, a second examination can only be carried out with the consent of the surviving spouse or relative of the deceased.[147] But this is not so. First, the statutory powers of coroners relating to post-mortem examinations,[148] and the powers to pay for them,[149] are not expressly limited to use on a single occasion only. There is no more reason to restrict them in this way than any other investigatory power of the coroner (e.g. to call a witness to give evidence). As a result, the courts have seen no difficulty in the coroner authorising a second post-mortem in appropriate circumstances.[150] Secondly, the statutory provision requiring "appropriate consent" does not apply to an examination made "under the authority of a coroner".[151]

Coroner's use of powers

8–43　　In practice, a coroner very frequently employs his power to request a post-mortem examination, although the number of such examinations, both as an absolute and as a percentage of total deaths reported to coroners, has been falling since the 1970s.[152] Almost invariably the coroner proceeds by standing agreement with a

---

[143] Home Office Circular No. 30 of 1999, *Memorandum of Good Practice re Early Release of Bodies in Cases of Suspicious Death.* See also 9–11, 9–14 above.

[144] All reports of forensic autopsies by forensic pathologists are in any event to include a "critical conclusions check" by another pathologist (*Code of practice and performance standards for forensic pathology in England, Wales, and Northern Ireland,* October 2012, para.7.1(d)), so the first autopsy ought to be sufficiently robust. But this is not always the case.

[145] *Dobson v North Tyneside Health Authority* [1996] 4 All E.R. 474, CA.

[146] *R v Winzar* [2002] EWCA Crim. 2950; see also *J Preston & Sons Ltd v Julie Hurst* [2012] EWHC 870 (QB); *Matthews v Collins* [2013] EWHC 2952 (QB).

[147] Hinchliff (1998) 148 N.L.J. 178.

[148] See 8–35 above.

[149] cf. Home Office Newsletter, May 8, 1985; the Local Government Association indicated that the cost of second examinations should be absorbed by relevant local authorities: Home Office Circular No. 30 of 1999, para.11. But this is not legally binding, and advance agreement is desirable. See 18–40.

[150] e.g. *R. v South London Coroner Ex p. Ridley* [1985] 1 W.L.R. 1347; *R. (McLeish) v North London Coroner* [2010] EWHC 3624 (Admin.) at [36].

[151] Human Tissue Act 2004 s.11.

[152] Down from 88 per cent in the 1970s to 41 per cent in 2013.

local pathologist or group of pathologists possessing appropriate specialist skills and facilities. As with other powers granted to the coroner, they are conferred for the purpose of advancing the coroner's inquiry, and may not be used for collateral purposes. The coroner may hence authorise photography (or video recording) as part of the examination where this would advance the inquiry, but not for other, unrelated purposes (e.g. for a television programme). The coroner may delegate the making of arrangements for the examination to his officers, but not the decision itself.[153]

Where a suitable practitioner is requested to make a post-mortem examination, **8–44** he may of course decline to carry it out, for example because he is too busy, or because the deceased was suffering from some highly contagious disease or condition, such as certain forms of hepatitis, HIV infection, acquired immune deficiency syndrome (AIDS),[154] or rabies.[155] In earlier times, when mortuary facilities were less modern, this sometimes resulted in a restricted or even no post-mortem report being available, so that an inquest had to be held and (possibly) an open verdict recorded.[156] Today, however, although mortuaries (and their staff) vary, and not all mortuaries are suitable for the reception of "infected" bodies, it is usually possible to find pathologists and mortuary facilities appropriate for high-risk examinations. Coroners are no longer restricted to premises in their own or the adjacent coroner area.[157]

Selection of a medical practitioner

The word "pathologist" is used to describe medical practitioners who have **8–45** different skills. The type of pathologist for a coroner's post-mortem is one who has training and experience in the performance of post-mortem examinations and the microscopic investigation of tissues (histopathologist). This is in contrast to pathologists who specialise in chemistry, immunology or other branches of pathology. The latter specialist pathologists may perform investigations relating to the post-mortem,[158] but do not themselves conduct autopsies. Where deaths of young children are concerned, however, it will normally be desirable to engage a paediatric pathologist who is an expert in the causes of childhood deaths.[159]

Within histopathology, there is a difference between those who restrict **8–46** themselves to routine post-mortem examinations, and those who are prepared to undertake so-called "forensic" or "special" post-mortem examinations (these may

---

[153] See 2–144, and also the Chief Coroner's Guidance No. 8, on *Pre-Signed Forms* para.10.

[154] See, e.g. *Re Thompson-Neil*, *The Times*, November 2, 1983, Walthamstow coroner; *Re Cairns*, *The Times*, January 16, 1985, Hammersmith coroner; *Re Phillips*, *The Times*, September 28, 1985, Southwark coroner.

[155] As to mortuary practice and safety in such cases, see the Royal Institute of Public Health and Hygiene's *A Handbook of Mortuary Practice and Safety for Anatomical Pathology Technicians*, 1991.

[156] As happened in *Re Cairns*, *The Times*, January 16, 1985. In *Re Thompson-Neil*, *The Times*, November 2, 1983, a verdict of accidental death was recorded, and in *Re Phillips*, a verdict of natural causes.

[157] See Coroners and Justice Act 2009, s.15(2); see 4–29, 8–11.

[158] See also the Brodrick Report paras 23–14 and 23–15.

[159] See Home Office Newsletter No. 22, December 1996. Thus, in cases of sudden infant death syndrome ("cot death"), coroners are advised to consult one of the panel of paediatric pathologists: Home Office Newsletter No. 4, para.6. The list was annexed to Home Office Newsletter No. 12. See also App.6.

involve contested criminal proceedings).[160] Coroners pay a higher fee for the latter than the former.[161] Most autopsies are done by NHS histopathologists, usually a consultant pathologist at a district general hospital or a member of an academic department of pathology at a university teaching hospital.[162] Both of these will have access to a mortuary suitable for the conduct of post-mortems and the storage of bodies, together with facilities for standard laboratory investigations. The coroner needs to be astute to select a pathologist with the appropriate qualifications for the job in hand. In case of difficulty in finding a suitable pathologist, coroners could consult the Royal College of Pathologists,[163] the Association of Clinical Pathologists,[164] the British Association in Forensic Medicine,[165] or the local health authority, which is responsible for hospital pathology.

8–47   In selecting a "suitable practitioner"[166] for the purpose of carrying out a post-mortem examination, the coroner must have regard to certain considerations. First of all, a post-mortem examination[167] may only be carried out by or under the direction of a person licensed by the Human Tissue Authority (usually, but not necessarily, the pathologist).[168] There is no longer a requirement that the person appointed should be a pathologist with suitable qualifications and experience, and have access to laboratory facilities.[169] Secondly (but rarely applicable), where the coroner is informed that the treatment of the deceased by a person was improper or negligent, and wholly or partly caused the death, that person must not make or assist at the examination,[170] although he or she is entitled to be represented at it.[171]

8–48   Thirdly, if the coroner is informed by a chief officer of police that a homicide offence[172] is suspected in connection with the death of the deceased, the coroner must consult the chief officer of police about who should make the post-mortem

---

[160] See *R. v Clarke and Morabir* [2013] EWCA Crim. 163, and App.6.
[161] See Coroners Allowances, Fees, and Expenses Regulations 2013 (SI 2013/1615) reg.8, Sch. para.6.
[162] See the Home Office's *Coroner Service Survey*, 1998 (Research Study 118), p.19, and the Royal College of Pathologists' *Guidelines on Autopsy Practice*, September 2002 para.4.2 (available at *http://www.rcpath.org* [Accessed June 6, 2014]).
[163] The address is 2 Carlton House Terrace, London, SW1Y 5AJ (Tel: 020 7451 6700; website *http://www.rcpath.org* [Accessed June 6, 2014]).
[164] The address is 189 Dyke Road, Hove, East Sussex, BN3 1TL (Tel: 01273 775700; website *http://www.pathologists.org.uk* [Accessed June 6, 2014].
[165] The address is the Medico-Legal Centre, Watery Street, Sheffield S3 7ES (Tel: 0114 273 8721; secretary, Prof. Christopher Milroy).
[166] Coroners and Justice Act 2009 s.14(3); see 8–35.
[167] A term not defined by law, but see 8–64—8–65 above.
[168] Human Tissue Act 2004 s.16 Sch.3.
[169] Coroners Rules 1984 r.6(1)(a). Home Office Circular No. 121 of 1951 suggested that, where the deceased was believed to have died as a result of a submarine or diving accident or an underwater explosion, the Director of Research, Royal Naval Medical School, Monckton House, Alverstoke, Hants, would be able to provide expert examination and advice on technique. The Royal Naval Medical School has gone, but the Medical Officer in Charge, The Institute of Naval Medicine (the successor to the School) may be able to assist. The address is Crescent Road, Alverstoke, Gosport, Hampshire PO12 2DL, and the telephone number is 023 9276 8000. The expertise in military diving equipment is now with QinetiQ Plc, Fort Road, Alverstoke, Gosport, Hampshire PO12 2DU (Tel: 023 9233 5879).
[170] Coroners and Justice Act 2009 s.14(4)(a).
[171] Coroners and Justice Act 2009 s.14(4)(b).
[172] Defined in the Coroners and Justice Act 2009 s.11 para.1(6). See 10–75.

examination.[173] In practice the pathologist will be on the Home Office List (or, in Scotland, the Crown Office List) of accredited forensic pathologists, and will probably have a contract with the relevant police force.[174] But the coroner is not *obliged* to use such a pathologist. In some cases other forensic skills, such as forensic anthropology or forensic botany may be needed too.

Recent history of pathology in England and Wales

The post-war period was expansionist for higher education: there was more money   **8–49** for existing universities, new universities were founded, and there were new disciplines, and new sub-disciplines; forensic pathology was one of these. Forensic pathologists thus had an academic base and a salary to begin with, which meant they were able to accept instructions from coroners to conduct post-mortem examinations at low, central government-authorised piecework rates.[175] And a steady supply of such post-mortem examinations (at a rate higher than almost everywhere else in the world)[176] enabled such pathologists to gain experience fast and attain a world-class reputation.

But the cuts in public spending in the 1970s led to retrenchment. Forensic   **8–50** pathology (not ordinary histopathology) was one of the first subjects to be downgraded. To some extent this was the result of pathologists' own achievement. Their success in attracting a second income from coroners' post-mortem examinations meant that they were envied by other less fortunate colleagues.[177] And (with some notable exceptions) they did not contribute so much to research and publications. So colleagues did not try too hard to defend them. First of all, chairs were not filled, then academic departments were amalgamated, or even closed, especially in London.[178] Partly as a consequence of the failure to support universities and medical schools, and partly because of competition for space on the medical undergraduate curriculum, nowadays it is rare for medical students to have much idea about forensic pathology, or indeed about how the medical profession interacts with the coroner service.

Next, and not surprisingly, there were shortages of forensic pathologists   **8–51** generally,[179] leading to a "crisis" in some specialist areas.[180] This meant that, particularly in London, the forensic pathology service was carried out more and more by medical practitioners in private practice. A Home Office Review in 1989 concluded that the "forensic pathology service of England and Wales consists of a group of independent medical practitioners who, *pro bono publico*, are willing to put

---

[173] Coroners (Investigations) Regulations 2013 reg.12.

[174] See Home Office Circular No. 9 of 1993. See also 8–52.

[175] Havard, (1990) 301 B.M.J. 943.

[176] Pounder et al., (2011) 104 J.R. Soc. Med. 19–24.

[177] Scottish pathologists seem to have particularly strong feelings in this respect: Pounder, (2002) 324 B.M.J. 1408; Pounder et al., (2011) 104 J.R.Soc. Med. 19–24. Compare Rutty et al., (2001) 54 J. Clin. Pathol. 279–284.

[178] See inter alia Knight, (1985) 291 B.M.J. 1145; Havard, (1990) 301 B.M.J. 943; Pounder, (2002) 324 B.M.J. 1408.

[179] Home Office, *Review of Forensic Pathology Services in England and Wales* (2003); *Shipman Inquiry, 3rd Report*, Ch.10, esp. 10.10.

[180] See Royal College of Paediatric and Child Health, *The Future of Paediatric Pathology Services* (2002) available at *http://www.rcpch.ac.uk/publications* [Accessed June 6, 2014], and also Pounder, "Forensic Pathology Services" (2002) 324 B.M.J. 1408, 1409.

their considerable expertise at the disposal of the police and the courts". On the other hand, this ad hoc system "cannot be relied upon to continue to meet the needs of the police in the 1990s and beyond".[181]

8–52   The problem was unwittingly intensified by the police. At the front line of response to criminal activity, and faced with a patchwork quilt of uneven service, they needed to ensure lines of supply. So police forces entered into contracts with pathologists.[182] This ensured big fees for special post-mortem examinations and further advice/evidence in court, which dwarfed then (and still dwarf) the fees which coroners are authorised by the Secretary of State to pay. While in terms of time, a special post-mortem examination may take more than six times as long, the fee which coroners are currently authorised to pay for a special examination is less than three times as much as a routine examination. Conversely, a police contract ensures fees of about 10 times what the coroner pays for a special post-mortem.[183]

8–53   Understandably, forensic pathologists going into private practice had to be or become more business-like than when they were employed by universities or the NHS. Given the enhanced fees from the police for special post-mortems, they were less interested in coroners' routine post-mortem examinations,[184] although of course they would do them where possible, particularly in the early years of practice. Anecdotal evidence from coroners suggests that even NHS pathologists are now much less interested in doing coroners' post-mortem examinations than previously. Autopsies today certainly suffer from various weaknesses,[185] probably as a result of these changes, but certainly as a result of lack of resources. In London, there is evidence that the privatisation of coroners' post-mortem examinations has led to a decline in the quality of the reports of such post-mortems (if not post-mortems themselves), and also a decline in the training available for the next generation.[186]

8–54   In law, coroners have the choice of pathologist,[187] and sometimes have informal agreements concerning routine autopsies. But, in cases where homicide is suspected, the coroner is obliged to consult the police,[188] and, because the police pay greatly enhanced fees for special autopsies, in effect in relation to these cases it is the police that really have the choice, and they enter into standing agreements with particular pathologists or teams of pathologists. If the agreement is with a team, the coroner may have to make do with the team member who is "on call" that day, rather than the one he would prefer.

8–55   Quality control is an issue. Before the Second World War, many post-mortem examinations were carried out by general practitioners, often at the deceased's

---

[181] Home Office, *Report of the working party on forensic pathology,* Chaired by Mr G.J. Wasserman (London: HMSO, 1989).

[182] Home Office *Review of Forensic Pathology Services in England and Wales* (2003).

[183] Although that must also cover scene visits, conferences with lawyers, attendance in court, etc.

[184] See Royal College of Pathologists Annual Report of 2007-08, 15, 17.

[185] See *The Coroner's Autopsy: Do we deserve better?* National Confidential Enquiry into Patient Outcome and Death Report, 2006.

[186] See Royal College of Pathologists Annual Report of 2006-07, 14; Royal College of Pathologists Annual Report of 2007-08, 15, 17.

[187] Coroners and Justice Act 2009 s.14.

[188] Coroners (Investigations) Regulations 2013 reg.12. See 8–48.

home, on the kitchen table.[189] The world has changed since then, but the basic qualification required by coroner legislation (to be a registered medical practitioner)[190] has not, although today other legislation fortuitously requires a person to be licensed by (or acting under the direction of a person licensed by) the Human Tissue Authority in order to carry out a post-mortem examination.[191] Some pathologists are admitted to the so-called Home Office Register of Pathologists.[192] They are those considered to have the knowledge and experience needed to carry out so-called forensic (or "special") post-mortem examinations.[193] However, whatever the media may think, they are not employed by the Home Office (or any part of the government),[194] and there is no legal rule that only those on the Home Office list can carry out special post-mortem examinations.

In the United Kingdom there is no national forensic science institute to set   **8–56** standards[195] and carry out post-mortem examinations and other tests in cases involving the public interest in the UK, as there should be,[196] and indeed as there is in most other developed countries. Nor are forensic pathologists even generally employed by the public service, where a hierarchy may enable proper assessment of their qualities. A policy of benign neglect[197] adopted by successive governments has driven forensic pathology into the private sector. Self-evidently, a lawyer coroner in particular (all coroners in the new system will be lawyers in future)[198] has to rely on others for assessment of the pathology skills provided to him or her.[199] He or she can tell if the pathologist is helpful, explains things well in court or to relatives, and seems knowledgeable and up to date. But, not being an expert, the coroner must defer to others with the requisite expertise. The government having failed to make other arrangements, it is up to it and the medical authorities[200] to ensure that only medical practitioners with the right expertise carry out post-mortem examinations. Accordingly, in 2013 the Pathology Delivery

---

[189] Hollman, "Postmortems on the Kitchen Table" (2001) 323 B.M.J. 1472.

[190] Coroners and Justice Act 2009 s.14(3)(a).

[191] See Human Tissue Act 2004, s.16(2)(b), Sch.3; see also 8–80, 8–87.

[192] See the Home Office Register of forensic pathologists, at *https://www.gov.uk/government/publications/home-office-register-of-forensic-pathologists-february-2013* [Accessed June 6, 2014], the criteria for registration, at *https://www.gov.uk/government/publications/pathology-delivery-board-criteria-registration* [Accessed June 6, 2014], and the Protocol for Home Office Registered Forensic Pathologists, at *https://www.gov.uk/government/publications/protocol-for-home-office-registered-forensic-pathologists* [Accessed June 6, 2014].

[193] See 8–46.

[194] Even some pathologists get this wrong: Pounder, (2002) 324 B.M.J. 1408, 1409. It is not much more than a mark of quality of certain skills, rather like being a Queen's Counsel is for a barrister.

[195] But see the *Code of practice and performance standards for forensic pathology in England, Wales and Northern Ireland*, published by the Home Office, The Forensic Science Regulator, the Department of Justice and the Royal College of Pathologists, October 2012.

[196] Havard, (1990) 301 B.M.J. 943. Scotland and Northern Ireland have more formal arrangements than England and Wales.

[197] More correctly, declining to resource.

[198] See 2–33.

[199] cf. Luce Report, Ch.13, para.32.

[200] Such as the National Policing Improvement Agency (formerly the Home Office Policy Advisory Board for Forensic Pathology), the Royal College of Pathologists, and the General Medical Council.

Board, an agency of the Home Office, became the designated organisation to oversee the revalidation of forensic pathologists within England and Wales.[201]

Time and place of post-mortem examination

8–57   A coroner who considers that a post-mortem examination should be made must request a suitable practitioner to make it as soon as reasonably practicable.[202] Any delay reduces the value of the post-mortem examination, and in certain cases may render the post-mortem examination unreliable. However, if it is considered that any persons are entitled and likely to wish to be represented at the post-mortem examination,[203] then, unless delay would jeopardise the value of the examination, it is desirable that the post-mortem examination should be deferred until they are in a position to be represented.

8–58   The rules which formerly existed regarding the premises for an examination[204] have gone and have not been replaced. They are no longer needed, since the Human Tissue Authority licenses mortuaries and inspects them.[205] However, a local authority[206] may, and if required by the Secretary of State, must, provide and maintain a post-mortem room and also a mortuary.[207] In fact most authorities do not so provide, and the overwhelming majority instead contract with NHS trusts for the coroner to use hospital mortuaries.[208] In contrast to the previous restrictive rule,[209] a body may be removed to any suitable place, within the coroner's area or elsewhere, for the purposes of the examination,[210] unless the person providing the place does not consent to the removal there.[211] But the requirement of consent does not apply to a place within the coroner's area provided by a district council, a county council, a county borough council or the Common Council of the City of London.[212] This change of rule has greatly assisted coroners who have no local specialist paediatric mortuary facilities; their paediatric cases may now be sent further away without breaking the law. It will also facilitate the removal of bodies to centres that can undertake cross-sectional imaging examinations.

Safety during examination

8–59   An important consideration in post-mortem examinations today is safety. Following death, bacteria, viruses and fungi may multiply in the body, and therefore

---

[201] Medical Profession (Responsible Officers) Regulations 2010 (SI 2010/2841), as amended by Medical Profession (Responsible Officers) (Amendment) Regulations 2013 (SI 2013/291).
[202] Coroners (Investigations) Regulations 2013 reg.11.
[203] See 8–61 above.
[204] Coroners Rules 1984 r.11.
[205] See Human Tissue Act 2004, s.16, Sch.3.
[206] This means the council of a district or London borough, the Common Council of the City of London, the Sub-Treasurer of the Inner Temple and the Under Treasurer of the Middle Temple: Public Health Act 1936 s.1(2).
[207] Public Health Act 1936 s.198.
[208] See the Home Office's *Coroner Service Survey*, 1998 (Research Study 181), pp.18–19. In 2001 the Home Office estimated that there were only 36 public mortuaries in England and Wales.
[209] Coroners Act 1988 s.22(1).
[210] Coroners and Justice Act 2009 s.15(1), (2). In the case of an examination by scanning, this will include premises with suitable scanning equipment: see 8–67, 8–68.
[211] Coroners and Justice Act 2009 s.15(3).
[212] Coroners and Justice Act 2009 s.15(4).

skilled and careful technique, and above all hygiene, are required during the examination in order to minimise the risk of infection. This is particularly so in relation to high-risk cases, such as anthrax, leptospirosis, spongiform-encephalop-athy, viral hepatitis and AIDS, and cases of chemical, biological, radiological, and nuclear (CBRN) contamination. The standards and precautions required in the handling of bodies and in the conduct of post-mortem examinations in such cases are beyond the scope of this work, but are discussed elsewhere.[213] Because post-mortem examinations today are usually carried out before full information is available (including the results of blood tests), pathologists tend routinely to adopt a method of working which exposes them and the mortuary staff to the least risk. The only sensible approach is to regard all cadavers as potentially infective and proceed accordingly.

Persons who should be informed of examination

Where a coroner has requested a suitable practitioner to make an examination, he **8–60** must notify certain persons of the date time and place of the examination,[214] unless it is impracticable to inform them or to do so would cause the examination to be unreasonably delayed.[215] These persons are:[216]

(a) the next of kin or the personal representative of the deceased or any other interested person[217] who has notified the coroner in advance of his desire to be represented at the examination;

(b) the deceased's regular medical practitioner, if he has notified the coroner of his desire to be represented at the examination;[218]

(c) if the deceased died in hospital, that hospital;

(d) if the death of the deceased may have been caused by an accident or disease which must be reported to an enforcing authority,[219] to that authority or the appropriate inspector or representative of that authority;[220]

---

[213] e.g., in the Royal Institute of Public Health and Hygiene's *A Handbook of Mortuary Practice and Safety for Anatomical Pathology Technicians* (1991) and the Royal College of Pathologists' *Guidelines on Autopsy Practice* (September 2002) (available at *http://www.rcpath.org* [Accessed June 6, 2014]).

[214] Coroners (Investigations) Regulations 2013 reg.13(1); formerly Coroners Rules 1984 r.7(1).

[215] Coroners (Investigations) Regulations 2013 reg.13(2).

[216] Coroners (Investigations) Regulations 2013 reg.13(3); formerly Coroners Rules 1984 r.7(2).

[217] As to this expression, see 8–22.

[218] See *Re Devine and Breslin's Application* [1988] 14 N.I.J.B. 10, HC (NI), Carswell J.

[219] This has the meaning given by the Health and Safety at Work etc. Act 1974 s.18(7): Coroners and Justice Act 2009 s.48(1).

[220] As to these accidents and diseases, see Ch.15. The relevant names and addresses were set out in Home Office Circular No. 3 of 1981.

(e) a government department which has notified the coroner of its desire to be represented at the examination;[221]

(f) if the chief officer of police has notified the coroner of his desire to be represented at the examination, the chief officer of police.

If the coroner believes that the deceased was under the age of 18, he must also notify the appropriate Local Safeguarding Children Board within three days of directing the examination,[222] and must provide all information to it.[223]

Entitlement to representation

8–61 Any of the persons or bodies listed in the previous paragraph are entitled to be represented at the examination by a medical practitioner,[224] although, exceptionally, the chief officer of police may be represented by a member of his own force,[225] and a person entitled to be represented at the examination who is also a medical practitioner may instead attend in person.[226] But this exceptional entitlement is for attendance at the examination and does not extend to taking part. Where there is a viewing room, the entitlement will be satisfied by viewing the examination from that room. In addition, where the coroner is informed that the treatment of the deceased by a person was improper or negligent and wholly or partly caused the death, that person is entitled to be represented at it.[227] In one case, a widow's representatives were informed so shortly before the post-mortem examination took place that she could not be represented at it, and in the circumstances the coroner was obliged to consent to a second post-mortem examination being carried out by her (the widow's) own pathologist.[228] The coroner may consent to

---

[221] In the case of death from a submarine or diving accident, or an underwater explosion, the coroner was asked by Home Office Circular No. 121 of 1951 to inform the Director of Research, Royal Naval Medical School. This institution has been succeeded by the Institute of Naval Medicine, Crescent Road, Alverstoke, Gosport, Hampshire PO12 2DL (Tel: 023 9276 8000). Where a person working at increased atmospheric pressure (e.g. a diver or tunnel worker) dies in an accident, coroners were asked by Home Office Circular No. 16 of 1975 to contact a member of the Medical Research Panel's Decompression Sickness Panel to permit him to attend the post-mortem examination.

[222] Coroners (Investigations) Regulations 2013 reg.24(1); formerly Coroners Rules 1984 r.57A(2).

[223] Coroners (Investigations) Regulations 2013 reg.24(2); formerly Coroners Rules 1984 r.57A(3). As to "information", see reg.24(3).

[224] Coroners (Investigations) Regulations 2013 reg.13(4). As to the meaning of medical practitioner, see the Medical Act 1983, s.55(1).

[225] Coroners (Investigations) Regulations 2013 reg.13(5)(a). This means that detectives investigating a homicide can be present.

[226] Coroners (Investigations) Regulations 2013 reg.13(4). Cf. *R. (Shaw) v Leicester City and South Leicestershire ADC* [2013] EWHC 386 (Admin.), affirmed [2014] EWCA Civ. 294.

[227] Coroners and Justice Act 2009 s.14(4)(b).

[228] *R. v South London Coroner Ex p. Ridley* [1985] 1 W.L.R. 1347, QBD; *R. (McLeish) v North London Coroner* [2010] EWHC 3624 (Admin.) at [25]; cf. *R. v North London Coroner Ex p. Lewy* Unreported July 31, 1995, CA (allegation that applicant not advised of examination, and so unable to be represented at it, insufficient to justify leave to move for judicial review).

any other person attending the post-mortem examination, including a trainee doctor, medical student or other medical practitioner.[229]

Two categories of person in particular are not mentioned in the statutory list, **8–62** and so can be represented at the examination only with the consent of the coroner. They are (i) the Independent Police Complaints Commission and (ii) those suspected of or charged with the homicide of the deceased. Both would be "interested persons" for the purposes of the investigation,[230] but neither is in the list for representation at the examination. As to the former, in the case of a managed or independent investigation by the IPCC into a death, the IPCC should indicate to the coroner the reasons why it is thought that their attendance might be useful, and the coroner should ordinarily accede to a request by the IPCC to attend the examination. Where the IPCC is still deciding what mode of investigation to undertake, giving their reasons is especially important. There may be rare cases where the coroner will rightly refuse an IPCC request.[231]

As to the latter, the police are understandably unhappy if a person suspected of **8–63** criminal responsibility for a death (particularly murder) is permitted to be present or represented at a coroner's post-mortem examination, when it is likely that the police will also be represented, with a view to obtaining information useful for any subsequent proceedings against the suspect. There is no presumption against the coroner allowing a suspect to be so represented. Each case must be considered on its merits. A suspect has no right as such (though he may have a right in another capacity) to be present or represented, and it is a matter for the coroner's discretion, to be exercised judicially. No doubt the circumstances in which it will be proper to permit a suspect himself to attend the autopsy will be very rare indeed. It will be more common to allow him to be represented by a medical practitioner, A second autopsy is never as satisfactory, from the point of view of obtaining information about the death, as the first. If in a given case it is right to allow a second autopsy, it is likely also to be appropriate instead to permit the suspect to be represented at the first.[232]

Definition of post-mortem examination

There is no legal definition of what constitutes a post-mortem examination. **8–64** Strictly speaking, the term includes both the limited examination of the body, which is non-invasive and confined to external phenomena, and also the "full", invasive examination of internal organs (technically called "autopsy" or "necropsy"). Unless there are good reasons for taking a different course, the coroner will ask the pathologist to exercise his skill and judgment with regard to the extent of the examination necessary to enable him to give an opinion about the cause of

---

[229] Coroners (Investigations) Regulations 2013 reg.13(5)(b); formerly Coroners Rules 1984 r.7(4). The power to consent is conferred for the purposes of the inquiry, and it would obviously be wrong to permit attendance for an improper purpose, e.g. mere entertainment. cf. *Marcel v Metropolitan Police Commissioner* [1992] Ch. 225, 237; *Scopelight Ltd v Chief Constable for Northumberland* [2010] Q.B. 938. See also *Smith v State Coroner* [1999] NSWSC 779.

[230] See 8–22.

[231] *R. (IPCC) v Inner North London Coroner* [2009] EWHC 2681 (Admin.).

[232] In practice it is unlikely that a charge will have been made before the examination, and it is more likely that a second examination will be sought on behalf of the accused: see 8–40 above.

death. In practice, in England and Wales, the coroner's post-mortem will therefore usually be of the "full", invasive kind.

8–65   As to what it includes, regard may usefully be had to the form prescribed under the old system which the pathologist had to complete in reporting to the coroner,[233] to the Royal College of Pathologists' *Guidelines for Autopsy Practice.*[234] In broad terms, it will involve:

(1) an external examination of the body;

(2) dissection of the three major body cavities (head, chest and abdomen), and examinations of the major organs; and

(3) taking samples for analysis and further investigation.[235]

8–66   In some cases it may be possible, or (for health and safety reasons) necessary, to limit the scope of the examination. But this is generally undesirable, as it considerably reduces the amount of information available about the deceased's medical state, and can lead to concurrent or contributory causes of death being missed. Nevertheless, out of deference to the feelings (both religious and secular) of relatives in many cases, coroners should not unthinkingly order a full post-mortem examination in every case, but should do so when (and because) it is in their view necessary. Their decisions will not be interfered with by the courts, unless *Wednesbury* unreasonable.[236]

8–67   There is now considerable experience in the United Kingdom[237] of carrying out post-mortem investigation by means of "scanning", whether magnetic resonance

---

[233] Coroners Rules 1984 r.10(1) and Sch.2. This form in 1980 replaced the 1953 form, which had been the subject of many complaints. As to the 1984 form, see *R. (Kasperowicz) v Plymouth Coroner* [2005] EWCA Civ. 44, para.14: "What is necessary and appropriate to complete must, I would have thought, be case-dependent."

[234] September 2002, ss.7 and 8 (since updated: available at *http://www.rcpath.org* [Accessed June 6, 2014]). Note that pathologists on the Home Office List are subject to tougher rules than are laid down by the Royal College of Pathologists. See also Knight, *The Coroner's Autopsy* (1983); Knight, *Forensic Pathology,* 2nd edn (1996) Ch.1; Burton and Rutty, *The Hospital Autopsy,* 2nd edn (2001). An Australian perspective is given by Ranson, in Selby (ed.), *The Inquest Handbook* (1988). Irish perspectives are given by Leckey and Greer, *Coroners' Law and Practice in Northern Ireland* (1998), Ch.6, and Farrell, *Coroners' Law and Procedure* (2000), Ch.9 (Republic of Ireland).

[235] See 8–69 ff (special examinations) and 8–72 ff above (retention of organs and tissue).

[236] *R. v Greater Manchester Coroner Ex p. Worch* [1988] Q.B. 513, CA; *Re Jacobs' Application for Judicial Review* (1999) 53 B.M.L.R. 21, CA; *R. (Kasperowicz) v Plymouth Coroner* [2005] EWCA Civ. 44; cf. *Abernethy v Deitz* Unreported July 3, 1996, CA of NSW (no further useful information capable of being obtained through examination); *Green v Johnstone* [1995] V.R. 176, Sup. Ct. Vic. (autopsy contrary to Aboriginal culture and religion); *Ronan v State Coroner* [2000] W.A.S.C. 260 (order that no post-mortem be performed); and cf. *Pope v State Coroner* [1998] S.A.S.C. 6526 (application for such an order dismissed).

[237] See Bissett and others, (2002) 324 B.M.J. 1423; Thali and others, (2003) 24(1) Am.J.For.Med.Pathol., 22–27; Rutty and others, "The Role of Mobile Computed Tomography in Mass Fatality Incidents" (2007) 52 *Journal of Forensic Science* 1343-1349; Aghayev and others, "CT Data-Based Navigation for Post-Mortem Biopsy—a Feasibility Study" (2008) 15 (6) *Journal of Forensic & Legal Medicine* 382-387; Roberts and others, "Diagnosis of Coronary Artery Disease Using a Minimally Invasive Autopsy: Evaluation of a Novel Method of Post-Mortem Coronary CT Angiography" (2011) 66 (7) Clin. Radiol. 645-650; Rutty and others, "Targeted Cardiac Post-Mortem Computed Tomography Angiography: a Pictorial Review" (2012) 8(1) *Forensic Medicine Science and Pathology* 40-47; Roberts and others, "Could Post-Mortem Imaging be an Alternative to Autopsy in the Diagnosis of Adult Deaths? A Validation Study" (2012) 379 (9811) *Lancet* 136-142; earlier material

imaging ("MRI"), or multislice computed tomography ("CT scan").[238] These are non-invasive, and hence more attractive than a conventional autopsy for those relatives with personal or religious objections to that course. MRI has been trialled in some coroner areas.[239] Research has shown however that CT scanning is more accurate, especially when combined with radiographic techniques to evaluate the coronary vasculature.[240] There can be no doubt that scanning as a process falls within the scope of the term "post-mortem examination".[241]

But there are difficulties. First, it is accepted by most radiologists that at present **8–68** the technology is not yet good enough to give as much detail as a conventional autopsy in all cases.[242] On the other hand, in some cases, imaging may produce better results than invasive techniques (e.g. intracranial pathology). In any event, samples of tissue and fluid may still need to be removed for examination and analysis. Second, there are very few facilities in the United Kingdom willing to scan dead bodies, and for the moment it has to be done privately, at a cost significantly exceeding what the coroner can pay under the current rules.[243] Third, the relevant expertise (involving a crossover between forensic pathology and radiology) is limited: accurate interpretation of the results is of course crucial.[244] All of these difficulties must be addressed if imaging techniques are to become a more widespread and reliable form of post-mortem examination. In October 2012 a joint statement on post-mortem imaging was issued by the Royal College of Radiologists and the Royal College of Pathologists.[245] It is for the Chief Coroner to set the appropriate qualifications for a "suitable practitioner" to carry out a post-mortem examination.[246] So far, he has not done so.

Special examination

Under the old system, in addition to, or in place of, the post-mortem examination, **8–69** the coroner might decide that a "special examination" was required. A special examination was an examination by way of analysis, test or otherwise of such parts or contents of the body or such other substances or things as ought, in the opinion of the coroner, to be submitted to analyses, tests or other special examinations which a view to ascertaining how the deceased came by his death.[247] Under the new system there is no need for separate "special examination", since it is clear that "post-mortem examination" can refer to any kind of examination specified by the

---

includes an article in *The Lancet* (26 October 1996, Vol.348 at 1139–1141) and correspondence in the B.M.J. (21 November 1998, Vol.317 at 1450; and 3 July 1999, Vol.319 at 56).

[238] See the Chief Coroner's Guidance No. 1, *The Use of Post-Mortem Imaging.*

[239] Indeed, some coroners have scanning protocols.

[240] Roberts and others, "Could Post-Mortem Imaging be an Alternative to Autopsy in the Diagnosis of Adult Deaths? A Validation Study" (2012) 379 (9811) *Lancet* 136-142.

[241] See *R. (Kasperowicz) v Plymouth Coroner* [2005] EWCA Civ. 44 at [13]–[15].

[242] One recent study gave a discrepancy rate from invasive autopsies of 32 per cent for CT scans and 43 per cent for MRI: Roberts and others, "Could Post-Mortem Imaging be an Alternative to Autopsy in the Diagnosis of Adult Deaths? A Validation Study" (2012) 379 (9811) Lancet 136-142.

[243] See 18–38 below.

[244] See e.g. Page, "Necro-Radiology" (2009) Aug-Sept. *Forensic Magazine.*

[245] Available at *http://www.rcr.ac.uk* [Accessed June 6, 2014].

[246] See 8–35.

[247] Coroners Act 1988 s.20(4).

coroner,[248] and the person who carries it out need not be a medical practitioner.[249] In any event, now that post-mortem examinations are almost invariably made by a pathologist with access to laboratory facilities, it is reasonable to expect less use to be made of special examinations and to expect the pathologist to undertake microscopic or other work as part of the post-mortem examination.

AFTER THE EXAMINATION

Circulation of examination reports

8–70   The person making a post-mortem examination must as soon as practicable report the result to the coroner in the form required by him.[250] This is a change from the old law, which specified the format.[251] The coroner may therefore decide whether to require a written or an oral report, or both. The post mortem examiner may not supply the report or a copy of it to any person without the coroner's written authority.[252] In 1999 the Home Office envisaged that the pathologist would do this in cases of suspicious death "in any event within 14 days".[253] Where an interested person[254] asks for disclosure of a post-mortem examination report, the coroner must provide it or a copy of it, or make it available for inspection by that person as soon as reasonably practicable.[255] The coroner may not charge a fee for doing so before or during an inquest.[256] Some coroners do not allow a clinician involved in treating the deceased to see the report until he or she has made his or her report to the coroner.

8–71   In practice, the coroner's officer will usually explain the main points of the report in summary terms to the relatives. Most relatives do not ask to see or have a copy. But a study in 2002 (relating to fetal and infant deaths) confirmed that relatives mostly view the post-mortem examination positively, as a useful and necessary tool in helping to discover the reasons for the death.[257] Following the publication of the Alder Hey Report,[258] the Home Office (a) recommended coroners to arrange for post-mortem examiners to record on the post-mortem

---

[248] Coroners and Justice Act 2009 s.14(2).

[249] Coroners and Justice Act 2009 s.14(3)(b); see 8–35.

[250] Coroners and Justice Act 2009 s.14(5); Coroners (Investigations) Regulations 2013 reg.16(1).

[251] Coroners Rules 1984 Sch.2.

[252] Coroners (Investigations) Regulations 2013 reg.16(2); formerly Coroners Rules 1984 rr.10(2), 13.

[253] Memorandum attached to Home Office Circular No. 30 of 1999, para.8. The memorandum was reissued by the Ministry of Justice in substantively the same terms in May 2008. In *R. (McLeish) v North London Coroner* [2010] EWHC 3624 (Admin.), Calvert-Smith J held that this was not a policy document for the purposes of *Gransden & Co Ltd v Secretary of State for the Environment* [1987] P. & C.R. 86, but that in any event the memorandum only concerned suspicious deaths, which the instant case did not.

[254] Coroners and Justice Act 2009 s.47; see 8–22.

[255] Coroners (Investigations) Regulations 2013 reg.23; Coroners (Inquests) Rules 2013 r.13(1)(2)(a).

[256] Coroners (Inquests) Rules 2013 r.16.

[257] See Rankin, Wright, Lind, "Cross sectional survey of parents' experience and views of the post-mortem examination" (2002) 324 B.M.J. 816–818; see also Brodie, Laing, Keeling, McKenzie, "Ten years of neonatal autopsies in tertiary referral centre: retrospective study" (2002) 324 B.M.J. 761–763.

[258] See 8–72.

report any retention of tissue from the body, but (b) exhorted coroners to supply copies of such reports to relatives "only after reference to the relevant [NHS] Trust, or otherwise with a clear statement that there was no guarantee that other material had not been removed and retained".[259]

Retention of organs and tissue

There has been intense interest in the subject of tissue and organ retention in recent times, and several reports containing recommendations and codes of practice have been published.[260] A new body, the Retained Organs Commission,[261] was established to oversee the cataloguing and return or disposal of organs and tissue retained by NHS pathology departments. It issued guidance to NHS Trusts but closed in 2004. Since 2005 specific legislative provision has been made, and the current position is as follows. Where a suitable practitioner conducts a post-mortem examination, and preserves or retains material[262] which, in his opinion, relates to the cause of death or identity of the deceased, he must so notify the coroner in writing,[263] identifying the material being preserved or retained, and explaining why he is of the opinion that it relates to the cause of death or identity of the deceased.[264] The notification may also specify the period or periods of time for which the material should be retained or preserved.[265]

8–72

On receiving that notification, the coroner must notify the suitable practitioner of the period for which he requires the material to be preserved or retained for his functions under the 2009 Act.[266] He must do the same to the police or prosecuting authority where he receives a request from a prosecuting authority, Provost Marshal or Director of Service Prosecutions to suspend an investigation, or becomes aware that a person has been charged with an offence in relation to the death of the

8–73

---

[259] Letter to coroners dated March 16, 2001.

[260] These include the Royal College of Pathologists' *Guidelines for the retention of tissues and organs at post-mortem examination* (March 2000: sent to coroners with Home Office Newsletter No. 32, April 26, 2000); the interim report of the *Inquiry into the management of care of children receiving complex heart surgery at the Bristol Royal Infirmary* (May 2000: available at *http://webarchive.nationalarchives.gov.uk/ +/www.dh.gov.uk/en/Publicationsandstatistics/Publications/PublicationsPolicyAndGuidance/DH_4005620* [Accessed June 6, 2014]); the Report of the *Inquiry into the Liverpool Children's NHS Trust (Alder Hey)* (January 2001: available at *http://www.rlcinquiry.org.uk* [Accessed June 6, 2014]); a Home Office letter to coroners dated March 16, 2001; the Chief Medical Officer's *Advice on the Removal, Retention and Use of Human Organs and Tissue from Post Mortem Examinations* (August 2001, available at *http:/ /collection.europarchive.org/tna/20060802143339/http://dh/gov.uk/prod_consum_dh/DH_ 4065047bab2.pdf* [Accessed June 6, 2014]); the Department of Health's *Use of Human Organs and Tissue: a Draft Interim Statement for Consultation*, (January 2002); the Department of Health's Draft Code of Practice on the Import and Export of Human Body Parts (July 2002, available at *http:/ /webarchive,nationalarchives.gov.uk/20130107105354/http://www.dh.gov.uk/prod_consum_dh/groupd/ dh_digitalassets/@dh/@en/documents/digitalasset/dh_4071139.pdf* [Accessed June 6, 2014]); the Department of Health's *The Isaacs Report* (May 2003).

[261] Website *http://collections.europarchive.org/tna/20060802143339/nhs.uk/retainedorgans/* [Accessed June 6, 2014].

[262] This is not defined for this purpose. The Human Tissue Act 2004 s.53, defines "relevant material" as "material, other than gametes, which consists of or includes human cells". But this is probably too wide for present purposes, since even urine and stomach contents will also include some cells.

[263] Coroners (Investigations) Regulations 2013 reg.14(1); formerly Coroners Rules 1984 r.9. cf. *R. (Marper) v Chief Constable of South Yorkshire, The Independent*, October 1, 2002, CA (retention of DNA samples from unconvicted person did not infringe human rights).

[264] Coroners (Investigations) Regulations 2013 reg.14(2).

[265] Coroners (Investigations) Regulations 2013 reg.14(3).

[266] Coroners (Investigations) Regulations 2013 reg.14(4).

deceased,[267] and to the chairman of a public inquiry where is informed that the inquiry is to be held instead of an inquest.[268] The coroner may from time to time vary a period so notified, but must notify the variation to both the suitable practitioner and any police, prosecuting authority or chairman notified of the original period.[269] A suitable practitioner who believes that the coroner should vary the time period may request that the coroner vary the period.[270]

8–74   The coroner must also notify, where known, the next of kin or personal representative of the deceased, and any other relative who has notified the coroner of his desire to be represented at the examination, (i) that material is being preserved or retained, (ii) the periods for which it is being retained, and (iii) the options for dealing with it once the periods have expired.[271] Those options are (a) disposal by burial, cremation or other lawful disposal by the suitable practitioner, (b) return to one of the next of kin, personal representative, or any other relative who has notified the coroner of his desire to be represented at the examination, or (c) retention for medical research or other purposes in accordance with the Human Tissue Act 2004, with the consent of one of the next of kin, personal representative, or any other relative who has notified the coroner of his desire to be represented at the examination.[272]

8–75   It is to be noted that this rule does not require the coroner to *obtain a decision*, only to *notify*. Thus it is possible that no decision is made. It is also possible that several different decisions are made. It not clear what happens if one of the persons so notified wishes to follow one option, and another or others of them wishes or wish to follow others. In practice the coroner is likely to do nothing until either the various persons have agreed, or the court has ruled. In effect, the coroner interpleads.[273] This creates a problem for the suitable practitioner. Where the time period for retention has expired, the suitable practitioner must record how the material has been dealt with,[274] and must retain the record.[275] The rules do not explain what the suitable practitioner must do if several inconsistent decisions have been made, or if none has. But no offence is committed under the statute merely by destroying the material; it is preservation without lawful authority that is the problem.

8–76   These rules do not apply to—and hence do not authorise the retention of—material which, in the suitable practitioner's opinion, does *not* bear upon the cause of death or the identity of the deceased. Nor do they confer any right on the practitioner independently of the coroner, in relation to such material. In removing and examining the material, the pathologist is acting as the coroner's agent, although he retains and preserves it pursuant to his statutory duty. If the pathologist

---

[267] Coroners (Investigations) Regulations 2013 reg.15(1).
[268] Coroners (Investigations) Regulations 2013 reg.15(2).
[269] Coroners (Investigations) Regulations 2013 reg.15(3).
[270] Coroners (Investigations) Regulations 2013 reg.15(4).
[271] Coroners (Investigations) Regulations 2013 reg.14(5).
[272] Coroners (Investigations) Regulations 2013 reg.14(6).
[273] Cf. *Borrows v Preston Coroner* [2008] EWHC 1387 (QB).
[274] Coroners (Investigations) Regulations 2013 reg.15(5).
[275] Coroners (Investigations) Regulations 2013 reg.15(6).

removes other material, it must be pursuant to some other power,[276] or it is unlawful. This has nothing to do with the coroner, and it is not for him to consent to it.

Quite apart from these rules, there is the problem of subsequent civil **8–77** proceedings, particularly where industrial disease is in issue. Where there has been an inquest conclusion of or including industrial disease, any communication to the deceased's family about the disposal of histological samples should contain advice that, if a claim in respect of the deceased's death is pending, they should consult their solicitor before giving authority for disposal.[277] It would be good practice also for solicitors instructed by claimants in fatal asbestos claims to advise both their clients and the coroner that disposal of histological samples should not be undertaken without confirmation from those solicitors that the samples are not required for the purposes of the claim.[278]

ORGAN TRANSPLANTS[279]

Regulation

Organ transplants fall within the remit of the Human Tissue Authority.[280] **8–78** Statutory provision is made for the removal of the organs or other tissues of the body of a deceased person for use for therapeutic purposes, or for the purposes of medical education or research.[281] Unless "done for purposes of functions of a coroner or under the authority of a coroner",[282] and subject to certain transitional provisions, removal from a dead body of "relevant material of which the body consists or which it contains"[283] without "appropriate consent" for the purposes of (inter alia) medical research or transplantation[284] is unlawful, and in most cases is a criminal offence.[285] In this context, "relevant material" means "material, other than gametes, which consists of or includes human cells".[286] Human gametes fall within the remit of the Human Fertilisation and Embryology Authority, and are dealt with later.[287]

"Appropriate consent" is elaborately defined separately for children[288] and for **8–79** adults.[289] In relation to transplantation, the position is this. For a child who is alive,

---

[276] e.g. Police and Criminal Evidence Act 1984 s.19 (if applicable on the facts). But this power does not permit retention of material once there is no longer any law enforcement reason for so retaining: *Gough v Chief Constable for West Midlands* [2004] EWCA Civ. 206.

[277] *Matthews v Collins* [2013] EWHC 2952 (QB) at [94].

[278] *Matthews v Collins* [2013] EWHC 2952 (QB) at [95].

[279] See generally, Kennedy and Grubb, *Medical Law,* 3rd edn (2000), pp.1832–1880; Mason, *Forensic Medicine for Lawyers,* 4th edn (2001), Ch.12.

[280] Human Tissue Act 2004 ss.13-15 Sch.2.

[281] Human Tissue Act 2004, replacing the Human Tissue Act 1961, itself replacing the more limited Corneal Grafting Act 1952.

[282] Human Tissue Act 2004 s.11.

[283] Human Tissue Act 2004 s.1(1)(c).

[284] Human Tissue Act 2004 Sch.1 paras 6, 7.

[285] Human Tissue Act 2004 s.5.

[286] Human Tissue Act 2004 s.53.

[287] See 8–90 ff.

[288] Human Tissue Act 2004 s.2.

[289] Human Tissue Act 2004 s.3.

it is his own consent, but if he has not made a decision or is incompetent to do so then it is the consent of a person with parental responsibility.[290] Where the child has died, the position is similar, except that if there was no person with parental responsibility immediately before he died, then it is the relative or friend who at that time had the highest-ranking "qualifying relationship"[291] to him.[292] For an adult who is alive, it is his own consent.[293] For an adult who has died, it is his own consent, the consent of a person appointed by him[294] to deal with the issue after his death, or if neither applies then it is consent of the relative or friend with the highest-ranking "qualifying relationship"[295] to him immediately before he died.[296]

8–80   Even assuming appropriate consent, the person making the removal must be licensed,[297] *except* where the removal is for the purpose of transplantation.[298] Acting without a licence is a criminal offence, unless the person reasonably believes that he has one or does not need one.[299] On top of all that, a person must not remove or use such material where he "knows, or has reason to believe, that" the body or the material "is, or may be, required for the purposes of functions of a coroner . . . except with the consent of the coroner".[300] Hence the practice of seeking the coroner's consent. The reference to *functions* of a coroner is in principle wider than the previous law, which referred only to an inquest or post-mortem examination.

8–81   In addition, both removal of material from the body of a living person and transplantation of that material are also offences in some circumstances.[301] This will cover the case of removal for transplantation *before* the patient dies and the coroner acquires jurisdiction. There are also provisions to permit retention and the taking of minimum steps for preservation of material until a decision can be taken as to whether removal for transplantation should take place,[302] but again only with the coroner's consent.[303]

Transplant operation procedures

8–82   Given that a common (and indeed essential) source of organs for transplant is persons who die suddenly or through acts of violence, e.g. in motor accidents, all of which are cases where the coroner will be involved, it is important for the coroner to be aware of the various procedures involved in a transplant operation.[304]

---

[290] Human Tissue Act 2004 s.2(2), (3).
[291] Human Tissue Act 2004 s.27(4).
[292] Human Tissue Act 2004 s.2(7).
[293] Human Tissue Act 2004 s.3(2).
[294] Human Tissue Act 2004 s.4.
[295] Human Tissue Act 2004 s.27(4).
[296] Human Tissue Act 2004 s.3(6).
[297] Human Tissue Act 2004 s.16 Sch.3. The reference to "includes" makes it very wide, and means that the definition strictly speaking includes urine, faeces and vomit.
[298] Human Tissue Act 2004 s.16(2)(c).
[299] Human Tissue Act 2004 s.25.
[300] Human Tissue Act 2004 s.11(2).
[301] Human Tissue Act 2004 s.33.
[302] Human Tissue Act 2004 s.43.
[303] Human Tissue Act 2004 s.43(5A).
[304] See, e.g. Pallis and Harley, *ABC of Brainstem Death,* 2nd edn (1996), Ch.10.

Given also that there is a major shortage of organs for transplantation,[305] it is equally important for him not to adopt an obstructive attitude.[306] But the coroner should bear in mind that he has no involvement in law unless or until there is a dead body.[307] Any informal indication pre-death can be no more than that.

The first objective is achieved through supply to coroners of up-to-date **8–83** information on transplant procedures. This includes a code of practice issued by the Human Tissue Authority in September 2009, *Donation of solid organs for transplantation*.[308] This code of practice was revised in March 2013, but the revision has not yet been approved by Parliament.[309] The code does not include guidance on the diagnosis of death. That guidance is given by the Academy of Royal Colleges' *A Code of Practice for the Diagnosis and Confirmation of Death*.[310] From this it will be seen that, since transplants, if to be carried out at all, must be carried out shortly after death of the donor, the coroner when approached for consent must be prepared to make rapid decisions.[311]

As for the second matter referred to, the Home Office some years ago gave **8–84** guidance[312] on the circumstances in which a coroner should delay or refuse giving his consent to removal of material. The Home Office view was that, since a coroner is an impartial legal officer, he should never refuse consent on moral or ethical grounds, but only where his own functions or other legal considerations were involved. Specifically, the Home Office considered only three cases in which refusal would be proper:

(1) where the material, consent to removal of which was sought, would have an evidential value in later criminal proceedings which the coroner is aware might take place;

(2) where the death was thought to have been caused, wholly or partly, by some malfunction in the organ or other material itself;

(3) where the coroner's own inquiries might be obstructed by such removal.

In the nature of things, material having evidential value in later criminal **8–85** proceedings is likely to be damaged in some way, and thus cases where removal of such material for transplantation is sought will be few and far between. Similarly, an organ which is defective and has caused the death is unlikely to be a desirable

---

[305] *Report of the Working Party on the Supply of Donor Organs for Transplantation*, 1987; public disquiet in recent years over unauthorised organ retention has had a negative impact (e.g. in the North Thames Region the rate of relative refusal more than doubled between 2000 and 2001).

[306] The *Report of the Working Party* in 1987 found "general praise for the attitude and helpfulness of coroners. Seldom has the need for a coroner's post-mortem examination prevented the donation of organs."

[307] As to which see 5–03, 5–14.

[308] Available at *http://www.hta.gov.uk* [Accessed June 6, 2014]; see the Human Tissue Act 2004 s.26.

[309] Under the Human Tissue Act 2004 s.26. Approval is expected to be sought during 2014.

[310] October 2008, available at *http://www.aomrc.org.uk* [Accessed June 6, 2014]; see App.5.

[311] As to whether the coroner is obliged to be available for this purpose at all times, see 2–75.

[312] Home Office Circular No. 65 of 1977. This guidance was criticised as insufficiently clear: see *The Times*, April 26, 1985.

candidate for transplant.[313] In practice, therefore, the only objection to consent which the coroner will normally be able to put forward consistently with the Home Office guidance is that in category (3) above. To the extent that this does not overlap with the other two categories, it seems to cover logistical problems (such as the need for a post-mortem examination) rather than medical or legal ones. In considering whether to object under this heading to the removal of organs, the coroner may need to consult with the pathologist and the doctor(s) who cared for the deceased before his death.

8–86 Although the coroner's discretion to consent or not appears to be absolute, there is little doubt that, as with any other coronial decision, it will be subject to judicial review.[314] The court in a proper case could quash the coroner's decision, but not (of course) substitute its own. In the nature of things, however, it is unlikely that there would be time to obtain a decision before the organ deteriorated, and the matter became academic. If a coroner persisted in making perverse decisions, the only solution would appear to be to remove him for misbehaviour.[315]

Anatomical Examination[316]

8–87 Anatomical examination of bodies for teaching or other educational purposes, or for research is permitted under certain strict conditions laid down by statute,[317] including the licensing by the Human Tissue Authority of both the person who is to carry out such examination and also the premises at which it is to be carried out.[318] Storage and use of a dead body for anatomical examination is lawful if done with "appropriate consent" and after relevant death certification formalities have been completed.[319] "Appropriate consent" is elaborately defined separately for children[320] and for adults.[321]

8–88 Acting without a licence is a criminal offence, unless the person reasonably believes that he has one or does not need one.[322] But a person must not store or use a body for anatomical examination where he "knows, or has reason to believe, that" the body "is, or may be, required for the purposes of functions of a coroner . . . except with the consent of the coroner".[323] The reference to *functions* of a coroner is in principle wider than the previous law, which referred only to an inquest or post-mortem examination.

---

[313] Yet the Stoke-on-Trent deputy coroner on one occasion prevented a heart transplant from going ahead on the ground that the heart's pre-existing condition "might be relevant to the jury inquest in due course": see *The Times*, December 17, 1983.

[314] See Ch.19.

[315] See 2–105 above.

[316] See generally Skegg (1991) Med. Sci. Law 345; Kennedy and Grubb, *Medical Law,* 3rd edn (2000), pp.2254–2263.

[317] See the Human Tissue Act 2004, replacing the Anatomy Act 1984.

[318] Human Tissue Act 2004 s.16 Sch.3.

[319] Human Tissue Act 2004 s.1(2), (3).

[320] Human Tissue Act 2004 s.2. See 8–79.

[321] Human Tissue Act 2004 s.3. See 8–79.

[322] Human Tissue Act 2004 s.25.

[323] Human Tissue Act 2004 s.11(2).

No doubt the coroner in deciding whether to give or refuse his consent (in those **8–89** cases where this is required) will be guided by similar considerations as those above mentioned in connection with organ transplants,[324] although there is clearly less urgency involved in anatomical examination, and no life stands directly to be saved or lost dependent upon the giving or refusing of consent.

HUMAN GAMETES

The Human Fertilisation and Embryology Authority is the authority dealing with **8–90** the treatment of human gametes, and is regulated by statute.[325] The Human Tissue Act 2004, and the consent and dealing arrangements put in place by hospitals and others under that legislation, do not apply to gametes.[326] In the coronial context, three questions arise: (1) Can gametes be lawfully retrieved from a dead body? (2) Can such gametes be lawfully stored? (3) Can such gametes be lawfully used?

As to (2) and (3), such gametes cannot be lawfully stored or used within the **8–91** United Kingdom without the effective consent of the deceased,[327] and the court cannot supply such consent.[328] On the other hand the Human Fertilisation and Embryology Authority appears to have statutory power to permit storage in the United Kingdom pending export and use of such gametes outside the United Kingdom.[329]

As to (1), the legislation does not cover the question,[330] and it is necessary to **8–92** consider the common law. But, at common law, the matter is uncertain.[331] Cases dealing with interference with the bodies of deceased persons (suggesting that personal representatives, surviving spouses or hospitals may authorise such actions) do not address the question of gamete removal, and those dealing with property in a body do not concern removal of body parts.[332] However, since the legislation does not cover the question, it does not make the removal criminal, and, if the only persons who can lawfully complain give their consent (including the coroner in whose possession the body lies), it is hard to see that the removal in itself can be in any meaningful way "unlawful".[333]

---

[324] See 8–84—8–85 above.
[325] Human Fertilisation and Embryology Act 1990.
[326] Human Tissue Act 2004 s.53 (definition of "relevant material").
[327] Human Fertilisation and Embryology Act 1990 s.4; *L v Human Fertilisation and Embryology Authority* [2008] EWHC 2149 (Fam.); [2008] 2 F.L.R. 1999 at [77].
[328] *L v Human Fertilisation and Embryology Authority* [2008] EWHC 2149 (Fam.); [2008] 2 F.L.R. 1999 at [100], [144]. But quaere whether it could if application were made to the court *before* death, at a time when the deceased was still alive but unable to consent for himself or herself.
[329] *L v Human Fertilisation and Embryology Authority* [2008] EWHC 2149 (Fam.); [2008] 2 F.L.R. 1999 at [129]–[130] (but this was a "preliminary view').
[330] *L v Human Fertilisation and Embryology Authority* [2008] EWHC 2149 (Fam.); [2008] 2 F.L.R. 1999 at [146].
[331] *L v Human Fertilisation and Embryology Authority* [2008] EWHC 2149 (Fam.); [2008] 2 F.L.R. 1999 at [155].
[332] *L v Human Fertilisation and Embryology Authority* [2008] EWHC 2149 (Fam.); [2008] 2 F.L.R. 1999 at [158].
[333] See 9–07.

Chapter 9

DISPOSAL OF HUMAN REMAINS

POSSESSION OF THE BODY

As already stated,[1] whenever the coroner is under a duty, or is considering whether   **9–01**
he is under a duty, to conduct an investigation into the death of a particular person
he has a right to possession of the body for the purpose of those enquiries.[2] This
right overrides all others, although, as stated, it will come to an end in certain
circumstances.[3] Secondly, certain rights to possession of a body for the purposes of
anatomical examination may arise in some circumstances.[4] Thirdly, tissue removed
at post-mortem may be retained in some circumstances and not returned to the
body.[5] But in this chapter the concern is not with those rights. Instead, it is with
the legal position *subject* to those rights. The starting point is what happens to a
person's property on death.

When a person dies, all his property immediately vests in the executors   **9–02**
appointed by his will, or (if he has made no valid will)[6] in the Public Trustee,[7]
pending appointment by the court of an administrator, who thereupon has all such
property vested in him.[8] An executor will need to have his appointment confirmed
by the court, by "proving the will", but, in principle, having been appointed by the
deceased, he is entitled to act in the affairs of the deceased's estate from the
moment of death.[9] An administrator, on the other hand, derives title from the
action of the court in appointing him, and has no legal power to act until then.[10]
The persons who may be appointed administrator are largely, but not exclusively,
members of the deceased's family.[11] Executors and administrators are known
generically as "personal representatives".[12]

---

[1] See 8–11.

[2] Para. 6–10 above. That he has this power even when he is merely considering whether he has a duty
is demonstrated by the fact that he has the power at this time to request a post-mortem examination
of the body: s.14(1)(b); see 8–13.

[3] See 8–11.

[4] Human Tissue Act 2004; see 8–87 above.

[5] See 8–72 ff above.

[6] Administration of Estates Act 1925 s.1 (realty); *Wind v Jekyl* (1719) 1 P. Wms 572; 24 E.R. 522;
Wentw. Off. Ex., 14th edn, 228; 11 Vin.Abr. 240.

[7] Administration of Estates Act 1925 s.9, as amended by the Law of Property (Miscellaneous
Provisions) Act 1994 s.14 (previously it vested in the President of the Family Division).

[8] Administration of Estates Act 1925 s.9. For cases where the Treasury Solicitor will act, see 9–19.

[9] *Wankford v Wankford* (1699) 1 Salk. 299; *Woolley v Clarke* (1822) 5 B. & Ald. 744.

[10] *Ingall v Moran* [1944] K.B. 160; *Long v Burgess* [1950] 1 K.B. 115.

[11] See 9–08—9–09.

[12] See also 8–29.

9–03   The question is how far personal representatives and others have rights in relation to the body of the deceased. It is often said, for example, that there is no "property" in the human body.[13] Plainly, this word is not being used in a physical sense, for a body is tangible matter having characteristics similar to other animal tissue, in which property rights can and do undoubtedly exist. On the other hand, in the legal sense, to have "property" in a thing means to have certain rights, powers, duties and liabilities in relation to it,[14] and in that sense it is clear that there *is* property in a body.[15] For example, parts of bodies have been held capable of theft,[16] cremated human remains preserved *in specie* have been led to be subject to the ordinary rights of property,[17] and human gametes destroyed by negligence have been held the subject of property rights.[18] For present purposes it is necessary only to consider one aspect of such "property", and that is the right to possession of the body. Questions relating to organ donation and the retrieval and use of human gametes have been dealt with elsewhere.[19]

9–04   The personal representatives of the deceased,[20] rather than members of the family as such, have the duty to arrange (and pay for) the appropriate disposal of the body, and for that purpose they also have the right to possession of it.[21] But if there are no personal representatives, a duty to dispose of the body is cast upon other persons, such as the father of a deceased infant child,[22] the person entitled to letters of administration to the deceased's estate, even before administration is applied for,[23] the occupier of the house where the person in question dies,[24] and ultimately (if the local authority is satisfied that no other suitable arrangements are

---

[13] 3 Co. Inst. 203; 2 Bl. Comm. 429; 4 Bl. Comm. 236; 2 East P.C. 652; *Williams v Williams* (1882) 20 Ch.D. 659 at 662–663; *Dobson v North Tyneside Health Authority* [1996] 4 All. E.R. 474 at 478, CA; *Buchanan v Milton* [1999] 2. F.L.R. 844 at 845; *AW v CW* [2002] NSWSC 301; *Re X* [2003] J.R.C. 111; Williams, Mortimer and Sunnucks, *Executors, Administrators and Probate*, 20th edn (2013) para.48–02.

[14] *Blade v Higgs* (1865) 11 H.L.C. 621, 11 E.R. 1474; *National Provincial Bank Ltd v Ainsworth* [1965] A.C. 1175 at 1247–1248, per Lord Wilberforce.

[15] See, generally, Matthews, "Whose Body? People as People" (1983) 36 *Current Legal Problems* 193; Magnussen, *Proprietary Rights in Human Tissue*, in Palmer and McKendrick (eds), *Interests in Goods*, 2nd edn (1998) Ch.2; Stern and Walsh (eds), *Property Rights in the Human Body* (Centre of Medical Law and Ethics, 1997).

[16] *R. v Kelly* [1999] Q.B. 621, CA; see also *DPP v Smith* [2006] EWHC 44 (Admin.).

[17] *Leeburn v Derndorfer* [2004] WTLR 867, [2004] V.S.C. 172 at [27].

[18] *Yearworth v North Bristol NHS Trust* [2009] EWCA Civ. 37.

[19] See 8–78 ff and 8–90 ff.

[20] In practice, administrators are unlikely to be involved, as they may not be appointed for some time, and only have title to act once appointed: see 9–02 above; *Warner v Levitt* (1994) 7 BPR 15,110, 15,113; *Dobson v North Tyneside Health Authority* [1996] 4 All E.R. 474, 478, CA; *Buchanan v Milton* [1999] 2 F.L.R. 844, 845.

[21] *Sharp v Lush* (1879) 10 Ch.D. 468, 472; *Williams v Williams* (1882) 20 Ch.D. 659; *Hunter v Hunter* (1930) 65 O.L.R. 586; *Dobson v North Tyneside Health Authority* [1996] 4 All. E.R. 474, 478, CA; *Smith v Tamworth City Council* (1997) 41 NSWLR 680, 691; *Buchanan v Milton* [1999] 2 F.L.R. 844, 845; *Ibuna v Arroyo* [2012] EWHC 428 (Ch.); *Takemore v Clarke* [2013] 2 NZLR 733, SC.

[22] *R. v Vann* (1851) 2 Den. 325; 169 E.R. 523. There was formerly a similar rule for husbands in relation to their deceased wives, but this no long obtains: *Rees v Hughes* [1946] K.B. 517, CA. For children in the care of a local authority, see the Children Act 1989 s.23(9) and Sch.2 para.20.

[23] *Holtham v Arnold* (1985) 2 B.M.L.R. 123, Hoffmann J; *Warner v Levitt* (1994) 7 BPR 15,110, 15,113; *R. (Haqq) v Inner West London Coroner* [2003] EWHC 3366 (Admin.); *Borrows v Preston Coroner* [2008] EWHC 1387 (QB); cf. *Buchanan v Milton* [1999] 2 F.L.R. 844 at 846 (but *Holtham v Arnold* was not cited). For details of the order of priority, see 9–09.

[24] *R. v Stewart* (1840) 12 Ad. & El. 773; 113 E.R. 1007; *University College Hospital Lewisham NHS Trust v Hamuth* [2006] EWHC 1609 (Ch.).

being made) the local authority.[25] Such a duty to dispose will naturally carry with it a right to possession of the body for the purpose of discharging that duty.[26] But there is no such duty cast on, and therefore no such right attaching to, the next of kin as such.[27]

However, where no application is made for probate or letters of administration **9–05** of the estate of the deceased, it is members of the deceased's family who in practice will arrange the funeral. In most cases, therefore, funeral and other arrangements for the disposal of the body of the deceased will be made *either* by the executors of the deceased, *or* (and of course they may well be the same persons) members of the deceased's family.[28]

Disputes over disposal[29]

Disputes may arise between, say, the personal representatives and others in relation **9–06** to three points. The first is *whether* the body should be disposed of at this time. The second is *how* it should be disposed of, and the third is *who* should make the arrangements. Dealing with the first of these, the rights to possession of an executor,[30] a parent of the deceased,[31] and the occupier of a house where the deceased dies,[32] are all rights conferred for the purpose of discharging the duty properly and decently to dispose of the body.[33] Similarly the statutory duty of the local authority is to bury or cremate the body.[34] A person holding an anatomy licence[35] is under a similar duty, after the conclusion of an anatomical examination, to ensure the disposal of the body in accordance with any wishes of the deceased or any surviving spouse or relative of his.[36]

So, on the face of it, the body must be disposed of. However, it seems that, once **9–07** such a person has possession of the body, but no one with a right to do so[37] complains that the duty to dispose of the body has not been discharged, there is

---

[25] Public Health (Control of Disease) Act 1984 s.46(1); *Secretary of State for Scotland v Fife County Council*, 1953 S.C. 257 (predecessor provision imposed *duty* rather than conferred *power*).

[26] *Dobson v North Tyneside Health Authority* [1996] 4 All E.R. 474 at 478, CA; cf. the right of a coroner to possession of the body, arising out of his duties in relation to it: 8–11.

[27] *Dobson v North Tyneside Health Authority* [1996] 4 All E.R. 474, CA; *Holtham v Arnold*, above, was not cited.

[28] For cases where the coroner may make funeral or other arrangements for disposal, see 9–19.

[29] See Conway, (2003) 23 Leg. Stud. 423.

[30] *Williams v Williams* (1882) 20 Ch.D. 659.

[31] *R. v Vann* (1851) 2 Den. 325; 169 E.R. 523.

[32] *R. v Stewart* (1840) Ad. & E1. 773; 113 E.R. 1007; *University College Hospital Lewisham NHS Trust v Hamuth* [2006] EWHC 1609 (Ch.).

[33] *Dobson v North Tyneside Health Authority* [1996] 4 All E.R. 474 at 478. CA.

[34] Public Health (Control of Disease) Act 1984 s.46(1).

[35] Under the Human Tissue Act 2004 s.16; see 8–87.

[36] Anatomy Regulations 1988, reg.4(1)(e).

[37] Presumably a person who would have the duty to bury or cremate the body if the person in possession did not do so; see, e.g. *Herring v Walrond* (1682) 2 Ch.Cas. 110; 22 E.R. 870; *R. v Vann* (1851) 2 Den. 325; 169 E.R. 523.

nothing to prevent the body remaining in such possession undisposed of,[38] or handed down from one generation to another,[39] or even given away[40] or sold.[41]

Funeral arrangements

9–08   The second and third questions can be dealt with together. The person who makes the arrangements generally has the right to decide on how (and where) the body should be disposed of. It is necessary to consider not only who has right of possession, but also who ultimately is responsible for the funeral and other expenses connected with the death. On both grounds, the executors are entitled to determine the mode and, within certain limits,[42] the place of disposal of a body, even where other members of the family object.[43] If there are no executors, then it is necessary to consider who is entitled to apply for a grant of letters of administration to the estate of the deceased. If the deceased was married or in a civil partnership, the deceased's spouse or civil partner is the person first entitled to such a grant,[44] at least until it is clear that he or she is incapable of acting[45] or does not intend to apply for such a grant.[46]

9–09   Subject to that, the other persons[47] able to apply for a grant should be treated as the persons to determine mode and place of disposal.[48] Establishing who this is may involve interstitial questions of some difficulty, such as the validity of a marriage, which may be impossible in summary proceedings.[49] However, the court has power where by reason of special circumstances it appears to be necessary or

---

[38] e.g. a body retained under the Human Tissue Act might remain in a medical museum.

[39] As happened in *Doodeward v Spence* (1908) 6 C.L.R. 406 (High Court of Australia).

[40] As the executor of Jeremy Bentham did with Jeremy Bentham's body, pursuant to a direction of his will: the skeleton is still in the possession of the original donee, University College London.

[41] As with human skeletons for medical students (though most these days are made of plastic or other artificial substances).

[42] *Holtham v Arnold* (1986) 2 B.M.L.R. 123, 125; *Grandison v Nembhard* (1989) 5 B.M.L.R. 140 at 144. Executors, being in the position of quasi-trustees for those ultimately beneficially entitled to the estate, must not in the absence of specific authority or consent expend more than reasonable amounts on funeral expenses, such as the cost of transporting the body to its final resting place: see Williams, Mortimer and Sunnucks, *Executors, Administrators and Probate*, 20th edn (2013), at para.48-13.

[43] *Williams v Williams* (1882) 20 Ch.D. 659; *Hunter v Hunter* (1930) 65 O.L.R. 586; *Holtham v Arnold* (1986) 2 B.M.L.R. 123, 125; *Grandison v Nembhard* (1989) 5 B.M.L.R. 140; *Takemore v Clarke* [2013] 2 NZLR 733, SC.

[44] Non-Contentious Probate Rules 1987 r.22(1)(a): see App.2; *Holtham v Arnold* (1985) 2 B.M.L.R. 123, Hoffmann J; *R. (Haqq) v Inner West London Coroner* [2003] EWHC 3366 (Admin.); *Borrows v Preston Coroner* [2008] EWHC 1387 (QB).

[45] When a grant of administration can be made to another for the spouse's use and benefit: Non-Contentious Probate Rules 1987 r.35.

[46] When he or she will either renounce the right to a grant (r.37), or be "cleared off" by citation to take one (r.47).

[47] Non-Contentious Probate Rules 1987 r.22. In summary, the list is as follows: (1) surviving spouse or civil partner, (2) children, (3) parents, (4) siblings, (5) half-siblings, (6) grandparents, (7) siblings of parents, (8) half-siblings of parents (but, in each preceding case, issue of a person otherwise entitled who has already died are entitled with the same priority), (9) the Treasury Solicitor (where bona vacantia is claimed), (10) creditors. See Williams, Mortimer and Sunnucks, *Executors, Administrators and Probate*, 20th edn (2013) para.19–02.

[48] *Holtham v Arnold* (1986) 2 B.M.L.R. 123, Hoffmann J (widow preferred to mistress); *Smith v Tamworth City Council* (1997) 41 N.S.W.L.R. 680, Young J (highest right to administration preferred); *Buchanan v Milton* [1999] 2 F.L.R. 844, Hale J; *Dodd v Jones* (1999) 73 SASR 328 (de facto wife preferred to father); *Borrows v Preston Coroner* [2008] EWHC 1387 (QB) at [28].

[49] See e.g. *Privet v Vovk* [2003] NSWSC 1038; *R. (Haqq) v Inner West London Coroner* [2003] EWHC 3366 (Admin.).

expedient to change the order of priority for a grant,[50] which may be limited as the court thinks fit.[51] In exercising this power the court must consider, first, whether there *are* special circumstances which may displace the order of priority, and, second, if there are, whether it is necessary or expedient by reason of those circumstances to displace the normal order.[52] This will be rare.[53] Coroners asked to release a body to a person who does not have priority under the general law should carry out a similar exercise.[54] Any decision which they make will be subject to legal challenge before the High Court, but the court will be slow to interfere.[55] As a matter of general law, the killer of a person is normally passed over as a personal representative of the deceased.[56] Where two or more persons rank equally, the court will resolve the dispute on a practical basis.[57] However, it has been held that one of several executors may make a decision which, at least once implemented, is binding on all.[58]

How far the discussion above is affected by human rights considerations is   **9–10**
unclear.[59] In an appropriate case, either or both of arts 8 (right to respect for family and private life)[60] and 9 (rights to religion and to manifest religion or beliefs)[61] may be engaged.[62] To the extent that the views of the deceased as to the funeral and other disposal arrangements that should be made must be taken into account,[63] they can be treated as possible "special circumstances",[64] potentially justifying a change in priority, so that someone else is given the duty of disposing the body. But if the priority is not changed, such views do not bind the personal representative.[65]

---

[50] Senior Courts Act 1981 s.116(1); *Buchanan v Milton* [1999] 2 F.L.R. 844; *Borrows v Preston Coroner* [2008] EWHC 1387 (QB); *Ibuna v Arroyo* [2012] EWHC 428 (Ch.); cf. *Holtham v Arnold* (1986) 2 B.M.L.R. 123.

[51] Senior Courts Act 1981 s.116(2).

[52] *Borrows v Preston Coroner* [2008] EWHC 1387 (QB) at [17].

[53] *Buchanan v Milton* [1999] 2 F.L.R. 844; *Borrows v Preston Coroner* [2008] EWHC 1387 (QB) at [17].

[54] *Borrows v Preston Coroner* [2008] EWHC 1387 (QB) at [29].

[55] *Borrows v Preston Coroner* [2008] EWHC 1387 (QB) at [29].

[56] *Re Crippen* [1911] P. 108. But an accused person may be able to delay disposal, e.g. to obtain a further post-mortem examination: see 8–40, 9–11, 9–16, 9–17, 14–18.

[57] e.g. *Calma v Sesar* (1992) 2 N.T.L.R. 37 (estranged parents; burial where body was); *Fessi v Whitmore* [1999] 1 F.L.R. 767 (burial of cremated remains where centre of family interests and history); *Leeburn v Derndorfer* [2004] WTLR 867; [2004] V.S.C. 172 (estranged sibling-executors: ashes left where they had been interred); *Hartshorne v Gardner* [2008] 2 FLR 1681; [2008] WTLR 837; [2008] Fam. Law 985; *Scotching v Birch* [2008] EWHC 844 (Ch.).

[58] *Leeburn v Derndorfer* [2004] WTLR 867; [2004] V.S.C. 172.

[59] *Ibuna v Arroyo* [2012] EWHC 428 (Ch.) at [50].

[60] *X v Federal Republic of Germany*, App no. 8741/79, 10 March 1981; DR 24, 137 (interference justified); *Dodsbo v Sweden* ECHR 2006 No. 5 (assumption that art.8 engaged; interference justified). See 21–29.

[61] See 21–49.

[62] *Borrows v Preston Coroner* [2008] EWHC 1387 (QB); *Ibuna v Arroyo* [2012] EWHC 428 (Ch.); *R. (the Plantagenet Alliance Ltd) v Secretary of State for Justice* Unreported 15 August 2013, Haddon-Cave J, [2014] EWHC 1668, DC.

[63] See e.g. *Privet v Vovk* [2003] NSWSC 1038 at [13].

[64] *Borrows v Preston Coroner* [2008] EWHC 1387 (QB) at [20].

[65] *Ibuna v Arroyo* [2012] EWHC 428 (Ch) at [50].

Consequences of release or non-release of a body

9–11   If the body is released to a person who disposes of it in a way or place disapproved
of by another person or persons who actually have the right to possession for that
purpose, the coroner or his officer may be liable in damages to such person or
persons for any loss[66] or injury to feelings[67] sustained. Or a person accused of
homicide may seek an injunction to restrain the coroner from releasing the body
to the family until a further post-mortem examination has been conducted.[68]
Moreover, there may be criminal consequences in releasing a body: it is, for
example, an indictable offence for a person having lawful custody of a body to sell
it for unauthorised anatomical examination.[69]

9–12   Conversely, a coroner may be liable for damages, or open to attack by way of
judicial review of his decision,[70] if he declines to release the body to a person
properly entitled, either on grounds of some supposed right to withhold
possession,[71] or because he claims that another person has a better right.[72] In
consequence, the coroner or his officer, in releasing a body after conclusion of the
coroner's inquiries, should take care to release the body only into the custody of
the person properly entitled to possession of it, or as directed by such person.[73] The
Home Office view was that any dispute had to be resolved by the person(s)
claiming the body, whether by judicial review or otherwise.[74]

Disposal of a Body

9–13   A body lying in England and Wales may generally be lawfully disposed of in one
of three ways: burial, cremation, or removal out of England and Wales for final
disposal elsewhere.[75] Of these three, cremation[76] is by far the most common.[77] As
the procedures in each case are different, it is necessary to consider them in turn.
There are some special rules for the disposal of body parts.[78] In addition, there are
certain exceptional cases, to which these procedures do not apply and these will be
referred to in due course.[79] The civil registration system has been modernised in
recent years. From the coronial point of view, the most significant reform is the
introduction of the medical examiner system,[80] previously forecast to take place in

---

[66] cf. misdelivery in the law of bailment: 16–10 below.
[67] *Owens v Liverpool Corporation* [1939] 1 K.B. 394; see also *Vigers v Cook* [1919] 2 K.B. 475.
[68] See 8–40, 9–11, 9–16, 9–17, 14–18.
[69] *R. v Cundick* (1822) D. & Ry. N.P. 13, 171 E.R. 900.
[70] e.g. *Re Jacobs' Application* (1999) 53 B.M.L.R. 21, CA; see Ch.19 below.
[71] *R. v Fox* (1941) 2 Q.B. 246; 114 E.R. 95 (gaoler claiming lien on body); *R. v Bristol Coroner Ex p.
Kerr* [1974] Q.B. 652 (coroner claiming to discharge duties).
[72] *R. v Hampshire Coroner Ex p. Horscroft, The Times,* October 3, 1985.
[73] e.g. to a named undertaker.
[74] See Home Office Newsletter to Coroners, August 29, 1990.
[75] Anatomical examination (see 8–87 above) is simply a staging post on the way to final disposal.
[76] See *R. v Price* (1884) 12 Q.B.D. 247; *R. (Ghai) v Newcastle City Council* [2010] EWCA Civ. 59.
[77] In 2011 it was used in about 78 per cent of cases in England and Wales, up from 1 per cent in 1931,
and 56.7 per cent in 1970 (cremations exceeded burials for the first time in 1968). The figures for
Scotland and Northern Ireland are lower (only 11 per cent in Northern Ireland).
[78] See 9–33 below.
[79] See 9–42—9–43 below.
[80] Coroners and Justice Act 2009 ss.18-21; see Ch.3.

October 2014.[81] What follows represents the current system, before the introduction of medical examiners.

A coroner must release a body for burial or cremation as soon as is reasonably **9–14** practicable.[82] In some but not all cases he can also issue a burial[83] or cremation[84] order.[85] This must be after he has begun an investigation,[86] but may be before any inquest is opened. In such a case the coroner must be careful to ensure sufficient evidence of identification and of the cause of death being available at the inquest.[87] The coroner must also bear in mind the possible need for further medical investigations in light of the results of the examination or any laboratory tests which may be commissioned, and these may be impeded or prevented if the body is disposed of. Normally the pathologist will indicate in his report (written or oral) of the post-mortem examination if he requires further access to the body, but if nothing is said expressly, the coroner would be wise to check with the pathologist before authorising disposal.[88]

Releasing body of unknown person

Where other methods of identifying a body have failed,[89] Missing People (formerly **9–15** the National Missing Persons Helpline) can sometimes assist.[90] If the coroner releases the body of an unknown person, clothing, personal property or other material, identifiable or not, should be carefully retained. Where a post-mortem examination is made, the coroner should consider asking for a DNA sample to be taken and preserved, so that, if a possible identity later comes to light, it can be tested against that.

Enquiries by other interested persons

Once a coroner realises that his making a burial or cremation order may affect **9–16** another person in some way, he "is almost certainly under a duty to give the person who may be affected by [the order] a chance of saying something about it".[91] There will be cases where a burial or cremation order should not be made until

---

[81] Letter of June 3, 2013 from Secretary of State for Health to the Chairman of the House of Commons Health Select Committee. But this appears to have been quietly dropped until after the 2015 general election.

[82] Coroners (Investigation) Rules 2013 (SI 2013/1629, r 20(1); see 8–11, 8–12. This does not apply to applications to remove a body out of England, because such bodies are not in the coroner's possession to begin with, so he does not 'release' them: see 9–36 ff.

[83] The form is prescribed by Coroners (Investigation) Rules 2013 (SI 2013/1629) r.21(2) and Sch. Form 3.

[84] The form is prescribed by Cremation (England and Wales) Regulations 2008 (SI 2008/2841) reg.18 Sch.1 Form 6.

[85] Coroners (Investigation) Rules 2013 (SI 2013/1629) r.21(1).

[86] See 9–21, 9–28 below.

[87] cf. *R. v Greater Manchester Coroner Ex p. Worch* [1987] Q.B. 627, DC (the point was not taken in the Court of Appeal).

[88] cf. *Howlett v Devon Coroner* [2006] EWHC 2570 (Admin.) at [20].

[89] Including DNA tests.

[90] Tel: 020 8392 4590; *http://www.missingpeople.org.uk* [Accessed June 9, 2014]; see Home Office Newsletter No. 26 (May 5, 1998) para.4 (giving an earlier number).

[91] *R. v Bristol Coroner Ex p. Atkinson* Unreported May 5, 1983, Forbes J. The judge appeared to rely to some extent on the provisions of s.14 of the Coroners (Amendment) Act 1926, and it was not brought to his attention that these provisions were repealed by the Coroners Act 1980, but it is submitted that the dictum cited is nonetheless correct in principle and represents the law.

other interested parties (such as a defendant charged with causing the death of the deceased) have had the opportunity to seek to make such enquiries or examinations as they wish.[92] On the other hand, delay in releasing the body for disposal can cause distress to relatives, and any potential sources of delay should be eliminated, both in the time taken for such examination to be carried out,[93] and in carrying out any second post-mortem examination.[94]

Decision on release and burial or cremation order subject to review

9–17   The decisions to release a body or not, and whether to issue or to refuse a burial or cremation order are, like every other coronial decision, subject in an appropriate case to judicial review by the High Court.[95] Failure to give an opportunity to an interested person of being heard, where this is appropriate, may lead to the decision being quashed for this reason alone.[96] Where a further examination of the body can be demonstrated to be necessary for a fair trial of a homicide charge, an injunction may be granted to restrain the release of the body.[97]

Burial or cremation order must avoid duplication of registrar's certificate

9–18   The coroner should try to ensure that he does not issue a burial or cremation order when a registrar's certificate for the disposal of the body[98] has been issued[99] in respect of the same body.[100] Under the old law, if he was satisfied that a certificate for the disposal of a body had been issued, he could not issue a burial or cremation order unless the certificate was surrendered to him, and he had thereupon to transmit it to the registrar of births and deaths who issued it, and to inform him of the issue of his own order.[101] But this obligation has not been carried over into the new law, as the Government considered that it was no longer required.

Default disposal arrangements

9–19   It is no part of the functions of the coroner to make arrangements for the actual burial or cremation of the body, unless he is authorised by, and acting as an agent of, the Treasury Solicitor, in cases where the Treasury Solicitor proposes to

---

[92] cf. *R. v Bristol Coroner Ex p. Kerr* [1974] Q. B. 652; *R. v Bristol Coroner Ex p. Atkinson* Unreported May 5, 1983, per Forbes J. See also 8–40, 9–11, 9–17, 14–18.

[93] Home Office Circular No. 5 of 1982: see also the debate in the House of Commons on delays in the release of bodies for burial, *Hansard*, HC, cols 1081–1086 (December 10, 1981).

[94] See Home Office Circular No. 30 of 1999, *Memorandum of Good Practice re Early Release of Bodies in Cases of Suspicious Death*. See also 8–41, 14–18.

[95] Ch.19; *R. v Greater Manchester Coroner Ex p. Worch* [1987] Q.B. 627, DC. cf. *R. v Bristol Coroner Ex p. Atkinson* Unreported May 5, 1983, per Forbes J, where the applicant was charged with the murder of the deceased and his advisers wished to be able to carry out a post-mortem examination of the deceased's body for defence purposes: the application for judicial review was rejected as premature, because the coroner had wisely indicated that he would consider representations on the applicant's behalf before he actually made a burial order.

[96] *Cooper v Wandsworth Board of Works* (1863) 14 C.B.N.S. 180; 143 E.R. 414; *Weinburger v Inglis* [1919] A.C. 606 at 616; *Ridge v Baldwin* [1964] A.C. 40.

[97] *Haydon v Chivell* (1999) 73 A.L.J.R. 1311, HC (Aus.), Gaudron J: injunction refused on facts.

[98] It is in fact a certificate of registration of the death, but by reg.48 of the Registration of Births and Deaths Regulations 1987 it is treated for the purposes of Pt XI of those Regulations (Disposal of Bodies of Deceased Persons) as a "certificate for disposal".

[99] Under the Births and Deaths Registration Act 1953 s.24(1).

[100] cf. Births and Deaths Registration Act 1953 s.24(1), proviso.

[101] Coroners Rules 1984 r.15, now revoked.

administer the estate of the deceased.[102] Where there are no executors or relatives of the deceased (or none can be discovered) and the Treasury Solicitor does not propose to administer the estate of the deceased, the coroner should inform the local authority,[103] which has a residual obligation properly to dispose of the body.[104]

Burial

Issue of burial order

Before the body of a deceased person[105] can be buried[106] in England or Wales, *either* a burial order must have been issued[107] by a coroner *or* a certificate for the disposal of the body[108] or of non-liability to register the death[109] must have been issued by the registrar of births and deaths.[110] This rule applies wherever the death took place. A similar rule applies to the burial of a stillborn child.[111] There is, however, no such requirement in the case of the interment of cremated human remains,[112] although such interment in or under a parish church requires a faculty.[113]

9–20

Although a coroner has a duty to release the body for burial or cremation as soon as is reasonably practicable, a coroner can issue a burial order[114] only once he no longer needs to retain the body for the purposes of the investigation.[115] There is no longer any rule that he can only do so if he has at least decided to open an

9–21

---

[102] The Treasury Solicitor will normally do so, pursuant to the Treasury Solicitor Act 1876, in cases where the deceased dies intestate with no relatives and an estate exceeding known liabilities: Home Office Circular No. 68 of 1955 para.17. If the coroner believes that he has such a case, he should contact the Treasury Solicitor for this purpose: Home Office Circular No. 68 of 1955 para.17. Where the assets of the estate are situate in (historic) Lancashire or the extra-Palatine liberties of the Duchy of Lancaster, the Solicitor to the Duchy of Lancaster replaces the Treasury Solicitor: Duchy of Lancaster Act 1920 s.3(3), Local Government Act 1972 s.272(5); and where the assets are in Cornwall it is the Solicitor to the Duchy of Cornwall who acts: *Solicitor of the Duchy of Cornwall v Canning* (1880) 5 P.D. 114.

[103] Home Office Circular No. 68 of 1955 para.18.

[104] Public Health (Control of Disease) Act 1984 ss.46(1), 48(1).

[105] This does not include a stillborn child: cf. Births and Deaths Registration Act 1926 s.5 (as amended).

[106] This expression includes interment by placing the body in a vault.

[107] It need not actually have been delivered to the person effecting the burial if there is a written declaration in the prescribed form that it has been issued: Births and Deaths Registration Act 1926 s.1(1), proviso.

[108] Births and Deaths Registration Act 1953 s.24(1): see the Registration of Births and Deaths Regulations 1987 reg.48, treating the certificate of registration of death as a certificate for disposal.

[109] Births and Deaths Registration Act 1953 s.24(2); Registration of Births and Deaths Regulations 1987 reg.32 Form 19.

[110] Births and Deaths Registration Act 1926 s.1(1). The person effecting the burial must notify the registrar within 96 hours of doing so: Births and Deaths Registration Act 1926 s.3(1).

[111] Births and Deaths Registration Act 1926 s.5 (as amended).

[112] But it is treated as a burial for the purposes of the Local Authorities Cemeteries Order 1977, regulating burial in cemeteries.

[113] *Re Kerr* [1894] P. 284. A right of burial in the parish churchyard includes the right to bury cremated remains: Church of England (Miscellaneous Provisions) Measure 1992 s.3(1).

[114] The form is prescribed by Coroners (Investigation) Rules 2013 (SI 2013/1629) r.21(2) and Sch. Form 3.

[115] Coroners (Investigation) Rules 2013 (SI 2013/1629) r.21(1); see 8–11, 8–12.

inquest.[116] However, the requirement that he no longer needs the body for the purposes of the investigation means that he must by then have come under a duty to conduct such an investigation. So the coroner cannot make a burial order in any case which he disposes of at the stage of preliminary inquiries, without ever having come under a duty to conduct one,[117] for instance where a body is repatriated for burial here but the deceased died a natural death.

Form of burial order

9–22   The form of burial order is prescribed by coroner legislation, and the regulations say that the coroner must use it.[118] On its face it does not apply to stillborn children.[119] As prescribed, it is so simple that it does not have any practical function. Accordingly the registrar of deaths has for many years issued a more complex and useful version, based on the statutory form. This is in three parts. Part A is a counterfoil, retained by the coroner, to prove that the order has been given. Part B is an expanded version (with notes) of the statutory form, containing all the information that that form requires (and more). Part C is a blank form of notification to the registrar that the burial has been completed. Parts B and C are normally given to the relative or undertaker arranging for the burial of the body. Part B is retained by the burial ground authority where the burial takes place. The person effecting the burial must complete Part C and send it to the Registrar within 96 hours after burial.[120]

Cremation

Prescribed forms

9–23   Cremation is regulated by statute.[121] The following account is based on the regulations currently in force. When the new medical examiner system is introduced, it will change. Application for cremation of the remains of a dead person is made in the prescribed form,[122] normally by the executor or the nearest relative of the deceased.[123] There is separate provision for the cremation of stillborn children[124] and body parts.[125] In addition to the application form, various

---

[116] Coroners Rules 1984 r.14.

[117] Similarly with cremation: 9–28. As to when the duty to conduct an investigation arises, see 8–18.

[118] Coroners (Investigation) Rules 2013 (SI 2013/1629) r. 21(2) and Sch. Form 3, replacing Coroners Rules 1984 Sch. Form 21 (which was not, however, compulsory).

[119] The coroner will usually have concluded during preliminary inquiries that he is dealing with a stillbirth, and so will never come under an obligation to conduct an investigation: see 8–13, 5–05.

[120] Births and Deaths Registration Act 1926 s.3(1); Registration of Births and Deaths Regulations 1987 reg.50.

[121] Cremation Act 1902; Cremation (England and Wales) Regulations 2008; see *R. (Ghai) v Newcastle City Council* [2010] EWCA Civ. 59 (not unlawful to cremate in open structure according to Hindu religion).

[122] Cremation (England and Wales) Regulations 2008 Sch.1, Form 1: see App.2. If the deceased died outside England and Wales, the prescribed form need not be used, but the same information must be given: Cremation (England and Wales) Regulations 2008 reg.14(2).

[123] Cremation (England and Wales) Regulations 2008 reg.15.

[124] See 9–32 below.

[125] See 9–33 below.

certificates are required.[126] If the coroner gives a cremation certificate,[127] it is simply the written authority of the medical referee.[128] If there is a certificate that the body has been subject to anatomical examination under a Human Tissue Act licence,[129] they are *either* a certificate of registration of death *or* a certified copy of an entry in the relevant register, *plus* (in either case) written authority of the medical referee.[130] In any other case, they are two separate medical certificates of the cause of death,[131] *either* a certificate of registration of death *or* a certified copy of an entry in the relevant register, and (in either case) the written authority of the medical referee.[132]

However these requirements do not apply to cremation of human remains   9–24 which are exhumed after being buried for at least one year,[133] though there may be other requirements or conditions to fulfil.[134] Where it would otherwise apply, the need to produce either a certificate of registration of death *or* a certified copy of an entry in the relevant register is dispensed with in certain cases.[135] These are (a) where a coroner's post-mortem examination has revealed the cause of death and the coroner does not think it necessary to continue the investigation,[136] (b) the coroner has begun an investigation,[137] or (c) the death occurred outside the British Islands[138] and no post-mortem examination or investigation is necessary.[139]

Forms 4 and 5

Both forms of certificate are lengthy documents which ask wide-ranging and often   9–25 searching questions. They cover not only the cause of death, but many other facts concerning the death and those involved. Any registered medical practitioner may give the first certificate, in Form 4.[140] But the confirmatory certificate, in Form 5, may only be given by a registered medical practitioner of at least five years' standing[141] who is not the first practitioner, nor a relative, partner or colleague in

---

[126] Cremation (England and Wales) Regulations 2008 reg.16(1).

[127] Cremation (England and Wales) Regulations 2008 reg.18 Sch.1 Form 6.

[128] Cremation (England and Wales) Regulations 2008 reg.23 Sch.1 Form 10.

[129] Cremation (England and Wales) Regulations 2008 Sch.1 Form 7.

[130] Cremation (England and Wales) Regulations 2008 reg.23 Sch.1 Form 10. See 9–30.

[131] Cremation (England and Wales) Regulations 2008 reg.17 Sch.1 Forms 4 and 5. The confirmatory certificate (Form 5) can be dispensed with in some cases: see 9–26.

[132] Cremation (England and Wales) Regulations 2008 reg.23 Sch.1 Form 10. See 9–30.

[133] Cremation (England and Wales) Regulations 2008 reg.16(2).

[134] Cremation (England and Wales) Regulations 2008 reg.21.

[135] Cremation (England and Wales) Regulations 2008 regs 16(1)(b), 18.

[136] See 8–36. The amendment of the Cremation (England and Wales) Regulations 2008 reg.18(a) by the Coroners and Justice Act 2009 (Commencement No. 15, Consequential and Transitory Provisions) Order 2013 (SI 2013/1869) art.4 and Sch. para.4, is defective, but this seems to be the sense of it.

[137] See 8–18.

[138] This means the United Kingdom, the Channel Islands and the Isle of Man: Interpretation Act 1978 s.5, Sch.

[139] A death outside England and Wales is not required to be registered (Births and Deaths Registration Act 1953 s.15; see 18–11), so if the body is brought into England and Wales there will only be a post-mortem or investigation if the statutory criteria in s.1 of the 2009 Act are satisfied: see 5–01.

[140] Cremation (England and Wales) Regulations 2008 reg.17(1).

[141] Defined by Cremation (England and Wales) Regulations 2008 reg.2(1) to mean someone who has been a fully registered person under the Medical Act 1983 s.55, for at least five years, and has held a licence to practise under that Act for at least five years or since the coming into force of the Medical Act 1983 (Amendment) Order 2002 Sch.1 para.10 (November 16, 2009).

the same practice or clinical team of the first practitioner, nor a relative of the deceased person.[142]

9–26 The confirmatory certificate is not needed where the deceased died as an in-patient in a hospital, and a registered medical practitioner who could have given that certificate made or supervised a post-mortem examination on the deceased, whose result was known to the first practitioner before the certificate in Form 4 was given.[143] For this purpose, "hospital" means any institution for the reception and treatment of persons suffering from illness or mental disorder, a maternity home and a convalescent home.[144]

9–27 If the applicant for cremation asks to inspect the two medical certificates (Forms 4 and 5), either personally or through a nominee, and has given a telephone number or numbers on which to be contacted, the cremation authority must make all reasonable efforts to notify the applicant or the nominee of the receipt of those certificates.[145] Within 48 hours of the notification the applicant or the nominee may inspect the certificates and make representations about anything contained in them or the inquiries made by the person giving the certificate.[146]

Form 6

9–28 Although a coroner has a duty to release the body for burial or cremation as soon as is reasonably practicable, a coroner can give a cremation certificate[147] only once he no longer needs to retain the body for the purposes of the investigation.[148] The coroner certifies that *either* (a) a coronial post-mortem has been carried out and no inquest is necessary, *or* (b) the coroner has opened an investigation into the death, *or* (c) the death occurred outside the British Islands[149] and no post-mortem examination or inquest is necessary. The coroner also certifies that in his opinion no further examination of the body is necessary. However, the statutory requirement that the coroner no longer needs the body "for the purposes of *the* investigation"[150] means that before he can give a certificate he must have come under a duty to conduct such an investigation. This is confirmed by the 2013 amendment made to the coroner's certificate, which in part now reads: "I have opened an investigation into the death of the deceased".[151] So the coroner cannot give a cremation certificate in any case which he disposes of at the stage of preliminary inquiries, without ever having come under a duty to conduct an

---

[142] Cremation (England and Wales) Regulations 2008 reg.17(2).

[143] Cremation (England and Wales) Regulations 2008 reg.17(3).

[144] Cremation (England and Wales) Regulations 2008 reg.17(4).

[145] Cremation (England and Wales) Regulations 2008 reg.22(1), (2).

[146] Cremation (England and Wales) Regulations 2008 reg.22(3).

[147] In the Coroners (Investigation) Rules 2013 (SI 2013/1629) r.21(1) it is called an "order", but in the Cremation (England and Wales) Regulations 2008 reg.18 Sch.1 Form 6 (where it is prescribed) it is called a "certificate".

[148] Coroners (Investigation) Rules 2013 (SI 2013/1629) r.21(1); see 8–11.

[149] This means the United Kingdom, the Channel Islands and the Isle of Man: Interpretation Act 1978 s.5, Sch.

[150] Emphasis supplied.

[151] Cremation Form 6, as amended by the Coroners and Justice Act 2009 (Commencement No. 15, Consequential and Transitory Provisions) Order 2013 (SI 2013/1869) art.4 and Sch. para.4(4)(a).

investigation.[152] This will include the case where a body is repatriated for burial here, but the deceased died a natural death.

Form 6 as printed is in three parts. Part 1 contains the details of the deceased and   **9–29**
the cause of death. Part 2 contains the coroner's certificate. Part 3 is to enable the registrar of cremations to send to the Registrar of Births and Deaths the prescribed notification[153] of the cremation of the remains of the deceased person to whom the Form 6 relates. Before issuing a Form 6, the coroner should fill in at the head of Part 3 the name of the deceased person to whose body the form relates, to prevent any use being made of that Part to notify the disposal of some other body than that of the deceased person in respect of whom the form was issued.[154] If the death took place outside England and Wales, it would be sufficient if the space were completed to show that the notification should be sent to the registrar of births and deaths for the sub-district in which the crematorium is situated.

Form 10

The final document required for a cremation of human remains to be carried out   **9–30**
is an authority from the medical referee of the cremation authority (known as "Form 10"),[155] who must certify his satisfaction that all requirements have been met, that the inquiry required to be made for certain certificates (including that of the coroner) was adequate, that the fact and cause of death have been definitely ascertained, and that at least 48 hours have passed since any notification to the applicant that the medical certificates were available for inspection,[156] and at least 24 since any inspection.[157] If a coroner has decided to hold an inquest, the medical referee may not authorise cremation until it has been opened.[158]

Where a person dies outside the British Islands[159] and the body is brought to   **9–31**
England and Wales for disposal, the application need not be made in the prescribed form, but must contain the same information.[160] If the death occurred in Scotland, Northern Ireland, the Isle of Man or the Channel Islands, applications for cremation supported by certificates in accordance with the law in force in the place of death, but fulfilling similar function as certificates in England, are acceptable.[161]

---

[152] In relation to burial, see 9–21; as to when the duty to conduct an investigation arises, see 8–18.
[153] See 9–35 below.
[154] For the purpose of notification of the cremation: see 7–27 below.
[155] Cremation (England and Wales) Regulations 2008 Sch. Form 10: see App.2.
[156] Subject to Cremation (England and Wales) Regulations 2008 reg.23(2), where the cremation authority has made all reasonable efforts but been unable to notify the applicant within 48 hours.
[157] Cremation (England and Wales) Regulations 2008 reg.23(1). Where a deceased person was fitted with a cardiac pacemaker, it must be removed before cremation, or else it is liable to explode and give off toxic fumes. DHSS Health Notice HN(83)(6). The Home Office asked that pacemakers should be removed and returned to the cardiac departments which implanted them for checking: Home Office Circular No. 99 of 1983. In practice this rarely happens.
[158] Cremation (England and Wales) Regulations 2008 reg.23(3).
[159] This means the United Kingdom, the Channel Islands and the Isle of Man: Interpretation Act 1978 s.5 Sch.
[160] Cremation (England and Wales) Regulations 2008 reg.14(2)(a).
[161] Cremation (England and Wales) Regulations 2008 reg.14(2).

Cremation of stillborn child

9–32   The coroner is not concerned in the procedure, and does not give a certificate for cremation. A stillborn child[162] may be cremated if an application is made in statutory form, a certificate of registration of stillbirth is given, a registered medical practitioner or registered midwife certifies after examination that the child was stillborn,[163] and the medical referee gives his authority.[164] But the medical referee may not authorise such a cremation unless he is satisfied that these requirements have been met, that the examination already made was adequate, and that there is no reason for further examination.[165] Where the stillbirth occurred outside England and Wales, a similar procedure operates, but a certificate given by a medical practitioner or midwife in the place where it occurred may be given instead of the statutory certificate.[166] No notification[167] of the cremation of a stillborn child is required.

Cremation of body parts

9–33   Body parts[168] may be cremated if:

(1) application has been made in the statutory form;[169]

(2) the death of the person concerned or the stillbirth has been duly registered;[170]

(3) *either* the authority holding the parts certifies that there is no reason for further inquiry and releases them for cremation, *or* evidence is produced that the body parts were removed during a post-mortem examination of the body of the deceased;[171] and

(4) the medical referee gives authority,[172] being satisfied that the foregoing requirements have been met.[173]

---

[162] This means a child born after the 24th week of pregnancy and which did not at any time breathe or show any other signs of life: Cremation (England and Wales) Regulations 2008 reg.2(1). It does not include fetal remains (which also are not "body parts": see 9–33 above), whose disposal is subject only to common law rules, e.g. on outraging public decency: see *R. v Gibson* [1991] 1 All E.R. 439, CA.

[163] Cremation (England and Wales) Regulations 2008 reg.20(2) permits this to be substituted by a declaration from a "qualified informant" (see Births and Deaths Registration Act 1953 s.1(2)) where no registered medical practitioner or registered midwife attended, or no certificate can be obtained from such a person.

[164] Cremation (England and Wales) Regulations 2008 reg.20(1).

[165] Cremation (England and Wales) Regulations 2008 reg.26.

[166] Cremation (England and Wales) Regulations 2008 reg.14(4).

[167] See 9–35.

[168] This means material consisting of or including human cells from a deceased person (whether the separation occurred before or after death) or a stillborn child: Cremation (England and Wales) Regulations 2008 reg.2(1).

[169] Cremation (England and Wales) Regulations 2008 reg.19(a).

[170] Cremation (England and Wales) Regulations 2008 reg.19(b).

[171] Cremation (England and Wales) Regulations 2008 reg.19(c).

[172] Cremation (England and Wales) Regulations 2008 reg.19(d).

[173] Cremation (England and Wales) Regulations 2008 reg.25.

Where the death concerned took place outside England and Wales, foreign **9–34** certificates will be accepted that give the necessary particulars.[174] Provisions relating to the cremation of body parts were introduced for the first time in 2000[175] only after it emerged that over many years, organs and other material removed during post-mortem examinations[176] had been retained, and that the existing regulations did not cover the cremation of body parts, the body itself having already been disposed of. Body parts not cremated under this procedure may be incinerated in accordance with a permit to that effect issued under special regulations for the disposal of clinical waste.[177]

After the cremation

Within 96 hours after a cremation has taken place, the registrar of the cremation **9–35** authority must notify the registrar of births and deaths for the sub-district of death (or, where the death took place outside England and Wales, where the crematorium is) of the fact.[178] But this does not apply to cremation of a body buried for at least one year.[179] The ashes must be handed over to the person who applied for the cremation, or his nominee, if he wishes,[180] or otherwise retained by the cremation authority.[181] In the absence of any special arrangement for burial or preservation, any such retained ashes must be decently interred or scattered.[182] The authority may not inter or scatter the ashes unless 14 days' notice of the intention to do so has been given to the applicant.[183] Ashes preserved *in specie* have been held to be subject to the ordinary rights of property.[184]

---

[174] Cremation (England and Wales) Regulations 2008 reg.14A(3).

[175] By the Cremation (Amendment) Regulations 2000 (SI 2000/58). See Home Office Circular No. 2 of 2000, circulated with Home Office Newsletter 32 (April 26, 2000).

[176] As to which, see 8–39 ff.

[177] Cremation (England and Wales) Regulations 2008 reg.29. See a letter from the Department of Constitutional Affairs dated January 24, 2006 to all cremation authorities and coroners which, inter alia, stated that "Incineration of body parts is not a matter for a cremation authority."

[178] Cremation (England and Wales) Regulations 2008 reg.32(2).

[179] Cremation (England and Wales) Regulations 2008 regs 32(2), 16(2).

[180] Cremation (England and Wales) Regulations 2008 reg.30(1). There are unlikely to be any ashes following the cremation of body parts or fetal remains.

[181] Cremation (England and Wales) Regulations 2008 reg.30(2).

[182] Cremation (England and Wales) Regulations 2008 reg.30(3). As to burial of ashes, see 9–20.

[183] Cremation (England and Wales) Regulations 2008 reg.30(4).

[184] *Leeburn v Derndorfer* [2004] WTLR 867; [2004] V.S.C. 172 at [27]; cf. *Fessi v Whitmore* [1999] 1 F.L.R. 767.

Removal of Bodies out of England and Wales[184a]

Requirement to give notice of intent to remove

9–36   Every person intending to remove the body[185] of a deceased person out of England and Wales[186] must give notice[187] of such intention "to the coroner within whose jurisdiction the body is lying".[188] No doubt, "jurisdiction"[189] is to be interpreted as "coroner area".[190] It is to be noted that, at this stage at least, the body is not in the possession of the coroner. A stillborn child is not a deceased person, and accordingly the coroner is not concerned with the removal from England and Wales of stillborn children. There is nothing in the regulations which requires the death to have been registered before notice is given to the coroner.

Procedure upon notice

9–37   The notice given to the coroner enables him to enquire into the circumstances surrounding the death, to consider whether an inquest or post-mortem examination is necessary,[191] and if necessary to take possession of the body for these purposes. Where the deceased person died in England or Wales and a certificate for the disposal of the body has been given to the registrar of births and deaths,[192] or a coroner's order for burial or certificate for cremation has been issued, then such certificate or order must be delivered to the coroner with the notice.[193]

9–38   The coroner on receiving such notice must forthwith send or deliver an acknowledgement of its receipt[194] to the sender or to the undertaker or other person designated by him for that purpose.[195] The coroner must also forthwith inform the registrar of births and deaths for the sub-district in which the death occurred or in which the dead body was found, that he has received such a notice

---

[184a] See Chief Coroner, *Release of the Body for Burial or Cremation*, 1 May 2014. [32]–[35].

[185] "Body" presumably includes the remains of a body which has been buried, but does not include cremated ashes: *Re Kerr* [1894] P. 284. As to bodies having a relevant association with a visiting force, or bodies of persons entitled to diplomatic or consular immunity, see 9–42, 9–43 above. See also the Department of Health's Draft Code of Practice on the Import and Export of Body Parts, July 2002, available at *http://webarchive.nationalarchives.gov.uk/20130107105354/http://www.dh.gov.uk/prod_consum_dh/groups/dh_digitalassets/@dh/@en/documents/digitalasset/dh_4071139.pdf* [Accessed June 9, 2014].

[186] Although the legislation refers only to England, a reference to Wales is included by virtue of the Interpretation Act 1978 Sch. 2 para.5(a).

[187] The form is set out in the Removal of Bodies Regulations 1954 Sch.I, and is known as Form 104 REV. See App.2. Notice may be given prior to registration.

[188] Removal of Bodies Regulations 1954 reg.4. Note that the regulation applies on the basis of presence of the body, and not death, within the coroner's area.

[189] This was the word used in the Coroners Act 1887, the Act in force at the time of the 1954 Regulations.

[190] See 2–30 above. As for concurrent jurisdiction, see 5–116 ff above.

[191] Home Office Circular No. 68 of 1955 para.24.

[192] Under s.24(1) of the Births and Deaths Registration Act 1953.

[193] Removal of Bodies Regulations 1954 reg.4. The regulation does not cover the rare case where a body has been brought into England and Wales for disposal and a certificate issued under s.24(2) of the 1953 Act, and the body is then removed out of England and Wales for disposal elsewhere.

[194] The form is set out in the 1954 Regulations Sch.2, and is known as Form 103. See App.2.

[195] Removal of Bodies Regulations 1954 reg.5(1)(a).

and, if the registrar has issued a certificate for the disposal of the body, return such certificate to him.[196]

Retention of burial order or certificate for cremation

The coroner's order for burial or certificate for cremation forwarded with the **9–39** notice of intention to remove a body must be retained by the coroner unless he is notified in writing by the person wishing to remove the body that it is intended that the body shall be removed to and cremated in Scotland, Northern Ireland, the Channel Islands or the Isle of Man. In the latter case, the coroner must endorse the certificate for cremation with the words to the effect that it is only valid for cremation in Scotland, Northern Ireland, the Channel Islands or the Isle of Man (as the case may be), and then return the certificate to the person to whom he sends his acknowledgement of receipt of the notice of intention to remove the body.[197]

Waiting period in absence of acknowledgement

Unless the coroner states in his acknowledgement of receipt of the notice of **9–40** intention to remove the body that after making due enquiry he is satisfied that no further enquiries by him are needed (in which case the body may be removed at any time thereafter), the body may not be removed out of England and Wales before the expiration of a period of four clear days after the day on which notice of intention to remove the body was received by the coroner.[198] However, this is subject to any lawful direction to the contrary which might be given in the meantime.[199] Removal of the body in contravention of the statutory provisions is an offence punishable on summary conviction by a fine not exceeding level 3 on the standard scale.[200]

Communication of notices

All the notices referred to may be sent by post.[201] In many cases the coroner finds **9–41** it possible to give permission for the removal of the body in a much shorter period than four days, especially where urgency exists. No additional fee is payable to the coroner for carrying out this function.[202] On the other hand, the rule that "a coroner must be available at all times"[203] is only in order to address matters relating to *an investigation* into a death which must be dealt with immediately and cannot wait until the next working day. Here, "investigation" refers to an investigation

---

[196] Removal of Bodies Regulations 1954 reg.5(1)(b).
[197] Removal of Bodies Regulations 1954 reg.5(2). A cremation certification issued by a coroner in England and Wales is accepted in Scotland, Northern Ireland, the Channel Islands and the Isle of Man.
[198] Removal of Bodies Regulations 1954 reg.6.
[199] e.g. that the coroner proposes to take possession of the body (as to which see 8–11 above) for the purpose of making an examination or further enquiries or in order to hold an inquest: see, e.g. *R. v Bristol Coroner Ex p. Kerr* [1974] Q.B. 652.
[200] Births and Deaths Registration Act 1926 s.4, as amended by the Criminal Justice Act 1982 ss.38, 46. Level 3 is currently £1,000.
[201] Removal of Bodies Regulations 1954 reg.7.
[202] Coroners and Justice Act 2009 s.23 Sch.3 para.18.
[203] Coroners (Investigations) Regulations 2013 (SI 2013/1629) reg.4; see 2–72 ff.

conducted under the 2009 Act.[204] Dealing with the removal of a body from England and Wales does not involve such an investigation, unless and until the coroner is satisfied that the statutory criteria for an investigation[205] are satisfied, and in that (rare) case the coroner will not allow the body to leave anyway.

Visiting forces

9–42   The above restrictions on, and formalities regarding, removal out of England and Wales of the body of a deceased person do not apply to the body of a person who at the time of his death had a relevant association[206] with a visiting force,[207] except in a case where the Lord Chancellor directs the coroner to conduct or to resume an investigation concerning the death of that person.[208] Where the restrictions do not apply, no disposal certificate will be issued by the registrar of deaths.[209] This is to ensure that unused disposal certificates are not in circulation.[210] Similarly, the coroner should not issue a burial order or Form 6 for cremation.[211]

Diplomatic immunity

9–43   Although the point is unclear, it seems likely that the above restrictions and formalities do not apply to the removal of the body of a person entitled to diplomatic immunity, or of the body of a member of his family,[212] but that they do apply to the removal of the body of a consular officer or employee not also entitled to diplomatic immunity.[213]

Burial at sea

9–44   Where the purpose of removing a body out of England and Wales is burial at sea, then, in addition to notifying the coroner of intention to remove the body, and awaiting either the acknowledgement of receipt of the notice of removal or the four-day period, a licence will be needed from the Secretary of State or (in respect of Wales) the Welsh Ministers.[214]

---

[204] Coroners (Investigations) Regulations 2013 (SI 2013/1629) reg.2(1).
[205] Coroners and Justice Act 2009 s.1(2); see 5–01.
[206] For the meaning of this expression, see 5–104 above.
[207] For the meaning of this expression, see 5–102 above.
[208] Visiting Forces Act 1952 s.7(4).
[209] Visiting Forces Act 1952 s.7(5).
[210] Home Office Circular No. 54 of 1981 para.13.
[211] Home Office Circular No. 54 of 1981 para.13.
[212] See 5–109 ff.
[213] See 5–113 ff above.
[214] Marine and Coastal Access Act 2009 ss.65, 66(1), 113(4), (8).

Part III

THE INQUEST

Chapter 10

THE INQUEST: PRELIMINARIES

STATUS OF THE COURT

The coroner's court today is an (inferior) court of record.[1] A court of record is one of which the acts and judicial proceedings are enrolled in its archives and are conclusive evidence of what is recorded. Amongst the incidents pertaining to a court of record are the power to commit a person to prison for contempt of court,[2] and immunity for the judge for acts done by him in the execution of his duty as a judge.[3] However, the coroner's court is a court of a peculiar kind, being *inquisitorial* in function rather than accusatorial.[4]   **10–01**

This gives rise to certain important differences in procedure, compared with the ordinary civil and criminal courts, some of which have already been referred to,[5] or which will be adverted to in due course.[6] There is also the consequence that the inquest verdict is not binding on any person raising the same issue in subsequent litigation.[7] A court endowed with a particular jurisdiction inherently has powers "which are necessary to enable it to act effectively within such jurisdiction".[8] This   **10–02**

---

[1] 1 Britton c. 2, ss.1, 17; 4 Co. Ins. 271; Com. Digest., *Officer*, G.5; *Garnett v Ferrand* (1827) 6 B. & C. 611; 108 E.R. 576; *Thomas v Churton* (1862) 2 B. & S. 475 at 478; *Chippett v Thompson* (1868) 7 N.S.W. S.C.R. 349; *R. v Hammond* (1899) 29 Ont. 211, 215; *Davidson v Garrett* (1900) 30 Ont. 653 at 656; *Halsbury's Laws of England* 4th edn, Vol.9(2) (reissue), para.802 at 917; *Faber v The Queen* (1975) 65 D.L.R. (3d) 423 (Sup.Ct. (Can.)); *Attorney General v BBC* [1981] A.C. 303 at 342, 355–356; *R. v West Yorkshire Coroner Ex p. Smith (No. 2)* [1985] Q.B. 1096, DC; cf. *Jewison v Dyson* (1842) 9 M. & W. 540, 586, 152 E.R. 288 at 247, per Lord Abinger CB.

[2] See 11–89 ff below.

[3] See 2–120 ff above.

[4] See 1–18 ff above.

[5] See 8–21 ff below.

[6] See 10–25, 10–64, 11–21, 12–61, 12–71, 12–106 below.

[7] See 20–02 below. The Irish Supreme Court has suggested that a coroner's court in holding an inquest is not exercising the judicial power of the state: *Morris v Dublin City Coroner* [2000] 3 I.R. 602 and [11], Irish Sup.Ct. But this seems wrong in principle.

[8] *Connelly v DPP* [1964] A.C. 1264 at 1301 per Lord Morris.

notion of inherent jurisdiction applies to inferior courts, such as the county court,[9] so there is no reason for it not to apply to the coroner's court.[10]

10–03   One important procedural difference is that there are no parties to an inquest, as there are to criminal or civil litigation. Instead, there are only "interested persons", who have greater rights at the inquest than do ordinary members of the public. In particular, they have the right to examine witnesses at an inquest, either in person or through a representative.[11] There is no definition of "representative", and it does not appear to be confined to a qualified lawyer, but the coroner is the master of his own procedure[12] and it will be for him to decide whether to hear a particular person as a representative of an interested person. The concept of the "interested person" has already been discussed.[13]

Opening and Adjourning the Inquest

10–04   Under the old system until 2013, the whole of the coroner's investigation was referred to as the "inquest". Once he had come under a duty to inquire, the first step taken by a coroner was to "open" the inquest, and then, in practice, immediately to adjourn it.[14] But it is different under the new system. The coroner who comes under a duty to inquire must as soon as practicable conduct an investigation,[15] which may or may not lead to a court hearing or hearings. It is that part of the investigation comprising the court hearing or hearings that is henceforward to be known as "the inquest".[16]

10–05   A senior coroner who conducts an investigation must as part of that investigation hold an inquest,[17] unless the investigation is discontinued,[18] or the investigation is transferred to another coroner[19] (but in the latter case, if there is to be an inquest, the other coroner will have to hold it). An inquest must be opened as soon as reasonably practicable after the date on which the coroner considers that the duty to hold one applies.[20]

10–06   In practice there are three classes of case. In the first class, the coroner is informed of a death in custody, or of certain kinds of violent death (e.g. from gunshot wounds, or a fall from a height). In such a case the coroner knows right from the beginning both that there is a duty to investigate, and also that the

---

[9] *Langley v North West Water Authority* [1991] 1 W.L.R. 697, CA.

[10] See e.g. *R. v North Humberside Coroner Ex p. Jamieson* [1995] Q.B. 1: the coroner "must set the bounds of the inquiry. He must rule on the procedure to be followed". And in *R. v Lincoln Coroner Ex p. Hay* [2000] Lloyd's Rep. Med. 264, the Divisional Court said: "it is for each coroner to decide how best he should perform his onerous duties in a way that is as fair as possible to everyone concerned".

[11] Coroners (Inquests) Rules 2013 (SI 2013/1616) r.19(1).

[12] See e.g. *R. v North Humberside Coroner Ex p. Jamieson* [1995] Q.B. 1, CA.

[13] See 8–21.

[14] See 12th ed, 10–01.

[15] See 5–01, 8–18.

[16] See 10–05.

[17] Coroners and Justice Act 2009 s.6. See Chs 11, 12.

[18] Coroners and Justice Act 2009 s.4. See 8–36.

[19] Coroners and Justice Act 2009, ss 2,3. See 4–22.

[20] Coroners (Inquests) Rules 2013 (SI 2013/1616) r.5(1).

investigation will not be capable of being discontinued. There will have to be an inquest, and the coroner must open one as soon as practicable.

In the second class, the coroner is informed of a possible violent or unnatural **10–07** death (e.g. a potential suicide or a road traffic accident). In some such cases the coroner will need to make further enquiries to establish that it was indeed a violent or unnatural death and not for example one with a natural cause (e.g. a stroke or heart attack at the wheel). So in such a case the coroner does not necessarily know that there will not be a discontinuance. He does not open an inquest until he knows that that will not happen, because after opening an inquest he loses the power to discontinue.[21] After a post-mortem examination and any other tests have been completed, he will usually know whether discontinuance will occur, and if it will not he must open an inquest as soon as practicable.

In the third class of case, the coroner is informed of a death of at present **10–08** unknown cause. This may be because no medical certificate of the cause of death is available, but certainly there will be no reason to suspect that the death occurred in custody or was violent or unnatural. Again, after post-mortem examination and other tests the coroner may discontinue, and there will be no inquest.[22] But if he does not discontinue, he will know that there must be an inquest, and must open one as soon as practicable thereafter.

The opening of the inquest is an important milestone. Proceedings are then **10–09** "live" for contempt purposes.[23] The coroner must open the inquest in public,[24] unless he does not have immediate access to a court room or other appropriate premises, in which case he may open it privately and then announce that it has been opened at the next inquest hearing held in public.[25] There is no requirement that the coroner notify anyone of his intention to open the inquest. Although the coroner must notify certain persons,[26] and keep a recording,[27] of every "inquest hearing", in the latter case including any pre-inquest review hearing, these rules do not apply to inquest *openings* which do not go on to deal with the substance of the case, because they are not "inquest hearings" within the rules.[28] If they did, it would be impractical, at least for those inquests permitted to be opened in private, because the court recording equipment is usually not easily transportable.

At the opening, the coroner must where possible set the dates for subsequent **10–10** hearings to take place.[29] In practice, where a coroner considers that the preparation for the inquest will (or may) be completed by a certain time he simply sets a date for the inquest to take place. This will usually be within the six-month time limit for the completion of inquests.[30] Where matters are too uncertain to do that (e.g.

---

[21] Coroners and Justice Act 2009 s.4(1)(a). See 8–36.
[22] Coroners and Justice Act 2009 s.4(3)(a). See 8–38.
[23] See 11–92 below.
[24] Coroners (Inquests) Rules 2013 (SI 2013/1616) r.11(1).
[25] Coroners (Inquests) Rules 2013 (SI 2013/1616) r.11(2).
[26] Coroners (Inquests) Rules 2013 (SI 2013/1616) r.9. See 10–22.
[27] Coroners (Inquests) Rules 2013 (SI 2013/1616) r.26. See 12–104.
[28] If they were, r.11(1) and (2) would be otiose. Also, r.26 specifically refers to pre-inquest review hearings, but not openings. The *Chief Coroner's Guide to the Coroners and Justice Act 2009*, November 2013 para.145, takes the same view. The Chief Coroner's Guidance No. 4, on *Recordings* para.1, however advises that recordings should be kept of openings as well, "where practicable".
[29] Coroners (Inquests) Rules 2013 (SI 2013/1616) r.5(2).
[30] Coroners (Inquests) Rules 2013 (SI 2013/1616) r.8. See 10–14.

because there may be criminal proceedings first, or because it is not clear who will be interested persons or what the issues are likely to be) he may at least fix a date or dates to review the case in court. This serves to focus minds on what needs to be done.

10–11   Apart from that, the further purposes of the opening will depend to some extent on the coroner. At its simplest, it is just to take evidence of identification of the deceased (including information needed for registration of the death), and to deal with any outstanding applications for the release of the body, if not already given.[31] If it is a homicide case[32] a police officer may attend to tell the coroner formally of the progress of the police enquiry, and may have something to say in relation to the question of release of the body.[33] Sometimes preliminary evidence of the medical cause of death is given as well, where it is desirable that this be made public at this stage.[34] Some coroners require more than this to be given in evidence, for example details of the original report of the death, details of the autopsy and of any tissue retention, and wishes for tissue disposal and funeral. But it is hard to see that it is appropriate either to admit some of this information as evidence at this stage (or in some cases at all),[35] or to make it public.[36]

10–12   A relative or other identifying witness may attend the opening to give the relevant evidence on oath, although usually the coroner's officer gives hearsay evidence[37]—oral or in statement form—of the identification to him by the identifying witness and the other information required by the coroner. It is not normally a lengthy or contentious hearing, and there is normally no need for representation. Once the relevant business has been transacted, the inquest hearing is adjourned to the next hearing date, or a date to be fixed. It is a convenient moment for the next of kin or personal representative to ask for and be given a certificate of the fact of death.[38]

10–13   The coroner's power to adjourn the inquest from time to time is considered in detail later[39]. But there are a number of cases where, whether an inquest has been opened or not, the coroner is obliged to suspend the investigation, and to adjourn any inquest being held as part of that investigation. For convenience, these cases are briefly mentioned now, and fully dealt with later in this chapter, since chronologically this is the point in time at which they are most likely to fall to be considered. They are (i) cases involving visiting forces,[40] (ii) cases where any criminal proceedings arising out of the death are pending or envisaged,[41] and (iii) cases where a public inquiry is to be held into the events surrounding the death.[42]

---

[31] See 9–11, 9–17, 14–18. But often these have already been dealt with.
[32] See Ch.14.
[33] See 14–18 below.
[34] See 7–02 ff.
[35] Since not relevant to the inquiry into who, how, when and where: cf. Coroners (Inquest) Rules 2013 (SI 2013/1616) r.19(2). The coroner does of course need to know all this, but not as part of the inquest.
[36] cf. 7–02 ff.
[37] See 12–79.
[38] See 8–20.
[39] See 11–36 ff.
[40] See 10–74.
[41] See 10–75—10–80.
[42] See 10–81.

The other cases of compulsory adjournment of the inquest[43] are likely to occur at or during the resumed inquest hearing itself, and are dealt with elsewhere.[44]

TIME OF INQUEST

Early cases held that a coroner must not permit a body to putrefy by delaying the holding of an inquest.[45] Nowadays, where the right to life[46] is engaged, the investigation and any inquest must "commence promptly and [be] pursued with reasonable expedition".[47] The statutory rule is that a coroner must complete an **inquest** within six months of the date on which he is made aware of the death, or as soon as reasonably practicable after that date.[48] It is an aspirational rather than an absolute obligation, and there will be cases where it is not possible to complete an inquest within six months, or even longer. However, if the **investigation** has not been completed or discontinued within a year, the coroner must notify the Chief Coroner of the fact, and then also notify him when it is completed or discontinued.[49]   **10–14**

An inquest must be held[50] on a working day, unless the coroner considers that there is an urgent reason for holding it on another day.[51] Circumstances that might justify such a decision are, for example, that one of the witnesses proposed to leave the country the following day. An inquest should not be held late in the evening or at any hour that may cause inconvenience to any of those such as jurors or witnesses who will have to attend.[52] It is a matter for the coroner as to how much time is set aside for the inquest.[53]   **10–15**

PLACE OF INQUEST

Formerly, the inquest had to be held within the district of the coroner originally having jurisdiction,[54] except where jurisdiction had been transferred from one coroner to another pursuant to statute,[55] when it had to be held within the district   **10–16**

---

[43] See 11–36 ff.

[44] See 11–36 ff.

[45] *Re Hull* (1882) 9 Q.B.D. 689.

[46] Under the European Convention on Human Rights art.2 (deaths through state agency or in state custody); see 21–15 ff below.

[47] *Jordan v United Kingdom* (2001) 11 B.H.R.C.1, ECtHR; *McShane v United Kingdom* Unreported May 28, 2002, ECtHR; *Re Morgan's Application for Judicial Review* [2006] NIQB 82.

[48] Coroners (Inquests) Rules 2013 (SI 2013/1616) r.8.

[49] Coroners and Justice Act 2009 s.16(1). See Coroners (Investigations) Regulations 2013, SI 2013, No. 1629, reg.26. See 2–51.

[50] It is assumed that "held" includes any part of the proceedings, including the opening (as to which see 10–01).

[51] Coroners (Inquests) Rules 2013 (SI 2013/1616) r.7, formerly Coroners Rules 1984 r.18. This rule does not apply to a coroner's ministerial acts: *Mackalley's Case* (1611) 9 Co. Rep. 650; so a burial or cremation order, or out of England order, can be given.

[52] See 13–11 below.

[53] *Re Chaudhari's Application* Unreported, September 10, 2001, Elias J.

[54] Coroners Act 1988 s.5(2); as to territorial jurisdiction, see Ch.4.

[55] Coroners Act 1988 s.14.

of the latter and not the former coroner.[56] This restriction was abolished on February 12, 2013,[57] and has not been repeated in the new coroner system. So a coroner for a particular area can hold an inquest anywhere in England and Wales. The choice of the particular place where the inquest is to be held is in principle at the discretion of the coroner,[58] and not, for example, at that of his funding local authority.[59] Even so, the coroner must "exercise his discretion judicially, bearing in mind that the inquest is to be held in public and the purpose of the inquest".[60] Thus, a decision infringing this principle would be liable to be quashed on an application for judicial review.[61]

Council provision of accommodation

10–17   Funding local authorities must provide or secure the provision of accommodation appropriate to the needs of coroners carrying out their functions.[62] This will include the holding of inquests. Even before 2013, however, it was usual in practice for the council also to provide the accommodation for the inquest.[63] However, this does not give the authority any power to determine where inquests should be held.[64]

Convenience of witnesses, and interested persons[65]

10–18   As stated above, the coroner may sit anywhere in England and Wales. In practice, the occasions on which he will sit outside his area will be rare,[66] unless he has his regular accommodation in a nearby area. Where the coroner's area is very large, the coroner may be able to sit conveniently near the witnesses and interested persons concerned, so as to save them expense and time in attending the inquest. In exceptional cases, however, where local feelings are running high, it may be desirable for the inquest to be held in some other part of the coroner's area.[67] Where the inquest is to be held with a jury,[68] and perhaps even where it is not, it may be undesirable to hold it in premises with excessive public accommodation, in

---

[56] Coroners Act 1988 ss.14(7), 5(2).

[57] Coroners and Justice Act 2009 s.178 Sch.23 Pt I, and Coroners and Justice Act 2009 (Commencement No. 11) Order 2013 (SI 2013/250) art.2, repealing Coroners Act 1988 s.5(2)(a); Chief Coroner's Guidance No. 2, *Location of Inquests.*

[58] Historically, in the case of a judicial execution it appears to have been the invariable practice to hold the inquest within the prison where the execution took place: cf. the Capital Punishment Amendment Act 1868 s.5.

[59] *R. v Inner London Coroner Ex p. Chambers, The Times,* April 30, 1983, Woolf J.

[60] *R. v Inner London Coroner Ex p. Chambers, The Times,* April 30, 1983, Woolf J.

[61] *R. v Inner London Coroner Ex p. Chambers, The Times,* April 30, 1983, Woolf J, and see Ch.19. See also *Aplin v McIntyre* [2002] Q.S.C. 288.

[62] Coroners and Justice Act 2009 s.24(1)(b), replacing Coroners Act 1988 s.31, itself replacing Local Government Act 1985 s.13(7), and before that London Government Act 1963 s.78(3).

[63] See the Home Office's *Coroner Service Survey* (Research Study 118) (1998), p.17.

[64] *R. v Inner London Coroner Ex p. Chambers, The Times,* April 30, 1983.

[65] As for jurors, see 10–42.

[66] cf., e.g. *St Edmundsbury & Ipswich Diocesan Board of Finance v Clark* [1973] Ch. 323 (whether the High Court Chancery Division should sit in a village hall outside London to hear the evidence of a frail witness).

[67] *R. v Inner London Coroner Ex p. Chambers, The Times,* April 30, 1983.

[68] For these cases, see 10–34 below.

case the atmosphere becomes emotionally charged or even oppressive to the jury (or coroner).[69]

Where no regular court room available

In areas where no regular courtroom is available, it has been usual in the past to **10–19** utilise schoolrooms, council offices, or a room in a hospital or other public institution, a hotel or even a private house.[70] Theoretically, an inquest can even be held in the open air. The sole constraint used to be that it could not be held in any licensed premises or in a room in a building part of which is licensed premises, if any other suitable place was provided,[71] but this rule was repealed in 2005.[72]

Change in location of proceedings

It is not necessary that all the proceedings of an inquest should occur at the same **10–20** place. Thus some part of the proceedings may occur in one place and the rest in another.[73]

NOTICE OF INQUEST[74]

Where an inquest hearing is to be held, the coroner must make details of the date, **10–21** time and place of the inquest hearing[75] *publicly available* before the hearing commences,[76] and must make the details of any alteration in those arrangements *publicly available* within one week of the decision to alter.[77] But making "publicly available" does not mean taking positive steps to notify anyone. The coroner may exhibit beforehand a public notice at the place of inquest or elsewhere, or post a notice on an internet website. In each case, it is possible that no one might pass by the building, or visit the website, and thus see the notice, though if anyone did so they should be able to find it. Similarly the coroner might simply arrange for his officer to give out the details in response to enquiries from the media, if any are made.[78] The details are just as "publicly available".

---

[69] See *R v Inner North London Coroner Ex p. Chambers*, above.
[70] See the Home Office's *Coroner Service Survey* (Research Study 118) (1998), p.17.
[71] Licensing Act 1964 s.190(3).
[72] Licensing Act 2003 Sch.7 para.1 (SI 2005/3056) (as from November 24, 2005).
[73] 2 Hawk. P.C. 19 s.25; cf. *R. v Hinde* (1844) 5 Q.B. 944.
[74] *Chief Coroner's Guide to the Coroners and Justice Act 2009* at [110]–[112].
[75] This does not apply to a pre-inquest hearing: cf. Coroners (Inquests) Rules 2013 (SI 2013/1616) rr.11(3), 26.
[76] Coroners (Inquests) Rules 2013 (SI 2013/1616) r.9(3).
[77] Coroners (Inquests) Rules 2013 (SI 2013/1616) r.10(2).
[78] Both the Brodrick Committee (15–19) and the Working Party on the Coroners Rules (2nd Report, April 30, 1980, paras 37–40) were urged by press representatives to recommend formalising and strengthening the informal arrangements which usually exist for the benefit of the media. Neither body so recommended, the Working Party saying that they "did not consider that the Press should be given a special position under the Coroners Rules". Nonetheless, the Home Office view was that the spirit of the existing informal position whereby the local media were normally informed of inquest arrangements should be given effect where possible: Home Office Circular No. 53 of 1980, paras 19 and 20. As to media relations with coroners in Australia, see Waterford, in Selby (ed.), *The Inquest Handbook* (1998), Ch.5.

Persons to receive notice

10–22   In addition to the requirement to make inquest details publicly available, a coroner must notify the next of kin or personal representative,[79] and any other interested persons[80] who have made themselves known to the coroner, of the date, time and place of the inquest hearing within one week of setting the date.[81] Under the old rules, the coroner had to give notice of the time and place of the inquest to any other person whose conduct was likely in the coroner's opinion to be called into question at the inquest.[82] But this rule has not been carried over into the new system, on the basis that such persons will be interested persons and notified anyway.[83] In this connection strict adherence to the letter of the rules does not necessarily mean that fairness has resulted.[84] The Home Office formerly encouraged coroners to make reasonable inquiries to establish contact with relatives with a proper interest in the death.[85]

10–23   In the case of death through certain industrial accidents or diseases, notification of the inquest has to be given to an inspector or enforcing authority.[86] Such persons too fall within the definition of "interested person".[87] In 1981 the Home Office made a blanket request to coroners to notify such persons of the opening of an inquest, and for that purpose supplied them with telephone numbers and addresses.[88] This request may have had some effect at the time, but cannot now satisfy the provisions referred to in the previous paragraph, and so put the coroner under an obligation to notify such persons of the opening of the inquest.[89] The coroner may (not must) also consider giving notice to any relevant trade union

---

[79] For the meaning of these expressions, see 8–29 ff.

[80] For the meaning of this expression, see 8–22.

[81] Coroners (Inquests) Rules 2013 (SI 2013/1616) r.9(1), (2); formerly Coroners Rules 1984 r.19(b). The Home Office supplied coroners with the addresses and telephone numbers of all relevant inspectors or enforcing authorities for this purpose (Home Office Circular No. 3 of 1981), but, whether or not this was a sufficient compliance with the old rule, it cannot be one for the purposes of the new. No one can claim to be an interested person before the death has occurred. If any person to be notified is in prison or other place of detention, the coroner should notify the prison governor (or similar person) as early as possible of the date of the inquest so that the necessary arrangements may be made; however, this need not be done where the inquest is to be opened and immediately adjourned under the Coroners (Amendment) Act 1926 s.20 (now the Coroners and Justice Act 2009 s.11 Sch.1 para.2, formerly Coroners Act 1988 s.16): Home Office Circular No. 68 of 1955 para.14; Home Office Circular No. 5 of 1972.

[82] Coroners Rules 1984 r.24. Indeed, in *R. v Davies* [2011] EWCA Crim. 871, the Court of Appeal in a manslaughter case held that "fairness" demanded that the coroner having formed a preliminary view on the papers that the likely conclusion would be unlawful killing should have informed the solicitors for the suspect of that view.

[83] Strictly this is not quite correct: to fall within the notification rule the person must have made himself known to the coroner; the old rule was absolute.

[84] *Re Price's Application* [1986] N.I. 390, CA (NI); *Re McKerr's Application* [1993] N.I. 249, CA (NI).

[85] See Home Office letter to coroners of April 30, 2002 (sent with Newsletter No. 38 of the same date): "this may entail making enquiries of a range agencies [*sic*] or organisations to which relatives may have given their contact details." Cf. 8–60 above (obligation to notify persons of post-mortem examination).

[86] See Ch.15.

[87] Coroners and Justice Act 2009 s.47(2)(l); see 8–22.

[88] Home Office Circular No. 3 of 1981.

[89] The request was made in relation to the earlier legislation. Moreover, no one can claim to be an interested person before a death has occurred. In any event the contact details will probably have changed in over 30 years.

representative,[90] although where the deceased's death may have been caused by an injury in the course of employment or by an industrial disease, and the deceased belonged to a trade union, such representative is an interested person,[91] and therefore entitled as of right to be notified, if he makes himself known to the coroner.[92]

There was formerly a provision that, where an accident occurred within Greater **10–24** London or the City resulting in death, and the accident was alleged to be due to the nature or character of a road or road surface, or to a defect in the design or construction of a vehicle or in the materials used in the construction of a road or vehicle, the coroner inquiring into the death had to notify the Secretary of State in writing of the time and place of holding the inquest.[93] But this has not been carried over into the new system. If such circumstances occur now, anywhere in England and Wales, the coroner may consider that the highway authority[94] or some other person responsible for the road surface or the construction of the road vehicle involved is an interested person,[95] and may be notified accordingly.

SUMMONING WITNESSES

Power to call witnesses

The coroner must also consider which persons should be called as witnesses, and **10–25** how best to secure their attendance at the inquest.[96] Unlike ordinary civil proceedings, where witnesses are called by the parties, and cannot be called by the judge except with their consent,[97] and criminal proceedings, where the judge *has* power (to be exercised sparingly)[98] to call witnesses but the parties themselves usually do so, at an inquest it is the coroner alone who has the power to call witnesses.

This is a consequence of the inquisitorial nature of the proceedings before the **10–26** coroner.[99] It is his or her duty to conduct an investigation, rather than to hear and determine issues raised by parties to litigation.[100] Hence the coroner, and no one

---

[90] Home Office Circulars No. 40 of 1956 and No. 18 of 1980.

[91] Coroners and Justice Act 2009 s.47(2)(g); see 8–22.

[92] Coroners (Inquests) Rules 2013 (SI 2013/1616) r.9(2); formerly Coroners Rules 1984 rr.19(b), 20(2)(e); see 10–22 above.

[93] Coroners Act 1988 s.18(1).

[94] See Highways Act 1980, ss 1–3.

[95] Coroners and Justice Act 2009 s.47(2)(f); see 8–22.

[96] See also 12–01 ff below.

[97] *Re Enoch and Zaretsky, Bock & Co.'s Arbitration* [1910] 1 K.B. 327.

[98] *R. v Edwards* (1848) 3 Cox C.C. 82; *R. v Cleghorn* [1967] 3 Q.B. 584; *R. v Grafton* [1993] Q.B. 101.

[99] Compare the procedural directions given by Lord Scarman in the *Red Lion Square Inquiry* (1974) (cited by Scott (1995) 111 L.Q.R. 596, 610–611): "First of all it is I, and I alone, who will decide what witnesses will be called. I also decide to what matters their evidence will be directed." This was endorsed by Lord Hutton at the opening of the *Hutton Inquiry into the Death of Dr David Kelly* on August 1, 2003.

[100] *R. v South London Coroner Ex p. Thompson*, 1–19 above; cf. *Jones v National Coal Board* [1957] 2 Q.B. 55 at 63.

else, decides which witnesses can give relevant evidence,[101] and hence shall be called.[102] This applies to the production of documents as to the giving of oral evidence. And notwithstanding that there may be an obligation at common law for all persons able to give evidence to attend at the inquest,[103] it is still for the coroner to decide who should be examined.[104] He will do this by reference to the proper scope of the inquiry.[105] Privilege to refuse to answer questions put[106] is not a conclusive reason for not calling a person as a witness.[107]

Medical evidence

10-27 Formerly it was held that the coroner should call a "surgeon" to give medical evidence in all cases of sudden or violent death, and particularly when a criminal charge was likely to be made.[108] There used to be special provisions for calling medical practitioners,[109] but these were little used, and have now been replaced by the general provisions already referred to above. In practice, medical evidence is given at every inquest, though sometimes in documentary form rather than orally: in some cases more than one medical witness may be desirable or necessary, particularly where the medical issues are complex and involve more than one medical speciality, or where complaint is made regarding medical treatment received or some allegation of negligence is made.[110] Even if the coroner is himself medically qualified, he cannot give expert evidence, and will need to call a suitably qualified medical expert in appropriate cases.[111] That does not, of course, mean that the coroner must call all the available experts: it is a matter for him.[112] In particular, where the coroner has called other witnesses with appropriate expertise, he is not obliged to call a particular expert who had prepared a report for an interested person.[113]

---

[101] *R. v West Yorkshire Coroner Ex p. Clements* (1993) 158 J.P. 17, DC; *Re Chaudhari's Application* Unreported September 10, 2001, Elias J. "Relevance" is determined by the scope of the inquest: see Ch.6.

[102] *McKerr v Armagh Coroner* [1990] 1 W.L.R. 649, HL; *R v East Sussex Coroner Ex p. Homberg* (1994) 158 J.P. 357, DC; *Re Bradley's Application* Unreported August 29, 1996, HC (NI), Kerr J; *Re Potter's Application* Unreported January 24, 1997, Harrison J; *Hay v Devon Coroner* (1997) 162 J.P. 96, CA; *Quinlan v Deputy State Coroner* [2000] NSWSC 434 (failure to call witness did not amount to insufficiency of inquiry); *R. (Al-Fayed) v Inner West London ADC* [2008] EWHC 713 (Admin.); *R. (Ahmed) v South and East Cumbria Coroner* [2009] EWHC 1653 (Admin.).) at [35]; *R. (Le Page) v Inner South London ADC* [2012] EWHC 1485 (Admin.).

[103] See 12–01 below.

[104] Coroners Act 1988 s.11(2) (not carried over expressly into the 2009 Act); *R. v West Yorkshire Coroner Ex p. Clements* (1993) 158 J.P. 17, DC; *R. v South Yorkshire Coroner Ex p. Stringer* (1993) 158 J.P. 453, DC; *Francis v Southwark Coroner's Office* [2013] EWCA Civ. 313 at [5].

[105] See Ch.6.

[106] See 12–94 below.

[107] cf. *R. v Lincoln Coroner Ex p. Hay* [2000] Lloyd's Rep. Med. 264 at [55].

[108] *R. v Quinch* (1831) 4 C. & P. 571; see also the first edition of this work (1829).

[109] Coroners Act 1988 s.21(1).

[110] *R. (Warren) v Northamptonshire Assistant Deputy Coroner* [2008] EWHC 966 (Admin.).

[111] *R. v Inner North London Coroner Ex p. Linnane (No. 2)* (1990) 155 J.P. 343, DC; *Nicholls v Liverpool Coroner* Unreported November 8, 2001, DC. As to the duties of expert witnesses, see *R. v T* [2010] EWCA Crim. 2439. See also *Re Siberry's Application for Judicial Review* [2008] N.I.Q.B. 147.

[112] See 10–25—10–26 above.

[113] *R. (Warren) v Northamptonshire Assistant Deputy Coroner* [2008] EWHC 966 (Admin.).

Challenge to coroner's decision on witnesses

But a coroner's decision to call[114] or not to call a particular witness, or to ignore   **10–28**
the possibility of evidence from a particular quarter, is not unassailable. It is clear
that where, at an inquest, the coroner refuses to seek to obtain relevant
documents,[115] or to hear potential witnesses having relevant evidence to give and
being available to give that evidence at the hearing,[116] or even where he declines
to call such witnesses (even expert)[117] and as a result makes an insufficient
inquiry,[118] the whole inquest is liable to be quashed.[119] Thus, although it is in the
discretion of the coroner as to who should be called and examined as witnesses,
there will be cases where any decision by the coroner *not* to call particular witnesses
will be quashed by the court and the coroner will be ordered to call such
witnesses.[120] As long as the coroner has made a definitive decision, it is unnecessary
to wait for the inquest to be held before challenging that decision.

Procedure for notification

Usually, notification to a witness is informal, but if the coroner considers that the   **10–29**
witness may not attend unless a formal coroner's notice is served, then such a
notice should be prepared and served. The procedure for obtaining evidence and
other information before the inquest and for calling witnesses has already been
described.[121] In summary, the coroner may by written notice require a person
(who may be a medical practitioner, a witness of fact or an expert), during the
investigation to provide evidence in the form of a statement, to produce relevant
documents in his custody or control, or produce for examination or testing
anything in his custody or control relevant to the investigation,[122] and may require

---

[114] See *Re Donaldson's Application* [2010] NIQB 144. See also *Re Siberry's Application for Judicial Review*
[2008] N.I.Q.B. 147 (coroner's decision to permit Prison Ombudsman to give evidence to jury of
all contents of his Report held *Wednesbury* unreasonable in relation to matters addressed in medical
expert reports).
[115] *Re O'Reilly* (1996) 160 J.P. 749, DC; cf. *Hay v Devon Coroner* (1997) 162 J.P. 96, CA; see 10–65
below.
[116] *R. v Carter* (1876) 45 L.J.Q.B. 711; *Dowler v North London Coroner* [2009] EWHC 3300 (Admin.);
R. (Le Page) v Inner South London ADC [2012] EWHC 1485 (Admin.). Cf. *Francis v Southwark
Coroner's Office* [2013] EWCA Civ. 313 at [5].
[117] *R. (Stanley) v Inner North London Coroner, The Times*, June 12, 2003, Silber J; *R. (Duffy) v
Worcestershire Deputy Coroner* [2013] EWHC 1654 Admin.
[118] *R. v Rothera Ex p. Chetwin, The Times*, July 25, 1930, DC; *R. (Hair) v Staffordshire (South) Coroner*
[2010] EWHC 2580 (Admin.); *R. (Mack) v Birmingham and Solihull Coroner* [2011] EWCA Civ. 712;
R. (Le Page) v Inner South London ADC [2012] EWHC 1485 (Admin.).
[119] See 19–30—19–31 below.
[120] cf. *R. v South London Coroner Ex p. Ridley* [1985] 1 W.L.R. 1347, QBD; *R. v Southwark Coroner Ex
p. Hicks* [1987] 1 W.L.R. 1624. See also *R. v Elliott Ex p. McKerr, The Independent*, December 21, 1988
(revsd. on other grounds, *sub. nom. McKerr v Armagh Coroner* [1990] 1 W.L.R. 649; *R. v Inner North
London Coroner Ex p. Linnane (No. 2)* (1990) 155 J.P. 343, DC; *R v West Berkshire Coroner Ex p. Thomas*
(1991) 155 J.P. 681; *R. v East Sussex Coroner Ex p. Homberg* Unreported June 14 1993, DC; *Re
Bradley's Application* Unreported August 29, 1996, HC (NI); *Re Mullan's Application* [2000] B.N.I.L.
14, HC (NI); *Nicholls v Liverpool Coroner* Unreported November 8, 2001, DC.
[121] See 7–12 ff. Where the witness is in prison, application may be made to the Secretary of State under
the Crime (Sentences) Act 1997 s.41 Sch.1 para.3, for the production of the witness at the inquest.
But this is a matter of discretion for the Secretary of State. An alternative procedure is to apply on
affidavit to a judge of the Queen's Bench Division for an order for the witness to be produced for
examination under s.9 of the Criminal Procedure Act 1853.
[122] Coroners and Justice Act 2009 s.32 Sch.5 para.1(2); see 7–13.

such a person to attend an inquest to give evidence or produce such documents or things.[123] There is a procedure for challenging such notices.[124] Disobedience to the notice is punishable summarily by the coroner at the inquest,[125] even without an appropriate sum by way of conduct money having been tendered or paid.[126]

10-30   Formerly, in order to enforce the attendance of a witness from outside the coroner's area, the coroner had to obtain a High Court or county court witness summons[127] (in the High Court, formerly called a writ of subpoena). But since 2013 a coroner's notice to summon a witness is effective throughout the whole of England and Wales. This means that a High Court or county court witness summons can no longer be issued in aid of a coroner's court in respect of witnesses in England and Wales.[128] The procedure for applying to set aside a coroner's notice has already been described.[129] The extent to which a witness may be protected by anonymity orders and by being screened from view whilst giving evidence is discussed later.[130]

JOINDER OF INQUESTS

Multiple deaths with factors in common

10-31   Where there has been an accident involving many deaths, for example a railway or mining disaster, it is common for the inquests to be held concurrently.[131] In such cases the inquest on each body is a separate inquest. Thus any jury will need to be sworn to inquire into each death, and a separate record of inquest[132] will be needed for each death. While evidence of identification will differ in each case and evidence of the cause of death may not be the same in all cases, much of the evidence will be common. If, however, there is not the nexus of a common accident or other occurrence, there is no justification for holding the inquests concurrently.[133] One other consideration is the uncertainty as to whether

---

[123] Coroners and Justice Act 2009 s.32 Sch.5 para.1(1); see 7–14. Although where the witness is a prisoner or "person confined in any gaol, prison or place", there is an alternative procedure under s.9 of the Criminal Procedure Act 1853, referred to above.

[124] See 7–16 above.

[125] See 7–17, 12–03 below.

[126] See 12–04—12–05.

[127] See the 12th edn of this work, paras 10–18—10–21 for the details of the procedure.

[128] Cf. CPR 34.3(3), defining an "inferior court or tribunal" as one that does not have the power to issue a witness summons in respect of proceedings before it; see further *Currie v Chief Constable of Surrey* [1982] 1 W.L.R. 215.

[129] See 7–12.

[130] See 12–22 ff.

[131] *R. v Durham County Council Ex p. Graham I* (1912) 76 J.P. 219; *Maksimovich v Attorney General* [1985] 4 N.S.W.L.R. 318, CA (NSW). Thus in recent years concurrent inquests have been heard following the Zeebrugge ferry disaster (1987), the King's Cross Underground fire (1988), the Marchioness river disaster (1989), the Clapham Junction rail crash (1990), the deaths of Diana, Princess of Wales and Dodi Al-Fayed (2007-08) and the July 7, 2005 bombings (2010).

[132] See Ch.13 below.

[133] *Re Mitchelstown Inquisition* (1888) 22 L.R. Ir. 279 (several persons shot by police during an affray, but at different places and at different times, single jury summoned; inquest quashed for this and other reasons). cf. the concurrent inquests held following the so-called "Hungerford massacre", where a gunman killed 15 people in different places and at different times before killing himself: *The Times*, September 25, 1987.

documentary hearsay can generally only be admitted if undisputed.[134] In an overseas death inquest, the bulk of the evidence will be documentary.[135] But if a person interested in inquest A, by disputing the documentary evidence, could in effect render conjoined inquests B, C, and D valueless, that would be a serious matter.[136]

Bodies in different areas

Where the various bodies lie in different areas, so that more than one coroner has   **10–32** jurisdiction, and it is nonetheless felt desirable to hold concurrent inquests, it can be arranged for all coroners save one to surrender jurisdiction to that one,[137] though it should be noted that this power does not permit a coroner to be deprived of jurisdiction over a body in his area without his consent. In an appropriate case, of course, a failure to exercise the power to transfer jurisdiction will be subject to judicial review.[138]

Summoning a Jury

Originally, every inquest was held with a jury, and the first step in the holding of   **10–33** an inquest was for the coroner to issue his warrant ordering a jury to be summoned.[139] Nowadays, with certain exceptions, a coroner may hold an inquest without a jury,[140] and the majority of inquests are now disposed of by the coroner sitting alone, pursuant to this power.

Circumstances where jury required

The circumstances in which a jury is still necessary are as follows. If the coroner has   **10–34** reason to suspect that:

(a) the deceased died while in custody or otherwise in state detention,[141] and that either (i) the death was violent or unnatural,[142] or (ii) the cause was unknown;[143] or that

---

[134] See 12–32 below.
[135] See 5–92.
[136] *R. v Coroner of the Royal Household Ex p. Al Fayed* Unreported July 18, 2000, Newman J. In some cases it may be possible to call "live" hearsay evidence, not caught by the documentary rule; or it may be that the documentary hearsay is treated as evidence in inquests B, C and D, but not A (this would not be possible in a jury inquest, of course).
[137] Coroners and Justice Act 2009 s.2; formerly Coroners Act 1988 s.14; see 4–19 ff above.
[138] See, e.g. *R. v Coroner of the Royal Household Ex p. Al Fayed* Unreported July 18, 2000, Newman J (challenge dismissed).
[139] See Coroners Act 1887 s.3(1) (repealed).
[140] Coroners and Justice Act 2009 s.7(2); formerly Coroners Act 1988 s.8(1).
[141] See 5–83 ff.
[142] See 5–70 ff.
[143] Coroners and Justice Act 2009 s.7(2)(a); formerly Coroners Act 1988 s.8(3)(a); see 5–80 ff.

(b) the death resulted from an act or omission of (i) a police officer, or (ii) a member of a police service force, in the purported execution of his duty;[144] or that

(c) the death was caused by an notifiable[145] accident, poisoning or disease;[146]

then the coroner must summon a jury.[147] Where the statutory conditions for a jury are met, the coroner has no discretion in the matter.[148]

10–35 Whether the coroner "has reason to suspect" is a more objective question than whether it appears to the coroner that he has reason to suspect. In the latter case his decision can only be overturned if he materially misdirects himself.[149] But the phrase "has reason to suspect" does not require positive proof, and any information giving "reason to suspect" will suffice.[150] Formerly there was a fourth, residual category, for cases where the death occurred in circumstances the continuance or possible recurrence of which was prejudicial to the health or safety of the public or any section of the public,[151] but this was not carried over into the 2009 Act.

10–36 The existence of the third category above (death caused by notifiable accident, etc.) is unfortunate in one respect, and that is that the reporting obligation can be (and has been) considerably extended for health and safety reasons by statutory instrument, without any thought as to the effect this would have upon coroners' inquests, and the anomalies thereby created.[152] Thus, for example, a death caused by a camp fire using a refillable gas cylinder must be reported; but a death caused by a similar fire using a *disposable* cylinder need not.[153] In consequence, the coroner must sit with a jury in the former case, but not in the latter. And whether a death on a railway is now reportable—hence requiring a jury inquest—formerly gave rise to a difficult question, but happily is now rendered much easier.[154]

---

[144] Coroners and Justice Act 2009 s.7(2)(b); formerly Coroners Act 1988 s.8(3)(b). See also *R. v West Berkshire Coroner Ex p. Thomas* (1991) 155 J.P. 681, DC.

[145] This means that notice is required to be given under any Act to (a) a government department, or (b) to any inspector or other officer of a government department or (c) to an inspector appointed under s.19 of the Health and Safety at Work, etc., Act 1974: Coroners and Justice Act 2009 s.7(4). In Wales, the reference to "government department" is a reference to the National Assembly: Government of Wales Act 1998 s.43(1).

[146] Coroners and Justice Act 2009 s.7(2)(c); formerly Coroners Act 1988 s.8(3)(c); see 10–26 below, and see further Ch.15.

[147] A jury is no longer necessary in a treasure inquest, but that question is dealt with later; see 16–45.

[148] *R. (Handley) v Birmingham Coroner* [2011] EWHC 3337 (Admin.).

[149] *R. v Inner North London Coroner Ex p. Linnane* [1989] 1 W.L.R. 395, DC.

[150] *R. v Inner North London Coroner Ex p. Linnane* [1989] 1 W.L.R. 395, DC; *R. (Aineto) v Brighton Hove Coroner* [2003] EWHC 1896 Admin., DC. See also *R. v South London Coroner Ex p. Weeks* Unreported December 6, 1996, Scott Baker J, referring to *Hussien v Chung Fook Kam* [1970] A.C. 942 at 949B; *R. (Canning) v Northampton Coroner* [2006] EWCA Civ. 1225 (dealing with "reasonable cause" under the 1988 Act; *R. (Gracey) v Cheshire Coroner* [2008] EWHC 957 (Admin.).

[151] Coroners Act 1988 s.8(3)(d). See, e.g. *R. (Takoushis) v Inner North London Coroner* [2006] 1 W.L.R. 461, CA; *R. (Paul) v Deputy Coroner of The Queen's Household* [2007] EWHC 408 (Admin.); *R. (Heseltine) v Coroner's Office* [2010] EWCA Civ. 267; *R. (Mack) v Birmingham and Solihull Coroner* [2011] EWCA Civ. 712; *Davey v Leicestershire Coroner* [2013] EWHC 840 (Admin.).

[152] See 15–09 ff below.

[153] Reporting of Injuries, Diseases and Dangerous Occurrences Regulations 2013 (SI 2013/1471) reg.11(1). See 15–10.

[154] See 15–13 ff below.

Finally, the existence of the coroner's power[155] to report matters to a person or authority having power to take action to prevent further fatalities, is "ancillary to the inquest procedure and not its mainspring".[156] Hence it is irrelevant to the question whether a jury is required.[157] Subject to these obligations, the coroner has power (but no duty) to summon a jury whenever it seems to him that there is reason so to do.[158] The mere fact that art.2 is engaged (if it is) cannot make any difference, since summoning a jury affects only the identity of the fact-finding tribunal, and not its function. After all, the civil law member states of the Council of Europe have to comply with art.2, but none of them uses a jury to do so.[159] The coroner's decision not to sit with a jury pursuant to this power can only be attacked (if at all) as a wrong exercise of discretion on normal *Wednesbury* principles.[160]

10–37

Equal validity of inquest with and without jury

It is further provided that, where an inquest hearing begins without a jury, but a jury is subsequently summoned, the validity of anything done by the coroner before the jury is summoned is still effective.[161] Plainly this covers the case where a coroner does not originally have reason to suspect that any of the compulsory jury conditions is satisfied, and so sits alone, but then later acquires such reason to suspect and comes under an obligation to sit with a jury. But it must at least be doubtful that it permits the coroner who, knowing that the jury condition is satisfied, proceeds to hold part of an inquest by himself before he summons a jury.[162]

10–38

In fact, it is not uncommon for a coroner who knows he will ultimately have to sit with a jury to open the inquest alone and then to adjourn to a date at which a jury will be summoned.[163] He does this because summoning juries has become more complex and time-consuming, and in practice it is not possible to keep a single jury together for weeks or months. Moreover, he can call *one* jury to sit for

10–39

---

[155] See 13–122 ff below.

[156] *Re Kelly* (1996) 161 J.P. 417, DC; Chief Coroner's Guidance No. 5, *Reports to Prevent Future Deaths* at [6].

[157] *R. v West Yorkshire Coroner Ex p. National Union of Mineworkers (Yorkshire Area)* (1985) 150 J.P. 58, DC.

[158] See e.g. *Re Berry's Application* Unreported May 30, 2002, Burton J (decision to sit with jury did not imply that coroner would not restrict conclusions left to them to those justified on evidence). By Home Office Circulars No. 35 of 1969 and No. 23 of 1981, the Secretary of State's view was set out that coroners should exercise their discretion in favour of holding an inquest and summoning a jury in every case where the death of a person in legal custody (including police custody) was reported to them, even though death might actually have occurred, e.g. in a hospital. Home Office Circular No. 109 of 1982 made clear that, to the extent that the summoning of a jury has not been made mandatory (see 10–34), the Home Secretary's view remained the same.

[159] See Ch.22.

[160] *R. v Ceredigion Coroner Ex p. Wigley* [1993] C.O.D. 364; *R. (Cairns) v Inner West London Deputy Coroner* [2011] EWHC 2890 (Admin.); *R. (Collins) v Inner South London Coroner* [2004] EWHC 2421 (Admin.); *R. (Francis) v Inner South London Deputy Coroner* [2005] EWHC 980 (Admin.); *R. (Kent CC) v Kent Coroner* [2012] EWHC 2768 (Admin.). See 19–31 below.

[161] Coroners (Inquests) Rules 2013 (SI 2013/1616) r.32; formerly Coroners Act 1988 s.8(5) (though with some changes of substance).

[162] *R. v Belfast City Coroner* Unreported March 31, 1969, HC (NI), Lowry J: inquisition quashed for want of jurisdiction; cf. *R. v Northamptonshire Coroner Ex p. Walker* (1988) 153 J.P. 289 (death through reportable railway accident, but coroner sat alone; defect not adverted to by court).

[163] cf. *R. v Surrey Coroner Ex p. Campbell* [1982] Q.B. 661 at 667, and see, e.g. *Re Jason Fitzsimmons, The Times*, August 6, 1985 (Merseyside coroner).

a period, hearing several cases consecutively, thus saving time, effort and money.[164] But this is not inconsistent with the rule, because the opening of an inquest is not an "inquest hearing".[165] Nor should a jury be summoned for a pre-inquest review hearing, where preparatory discussions, preliminary applications and submissions on points of law are dealt with.[166]

Composition of jury

10–40 A coroner's jury must be composed of between 7 and 11 persons.[167] Persons are qualified to serve as jurors at a coroner's inquest only if qualified to serve as jurors in the Crown Court, the High Court and county courts.[168] There are limited disqualifications,[169] and it is an offence for a person to serve who knows he is disqualified.[170] However, persons otherwise qualified to serve may be excused from jury service in certain circumstances.[171]

10–41   Challenge of prospective jurors at the inquest,[172] and discharge of a juror once sworn,[173] are dealt with later. The rules on judicial bias undoubtedly apply to jurors[174] as they do to coroners.[175] Whilst it is no doubt right that a coroner can decline to empanel a juror who cannot be seen to be impartial,[176] a coroner's officer summoning a jury is unlikely to have any basis upon which at that stage he could properly so conclude, assuming the proper delegation to him of appropriate power.[177] Declining to call for jury service persons otherwise qualified is unlawful and open to challenge.[178]

---

[164] See 10–43 above.

[165] See 10–09.

[166] *R. (Coker) v Inner South London Coroner* [2006] EWHC 614 (Admin.).

[167] Coroners and Justice Act 2009 s.8(1); formerly Coroners Act 1988 s.8(2)(a); before 1926 it was 12 to 23, following the grand jury: see Stephen, *A Digest of the Law of Criminal Procedure in Indictable Offences* (1883) art.212.

[168] Coroners and Justice Act 2009 s.8(4); formerly Coroners Act 1988 s.9. This means being qualified in accordance with the Juries Act 1974 s.1, i.e.: (i) aged between 18 and 70 years; and (ii) registered as a parliamentary or local government elector; and (iii) resident in the UK, Channel Islands or Isle of Man for five years since the age of 13; and (iv) not ineligible (under Sch.1, Pt I) or disqualified (Pt II).

[169] Juries Act 1974 s.1 Sch.1 (as substituted in 2004 by the Criminal Justice Act 2003 Sch.33 para.15). These fall into the following two main categories: (i) persons liable to be detained under the Mental Health Act 1983 or resident in hospital through mental disorder, under guardianship or subject to a community treatment order under the 1983 Act, or lacking capacity under the Mental Capacity Act 2005 to serve as a juror; (ii)(a) persons on bail in criminal proceedings within the Bail Act 1976, or (b) who have at any time been sentenced in the UK, Channel Islands or Isle of Man to a term of imprisonment or detention for life, at pleasure, or for at least five years, or for public protection, or to certain extended sentences, or (c) who have within the last 10 years in the UK, Channel Islands or Isle of Man served a term of imprisonment or detention, or been sentenced to such a term suspended, or had made in respect of them (in England and Wales) certain community or drug testing orders, or (in the rest of the UK, the Channel Islands and the Isle of Man) any corresponding orders. Lawyers, judges and others connected with the justice system are no longer disqualified.

[170] See Coroners and Justice Act 2009 Sch.6 para.1(1) (level 5 on the standard scale: para.1(2)).

[171] See 10–48 below.

[172] See 11–14 below.

[173] See 11–21 below.

[174] *R. v Kingston upon Hull Coroner Ex p. Dawson* [2001] A.C.D. 68, Jackson J; *R. v Abdroikov* [2007] UKHL 37; *Khan v R.* [2008] EWCA Crim. 531. See 11–15.

[175] See 5–66 ff above.

[176] See 11–14 below.

[177] See 2–139 ff above.

[178] *R. v Surrey Coroner Ex p. Campbell* [1982] Q.B. 661 (men only summoned).

Considerations in summoning jurors

The person (usually the coroner's officer) who actually summons jurors was **10–42** formerly obliged to have regard to the convenience of the jurors and to their respective places of residence, and in particular to the desirability of selecting jurors within reasonable daily travelling distance of the place where they were to attend.[179] But under the new system this formal rule has now gone. Instead, the rule is simply that the coroner may summon persons (whether within or without the coroner area for which he is appointed) to attend at the time and place stated in the summons.[180] In practice it is still usual for jurors to be drawn from the neighbourhood.

Procedure for summoning of jurors

The procedure for summoning jurors under the old system was held to be **10–43** mandatory, and a failure to follow it meant that proceedings before an irregularly summoned jury were a nullity.[181] This is probably equally true under the new system, though the relevant statutory requirements are fewer. Most coroners hold all their jury inquests together from time to time, in a period of a few weeks, in order to minimise inconvenience and reduce the number of jurors required. The process begins when the coroner issues his warrant[182] to his officer and to all the constables for the area in which the coroner's jurisdiction is comprised. It sets out the number of jurors to be summoned.

On receipt of the warrant the coroner's officer will make out the summons[183] **10–44** to be served on the persons selected as jurors. Usually, the names are taken from a list provided by the Jury Summoning Officer,[184] being the list used to summon juries for other courts. The selection by the coroner's officer should be at random, for it is contrary to the principle of the jury system to have a small panel of regular jurors.[185] Summonses should not, of course, be sent to those known to be ineligible by reason of age[186] (which the jury list will show).[187] Certainly, the coroner should not personally interfere with the summoning of the jurors as this may be a ground for quashing the inquisition.[188]

The summons in statutory form[189] must be sent by post with a return envelope **10–45** to the juror or delivered by hand at his or her address as shown in the electoral register.[190] However, if it appears that the jury will be, or probably will be,

---

[179] Coroners Rules 1984 r.44.
[180] Coroners and Justice Act 2009 s.8(2).
[181] *R. v Merseyside Coroner Ex p. Carr* [1994] 1 W.L.R. 578, DC.
[182] This is no longer statutory: see formerly Coroners Act 1988 s.9(2); Coroners Rules 1984 Sch.4 Form 3.
[183] Coroners (Inquests) Rules 2013 (SI 2013/1616) r.29(1) Sch. Form 1; formerly Coroners Rules 1984 Sch.4 Form E.
[184] Jurors in criminal cases at Crown Courts in England and Wales are now summoned centrally by the Jury Central Summoning Bureau, 8 Pocock Street, London SE1 0BJ; tel 0845 803 8003; email jurysummoning@hmcts.gsi.gov.uk.
[185] *R. v Divine Ex p. Walton* [1930] 2 K.B. 29.
[186] Juries Act 1974 s.1(1)(a) (below 18 or above 70 years old).
[187] Home Office Circular No. 108 of 1983.
[188] *Re Mitchelstown Inquisition* (1888) 22 L.R. Ir. 279.
[189] Coroners (Inquests) Rules 2013 (SI 2013/1616) r.29(1) Sch. Form 1.
[190] Coroners (Inquests) Rules 2013 (SI 2013/1616) r.29(2); formerly Coroners Rules 1984 r.45.

incomplete, the coroner may require any persons up to the number needed who are in, or in the vicinity of, the place of the inquest hearing to be summoned (without any written notice) for jury service.[191]

10–46 Formerly the person designated by the coroner as the "appropriate officer" (usually the coroner's officer)[192] had express powers in the rules to withdraw or amend the summons in certain cases,[193] to discharge a potential juror where he had doubts as to his capacity to act effectively as a juror,[194] and to excuse from attending a juror who showed good reason for being excused.[195] He had a duty to excuse a juror who showed he was entitled to be excused by virtue of his age, office or profession,[196] or that he had previously done jury service fulfilling certain conditions.[197]

10–47 None of this, however, has been carried over expressly into the new rules. It has therefore been suggested that the regime applicable to jurors in the Crown Court, High Court or county court somehow applies to coroners' juries too. This is wrong. That regime[198] is expressly limited to jurors summoned (by the Lord Chancellor) "under this Act", i.e. the Juries Act 1974.[199] But coroners' jurors used to be summoned (by the coroner) under the Coroners Act 1887,[200] and then the Coroners Act 1988,[201] and they are now summoned under the Coroners and Justice Act 2009.[202] Moreover, for the purposes of the Juries Act, "court" is defined to mean only the Crown Court, the High Court and the county court.[203] That is why it was necessary for the Coroners Rules 1984 to make express provision for excusal and discharge of jurors. The Coroners and Justice Act 2009 could have amended the Juries Act 1974 to apply its provisions for the future to coroners' juries. But it did not.

10–48 Instead, the coroner must fall back on the new rules and the statutory form prescribed. As already stated, the rules provide that jurors *must* be summoned using the statutory summons form,[204] but confer no other power of excusal or discharge. But the prescribed text of this form itself[205] informs the recipient that the coroner or authorised officer may excuse the potential juror "on the grounds of poor health, illness, physical disability, insufficient understanding of English, holiday arrangements or any other good reason". It also states that a potential juror may be

---

[191] Coroners (Inquests) Rules 2013 (SI 2013/1616) r.30; formerly Coroners Rules 1984 r.48.

[192] But not necessarily; the Home Office suggested that, where he has no permanent officer, the coroner should appoint another person as "the appropriate officer": Home Office Circular No. 108 of 1983.

[193] Coroners Rules 1984 r.47.

[194] Coroners Rules 1984 r.52.

[195] Coroners Rules 1984 r.51(2). See Home Office Circular No 32 of 2004, dated June 1, 2004.

[196] i.e. those persons set out in the Juries Act 1974 s.1 Sch.1 Pt.III: repealed in 2004.

[197] Coroners Rules 1984 r.49. This would normally be shown by production of a certificate of attendance at the previous proceedings: the coroner's form of certificate was prescribed by the Coroners Rules 1984 Sch.4 Form 6, now repealed.

[198] Juries Act 1974 ss.8, 9, 9A, 9B and 10.

[199] Section 2.

[200] Section 3.

[201] Section 8(2).

[202] Section 8.

[203] Juries Act 1974 s.23(2).

[204] Coroners (Inquests) Rules 2013 (SI 2013/1616) r.29(1).

[205] Coroners (Inquests) Rules 2013 (SI 2013/1616) r.29(1) Sch. Form 1.

discharged if there is doubt as to his capacity to serve on a jury "because of physical disability or insufficient understanding of English". It is therefore implied in the new rules that the coroner and the appropriate officer have these powers (but not the others which they formerly had).[206] It is an offence to make or cause to be made any false representation with the intention of evading or enabling another to evade jury service.[207]

Provision of information on jury composition

There is no obligation to supply a list of jurors to interested persons,[208] much less **10–49** a list of those who have been excused or discharged from attendance.

Expenses of jurors

Coroners' jurors are entitled for their attendance at court to allowances at **10–50** prescribed rates for travelling and subsistence, and for financial loss such as loss of earnings or social security payments.[209]

LEGAL AID

The legal aid system dating back to 1949[210] was replaced in 1999[211] by the **10–51** Community Legal Service and the Criminal Defence Service, both run by the Legal Services Commission.[212] That in turn has now been replaced,[213] as from April 1, 2013, by a new system, in which the Legal Services Commission has been abolished,[214] and the legal aid service brought back under the control of the Lord Chancellor,[215] though with the interposition of a senior civil servant, the Director of Legal Aid Casework ("the Director").[216]

   In the new scheme, "legal services" means providing advice as to how the law **10–52** applies in particular circumstances, providing advice and assistance in relation to legal proceedings, providing other advice and assistance in relation to preventing or settling legal disputes and in relation to enforcement of legal decisions.[217] They include advice and assistance by way of representation, mediation and other dispute resolution.[218] "Civil legal services" means any legal services which do not fall

---

[206] As to the exercise of these powers, see the *Guidance for summoning officers*, published by HM Court Service (as it then was) in 2009.

[207] Coroners and Justice Act 2009 s.33 Sch.6 paras 3, 4 (maximum penalty a fine at level 3 on the standard scale).

[208] *Re McKerr's Application* Unreported June 2, 1992, Carswell J, HC (NI). See also *R. v Comerford* [1998] 1 W.L.R. 191, CA.

[209] Coroners and Justice Act 2009 s.34 Sch.7 para.1; Coroners Allowances, Fees and Expenses Regulations 2013 (SI 2013/1615); formerly Coroners Act 1988 s.25. See 18–50.

[210] Legal Advice and Assistance Act 1949; Legal Aid Act 1988.

[211] Access to Justice Act 1999.

[212] Access to Justice Act 1999 s.1(1), replacing the Legal Aid Board.

[213] Legal Aid, Sentencing and Punishment of Offenders Act 2012 Pt I.

[214] Legal Aid, Sentencing and Punishment of Offenders Act 2012 s.38(1).

[215] Legal Aid, Sentencing and Punishment of Offenders Act 2012 ss.1-3.

[216] Legal Aid, Sentencing and Punishment of Offenders Act 2012 s.4.

[217] Legal Aid, Sentencing and Punishment of Offenders Act 2012 s.8(1).

[218] Legal Aid, Sentencing and Punishment of Offenders Act 2012 s.8(2).

within the scope of criminal legal aid.[219] Such services are to be available to an individual only if they are both set out in a statutory list and the individual has been determined to qualify for them on the basis of a means test.

10–53   The statutory list[220] sets out a number of civil legal services, in each case subject to a complex series of exclusions. The Lord Chancellor has power to add services to the statutory list, or to vary or omit them from it.[221] Two of the services in the list as it stands are most relevant to coroners. The first is civil legal services in relation to judicial review.[222] These services are subject to general exclusions for various kinds of legal services,[223] and specific exclusions for services that do not have the potential to produce a benefit for the individual, a member of his family[224] or the environment.[225] But they otherwise include advocacy services in the High Court, Court of Appeal and Supreme Court.[226]

10–54   It is not clear whether a claim under s.13 of the Coroners Act 1988[227] is included in the phrase "judicial review". It includes any procedure in which the High Court, Court of Appeal or Supreme Court is required by an enactment to make a decision applying the principles applicable to judicial review.[228] But s.13 cases are wider than judicial review in the strict sense.[229] Nevertheless, since they are a complementary way of dealing with appeals from coroner or inquest decisions, the better view is that the phrase "judicial review" should cover a s.13 application.

10–55   The second civil legal service relevant to coroners is that "provided to an individual in relation to an inquest under the Coroners Act 1988 into the death of a member of the individual's family".[230] There are a number of points to make in relation to this service. The first is that, strictly speaking, since July 25, 2013 there can be no inquest so conducted, since inquests into death are now conducted under the Coroners and Justice Act 2009. But, at the time of enactment of the legal aid legislation, it was the 1988 Act and not the 2009 Act that was in force, and so presumably the reference to the 1988 Act will now be interpreted as one to the 2009 Act.[231] The next point is that this service is subject to various exclusions, of

---

[219] Legal Aid, Sentencing and Punishment of Offenders Act 2012 s.8(3).
[220] Legal Aid, Sentencing and Punishment of Offenders Act 2012 Sch.1 Pt I.
[221] Legal Aid, Sentencing and Punishment of Offenders Act 2012 s.9(2).
[222] Legal Aid, Sentencing and Punishment of Offenders Act 2012 Sch.1 Pt I para.19. As to the meaning of "judicial review" see Legal Aid, Sentencing and Punishment of Offenders Act 2012 Sch.1 Pt I para.19(10).
[223] Legal Aid, Sentencing and Punishment of Offenders Act 2012 Sch.1 Pt I para.19(2).
[224] As to which see Legal Aid, Sentencing and Punishment of Offenders Act 2012 Sch.1 Pt I para.19(9).
[225] Legal Aid, Sentencing and Punishment of Offenders Act 2012 Sch.1 Pt I para.19(3), but subject to para.19(4).
[226] Legal Aid, Sentencing and Punishment of Offenders Act 2012 Sch.1 Pt 1 para.2(b), Pt 3 paras 1-3.
[227] See 19–05 ff.
[228] Legal Aid, Sentencing and Punishment of Offenders Act 2012 Sch.1 Pt 1 para.19(10).
[229] See 19–12—19–13.
[230] Legal Aid, Sentencing and Punishment of Offenders Act 2012 Sch.1 Pt 1 para.41(1). As to the meaning of "member of an individual's family", see Legal Aid, Sentencing and Punishment of Offenders Act 2012 Sch.1 Pt 1 para.41(3).
[231] cf. Interpretation Act 1978 s.17(2)(a). See also Legal Aid, Sentencing and Punishment of Offenders Act 2012 Sch.1 Pt 4 para.2.

which the most significant is advocacy.[232] The other exclusions relate to services relating to various areas of law, with the exception of personal injury or death.[233] The result is that this service is for the provision of advice and even representation in relation to an inquest, but *not* advocacy services.

In addition, there is provision for two exceptional cases,[234] both of which are **10–56** relevant to coroners. The first is where, in addition to an individual satisfying the means test, the Director has made a determination (called "an exceptional case determination")[235] that (a) it is necessary to make certain services (which could include advocacy) available to the individual to avoid *either* a breach of that individual's ECHR rights under the Human Rights Act 1998,[236] *or* a breach of any enforceable EU rights to those services, or (b) it is appropriate to do so in the particular circumstances, having regard to the risk that any failure would be such a breach.[237] This is intended to cover cases where, for example, art.2 of the ECHR is engaged following the death, and it would or might be a breach of the ECHR not to provide legal aid to cover representation (perhaps including advocacy) at the inquest.[238] The Director must have regard to the Lord Chancellor's Exceptional Funding Guidance (Inquests).[239]

The second case is where the services concerned are advocacy services at an **10–57** inquest under the 1988 Act[240] into the death of a member of the individual's family,[241] the Director has made a "wider public interest determination", and the individual satisfies a means test.[242] For this purpose a "wider public interest determination" is one that in the circumstances the provision of advocacy for the individual at the inquest is likely to produce significant benefits for a class of person other than the individual and his family.[243]

The result is that legal aid at inquests will normally be confined to advice and **10–58** representation, but not advocacy, unless the ECHR is engaged or a wider public interest determination has been made. Where legal aid is not available (whether at the inquest itself or in review proceedings), it is sometimes possible to obtain assistance from other sources, such as law centres or the Bar Pro Bono Unit.[244]

---

[232] Legal Aid, Sentencing and Punishment of Offenders Act 2012 Sch.1 Pt 1 para.41(2)(b), Pt 3.
[233] Legal Aid, Sentencing and Punishment of Offenders Act 2012 Sch.1 Pt 1 para.41(2)(a), Pt 2.
[234] Legal Aid, Sentencing and Punishment of Offenders Act 2012 s.10(1).
[235] Legal Aid, Sentencing and Punishment of Offenders Act 2012 s.10(2).
[236] *Re Hemsworth's Application* [2003] N.I.Q.B. 5, Kerr J; *Re Hemsworth (No. 2)* [2004] N.I.Q.B. 26, Weatherup J; *R. (Khan) v Secretary of State for Health* [2003] EWCA Civ. 1129.
[237] Legal Aid, Sentencing and Punishment of Offenders Act 2012 s.10(3).
[238] See e.g. *R. (Humberstone) v Legal Services Commission* [2010] EWCA Civ. 1479, for similar criteria under the previous system
[239] *http://www.justice.gov.uk/downloads/legal-aid/funding-code/chancellors-guide-exceptional-funding-inquests.pdf* [Accessed June 9, 2014].
[240] See 10–55 above in relation to the possibility of treating the reference to the 1988 Act as one to the 2009 Act.
[241] This means they are relatives, cohabitants, or one has parental responsibility for the other: Legal Aid, Sentencing and Punishment of Offenders Act 2012 s.10(6).
[242] Legal Aid, Sentencing and Punishment of Offenders Act 2012 s.10(4).
[243] Legal Aid, Sentencing and Punishment of Offenders Act 2012 s.10(5). See, e.g. *R. (Patel) v Lord Chancellor* [2010] EWHC 2220 (Admin.) for similar criteria under the old system.
[244] Tel: 020 7831 9711; *http://www.barprobono.org.uk* [Accessed June 9, 2014].

10–59   Coroners may be asked to make representations to the legal aid authorities in connection with applications for legal aid, and any views expressed will be considered. Usually the coroner is asked to say that the inquest will engage ECHR art.2 (and will therefore be a *Middleton* inquest), and that it is necessary that the family need to be represented in order to avoid a breach of the procedural obligation inherent in art.2. The first point is plainly a question of law, which the coroner at some stage may have to decide. In cases where other interested persons contend that art.2 is not engaged at all, and the coroner does not yet have all the material relevant to the art.2 decision, it will usually be impossible to state that art.2 is engaged at that stage. Even in other cases it will sometimes be difficult.

10–60   The second point, however, is more for the Legal Aid Agency than the coroner. The art.2 obligation lies on the state, not on the coroner.[245] The coroner is merely one of the means by which the state discharges its art.2 obligation.[246] The Agency is another. It is not the coroner's function under domestic law to ensure that the family of the deceased have funding for inquests where this is necessary to avoid a breach of art.2.[247] That is the function of the Agency. It is the coroner's function under domestic law to hold inquests timeously[248] and according to the rules laid down for that purpose (designed and certified to be ECHR-compliant). Accordingly, coroners have no obligation to adjourn inquests to enable applications to be processed.

10–61   Indeed coroners have no legal obligation to make representations to the Agency at all. Nevertheless, if requested, the coroner should assist the Agency with a view on relevant issues, where this is possible within the limits of the resources available. The coroner can properly take the view that it would be desirable, even necessary, for an interested person to be represented in order for a full inquiry to take place, without necessarily committing to the view at that stage that art.2 is engaged on the facts of the case.

10–62   For this purpose, the coroner may consider and could properly refer where appropriate to (inter alia) the amount of documentation involved, the complexity of the issues (legal and factual), the technical nature of the evidence (e.g. medical or scientific) likely to be given, the existence of legal representation for other interested persons, and any relevant vulnerabilities of the family (e.g. mental illness). He or she can also properly say (if it be the case) that it will be a *Middleton* inquest in any event, even if the art.2 point has not yet been decided.

10–63   The most weight will be given by the Agency to a coroner's view that not merely confirms that in his or her view (i) the case engages ECHR art.2, and (ii) the family requires representation to participate effectively in the proceedings, but also explains (iii) *why* this is so in both cases. But, given misunderstandings in the past by the legal aid authorities of inquest proceedings, where the coroner is not able to give all or some of these confirmations and explanations, it will be

---

[245] *R (Antoniou) v Central and North West London NHS Foundation Trust* [2013] EWHC 3055 (Admin), [24], DC.

[246] See 21–16.

[247] Indeed, under the Coroners and Justice Act 2009, it was dealt with by s.51. But this was repealed before coming into force.

[248] Coroners (Inquests) Rules 2013 (SI 2013/1616) r.8; Coroners (Investigations) Regulations 2013 (SI 2013/1629) reg.26; see 10–14.

important nevertheless to confirm (a) that there will in any event be an inquest (with a jury, if that is the case), and that the coroner has no power to dispense with one, and (b) that some one or more members of the family is or are interested persons with rights of participation in the investigation and inquest.

PREPARATION FOR THE HEARING

Since the proceedings are inquisitorial in nature,[249] there are no issues to be litigated between parties. Indeed, there are no "parties", merely "interested persons".[250] The court undertakes an inquiry, without the need for any equivalent to statements of case (pleadings) in civil proceedings or an indictment or an information in criminal proceedings.[251] On the contrary, an inquiry requires an open mind, not a pre-formed "case". In complex cases, the coroner is often assisted by the engagement of counsel (and sometimes solicitors) to the inquest.[252] **10–64**

The coroner prepares for the inquest by obtaining statements from the available witnesses,[253] and other relevant documents and information from appropriate agencies and third parties, and for this purpose he has the power to issue and serve a notice requiring this information to be supplied.[254] It is the duty of the police to supply to the coroner for the purposes of the inquest all the material in their possession concerning the cause and circumstances of the death.[255] In practice, prisons, hospitals and others supply relevant documents and reports without the need for a coroner notice.[256] So does the family of the deceased in most cases.[257] **10–65**

The coroner must not confine himself to his witness statements and ignore material from third parties. On the other hand, it is for him to decide how best to allocate his limited resources between the various inquests with which he has to deal, and hence he is not to be criticised in a particular case if he does not pursue every possible source of information or personally peruse every document available, provided that he has made reasonable and appropriate efforts to obtain the information and evidence which he reasonably considers that he needs for the inquest in question.[258] **10–66**

Where a witness who is abroad will not come to England for the inquest or provide a statement, the coroner may ask the judicial authorities of the relevant state to provide it in accordance with their own rules. This is done by way of a **10–67**

---

[249] See 1–18 ff.
[250] See 8–21 ff, 10–03 above.
[251] See 1–19—1–21.
[252] See 11–29—11–30.
[253] See 10–25 ff.
[254] Coroners and Justice Act 2009 s.32 Sch.5 para.1. See 7–12 ff.
[255] *Peach v Metropolitan Police Commissioner* [1986] 2 All E.R. 129 at 138; *R. v Derby Coroner Ex p. Hart* (2000) 164 J.P. 429 at [93]; *Re Maddison* [2002] EWHC 2567 (Admin.), DC; *McCaughey & Anor, Re Application for Judicial Review* [2004] N.I.Q.B. 2; *Chief Constable of PSNI, Re Application for Judicial Review* [2010] N.I.Q.B. 66.
[256] This usually includes internal inquiry reports and the like. As to the notice, see 7–13 ff.
[257] Cf. *R. (Sutovic) v North London Coroner* [2006] EWHC 1095 (Admin.). at [57]–[58].
[258] See, e.g. *R. (Ahmed) v South and East Cumbria Coroner* [2009] EWHC 1653 (Admin.). at [35].

formal "letter of request".[259] Evidence may also be obtained by video-link from a witness who cannot or will not travel.[260] The coroner is the master of his own procedure.[261] Hence, where he considers it appropriate, the coroner may hold a pre-inquest hearing with such of the interested persons as may think proper, to discuss the preparations for the resumed inquest and to hear preliminary applications and receive submissions on points of law, or to make public the post-mortem examination report, where this is appropriate.[262]

Disclosure to interested persons by coroners

10–68   The law of disclosure by coroners to interested persons has developed exponentially in recent years. Originally there was little or no duty on coroners to provide information before the inquest hearing.[263] Then the Human Rights Act 1998 enabled the European Convention on Human Rights to be taken more directly into account.[264] The European Court of Human Rights criticised the lack of advance disclosure of witness statements in inquests as contributing to a failure to comply with the procedural obligation[265] under art.2 (the right to life),[266] where that was engaged.[267] But a similar approach was then adopted in non-art.2 cases.[268] As a result, there was a presumption in favour of disclosure, and the burden was on the coroner to explain why it was not needed.[269] But the European approach has not always been adopted.[270] Since 2013, however, there is a statutory system of disclosure to interested persons, which has already been described.[271] It applies not only for the purposes of inquests but also for the purpose of investigations generally.

Disclosure to interested persons by others

10–69   So far as interested persons are concerned, because the coroner's investigation is an *inquiry*, rather than *litigation*, there is no process in the coroner's court for interested persons to obtain sight or copies of relevant documents in the hands of others before the hearing (such as the process of disclosure in civil proceedings).[272] Like any inquiry, only the coroner himself has the power to call witnesses and to compel production of documents by notice,[273] although the exercise of (or failure to

---

[259] See 5–94—5–95.

[260] See 12–29.

[261] See *R v North Humberside Coroner, ex p Jamieson* [1995] QBI, 26 (14).

[262] *R. (Coker) v Inner South London Coroner* [2006] EWHC 614 (Admin.).

[263] *R. v Lincoln Coroner Ex p. Hay* [2000] Lloyd's Rep. Med. 264, DC.

[264] See 21–01.

[265] i.e. the obligation in some cases to investigate the death; see 21–18 below.

[266] *Jordan v United Kingdom* (2001) 11 B.H.R.C.1 at [133], [134], [142]; *McShane v United Kingdom* Unreported May 28, 2002 at [122]–[123], ECtHR.

[267] See 21–15 below.

[268] *R. v Avon Coroner Ex p. Bentley*, (2001) 166 J.P. 297, Sullivan J.

[269] *R. (Ahmed) v South and East Cumbria* [2009] EWHC 1653 (Admin.); *R. (Butler) v Black Country District Coroner* [2010] EWHC 43 (Admin.).) at [78]–[79]; cf. *R. (McLeish) v North London Coroner* [2010] EWHC 3624 (Admin.).

[270] *R. (Green) v Police Complaints Authority* [2002] UKHRR 985 (complaint to the Police Complaints Authority about, and their investigation into, allegedly racist behaviour by a police officer resulting in personal injury, though not death).

[271] See 7–24 ff.

[272] *R. v Southwark Coroner Ex p. Hicks* [1987] 1 W.L.R. 1624.

[273] See 10–25, 10–65 below.

exercise) such powers will be open to review in appropriate cases. Moreover it is for the coroner alone to decide what documents should be placed before a jury.[274] At the hearing of the inquest interested persons will be entitled to see documents put in evidence,[275] and also to see any document used by a witness to refresh his memory.[276]

Where a person dies in prison, the prison service[277] has a power, but no duty,   **10–70** to supply copies of relevant documents to the deceased's family in advance of the inquest, but the exercise of this power will not be reviewed in the absence of appropriate circumstances.[278] In fact, the Prisons and Probation Ombudsman (whose office investigates the deaths of all prisoners in UK prisons) has operated a policy of routinely (and voluntarily) disclosing to the family of a deceased prisoner before the inquest the findings of his inquiry reports following the death.[279] A similar policy applies in relation to deaths in police custody.[280] But even where art.2 of the ECHR applies, that does not mean that an "interested person" is entitled to see the police file.[281] In each case it is the authority concerned, rather than the coroner, which is responsible for any disclosure, although the coroner will be consulted to ensure that disclosure does not interfere with the inquest itself.

The relatives of a deceased person may also have rights to obtain documents and   **10–71** information which may be relevant to the inquest's purposes, but entirely outside the inquest procedure. They may, for example, be entitled to see medical and other records relating to the deceased pursuant to the Access to Medical Reports Act 1988, the Access to Health Records Act 1990, or the Data Protection Act 1998.[282] Or they may seek pre-action disclosure against a potential defendant to civil proceedings.[283] It is no objection to seeking such disclosure that the inquest has not yet been held.[284]

One final point relates to the confidentiality of any documents or other   **10–72** information disclosed. Where disclosure is given compulsorily, for a specific and limited purpose, the general principle is that it is subject to a duty of confidentiality such that it may not be used or revealed except to further the specific purpose.[285] But where (as may be the case at an inquest) it is given voluntarily, there is no such duty imposed by the general law. Accordingly, written undertakings, based on

---

[274] *Re McKerr's Application* Unreported June 2, 1992, HC (NI), Carswell J.

[275] See 7–24 ff.

[276] *Re McKerr's Application* Unreported May 28, 1993, CA (NI).; cf. *R. v Davies* [2011] EWCA Crim. 871 at [69]; see 12–65 below.

[277] Part of the National Offender Management Service, an executive agency of the Ministry of Justice.

[278] *R. v Home Secretary Ex p. O'Grady* Unreported October 1, 1991, Kennedy J.

[279] See *R. (Hair) v Staffordshire (South) Coroner* [2010] EWHC 2580 (Admin.), where the failure to disclose documents until during the inquest had serious consequential effects, leading to the quashing of the inquest.

[280] See Home Office Circular No. 20 of 1999, replaced by No. 31 of 2002. The Police Complaints Authority has been replaced by the Independent Police Complaints Commission under the Police Reform Act 2002.

[281] *Re Wright's Application for Judicial Review* [2003] N.I.Q.B. 17, Kerr J; cf. *R. (Lagos) v City of London Coroner* [2013] EWHC 423 (Admin.) (not art.2).

[282] As to this Act, see 7–33 ff.

[283] Under the Senior Courts Act 1981 s.33, or the County Court Act 1984 s.52, and CPR r.31.16.

[284] *Stobart v Nottingham Health Authority* [1992] 3 Med. L.R. 284.

[285] See, e.g. *Marcel v Metropolitan Police Commissioner* [1992] Ch. 225 at 237. See also *R. v Derby Coroner Ex p. Hart* (2000) 164 J.P. 429 at [95].

those implied in civil litigation disclosure,[286] should be specifically sought and obtained. Requiring such undertakings does not infringe the European Convention on Human Rights.[287]

COMPULSORY SUSPENSION OF INVESTIGATION AND ADJOURNMENT OF INQUEST

10–73   As mentioned earlier,[288] in a number of cases the coroner must suspend an investigation and adjourn any inquest being held as part of it.[289] These cases involve (i) visiting forces, (ii) pending criminal proceedings, and (iii) public inquiries. They are dealt with in detail here. Other cases of compulsory adjournment, arising during the inquest hearing, are dealt with later,[290] as are cases of *discretionary* adjournment.[291] (There is also a *power* to suspend an investigation where considered appropriate to do so. This was dealt with earlier.)[292]

Visiting forces

10–74   In the first group there are two cases. The first is where the coroner is satisfied that the deceased had a relevant association[293] with a visiting force:[294] unless the Secretary of State otherwise directs, the coroner must suspend the investigation, adjourn any inquest opened and discharge any jury summoned.[295] The second is where the coroner is satisfied that a person subject to the jurisdiction of the service courts of a country within the visiting forces legislation has been charged before a court of that country with the homicide of the deceased, or is being detained by that country's authorities with a view to being so charged. In this case too, the coroner must suspend the investigation, adjourn any inquest and discharge any jury. In either case he or she may furnish the registrar of deaths with a certificate of particulars for registration of the death so far as ascertained.[296]

Pending criminal proceedings

10–75   The next group contains three cases. The first relates to possible future criminal charges, and the second and third to charges that have been made. For these purposes, the legislation uses three important defined terms. The first is "homicide offence". This means[297] (a) murder,[298] manslaughter,[299] corporate manslaughter[300]

---

[286] See generally, Matthews and Malek, *Disclosure,* 4th edn (2012), Ch.19; cf. the suggested notice at 7–29.
[287] *Re Jordan's Application* Unreported September 4, 2001, HC (NI), Kerr J.
[288] See 10–13 above.
[289] *Chief Coroner's Guide to the Coroners and Justice Act 2009,* [88] ff.
[290] See 11–44 ff.
[291] See 11–36 ff.
[292] See 8–18.
[293] As to which see 5–104 above.
[294] As to which see 5–102 above.
[295] Visiting Forces Act 1952 s.7(1): 5–99 above.
[296] As to which see paras 5–98—5–99.
[297] Coroners and Justice Act 2009 s.11 Sch.1 para.1(6).
[298] See 14–37 ff.
[299] See 14–42 ff.
[300] See 14–52 ff.

or infanticide,[301] (b) the road traffic offences of causing death by dangerous driving,[302] by careless or inconsiderate driving,[303] by careless driving when under the influence of drink or drugs,[304] and by driving when unlicensed, disqualified or uninsured,[305] (c) encouraging or assisting suicide,[306] and (d) causing or allowing the death of a child or vulnerable adult.[307]

The second term is "related offence". This means[308] an offence that *either* **10–76** involves the death of the deceased but is not a homicide offence or the service equivalent of a homicide offence, *or* involves the death of a person other than the deceased and is committed in circumstances connected with the death of the deceased. So a "related offence" will typically be an offence less than homicide (e.g. an assault offence) but which involved the death of the deceased, or a homicide offence directed at someone other than the deceased but connected with the death of the deceased (such as a bomb explosion killing the deceased and others).

The third term is "the service equivalent of a homicide offence". This means[309] **10–77** offences under the armed forces legislation[310] corresponding to a homicide offence.

The first case is where a prosecuting authority[311] requests the coroner to suspend **10–78** an investigation on the ground that a person may be charged *either* with a homicide offence involving the death of the deceased *or* an offence alleged to be a related offence.[312] This also applies where a Provost Marshal or the Director of Service Prosecutions similarly requests in relation to *either* the service equivalent of a homicide offence *or* a service offence[313] alleged to be a related offence.[314] In such cases the coroner must suspend the investigation[315] (and adjourn any inquest,[316] discharging any jury if he thinks fit)[317] for 28 days[318] or any longer period specified by the coroner.[319] This period may be extended or further extended.[320]

The second case is where a coroner becomes aware that a person (i) has appeared **10–79** or been brought before a magistrates' court charged with a homicide offence

---

[301] See 14–69.
[302] See 14–62 ff.
[303] See Road Traffic Act 1988, s.2B.
[304] See 14–67, 14–68.
[305] See Road Traffic Act 1988, s.3ZB; *R v Hughes* [2013] 1 WLR 2461, SC.
[306] See 14–76 ff.
[307] See Domestic Violence, Crime and Violence Act 2004, s.5.
[308] Coroners and Justice Act 2009 s.11 Sch.1 para.1(6).
[309] Coroners and Justice Act 2009 s.11 Sch.1 para.1(6).
[310] Armed Forces Act 2006 s.42; Army Act 1955 s.70; Air Force Act 1955 s.70; Naval Discipline Act 1957 s.42.
[311] That is, the Director of Public Prosecutions, or a person of a description prescribed by an order made by the Lord Chancellor: Coroners and Justice Act 2009 s.48(1).
[312] Coroners and Justice Act 2009 s.11 Sch.1 para.1(2).
[313] This has the meaning given by the Armed Forces Act 2006 s.50(2), that is, any of various offences under that Act, and under some earlier legislation, but also includes an offence under the earlier services legislation: Coroners and Justice Act 2009 s.48(1).
[314] Coroners and Justice Act 2009 s.11 Sch.1 para.1(3).
[315] Coroners and Justice Act 2009 s.11 Sch.1 para.1(1).
[316] Coroners and Justice Act 2009 s.11 Sch.1 para.6(1).
[317] Coroners and Justice Act 2009 s.11 Sch.1 para.6(2).
[318] Coroners and Justice Act 2009 s.11 Sch.1 para.1(4)(a).
[319] Coroners and Justice Act 2009 s.11 Sch.1 para.1(4)(b).
[320] Coroners and Justice Act 2009 s.11 Sch.1 para.1(5).

involving the death of the deceased,[321] or (ii) has been charged on an indictment with such an offence without having so appeared or been brought before such a court, or (iii) has been charged with the service equivalent of a homicide offence involving the death of the deceased.[322] The coroner must suspend the investigation[323] (and adjourn any inquest,[324] discharging any jury if he thinks fit),[325] unless (in cases (i) and (ii)) the prosecuting authority or (in case (iii)) the Director of Service Prosecutions informs the coroner that there is no objection to the investigation continuing, or (in any case) the coroner thinks there is an exceptional reason for not suspending the investigation.[326] The suspension comes to an end if a person is thereafter charged with such an offence but the prosecuting authority or the Director of Service Prosecutions (as appropriate) informs the coroner that there is no objection to the investigation continuing and the coroner decides not to suspend the investigation.[327]

10–80   The third case is where *either* (i) a prosecuting authority informs a coroner that a person (a) has appeared or been brought before a magistrates' court charged with an offence alleged to be a related offence,[328] or (b) has been charged on an indictment with such an offence without having been sent for trial for it,[329] *or* (ii) the Director of Service Prosecutions informs a coroner that a person has been charged with the service equivalent of a homicide offence involving the death of the deceased,[330] and the prosecuting authority or Director requests the coroner to suspend the investigation.[331] In either case the coroner must suspend the investigation[332] (and adjourn any inquest,[333] discharging any jury if he thinks fit),[334] unless (in cases (i) and (ii)) the prosecuting authority or (in case (iii)) the Director of Service Prosecutions informs the coroner that there is no objection to the investigation continuing, or (in any case) the coroner thinks there is an exceptional reason for not suspending the investigation.[335]

---

[321] Coroners and Justice Act 2009 s.11 Sch.1 para.2(2)(a).

[322] Coroners and Justice Act 2009 s.11 Sch.1 para.2(3).

[323] Coroners and Justice Act 2009 s.11 Sch.1 para.2(1).

[324] Coroners and Justice Act 2009 s.11 Sch.1 para.6(1).

[325] Coroners and Justice Act 2009 s.11 Sch.1 para.6(2).

[326] Coroners and Justice Act 2009 s.11 Sch.1 para.6(6). See *Pereira v Inner South London Coroner* [2007] EWHC 1723 (Admin.), concerning the words "in the absence of reason to the contrary" in the predecessor provision, Coroners Act 1988 s.16(1) (if there is such reason, the coroner has a discretion whether to adjourn, to be exercised judicially).

[327] Coroners and Justice Act 2009 s.11 Sch.1 para.2(7).

[328] Coroners and Justice Act 2009 s.11 Sch.1 para.2(4)(a).

[329] Coroners and Justice Act 2009 s.11 Sch.1 para.2(4)(b).

[330] Coroners and Justice Act 2009 s.11 Sch.1 para.2(5).

[331] Coroners and Justice Act 2009 s.11 Sch.1 para.2(4), (5).

[332] Coroners and Justice Act 2009 s.11 Sch.1 para.2(1).

[333] Coroners and Justice Act 2009 s.11 Sch.1 para.6(1).

[334] Coroners and Justice Act 2009 s.11 Sch.1 para.6(2).

[335] Coroners and Justice Act 2009 s.11 Sch.1 para.6(6). See *Pereira v Inner South London Coroner* [2007] EWHC 1723 (Admin.), concerning the words "in the absence of reason to the contrary" in the predecessor provision, Coroners Act 1988 s.16(1) (if there is such reason, the coroner has a discretion whether to adjourn, to be exercised judicially).

Pending inquiry

Unless there appears to be an exceptional reason for not doing so,[336] a coroner   **10–81**
must suspend an investigation if the Lord Chancellor requests the coroner to do so
on the ground that the cause of death is likely to be adequately investigated by an
inquiry under the Inquiries Act 2005 that is being or is to be held, a senior judge[337]
has been appointed as chairman of the inquiry, and the Lord Chief Justice has
approved of that appointment.[338] If the investigation is already suspended under the
first case of pending criminal proceedings set out above,[339] it is thereafter treated
as suspended under this heading for certain purposes.[340] The terms of the inquiry
must include among its purposes the ascertainment of the matters needed to be
ascertained at an inquest.[341]

Certificates

Where the coroner suspends an investigation within any of the criminal charge or   **10–82**
inquiry cases, he must furnish the registrar of deaths with the particulars
necessary[342] for the registration of death.[343] This is commonly done by way of a
certificate[344] supplied by the Registrar General.

Resumption of inquest[345]

Where an investigation is resumed, the coroner must resume any inquest that was   **10–83**
adjourned as part of it.[346] The question of the resumption of an investigation
suspended by reason of the visiting forces provisions has already been considered.[347]
As for the first of the three cases of pending criminal charges,[348] an investigation
adjourned for 28 days or longer must be resumed once the period expires (unless
the suspension continues under a different provision).[349] In that case the coroner
must notify the next of kin or personal representative of the deceased and any other
interested persons who have made themselves known to the coroner of the
resumption and the reason for the resumption.[350]

---

[336] Coroners and Justice Act 2009 s.11 Sch.1 para.3(2).
[337] This means a judge of the High Court, Court of Appeal or Supreme Court: Coroners and Justice
Act 2009 s.11 Sch.1 para.3(1).
[338] Coroners and Justice Act 2009 s.11 Sch.1 para.3(1).
[339] See 10–75.
[340] Coroners and Justice Act 2009 s.11 Sch.1 para.3(3).
[341] Coroners and Justice Act 2009 s.11 Sch.1 para.4; see 6–01, 13–01.
[342] Where the death occurred outside England and Wales it is not registrable (Births and Deaths
Registration Act 1953 s.15) and consequently no certificate need be furnished to the registrar.
[343] Coroners (Investigations) Regulations 2013 (SI 2013/1629) reg.8; formerly Coroners Act 1988
s.16(4). The limit of five days from adjournment in which to do this under Coroners Rules 1984
r.29, has however gone.
[344] Known as Form 120. It is divided into two sheets, Pts A and B. Pt A gives most of the information.
Pt B requests details of the incident leading to the death. See Home Office Circular, No. 12 of
1993.
[345] *Chief Coroner's Guide to the Coroners and Justice Act 2009*, [96] ff.
[346] Coroners and Justice Act 2009 s.11 Sch.1 para.11(1).
[347] See 5–108.
[348] See 10–75.
[349] Coroners and Justice Act 2009 s.11 Sch.1 para.7.
[350] Coroners (Investigations) Regulations 2013 (SI 2013/1629) reg.10.

10–84   As to the other cases of pending criminal charges, the investigation must not be resumed so long as proceedings are continuing before the court of trial in respect of a homicide offence (or the service equivalent) or the related offence,[351] unless the relevant prosecuting authority[352] or Director of Service Prosecutions (as appropriate) informs the coroner that there is no objection to the resumption.[353] Subject to that, the coroner may resume the investigation only if he thinks there is sufficient cause for resuming it (and then must do so).[354] But there is no obligation to notify anyone of the resumption or of the reason.[355]

10–85   In considering whether there is sufficient cause to resume an adjourned inquest,

> "the coroner must direct his attention to the question whether it has been sufficiently established who the deceased was, and how, when and where he came by his death. If the coroner, after looking at the facts of the case, considers that these matters have already been sufficiently established in public proceedings, he is quite justified in taking the view that an inquest is not necessary. The fact that the next-of-kin of a deceased person may thus not obtain the opportunity to cross-examine witnesses or tender more evidence does not itself make it necessary for him to hold an inquest. What is material is whether the relevant matters have been established in a manner in which the public interest has been adequately served."[356]

The relevant matters are who the deceased was, and when, where and how he or she came by his or her death.[357] Except in art.2 cases, "how" means "by what means".[358]

10–86   Thus where the criminal proceedings have already gone thoroughly into the facts surrounding the death, as in, e.g. a murder trial that goes to the jury (whatever the result), the coroner may well consider that no useful purpose would be served by resuming the inquest.[359] But if the criminal proceedings did not reach a substantive conclusion, or terminated on technical grounds, so that the evidence relating to the death itself was not heard, the matter may be otherwise.[360] A coroner is not obliged to take into account UK international law obligations in exercising the discretion as to whether to resume an investigation (and inquest).[361]

---

[351] Coroners and Justice Act 2009 s.11 Sch.1 para.8(2).

[352] This means the authority responsible for the prosecution or the request to suspend, as the case may be: Coroners and Justice Act 2009 s.11 Sch.1 para.8(4).

[353] Coroners and Justice Act 2009 s.11 Sch.1 para.8(3).

[354] Coroners and Justice Act 2009 s.11 Sch.1 para.8(1).

[355] cf. Coroners (Investigations) Regulations 2013 (SI 2013/1629) reg.10; see 10–83.

[356] *Re Downes' Application* [1988] 4 N.I.J.B. 91, HC (NI), Carswell J; see also *R. (Hurst) v North London Coroner* [2007] 2 AC 189, HL.

[357] See 6–01, 13–01.

[358] See 6–05 ff, 6–14 ff.

[359] See, e.g. *R. v Coroner for Inner West London Ex p. Walsh* Unreported 12 July 1993, Harrison J; *R. (Amin) v Home Secretary* [2002] 3 W.L.R. 505, CA; see also *R. (Southall Black Sisters) v West Yorkshire Coroner* [2002] EWHC 1914 (Admin.), Jackson J.; *Fraser v North West Wales Coroner* [2010] EWHC 1165 (Admin.); *R. (Palmer) v Worcestershire Coroner* [2011] EWHC 1453 (Admin.); *Re McMahon's Application* [2013] NIQB 22.

[360] cf. *R. v Inner West London Coroner Ex p. Dallaglio* [1994] 4 All E.R. 139, CA.

[361] *Metropolitan Police Commissioner v Hurst* [2007] 2 AC 189.

If the inquest is a *Jamieson* inquest,[362] its more limited scope means that in some cases the *Middleton* purpose of expressing conclusions on key issues on the broad circumstances of the death[363] cannot be satisfied, and there would be no point in the resumption of the inquest.[364] If it is a *Middleton* inquest, the matter may be otherwise.[365]

If an inquest is resumed after pending criminal proceedings have concluded, the   **10–87** determination must not be inconsistent with the outcome of the proceedings which caused the suspension of the investigation or any proceedings which had to be concluded before the investigation could be resumed.[366]

Where an investigation is suspended because of an inquiry, the general rule is   **10–88** that the coroner may resume only if he thinks there is sufficient cause for resuming it (and then must do so),[367] but must not do so within 28 days of the conclusion of the inquiry (if notified by the Lord Chancellor) or otherwise of the day on which its findings were published.[368] If criminal proceedings have also been taken of which he is aware, the coroner must also not resume until those proceedings are concluded, unless the prosecuting authority or Director of Service Prosecutions (as appropriate) informs the coroner that there is no objection to the resumption.[369] Any determination at a resumed inquest must not be inconsistent with the outcome of the inquiry or of any proceedings which had to be concluded before the investigation could be resumed.[370]

Where an inquest is resumed under these provisions, the ordinary provisions for   **10–89** requiring a jury[371] do not apply.[372] Instead, the resumed inquest may be held with a jury if the coroner thinks there is sufficient reason for it to be held with one.[373] If the adjourned inquest was held with a jury and the coroner decides to hold the resumed inquest with one, then, if at least seven members of the original jury are available to serve at the resumed inquest, it must be held with a jury consisting of those persons.[374] If they are not, or if the original jury was discharged, a new jury must be summoned.[375]

---

[362] See 6–05.

[363] See 6–14.

[364] *Metropolitan Police Commissioner v Hurst* [2007] 2 AC 189.

[365] *R. (Moss) v Durham and Darlington Coroner* [2008] EWHC 2940 (Admin.).

[366] Coroners and Justice Act 2009 s.11 Sch.1 para.8(5).

[367] Coroners and Justice Act 2009 s.11 Sch.1 para.9(1)(a). In the case of the inquest into the death of Dr David Kelly, the Oxfordshire Coroner held a hearing on March 16, 2004 in order to decide whether to resume the inquest under s.17A(4). His view was that probably an "exceptional reason" to resume the inquest would be if the public inquiry had not investigated the cause of death adequately, which he was unable to say was the case here.

[368] Coroners and Justice Act 2009 s.11 Sch.1 para.9(1)(b), (2).

[369] Coroners and Justice Act 2009 s.11 Sch.1 para.9(4), (6), (8), (10).

[370] Coroners and Justice Act 2009 s.11 Sch.1 para.9(11).

[371] Coroners and Justice Act 2009 s.7; see 10–34.

[372] Coroners and Justice Act 2009 s.11 Sch.1 para.11(2).

[373] Coroners and Justice Act 2009 s.11 Sch.1 para.11(3).

[374] Coroners and Justice Act 2009 s.11 Sch.1 para.11(4)(a).

[375] Coroners and Justice Act 2009 s.11 Sch.1 para.11(4)(b).

Pre-Inquest Review

10–90   A coroner may at any time during the course of an investigation and before an inquest hearing hold a pre-inquest review hearing.[376] This may be for the purpose of hearing one or more applications which can best be dealt with by way of a courtroom hearing, rather than on paper. Or it may be for the purpose of reviewing the preparations for the forthcoming inquest hearing. No evidence will be given at a pre-inquest review hearing, and even if the case requires a jury, no jury will be summoned for it.

10–91   Many of the rules applicable to the inquest hearing also apply to a pre-inquest review. Thus, any pre-inquest hearing must be held in public[377] unless the coroner considers that the public should be excluded from it in the interests of justice or national security.[378] The coroner must make and keep a sound recording of a pre-inquest review.[379] In holding a pre-inquest view the coroner is holding a court, and the ordinary rules on reporting[380] and on contempt of court[381] will apply.

10–92   The rules about making details of inquest hearings publicly available and of notifying interested persons[382] do not in terms apply to pre-inquest reviews, but in practice the coroner will notify whoever needs to be informed, and (since in principle such reviews are public) will normally make details publicly available. Under the new coroner system there are no longer any restrictions on where in England and Wales an inquest hearing is held,[383] and the same must apply to pre-inquest reviews. In principle there is no reason why a pre-inquest review cannot be conducted by telephone in an appropriate case.[384]

10–93   Where a pre-inquest review is held to review the preparations for an inquest, and it is appropriate to do so,[385] the coroner should prepare and supply in advance to the interested persons a written agenda, in appropriate cases containing his provisional views, on some or all of the following topics: who are the interested persons, the proposed witnesses, the issues likely to arise, the scope of the evidence, whether a jury should be summoned, whether ECHR art.2 is engaged, any disclosure issues, and the date of the inquest hearing.[386] The coroner should also

---

[376] Coroners (Inquests) Rules 2013 (SI 2013/1616) r.6.

[377] Coroners (Inquests) Rules 2013 (SI 2013/1616) r.11(3). See also 11–04—11–06.

[378] Coroners (Inquests) Rules 2013 (SI 2013/1616) r.11(5); formerly Coroners Rules 1984 r.17. But note the additional exception for "the interests of justice".

[379] Coroners (Inquests) Rules 2013 (SI 2013/1616) r.26. The coroner should take reasonable steps to ensure that the recording equipment is working well, and that those who speak in court do so in such a way that the recording can be fully and accurately transcribed: *Brown v Norfolk Coroner* [2014] EWHC 187 (Admin.) at [38].

[380] See 11–70 ff.

[381] See 11–89 ff.

[382] See 10–21—10–24.

[383] See 10–16—10–20.

[384] cf. the provisions of para.6 of Practice Direction 23A to the Civil Procedure Rules 1998, in relation to interlocutory applications in civil litigation. In practice it may be unnecessary to apply all the procedures there set out for the purposes of a coronial inquiry.

[385] Some matters may be dealt with by application letter, or written submissions, for example.

[386] *Brown v Norfolk Coroner* [2014] EWHC 187 (Admin.) 39–40.

ensure that as far as possible the interested persons have all the disclosure necessary to enable their full participation in the hearing.[387] After the review is over, the coroner should circulate a memorandum of what was decided.

---

[387] *Brown v Norfolk Coroner* [2014] EWHC 187 (Admin.) 41.

Chapter 11

PROCEDURE AT THE INQUEST: PART I

Publicity, Jury, Adjournment, Advocacy, Reporting, Contempt

HOLDING/RESUMING THE INQUEST

There is no requirement that the Court in holding or resuming the inquest hearing do so formally.[1] In a few courts it is still done by proclamation,[2] but in most cases the coroner's officer or the usher will simply call "Silence", "Court rise" or "All stand" as the coroner enters. The important thing is that it is made clear that the court is now sitting and that courtroom rules apply. **11–01**

Many coroners make a brief opening statement, not only to describe what will happen, but often also to manage expectations.[3] In jury cases, once the jury is sworn, it is appropriate to give a brief address to the jury as to the inquest's functions. This will be helpful both to inform the jury as to what they should be looking out for, and to give them certain warnings.[4] It will also be desirable to ask the representatives of interested persons (or the interested persons themselves, if unrepresented) to identify themselves at the outset. This may be important in cases where several members of the deceased's family attend, and they are not all of the same view.[5] **11–02**

It is usual for the coroner's officer or someone similar throughout the inquest to carry out the functions of both court clerk and usher, although sometimes when a courtroom is borrowed for an inquest the usual ushers continue to act in that capacity. The coroner's officer or other person will also check that the recording system is operating correctly. **11–03**

---

[1] cf. Coroners Rules 1984 r.16 (repealed).
[2] For forms of proclamation (nowadays rather old-fashioned), see App.3, Forms 5 and 6.
[3] See e.g. the Chief Coroner's Guidance No. 12, *The Inquest Checklist*.
[4] See the Chief Coroner's Guidance No. 10, *Warnings to Juries*, and also 11–18.
[5] See also the Home Office letter to coroners dated April 30, 2002 (sent with Newsletter No. 38, of the same date).

PUBLICITY

Hearing in public

11–04   An inquest hearing[6] must be held in public[7] unless the coroner considers that the public should be excluded (from the inquest hearing or any part of it) in the interests of national security.[8] This is a departure from the common law rule that the coroner had a discretion to decide on the degree of publicity allowed at the inquest.[9] But issues of national security are not involved merely because the deceased is alleged to have worked for the security services.[10]

11–05   The rules do not however allow the coroner to exclude some or all of the interested persons or their representatives on the grounds of national security; the coroner has no power to receive "closed material" in a "closed inquest", even in order to further the objective of the inquest.[11] Legislation[12] now permits so-called "closed material" hearings in civil litigation generally, which will include applications for judicial review of coroners' decisions,[13] but not inquests themselves.[14] Applications for the coroner's court to sit in private will often themselves have to be heard, at least in part, in private, though coroners should strive to hear as much as possible in public, and any decision on such an application should be given in open court.[15] The coroner's decision is of course subject to judicial review in an appropriate case.[16]

11–06   There is no breach of the rule requiring an inquest to be held in public merely because the limited accommodation is filled, and other members of the public cannot gain admission.[17] Nor is the rule breached by permitting the use of a screen to protect the identity of a witness in a proper case.[18]

---

[6] This does not include the opening of the inquest, which is covered by a different provision: see 10–09. As to pre-inquest reviews, see 10–90 ff.

[7] Coroners (Inquests) Rules 2013 (SI 2013/1616) r.11(3), cf *Scott v Scott* [1913] AC 417; *R (Guardian News and Media Ltd) v City of Westminster Magistrates Court* [2013] QB 618, CA (11–70).

[8] Coroners (Inquests) Rules 2013 (SI 2013/1616) r.11(4); formerly Coroners Rules 1984 r.17.

[9] *Garnett v Ferrand* (1827) 6 B. & C. 611; 108 E.R. 576; cf. *R. v Richards* (1998) 163 J.P. 246, CA (criminal trial).

[10] *R. v McHugh Ex p. Trelford* Unreported March 22, 1984, DC.

[11] *R. (Home Secretary) v Inner West London Assistant Deputy Coroner* [2010] EWHC 3098 (Admin.).

[12] Justice and Security Act 2013 Pt 2.

[13] cf. *R. v Chief Registrar of Friendly Societies Ex p. New Cross Building Society* [1984] Q.B. 227, CA.

[14] See the definition of "relevant civil proceedings" in the Justice and Security Act 2013 s.6(11).

[15] *R. v Ealing Justices Ex p. Weafer* (1982) 74 Cr.App.R. 204; *R. v Tower Bridge Justices Ex p. Osborne* (1989) 88 Cr.App.R. 28, DC (criminal cases).

[16] *R. v McHugh*, above; see Ch.19.

[17] *R. v Secretary of State Ex p. Devine* (1988) 14 N.I.J.B. 10, HC (NI), Carswell J; cf. *R. v Inner North London Coroner Ex p. Chambers, The Times*, April 30, 1983.

[18] *R. v Newcastle upon Tyne Coroner Ex p. A* (1998) 162 J.P. 387, Tucker J; see further, 12–26—12–27.

The Jury

Adjournment after formal opening

Only a minority of cases nowadays require a jury to be summoned for the inquest   **11–07**
hearing.[19] The formal opening of the inquest is not the "inquest hearing",[20] and
therefore, even where a jury is required to be summoned for the inquest hearing,
the coroner sits alone at the formal opening of the inquest, which is then
adjourned to a later date.[21] There may then be pre-inquest hearings,[22] followed in
due course by the inquest hearing itself. The jurors are summoned only for *that*
hearing, at which the evidence is given.

Check on attendance

If a jury has been summoned, the officer checks the attendance of each juror in   **11–08**
waiting. This could be done in open court, but will normally be done in private,
before the court hearing. There is no rule that the names of the jurors must be
made public.[23] There are two problem cases to deal with: those who do not attend
to serve when they should, and those who attend to serve when they should
not.

At common law the coroner had no power to fine an absent juror, and had to   **11–09**
return him to what used to be the assizes or quarter sessions (and is now the Crown
Court)[24] to be punished.[25] But now by statute, where a person duly summoned as
juror at least 14 days before his attendance at an inquest is required fails without
reasonable excuse to attend in accordance with the summons, or attending, refuses
without reasonable excuse to serve as juror, the coroner may impose upon such
person a fine not exceeding £1,000.[26]

Before imposing any penalty upon an absent juror,[27] the coroner should   **11–10**
examine the summoning officer upon oath there and then as a preliminary issue[28]
as to service of the summons, for the coroner cannot properly impose any penalty
upon an absent person, juror or witness, for non-attendance until he has proof of

---

[19] Coroners and Justice Act 2009 s.7(2), (3); see 10–34.

[20] See 10–09.

[21] See 10–10.

[22] See 10–90.

[23] *Re McKerr's Application* Unreported June 2, 1992, HC (NI), Carswell J; *R. v Comerford* [1998] 1 W.L.R. 191, CA (criminal trial).

[24] See 5–126—5–127 above.

[25] 2 Hale P.C. 62; 2 Co. Inst. 136; Bacon's Abr., Tit. "Fine for Contempt" 8; Umfreville, *Lex Coronatoria*, Ch. XV paras 81, 83; contrast the position for absent witnesses; 12–03 ff.

[26] Coroners and Justice Act 2009 s.33 Sch.6 para.5; formerly Act 1988 s.10(1), (4), as amended by the Criminal Justice Act 1991 s.17(3) and Sch.4, Pt I. Such a fine is treated for the purpose of its collection, enforcement or remission as having been imposed by the magistrates' court for the area in which the coroner's court was held: Criminal Justice Act 1988 s.67. The coroner must give particulars of the fine to the clerk of that magistrates' court as soon as practicable after imposition: Criminal Justice Act 1988 s.67. The form of certificate was prescribed by the Coroners Rules 1984 Sch.4 Form 11, now repealed; the current rules are silent on this.

[27] But it is probably better to fine only in those few cases where it appears that the evasion of jury service is wilful and deliberate; otherwise, if there are sufficient jurors without the defaulter, it probably meets the justice of the situation if he is.

[28] For a form of oath, see App.3, Form 10.

that person having been duly summoned to attend.[29] There is no requirement that jurors be offered conduct money before coming to court.[30]

11–11　　As to the other problem, it is an offence, punishable on summary conviction (not before the coroner) by a fine not exceeding level 5 on the standard scale,[31] for a person to serve on a jury at an inquest if he knows he is disqualified from jury service.[32] The coroner may put to a person summoned any questions that appear necessary to establish whether or not the person is qualified to serve as a juror.[33] A person refusing without reasonable excuse to answer any such question, or knowingly or recklessly giving a materially false answer to such a question, commits an offence, and on summary conviction (not before the coroner) is liable to a fine not exceeding level 3 on the standard scale.[34]

11–12　　It is always a risk for the coroner in summoning a jury that there are not enough qualified jurors to hold the inquest hearing. Accordingly, if it appears to the coroner that a jury will be, or probably will be, incomplete, the coroner may require any persons up to the number needed who are in, or in the vicinity of, the place of the inquest hearing to be summoned (without any written notice) for jury service.[35] But the use of the word "incomplete" means that this power cannot be used to summon the whole jury.[36] At least some members must be summoned regularly by written notice.[37]

Personation of a juror

11–13　　It is a common law offence to personate a juror: no corrupt motive or reward is necessary other than the intention to enter the jury box and to take the oath in the name of another.[38] The coroner should report any such offence to the police.

Coroner's power to refuse to swear a person as juror

11–14　　Interested persons attending an inquest have no power to challenge jurors.[39] But the coroner himself is entitled to refuse to swear a particular person as juror if there is a proper objection,[40] such as that the juror is not qualified[41] or that he cannot be seen to clearly impartial, as where he is employed by an interested person,[42] or related to the deceased.[43] An interested person may apply to the coroner to exercise

---

[29] The clerk must then notify the offender of the amount of the fine and the date and place when and where payment must be made, before a warrant of distress or commitment may be issued: Magistrates' Courts Rules 1981 (SI 1981/552) r.46.

[30] As to witnesses, see 12–04—12–05.

[31] Coroners and Justice Act 2009 s.33 Sch.6 para.1(2).

[32] Coroners and Justice Act 2009 s.33 Sch.6 para.1(1).

[33] Coroners and Justice Act 2009 s.8(5).

[34] Coroners and Justice Act 2009 s.33 Sch.6 para.2.

[35] Coroners (Inquests) Rules 2013 (SI 2013/1616) r.30, formerly Coroners Rules 1984 r.48. As to excusals, see 10–48 above.

[36] *R v Solomon* [1958] 1 Q.B. 203.

[37] *R v Merseyside Coroner Ex p Carr* [1974] 1 W.L.R. 578, DC.

[38] *R. v Clark* (1918) 82 J.P. 295.

[39] *Mirror of Justices,* Ch.13 (7 *Selden Society* 30); Fitzherbert and Crompton, *Justices de Peace* (1584) fol.177a.

[40] Umfreville, *Lex Coronatoria,* Ch.XV paras 84–89.

[41] As in *Sir William Withipole's case*(1628) Cro Car 134, where one of the jurors was an outlaw: cf. 10–40 above.

[42] Umfreville, *Lex Coronatoria,* Ch.XV para.87.

[43] Umfreville, *Lex Coronatoria,* Ch.XV para.88.

his power not to swear a particular juror. For this reason, the empanelling of the jury should take place in open court.[44] If the coroner does not take a proper objection, the inquisition will be quashed.[45]

The question of bias has already been discussed in relation to the coroner.[46] The **11–15** same principles apply to the coroner's jury, in cases where there is one.[47] Coroners should therefore have a mechanism for ascertaining whether there is likely to be a problem of possible bias, for example by asking jurors before they are sworn whether they know any of the persons involved in the case (including the deceased), or have an employment or other background which may be significant (e.g. with the Prison Service in the case of a prison death).

On the other hand, coroners ought not to discharge jurors, or refuse to swear **11–16** potential jurors, merely because of an assertion of some fact which might indicate a potential problem. They should inquire into the facts (in the absence of the other jurors) before reaching a decision. The mere fact that a juror comes from the same background as an important witness (or the deceased) is not likely to be decisive. But it may be different where for example there is an acute conflict of evidence on an important point in the case between two witnesses and the juror shares the background of one of them,[48] or where there is a danger of unconscious bias.[49]

Administration of oath

The jurors' oath[50] or affirmation may be administered[51] to and repeated by all the **11–17** jurors simultaneously,[52] or by the jurors in turn. The jury must be sworn "by or before" the coroner to inquire into the death of the deceased and to give a true determination according to the evidence.[53] An oath administered in the absence of the coroner by or before some other person such as a clerk has no effect,[54] but it is common for the jury to be sworn by the coroner's officer in the presence of the coroner.[55]

Once the jury is sworn, the coroner should give them clear instructions for how **11–18** to conduct themselves. This will include warnings[56] to decide the case only on the basis of the evidence, which they should not discuss with anyone else, e.g. family

---

[44] *Re McKerr's Application (No. 2)* Unreported December 21, 1992, HC (NI), Nicholson J.
[45] *Sir William Withipole's case*, above; 1 Hale P.C. 60.
[46] See 5–66 ff.
[47] *R. v East Riding and Kingston-upon-Hull Coroner Ex p. Dawson* [2001] EWHC Admin. 352; [2001] A.C.D. 68, Jackson J.
[48] cf. *Hanif and Khan v United Kingdom*, 20 December 2011, ECtHR.
[49] *R. v Pouladian-Kavi* [2013] EWCA Crim. 158.
[50] The form used to be prescribed by the Coroners Rules 1984 Sch.4 Form 7, now repealed. The form may be modified for a person who wishes to affirm: see the Oaths Act 1978 ss.5, 6, and cf. App.3 Form 15.
[51] The manner is set out in the Oaths Act 1978 s.1, but this may be modified for a person wishing to swear in the Scottish manner: Oaths Act 1978 s.3; and for a person who is neither a Christian nor a Jew, "the oath shall be administered in any lawful manner"; Oaths Act 1978 s.1(3). See in more detail 12–38 ff below.
[52] i.e., all those swearing do so together on one occasion, and all those affirming on another.
[53] Coroners and Justice Act 2009 s.8(3); formerly Coroners Act 1988 s.8(2)(b).
[54] *R. v Ferrand* (1819) 3 B. & Ald. 260; 106 E.R. 659.
[55] Such officer is regarded as a "person duly authorised to administer oaths" within the Oaths Act 1978 s.1(4); cf. *R. v Hallett* (1851) 2 Den. 237.
[56] See the Chief Coroner's Guidance No. 10, *Warnings to Juries*.

or friends, or on social media, and not to carry out independent research on the case, e.g. through use of the internet.[57]

Adjournments requiring dismissal of jury

11–19   After the jurors have been sworn, it would normally be irregular to dismiss them without proceeding with an inquest which is capable of being pursued.[58] However, the coroner has power to discharge the jury where the inquest is adjourned because of potential or actual criminal charges connected with the death,[59] and a duty to discharge the jury where the inquest is adjourned pursuant to the visiting forces provisions.[60]

11–20   Moreover, if the inquest becomes impossible to carry on before the same jury (as where the number of jurors drops below the minimum,[61] or an adjournment is required of such a long period that the jury could not properly be expected to resume the hearing after it,[62] or the jury have compromised their integrity by carrying out private research, contrary to the coroner's direction,[63] such that they cannot be trusted to decide the case solely on the evidence),[64] the coroner will be obliged to discharge the jury and summon a fresh one. It seems that a decision to discharge the jury is not open to review.[65]

Power to discharge individual juror

11–21   Unlike the position in a criminal trial,[66] there is no statutory power to discharge an *individual* juror at a coroner's inquest. However, historically the coroner's jury followed the pattern of the Grand Jury: up to 23 jurors were empanelled, but the votes of only 12 were needed for a verdict.[67] Since it was unlikely that more than 11 of the 23 would drop out along the way, there was no need to provide expressly for a reduced jury to continue.

11–22   The minimum number of jurors is now seven,[68] and therefore the coroner may discharge a juror and continue the inquest, as long as the number of jurors does not fall below that number.[69] For example, it would be proper to discharge a juror who was unwilling to reach any verdict,[70] or who misbehaved, or showed bias.[71] Other proper cases may include illness or other unavoidable absence (particularly where the inquest has overrun its time estimate). In some cases, however, it may be

---

[57] *R. v Thompson* [2010] EWCA Crim. 1623 (not a coroner's case); *R v Mpelenda* [2011] EWCA Crim 1235 (not a coroner's case); Criminal Practice Directions [2013] EWCA Crim 1631, 39 G.3.

[58] *Re Ward* (1861) 3 De G. F. & J. 700.

[59] Coroners and Justice Act 2009 s.11 Sch.1 Pt 1; formerly Coroners Act 1988 s.16(1); see 10–75 ff.

[60] See 10–74 above.

[61] cf. *R. v Merseyside Coroner Ex p Carr* [1974] 1 W.L.R. 578, DC.

[62] cf. *Re Devine and Breslin's Application* [1988] 14 N.I.J.B. 10, HC (NI), Carswell J.

[63] See 11–18.

[64] cf. *R. v McDonnell* [2011] 1 Cr. App. R. 28, CA.

[65] cf. *Winsor v R.* (1866) LR 1 Q.B. 289; *R. v Lewis* (1909) 2 Cr. App. R. 180, CCA (criminal cases).

[66] Criminal Justice Act 1925 s.15; *R. v Hamberry* [1977] Q.B. 924, CA.

[67] See the Coroners Act 1887 s.3(1), (3), as originally enacted.

[68] See 10–40.

[69] *R. v Merseyside Coroner Ex p. Carr* [1994] 1 W.L.R. 578, DC.

[70] *R. v Schot and Barclay* (1997) 161 J.P. 473, CA (criminal trial).

[71] See 10–41.

possible to adjourn the inquest for a limited time so as to deal with a particular juror's absence. It must depend on the facts.

Swearing new juror after existing jury hear evidence

It is improper, and a ground for quashing the inquisition, for another juror to be   **11–23**
sworn and to take part in the proceedings after the existing jury have heard some of the evidence; it makes no difference that the new juror has all the evidence already taken read over to him; nor that there was a sufficient number of jurymen without the one in question.[72]

COMPOSITION OF THE BENCH

The coroner normally sits alone on the bench. But, in circumstances increasingly   **11–24**
rare today, he may be accompanied. This is to be distinguished from the case where the coroner is assisted by counsel to the inquest, discussed below.[73]

Invitation to expert to act as assessor

Where particular expertise will be required even to understand the significance of   **11–25**
the evidence, a coroner might invite an appropriate expert to sit with him as an assessor.[74] However, in that case the coroner must be careful to avoid any suggestion that the decisions or conclusions are being made by such assessor. The assessor may even, under the coroner's control, ask questions within his expertise of an expert witness. But he should not himself give expert evidence.[75] The coroner should not appoint an assessor unless it is clear that the cost will be met by the local authority.[76]

Provision was formerly made by statute for the coroner to sit with an assessor,   **11–26**
appointed by the Secretary of State to assist in holding an inquest on the death of a person occasioned by a railway accident: the person so appointed also made a report to the Secretary of State which was later made public.[77] It should also be noted that the High Court on at least one occasion where an inquisition was quashed suggested that an assessor might sit with the coroner at the subsequent inquest.[78]

Other persons accompanying coroner

If other persons, such as colleagues or visitors,[79] accompany the coroner onto the   **11–27**
bench, they should be careful not to take part in the proceedings, nor to do

---

[72] *R. v Yorkshire Coroner* (1863) 9 L.T. 424, 9 Cox C.C. 373.
[73] See 11–29.
[74] Home Office Circular No. 61 of 1997 para.11.
[75] *R. v Surrey Coroner Ex p. Wright* [1997] Q.B. 786; affirmed CA (1996) 35 B.M.L.R. 57; see also *Owners of the Bow Spring v Owners of the Manzanillo II* [2004] EWCA Civ. 1007.
[76] See 18–40. Coroners Allowances, Fees and Expenses Regulations 2013, SI 2013 No.1615 reg.7 requires the coroner to notify the authority in advance, as it is an unusual expense.
[77] Regulation of Railways Act 1871 s.8, repealed by the Railway Safety (Miscellaneous Provisions) Regulations 1997; see Home Office Circular No. 61 of 1997 para.11.
[78] See, e.g. *R. v Carter* (1876) 34 L.T. 847; 45 L.J.Q.B. 711 (the "Bravo Case"), where the coroner had a legal assessor at the second inquest, provided for out of public funds.
[79] e.g. a new assistant gaining experience, or a county dignitary.

anything to give rise to supposition that they have done so. If government ministers or others not connected with the coroner service are permitted to make public statements from the coroner's bench, even on non-controversial issues,[80] it must inevitably compromise the coroner's judicial independence in the eyes of the public. Accordingly, such activities should be avoided.

Coroner should not seek anonymity

11–28   A coroner should not sit, or attempt to sit, anonymously, shielding his identity from the public.[81] The position of the jury is (or may be) different.[82]

Counsel to the Inquest

11–29   It is not uncommon in complex cases nowadays for the coroner to engage a barrister or solicitor to act as counsel to the inquest, rather like an *amicus curiae*, or counsel to a public inquiry.[83] Rather than sit with the coroner on the bench, such counsel sit in court with the other advocates and make their contributions openly rather than in private.[84] In this way there can be no suggestion that they are usurping the coroner's function, whilst at the same time providing him with the benefit of a disinterested viewpoint.

11–30   It is also common for counsel to the inquest to examine the witnesses on the coroner's behalf, before the other interested persons do so, and this is unobjectionable.[85] The costs of such counsel will be an unusual expense, and so must be reported to the funding local authority, in advance where possible.[86] Their engagement has survived criticism in at least one "controversial" inquest.[87] In the largest cases there may be a team of counsel and solicitors performing this role.[88]

Views

View of the body

11–31   Originally the body lay before the coroner and the jury during the whole inquest, and was itself evidence.[89] Later the requirement was simply that both coroner and jury view the body, otherwise they had no jurisdiction to hold the inquest at all.[90]

---

[80] As happened at the inquests held after the bombing of the Grand Hotel, Brighton, when the chairman of the Conservative Party made a statement paying tribute to those who had died in the explosion: *The Times*, October 16, 1984.

[81] cf. *R. v Felixstowe Justices Ex p. Leigh* [1987] Q.B. 582, DC.

[82] See 11–08 above.

[83] e.g. the *Arms for Iraq* inquiry conducted by Sir Richard Scott, which reported in 1995.

[84] cf. *Clark v Kelly* [2004] 1 A.C. 681, PC.

[85] cf. *R v Derby Coroner Ex p Hart* (2000) 164 J.P. 429 at [120].

[86] Coroners Allowances, Fees and Expenses Regulations 2013 (SI 2013/1615) reg.7; see 18–40.

[87] *Re Devine and Breslin's* Application [1988] 14 N.I.J.B. 10, HC (NI), Carswell J.

[88] e.g. in the inquests into the deaths of Diana, Princess of Wales and Dodi Fayed, and the deaths of the victims of the July 2005 London bombings.

[89] *R. v Ferrand* (1819) 3 B. & Ald. 260.

[90] *R. v Ferrand* (1819) 3 B. & Ald. 260.

The need to view the body was abolished for the jury in 1927[91] and for the coroner only in 1980.[92]

Although there is no legal impediment to viewing the body at a modern inquest   **11–32**
if it is still available, it will normally have been released for disposal by that time, and in practice it never happens. If there is some need for the jury to see the body, it is more common for this to be done by way of photographs. But it should be borne in mind that by introducing photographs into evidence all interested persons will be aware of documents which they are entitled to inspect or have copies of.[93]

View of scene or instruments relating to death

In some cases the coroner (or the jury) may gain an improved understanding of the   **11–33**
facts by actually inspecting, say, the place of finding of a body, or the scene of an accident, or by examining a motor vehicle or other machine that may have been involved in causing a death. The decision whether to make such an inspection is for the coroner alone, although subject, in an appropriate case, to judicial review.[94] The coroner must report to his authority, in advance if possible, any unusual expenses that will be incurred.[95]

So far as view or inspection by himself is concerned, the coroner will probably   **11–34**
meet with no difficulty,[96] but care must be exercised in the case of the jurors. They can undertake a view only after they have been sworn as a jury.[97] They must be kept away from others, (including any witness, lawyer or interested person) while they are viewing and to ensure regularity they should be placed in the care of the coroner's officer. The officer himself should not discuss the matter with them during the view.

Presence of interested persons at view

It is within the discretion of the coroner whether he allows others interested or   **11–35**
their representatives to be present with the jury at a view.[98] In one old case specifically dealing with inquests, it was said that the coroner himself should not normally be present.[99] But more recent cases (involving criminal prosecutions) have restated the need for the judge to be present to control procedure, particularly where witnesses are to be present as well.[100] The preferable course is for the coroner to attend. In that case, of course, the coroner should not discuss the case with the jury, except after appropriate discussion with the interested persons or

---

[91] Coroners (Amendment) Act 1926 s.14(1).
[92] Coroners Act 1980 s.1(b); later Coroners Act 1988 s.11(1) (not replicated in 2009 Act). After 1926 the jury had a right to see the body if a majority of them so desired, or a duty to do so if the coroner so directed (Coroners (Amendment) Act 1926 s.14(1)), but this provision was repealed in 1980 (Coroners Act 1980 Sch.2).
[93] See 7–25. As to publication of such photographs by interested persons, see 7–29.
[94] On which see Ch.19 below. The proposition in the text was approved by Carswell J in *Re Devine and Breslin's Application* [1988] 14 N.I.J.B. 10, HC (NI).
[95] Coroners Allowances, Fees and Expenses Regulations 2013 (SI 2013/1615) reg.7; see 18–40.
[96] cf. *Salsbury v Woodland* [1970] 1 Q.B. 324, CA (view by judge alone in civil action held to be in order) with *Parry v Boyle* (1986) 83 Cr.App.R. 310, DC (held undesirable for lay magistrates to view scene without the parties present).
[97] *R. v Divine Ex p. Walton* [1930] 2 K.B. 29.
[98] *R. v Divine Ex p. Walton* [1930] 2 K.B. 29.
[99] *R. v Divine Ex p. Walton* [1930] 2 K.B. 29.
[100] *Tameshwar v R.* [1957] A.C. 476, PC; *R. v Hunter* [1985] 1 W.L.R. 613, CA.

their representatives (e.g. to point out something which otherwise they might miss).

Adjournment of Inquest

11–36   In some cases the coroner is obliged to suspend an investigation.[101] He also has a *power* to suspend one if it appears to him to be appropriate to do so.[102] If he does suspend an investigation, he will also have to adjourn any inquest that has been opened as part of that investigation, and provide the registrar of deaths with the particulars required to register the death.[103] But there will be other cases, where the coroner has not suspended the investigation, but has opened an inquest. In such cases, a coroner may adjourn an inquest if he is of the opinion that it is reasonable to do so.[104] The High Court will not interfere with the decision unless it is clear that the coroner has misdirected himself or his decision is unreasonable.[105]

11–37   If the coroner does adjourn, he must as soon as practicable inform the next of kin or personal representative[106] and any other interested persons[107] who have made themselves known to him of (i) the decision to adjourn, (ii) the date of and the reason for the decision,[108] and (iii) the date, time and place for the resumption.[109]

11–38   Thus the coroner may open an inquest and take evidence of identification, issue the order for disposal of the body and adjourn until a suitable date (or to a date to be fixed) or to a more convenient place.[110] At the resumed inquest hearing, the coroner will adjourn from time to time during the day as necessary, and, where it exceeds one day, from day to day. In addition, the power to adjourn should be exercised if it becomes apparent during the hearing that there is a gap in the evidence, in order to enable the relevant evidence to be obtained.[111] In some cases it may be desirable to adjourn so as to hear a number of aspects of a case together.[112]

11–39   On the other hand, refusals to exercise the power to adjourn have been upheld.[113] Indeed, excessive exercise of the power to adjourn may in some cases amount to an irregularity justifying quashing the verdict,[114] and the length of the

---

[101] See 10–73 ff, 11–47 ff.
[102] Coroners and Justice Act 2009 s.11 Sch.1 para.5; see 8–18.
[103] Coroners (Investigations) Regulations 2013 (SI 2013/1629) reg.8. See 8–18.
[104] Coroners (Inquests) Rules 2013 (SI 2013/1616) r.25(1).
[105] *Re Doyle's Application* Unreported April 18, 2005, Sullivan J; see also *R. (Butler) v Black Country District Coroner* [2010] EWHC 43 (Admin.) at [80].
[106] For these expressions see 8–29 ff.
[107] For this expression see 8–21 ff.
[108] Coroners (Inquests) Rules 2013 (SI 2013/1616) r.25(2).
[109] Coroners (Inquests) Rules 2013 (SI 2013/1616) r.25(3).
[110] See 10–09 ff above.
[111] *R. v Southwark Coroner Ex p. Hicks* [1987] 1 W.L.R. 1624, DC; *R. v Lincoln Coroner Ex p. Hay* [2000] Lloyd's Rep. Med. 264, DC; *Nicholls v Liverpool Coroner* Unreported November 8, 2001, Sullivan J.
[112] *Re Jordan's Application* Unreported March 8, 2002, HC (NI), Kerr J.
[113] *R. (Cairns) v Inner West London Deputy Coroner* [2012] EWHC 2890 (Admin.).
[114] *Re Devine and Breslin's Application* [1988] 14 N.I.J.B. 10, HC (NI).

adjournment between opening and resuming an inquest has sometimes been criticised.[115]

A particular problem concerns the question of adjournment for the purpose of **11–40** seeking judicial review of some interlocutory decision. A coroner faced with an application for such an adjournment may feel that it is fairer to adjourn than not to.[116] But, certainly where a jury is concerned, and evidence has already been heard, it is usually better to proceed to a conclusion.[117] In that way, the High Court on a judicial review application will have the benefit of knowing the whole of the evidence, the coroner's summing up, and the jury's verdict.[118] The court will be better able to judge what difference any error of law might have made.[119]

If the inquest is interrupted, the jury are left in the difficult position of having **11–41** to pick up the threads again weeks or months later,[120] and the reviewing court must be very careful in what it says about the facts for fear of prejudicing the decision.[121] But even in a non-jury case it is not desirable to adjourn merely because a point of law arises which, if decided a particular way, might save time or expense.[122] Not uncommonly, the result of taking a "preliminary issue" approach is the opposite of that intended.[123] Accordingly, challenges at an interlocutory stage should not normally be entertained by the High Court.[124]

Interim certificate

Where a coroner has begun, but not yet completed or discontinued, an **11–42** investigation, he may—but is not obliged to—issue an interim certificate of the fact of death[125] if asked to do so by the next of kin or personal representative of the deceased[126] (registration of death not being possible until the conclusion of the investigation, including any inquest). The form of the certificate is prescribed.[127] Unlike under the former rules, this certificate can now be issued even when there has not been an adjournment. Strictly, there is no obligation to provide more than one such certificate, though it is common for the coroner to be asked to provide multiple copies.

---

[115] *R. v South Glamorgan Coroner Ex p. BP Chemicals Ltd* (1987) 151 J.P. 799 (three years).

[116] *R. (Khan) v West Hertfordshire Coroner* [2002] EWHC 302 (Admin.) at [3].

[117] *Re applications by Officers C, D, H and R* [2012] NICA 47; *R. (Cooper) v North East Kent Coroner* [2004] EWHC 586 (Admin.). See also *Re McDonnell's Application* [2014] NIQB 66.

[118] *Re applications by Officers C, D, H and R* [2012] NICA 47; *R. (Khan) v West Hertfordshire Coroner* [2002] EWHC 302 (Admin.) at [3].

[119] *R. (Khan) v West Hertfordshire Coroner* [2002] EWHC 302 (Admin.) at [3]. cf. *R. v West Yorkshire Coroner Ex p. National Union of Mineworkers (Yorkshire Area)* (1985) 150 J.P. 58, DC; *R. v St Pancras Coroners' Court Ex p. Higgins* (1988) 152 J.P. 637, DC; and see 11–65 ff, 19–64.

[120] cf. *Re Devine and Breslin's Application* [1988] 14 N.I.J.B. 10, HC (NI), Carswell J.

[121] *R. v Inner North London Coroner Ex p. Diesa Koto* (1993) 157 J.P. 857, DC.

[122] *R. v East Kent Coroner Ex p. Spooner* (1987) 152 J.P. 115, DC; *R. v Inner North London Coroner Ex p. Diesa Koto* (1993) 157 J.P. 857, DC.

[123] See, e.g. *Tilling v Whiteman* [1980] A.C. 1 at 17, 25 (not a coroner's case).

[124] *Re applications by Officers C, D, H and R* [2012] N.I.C.A. 47; *R. (Cooper) v North East Kent Coroner* [2004] EWHC 586 (Admin.) at [17].

[125] Coroners (Investigations) Regulations 2013 (SI 2013/1629) reg.9(1); formerly Coroners Rules 1984 r.30. As to whether this may pre-empt the decision of the inquest in the future, see *R. (Coker) v Inner South London Coroner* [2006] EWHC 614 (Admin.) at [31]–[32].

[126] As to this expression, see 8–29 ff.

[127] Coroners (Investigations) Regulations 2013 (SI 2013/1629) reg.9(2) Sch. Form 1; formerly Coroners Rules 1984 Sch.4 Form 14. See App.2.

Formal process

11–43   Formerly, it was provided that every adjournment had to be made in a formal manner,[128] but this rule has now gone, being considered unnecessary. In practice, the coroner will still announce at the hearing that the inquest is adjourned, whether to a particular date and time, or to a date and time to be fixed.

Compulsory adjournment

11–44   In some cases the coroner is obliged to adjourn the inquest. These cases were dealt with above.[129] Here we deal with two further cases, one of which formerly involved compulsory adjournment, but which no longer does so.

11–45   **Persons whose conduct is called into question.** Under the old rules, if the conduct of any person was called into question at an inquest on grounds which the coroner thought substantial, and the criticism was relevant to the matters to be inquired into at the inquest, then unless such person had previously been given notice of the inquest, the coroner had to adjourn the inquest so as to enable that person to attend if he so desires.[130]

11–46   This provision has not been replicated in the new rules, because in most cases the person concerned will have been summoned as a witness or otherwise given notice of the inquest as an interested person.[131] In exceptional cases, however, the conduct of a person will be criticised unexpectedly and the coroner will then have to decide whether or not to adjourn under the power conferred for this purpose.[132] The coroner must not adjourn merely because criticism has been levelled. He has to consider whether the interests of justice demand an adjournment.

11–47   **Coroner's consideration of pending charges.** The coroner must adjourn the inquest and notify the DPP if it appears to the coroner during the course of the inquest itself that the death is likely to have been due to a homicide offence[133] and that a person may be charged in relation to that offence.[134]

11–48   According to the Home Office, the purpose of adjournment is not to prevent proper enquiry being made, but to ensure that as little prejudice as possible attaches to any person suspected of involvement in the death and that the coroner's proceedings remain neutral and do not become accusatorial.[135]

11–49   Clearly it will be difficult for the coroner to know when the duty to adjourn arises: he must obviously hear enough evidence to know that a reference to the DPP is justified (with all the prejudicial connotations that that implies), yet not so

---

[128] Coroners Rules 1984 r.16.

[129] See 10–73 ff above.

[130] Coroners Rules 1984 r.25. See e.g. *Dowler v North London Coroner* [2009] EWHC 3300 (Admin.).

[131] See 10–22.

[132] See 11–36.

[133] See 10–75.

[134] Coroners (Inquests) Rules 2013 (SI 2013/1616) r.25(4); formerly Coroners Rules 1984 r.28(1). This is a duty, and not a power, to adjourn: see, e.g. *Re Leslie Hoggett, The Independent,* December 20, 1986 (Isle of Wight coroner). See also *Attorney General v Maksimovich* [1985] 4 N.S.W.L.R. 300, CA (NSW).

[135] Home Office Circular No. 187 of 1977, App.C para.8.

much evidence as will unfairly prejudice any suspected person. Thus the Home Office suggested that, once the coroner is aware that the inquest if continued is likely to lead to a serious suggestion of guilt against an individual, the duty to adjourn and refer the matter should be engaged, the decision so to do being announced in open court.[136]

An example of this would be where, although it is clear that death was due to **11–50** homicide, no sufficient evidence to charge a person emerges until part of the way through the inquest: at that point the inquest should be adjourned. Similarly where a death is not thought to be due to homicide when the inquest opens, but evidence subsequently is given which not only suggests that it was homicide but also who was responsible: for instance, where the death involved two persons only and was either misadventure or homicide,[137] and evidence is given suggesting homicide, the inquest should be adjourned.[138]

Where the person who is or would be implicated in the death if the inquest **11–51** continued is himself dead, there is clearly no point in adjourning the inquest to refer the case to the DPP or CPS.[139] The view of the Working Party on the Coroners Rules[140] (disagreeing with the Brodrick Committee)[141] was that in such cases the coroner must balance the reputation of the dead against the possibility of unjust suspicion against other living persons and it may be better for the coroner to indicate that police enquiries into the death have ceased because a person whom they wanted to question is also dead; the Home Office takes the same view.[142]

Formerly it was expressly provided that, if criminal proceedings were instituted **11–52** arising out of the death of the deceased, and the circumstances did not fall within any of the cases set out above where it was obligatory to adjourn the inquest (e.g. they were summary proceedings only),[143] the inquest should not be adjourned solely by reason of the institution of such proceedings.[144] Furthermore, it was held that any such proceedings should not normally be heard or determined until the inquest was concluded, in order to prevent or lessen the risk of two tribunals coming to inconsistent results in relation to the same set of facts.[145] But this was not an absolute rule of law.[146]

The express rule has now gone. There is now provision that the coroner need **11–53** not suspend an investigation (and therefore adjourn any inquest) in certain circumstances, notably when prosecuting authorities bringing criminal charges have no objection to the investigation continuing, or the coroner thinks there is exceptional reason for not suspending the investigation.[147] This makes the same point obliquely. Where the compulsory grounds of suspension or adjournment do

---

[136] Home Office Circular No. 187 of 1977, App.C para.9.
[137] cf. *R. v Durham Coroner Ex p. Attorney-General*, *The Times*, June 29, 1978, DC.
[138] Home Office Circular No. 187 of 1977, App.C para.10.
[139] See, 11–47 above.
[140] Home Office Circular No. 187 of 1977, App.C para.10.
[141] Brodrick Report para.16–24.
[142] Home Office Circular No. 187 of 1977, App.C para.11.
[143] *Smith v DPP* [2000] R.T.R. 36, DC.
[144] Coroners Rules 1984 r.32.
[145] *Re Beresford* (1952) 36 Cr.App.R. 1, per Devlin J; *Smith v DPP* [2000] R.T.R. 36, DC; see also *Sylvester v DPP* Unreported May 21, 2001, DC.
[146] *Smith v DPP* [2000] R.T.R. 36, DC.
[147] Coroners and Justice Act 2009 s.11 Sch.1 para.2(6); see 10–79.

not apply, there is no presumption in favour of suspension or adjournment merely because other criminal proceedings have been instituted. The coroner has a discretion, to be exercised judicially. The risk of inconsistency between two tribunals remains, and must be resolved on a sensible basis.

11–54   The problem for prosecuting authorities was that, if they successfully prosecuted for a non-homicide offence, and thereafter the inquest resulted in an unlawful killing conclusion, a manslaughter conviction might not be possible to obtain, because of the principle of double jeopardy.[148] So they tended to wait until after the inquest was over, which made it more difficult for the coroner to conduct his inquiry. The privilege against self-incrimination recognised, but did not entirely protect against, the risk of prejudice to a witness at risk of prosecution by an authority which used the inquest process to gather further material. But some prosecuting authorities, such as the Health and Safety Executive, have in recent years changed their approach, and in cases where an unlawful killing conclusion is regarded as of minimal likelihood a prosecution may now take place before the inquest.[149]

Power to require recognisances

11–55   The coroner has power at common law, on the adjournment of an inquest, to require the witnesses and jurors to enter into oral undertakings, called recognisances, to forfeit a stated sum of money to the Crown if they fail to attend at the adjourned time and place.[150] They are almost never required in practice nowadays.[151] If any is, a note of it should be made on the notes of evidence made by the coroner.

11–56   A recognisance will automatically become void if the witness or juror is notified that the inquest will not be resumed, or if the witness is notified that his attendance at the resumed inquest is not required.[152] If the witness or juror has not been so notified, and fails to attend on the resumed inquest, the recognisance is forfeited, and the coroner should proceed as if he had imposed a fine for failure to appear.[153]

Inquest not resumed

11–57   The old cases held that if an inquest adjourned to a stated date was not resumed on that date, it would simply come to an end, and any inquisition resulting from what

---

[148] *R. v Beedie* [1998] Q.B. 356, CA (HSE prosecution). The rules on double jeopardy have since been modified, by the Coroners and Justice Act 2009, Pt 10.

[149] See e.g. the *HSE Enforcement Guide*, Coroners' Inquests, paras 24–36, at *http://www.hse.gov.uk/enforce/enforcementguide/index.htm* [Accessed June 10, 2014].

[150] See the first edition of this work (1829), at 293, 398. There was no express rule to this effect (though the power was recognised by Coroners Rules 1984 r.34); the form was formerly prescribed by the Coroners Rules 1984 Sch.4 Form 12.

[151] Jurors are now summoned to appear on a specific date "as a juror . . . until [they] are no longer needed": Coroners (Inquests) Rules 2013 (SI 24013/1616) r.29(1) Sch. Form 1.

[152] This was so stated by Coroners Rules 1984 r.34 (repealed), but the form of the recognisance itself so provides.

[153] Criminal Justice Act 1988 s.67(2); see Coroners Rules 1984 Sch.4 Form 19 (now repealed); 12–03 ff.

purported to be a resumption at a later date would be quashed,[154] as being taken before a person who no longer had judicial authority in respect of that case.[155] It must be doubted that this represents the modern law. A coroner must be allowed after adjournment to change the date of resumption without the necessity of holding a formal court to do so, provided at least that he complies with the rules on notifying third parties of the change of date of resumption.[156]

REPRESENTATION AND ADVOCACY

An interested person may wish to be represented at the inquest by someone to speak for him or her and ask questions on his or her behalf. The rules on rights of audience in court have changed significantly in recent years, becoming more complex in the process. In relation to such rights, the previous system of "authorised advocates"[157] has been replaced by a new system of "authorised" and "exempt" persons.[158] In broad terms, legal professionals such as barristers and solicitors will be authorised persons, and parties to proceedings will be exempt persons.[159] A right of audience for this purpose includes the rights to appear before and to address a court, and to call witnesses and examine them.[160]   **11–58**

The new scheme is not quite apt for coroners' inquests, where only the coroner has the right to call witnesses,[161] and there are no parties, only "interested persons".[162] Moreover, express provision for advocacy is made by the rules. Any interested person[163] who so requests is entitled to examine witnesses at an inquest, either in person or by a "representative" (not defined).[164] The old rule restricted advocacy (if not carried out by the individual) to "authorised advocates";[165] the current rule does not. But it has always been possible for the coroner in a particular case to permit an unqualified person to represent a person entitled to examine witnesses, under the common law principle that the courts may give the right of audience to whomever they think appropriate.[166]   **11–59**

---

[154] *R. v Payn* (1864) 34 L.J.QB 59; 11 L.T. 488 (sub nom. *R. v Dover Coroner*); *R. v Margate Coroner* (1865) 10 Cox C.C. 64; 11 L.T. 707.

[155] This is usually described by the Latin phrase "*coram non judice*".

[156] See 10–22.

[157] Within the Courts and Legal Services Act 1990 s.119(1), i.e. a person with a right of audience granted by an authorised body. This included a barrister or solicitor, or a Fellow of the Institute of Legal Executives who had obtained the right of audience: see the Institute of Legal Executives Order 1998 (SI 1998/1077); and also a registered European lawyer: European Communities (Lawyers' Practice) Regulations 2000 (SI 2000/1119) reg.11.

[158] Legal Services Act 2007 ss.18 (authorised persons), 19 (exempt persons).

[159] Under the previous regime it was held that parties could not delegate their personal right of audience to others who were otherwise unqualified, even by power of attorney: *Gregory v Turner* [2003] 1 W.L.R .1149, CA.

[160] Legal Services Act 2007 s.12 Sch.2 para.3(1).

[161] See 10–25.

[162] See 8–21.

[163] See 8–22.

[164] Coroners (Inquests) Rules 2013 (SI 2013/1616) r.19(1); formerly Coroners Rules 1984 r.20(1). This means an authorised advocate.

[165] See 11–58.

[166] See *Abse v Smith* [1986] Q.B. 322, CA; *D v S (Rights of Audience)* [1997] 1 F.L.R. 724, CA; *Clarkson v Gilbert* [2000] 2 F.L.R. 839, CA; *Francis v Barton Bridging Capital Ltd* [2010] EWHC 1525 (Ch).

11–60   Thus the new rule does not confer a right of audience on an otherwise unqualified representative; it merely formalises the existing position. Since the coroner is the master of his own procedure,[167] in an appropriate case he may properly refuse to hear someone who is not an authorised or exempt person.[168] Under the old regime it was held not a breach of the Human Rights Act 1998 so to refuse.[169] In any event, a person entitled to address the court or examine witnesses can, of course, be accompanied by a friend or other person to take notes and quietly advise him, a so-called "McKenzie friend".[170]

11–61   In a case where art.2 of the European Convention on Human Rights is engaged,[171] the absence of legal representation for the family at the inquest may result in a breach of that article.[172] In such cases coroners should therefore encourage the family to obtain representation. Subject to that, however, there is no duty upon the coroner to advise interested persons of their rights to be legally represented and to examine witnesses.[173] Unfortunately not all families are a cohesive single entity. Sometimes different members of the family take different stances.[174] In such cases the coroner should pay close attention to the wording of the rules.

Examination by police and others

11–62   Formerly, where the police took part in an inquest in an official capacity, they had to be represented by an authorised advocate. If a police officer was personally concerned in the inquest, however, he was to be treated like any other properly interested person and allowed to examine witnesses in person (unless he himself wished to be represented by an authorised advocate).[175] But it is no longer necessary for the police to be represented only by an authorised advocate.

11–63   The definition of "interested person" is wide enough to include *persons appointed by*, or *representatives of* an "enforcing authority",[176] and (in the case of deaths which may have been caused by injuries in the course of employment or industrial disease) *a representative of* a trade union of which the deceased was a member at the time of death. This puts such persons or representatives in a privileged position, as

---

[167] See *R v North Humberside Coroner, ex p. Jamieson* [1995] QB 1, 26 (14).

[168] *R. (Chaudhari) v Walthamstow Coroner's Court* Unreported March 26, 2002, Sedley LJ.

[169] *Re Chaudhari's Application* Unreported September 10, 2001, Elias J; see also *Francis v Barton Bridging Capital Ltd* [2010] EWHC 1525 (Ch).

[170] *McKenzie v McKenzie* [1971] P. 33, CA; *R. v Leicester Justices Ex p. Barrow* [1991] Q.B. 260, CA; *R. v Bow County Court Ex p. Pelling* [1999] 3 All E.R. 751, CA. See also *Practice Guidance: McKenzie Friends: Civil, Family Courts* [2010] 1 W.L.R. 1881.

[171] See 21–15 ff.

[172] *R. (Wright) v Home Secretary* [2001] U.K.H.R.R. 1399 at [60].

[173] *R. v Central Cleveland Coroner Ex p. Dent* (1986) 150 J.P. 251; *R. v North London Coroner Ex p. Lewy* Unreported July 31, 1995, CA; see also *Maksimovich v Attorney General* [1985] 4 N.S.W.L.R. 318, CA (NSW), and *Re Price's Application* (1986) 15 N.I.J.B. 84, CA (NI).

[174] See, e.g. *R. v South London Coroner Ex p. Driscoll* (1993) 159 J.P. 45, DC.

[175] Coroners Rules 1984 r.20(1), proviso (a). For examples, see *R. v Inner North London Coroner Ex p. GLC and others*, The Times, April 30, 1993, Woolf J, and *R. v Derby Coroner Ex p. Hart* (2000) 164 J.P. 429. As to "authorised advocate", see 11–58.

[176] This expression has the meaning given by the Health and Safety at Work etc Act 1974 s.18(7), i.e. the Health and Safety Executive or any other authority which is made responsible for the enforcement of any provisions of the 1974 Act.

interested persons are themselves given the right personally to speak at and ask questions of witnesses at an inquest.[177]

Power of coroner to disallow questions

The right of an interested person to ask questions is subject to the duty of the **11–64** coroner to disallow any question put to the witness which he considers irrelevant.[178] This would include questions which go to matters falling outside the scope of the inquest,[179] questions which are oppressive or unnecessarily intrusive,[180] or which are asked, not for the purposes of the inquest, but for some purpose collateral to it.[181]

APPLICATION BY INTERESTED PERSONS

In addition to the matters which have already been referred to, the coroner must **11–65** be ready to consider any applications or other matters which interested persons wish to raise during the course of the inquest. Assuming that the person concerned has a sufficient interest in the subject-matter of the application,[182] it is the duty of the coroner to deal judicially[183] and (normally) in open court, with all such applications as may be made to him during the inquest.[184]

These might include applications by a potential witness to be called or by an **11–66** interested person for the coroner to call a particular person as a witness,[185] applications for documents to be produced at the hearing[186] and applications to order a view (e.g. of the place of death)[187] or to adjourn the inquest. A refusal to hear legal submissions is a breach of natural justice and may give grounds for quashing the inquisition.[188] No one has the right, in the guise of making an application, to address the court as to the facts.[189] But that does not prevent appropriate reference being made to the evidence given or to be given, so far as that is necessary for the purposes of the application.

In other contexts, where a tribunal or other body makes a decision affecting the **11–67** rights or obligations of persons before it, the tribunal must give reasons for its

---

[177] See 12–58, 12–106.
[178] Coroners (Inquests) Rules 2013 (SI 2013/1616) r.19(2); formerly Coroners Rules 1984 r.20(1), proviso (b).
[179] See Ch.6.
[180] See 12–63, 12–66 below.
[181] Coroners (Inquests) Rules 2013 (SI 2013/1616) r.19(2); formerly Coroners Rules 1984 r.20(1), proviso (b).
[182] As to which see 19–37 ff in the context of judicial review, and paras 8–21 ff above as to who is an "interested person".
[183] Particularly keeping in mind the rules of natural justice: see *Annetts v McCann* (1990) 65 A.L.J.R. 167, HC (Aus).
[184] As to applications made before the inquest hearing, see 10–90.
[185] See 10–25 above.
[186] *R. v Southwark Coroner Ex p. Hicks* [1987] 1 W.L.R. 1624, CA.
[187] See 11–31 ff above.
[188] *R. v East Berkshire Coroner Ex p. Buckley* (1992) 157 J.P. 425, DC.
[189] Coroners (Inquests) Rules 2013 (SI 2013/1616) r.27; formerly Coroners Rules 1984 r.42. But, in Australia, see *Annetts v McCann* (1990) 170 CLR 596, HC (Aus), and *R. v Tennent Ex p. Jager* [2000] TASSC 64.

decisions.[190] Indeed, the European Court of Human Rights has interpreted art.6 of the European Convention as imposing a duty to give reasons,[191] but art.6 does not normally apply to an inquest, because it does not determine anyone's rights or obligations.[192]

11–68   At common law there was no legal requirement that coroners give reasons for their decisions.[193] Nonetheless it is usually desirable to do so,[194] sometimes (in complex cases) in writing. And, in cases where art.2 of the ECHR is engaged, it has been held that there is an obligation on a coroner to give reasons for his decision as to what verdicts they were prepared to leave to juries.[195] In such cases the High Court might well remit the case to the coroner for reasons to be given, rather than simply quash the decision for giving none.[196]

11–69   An interested person who fails in an application to the coroner may seek an adjournment of the inquest in order to apply for judicial review of the coroner's decision. But it is not normally appropriate to adjourn at that stage and interrupt the flow of the inquest.[197] The question of such an adjournment has already been dealt with.[198]

REPORTING RESTRICTIONS

11–70   As a general rule, the media are not entitled to any more (or any less) information about legal proceedings or a public inquiry than are the public generally.[199] But any court has power at common law to accede to the request of a journalist to see written documents supplied to the court for the purposes of proceedings and referred to publicly (but not read out) in court. Where there are good reasons for such access to be provided (e.g. to enable the journalist to understand the arguments being made) and there is neither risk of harm to any party nor great burden placed on the court, the request should be granted.[200]

---

[190] e.g. *R. v Knightsbridge Crown Court Ex p. International Sporting Club* [1982] Q.B. 364; *R. v Lambeth LBC Ex p. Walters* (1993) 26 H.L.R. 170; *Flannery v Halifax Estate Agencies Ltd, The Independent,* February 26, 1999, CA; *Gupta v General Medical Council, The Times,* January 9, 2002, PC; *R. (Wooder) v Feggetter, The Independent,* May 3, 2002; *The Times,* May 28, 2002, CA; *English v Emery Reinbold & Strick Ltd* [2002] 1 W.L.R. 2409, CA; *Burns v Royal Mail Group plc (No. 2), The Times,* June 24, 2004, EAT; *R. (T) v Legal Aid Agency* [2013] EWHC 960 (Admin.).

[191] See 21–22 ff below.

[192] See 21–22 below.

[193] Nor does an absence of reasons justify the inference that there are none: *R. (Farrakhan) v Home Secretary* Unreported April 30, 2002, CA at [7].

[194] *R. (Cooper) v North East Kent Coroner* [2004] EWHC 586 (Admin.) at [20]–[21].

[195] *R. (Stanley) v Inner North London Coroner* [2003] EWHC 1180 (Admin.). See also *R. (Kent CC) v Kent Coroner* [2012] EWHC 2768 (Admin.), where art.2 was held not to be engaged, but the High Court held that "the coroner's reasons could have been fuller" (at [33]).

[196] *Re B (A Child)* Unreported May 20, 2003, CA.

[197] *Re applications by Officers C, D, H and R* [2012] N.I.C.A. 47; *R. (Cooper) v North East Kent Coroner* [2004] EWHC 586 (Admin.).

[198] See 11–40—11–41 above.

[199] Decision of Dame Janet Smith, Chairman, *The Shipman Inquiry,* October 25, 2001 para.52 (available at http://webarchive.nationalarchives.gov.uk/20090808154959/http://www.the-shipman-inquiry.org.uk/reports.asp).

[200] *R. (Guardian News and Media) v Westminster Magistrates* [2012] EWCA Civ. 420.

Anyone may take a note of court or inquiry proceedings except where there are **11–71** specific prohibitions by law, or the interests of justice so require.[201] Article 10 of the European Convention on Human Rights[202] protects freedom of expression, but it does not support a right (without consent) to film or record proceedings,[203] and art.6 (supporting public hearings) does not in terms apply to an inquiry (such as an inquest) which does not determine civil rights and obligations.[204] But where a matter is not given in evidence at all (e.g. as where persons involved in the facts, not being witnesses, are referred to by initials rather than by name), there is generally no need to consider reporting restrictions, for it will not be harmful to report that which has been given in evidence.

Even where a coroner's inquest is held (as it normally is) in public,[205] and **11–72** evidence is therefore given in public, there are occasions on which it is undesirable for evidence to be reported and published in the media. In such cases, it may be found that a request to the media not to publish some fact is observed if the request be made for a good cause. But the courts have no power at common law to restrain the publication of a report of proceedings conducted in open court, even though such publication, in prejudicing the administration of justice, might give rise to proceedings for contempt of court.[206] It is unwise for a coroner to discuss with the media, privately or "off the record", any aspect of inquest proceedings before him.[207]

Two statutory restrictions on publication arise from the law relating to contempt **11–73** of court. First, in any legal proceedings held in public (such as an inquest hearing) the court may, where it appears to be necessary for avoiding a substantial risk of prejudice to the administration of justice in those proceedings, or in any other proceedings pending or imminent, order that the publication of any report of the proceedings, or any part of the proceedings, be postponed for such period as the court thinks necessary for that purpose.[208]

Second, a court having power to allow a name or other matter to be withheld **11–74** from the public in proceedings before the court (as the coroner may do, in a proper case, by permitting a witness or other matter to remain anonymous)[209] may by

---

[201] Decision of Dame Janet Smith, Chairman, *The Shipman Inquiry*, October 25, 2001 para.61 (available at *http://webarchive.nationalarchives.gov.uk/20090808154959/http://www.the-shipman-inquiry.org.uk/reports.asp*).

[202] See below 21–42.

[203] Decision of Dame Janet Smith, above, Chairman, *The Shipman Inquiry*, October 25, 2001 para.60 (available at *http://webarchive.nationalarchives.gov.uk/20090808154959/http://www.the-shipman-inquiry.org.uk/reports.asp*) following *Leander v Sweden* (1987) 9 E.H.R.R. 433 para.74. See also para.10 of the ruling dated August 5, 2003 of Lord Hutton (available at *http://www.the-hutton-inquiry.org.uk* [Accessed June 10, 2014]) in the context of his Inquiry into the death of Dr David Kelly, agreeing with the decision of Dame Janet Smith. As to making sound recordings of inquest proceedings, see 11–85 ff.

[204] Decision of Dame Janet Smith, above, Chairman, *The Shipman Inquiry*, October 25, 2001 para.40 (available at *http://webarchive.nationalarchives.gov.uk/20090808154959/http://www.the-shipman-inquiry.org.uk/reports.asp*); see 21–22 below.

[205] See 11–04.

[206] *Independent Publishing Co Ltd v Attorney General of Trinidad and Tobago* [2004] UKPC 26; [2005] 1 A.C. 190.

[207] *R. v Inner West London Coroner Ex p. Dallaglio* [1994] 4 All E.R. 139, CA.

[208] Contempt of Court Act 1981 s.4(2). See *McLuckie v Coroner for Northern Ireland* [2011] N.I.C.A. 34 (coroner's refusal to make an order quashed).

[209] See 12–23.

direction prohibit publication of the name of the witness so far as is necessary for the purpose for which it was withheld.[210] This will allow the coroner in an appropriate case to prohibit the publication of details identifying the witness.

11-75   In addition, by separate statutory provision, the court has power to prohibit the publication of the name, address or school of any child or young person who is a witness and of any particulars calculated to lead to their identification.[211] In deciding whether to exercise the power under the coroner must weigh the interest in the full reporting of the events concerned against the need to protect the children involved from further harm.[212]

11-76   If the child concerned is not a witness, the matter is more complicated. Before the Human Rights Act 1998, where the local authority was concerned that the child should be protected from being identified at the inquest, it could apply to the High Court for the child to be warded, so that (if the order was made) that court would have jurisdiction to grant an injunction restraining the media from publishing details of the child calculated to lead to his identification as being involved in the events leading to the inquest.[213]

11-77   Since the Human Rights Act, the High Court now also has power to protect the art.8 rights of the child in freestanding proceedings, whether in relation to pending criminal proceedings[214] or indeed an inquest.[215] But the court must balance the art.8 rights against the art.10 rights of the media. An intense focus on the comparative importance of the specific rights being claimed in the individual cases is necessary before the ultimate balancing test in terms of proportionality is carried out.[216]

Defamation and privilege

11-78   So far as the law of libel is concerned, absolute[217] privilege attaches to fair and accurate reports of public proceedings in (amongst others) "any court in the United Kingdom".[218] The statutory privilege was extended to publication by broadcasting stations (including cable and satellite services) within the United Kingdom.[219] By contrast, there is no such privilege for reports of proceedings held

---

[210] Contempt of Court Act 1981 s.11; *R v Westminster City Council Ex p P* (1998) 31 H.L.R. 154, 161-163. This power is only exercisable, however, if such facts and matters are indeed withheld: *R. v Arundel Magistrates Ex p. Westminster Press Ltd* [1985] 1 W.L.R. 708, DC. cf. *R. v South Powys Coroner's Court Ex p. Jones* [1991] C.O.D. 14, DC (submissions in absence of jury on privilege against self-incrimination report in local press); *Birmingham Post and Mail Ltd v Birmingham City Council, The Times,* November 25, 1993, DC.

[211] Children and Young Persons Act 1933 s.39; *Re S (FC) (A Child)(Appellant)* [2004] UKHL 47 at [7]; for examples in coroners' courts, see, e.g. *Re Joseph Stickland* (1987) 131 S.J. 856; *Re Charlotte Whitby, The Times,* August 13, 1992; *Re Odette Coulson, The Daily Telegraph,* September 28, 2001.

[212] *R. v Central Criminal Court Ex p. Godwin and Crook* [1995] 1 W.L.R. 139, CA.

[213] The Court of Appeal made such an order in one coroner's case in July 1995, and there have been others.

[214] *Re S* [2005] 1 A.C. 593.

[215] *Re LM (Reporting Restrictions: Coroner's Inquest)* [2007] EWHC 1902 (Fam.).

[216] *A Local Authority v W and others* [2006] 1 F.L.R. 1 at [53].

[217] Before the Law of Libel (Amendment) Act 1888; s.3, at common law privilege was *qualified: Usill v Hales* (1878) 3 C.P.D. 319; cf. *McCarey v Associated Newspapers Ltd* [1964] 1 W.L.R. 855.

[218] Defamation Act 1996 s.14.

[219] Broadcasting Act 1990 Sch.20 para.2, now subsumed in the Defamation Act 1996 s.14.

in camera.[220] Whether the absolute privilege applies to coroner's courts is unclear.

"Court" includes any tribunal or body "exercising the judicial power of the **11–79** state".[221] There is Irish authority for saying that the coroner's court, because it does not *decide* anything, but instead *inquires*, does not exercise the judicial power of the state.[222] Reports of the proceedings of *inquiries* attract qualified privilege only.[223] But earlier English authority has assumed that the coroner's court exercises "the judicial power of the state" for the purposes of other legislation,[224] and it is submitted that this is correct.[225]

However, particular comments on the proceedings at an inquest which prejudice **11–80** issues arising in, or are calculated to interfere with, subsequent litigation, and particularly the fair trial of a person then or thereafter charged with an offence, may itself amount to an indictable offence,[226] or to a contempt of court.[227] Other comments on proceedings of inquests may be improper, but it does not appear that proceedings in respect of them could be taken.[228] A press report which names a person as having caused a death is no more prejudicial than naming a person as having been charged with an offence.[229]

Photography or graphic reproduction of proceedings

It is an offence to take, or attempt to take, in court any photograph, or with a view **11–81** to publication to make, or attempt to make, in court any portrait or sketch of the judge, or of a juror or witness in or a party to any proceedings before the court, or to publish any such photograph, portrait or sketch so taken or made, or any reproduction of it.[230] The maximum penalty is a fine at level 3 on the standard scale.[231] The coroner has no power to deal with this offence summarily, unless it also amounts to a contempt in the face of the court,[232] and therefore should report any offence to the police.

This provision expressly applies to the court of the coroner, treating the coroner **11–82** as the judge.[233] The prohibition extends beyond the courtroom itself, to the building in which the court is held, and to its precincts, and includes the taking or making of a photograph, portrait or sketch of the person entering or leaving the court building or precincts.[234] It is subject to certain exceptions provided for in

---

[220] *Scott v Scott* [1913] A.C. 417 at 452.
[221] Defamation Act 1996 s.14(3).
[222] *Morris v Dublin City Coroner* [2000] 3 I.R. 603 at [11], Irish Sup. Ct.
[223] Defamation Act 1996 s.15(1) Sch.1 paras 3, 11(1)(c)–(e).
[224] See 11–86.
[225] The judicial power of the state is not merely to decide questions of law between two parties, but by judicial reasoning to establish facts on the basis of evidence being given and tested in a public hearing. This is what an inquest does.
[226] *R. v Tibbits and Windust* [1902] 1 K.B. 77; *R. v Parke* [1903] 2 K.B. 432.
[227] *Attorney General v Times Newspapers Ltd* [1974] A.C. 273, HL. See 11–89 ff below.
[228] *Weldon v Moignard* (1889) 87 L.T. Jo. 356.
[229] *R. v West Yorkshire Ex p. Syed* Unreported December 4, 2001, Collins J.
[230] Criminal Justice Act 1925 s.41(1).
[231] Criminal Justice Act 1925 s.41(1); Criminal Justice Act 1982 ss.38, 46; level 3 is currently £1,000. *R. v D (Contempt of court: Illegal photography)* [2004] EWCA Crim. 1271.
[232] See *R. v D (Contempt of court: Illegal photography)* [2004] EWCA Crim. 1271, and 11–89 ff below.
[233] Criminal Justice Act 1925 s.41(2)(a),(b).
[234] Criminal Justice Act 1925 s.41(2)(c).

recent legislation.[235] Those exceptions now cover the video recording and broadcasting of appeals in the Court of Appeal,[236] but there is no exception so far for the coroner's court.

11–83   The prohibition on photography as originally enacted extends to the televising of the proceedings, or of persons taking part as they enter or leave the court building,[237] and also to the videotaping of proceedings in court.[238] Moreover, public filming amounting to a significant interference with private life can infringe art.8 (right to respect for private and family life) of the European Convention on Human Rights,[239] as can secret filming in a place to which the public have access.[240]

11–84   The legislative prohibition on sound recording, described below, contains provision for the court to consent to such recording in an appropriate case.[241] But, where television is concerned, it has been held that the court has no power to waive or dispense with the prohibition, even if it is otherwise desirable so to do.[242] It is submitted that this is wrong, and, the rule being enacted for the benefit of justice, the court may in an appropriate case consent to actions otherwise within the rule if justice is not impaired.[243] But public inquiries are not caught by these rules. The Shipman Inquiry produced two broadcasting protocols[244] for the oral hearings in Phase 2 of the Inquiry. On the other hand, the Hutton Inquiry into the death of Dr David Kelly in August 2003 refused permission for broadcasting of its proceedings.[245]

Sound recording

11–85   As will be seen later, the coroner must make a sound recording of all inquest hearings.[246] It is a contempt of court for anyone else to bring a tape recorder or other instrument for sound recording into a court for use there, or to use such instrument there, without the leave of the court.[247] Leave may be given subject to conditions,[248] and contravention of such conditions of any recording made is

---

[235] Crime and Courts Act 2013 s.32.

[236] Court of Appeal (Recording and Broadcasting) Order 2013 (SI 2013/2786).

[237] *Re St Andrews, Heddington* [1978] Fam. 121 (Salisbury Consistory Court).

[238] *J. Barber & Sons (a firm) v Lloyd's Underwriters* [1987] Q.B. 103; *R. v Loveridge* [2001] 2 Cr.App.R. 29, CA.

[239] *Von Hannover v Germany* (2004) 40 E.H.R.R. 1, ECtHR; *Von Hannover v Germany (No. 2)* (2012) 55 E.H.R.R. 15, ECtHR, Grd Chr.

[240] *R. v Broadcasting Standards Commission Ex p. BBC* [2000] 3 All E.R. 989, CA; *R. v Loveridge* [2001] 2 Cr.App.R. 29, CA.

[241] See 11–85 ff.

[242] *Re St Andrews, Heddington* [1978] Fam. 121 at 124.

[243] cf. the decision dated October 25, 2001, of Dame Janet Smith, Chairman, the Shipman Inquiry, in relation to an application by CNN to record the proceedings (available at *http://www.the-shipman-inquiry.org.uk*). See also *The Daily Telegraph*, June 25, 2002 (Plymouth and South West Devon coroner).

[244] April and September 2002, available on the Inquiry website, at *http://webarchive.nationalarchives.gov.uk/20090808154959/http://www.the-shipman-inquiry.org.uk/reports.asp*.

[245] The written reasons are available on the Inquiry's website at *http://www.the-hutton-inquiry.org.uk* [Accessed June 10, 2014].

[246] See 12–104.

[247] Contempt of Court Act 1981 s.9(1)(a).

[248] Contempt of Court Act 1981 s.9(2).

similarly a contempt,[249] as is publishing a recording (or any derived recording) by playing it to the public or a section of the public.[250] In addition to other penalties for contempt,[251] the court may order the instrument and any recording made to be forfeited.[252]

As with defamation privilege,[253] there is an obscurity in the legislation, as **11–86** "court" includes any tribunal or body "exercising the judicial power of the state",[254] and there is a doubt that the coroner's court does this.[255] But it has been assumed that the coroner's court is a "court" for the purpose of this legislation,[256] and this is the better view.[257] The ban on sound recording is subject to the same exceptions as provided for in relation to video-recording in recent legislation,[258] which now cover appeals in the Court of Appeal,[259] but not proceedings in the coroner's court.

The Home Office recommended that applications for leave to use tape- **11–87** recorders from parties or their legal representatives, or from bona fide journalists, be sympathetically treated, as in its view there was in principle no objection to their use. On at least one occasion in the past, a coroner has consented to a tape-recording being made of proceedings, which was subsequently broadcast on television as part of a programme.[260]

Factors militating against leave and in favour of revoking or suspending existing **11–88** leave have included impact on the sensitive nature of the proceedings caused by use of the machine.[261] Another would be the more widespread dissemination of intimate personal details relating to the deceased.[262] But the court will not give leave simply because the litigant or journalist asks for it; it is necessary to demonstrate a real need for the recording to be made.[263]

CONTEMPT OF COURT

In addition to specific powers to deal with particular situations, such as recalcitrant **11–89** witnesses or absent jurors,[264] the coroner has power summarily to punish contempt

---

[249] Contempt of Court Act 1981 s.9(1)(c).
[250] Contempt of Court Act 1981 s.9(1)(b).
[251] As to which see 11–97 below.
[252] Contempt of Court Act 1981 s.9(3).
[253] See 11–78 above.
[254] Contempt of Court Act 1981 s.19.
[255] See 11–79 above.
[256] *Peacock v London Weekend Television Ltd* (1985) 150 J.P. 71, CA; *Turnbull v BBC* Unreported June 30, 1992, CA.
[257] See also *General Medical Council v BBC* [1998] 1 W.L.R. 1573, CA.
[258] Crime and Courts Act 2013 s.32.
[259] Court of Appeal (Recording and Broadcasting) Order 2013 (SI 2013/2786).
[260] *Cutting Edge*, "Sudden Death" (Channel 4, January 11, 1993): see *The Times, Saturday Review,* January 9, 1993, pp. 10–11.
[261] Home Office Circular No. 79 of 1981. These recommendations were in line with the Practice Direction issued for the High Court which (by direction of the Lord Chancellor) applies also to county courts (but not to inquests): [1981] 1 W.L.R. 1526.
[262] See the decision of Dame Janet Smith, referred to in 11–84, at para.88.
[263] *Lewy v Lord Chancellor's Department* [2001] EWCA Civ. 600 at [16]–[17].
[264] See 11–09 (jurors) and 12–03 (witnesses) below.

committed in the face of the court,[265] whether by fine or by committal to prison.[266] Contempt "in the face of the court" includes photography in court,[267] and is not limited to cases where intervention is necessary to preserve the integrity of the hearing in progress or about to begin, but extends to the case of an attack on another party or a lawyer while judgment is being given.[268]

11–90   It is not confined to conduct which the judge sees with his own eyes, but extends to all contempt "in the cognisance of the court", i.e. in the courtroom though not seen by the judge, and even outside it.[269] But it is a power only exercisable when it is imperative to act immediately.[270] The common law on contempt in the face of the court has now developed to a point where the European Convention on Human Rights adds nothing to it.[271]

11–91   As the coroner's court is an inferior court of record,[272] the coroner has no power to punish contempt committed out of court,[273] as for example by the writing or publication of articles which reflect on the conduct of the coroner,[274] or which otherwise tend to interfere with the proceedings of the inquest.[275] In the last case, the test is whether publication created a substantial risk of serious prejudice to the course of justice,[276] in proceedings which are active at the time of publication.[277]

11–92   Proceedings before a coroner are active for this purpose as soon as the inquest is opened, even if only to establish non-contentious matters such as the fact of death and the identity of the deceased, and the inquest is then adjourned pending further or alternative investigations.[278] There is considerable case law on what constitutes "a substantial risk of serious prejudice".[279] In all these cases, the coroner should not proceed with the inquest (because of the risk of prejudice), and instead refer the matter to the Attorney General, who has the power to institute proceedings before the Divisional Court.[280]

---

[265] *R. v West Yorkshire Coroner Ex p. Smith (No. 2)* [1985] 1 Q.B. 1096, DC; as to what constitutes such contempt, see *R. v Powell, The Times*, June 3, 1993, CA (wolf-whistle at juror); *R. v Schot and Barclay* (1997) 161 J.P. 473, CA (contumacious refusal by juror to reach any verdict may be contempt).

[266] For a form of warrant of committal, see App.3 Form 18.

[267] *R. v D (Contempt of court: Illegal photography)* [2004] EWCA Crim. 1271 (12-month sentence imposed for contempt of court on a man who had used his mobile telephone to take three photographs in the court complex, two of them in the courtroom during the trial of his brother).

[268] *Wilkinson v S* [2003] 1 W.L.R. 1254, CA.

[269] *Balogh v St Albans Crown Court* [1975] Q.B. 73 at 84.

[270] *Balogh v St Albans Crown Court* [1975] Q.B. 73 at 85, 93.

[271] *R. v Dodds* [2002] EWCA Crim. 1328; *R. v MacLeod* Unreported November 29, 2000; *Wilkinson v S* [2003] 1 W.L.R. 1254, CA.

[272] See 10–01 above.

[273] *Ex p. Pater* (1864) 5 B. & S. 219; *R. v Lefroy* (1872) L.R. 8 Q.B. 134.

[274] *Bush v Green* [1985] 1 W.L.R. 1143, CA (county court judge); see also generally *Civil Aviation Authority v Australian Broadcasting Commission*, No. CA 40195/94, Sup Ct NSW (summons for declarations that contempt of coroner's inquest by broadcasting radio programme).

[275] As to which see the Contempt of Court Act 1981 ss.1–7, Sch.1 para.12.

[276] Contempt of Court Act 1981 s.2(2).

[277] Contempt of Court Act 1981 s.2(3).

[278] *Peacock v London Weekend Television Ltd* (1985) 150 J.P. 71, CA. As to whether the coroner's court is a "court" at all for these purposes, see 11–86.

[279] *Attorney General v MGN Ltd* [1997] 1 All E.R. 456; *Attorney General v Birmingham Post and Mail Ltd* [1997] 1 W.L.R. 361, DC; *Attorney General v Guardian Newspaper Ltd* [1999] E.M.L.R. 904, DC.

[280] See, e.g. *Attorney General v B.B.C.* [1981] A.C. 303, HL.

Alternatively, and if the article has not yet been published, the coroner, or **11–93** another person with a sufficient interest, may seek an injunction to restrain the commission of what would otherwise be a contempt of court.[281] Although contempt proceedings themselves require the consent of the Attorney General,[282] injunction proceedings to restrain a threatened contempt do not.[283] The contempt legislation does not, however, apply to proceedings in Parliament. On the other hand the so-called "sub judice" rule prevents debates on matters which are going to be the subject of judicial determination, including matters at coroners' inquests, although there is an exception for what are called "matters of national importance".[284]

Where the coroner has power to deal summarily with a contempt of court, he **11–94** should not decline to do so merely because the facts or matters amounting to such contempt do or may also amount to a separate criminal offence which is dealt with by different means.[285] Nor should he adjourn the question of contempt to the conclusion of the inquest proceedings unless he is certain that the alleged contemnor will remain, for he has no power to detain the latter till then, even in the case of contempt in the face of the court.[286]

The requirement of fairness

In dealing with a case of contempt committed in the face of the court, the coroner **11–95** must be seen to act fairly, even though summarily.[287] So far as applicable, he should act consistently with the Practice Direction relating to magistrates' courts,[288] even though such courts enjoy greater powers to deal with contempt in the face of the court.[289] He should attempt to arrange some form of legal representation for the offender,[290] e.g. from amongst the lawyers who may be in the vicinity of the court for other inquests. Where the offender is unrepresented, special precautions should be taken, such as warning of the punishment that may be imposed, asking whether he wishes to call witnesses or other evidence, and giving him an opportunity to

---

[281] See, e.g. *Peacock v London Weekend Television Ltd* (1985) 150 J.P. 71, CA; *Turnbull v BBC* Unreported June 30, 1992, CA (no substantial risk that course of justice in proceedings would be seriously impeded or prejudiced-injunction discharged upon undertakings). cf. *General Medical Council v BBC* [1998] 1 W.L.R. 1573, CA (professional conduct committee of General Medical Council not "court" for purposes of 1981 Act).

[282] Contempt of Court Act 1981 s.7.

[283] *Peacock v London Weekend Television Ltd* (1985) 150 J.P. 71, CA.

[284] Resolution HC 15 November 2001, CJ (2001-06) 194-51; Report of House of Commons Procedure Committee, 22 August 2006, HC 714. See Erskine May, *Parliamentary Practice*, 24th edn (2011), 441-443.

[285] *Caprice v Boswell* (1985) 149 J.P. 703, CA.

[286] cf. *Delaney v Delaney* [1996] Q.B. 387, 401, CA, and see also *Wilkinson v S* [2003] 1 W.L.R. 1254, CA. For magistrates' courts, see the Contempt of Court Act 1981 s.12, and *Practice Direction (Magistrates' Courts: Contempt)* [2001] 1 W.L.R. 1254.

[287] *Wilkinson v S* [2003] 1 W.L.R. 1254, CA.

[288] *Practice Direction (Magistrates' Court: Contempt* [2001] 1 W.L.R. 1254.

[289] Contempt of Court Act 1981 s.12.

[290] *R. v Chowdhury; R. v Crone, The Times*, March 29, 1984, CA; *R. v Bromell, The Times*, February 9, 1995, CA; *R. v Tyne Tees Television Ltd, The Times*, October 20, 1997, CA; *Wilkinson v S* [2003] 1 W.L.R. 1254, CA.

address the court before sentence.[291] Where the contempt affects the coroner personally, it is probably better to refer the matter to the Attorney General.

11–96   On mature reflection and after hearing submissions in mitigation, the coroner might well decide that the action concerned did not amount to a contempt at all,[292] or that, if it did, an apology and future compliance will suffice. Or that it merited only a reprimand rather than a fine or imprisonment.[293] If the coroner does decide to impose a penalty, he should first enquire into the offender's personal circumstances, to ensure that the particular penalty does not have a disproportionate effect upon him.

Limitation on power to punish

11–97   The coroner's power to punish for contempt is limited, however. Any sentence of imprisonment must be for a fixed term (although without prejudice to the court's power to order an early discharge), and must not exceed one month.[294] The maximum fine which may be imposed by the coroner in respect of contempt of court is £2,500 on one occasion.[295]

It should be noted that, unlike the superior courts, the coroner does not have the power to make a hospital order or guardianship order[296] in the case of a person suffering from mental illness or severe abnormality who could otherwise be committed to prison for contempt of court.[297]

Appeal from finding of contempt of court

11–98   A person may appeal from an order or decision of the coroner in the exercise of his jurisdiction to punish for contempt of court to a Divisional Court of the Queen's Bench Division of the High Court.[298] It appears that, at least where a committal order is made, permission to appeal is not required,[299] but otherwise it may be.[300] With the leave of the Divisional Court or of the Supreme Court, there is a further appeal to the Supreme Court, but such leave can only be granted if it is certified by the Divisional Court that a point of law of general public importance is involved in the decision and that it appears to the Divisional Court that the point is one that ought to be considered by the Supreme Court.[301]

---

[291] *Bailiffs of Shoreditch County Court v De Medeiros, The Independent*, February 23, 1988; *Wilkinson v S* [2003] 1 W.L.R. 1254, CA.

[292] See *Re Dr A.S. Rayan* (1984) 148 J.P. 569, DC; *Attorney General v Independent Television News Ltd* [1995] 2 All E.R. 370, DC.

[293] cf. *R. v Powell, The Times*, June 3, 1993, CA; *R. v Schot and Barclay* (1997) 161 J.P. 473, CA.

[294] Contempt of Court Act 1981 s.14(1). A person under the age of 17 years, however, may not be imprisoned at all; Contempt of Court Act 1981 s.14(3). As to the principles to be applied in imprisoning for contempt, see *R. v Moran* (1985) 81 Cr.App.R. 51, CA; and see *Re John Mikkelsen, The Independent*, February 11, 1987 (Hornsey coroner), where a witness who refused to take the oath, affirm, or answer any question, was sentenced to one month's imprisonment.

[295] Contempt of Court Act 1981 s.14(2), as amended by the Criminal Justice Act 1991.

[296] See the Mental Health Act 1983 ss.37, 40.

[297] As to which see 11–89 above.

[298] Administration of Justice Act 1960 s.13. As to legal aid, see 10–51 ff.

[299] cf. CPR r.52.3(1)(a)(i).

[300] *Government of Sierra Leone v Davenport* Unreported January 23, 2002, CA.

[301] Administration of Justice Act 1960 ss.13(4), 1(2).

The court to which an appeal is brought may reverse or vary the order or **11–99** decision of the court below, and make such other order as it considers just.[302] Pending the hearing of the appeal, a person imprisoned for contempt of court may be released on bail.[303] A court hearing an appeal against a finding of contempt of court has no power to award costs out of central funds to a successful applicant.[304] If objection is taken to the decision of the coroner to punish for contempt on the grounds of jurisdiction,[305] or of breach of the rules of natural justice (such as not being told that the coroner intended to deal with certain action as a contempt or failing to give adequate opportunity to explain conduct), or of treating as a contempt action which as a matter of law it could not so constitute,[306] proceedings may be brought by way of judicial review for the coroner's decision to be quashed.[307]

Enforcement of coroner's decision on contempt of court

Until 1988 it was not quite clear what was the proper means of enforcing a decision **11–100** of the coroner to impose a fine with respect to the contempt of court properly punishable by him.[308] Since 1988 the proper course of action in such cases is for the coroner to certify to the clerk to the justices for the area in which his court is situated that he has imposed the fine in question, and for the magistrates' court to enforce payment of the fine in the usual manner.[309]

Bias and perverting the course of justice

The question of bias, apparent or real, on the part of the coroner, and its **11–101** consequences, have already been dealt with,[310] and need not be repeated here. The offence of doing acts tending and intended to pervert the court of justice, which can be committed in relation to an inquest, has also been considered.[311] It can be committed not only in acts done before an inquest, but also at the hearing, as when a witness lies in giving evidence.[312]

---

[302] Administration of Justice Act 1960 s.13(3).

[303] Administration of Justice Act 1960 s.13(3).

[304] *R. v Moore (Peter)*, *The Times*, May 15, 2003, CA.

[305] e.g. *R. v West Yorkshire Coroner Ex p. Smith (No. 2)* [1985] Q.B. 1096, DC.

[306] *Re Dr A.S. Rayan* (1984) 148 J.P. 569, DC.

[307] On judicial review, see generally Ch.19 below. *Dr Rayan's* case was in fact an application under s.13 of the Administration of Justice Act 1960, rather than a judicial review, but it is conceived that the principle is the same.

[308] See *R. v West Yorkshire Coroner Ex p. Smith (No. 2)* [1985] Q.B. 1096, DC, where the point was ultimately not pursued, although Stephen Brown LJ stated (at 1108): "I feel it right to add that it would be remarkable indeed if a fine having been properly imposed by the coroner there should not be a machinery to collect it". It may have been the sheriff's duty to enforce the payment of the fine: see Dalton, *Sheriffs*, pp.146a–146b.

[309] Criminal Justice Act 1988 s.67(1).

[310] See 5–66 above.

[311] See 7–23.

[312] See also *Gosai v General Medical Council* [2003] UKPC 31, where the appellant had been struck off the medical register for serious professional misconduct in (a) failing adequately to treat a patient, who subsequently died, and (b) lying to the inquest into the patient's death so as to cover up the inadequate treatment. The Privy Council dismissed an appeal from a decision of the Professional Conduct Committee of the GMC that the appellant's right to apply for restoration of his name to the medical register be suspended indefinitely.

Chapter 12

PROCEDURE AT THE INQUEST: PART II

Witnesses, Evidence, Summing Up

WITNESSES

Securing attendance

It is said that at common law every person who is able to give evidence is bound **12–01** to attend at the coroner's court, and if he absents himself he does so at his peril.[1] In practice, the attendance of the relevant witnesses is secured either by an informal request, or by a formal coroner's notice.[2] There are special rules for prisoners,[3] and also for evidence to be given by videolink.[4]

Exemption from arrest

A person who has been summoned as a witness, or who is under recognisance to **12–02** attend as a witness, is exempt from civil (but not criminal) arrest when going to or returning from a coroner's court, and also while at the court.[5] But civil arrest is almost unknown nowadays.[6]

Failure to appear or refusal to answer questions

Where a person duly required[7] to attend to give evidence at an inquest, or to **12–03** produce documents relevant to the inquest, or to produce for inspection, examination or testing anything relating to a matter relevant to an inquest[8] without reasonable excuse fails so to attend, or attends but fails to answer a question put to

---

[1] See the 7th edn of this work, p.46, the 8th edn, p.85 and the 9th edn, p.147. cf. *R. v Wilkins* [1985] Crim.L.R. 222, CA: robbery victim, as a citizen, was under a duty to give evidence, and committed contempt if refused to do so. The sentence in the text was cited with apparent approval by the Northern Ireland Court of Appeal in *R. v Secretary of State Ex p. McKerr* Unreported December 20, 1988 (reversed on other grounds, [1990] 1 W.L.R. 649).

[2] See 10–29—10–30.

[3] See 10–29.

[4] See 12–29.

[5] See the 9th edn of this work, p.148.

[6] For a rare example, see the Insolvency Act 1986 s.364.

[7] As to the procedure, and the modes of challenge, see 7–12 ff. If the witness is not formally summoned no fine can be imposed: *Re Dr AS Rayan* (1984) 148 JP 569, DC.

[8] Coroners and Justice Act 2009 s.32 Sch.5 para.1(1); see 7–14.

him, produce documents or some thing, the coroner may impose upon such person a fine not exceeding £1,000.[9]

12–04 As with absent jurors,[10] the coroner should not inflict any penalty on an absent witness without first receiving proper evidence of the due service of the formal notice upon him. But it may be more efficient to issue a "bench warrant", as described below. Whether the coroner may commit the recalcitrant witness without proof of the tender of conduct money is an unresolved question. Such tender was held necessary in the case of an ordinary subpoena,[11] and it was equally held to be necessary in the case of other statutory requirements to attend at court, even where the statute concerned made no mention of it.[12] But they were cases where one party sought the attendance of another party.

12–05 In an inquest there are no parties,[13] and it is the coroner alone that calls the witnesses,[14] who are entitled by statute to allowances from the coroner for their attendance.[15] The state is in a different position from private parties to civil litigation, at least when it is enforcing public law rather than private law obligations,[16] and it is therefore submitted that there is no requirement for proof of tender of conduct money by the coroner before the witness can be attached for failure to attend.

Power to commit for contempt of court or to issue bench warrant

12–06 In addition to his statutory powers, the coroner may at common law commit for contempt of court[17] a witness duly summoned under the coroner's statutory power[18] who refuses to appear or who without lawful authority refuses to answer

---

[9] Coroners and Justice Act 2009 s.33 Sch.6 para.6; formerly Coroners Act 1988 s.10(2), as amended by the Criminal Justice Act 1991 s.17(3) and Sch.4 Pt I. Under the old law there was no defence of "reasonable excuse". Such a fine is treated for the purpose of its collection, enforcement or remission as having been imposed by the magistrates' court for the area in which the coroner's court was held: Criminal Justice Act 1988 s.67. The coroner must give particulars of the fine to the clerk of that magistrates' court as soon as possible after imposition: Criminal Justice Act 1988 s.67. The form was formerly prescribed by the Coroners Rules 1984 Sch.4 Form 11, but there is no equivalent in the new system. The clerk must then notify the offender of the amount of the fine and date and place when and where payment must be made, before a warrant of distress or commitment may be issued: Magistrates' Courts Rules 1981 (SI 1981/552) r.46 (which, however, still refers to s.19(5) of the Coroners Act 1887).

[10] See 11–10.

[11] *Fuller v Prentice* (1788) 1 Blackstone (H.) 49; *Brocas v Lloyd* (1856) 23 Beav. 129. See now Senior Courts Act 1981 s.36(4), and CPR r.34.7 (in relation to witness summonses)

[12] See e.g. *Re Harvey* [1907] P. 239; cf. *Re Wyatt* [1898] P. 15.

[13] See 10–03.

[14] See 10–25.

[15] See 18–36.

[16] cf., e.g. the Crown's position on applications for injunctions: *F Hoffmann-La Roche & Co AG v Secretary of State for Trade and Industry* [1975] A.C. 295, HL.

[17] As to which see 11–89 ff above; cf. the *Chief Coroner's Guide to the Coroners and Justice Act 2009*, [132].

[18] See 7–14. The coroner no longer has power to apply for the issue of a High Court or county court witness summons.

questions.[19] His common law power in the case of a duly summoned absent witness extends to issuing a warrant, often called a "bench warrant",[20] addressed to police officers to bring the witness in question before the court.[21] In most cases this will advance the inquest proceedings more quickly than committing the witness to prison for contempt. But the warrant cannot be backed for bail.[22]

The coroner may not, however, exercise both his statutory and his common law **12–07** powers in respect of the same default.[23] An alternative is for the coroner to apply directly to the High Court (or for him to ask the Attorney General so to apply) for an order committing the recalcitrant witness to prison for contempt. If the application hearing and the resumed inquest hearing are correctly timed, it may be possible for the witness to be imprisoned for a short period and taken to the coroner's court immediately before the end of that period.[24]

Types of evidence

There are two kinds of evidence: evidence of fact, and expert evidence. A **12–08** professional witness may be either a witness of fact (e.g. a treating doctor) or an expert (e.g. a consultant so retained), or both (e.g. a forensic pathologist). An expert witness is exceptional in being able to give evidence of his *opinion* and not merely of primary facts.[25] A professional witness (whether of fact or opinion) is also entitled to be remunerated.

Remuneration of professional and expert witness

Professional witnesses, such as doctors, are paid according to scales set by the **12–09** Secretary of State.[26] The remuneration of expert witnesses is at the discretion of the coroner, and depends on the actual work done.[27] A professional who gives both factual and opinion evidence could in theory receive two fees, but in practice the coroner is unlikely to exercise his discretion to pay an opinion fee if a sufficient factual fee has been paid.

---

[19] Umfreville, *Lex Coronatoria*, 303; *R. v Clement* (1821) 4 B. & Ald. 218; *R. v Little* [1925] 2 W.W.R. 762; *R. v Judge* [1931] 2 K.B. 422; *Re John Mikkelsen, The Independent*, February 11, 1987 (Hornsey coroner) (witness sentenced to one month's imprisonment). The sentence in the text was cited with apparent approval by the Northern Ireland Court of Appeal in *R. v Secretary of State Ex p. McKerr* Unreported December 20, 1988. cf. Britton (ed. Nichols, 1865), Vol.1 Ch.II, para.4, and Fitzherbert and Crompton, *Justices de Peace,* 1584, fol.176a, which express the view that the coroner had no power to fine anyone for any default.

[20] See *Zakharov v White* [2003] EWHC 2463 (Ch.); *Westwood v Knight* [2012] EWPCC 14. As to the form of such a warrant, see App.3, Form 11.

[21] Stephen, *Digest of the Law of Criminal Procedure in Indictable Offences* (1883), art.224 (pp.144-145): "The coroner at the inquest may summon any person to give evidence, and if necessary may issue a warrant directing a peace officer to bring anyone before him as a witness. And if such person resists such warrant or refuses without sufficient reason to give evidence, the coroner may commit him to prison for contempt."

[22] Because the Magistrates' Courts Act 1980 s.117, does not apply to coroners.

[23] cf Coroners Act 1988 s.10(3), which made the matter clear under the 1988 Act. There is no equivalent in the 2009 Act, but the principle is the same.

[24] As happened in *Kent Coroner v Terrill* [2000] Inq. L.R. 16; [2001] A.C.D. 5, DC.

[25] See 12–90.

[26] See 18–37, 18–38.

[27] See 18–39 below.

Witnesses to be examined

12–10   Formerly the coroner had to examine on oath all persons who tendered their evidence respecting the facts, and all persons having knowledge of the facts whom he thought it expedient to examine.[28] In practice it always was the coroner's decision as to whom to call and to examine, and this remains the position.[29] Witnesses whose evidence is in favour of any suspected person must be examined equally with witnesses whose evidence may be adverse.[30]

Evidence by persons lacking capacity

12–11   A person lacking capacity (within the meaning of the Mental Capacity Act 2005) may give evidence at common law if the coroner nonetheless takes the view that the witness understands both the nature of an oath and what he is being asked to do: if he does, it is then up to the jury (if there is one) or the coroner (if there is not) to say what weight should be given to the evidence of such a witness.[31] In *criminal* cases, however, the position is now by statute slightly different.[32]

Deaf and dumb witnesses

12–12   Deaf and dumb persons, if otherwise competent witnesses and able to communicate their ideas, may be admitted and examined through the intervention of an interpreter.[33]

Child as witness[34]

12–13   At common law the competence of a child to give evidence depended not on his age but on his ability to understand the nature of an oath, and in particular that it involves an obligation to tell the truth over and above the ordinary duty of doing so.[35] The position is now different in the coroner's court. In an inquest a child who is under the age of 14 years, or who is considered by the coroner to be unable to understand the nature of an oath of affirmation may, on promising to tell the truth, be permitted to give unsworn evidence.[36] In addition, the coroner is able to receive hearsay evidence,[37] and therefore in an appropriate case may call as a witness a person who has interviewed the child concerned. Screens and videolinks are

---

[28] Coroners Act 1988 s.11(2).

[29] See 10–25.

[30] *R. v Storey* (1748) 1 Leach (4th edn), p.43; *R. v Colmar* (1864) 9 Cox C.C. 506.

[31] *R. v Hill* (1851) 2 Den. 254; *Spittle v Walton* (1871) L.R. 11 Eq. 420; *R. v Bellamy* (1985) 82 Cr.App.R. 222, CA.

[32] See the Youth Justice and Criminal Evidence Act 1999 s.53(3): whether witness can understand questions put and can give answers which can be understood.

[33] *R v Ruston* (1786) 1 Leach C.C. 408. As to interpreters of foreign languages, see 12–42, 12–43.

[34] As to when a child witness should be summoned, see *Re P* [1977] 2 F.L.R. 447, CA.

[35] *R. v Brasier* (1779) 1 Leach 199; *R v Whitehead* (1866) L.R. 1 C.C.R. 33; *R v Imrie* (1917) 12 Cr.App.Rep. 282; *R v Hayes* [1977] 1 W.L.R. 234; cf. *R. v Bellamy* (1985) 82 Cr.App.R. 222, CA. See also Dickens, *Bleak House*, Ch.11.

[36] Coroners (Inquests) Rules 2013 (SI 2013/1616) r.20(2). In criminal cases the position is governed by the Youth Justice and Criminal Evidence Act 1999 s.55(2): a child under 14 years cannot be sworn, but can still give evidence.

[37] See 12–72 below

considered later.[38] Restrictions on publication of a child's details have already been considered.[39]

Other witnesses

Subject to any stated limitations, all persons are competent witnesses before the coroner. Statute makes special provision in criminal cases for vulnerable or intimidated witnesses, but this does not apply to inquests.[40] However, the coroner has power to use screens and videolinks where appropriate.[41]   **12–14**

Compellability of competent witness

The general rule is that all persons who are *competent* witnesses are also *compellable*. In particular, a person cannot refuse to be a witness merely because he might subsequently be charged with an offence arising out of or connected with the death.[42] However, once he is sworn and in the witness box, he may of course refuse to answer particular questions on the grounds of self-incrimination.[43] Similarly, although the spouse or civil partner of an accused person is in a few cases not compellable as a witness in criminal proceedings,[44] the inquest is not criminal proceedings, and neither is a person merely suspected an "accused".[45]   **12–15**

Exceptions to compellability

Notwithstanding the general rule, however, there are a few exceptional cases where a competent witness cannot be compelled to give evidence to the coroner's court.   **12–16**

Sovereign or head of state. First, neither our own nor any other sovereign or head of state can be so compelled.[46]   **12–17**

Diplomatic and consular officials. Secondly, heads of foreign missions and members of diplomatic staff (and their families),[47] consular officers,[48] persons in   **12–18**

---

[38] See 12–26 ff.

[39] See 11–75.

[40] Youth Justice and Criminal Evidence Act 1999 s.16.

[41] Coroners (Inquests) Rules 2013 (SI 2013/1616) rr.17, 18; see 12–26 ff.

[42] *Wakley v Cooke* (1847) 4 Ex. 511; *Boyle v Wiseman* (1855) 10 Ex. 647. If it is at all likely that he will be charged, the coroner will probably adjourn the inquest anyway: 11–44. The first two sentences in this paragraph were cited with apparent approval by the Northern Ireland Court of Appeal in *Ex p.McKerr*, above, although the House of Lords in reversing that decision ([1990] 1 W.L.R. 649) held that the position in Northern Ireland was different from that in England, being governed by express statutory provision. See also *R. v Attorney-General for Northern Ireland Ex p.Devine* [1992] 1 W.L.R. 262, HL.

[43] See 7–62 ff, 12–94 ff.

[44] See now the Police and Criminal Evidence Act 1984 s.80, as amended by the Youth Justice and Criminal Evidence Act 1999 s.67(1) Sch.4 para.13, and the Civil Partnership Act 2004 s.261 Sch.27 para.97.

[45] *Wakley v Cooke* (1847) 4 Ex. 511.

[46] *Halsbury's Law of England*, 5th edn Vol.61 [243], [244]–[245], [263]; State Immunity Act 1978 s.21.

[47] Diplomatic Privileges Act 1964 s.2 and Sch.1 arts 31, 37. As for domestic staff see Diplomatic Privileges Act 1964 Sch.1 art.37 para.4.

[48] Consular Relations Act 1968 s.1 Sch.1 art.44. Consular employees and members of the consular staff are in a different position: Consular Relations Act 1968 s.1 Sch.1 art.44.

similar service of a commonwealth country or the Republic of Ireland,[49] and the staff of various international organisations (in some cases)[50] are exempt from process to compel their attendance at the coroner's court.[51]

12–19   **Judges.** Thirdly, judges cannot be compelled to give evidence on any matter affecting the substance of any proceedings in which they have been engaged judicially.[52] However, the exception does not extend to matters collateral to the proceedings,[53] so that presumably if a person dies in court in the presence of a judge, the judge is a compellable witness as to the circumstances of the death. Neither does the exception apply to judges of inferior courts,[54] such as coroners themselves.[55] But in no case will the coroner investigate the correctness in law of any decision made by the witness.[56]

12–20   **Members of Parliament.** Fourthly, members of both Houses of Parliament are not compellable witnesses during the session of Parliament, although the privilege may be waived and leave of absence granted.[57] Any process to compel attendance may be set aside if no such leave has been given.[58] No similar claim to privilege appears to be made in respect of the members of the National Assembly for Wales[59] or the Scottish Parliament.[60]

12–21   **Other exceptions.** There is no right to refuse to attend to give evidence conferred upon a person by the visiting forces provisions,[61] although it is of course possible that national security or other state considerations may prevent some questions being asked or lines of questioning being pursued,[62] as indeed with any witness.

Anonymity and screening of witnesses

12–22   In the past it was doubted how far the coroner generally had the power to withhold facts and matters (such as the names or addresses of witnesses) from the public in proceedings before the court,[63] but the coroner has the inherent right (so far as not

---

[49] Consular Relations Act 1968 s.12; Diplomatic and Other Privileges Act 1971 s.4.
[50] International Organisations Act 1968 s.1 Sch.1.
[51] Diplomatic and other immunities may of course be waived by the state concerned, whatever the view of the potential witness: see 5–114 above. On establishing claims to immunity, see 5–115 above.
[52] *R. v Gazard* (1838) 8 C. & p.595, 173 E.R. 633; *Warren v Warren* [1977] QB 488, CA.
[53] *R. v Thanet* (1799) 27 St.Tr. 821 (escape of prisoners from courtroom).
[54] *R. v Harvey* (1858) 8 Cox C.C. 99; *McKinley v McKinley* [1960] 1 W.L.R. 120.
[55] It is, however, incompatible with the judicial status of a coroner that he should appear as an *expert* witness before another coroner: 2–156. Nor should a coroner give evidence to himself, even formal: *Re Sutherland* [1994] 2 N.Z.L.R. 242.
[56] See 6–11.
[57] *Halsbury's Laws of England*, 5th edn Vol.78 at [1087].
[58] *Hansard*, HC Vol.521, cols 957–959, 961 (December 1, 1953).
[59] See the Government of Wales Act 1998.
[60] See the Scotland Act 1998.
[61] See 5–98 ff
[62] See Ch.6, 12–63 ff.
[63] *R. v Socialist Worker Printers and Publishers Ltd Ex p. Attorney General* [1975] Q.B. 637, DC; *R. v Hove Justices Ex p. Gibbons, The Times*, June 19, 1981.

abrogated by legislation) to regulate his own proceedings,[64] and it is now accepted that he may, in a proper case, permit a witness to remain anonymous, or even to give evidence from behind a screen. Indeed, the latter is now regulated by express rule.[65]

As for anonymity, this was first held part of the coroner's inherent power of control of the proceedings in 1995.[66] It was made clear that, if anonymity were granted, the coroner must know the identity of the witness.[67] But any departure from open justice must be a stringently regulated exception.[68] An objective reason for anonymity must first be established. The fear must be for personal or family safety. But a wholly irrational fear is not enough. Neither are vague, unspecific threats. The fact that all interested persons consent to anonymity for the witness does not lessen the court's task, but instead increases the need for vigilance.[69]   **12–23**

At common law, the test is whether the procedure adopted was fair, bearing in mind the subjective fears of the witness, the degree to which those fears are objectively justified,[70] and the effect of anonymity on (i) the witness and (ii) the inquiry itself.[71] It is for the court[72] to carry out a balancing act. In considering whether the procedure is fair, however, it must be borne in mind that the coroner's inquest is not adversarial litigation, but an *inquiry*, and what may be unfair in the former may not necessarily be in the latter.[73]   **12–24**

Since the coming into force of the Human Rights Act 1998, in cases where art.2 of the ECHR is engaged, the test has not been whether there are subjective fears objectively justified, but whether there is a "real and immediate risk" of death to the witness.[74] For this purpose "a real risk is one that is objectively verified and an immediate risk is one that is present and continuing".[75] In a case looking at a risk that has not yet matured, a real and immediate risk is one which is neither fanciful nor trivial but is present (or will be if action is not taken).[76] But "the state is not expected to undertake an unduly burdensome obligation: it is not obliged to satisfy   **12–25**

---

[64] See *Attorney General v Leveller Magazine Ltd* [1979] A.C. 440, HL; *R. v Evesham Justices Ex p. McDonagh* [1988] Q.B. 553, DC; *R. v Bedford Coroner Ex p. Local Sunday Newspapers Ltd* (1999) 164 J.P. 283; decision of Dame Janet Smith, Chairman, *The Shipman Inquiry*, October 25, 2001 para.58 (available at *http://webarchive.nationalarchives.gov.uk/20090808154959/http://www.the-shipman-inquiry.org.uk/reports.asp*); *R. (A) v Lord Saville of Newdigate* [2002] 1 W.L.R. 1249 at [7], CA.

[65] See 12–27.

[66] *Re Jordan's Application* Unreported December 11, 1995, HC (NI), Carswell L.J.; affirmed CA, June 29, 1996.

[67] See the Court of Appeal of Northern Ireland's decision of June 29, 1996.

[68] *Attorney General v Leveller Magazine* [1979] A.C. 440 at 450; *R. v Legal Aid Board Ex p.Kaim Todner* [1998] 3 All E.R. 541 at 549; *R. v Bedford Coroner Ex p.Local Sunday Newspapers Ltd* (1999) 164 J.P. 283.

[69] cf *R v Westminster City Council Ex p. P* (1998) 31 H.L.R .154, 161-163.

[70] See *R. (Officer A) v Inner South London Coroner* [2004] EWCA Civ. 1439.

[71] See *R. (A) v Lord Saville of Newdigate* [2002] 1 W.L.R. 1249, CA.

[72] The decision is one for the court alone: *Rockett v Smith* (1991) 55 A. Crim. R. 79 at 85.

[73] *Re K (Infants)* [1965] A.C. 201, 240-241; *Roberts v Parole Board* [2005] 2 A.C. 738, HL; *Re Applications by Officers C, D, H, and R* [2012] N.I.C.A. 47. But procedural anonymity and screening can only be challenged afterwards if they have an impact on the verdict: *Re McDonnell's Application* [2014] NIQB 66.

[74] *Osman v United Kingdom* (1998) 29 E.H.R.R. 245, at [115]–[116], as interpreted in subsequent cases; see 21–16.

[75] *Re W's Application* [2004] N.I.Q.B. 67 at [17], approved in *Re Officer L* [2007] 1 W.L.R. 2135 at [20], HL.

[76] *Re Applications by Officers C, D, H, and R* [2012] N.I.C.A. 47.

an absolute standard requiring the risk to be averted, regardless of all other considerations."[77]

12–26   A further question concerns the screening of witnesses from the public. This is essentially an extension of the anonymity considered above. Not only the names, but the features of the witness's appearance, are withheld from the public (although again, not from the tribunal—nor, perhaps, the advocates). Screens have been used in criminal cases for many years,[78] and it was finally established also that "a coroner has an inherent power to order the screening of witnesses in exceptional cases if the administration of justice so requires".[79] If the coroner, jury, and the interested persons and their advocates, can see the witness, the fact that the general public and the media cannot will not, it seems, breach art.2 of the European Convention on Human Rights.[80]

12–27   The current rule for inquests is statutory. A coroner may, on his own initiative, or on the application of a witness (or his parent or legal guardian) or an interested person,[81] direct that a witness may give evidence at an inquest hearing[82] from behind a screen,[83] if the coroner determines that so doing would be likely to improve the quality of the evidence so given or allow the inquest to proceed more expediently.[84] In so determining, the coroner must consider all the circumstances, including in particular views expressed by the witness or interested persons, whether it would serve justice or national security, and whether it would impede the effective questioning of the witness by an interested person or his representative.[85]

Witness physically unable to attend

12–28   If a witness is physically unable to attend the coroner's court, and the coroner is unwilling to adjourn until the witness is able to do so, there is no objection to the inquest being adjourned to the place where the witness is (within England and Wales) so that he can give his evidence forthwith.[86] Formerly the only expedient open to the coroner was to receive the sworn evidence of another person such as a police officer to whom the witness had made a statement.[87]

12–29   An alternative, particularly where the witness is abroad, is to take the evidence by live video-link. (It may also be useful for a child (or other vulnerable) witness who might be overwhelmed by being in a courtroom.) This has been done by coroners in a number of cases hitherto using their common law powers as masters

---

[77] *Re Officer L* [2007] 1 W.L.R. 2135 at [21], HL; *Van Colle v United Kingdom* (2013) 56 E.H.R.R. 23.
[78] *R v Schaub and Cooper, The Times*, December 3, 1993, CA; *R. v Itani and Shah* [2003] EWCA Crim. 935.
[79] *R v Newcastle upon Tyne Coroner Ex p A* (1998) 162 J.P. 387; see also *Morris v Dublin City Coroner* [2000] 3 I.R. 603, Irish Sup. Ct.
[80] In *McCann v UK* (1995) 21 E.H.R.R. 97, ECtHR, some witnesses at the original inquest were screened, but the European Court found no breach on that account; see also *X v UK* (1993) 15 E.H.R.R. C.D. 113.
[81] Coroners (Inquests) Rules 2013 (SI 2013/1616) r.18(4).
[82] This does not include the inquest opening: 10–09.
[83] Coroners (Inquests) Rules 2013 (SI 2013/1616) r.18(1).
[84] Coroners (Inquests) Rules 2013 (SI 2013/1616) r.18(2).
[85] Coroners (Inquests) Rules 2013 (SI 2013/1616) r.18(3).
[86] *St Edmundsbury and Ipswich Diocesan Board of Finance v Clark* [1973] Ch. 323 (not a coroner's case)
[87] This will be hearsay evidence, but that is no objection in the coroner's court: 12–72.

of their own procedure.[88] But the present rule is statutory. A coroner may, on his own initiative, or on the application of a witness (or his parent or legal guardian) or an interested person,[89] direct that a witness may give evidence at an inquest hearing[90] through a live video link,[91] if the coroner determines that so doing would be likely to improve the quality of the evidence so given or allow the inquest to proceed more expediently.[92] In so determining, the coroner must consider all the circumstances, including in particular views expressed by the witness or interested persons, whether it would serve justice or national security, and whether it would impede the effective questioning of the witness by an interested person or his representative.[93]

Admission of documentary evidence

There is no provision in the rules for the taking on commission of the evidence of a potential witness.[94] However, there is an alternative to calling a witness to give live evidence. *Written* evidence (such as a letter, report or statement) is admissible in four quite different situations. Three are provided by the statutory rules, and one by the common law. These powers to admit written evidence are not confined to evidence from witnesses who are ill, but extend to all kinds of witnesses, whether present in court or not.   **12–30**

The first situation concerns written evidence from a living person as to who the deceased was, and how, when and where he came by his death. This is admissible if *any* of four conditions is or are satisfied.[95] They are (a) the maker cannot give evidence at the inquest hearing at all or within a reasonable time;[96] (b) there is a good and sufficient reason to believe that the maker will not attend the inquest hearing;[97] (c) there is a good and sufficient reason why the maker should not attend the inquest hearing;[98] (d) the evidence is unlikely to be disputed.[99]   **12–31**

But, before admitting such evidence (whether in full or as redacted), the coroner must announce at the inquest hearing (not necessarily at the beginning)[100] the nature of the evidence, the full name of the maker, and that any interested person may see a copy if he so wishes, and may object to its admission.[101] The express terms of these provisions are silent as to whether the objection by an interested   **12–32**

---

[88] See *R v North Humberside Coroner, ex p Jamieson* [1995] QB 1, 26, (14).
[89] Coroners (Inquests) Rules 2013 (SI 2013/1616) r.17(4).
[90] This does not include the inquest opening: 10–09.
[91] Coroners (Inquests) Rules 2013 (SI 2013/1616) r.17(1).
[92] Coroners (Inquests) Rules 2013 (SI 2013/1616) r.17(2); *Chief Coroner's Guide to the Coroners and Justice Act 2009*, [135]–[136].
[93] Coroners (Inquests) Rules 2013 (SI 2013/1616) r.17(3).
[94] Unlike in High Court and county court proceedings: CPR rr.34.8–34.12.
[95] Coroners (Inquests) Rules 2013 (SI 2013/1616) r.23(1).
[96] Coroners (Inquests) Rules 2013 (SI 2013/1616) r.23(1)(a).
[97] Coroners (Inquests) Rules 2013 (SI 2013/1616) r.23(1)(b).
[98] Coroners (Inquests) Rules 2013 (SI 2013/1616) r.23(1)(c).
[99] Coroners (Inquests) Rules 2013 (SI 2013/1616) r.23(1)(d).
[100] cf. Coroners Rules 1984 r.37(3) (repealed).
[101] Coroners (Inquests) Rules 2013 (SI 2013/1616) r.23(2), formerly Coroners Rules 1984 r.37(3). The need to observe the formalities in the old rules was emphasised in *R. v City of London Coroner Ex p. Calvi, The Times,* April 20, 1983, DC; *R. v West Berkshire Coroner Ex p. Thomas* (1991) 155 J.P. 681, DC; *R. (Sutovic) v North London Coroner* [2006] EWHC 1095 (Admin.), DC; *Howlett v Devon Coroner* [2006] EWHC 2570 (Admin.).

person to the admission of written evidence can be overridden by the coroner, as it could under the previous regime.[102] In the context of an intended liberalisation of the position, this would be a surprising result, and the better view must be that the objection *can* be so overridden.[103]

12–33 The second situation is where the coroner is of the opinion that a document made by a deceased person (not necessarily the deceased whose death is the subject of the inquest) is relevant to the purposes of the inquest. In this case the coroner has no discretion:[104] he *must* admit the document as evidence, and despite objection by any interested person. In further contrast with the first category of documentary evidence, there are *no* requirements as to formalities before he does so.

12–34 In relation to either the first or the second category of case, the coroner may do one of two things. First, he may redact the document to exclude irrelevant material. A coroner might properly redact a suicide note, for example, to omit material not bearing on the questions relevant to the inquest.[105] Indeed, in some cases he may have to, in order to comply with art.8 of the European Convention on Human Rights.[106] Second, he may direct that all or parts only of the written evidence (whether in full or as redacted) be read aloud at the inquest hearing.[107]

12–35 The third situation is where the coroner considers that the findings of an inquiry[108] are relevant to the purposes of the inquest.[109] In that case the coroner may admit them, after announcing (not necessarily at the beginning of the inquest hearing) that they may be admitted as evidence, giving details of the inquiry, date of publication and a brief account of the findings, and that any interested person is entitled to see a copy.[110] There is no provision for any objection by an interested persons, and no requirement that the findings be read aloud.[111]

12–36 The fourth situation is where the maker of the document, or some other person who has had sufficient contact with it to be able to produce it to the court, is present at the inquest. In this case that person can be called to put it in evidence.[112] Alternatively, if the document records an interview between two or more persons, and a person other than the maker was present, that other person can give evidence of what was said.[113] In such cases, there is no need to rely on the statutory provisions.

---

[102] Coroners Rules 1984 r.37(2) (repealed); see *R. (Butler) v Black Country District* [2010] EWHC 43 (Admin.) at [76].

[103] See the *Chief Coroner's Guide to the Coroners and Justice Act 2009*, [139]–[142].

[104] In contrast with the old rule: see e.g. *Re Palmer's Application* Unreported December 10, 1997, CA.

[105] cf. Home Office Circular No. 53 of 1980 para.14.

[106] See 21–29 ff below.

[107] Coroners (Inquests) Rules 2013 (SI 2013/1616) r.23(4), formerly Coroners Rules 1984 r.37(6).

[108] Including an inquiry under the Inquiries Act 2005.

[109] Coroners (Inquests) Rules 2013 (SI 2013/1616) r.24(1), formerly Coroners Rules 1984 r.37A(1).

[110] Coroners (Inquests) Rules 2013 (SI 2013/1616) r.24(2), formerly Coroners Rules 1984 r.37A(2). cf. 12–90, fn.251 and Chief Coroner's Guidance No. 13.

[111] cf. Coroners Rules 1984 r.37A(3) (repealed).

[112] *Assistant Deputy Coroner for Inner West London v Paul and Ritz Hotel* [2007] EWCA Civ. 1259.

[113] *R. v Lincoln Coroner Ex p.Hay* [2000] Lloyd's Rep. Med. 264, DC.

Witness evidence to be given on oath or affirmation

It was formerly held that an inquisition would not be quashed on the grounds that [114] at any rate unless it appeared **12–37** that the verdict has been influenced by such unsworn evidence.[115] But now every witness providing evidence at an inquest hearing[116] (including one giving evidence by video-link)[117] shall be examined by the coroner on oath or affirmation,[118] except that a child under 14 years or one who is considered by the coroner to be unable to understand the nature of an oath or affirmation may on promising to tell the truth be permitted to give unsworn evidence.[119]

Form of oath

The form of oath for use by a witness was prescribed under the old rules[120] but not **12–38** under the new. In practice it will be the same. But it will need modification in the case of a person who desires to affirm[121] or to be sworn in the Scottish form.[122] In general a witness may take whatever form of oath he deems to be binding upon him.[123] The questions for the court are simply (a) whether the oath appears to the court to be one binding on the witness's conscience, and (b) whether it is one which the witness considers to be so binding.[124]

A Christian is sworn upon the New Testament, a Jew upon the Old **12–39** Testament.[125] In the case of a person who is neither Christian nor Jew, the oath is to be administered "in any lawful manner".[126] In the case of a Muslim this would normally[127] involve holding a copy of the Koran, in the case of a Hindu, the Gita, in the case of a Sikh, the Adi Grantu, and in the case of other religions their respective sacred books.[128]

Where a copy of the relevant holy book is not available, it is probably better for **12–40** the witness to affirm rather than to use another book.[129] Coroners should accommodate requests from witnesses from some religions who ask to be able to

---

[114] *R. v Ingham* (1864) 5 B. & S. 257, 122 E.R. 827.

[115] *R. v Staffordshire Coroner* (1864) 10 L.T. 650; *R. v Divine Ex p. Walton* [1930] 2 K.B. 29 at 36.

[116] This appears not to apply to a person who merely produces a document to the court pursuant to a coroner's notice (see 7–14) or witness summons, without being examined: *Summers v Moseley* (1834) 2 Cr. & M. 477; *Perry v Gibson* (1834) 1 Ad. & El. 48; *Rush v Smith* (1834) 1 Cr. M. & R. 94.

[117] *R v Sharman* [1998] 1 Cr. App.R. 406; [1998] 1 F.L.R. 785 (not a coroner's case).

[118] Coroners (Inquests) Rules 2013 (SI 2013/1616) r.20(1), formerly Coroners Act 1988 s.11(2), replacing the Coroners Act 1887 s.4(1).

[119] Coroners (Inquests) Rules 2013 (SI 2013/1616) r.20(2).

[120] Coroners Rules 1984 Sch.4 Form 9 (repealed).

[121] Oaths Act 1978 ss.5, 6: see App.3 Form 15. As to questioning a person who desires to affirm, see *R. v Mehrban* [2002] 1 Cr.App.R. 561; [2002] EWCA Crim. 2627.

[122] Oaths Act 1978 s.3: see App.3 Form 14.

[123] Oaths Act 1978 s.4(1). The fact that a witness to whom an oath was administered had at the time of taking the oath no religious belief does not affect the validity of the oath; Oaths Act 1978 s.4(2).

[124] *R. v Kemble* (1990) 91 Cr.App.R. 178, CA (criminal trial).

[125] Oaths Act 1978 s.1(1).

[126] Oaths Act 1978 s.1(3).

[127] But not all adherents use these works.

[128] See *Phipson on Evidence,* 18th edn (2013) para.9–34.

[129] See para.4 of the Judicial Studies Board *Occasional Paper 1: Oaths and Oath-taking* (November 11, 1992), sent to coroners with Home Office Newsletter No. 20, dated April 4, 1996.

wash their hands (or other parts of the body) before taking the oath,[130] or who ask to remove their shoes and cover their heads when taking the oath.[131]

A witness who has taken an oath or affirmed is liable to a charge of perjury

12–41   When a witness has taken or affected to take an oath, or has affirmed,[132] he becomes liable to a charge of perjury upon its violation. It should be noted, however, that perjury can be committed only in relation to evidence that is material to the coroner's inquiry.[133] Provision is made for the coroner (since he is a person presiding in a court of record) to order the prosecution of a witness for perjury and then and there to commit him for trial and grant bail.[134] But this course should seldom, if ever, be taken. It is desirable that any question of such importance as a prosecution for perjury should be investigated and considered by the police and the Crown Prosecution Service before proceedings are taken.

Witnesses not sufficiently fluent to take oath in English

12–42   If a witness professes or appears not to understand the English language, he should be examined through an interpreter. The interpreter is sworn[135] well and truly to interpret the oath and the questions which will be put to the witness by the coroner (and jury), and also the answers which the witness gives.[136] In non-contentious cases, a coroner may ask a friend or relative of the witness to interpret. Indeed, if the coroner is sitting alone, and is proficient in the language, an interpreter may not be needed at all. But the coroner in such a case should always say out loud (in English)[137] what he understands by the witness's words, and should not act as an interpreter for others' questions.

12–43   In other cases the interpreter is a professional, paid according to the schedule of fees.[138] At inquests held in Wales, any persons (and not merely witnesses) may use the Welsh language if they wish.[139] But if the coroner uses Welsh he will have to repeat himself in English for the benefit of any non-Welsh speaker in court. An interpreter may also be needed to enable interested persons to play a full part in the proceedings, especially where Article 2 of the European Convention on Human Rights is engaged.[140]

---

[130] Judicial Studies Board Occasional Paper 1: *Oaths and Oath-taking* para.7.

[131] Judicial Studies Board Occasional Paper 1: *Oaths and Oath-taking* para.8.

[132] There may be cases where it is permissible for a witness who might have been expected to take the oath but who in fact affirmed to be cross-examined on why he did so: *R. v Mehrban* [2002] 1 Cr.App.R. 561; [2002] EWCA Crim. 2627 (criminal trial).

[133] Perjury Act 1911 s.1.

[134] Perjury Act 1911 s.9.

[135] See 12–38 ff.

[136] For a form of oath see App.3 Form 16.

[137] At least in England.

[138] See Home Office Circular No. 176 of 1955 para.11. For the schedule of fees, see 18–36 below. They should be treated as expert witnesses and hence compensated in the coroner's discretion pursuant to para.(3) of the Schedule: essentially an interpreter uses expert skill to interpret primary facts (i.e. what the witness says in a foreign language) for the court.

[139] Welsh Language Act 1993 s.22(1); see also ss.23 (translations of oaths and affirmations) and 24 (provision of interpreters).

[140] See 21–18.

Order of witnesses

The actual order of calling the witnesses lies entirely within the discretion of the **12–44**
coroner.[141] It is usual and proper for the first witness to be the one who is to give
evidence of the identification of the deceased, if the body has been identified, or
the witness who can speak to the finding of the body, if it is unidentified. It is also
common for a person whose conduct may be called into question (e.g. in a road
accident inquest, the driver of the vehicle concerned) to give evidence last. Subject
to that, it is usually found convenient to follow a more or less regular or expected
order, so that the evidence of the witnesses is given as far as may be in the same
chronological order as the actual occurrence of the events.

Thus, in any inquest arising from a street accident, after the identifying witness **12–45**
had been called first, there may be called the witness (who is often a police officer)
who has prepared a plan or produced photographs of the scene of the accident (as
is often done); he would be followed by independent witnesses, so far as possible
in an order which gives point to their successive accounts of the occurrence. They
may be followed by the police officer who attended (if one did), who can describe
the scene as he found it. If a gap in the evidence is revealed at the hearing, there
should be an adjournment to obtain such evidence, even if this is inconvenient.[142]

Medical evidence may present a problem. Where the only such evidence is from **12–46**
a pathologist, his opinion as to the cause of death will usually be enhanced in
difficult or borderline cases by his giving evidence last (or perhaps penultimately),
after all the evidence of fact has been given. After all, his evidence in court is not
confined to his opinion on matters arising out of his examination of the body
(which might exclude listening to other evidence), but extends to the wider
question of how the deceased came by his death.[143]

However, care must be taken, for if he does revise his opinion from that **12–47**
expressed in his post-mortem examination report, interested persons who have
seen the report before the inquest may have grounds for complaining that the
inquest hearing was conducted on a false basis.[144] This is usually avoided by
requiring the pathologist to notify the coroner if he changes his opinion before the
hearing.[145] If the change of mind occurs during the hearing, it may in some cases
be necessary to adjourn the inquest to obtain further expert evidence on the
point.[146]

On the other hand, in cases where there is a danger of the examination of **12–48**
witnesses being taken unnecessarily into irrelevant areas, it may be helpful in trying
to concentrate the evidence on the important points to take the pathologist's
evidence at or near the beginning.[147] The disadvantage of this course is that it
involves the pathologist in making assumptions as to (possibly disputed) matters of

---

[141] *Re Devine and Breslin's Application* [1998] 14 N.I.J.B. 10, HC (NI).
[142] *R. v Southwark Coroner Ex p.Hicks* [1987] 1 W.L.R. 1624, DC.
[143] cf. Coroners Act 1988 s.20(2) (repealed).
[144] *R. v Maidstone Coroner's Court Ex p. Johnstone* (1994) 158 J.P. 1115, DC.
[145] cf. *The Ikarian Reefer* [1993] 2 Lloyd's Rep. 68 at 82.
[146] *R. v Maidstone Coroner's Court Ex p.Johnstone* (1994) 158 J.P. 1115, DC.
[147] e.g. whether the deceased was struck on the head by another person, or fell to the floor and hit his
head.

fact *before* the relevant witnesses have given evidence.[148] In addition it is unsatisfactory for the jury to hear "evidence" of the facts for the first time in the assumptions made by (or instructions given to) the pathologist.[149] If there are other experts to give evidence they cannot in practice do so until the factual witnesses have been heard,[150] and the pathologist will normally give his evidence then as well.

Attendance of witnesses in court until called

12–49   Unless there is likely to be a conflict of evidence, or credible evidence of collusion, or there is some other proper objection, it is usual for witnesses at an inquest to sit in court until they are called to give evidence.[151] After giving evidence, witnesses may be released by the coroner, and may then leave the court. If not released, witnesses should remain in court.

12–50   Other than in wholly exceptional circumstances, a formal, professional or scientific witness is never excluded before giving evidence. Normally, neither is any person whose conduct may be called into question. Indeed, the usual course is that all witnesses are present and in a position to hear what is said throughout. The decision whether witnesses hear other evidence lies in the coroner's discretion.[152]

Exclusion of witness whose evidence may conflict or is likely to be tested

12–51   A difficulty can arise where there is likely to be a conflict of evidence, or credible evidence of collusion, or it is desired to test evidence to be given by each of several witnesses in a group, and it is sought to exclude those witnesses from court before giving evidence, although their conduct may be brought into question. In such a case the coroner's statutory duty to find out the truth must prevail over any apparent unfairness to individual witnesses.[153] It must be remembered that a coroner has a duty to adjourn the inquest if he considers from the evidence given that a person may be charged with one of certain criminal offences.[154]

Privilege of jury to recall witnesses

12–52   Subject to the overriding discretion of the coroner to ensure a properly conducted and fair proceeding, it is the privilege of the jurors, at any time during the investigation, to call back before them and to re-examine any witness who has

---

[148] *Alpina Zurich Insurance Co v Bain Clarkson Ltd, The Times,* January 23, 1989; see also *The Ikarian Reefer* [1993] 2 Lloyd's Rep. 68 at 81 (expert opinion should state the factual assumptions on which it is based).

[149] Indeed, at common law the strict rule of evidence was that an expert could not give hearsay evidence of the facts forming the basis of his opinion *(English Exporters (London) Ltd v Eldonwell Ltd* [1973] Ch. 415; *R. v Abadom* [1983] I W.L.R. 126, CA), which facts must be strictly proved by direct evidence *(R. v Jackson* [1996] 2 Cr.App.R. 420, CA).

[150] See e.g. *Alpina Zurich Insurance Co v Bain Clarkson Ltd, The Times,* January 23, 1989; *Chancery Guide* para.9.17; *Commercial Court Guide* para.H2.31; Phipson, *Evidence,* 18th edn (2013) para.33–42.

[151] cf. *Moore v Lambeth County Court Registrar* [1969] 1 W.L.R. 141 at 142, CA (county court); *Tomlinson v Tomlinson* [1980] 1 W.L.R. 322 (magistrates' court).

[152] *Re Devine and Breslin's Application* [1988] 14 N.I.J.B. 10, 26, HC (NI), Carswell J.

[153] cf. *R. v Surrey Coroner Ex p.Campbell* [1982] Q.B. 661 at 676. But a witness excluded from court beforehand may be more inclined to rely on the right to refuse to answer potentially incriminating questions.

[154] See 11–47 ff above.

already been examined, in order to ask further questions, perhaps arising out of other evidence[155] (but if the witness has been released, it is, strictly speaking, necessary to re-summon him formally).

Witness in custody

The procedure for summoning a witness in custody has already been discussed.[156] **12–53** The question whether such a witness should give evidence whilst manacled or handcuffed is one for the coroner alone, and not for the police or prison authorities.[157] Particularly where a jury is involved, the witness should not be seen to be under restraint in giving evidence.[158] Usually it is possible to provide sufficient security by other means.[159]

Procedure for examination

Unless the coroner otherwise determines, a witness at an inquest must be examined **12–54** first by the coroner, then by any interested person who has asked to examine him, and lastly, if the witness is represented at the inquest, by the representative.[160]

Examination by coroner. The coroner will probably have before him a **12–55** statement by, or about, the witness, on which to base his questions and it is usual for him to conduct the first (and most important) examination. The coroner should permit the witness to read his statement before giving evidence.[161] If there is any inconsistency between the written statement of a witness and his oral evidence, and the interested persons are not aware of the inconsistency, the coroner must explore and deal with it himself.[162]

Because the inquest is an inquiry, rather than litigation, the examination is **12–56** neither an examination-in-chief nor a cross-examination.[163] Nevertheless, on contentious matters, the coroner should avoid asking leading questions which suggest the answer,[164] although he may of course direct the witness's attention to a particular subject. For the same reason, he should not read a witness's statement out and then ask the witness whether he or she adopts it. Previous inconsistent statements may be put to the witness.[165] Before asking questions about sensitive subjects such as previous convictions of the deceased, the coroner should inform interested persons of his intentions (in the absence of the jury, if there is one).[166]

---

[155] cf. *R. v Sullivan* [1923] 1 K.B. 47; *R. v McKenna* (1956) 40 Cr.App.R. 65; *Phelan v Black* [1972] 1 W.L.R. 273, DC (all criminal cases).
[156] See 10–29.
[157] *R. v Cambridgeshire Justices Ex p.Peacock* (1992) 152 J.P. 895, DC (criminal case).
[158] *R. v Mullen* [2000] Crim.L.R. 873, CA (criminal case).
[159] *R. v Mullen* [2000] Crim.L.R. 873, CA.
[160] Coroners (Inquests) Rules 2013 (SI 2013/1616) r.21; formerly Coroners Rules 1984 r.21.
[161] *R. v Davies* [2011] EWCA Crim. 871 [69] (criminal appeal, but dealing with what happened at inquest).
[162] *Re Cohen* (1993) 158 J.P. 644, DC.
[163] See 12–61 below.
[164] cf. the Brodrick Report, paras 16–29—16–70.
[165] Criminal Procedure Act 1865 ss.3–5 (which apply also to inquests.).
[166] *R. (Stanley) v Inner North London Coroner* [2003] EWHC 1180 (Admin.) at [52].

12–57   At the beginning of such examination the coroner should ascertain or check the name and occupation of the witness[167] and, if he is the identifying witness, the registrable particulars of the deceased.[168] These details should normally be given openly,[169] though there may be cases (e.g. where there is a reasonable fear of retaliation)[170] in which a witness's details can be written down and passed to the coroner.[171] The coroner has power, in appropriate cases, to permit witnesses not to be fully identified and to give evidence shielded from public view (but not from that of the coroner, the jury or the lawyers) by screens.[172] It is, however, wrong to take evidence in private.[173]

12–58   **Examination by interested persons.** After the coroner's examination is concluded, the coroner must allow any interested person[174] who so requests to examine the witness either in person or by his or her representative.[175] If it is appropriate to the room in which the inquest is being held, the examiner should stand up to ask his questions. It is not clear whether an interested person should be permitted to cross-examine a witness who gives evidence *favourable* to that person.[176] In principle, since an inquest is an inquiry and not litigation,[177] the better view is to allow any question that is relevant and proper.[178]

12–59   Unless the coroner otherwise determines, the witness's own representative (if he has one) should examine him last of all.[179] If there are other interested persons, the coroner must decide on the order in which they should examine the witness, although very often they or their representatives can agree amongst themselves as to this.

12–60   If an interested person who is not represented by counsel or a solicitor wishes to ask questions, the coroner may have to assist in their formulation. An inability on the part of an interested person to examine witnesses is not a ground for complaint if it arises because he and his legal representative have withdrawn in protest at an allegedly wrong decision by the coroner.[180]

---

[167] *Re Jordan's Application* Unreported June 28, 1996, CA (NI); there have been rare cases where this did not happen: e.g. the SAS soldiers involved in the Iranian embassy siege in 1980 remained unidentified (even to the coroner) throughout the subsequent inquest.

[168] See 13–115 below.

[169] *R. v Evesham Justices Ex p. McDonagh* [1988] Q.B. 553, DC; *Re Ian Bennett, The Independent*, April 28, 1992 (West Yorkshire coroner).

[170] See *Re Colin Atkins and Dale Robson, The Times*, February 2, 1991.

[171] See 12–23; as to power to withhold such details from the public, see 11–73, 11–74 above.

[172] See 12–26 ff.

[173] *Matthews v Hunter* [1993] 2 N.Z.L.R. 683, HC (NZ).

[174] See 8–21 above.

[175] Coroners (Inquests) Rules 2013 (SI 2013/1616) rr.19(1), 21(b).

[176] See *Dryden v Surrey CC* [1936] 2 All E.R. 535 at 538; *Sierra 4 v Moles* Unreported March 31, 1994, Sup. Ct. Tas.

[177] See 1–19.

[178] cf. 12–63, 12–66.

[179] Coroners (Inquests) Rules 2013 (SI 2013/1616) r.21(c); formerly Coroners Rules 1984 r.21.

[180] *R. v East Sussex Coroner Ex p. Homberg* Unreported June 14, 1993, DC, and subsequently (1994) 158 J.P. 357. See also *Re Arthurs' Application for Judicial Review* Unreported May 24, 1996, HC (NI).

Examination in inquisitorial proceedings

In exercising the right to examine a witness, regard must be had to the inquisitorial   **12–61**
nature of the proceedings: an inquest is not a trial. Thus, in one case, the judge
said:

> "It is quite true that the coroner must allow interested parties to examine a
> witness called by the coroner. But that must be for the purpose of assisting in
> establishing the matters which the inquest is directed to determine. It is not
> intended by rule 16 [now rule 19] to widen the coroner's inquest into adversarial
> fields of conflict."[181]

Another judge, extra-curially, has said: **12–62**

> "In an inquisitorial Inquiry, the questioning of the witnesses by the Inquiry is
> not an examination-in-chief, nor is it a cross-examination. Hearsay evidence
> may be sought. Opinions, whether or not expert, may be sought. Questions to
> which the questioner does not know the answer will frequently be asked—and,
> indeed, will be asked *because* the questioner does not know the answer. The
> techniques of questioning witnesses in adversarial litigation can be set aside. The
> questioning process is, or should be, a part of a thorough investigation to
> determine the truth. It is not a process designated either to promote or to
> demolish a 'case'."[182]

Improper or irrelevant questions, insulting behaviour, unfounded accusations

It should be noted that the coroner has a positive duty to disallow any question   **12–63**
which he considers to be irrelevant.[183] Relevance is of course to be established by
reference to the proper scope of the investigation.[184] In addition, the coroner
should protect witnesses from humiliating, intimidating or abusive questions.[185]

A further problem is that of behaviour by interested persons or their advocates   **12–64**
which goes beyond proper limits, to become insulting or belligerent, or which
involves unfounded accusations of bias or discrimination. The coroner, like any
other judicial officer, must be prepared for this, and be able to rise above it. Hasty
words said in the heat of the moment can often be simply ignored. Where the
tension rises too far, it may be defused by a short adjournment. Sometimes an
invitation to the person concerned to withdraw the comments if they cannot be
justified solves the problem; if the comments are withdrawn, the hearing can
normally continue. A coroner should avoid making an immediate order without

---

[181] *R. v Hammersmith Coroner Ex p. Peach* [1980] Q.B. 211, 220, per Griffiths J; *R. v Secretary of State Ex p. Devine* Unreported September 9, 1988, HC (NI), Carswell J.; *R. v Derby Coroner Ex p. Hart* (2000) 164 J.P. 429 at [95], [99].
[182] Sir Richard Scott, VC, "Procedures at Inquiries—the Duty to be Fair" (1995) 111 L.Q.R. 596 at 610.
[183] Coroners (Inquests) Rules 2013 (SI 2013/1616) r.19(2); formerly Coroners Rules 1984 r.20(1), proviso (b).
[184] As to which see Ch.6.
[185] cf. *R. v Brown* [1998] 2 Cr.App.R. 364, CA (criminal case).

giving the person concerned an opportunity to reflect, and in particular on what the coroner has in mind to do. The most important thing is not to overreact.[186]

Examination by legal representative

12–65   All that said, it is nonetheless perfectly proper for a legal representative to test opinions given in evidence, and to suggest that a witness is wrong.[187] Moreover, he is entitled to inspect any document used by the witness to refresh his memory;[188] if neither the coroner nor the witness has it in his possession at the court, the coroner may require production of the document by means of a witness notice.[189] Inspecting a document used to refresh memory does not normally put it into evidence.[190]

The propriety of questions in examination

12–66   As to the propriety of particular questions, a coroner must be careful not to allow the inquisitorial nature of the proceedings to become oppressive and an intrusion into the privacy of individuals' lives.[191] For example, in suicide cases the coroner should not as a matter of course extend his enquiries into a general or detailed survey of the matrimonial or financial problems of the deceased, even though in exceptional cases this might properly be considered relevant to intent.

12–67   In some cases, criminal convictions of the deceased may be relevant and so admissible in evidence,[192] but in others they may be irrelevant and so inadmissible.[193] Similarly, information as to the decision of the CPS to prosecute or not to prosecute persons involved in the death may sometimes be relevant, and irrelevant at others. But even if relevant it may be so prejudicial that it should not be admitted.[194] At the same time it is quite proper, and not an abuse of power, for the police to examine witnesses in aid of the inquest process in order to investigate suspected crime.[195]

12–68   Other kinds of questions which may be improper are those which are designed, not so much to elicit the true facts relating to the death in question, but to provide a platform for the airing of particular (often political) views not directly connected with it or for criticising the behaviour of particular persons or organisations.

Seeking justification where relevance is unclear

12–69   Where the coroner considers that a question may not be relevant or proper, he should seek a justification for it, or for the line of questioning of which it forms part, and should not permit the examination to continue until the matter has been

---

[186] *Bennett v Southwark LBC* [2002] I.R.L.R. 407, CA (civil case); Davies [2002] 13 L.S.Gaz. 29.
[187] *Re Adam Bithell* (1986) 150 J.P. 273.
[188] *Re McKerr's Application (No. 2)* [1993] N.I. 249, CA (NI); *Senat v Senat* [1965] P. 172 at 177 (civil case).
[189] See 7–14.
[190] cf. *R. v Virgo* (1978) 67 Cr.App.R. 232, CA (criminal case).
[191] See Ch.6. Cf., e.g. *Tristram v The Moon Life Assurance Co* in Herbert, *Uncommon Law* (1969), p.261.
[192] *R. v Inner South London Coroner Ex p. Fields* (1998) 162 J.P. 411.
[193] *R. (Stanley) v Inner North London Coroner* [2003] EWHC 1180 (Admin.), Silber J.
[194] cf. *R. (Stanley) v Inner North London Coroner* [2003] EWHC 1180 (Admin.), Silber J, where two police officers had shot and killed the deceased in alleged self-defence.
[195] *R. v Derby Coroner Ex p.Hart* (2000) 164 J.P. 429, Newman J at [119]–[120].

resolved. If the inquest is being held with a jury, it is usually better that they retire during the argument, so that they are not influenced by matters or questions which ultimately it may be decided that they ought not to hear.[196] Where the issue of relevance or propriety is raised, a careful note must be made, not only of the question or questions concerned, but also of the justification advanced and of the coroner's decision upon the matter.

EVIDENCE

Common law restrictions

At common law there were considerable restrictions on the types and forms of **12–70** evidence that could be received by a court of law. Those restrictions were largely, if not entirely, the result of the accusatorial nature of both civil and criminal proceedings, whereby one party put forward a series of pre-formed allegations against another party and then proceeded to try and prove them, and of the nature of the consequences that would flow from success or failure in so doing. In recent years many of those restrictions have disappeared, both in civil and in criminal proceedings.

The requirements of an inquisitorial process

In theory at least, the coroner's inquest, being an *inquisitorial* proceeding, designed **12–71** for the coroner (and his jury) to start with no preconceptions and to elicit the true facts regarding the incident in question, had no need for such restrictions. The aim was to find out that objective truth in the public interest, and not the limited "truth" as between and for the purposes of two or more parties.[197]

The result is that the coroner's court has never been bound by the strict laws of **12–72** evidence.[198] In particular, this means that "hearsay" evidence, even of a documentary nature,[199] can be admitted.[200] It should also mean that opinion evidence can be admitted, even in cases where it would not have been at common law.[201] This can be compared with the exercise of the paternal jurisdiction in relation to wards of court, children and mental patients, which again is not accusatorial in

---

[196] cf. *R. v East Berkshire Coroner Ex p.Buckley* (1992) 157 J.P. 425, DC (submissions of law ought to be made to coroner in jury's absence).

[197] Sir Richard Scott, VC, "Procedures at Inquiries—the Duty to be Fair" (1995) 111 L.Q.R. 596, at 605.

[198] *R. v Davies, The Times*, March 18, 1890, per Wills J; *R. v Divine Ex p. Walton* [1930] 2 K.B. 29 at 36; *R. v South London Coroner Ex p. Thompson, The Times*, July 9, 1982, DC; *R. v Greater Manchester Coroner Ex p. Tal* [1985] Q.B. 67 at 84.

[199] As to the procedural rules governing the admissibility of documentary hearsay, see 12–30 ff, 12–101 ff

[200] *R. v Greater Manchester Coroner Ex p. Tal* [1985] Q.B. 67, 84-85; *R. v Attorney-General for Northern Ireland Ex p. Devine* [1992] 1 W.L.R. 262, HL; *R. v Lincoln Coroner Ex p. Hay* [2002] Lloyd's Rep. Med. 264, DC.

[201] e.g. where the rule in *Hollington v Hewthorn* applies: see 12–90.

nature, and where the courts have the power to receive and act upon evidence not complying with the strict rules for accusatorial proceedings.[202]

Historical power to charge with homicide offence

12–73   Until 1977 it was possible for a coroner's inquisition to charge a named person with a homicide offence, such as murder.[203] The inquisition did not determine guilt or innocence, but merely—like the old grand jury, or examining justices-—whether there was a case to answer.[204] This meant that a suspected person attending a coroner's court could not be considered a party accused (and therefore the proceedings were not criminal proceedings) until *after* a verdict had been found against him.[205] Nonetheless the proceedings might take on an accusatorial air, and in practice coroners tended more or less to follow the restrictions on evidence observed in criminal courts.

Verdict framed so as not to determine issues of liability

12–74   Whatever the theory of the matter, however, since 1977 the possibility of an inquisition operating so as to charge a person with any offence has disappeared.[206] The determination (formerly verdict) nowadays must be framed so as not to appear to determine any question of criminal liability of a named person or any question of civil liability.[207] It may therefore be considered less important now for the coroner to be bound by the restrictive rules of evidence: the purpose of the inquiry is to find out certain facts about the deceased, in the public interest, and nothing more. But some judges persist in measuring the conduct of inquests against criminal trials,[208] and in any event the use of words such as "neglect" is sometimes argued to offend against the principle.[209]

Outlines of rules of evidence

12–75   But in matters of evidence, as in others, a coroner must act in a manner which is fair,[210] and just because particular evidence (e.g. double hearsay) is technically admissible, does not make it satisfactory in all circumstances.[211] It is therefore desirable for coroners to be aware of the main rules of evidence, so as to reduce so far as possible the number of occasions upon which it is necessary to depart from

---

[202] *Official Solicitor v K* [1965] A.C. 201, HL. Similarly with some statutory tribunals and other bodies: *R. v Commission for Racial Equality* [1980] 1 W.L.R. 1580; *R. v Deputy Industrial Commissioner Ex p. Moore* [1965] 1 Q.B. 456. See also *Re L (A Minor)* [1997] A.C. 16, HL.

[203] See 1–28 above.

[204] *R. v Davies, The Times,* March 18, 1890, per Wills J, reprinted in the 7th edn (1927), of this work, pp.254–256, the 8th edn (1946), pp.296–298, and the 9th edn (1957), pp.508–510.

[205] *Wakley v Cooke* (1849) 4 Exch. 511 at 518.

[206] See 1–28 above.

[207] Coroners and Justice Act 2009 s.10(2); formerly Coroners Rules 1984 r.42; 12–112, 13–57, 13–103.

[208] E.g. *Clayton v South Yorkshire Coroner* [2005] EWHC 1196 (Admin.) at [9]; *R. (Sharman) v Inner North London Coroner* [2005] EWCA Civ. 967 at [34]; *R. v Davies* [2011] EWCA Civ. 871. cf. *R. (Bennett) v Inner South London Coroner* [2007] EWCA Civ 617.

[209] See 13–34, 13–103.

[210] *Re McKerr's Application (No. 2)* [1993] N.I. 249, CA (NI); *R. v Avon Coroner Ex p. Bentley, The Times,* March 23, 2001.

[211] *Re Sutherland* [1994] 2 N.Z.L.R. 342 at 347, HC (NZ).

them. Consequently, there now follows a (necessarily brief) outline of the major rules on the admissibility of evidence at common law.[212]

Relevant facts to be proved by best evidence

First, it has long been a general principle that any fact that is relevant and in evidence should be proved by the best evidence: that is, if a particular person has heard some admissible statement, or has made or seen some relevant event occur, evidence as to this should come from him. Similarly, if it is desirable to produce a document in evidence, it is necessary to produce the original document, unless it can be proved not to be available, when secondary evidence of its contents may be given.[213] But the "best evidence" rule, like so many fundamentals of the English law of evidence, has been so whittled down by exceptions that is is unclear how far it remains a principle today at all.[214]

12–76

Only relevant evidence is admissible

Secondly, *all* evidence relevant to issues before the court is admissible, and *only* that evidence. All irrelevant evidence should be excluded.[215] For this purpose "relevant" means that

12–77

> "any two facts to which it is applied are so related to each other that according to the common course of events one either taken by itself or in connection with other facts proves or renders probable the past, present, or future existence nor non-existence of the other."[216]

Exceptions to the general rule. But the general rule is subject to a number of important exceptions at common law, which exclude from the court's attention evidence which is relevant and otherwise admissible, such as hearsay, opinion, character, and evidence of conduct on other occasions. Evidence of marginal relevance, or obtained unfairly, or whose probative value is outweighed by its prejudicial effect, may also be excluded. It is important to notice that in both civil and criminal proceedings the common law rules of evidence have been considerably liberalised in recent years. But inquests are neither civil nor criminal proceedings, and the statutory changes do not apply to them.[217]

12–78

Hearsay evidence. From the coroner's point of view, the most important of these excluded categories is that for hearsay. With certain exceptions,[218] *oral*

12–79

---

[212] For a full treatment see *Cross & Tapper on Evidence,* 12th edn (2010); *Phipson on Evidence,* 18th edn (2013).
[213] *Brewster v Sewell* (1820) 3 B. & Ald. 296; 106 E.R. 672; *Mills v Oddy* (1834) 6 C. & P. 728; *Garton v Hunter* [1969] 2 Q.B. 37, CA.
[214] *Phipson on Evidence,* 18th edn (2013), paras 7-40–7-41.
[215] *Hollington v Hewthorn & Co Ltd* [1943] K.B. 587 at 594, per Goddard L.J.; *Cross & Tapper on Evidence,* 12th edn (2010), p.64.
[216] Stephen, *Digest of the Law of Evidence,* 12th edn, art.1; *Cross & Tapper on Evidence,* 12th edn (2010), p.65; *Phipson on Evidence,* 18th edn (2013), 7–08.
[217] See below 12–89.
[218] See the Police and Criminal Evidence Act 1984 Pt VIII.

hearsay evidence is still inadmissible in the criminal courts.[219] *Documentary* hearsay is now admissible in those courts under certain conditions.[220] By "hearsay" is meant an oral or written statement other than one made by a person giving oral evidence in the court proceedings in question: this is inadmissible as evidence of any fact or opinion expressed in the statement. Thus, a witness in the proceedings would not be permitted to relate what some other person was heard to say on an earlier occasion. However, the evidence of a person who saw a videotape recording has been held not to be hearsay evidence of the truth of the events which are there depicted.[221] Similarly with photographs,[222] audio recordings[223] and at least some computer records.[224]

12–80   The objections to the admissibility of hearsay at common law were summed up by Lord Normand as follows:

> "The rule against the admission of hearsay evidence is fundamental. It is not the best evidence, and it is not delivered on oath. The truthfulness and accuracy of the person whose words are spoken by another witness cannot be tested by cross-examination and the light which his demeanour would throw on his testimony is lost."[225]

12–81   It should be emphasised that the common law rule prohibits the adducing of hearsay evidence of a particular statement to prove the truth of facts contained in that statement: it does *not* prevent such evidence being adduced for any other purpose, such as proving that the statement was made at all,[226] or proving *what* the contents of the statement were[227] (as opposed to whether or not they were true), or what was the state of mind of the person making the statement at that time.[228]

12–82   **Exceptions to the hearsay rule.** It may be of assistance briefly to set out the exceptions to the strict hearsay rule at common law. The first is the principle of *"res gestae"*.[229] By this is meant that the statement, evidence of which is otherwise excluded by the hearsay rule, is so spontaneous and contemporaneous with facts and events which are the immediate subject of the legal proceedings in question as to preclude the possibility of concoction or distortion. These may be statements

---

[219] The rules are codified in the Criminal Justice Act 2003 Pt II c.2. Since the Civil Evidence Act 1986 there have been quite different (and more liberal) rules for civil proceedings on this subject: see now the Civil Evidence Act 1995; *Cross & Tapper on Evidence*, 12th edn (2010), Ch.XIII; *Phipson on Evidence*, 18th edn (2013), Ch.29.

[220] Criminal Justice Act 2003 ss.116-120. For the rules in coroners' courts, see 12–30—12–36.

[221] *Taylor v Chief Constable of Cheshire* [1986] 1 W.L.R. 1479.

[222] *R. v Tolson* (1864) 4 F. & F. 103.

[223] *R. v Ali and Hussain* [1966] 1 Q.B. 688, CCA.

[224] *R. v Wood* (1982) 76 Cr.App.R. 23, CA.

[225] *Teper v R.* [1952] A.C. 480 at 486; see also per Lord Bridge in *R. v Blastland* [1986] A.C. 41 at 54.

[226] *R. v Chapman* [1969] 2 Q.B. 346, CA.

[227] *R. v Willis* [1960] 1 W.L.R. 55, CCA; *Ratten v R.* [1972] A.C. 378, PC.

[228] *Subramaniam v Public Prosecutor* [1956] 1 W.L.R. 965, PC.

[229] This is preserved in criminal cases by the Criminal Justice Act 2003 s.118(1), category 4.

accompanying and explaining relevant acts,[230] spontaneous statements by participants in or observers of events,[231] or contemporaneous declarations of the physical or mental state of the speaker.[232] Where the statements fall into this category, hearsay evidence of them may be admitted for the purpose of proving the truth of their contents.[233]

The second exception relates to declarations made by persons who have since **12–83** died, being cases in which the application of the hearsay rule might be considered altogether unfortunate. Accordingly, hearsay evidence of certain categories of such declarations is admissible. These include declarations on matters of public concern, declarations made against the interest of the maker,[234] declarations made by persons which were recorded in the course of their duty so to act,[235] and dying declarations made by the victim of a homicide offence (though these are admissible only in relation to proceedings for such offence).[236]

A third exception at common law to the hearsay rule concerns statements made **12–84** in public documents. These are admissible evidence of the facts stated in them.[237] For this purpose, "public documents" includes public papers (such as royal proclamations or parliamentary papers; though not *Hansard*), public registers and records (such as birth, marriage and death registers), public inquisitions or surveys (such as a coroner's inquisition or determination, or the findings of a public inquiry), official certificates (e.g. from the government recognising a foreign state), company books, and published public works such as maps, dictionaries and scientific tables.

A fourth common law exception to the hearsay rule governs the admissibility of **12–85** informal admissions made by a party to proceedings against his own interest.[238] However, such admissions are evidence only against their maker and against any other person who may be affected by them. Admissions relevant to the question of guilt in criminal proceedings are usually called "confessions", and are subject to a stringent restriction on admissibility.

This is that, where a confession may have been obtained by oppression of the **12–86** person who made it, or in consequence of anything said or done which was likely to render unreliable any confession that might thereby be made, the confession is only admissible if it is proved that it was *not* so obtained.[239] For this purpose, a confession includes any statement wholly or partly adverse to the maker, whether

---

[230] *Rouch v Great Western Railway Co* (1841) 1 Q.B. 51: *R. v McCay* [1990] 1 W.L.R. 645, CA.

[231] *Ratten v R.* [1972] A.C. 378, PC; *R. v Andrews* [1987] A.C. 281, HL.

[232] *R. v Conde* (1868) 10 Cox C.C. 547.

[233] Although cf. Lord Atkinson in *R. v Christie* [1914] A.C. 545 at 553.

[234] *Coward v Motor Insurers' Bureau* [1963] 1 Q.B. 259.

[235] *Mills v Mills* (1920) 36 T.L.R. 772; *Simon v Simon* [1936] p.17; *R. v McGuire* (1985) 81 Cr.App.R. 323, CA.

[236] *R. v Woodcook* (1789) 1 Leach 500. This category is not preserved as such by the Criminal Justice Act 2003, but see s.116.

[237] *Irish Society v Bishop of Derry* (1846) 12 C. & F. 641; *Sturla v Freccia* (1880) 5 App. Cas. 623. This is preserved in criminal cases by the Criminal Justice Act 2003 s.118(1), category 1.

[238] This is preserved in criminal cases by the Criminal Justice Act 2003 s.118(1), category 5.

[239] Police and Criminal Evidence Act 1984 s.76.

made to a person in authority or not, and whether made in words or otherwise.[240]

12–87   The admissibility of a confession, if challenged, is tried as a preliminary issue[241] in a criminal trial by the judge alone in the absence of the jury. More stringent rules apply to confessions made by mentally handicapped persons.[242] Confessions must be distinguished from agreed or admitted facts (sometimes called "admissions"), which may be admitted at an inquest under the rules.[243]

12–88   The final common law exception to the hearsay rule to which it is necessary to refer is that which permits the reception of evidence of statements made in the presence of a party, in order to explain the reaction of that party to those statements or (if he admits their truth) to explain the adverse admissions being made.[244] A party's silence in the face of such statements will only exceptionally constitute an admission by the party of the truth of such statements.[245]

12–89   **Statutory exceptions to the hearsay rule.** Apart from the common law exceptions, there have been a number of minor exceptions made by statute[246] for the purposes of criminal proceedings. In relation to civil proceedings, on the other hand, the whole framework of the hearsay principle has been superseded by statute.[247] However, even if the hearsay principle applied, none of these statutory changes would be relevant for proceedings in coroners' courts.[248]

12–90   **Opinion evidence.**[249] The other main exceptions to the general rule that all relevant evidence is admissible at common law can be taken more shortly. Expert witnesses can give opinion evidence within the scope of their expertise. Opinion evidence given by non-experts is generally excluded because a non-expert witness may not give his opinion on matters calling for special expertise, and he may not give his opinion on other matters if the facts on which the opinion is based can be stated without reference to it in such a way as to lead equally well to discovery of

---

[240] Police and Criminal Evidence Act 1984 s.82(1); and see *Commissioners of Customs & Excise v Harz* [1967] 1 A.C. 760 at 817–818, per Lord Reid.

[241] The "voir dire", as it is called.

[242] Police and Criminal Evidence Act 1984 s.77.

[243] Coroners (Inquests) Rules, 2013 (SI 2013/1616) r.23; *Chief Coroner's Guide*, para.141.

[244] *R. v Christie* [1914] A.C. 545, HL. This category is not preserved by the Criminal Justice Act 2003.

[245] *Hall v R.* [1971] 1 W.L.R. 298, PC.

[246] Most recently by the Police and Criminal Evidence Act 1984, the Criminal Justice Act 1988, and the Criminal Procedure and Investigations Act 1996 s.68 and Sch.2, and the Criminal Justice Act 2003 Pt II.

[247] Civil Evidence Act 1995; *Cross & Tapper on Evidence,* 12th edn (2010) Ch.XIII; *Phipson on Evidence,* 18th edn (2013) Ch.29.

[248] The Civil Evidence Act 1995 does not apply because an inquest is not "civil proceedings before any tribunal, in relation to which the strict rules of evidence apply": Civil Evidence Act 1995 s.11. The Police and Criminal Evidence Act 1984 does not apply because an inquest is not "proceedings" within the meaning of ss.72(1) and 82(1) of that Act (both defining it as meaning "criminal proceedings": cf. *Wakley v Cooke* (1849) 4 Exch. 511). The Criminal Justice Act 2003 (so far as relates to hearsay) only applies to "criminal proceedings".

[249] See *Phipson on Evidence,* 18th edn (2013) Ch.33; *Cross & Tapper on Evidence,* 12th edn (2010) Ch.XI. Expert evidence is a category preserved in criminal cases by the Criminal Justice Act 2003 s.118(1) category 8.

the truth.[250] So at common law, decisions made by other courts or tribunals are not admissible because they represent the *opinion* of the judge or tribunal as to what happened, rather than direct evidence.[251]

Expert witnesses must provide the tribunal with all the necessary information to enable it independently to test the accuracy of their conclusions,[252] and it must be made clear how far a conclusion is subjective and based on experience or other factors which are expressed.[253] Experts do not give evidence of the *facts*, even though they refer to them as the basis of their opinions.[254] The facts must be established by direct evidence.[255]   **12–91**

Evidence as to character and behaviour. Finally, a person's character, and evidence of his behaviour on other occasions, may be thought relevant to the question whether he did a particular thing, the subject of the present proceedings, but in general it is not permitted to give evidence of either of these matters.[256]   **12–92**

Following the very brief outline of some of the more important rules of evidence set out above, there is the question how far a witness who is asked a particular question is obliged to answer it. First of all, it should be recalled that the coroner is obliged to disallow any question which is not relevant to the issues to be determined.[257] Secondly, there is the question of privilege. The rules of privilege have already been discussed.[258] But it is necessary to consider in particular the procedure for claiming the privilege against self-incrimination during an inquest hearing.   **12–93**

Procedure for a witness claiming privilege against self-incrimination.[259]   **12–94**
A witness cannot refuse to go into the witness box on the ground that he might incriminate himself: he can only claim the privilege after he is sworn and the question put.[260] The witness must pledge his oath that he honestly believes that that answer will, or may tend to, incriminate him.[261] It is not enough that he

---

[250] *Sherrard v Jacob* [1965] N.I. 151.

[251] *Hollington v F Hewthorn & Co Ltd* [1943] KB 587, CA; *Land Securities plc v Westminster City Council* [1993] 1 WLR 286. But coroners' courts are not bound by the strict rules of evidence (see 12–72). Moreover, it is at least arguable that proceedings under the Children Act 1989 constitute an exception to the rule in *Hollington v F Hewthorn & Co Ltd*: cf. *Aaron v Secretary of State for Business, Enterprise and Regulatory Reform* [2008] EWCA Civ. 1146. See the Chief Coroner's Guidance No. 13. See also 12–35, in relation to the findings of other inquiries.

[252] *Davie v Edinburgh Magistrates* 1953, S.C. 34 at 40, per Lord President Cooper.

[253] *R. v T* [2010] EWCA Civ. 2439.

[254] *English Exporters (London) Ltd v Eldonwell Ltd* [1973] Ch. 415; *R. v Abadom* [1983] 1 W.L.R. 126, CA; *R. v Bradshaw* (1988) 82 Cr.App.R. 79, CA.

[255] *R. v Jackson* [1996] 2 Cr. App. R. 420, CA.

[256] There are some exceptions, but these are unlikely to be at all significant in coroners' proceedings: see generally, *Cross & Tapper on Evidence,* 12th edn (2010) Chs VII and VIII; *Phipson on Evidence,* 18th edn (2013) Chs 17-22. Aspects of these are preserved in criminal cases by the Criminal Justice Act 2003 s.118(1) category 2.

[257] See 12–63.

[258] See 7–60 ff.

[259] This paragraph and the three following in the 11th edn were approved by the Divisional Court in *R. v Lincoln Coroner Ex p. Hay* [2000] Lloyd's Rep. Med. 264. The substantive law is dealt with at 7–62 ff.

[260] *Wakley v Cooke* (1847) 4 Ex. 511; *Boyle v Wiseman* (1855) 10 Ex. 647.

[261] *Webb v East* (1880) 5 Ex.D. 108; *Lamb v Munster* (1883) 10 Q.B.D. 110; *Downie v Coe, The Times,* November 28, 1997, CA.

believes it will expose him to civil liability, nor that it will incriminate someone else.[262] Similarly, the coroner cannot refuse to allow incriminating questions to be put to the witness.[263]

12–95   It is for the coroner to decide whether or not the witness is entitled to the privilege. He must first satisfy himself that the answer would tend to incriminate the witness.[264] At common law, he must go on to consider whether it was at all likely that the charge or other proceedings would in fact be brought,[265] but under the Coroners Rules it appears that the coroner is not obliged to consider this at an inquest.[266] This seems a surprising result. Since an inquest is not a trial,[267] and the witness is not a defendant, it may seem that there is no need for the jury to be sent out while the argument over admissibility is heard.[268] But legal submissions (concerning the summing-up) should be made to the coroner in the absence of the jury.[269]

12–96   **Procedure where witness is asked incriminating questions.** Where it appears to the coroner that a witness has been asked an incriminating question, the coroner must inform the witness that he may refuse to answer.[270] The witness or his representative must, however, take the objection himself,[271] and, if he chooses to answer an incriminating question, he waives his privilege.[272] The coroner should also add that if the witness does answer, he must tell the truth. However, if a series of incriminating questions is deliberately asked, then it is open to the coroner to forbid them to be put as not "proper" questions, or as oppressive.[273]

12–97   If objection is taken to a question, the coroner should make a note of the wording of the question and of the fact that objection was taken to it. It is the witness who is privileged, and not the evidence which he could give. Thus, the evidence which he is entitled to refuse to give may be proved in other ways, for example, by other witnesses who are not covered by the privilege. Since it is the right of a person asked an incriminating question to decline to answer, neither the coroner nor any jury is entitled to draw any inference adverse to the witness from the exercise of the right.

---

[262] cf. the Civil Evidence Act 1968 s.14(1)(b), for civil proceedings only.

[263] *R. v Lincoln Coroner Ex p.Hay* [2000] Lloyd's Rep. Med. 264, DC.

[264] *Re Reynolds Ex p. Reynolds* (1882) 20 Ch.D. 294.

[265] *R. v Boyes* (1861) 1 B. & S. 311.

[266] See 12–74 above. Nevertheless, coroners do do this: see e.g. *R. v Beedie* [1998] Q.B. 356, 359.

[267] See 12–74 above.

[268] cf. *R. v Hendry* (1989) 153 J.P. 166, CA.

[269] *R. v East Berkshire Coroner Ex p. Buckley* (1992) 157 J.P. 425, DC.

[270] Coroners (Inquests) Rules 2013 (SI 2013/1616) r.22(2); formerly Coroners Rules 1984 r.22(2).

[271] *Thomas v Newton* (1827) 2 C. & P. 606; *R. v Sloggett* (1856) Dears. C.C. 656; *R. v Coote* (1873) L.R. 4 P.C. 599 at 607.

[272] *R. v Lincoln Coroner Ex p. Hay* [2000] Lloyd's Rep. Med. 264, DC; see also the cases cited in *R. v Coote,* above, especially *R. v Chesham,* cited at p.606. cf. *Re John Rudderham, The Daily Telegraph,* August 30, 2001, North Yorkshire East coroner (witness statement read, witness declining to give evidence).

[273] See 12–66 ff above.

DOCUMENTARY EVIDENCE

No power for coroner to order production of documents

Under the old system it was held that a coroner by himself had no power to order **12–98**
the production of documents,[274] and that he could only compel such production
by means of what is now a High Court or county court witness summons.[275]
Under the new system the position is different, and the coroner may by notice
require a person to attend at a stated time and place and produce documents (or any
other thing) in his custody or control relating to a matter relevant to an
inquest.[276]

Privilege in relation to documents

But, however the documents are obtained, the same privileges and immunities **12–99**
apply to witness or evidence (as the case may be) in relation to documents as to oral
evidence.[277] Thus, for example, a hospital authority may not refuse to produce
medical records which may be relevant to the inquest's purposes on the grounds of
some supposed privilege for the doctor-patient relationship,[278] or merely on the
grounds that they are confidential.[279] Conversely, a written notice may be varied
or set aside,[280] for example on the basis of public interest immunity.[281]

Use of original documents and copies

The general rule is that an original document, and not a copy, must be given in **12–100**
evidence, but secondary evidence (such as a copy) may be given on proof of non-
availability of the original to the party wishing to put it in evidence.[282] Certain
public documents can however be proved by copies, such as Acts of Parliament,
by-laws, and records in the Public Record Office,[283] and there are special
provisions for entries in bankers' books to be similarly proved.[284]

ADMISSION OF DOCUMENTS

At common law, documentary hearsay evidence was admissible before the **12–101**
coroner's court. Those rules have now been replaced by express provisions for

---

[274] *R. v Southwark Coroner Ex p.Hicks* [1987] 1 W.L.R. 1624 at 1629; *Re McKerr's Application* [1993] N.I.
249.
[275] See 7–12 above, and *Assistant Deputy Coroner for Inner West London v Channel 4 Television Corporation*
[2007] EWHC 2513 (QB).
[276] Coroners and Justice Act 2009 s.32 Sch.5 para.1(1); see 7–13.
[277] Coroners and Justice Act 2009 s.32 Sch.5 para.2; see 7–15.
[278] See 7–71 above.
[279] Neither the Access to Medical Reports Act 1988 nor the Access to Health Records Act 1990 applies
in this context. The coroner's rights derive from the use of the witness notice.
[280] Coroners and Justice Act 2009 s.32 Sch.5 para.1(4); see 7–16.
[281] *Re Toman and others* Unreported July 11, 1994, HC (NI), Nicholson J.
[282] See 12–101 above.
[283] See *Cross & Tapper on Evidence,* 12th edn (2010) pp. 671–673; *Phipson on Evidence,* 18th edn (2013)
paras 32-55–32-107.
[284] Bankers' Books Evidence Act 1879; *Cross & Tapper on Evidence,* 12th edn (2010) pp. 673–674;
Phipson on Evidence, 18th edn (2013) paras 32-108–32-117.

admission at an inquest, without calling a witness to prove it, of three kinds of documentary evidence. These are (1) written evidence as to who the deceased was and how, when and where he came by his death, where the coroner is satisfied that the maker cannot give evidence within a reasonable time, there is sufficient reason why the maker should not attend (or to believe that he will not attend) the hearing, or it is unlikely to be disputed,[285] (2) the findings of an inquiry,[286] if the coroner considers them relevant to the inquest's purposes,[287] and (3) any document made by a deceased person where the coroner is of the opinion that the contents are relevant to the inquest's purposes.[288] These rules have already been discussed.[289]

12–102   Documentary evidence falling outside these provisions must be proved by a witness called for the purpose, although it is not necessary to call the maker of the document, as hearsay is admissible.[290] Otherwise, the admissibility of documentary evidence is restricted by similar rules as that of oral evidence.[291] Any material on which the coroner intends to rely at the inquest must be made available to interested persons; it is improper for the coroner to use material which is not shown and made available at the hearing.[292]

Exhibits in evidence

12–103   Formerly every exhibit produced in evidence, documentary or otherwise, had to be marked with an exhibit number, each preceded by the letter "C".[293] This is not required in the new system, but it is a sensible practice, for the avoidance of any doubt as to what was the exhibit. Once put in evidence an exhibit becomes subject to the rules under which documents may be provided for inspection to interested persons.[294] Copies of all documents retained by the coroner should be provided to the person otherwise entitled to their possession at such person's request, except in special circumstances.[295]

OTHER PROCEDURAL MATTERS

The taking of notes, or recording of proceedings by coroner

12–104   There is no longer an obligation for the coroner to take notes of the evidence given at the inquest,[296] although in practice it is sensible to do so, both because questions

---

[285] Coroners (Inquests) Rules 2013 (SI 2013/1616) r.23(1); formerly Coroners Rules 1984 r.37(1); see 12–30 ff above.

[286] Including any inquiry under the Inquiries Act 2005.

[287] Coroners (Inquests) Rules 2013 (SI 2013/1616) r.24; formerly Coroners Rules 1984 r.37A; see 12–35 above.

[288] Coroners (Inquests) Rules 2013 (SI 2013/1616) r.23(3); formerly Coroners Rules 1984 r.37(5). See 12–33 above.

[289] See 12–30—12–36.

[290] *Assistant Deputy Coroner for Inner West London v Paul and Ritz Hotel* [2007] EWCA Civ. 1259.

[291] Including those for privilege and immunity; 7–60 ff.

[292] *R. v Ceredigion Coroner Ex p. Wigley* [1993] C.O.D. 364, DC. As to "closed material" hearings, see the Justice and Security Act 2013 (which does not apply to inquest hearings); see 11–05.

[293] Coroners Rules 1984 r.38 (repealed).

[294] See 7–24 ff, 18–53.

[295] See *Arias v Metropolitan Police Commissioner* (1984) 128 S.J. 784, CA.

[296] Coroners Rules 1984 r.39 (repealed).

may arise as to what a particular witness said and also (if the coroner is sitting with a jury) he will need to prepare a summing-up for them. In the new system there is an obligation to make and keep a sound recording of every inquest hearing.[297] The coroner should take reasonable steps to ensure that the recording equipment is working well, and that those who speak in court do so in such a way that the recording can be fully and accurately transcribed.[298]

Written notes of evidence are likely to vary with the type of case: in some, the **12–105** notes will be fuller than in others. Sometimes such notes have been criticised for not adequately representing all that was said.[299] It is desirable that the coroner's notes should identify who asked particular questions of witnesses.[300] There is no obligation on the coroner to read over the note of a witness's evidence to that witness at the conclusion of the evidence.[301]

Facts in evidence and matters of law

No one is permitted to address the coroner or any jury as to the facts in evidence **12–106** at an inquest.[302] This rule is not incompatible with art.2 of the European Convention on Human Rights.[303] On the other hand, any interested person or his representative may address the coroner as to relevant matters of law. These include submissions as to the possible conclusions (in lay terms, "verdicts") to be left to the jury. Failure to allow such submissions may lead to the inquisition being set aside.[304] In making such a submission, it will usually be necessary to refer to the evidence given—or to be given—but this does not contravene the prohibition against addresses on the facts. Nor does a submission as to the areas of factual investigation to which the inquest should address itself.[305]

Where the coroner is sitting with a jury, it is usually desirable that they retire **12–107** during legal submissions, and this is essential when such submissions relate to the summing-up to be given by the coroner.[306]

Summing up

Once the evidence and legal submissions have been completed, and any rulings **12–108** have been made, the coroner if sitting with a jury must sum up the evidence to the jury, and direct them on all points of law that have arisen,[307] relating the directions

---

[297] See 7–74. Coroners (Inquests) Rules 2013 (SI 2013/1616) r.26; cf. *R. v South London Coroner Ex p. Thompson, The Times,* July 9, 1982, DC; *R. (Cash) v Northamptonshire Coroner* [2007] EWHC 1354 (Admin.). See also Chief Coroner's Guidance No. 4, *Recordings; Chief Coroner's Guide,* para.144.

[298] *Brown v Norfolk Coroner* [2014] EWHC 187 (Admin.) at [38].

[299] *R. v Ceredigion Coroner Ex p. Wigley* [1993] C.O.D. 364, DC.

[300] *Re Cohen* (1993) 158 J.P. 644, DC.

[301] *R. v Divine Ex p. Walton* [1930] 2 K.B. 29 at 39; *R. v Secretary of State for Northern Ireland Ex p. Devine* Unreported September 9, 1988, HC (NI).

[302] Coroners (Inquests) Rules 2013 (SI 2013/1616) r.27; formerly Coroners Rules 1984 r.40; *Chief Coroner's Guide to the Coroners and Justice Act 2009,* [150].

[303] *R. (Hair) v Staffordshire (South) Coroner* [2010] EWHC 2580 (Admin.); see also see *Annetts v McCann* (1990) 170 C.L.R. 596, HC (Aus), and *R. v Tennent Ex p Jager* [2000] TASSC 64.

[304] *R. v Southwark Coroner Ex p.Hicks* [1987] 1 W.L.R. 1624, DC; *R. v East Berkshire Coroner Ex p.Buckley* (1992) 157 J.P. 425, DC.

[305] *R. (Syed) v Bradford Council* Unreported December 4, 2001, Collins J.

[306] *R. v East Berkshire Coroner Ex p.Buckley* (1992) 157 J.P. 425, DC; *R. v East Sussex Coroner Ex p.Homberg* (1994) 158 J.P. 357; cf. Thurston's *Coronership,* 3rd edn (1985) para.20–06.

[307] Coroners (Inquests) Rules 2013 (SI 2013/1616) r.33; formerly Coroners Rules 1984 r.41.

to the evidence in the case.[308] This is particularly important where there are alternative theories of how the death occurred, which the jury is asked to decide between.[309] The coroner must direct the jury with care, and in particular on causation (e.g. where neglect applies) and also on the standard of proof.[310] Summing up to a jury in an art.2 case is inherently difficult.[311] Where the medical evidence is inconclusive, the jury should be directed that their duty is not to judge scientifically or with scientific certainty. They must take full account of the medical or scientific evidence, but at the same time must judge on the *whole* of the factual evidence "so that as sensible people you feel sure".[312] An inadequate summing-up is a ground for quashing the inquisition,[313] as is a failure to sum up at all.[314]

12–109   There is nothing wrong in the coroner's reading out witness statements to the jury, provided that either the statement has been properly admitted,[315] or that the witness in question has confirmed the contents in giving oral evidence.[316] Where documentary evidence has been admitted in the absence of the maker,[317] it is desirable that the coroner should warn the jury to take care. One reason is that no cross-examination of the maker of the statement has been possible.[318] Others are that the maker is not on oath, and that the jury cannot observe the demeanour of the maker in giving evidence.

12–110   In the course of summing up, a coroner should remind the jury not to carry out any further research of their own (e.g. through the internet),[319] and should warn the jury against adding any riders to the conclusion as to death (the layman's "verdict").[320] He must also explain to them the scope of the inquest[321] and warn them against making comments which are outside that scope. In particular, the jury must not seek to make any recommendations.[322] Although the coroner himself has a duty (formerly a power) in some cases to report matters to the appropriate

---

[308] *R. v Reading Coroner Ex p. West Berkshire Housing* Unreported July 11, 1995, Popplewell J.

[309] *R. v West Berkshire Coroner Ex p. Thomas* (1991) 155 J.P. 681 at 696–697, DC.

[310] *R. v Southwark Coroner's Court Ex p. Epsom Health Care NHS Trust* (1994) 158 J.P. 973, DC. See also *Bailey v Ministry of Defence* [2008] EWCA Civ. 883 (civil case where the defendant was held liable in damages for serious brain damage suffered by the claimant as a result of a want of care in a hospital managed by the defendant); *R. (Allen) v Inner North London Coroner* [2009] EWCA Civ. 623 at [40] (causation is important even in an art.2 (*Middleton*) inquest), and *R. (Lewis) v Mid and North Shropshire Coroner* [2009] EWCA Civ. 1403 (coroner has power but no duty in art.2 inquest to leave non-causative matters to jury). On the scope of the inquest, see Ch.6.

[311] *R. (P) v Avon District Coroner* [2009] EWCA Civ 1367, [25].

[312] *R. v Inner North London Coroner Ex p. Diesa Koto* (1993) 157 J.P. 857, DC, applying *R. v Dawson* (1979) 68 Cr.App.R. 44, CA.

[313] *R. (Hair) v Staffordshire (South) Coroner* [2010] EWHC 2580 (Admin.).

[314] *R. v Antrim Coroner* [1980] N.I. 123, HC (NI).

[315] See 12–101 ff.

[316] *R. v South London Coroner Ex p. Thompson, The Times,* July 9, 1982, DC. But it is not generally desirable to leave copies of the statement (or transcripts of a recording) with the jury, because that tends to overemphasise it at the expense of the other oral evidence.

[317] See 12–101 above.

[318] *R. v Curry, The Times,* March 23, 1998, CA (criminal case).

[319] *R. v Thompson* [2010] EWCA 1623 (criminal case).

[320] The power of the jury to add a rider has been abolished: Coroners (Amendment) Rules 1980 r.11.

[321] See Ch.6.

[322] *R. v Shrewsbury Coroner's Court Ex p. British Parachute Association* (1987) 152 J.P. 123, DC.

authority with a view to preventing similar fatalities in future,[323] the jury should be advised to limit themselves to the facts of the case and to answer the questions which are set out in the inquisition form.[324]

"Standard" directions to the jury[325] have been prepared in the past by the **12–111** Coroners' Society of England & Wales,[326] but ultimately it is up to the coroner to decide how to do this. The coroner, like the jury, is prohibited from uttering any unnecessary "extra" opinions,[327] which in any case may prejudice future legal proceedings.[328] It was formerly said that coroners should give written directions to a jury sparingly.[329] But more recently it has been said that, in complex cases, coroners should prepare (in advance of summing up) a statement of the requirements of each possible conclusion, which can be considered by lawyers attending, and be the subject of submissions. It can then be handed to the jury prior to commencing the summing-up.[330]

It is a matter for the coroner how best to elicit the jury's views on the issues **12–112** which arise, and so long as he does not do so in a *Wednesbury* unreasonable way his approach cannot be challenged.[331] The various conclusions that might be returned by the jury[332] should be described by the coroner, but it should be made clear that the jury are the final arbiters on the matter and that they are free to come to whichever of the described conclusions that they choose, subject to its not being framed in such a way as to appear to determine any question of criminal liability of a named person or civil liability generally.[333] A conclusion of death "as a result of a violation of his right to life contrary to Article 2 of the European Convention on Human Rights" is not permitted.[334] But a conclusion of accident will not contravene the rules so far as concerns an insurer bound to pay on a policy in the event of an accidental death.[335]

In a *Middleton* (ECHR art.2) case, it is a misdirection to tell a jury in effect that **12–113** they can only return a narrative verdict if they do not return a conclusion of suicide or accident, i.e. that they are alternatives.[336] It does not infringe ECHR art.8 to return a conclusion of unlawful killing merely because the evidence and the

---

[323] Coroners and Justice Act 2009 s.32 Sch.5 para.7; formerly Coroners Rules 1984 r.43; see 13–122 ff below.

[324] As to which, see Ch.13 below, though see also *R. (Lewis) v Mid and North Shropshire Coroner* [2009] EWCA Civ. 1403 at [27].

[325] See *R. v Inner South London Coroner Ex p. Douglas-Williams* [1999] 1 All E.R. 344; *R. v Lincoln Coroner Ex p. Hay* [2000] Lloyd's Rep. Med. 264, DC.

[326] See *A Coroner's Bench Book*, June 1999, though see *R. (Davies) v Birmingham Deputy Coroner* [2003] EWCA Civ. 1739.

[327] Coroners Rules 1984 r.36(2).

[328] *R. v Southend Magistrates Ex p. Paskin* Unreported July 11, 1991, DC.

[329] *R. v West London Coroner Ex p. Gray* [1988] Q.B. 467, DC.

[330] *R. v Inner South London Coroner Ex p. Douglas-Williams* [1999] 1 All E.R. 344 at 355.

[331] *R. (D) v Inner South London Assistant Deputy Coroner* [2008] EWHC 3356 (Admin.).

[332] These are discussed in Ch.13.

[333] Coroners and Justice Act 2009 s.10(2), formerly Coroners Rules 1984 r.42; *Hay v Devon Coroner* (1998) 162 J.P. 96, CA.

[334] *R. (Metropolitan Police Commissioner) v South London Coroner* [2003] EWHC 1829 (Admin.) at [16].

[335] *Re Sheppard* Unreported April 28, 1991, DC.

[336] *R. (P) v Avon District Coroner* [2009] EWCA Civ. 1367.

circumstances in a case are such that the conclusion must relate to the conduct of a person who is not named[337] but who is in fact identifiable.[338]

12–114 The coroner must not allow a particular conclusion as to death to be left to the jury if there is no evidence for that conclusion, or if the evidence presented, taken at its highest, is such that a jury properly directed could not properly reach that conclusion.[339] In such a case the coroner should not normally discuss such a conclusion with the jury.[340] But if there is some evidence, and its strength and weakness depends on the view taken of the witness's reliability or other matters within the jury's province, then normally it must be left to them.[341]

12–115 However, exceptionally there may be cases where, although there is some evidence for a particular conclusion, it is not in the interests of justice to leave that conclusion to the jury, and it is sufficient to leave only "those conclusions which realistically reflect the thrust of the evidence as a whole. To leave all possible [conclusions] could in some situations merely confuse and overburden the jury."[342] Indeed, the coroner should also ask whether it would be safe for a criminal jury to convict on the evidence before it.[343] In this context the coroner should bear in mind the scope of the inquest.[344] At the other extreme, it is occasionally possible to have a case where the evidence will only justify one conclusion. In such a case the coroner must direct the jury accordingly.[345]

12–116 If there is any likelihood that the jury may return a (short form) open verdict, it is desirable to ask them to agree as far as possible on the rest of the determination and findings. Thus the jury may be able to agree on the registrable particulars[346]

---

[337] In accordance with Coroners and Justice Act 2009 s.10(2), formerly Coroners Rules 1984 r.42.

[338] *R. (Evans) v Cardiff and Vale of Glamorgan Coroner* [2010] EWHC 3478 (Admin.); affirmed [2011] EWCA Civ. 719.

[339] *R. v Galbraith* [1981] 1 W.L.R. 1039, CA (criminal case); *R. v Inner North London Coroner Ex p. Diesa Koto* (1993) 157 J.P. 857, DC; *R. v Inner North London Coroner Ex p. Keogh* Unreported July 31, 1995, CA; *Re Palmer's Application* Unreported December 10, 1997, CA; *R. v Inner South London Coroner Ex p. Douglas-Williams* [1999] 1 All E.R. 344, CA; *R. v Worcester Coroner Ex p. UK Detention Services Ltd* Unreported February 18, 1998, Ognall J; *R. (Khan) v West Hertfordshire Coroner* Unreported March 7, 2002 at [43], Richards J; *Re Berry's Application* Unreported May 30, 2002, Burton J; *R. (Metropolitan Police Commissioner) v South London Coroner* [2003] EWHC 1829 (Admin.); *R. (Longfield Care Homes Ltd) v Blackburn Coroner* [2004] EWHC 2467 (Admin.); *R. (Sharman) v Inner North London Coroner* [2005] EWCA 967, CA; *R. (Bennett) v Inner South London Coroner* [2006] EWHC 196 (Admin.); *R. (Brown) v Neath and Port Talbot Coroner* [2006] EWHC 2019 (Admin.); *R. (W) v Northants Deputy Coroner* [2007] EWHC 1649 (Admin.); *R. (Le Page) v Inner South London Coroner* [2012] EWHC 1485; *R. (Secretary of State for Justice) v West Yorkshire (Eastern District) Deputy Coroner* [2012] EWHC 1634 at [23]. See also Chief Coroner's Law Sheet No. 2, *Galbraith Plus*.

[340] *R. v Inner North London Coroner Ex p. Diesa Koto* (1993) 157 J.P. 857, DC, per Blofeld J in argument.

[341] *R. v Inner North London Coroner Ex p. Diesa Koto* (1993) 157 J.P. 857, DC; *R. (Cash) v Northamptonshire Coroner* [2007] EWHC 1354 (Admin.); *R. (Bennett) v Inner South London Coroner* [2006] EWHC 196 (Admin.).

[342] *R. v Inner South London Coroner Ex p. Douglas-Williams* [1999] 1 All E.R. 344 at 349, CA; *R. (Scott) v Inner West London Coroner* (2001) 165 J.P. 417, DC; *R. (Dawson) v East Riding and Hull Coroner* [2001] EWHC 352 (Admin.); *R. (Anderson) v Inner North London Coroner* [2004] EWHC 2729 (Admin.) at [42]; *R. (Bennett) v Inner South London Coroner* [2006] EWHC 196 (Admin.) at [47].

[343] *R. (Secretary of State for Justice) v West Yorkshire Coroner (Eastern District)* [2012] EWHC 1634 (Admin.); Chief Coroner's Law Sheet 2, *Galbraith Plus*.

[344] As to which see Ch.6.

[345] *R. v West Berkshire Coroner Ex p. Thomas* (1991) 155 J.P. 681 at 697–698, DC.

[346] As to these, see 13–115 below.

even though they disagree in their conclusion as to death.[347] What happens if they disagree is dealt with elsewhere.[348]

It has been held in a criminal case that counsel for all parties are under a duty **12–117** to assist the court by pointing out defects in the summing-up that would provide a basis for a successful appeal.[349] There is no reason why a similar rule should not apply to inquests; indeed, in some respects the matter is all the stronger. Drawing attention to possible mistakes in the summing-up may prevent the need to seek judicial review.[350]

Hearings with no jury. If there is no jury, there may strictly be no legal **12–118** necessity for the coroner to sum up the evidence. Even when sitting alone, however, it is common practice for the coroner to refer as shortly as may be to the evidence that has been given before him[351] and to state publicly what conclusion[352] he proposes to record. Although there is no authority upon this latter point, it is clearly consistent with the general principles of our legal system that a public pronouncement of the conclusion should be made in each case.

As to the former, if the coroner sums up the evidence, he should be careful not **12–119** to contravene any other relevant rules, such as that which prohibits a determination from naming a person in respect of criminal liability.[353] It was held arguable that there was a breach of this rule when the coroner after a non-jury inquest produced a single document containing a summing-up of the evidence (which referred to the claimant by name as having carried out the act which killed the deceased) and also—without a break—the formal certification in the form of an inquisition containing a conclusion of unlawful killing (which did not, however, name the claimant).[354]

Particular care should be taken where the coroner makes comments which go **12–120** beyond the statutory questions for the inquest. Comments may be declared unlawful where they (i) do not relate to any of the statutory questions in any way; (ii) are matters of opinion; and (iii) are sufficiently unfairly critical and offensive of any party.[355]

It is not normally appropriate for the coroner to adjourn the inquest before the **12–121** jury retirement so as to enable an interested person to challenge a coronial ruling.[356]

---

[347] Indeed, in *R. v St. Pancras Coroner's Court Ex p.Higgins* (1988) 152 J.P. 637, DC. Parker LJ said that the registrable particulars were all that were necessary for the inquisition, although this is inconsistent with the form then prescribed by the Coroners Rules 1984 Sch.4, and now by Coroners (Inquests) Rules 2013 r.34 and Sch. Form 2.

[348] See 13–17.

[349] *R. v Langford, The Times,* January 12, 2001, CA.

[350] *R. (Marshall) v Coventry Coroner* Unreported October 22, 2001 at [33], Hooper J.

[351] Thurston's *Coronership,* 3rd edn (1995) para.20–01, suggests that a coroner would be "failing in his duty" if he did not do this, although elsewhere it is made clear that this is not a legal duty.

[352] As to possible conclusions, see Ch.13.

[353] Coroners and Justice Act 2009 s.10(2), formerly Coroners Rules 1984 r.42; see 12–112, 13–57.

[354] *R. (Evans) v Cardiff and Vale of Glamorgan Coroner* [2010] EWHC 3478 (Admin.); cf. *My Care (UK) Ltd v Coventry Coroner* [2009] EWHC 3630 (Admin.).

[355] *R. (Farah) v Southampton Coroner* [2009] EWHC 1605 (Admin.); see also *R. (Mowlem plc) v Avon Assistant Deputy Coroner* [2005] EWHC 1359 (Admin.).

[356] See 11–40, 11–41.

Chapter 13

DETERMINATION AND RECORD OF INQUEST

DETERMINATION AND FINDINGS

After the summing-up, the coroner, or the jury if there is one, must make a **13–01** determination and findings. The **determination** is of *who* the deceased was, and *by what means*, *when* and *where*, and (in ECHR art.2 cases) *in what circumstances* the deceased came by his or her death.[1] The **findings** are of the particulars needed for the registration of the death, if it is one which requires to be registered.[2] Both determination and findings are recorded in a document formerly called the "inquisition", but now known as the "record of the inquest".

The form of the record of inquest is prescribed.[3] It requires the following to be **13–02** recorded as having been found:

(1) the name of the deceased (if known);

(2) the medical cause of death;

(3) how, when and where and (in ECHR art.2 cases) in what circumstances the deceased came by his or her death;

(4) the conclusion of the coroner or (as it may be) jury as to the death;

(5) the registration particulars.

Under the old system, laymen and the media used the term "verdict" to refer **13–03** merely to the answer to item (4), but that that was only a small part of the information to be recorded in the inquisition. The same is true of the record of the inquest. Moreover, it is critical that the facts found (and recorded) in (1), (2) and (3) disclose a factual basis for the conclusion in (4). If they do not, then that conclusion cannot be supported.[4] Although the registration particulars are included in the record of the inquest the statutory requirement to find and record them is technically separate from the obligation to make a determination.[5]

---

[1] Coroners and Justice Act 2009 s.5(1), s.10(1)(a).
[2] Coroners and Justice Act 2009 s.5(1)(c), s.10(1)(b).
[3] Coroners (Inquests) Rules 2013 (SI 2013/1616) r.34 Sch. Form 2.
[4] See 13–22 ff below.
[5] Coroners and Justice Act 2009, ss 5(1)(c), 10(1)(b), formerly Coroners Act 1988 s.11(3)(b), (4)(b). See also 13–115.

JURY CASES

Management of jury

13–04   Jury management questions in coroners' inquests should be dealt with in similar fashion to those arising in criminal courts.[6] In a criminal case the jury should deliberate only when they were all together in the jury room, and not when, e.g., one of their number was late in attending court.[7] Nor should the jury carry out any of their own research, e.g. on the internet,[8] or discuss the case with others, e.g. via social media.[9]

13–05   At common law a criminal jury could not separate once the trial had begun.[10] In 1897 the court was empowered to permit a jury to separate if it had not yet been directed to consider a verdict.[11] But normally any separation thereafter was a material irregularity justifying discharge of the jury and a retrial.[12] The criminal court's power to permit a jury to separate has now been extended to the period *after* being directed to consider its verdict.[13] The coroner's jury is unaffected by these statutory changes. But it was the functional equivalent of the grand jury, who considered whether a case should go to trial, rather than of the petty jury, which actually tried cases.[14] So there is no need to apply the common law rule for petty juries to coroners' juries,[15] provided that appropriate steps are taken to minimise any possible interference with the jury.

13–06   Directions to be given to a criminal jury permitted to separate after retirement,[16] with any necessary modifications, could be used also in the case of a coroner's jury permitted to separate. In substance, these are that:

> (1) the jury must decide the case on the evidence seen and heard in court, and not on anything they might have seen or heard, or might see or hear, outside court;
>
> (2) once the evidence has been completed it would be wrong for any juror to seek to receive further evidence or information about the case;
>
> (3) the jury must not talk to anyone about the case, or allow anyone else to talk to them about the case, except other members of the jury, and then only when deliberating in the jury room;

---

[6] *Clayton v South Yorkshire Coroner* [2005] EWHC 1196 Admin., DC at [9]. See also *R. (Sharman) v Inner North London Coroner* [2005] EWCA Civ. 967 at [34].

[7] *R. v Hastings, The Times,* December 12, 2003, CA; see Chief Coroner's Guidance No. 10, *Warnings to Juries,* para.2.

[8] *R. v Thompson* [2010] EWCA Crim. 1623; *R. v Karakaya, The Times,* February 28, 2005, CA; Criminal Practice Directions [2013] EWCA Crim. 1631, 39G.3, ii; see Chief Coroner's Guidance No. 10, *Warnings to Juries,* para.4.

[9] *Attorney General v Fraill* [2011] EWCA Crim. 1570; Criminal Practice Directions [2013] EWCA Crim. 1631, 39G.3, iii.

[10] Co. Litt. 227b.

[11] Detention of Juries Act 1897 s.1.

[12] *R. v Goodson* [1975] 1 W.L.R. 549.

[13] Criminal Justice and Public Order Act 1994 s.43.

[14] See 1–29 above.

[15] *Re Devine and Breslin's Application* [1988] 14 N.I.J.B. 10, 24, HC (NI), Carswell J.

[16] *R. v Oliver* [1996] 2 Cr.App.R. 514.

(4) when they leave the court building they should try to put the case on one side until they return to court and retire to their jury room to continue the process of deliberating about their verdict.

These directions should be given in full on the first dispersal by the jury, and then a brief reminder at each subsequent dispersal.

Consideration of verdict in private

The jury should consider their verdict all together[17] in private without either the **13–07** coroner or anyone else present,[18] and it is therefore essential for them to retire from the court to a suitable room for the purpose of deliberation. The jury bailiff (usually the coroner's officer) should be responsible for ensuring that they remain together and that no person communicates with them during their private deliberation.[19] They may usefully take with them exhibits, such as plans, for detailed consideration. However, once they have retired they should not be given any additional evidence, matter or material to assist them,[20] except such as may be given to them by the coroner in open court, after all interested persons have had an opportunity to comment.

No communication with jury whilst out of court

It is improper for the coroner or (a fortiori) any other person to communicate **13–08** privately with the jury while they are out of court, or to accompany them to their room.[21] Furthermore, it is a contempt of court to obtain or seek to obtain (or, having obtained, to disclose)[22] any particulars of statements made, opinions expressed, arguments advanced or votes cast by members of the jury,[23] except to enable the jury to arrive at a verdict or to assist in delivery of it.[24] This does not prevent the consideration of allegations of misconduct by persons not part of the jury (e.g. a jury bailiff alleged to have put pressure on the jury).[25] Allegations relating to the (internal) conduct of juries are generally immune from investigation, even after the Human Rights Act 1998,[26] and the same applies in coroners' cases.[27]

---

[17] *R. v Hastings, The Times,* December 12, 2003, CA.
[18] *R. v Fitzgerald Ex p. O'Brien and Bourchier* (1883) 17 I.R. L.T. 34 at 36.
[19] Sometimes an oath is administered to him, although this is not required by law: see App.3 Form 19.
[20] *R. v Davis* (1975) 62 Cr.App.R. 194; *R. v Oliver* [1996] 2 Cr.App.R. 514, CA; *R. v Karakaya, The Times,* February 28, 2005, CA (information gathered from internet by juror after retirement; criminal appeal allowed).
[21] *Re The Mitchelstown Inquisition* (1988) 11 L.R.I.R. 279; *R. v Wood Ex p. Anderson* [1928] 1 K.B. 302.
[22] "Disclose" means "disclose generally", and hence includes publication of a newspaper article revealing statements, opinions and arguments during jury deliberations: *Attorney General v Associated Newspapers Ltd* [1994] 2 A.C. 338, HL.
[23] Contempt of Court Act 1981 s.8(1).
[24] Contempt of Court Act 1981 s.8(2).
[25] *Clayton v South Yorkshire Coroner* [2005] EWHC 1196 Admin., DC at [9]; *R. v Mole* [2013] EWCA Crim. 2420.
[26] *R. v Lewis, The Times,* April 26, 2001, CA; *R. v Qureshi, The Times,* September 11, 2001, CA.
[27] See *Clayton v South Yorkshire Coroner* [2005] EWHC 1196 Admin., DC at [11].

13–09   But in criminal cases it has been held that there are two narrow exceptional circumstances in which it is appropriate to examine what happened in the jury room.[28] These are where (1) "there has been a complete repudiation of the oath taken by the jurors to try the case according to the evidence; examples include a decision arrived at by the casting of lots or the toss of a coin, or the well-known case of the use, or rather misuse, of an Ouija board", or (2) "extraneous material has been introduced into the jury deliberations" such as "telephone calls into or out of the jury room, papers mistakenly included in the jury bundle, discussions between jurors and relatives or friends about the case, and in recent years, information derived by one or more jurors from the internet."[29] It is likely that the same exceptions will apply to coroners' juries.

13–10   If it is necessary for the coroner to communicate with the jury or to answer any question propounded by them during the course of their deliberations, this must be done in open court.[30] In one case it was held to be sufficient compliance with this rule where the foreman of the jury came back into the court room and had a private discussion with the coroner on the bench, but in full view of the court: if the discussion was inaudible, the remedy was to ask for the words to be repeated.[31]

Reasonable period for deliberation of jury

13–11   The coroner may detain the jury for a reasonable period to see if they can reach agreement. What is a reasonable period must vary according to the circumstances. In one case where the jury did not retire until 8.20 p.m. and returned a majority verdict at 10.00 p.m. (some 12 hours after the inquest began) the Divisional Court quashed the inquisition for various reasons, among them the lateness of the verdict and length of the proceedings on a single day.[32] In another case the inquisition was quashed where the jury sat from 10.49 a.m. to 4.41 p.m., with no lunch or other refreshment, and a single break of 15 minutes.[33]

13–12   In cases which have lasted several days, a reasonable time for jury deliberations may be several hours. In cases which have lasted several weeks, it may be two or three days. In one coroner case, an allegation that the coroner's officer told the jury that they must reach a verdict by 5.00 p.m. would, if made out (though on the facts it was not) have justified quashing the verdict and ordering a fresh inquest.[34]

Unanimous and majority decisions

13–13   At common law and under the Coroners Act 1887 there was no need for unanimity amongst the coroner's jury (of up to 23 members) as long as at least 12

---

[28] See *R. v Mirza* [2004] 1 A.C. 1118, HL; *R. v Smith (No. 2)* [2005] UKHL 12.

[29] *R. v Thompson* [2010] EWCA Crim. 1623 at [4]–[5].

[30] *R. v Wood Ex p. Anderson* [1928] 1 K.B. 302; *R. v West London Coroner Ex p. Gray* [1988] Q.B. 467, DC.

[31] *R. v Greater Manchester Coroner Ex p. Tal* [1985] Q.B. 67 at 85, DC.

[32] *R. v City of London Coroner Ex p. Calvi*, *The Times*, April 2, 1983, DC.

[33] *R. v Southwark Coroner Ex p. Hicks* [1987] 1 W.L.R. 1624, DC; cf. *R. v West Yorkshire Coroner Ex p. Clements.*

[34] *Clayton v South Yorkshire Coroner* [2005] EWHC 1196 Admin., DC. cf. *Morrison v Chief Constable of the West Midlands*, *The Independent*, February 28, 2003, CA (no reasonable apprehension of improper pressure where judge in civil case told deadlocked jury that they would have to be discharged, and they asked for more time, and then produced majority verdict).

were agreed.[35] This was the same as the grand jury, whose function was to decide whether to commit a person for trial.[36] In 1926 the number of coroner's jurors was reduced to the current maximum of 11,[37] and it was expressly provided that the coroner might accept a majority verdict where the minority consisted of not more than two.[38]

The current rule requires a unanimous determination or finding,[39] *unless* only   **13–14**
one or two members do not agree on it, *and* the jury has deliberated for a period of time which the coroner thinks reasonable in view of the nature and complexity of the case.[40] In that exceptional case, the coroner must require one of the jury to announce publicly how many of them agreed and how many did not.[41] A determination and a finding are separate matters. So unanimity (or a majority, where allowed) is required in respect of each. Hence a different majority could conceivably agree separately on a determination and on a finding. But each of a determination and a finding is composed of several elements. However, there is no warrant for saying that there can be different majorities for separate elements *within* a determination or finding.

Because of the requirement that a jury must have deliberated for a period of time   **13–15**
which the coroner thinks reasonable, a coroner should never give a majority direction in the original summing-up, but instead should wait until there has been a sufficient deliberation by the jury to show that a unanimous decision is unlikely to be achieved. Once the majority direction has been given, and it is clear that the jury is having difficulty in reaching even a majority decision, the coroner can give a so-called *Watson* direction.[42]

This is as follows: **13–16**

"Each of you has taken an oath to return a true verdict according to the evidence. No one must be false to that oath, but you have a duty not only as individuals but collectively. That is the strength of the jury system. Each of you takes into the jury box with you your individual experience and wisdom. Your task is to pool that experience and wisdom. You do that by giving your views and listening to the views of others. There must necessarily be discussion, argument and give and take within the scope of your oath. That is the way in which agreement is reached. If, unhappily, [10[43] of] you cannot reach agreement you must say so."

---

[35] Coroners Act 1887 s.4(5) (as originally enacted); see *Cobat's* case, 2 Hale P.C. 161n., 4 Bl. Comm. 301, cited by Huband, *A Practical Treatise on the Law relating to the Grand Jury in Criminal Cases, the Coroner's Jury and the Petty Jury in Ireland* (1896) p. 255; Stephen, *A Digest of the Law of Criminal Procedure in Indictable Offences* (1883) art.212.
[36] See 1–29 above.
[37] Coroners (Amendment) Act 1926 s.30 and Sch.2.
[38] Coroners (Amendment) Act 1926 s.15(1), later the Coroners Act 1988 s.12(2).
[39] Coroners and Justice Act 2009 s.9(1).
[40] Coroners and Justice Act 2009 s.9(2), formerly Coroners Act 1988 s.12. See also *R. v Merseyside Coroner Ex p. Carr* [1993] 4 All E.R. 65; *Re Bradley's Application* Unreported April 7, 1995, HC (NI); *R. v Northampton Coroner Ex p. Tompkinson* (1995) 160 J.P. 69, DC; and *R. v West Yorkshire Coroner Ex p. Clements* (1993) 158 J.P. 17, DC.
[41] Coroners and Justice Act 2009 s.9(2).
[42] From *R. v Watson* [1988] Q.B. 690.
[43] In the coronial context this will be the number of jurors actually present, less two.

13–17   But this direction must not be combined with the majority direction, and must not be modified or added to in any way.[44] Moreover, no other pressure must be put on the jury, e.g. by telling them that they must reach a verdict by a certain time.[45] If there is not a sufficient majority for a decision after a reasonable period for deliberation, the coroner may discharge the jury, summon another, and proceed with the inquest afresh.[46] The coroner is however obliged to accept a unanimous or a majority decision,[47] however perverse or inane it may be, if the jury after suitable explanation persist in their view.[48]

RECORD OF INQUEST

13–18   The formal record of the inquest, containing the determination and findings, is called the record of the inquest, formerly the inquisition. This should be drawn up immediately the decision is given[49] and signed by the coroner and, if there is a jury, by those members of the jury who agree with it.[50] It is not wrong, and may sometimes be sensible, for the coroner to question the jury (through the foreman) in order to remove any ambiguity or uncertainty in the answers which they give to the specific questions asked of them.[51] This will avoid the need to seek to correct any misunderstandings or mistakes later.[52] There should not, save for exceptional reasons, be an adjournment before the signing of the record.[53]

13–19   The form of record consists of three parts. These are the caption, the facts found (i.e. the statutory determination and the findings) and the attestation by the coroner (and the jury, if there is one). Previously all three parts were prescribed by the rules.[54] Now only the second and third are.[55]

Caption

13–20   The caption (which is not prescribed by the rules) sets out the essential facts necessary to give the coroner jurisdiction to hold the inquest. To begin, it is helpful also to mention the date on which the investigation started, because it will serve to remind the coroner in cases where the investigation concludes over a year after it

---

[44] *R. v Buono* (1992) 95 Cr.App.R. 338; *Clayton v South Yorkshire Coroner* [2005] EWHC 1196 Admin., DC.

[45] *R. v Rose* [1982] A.C. 822; *De Four v The State* [1999] 1 W.L.R. 1731; *Clayton v South Yorkshire Coroner* [2005] EWHC 1196 Admin., DC.

[46] Coroners and Justice Act 2009 s.9(3), formerly Coroners Act 1988 s.12(3).

[47] Coroners and Justice Act 2009 s.9(3); cf. Coroners Act 1988 s.12(2) ("the coroner *may* accept . . . ").

[48] *Smith's Case* (1696) Comb. 386. As to mistakes in pronouncing the verdict, see *R. v Andrews* (1985) 129 S.J. 869, CA; *Lalchan Nanan v State* [1986] A.C. 860, PC, and *R. v Tantram* [2001] Crim.L.R. 824, CA.

[49] Sometimes the formal parts are filled out in advance: see 13–30.

[50] See 13–116 below.

[51] *R. v West Yorkshire Coroner Ex p. Clements* (1993) 158 J.P. 17, DC.

[52] See 13–120 below.

[53] *R. v Mallett and Chilcote* (1846) 1 Cox. C.C. 336.

[54] Coroners Rules 1984 Sch.4 Form 22: App.2 (repealed).

[55] Coroners (Inquests) Rules 2013 (SI 2013/1616) r.34 Sch. Form 2.

started that he or she must notify the Chief Coroner.[56] Then the record sets out where the inquest was held and by or before whom. The record will be quashed if the coroner holding the inquest did not have jurisdiction for so doing.[57] The place where the inquest is held will normally be within the coroner's district, though this is no longer legally necessary.[58] The date or dates of the inquest, including any adjournment, is or are also set out.

The record may need modification according to whether the inquest is held   **13–21** with or without a jury, or partly with and partly without a jury. Home Office advice (now rather old) distinguishes between inquests held without a jury, when the caption should describe the inquest as being taken "by" the coroner alone, and inquests held with a jury, when the caption should describe the inquest as being taken "before" the coroner and the reference to the jury included. If the inquest is held partly with and partly without a jury, the caption should describe the inquest as being taken "by and before" the coroner and the jury.[59] It is not necessary, however, to specify at which hearing the jury was present. If it turns out that the body is that of a stillbirth, reference in the caption to its being a record of an inquest touching a death will have to be omitted, and reference to its being a record concerning a stillbirth substituted.

Facts found

Paragraph (1) of the facts found in the prescribed form of record requires the full   **13–22** name of the deceased to be given. This refers to the name that the deceased was known by at death (since in English law the name of a person is the name by which he or she is known, and not necessarily the name given at birth),[60] and not to any previous name or names. Thus a person who enters the country under a false identity and dies without the original name being known should be recorded here under the new name, because it is the one by which he or she was known. If no name is known, at least the sex of the deceased should be given. If the sex cannot be determined, it should be stated to be "undetermined."[61]

Paragraphs (2) and (3) of the facts found require particulars of the death to be   **13–23** given. Paragraph (2) is concerned with the medical cause of death. In most cases this is not itself controversial. Occasionally two doctors may disagree as to the cause of death, and the coroner (or jury) will have to decide. Such information should be given under paragraph (2) as to the cause of death as enables a clear picture of that cause to be obtained. For this purpose not only the immediate cause of death but also the morbid conditions giving rise to the immediate cause of death should be stated.[62] Where the death was violent, particulars of the injury should be given.

---

[56] Coroners (Investigations) Regulations 2013 (SI 2013/1629) reg.26. See 10–14.
[57] *Foxhall v Barnett* (1853) 2 E. & B. 928.
[58] See 10–16 ff above
[59] Home Office Circular No. 68 of 1955 App.4 fn.1.
[60] See e.g. *Halsbury's Laws of England*, 5th edn Vol.35 para.1272. A deed poll, or a statutory declaration, is simply *evidence* of the name by which a person is known, and is not a legal requirement for a change of name.
[61] It was formerly usual in such cases to give the sex as male.
[62] *Ex p. Minister of Justice* [1964] N.S.W.R. 1598. Further assistance on this point can be derived from the notes to the coroner's certificate after inquest issued by the Registrar General.

In the case of deaths from poison (including drugs), the poison should be specified.

13–24   Paragraph (3) is concerned with the time, place and means—or circumstances—at or by or in which the deceased came by his or her death. In most cases the questions of time and place are not difficult. Where the evidence does not give precise information, the range indicated by the evidence can be given, or otherwise the time and place that the body was found can be given. As to the question how, this means "by what means", except in cases where ECHR art.2 is engaged, when it means "by what means and in what circumstances".

13–25   Paragraph (3) is also the place for the so-called "narrative verdict".[63] This is not confined to art.2 cases, but is useful in other inquiries, for example where death results from two or more causes of different types.[64] The coroner is not obliged to invite the jury to compose and insert such a verdict.[65] Indeed, if there is to be one, that is a factor in favour of the coroner's deciding (as a matter of discretion) not to sit with a jury.[66]

13–26   The courts have expressed a number of views about what such verdicts should contain. On the one hand, it has been said that it should be both brief and factual, expressing no judgment or opinion.[67] On the other, it was held to be wrong for the coroner to direct the jury that any narrative verdict should be "entirely descriptive, neutral, [and] non-judgmental", as the resultant narrative was so anodyne as not to give conclusions on any of the key factual issues raised.[68]

13–27   To give the narrative some focus, it has been said that "Narrative verdicts may have a particular relevance in cases where the jury record particular breaches of duties, or particular failures to foresee risks, which should be recorded so that the industry can be alerted and all others concerned with the tragedy in this case can learn lessons for the future."[69]

13–28   But, by way of limitation, it has also been said that:

> "it was not incumbent on the coroner to investigate, still less to state his conclusion in relation to, every issue raised by the claimant, however peripheral to the main questions to be determined. In *Middleton* at [36], Lord Bingham of Cornhill said in relation to an article 2 inquest: 'it must be for the coroner, in the exercise of his discretion, to decide how best, in the particular case, to elicit the jury's conclusion *on the central issue or issues*' (emphasis added). The coroner

---

[63] *R. v West Yorkshire Coroner Ex p. Stringer* (1993) 158 J.P. 453, DC; *R. (Longfield Care Homes Ltd) v Blackburn Coroner* [2004] EWHC 2467 (Admin.). See also note (ii) to Form 2, in the Coroners (Inquests) Rules 2013 (SI 2013/1616) r.34 Sch.
[64] *R. (Longfield Care Homes Ltd) v Blackburn Coroner* [2004] EWHC 2467 (Admin.).
[65] *R. v East Sussex Coroner Ex p Homberg* (1994) 158 J.P. 357, DC.
[66] *R. (Collins) v Inner South London Coroner* [2004] EWHC 2421 (Admin.).
[67] *R. v East Sussex Coroner Ex p Homberg* (1994) 158 J.P. 357, DC; *R. v North Humberside Coroner Ex p. Jamieson* [1995] Q.B. 1, CA; *Re Bradley's Application* Unreported April 7, 1995, HC (NI), Carswell LJ); see also *Clayton v South Yorkshire Coroner* [2005] EWHC 1196 Admin., DC.
[68] *R. (Cash) v Northamptonshire Coroner* [2007] EWHC 1354 (Admin.).
[69] *R. (Bodycote HIP Ltd) v Herefordshire Coroner* [2008] EWHC 164 (Admin.). But this does not include the bald statement that the deceased died "as a result of violation of his right to life": *R (Metropolitan Police Commissioner) v South London Coroner* [2003] EWHC 1829 (Admin), [16]. See 12–112.

was, therefore, required to do no more than focus the investigation and the inquisition on the central issue or issues in the case."[70]

The time, place and circumstances of the injury being sustained should be stated **13–29** as accurately as possible. Thus, in road accident cases the name of the driver of the vehicle may be stated (subject to not appearing to determine any question of liability)[71] or, if that is not known, it should be stated that the car was driven by a person unknown. The Motor Insurers' Bureau (which deals with indemnity, and may therefore be an interested person, in such a case) will find this information helpful.[72]

Details of time, place and circumstances are often uncontroversial, and in the past **13–30** were sometimes completed before the inquest began.[73] But they are part of the determination and, in a jury case, such details are a matter for them.[74] It should not appear that coroners are seeking to erode the jury's function, and thus they should refrain from pre-filling in these details, or even providing the jury with a draft for consideration.[75] However, if there is no controversy over such facts, an inquisition will not be quashed because of a technical failure in this respect.[76]

Paragraph (4) of the facts found relates to the conclusion of the coroner or jury **13–31** as to death. Under the old system this paragraph was often colloquially called the "verdict", although strictly the verdict consisted in the whole of the facts found. The notes to the 2013 prescribed form of record[77] give a list of suggested, rather than compulsory,[78] conclusions. The object of this list is to standardise conclusions over the whole country and to make the statistics based on the Annual Return more reliable by avoiding as far as possible any overlap or gaps between the different conclusions.[79]

The 2013 list is as follows: **13–32**

   I Accident/misadventure.

   II Alcohol/drug related (seemingly replacing "dependence on drugs/non-dependent abuse of drugs" in the old list).

   III Industrial disease.

---

[70] R. (Allen) v Inner North London Coroner [2009] EWCA Civ. 623. See R. (Lewis) v Mid and North Shropshire Coroner [2009] EWCA Civ. 1403, and Ch.6 generally.

[71] See 13–57 and 13–103 ff.

[72] See Home Office Circular 68 of 1995, 10–12.

[73] cf. R. v Surrey Coroner Ex p. Campbell [1982] Q.B. 661, DC; R. v West Berkshire Coroner Ex p. Buckley (1992) 157 J.P. 425, DC.

[74] R. v West Berkshire Coroner Ex p Thomas (1991) 155 J.P. 681, DC.

[75] Re Bradley's Application Unreported April 7, 1995, HC (NI), Carswell LJ; R. (Mowlem plc) v Avon Assistant Deputy Coroner [2005] EWHC 1359 (Admin.).

[76] R. v East Berkshire Coroner Ex p Buckley (1992) 157 J.P. 425, DC.

[77] Coroners (Inquests) Rules 2013 (SI 2013/1616) r.34 Sch. Form 2; formerly Coroners Rules 1984 Sch.4 Form 22 (repealed): see 13–19 above.

[78] R. v Southwark Coroner Ex p Kendall [1988] 1 W.L.R. 1186, DC (in relation to the 1984 form). Indeed, the similar notes to the predecessor Form 18 in Sch.3 to the Coroners Rules 1953 were held not to be part of those Rules: R. v Turnbull Ex p. Kenyon Unreported March 15, 1984, DC. See also R. (Wilkinson) v Greater Manchester South Coroner [2012] EWHC 2755 (Admin.) at [65].

[79] See R. v South Glamorgan Coroner Ex p. BP Chemicals Ltd (1987) 151 J.P. 799, DC; R. v Northampton Coroner Ex p. Tomkinson (1995) 160 J.P. 69 at 73, DC.

    IV Lawful/unlawful killing.

    V Natural causes.

    VI Open.

    VII Road traffic collision.

    VIII Stillbirth.

    IX Suicide.

13–33   Four other conclusions which appeared in the notes to the 1984 form (as amended) but do not in the notes to that of 2013 are:

1. Want of attention at birth.

2. Attempted/self-induced abortion.

3. Death in the [*name*] disaster *(having been the subject of a public inquiry)*.

4. Execution of sentence of death.

13–34   In addition, note (4)(a) to the 1984 form suggested that each of natural causes, industrial disease, dependence on drugs/non-dependent abuse of drugs and want of attention at birth might, in appropriate circumstances, be qualified as being causes of death "aggravated" by lack of care (now called "neglect") or self-neglect. This note is not replicated in the 2013 form, and there is no mention of neglect. It relates to a difficult and controversial area, and is dealt with later.[80] It is also necessary to mention the possibility of a conclusion that the deceased died on or as a result of active service. This too is discussed later.[81]

13–35   Despite the existence of an "official" list of suggested conclusions, there is no statutory requirement that a "conclusion as to death" be in any particular form; all that is needed is that it should be expressed in concise and ordinary language so as to indicate how the deceased came by his death.[82] The Chief Coroner intends to issue further guidance on conclusions.[83] For now, however, all these suggested conclusions require further explanation. Comments on the various conclusions referred to above therefore follow.

---

[80] See 13–83—13–110 below.
[81] See 13–78 ff.
[82] *R. v Southwark Coroner's Court Ex p. Kendall* [1988] 1 W.L.R. 1186, DC; *R. v Birmingham Coroner Ex p. Home Secretary* (1990) 155 J.P. 107 at 122.
[83] *Chief Coroner's Guide*, para.170.

"Official" list

I *"Accident/misadventure"*[84]

Blackstone defined as "misadventure" a form of excusable homicide, as follows: **13–36**

> "HOMICIDE *per infortunium*, or *misadventure*, is where a man, doing a lawful act, without any intention of hurt, unfortunately kills another: as where a man is at work with a hatchet, and the head thereof flies off and kills a stander by; or, where a person, qualified to keep a gun, is shooting at a mark, and undesignedly kills a man: for the act is lawful, and the effect is merely accidental. So where a parent is moderately correcting his child, a master his servant or scholar, or an officer punishing a criminal, and happens to occasion his death, it is only misadventure; for the act of correction was lawful: but if he exceeds the bounds of moderation, either in the manner, the instrument, or the quantity of punishment, and death ensues, it is manslaughter at least, and in some cases (according to the circumstances) murder; for the act of immoderate correction is unlawful."[85]

But this is a discussion about possible criminal liability. In modern times, for   **13–37** coronial purposes no distinction is drawn between accident and misadventure in the conclusion. It is sometimes suggested that "accident" connotes something over which there is no human control, or an unintended act, while "misadventure" indicates some deliberate (but lawful) human act which has unexpectedly taken a turn that leads to death.[86] Thus misadventure, apparently involving the taking of a risk, is seen as morally more blameworthy than accident.

Even if this distinction exists in logic, it is clear that coroners have not observed   **13–38** it in practice,[87] and, for statistical purposes, these conclusions are treated as being the same. The Divisional Court has encouraged this trend, treating the distinction between accident and misadventure as "without purpose or effect", and suggesting

---

[84] This paragraph in the 11th edn was cited with approval in *R. v Birmingham and Solihull Coroner Ex p. Benton* (1997) 162 J.P. 807, 8 Med.L.R. 362.

[85] 4 Bl. Comm. 182 (notes omitted).

[86] See Burton, Chambers and Gill, *Coroners' Inquiries* (1985) p.84. See *Re Stuart Rushton and Adam Rushton, The Daily Telegraph*, May 30, 2002 (father and nine-year-old son drowned after father "recklessly" took son for walk along shore: misadventure conclusion for father; accident for son).

[87] Thus the verdict on one coach crash was accidental death (*Re Dalicia Moss, The Times*, October 14, 1983 (Exeter coroner)) whilst the verdict on another was misadventure (*Re M4 coach crash, The Times*, November 9, 1983 (Swindon coroner)); the verdict on one death as a result of a non-deliberate explosion was an accident (*Re Abbeystead disaster, The Times*, October 31, 1984 (Lancaster coroner)) and on another was misadventure (*Re Putney gas explosion, The Times*, April 3, 1985 (Westminster coroner)); and on one death from an injection that proved unintentionally fatal the verdict was accidental death (*Re Hannah McCarthy, The Times*, July 28, 1984 (Beaconsfield coroner)) and on another it was misadventure (*Re Julia Clegg, The Times*, October 4, 1984 (Exeter coroner)).

the suppression of the latter in favour of the former.[88] It is thus necessary to explain to the jury that recording "accident" does not deprive any person of any civil remedy he might otherwise have.

13–39   The distinction between natural causes and accidental death/misadventure in the medical context has been described as follows:

> "The first is where a person is suffering from a potentially fatal condition and medical intervention does no more than fail to prevent death. In such circumstances the underlying cause of death is the condition that proved fatal and in such a case, the correct verdict would be death from natural causes. This would be the case even if the medical treatment that had been given was viewed generally by the medical profession as the wrong treatment. All the more so is this the case where such a person is not treated at all, even if the failure to give the treatment was negligent . . . [89]
>
> On the other hand, where a person is suffering from a condition which does not in any way threaten his life and such person undergoes treatment which for whatever reason causes death, then assuming that there is no question of unlawful killing the verdict should be death by accident/misadventure. Just as the recording of death by natural causes does not absolve the doctors of fault so the recording of death by accident/misadventure does not imply fault."[90]

13–40   In non-medical cases, the accidental and non-natural ingestion of pathogens leading to a disease which kills is better recorded as accidental death, rather than natural causes.[91] But where the pathogens are transmitted by natural, including normal social, means, without intending to cause or create a risk of transmission, then death from such a disease is better recorded as natural causes.[92] Deliberate or reckless transmission of pathogens causing death may, in appropriate cases, amount to unlawful killing.[93] But where the causes of the fatal disease are chemical rather than pathogenic, it may be better to record this as "alcohol/drug related", as set out below.

---

[88] *R. v Portsmouth Coroner's Court Ex p. Anderson* [1987] 1 W.L.R. 1640, citing the earlier part of this paragraph in the 11th edn with apparent approval; *R. v Southwark Coroner Ex p. Kendall* [1988] 1 W.L.R. 1186, 1192, DC; *R. v Inner North London Coroner Ex p. Diesa Koto* (1993) 157 J.P. 857, DC; *R. v Lincoln Coroner Ex p. Hay* [2000] Lloyd's Rep. Med. 264 at [81]; cf. *Attorney General v South London Coroner* (1987) 152 J.P. 641, QBD and *R. v Wolverhampton Coroner Ex p. McCurbin* [1990] 1 W.L.R. 719 at 728, referring to the possibility of misadventure verdicts, though without citation of *Ex p. Anderson* or *Ex p. Kendall*. cf. Farrell, *Coroners: Practice and Procedure* (2000) para.15–12.

[89] Cf. *Re Deepak Patel*, *Daily Telegraph*, November 2, 2001, Hornsey Coroner (antibiotics to treat meningoccal septicaemia given by mistake to another patient; conclusion of natural causes).

[90] *R. v Birmingham and Solihull Coroner Ex p. Benton* (1997) 1962 J.P. 807; 8 Med.L.R. 362.

[91] *Re Roger Russell*, *Daily Telegraph*, February 15, 2002, Surrey coroner (test of spa bath at garden centre accidentally released Legionnaires' disease pathogens: accidental death).

[92] See para.[13–60].

[93] cf. *R. v Clarence* (1888) 22 Q.B.D. 23, CCR, as overtaken by *R. v Wilson* [1984] A.C. 242 at 260 and *R. v Burstow* [1997] 4 All E.R. 225, HL.

II *"Alcohol/drug related"* (formerly *"Dependence on drugs/non-dependent abuse of drugs"*)

In the notes to the equivalent 1953 form,[94] there were suggested conclusions of   **13–41**
"chronic alcoholism" and "addiction to drugs", but in the notes to the 1984 form
the former was omitted and the latter became "dependence on drugs/non-
dependent abuse of drugs". Now in the 2013 form the new wording is instead
"alcohol/drug related".

"Dependence on drugs" in the notes to the 1984 form referred only to the case   **13–42**
of the death of a confirmed drug addict from the poisoning effect of the drugs, just
like "chronic alcoholism" (in relation to alcohol) and "addiction to drugs" in the
1953 form.[95] A death resulting from an exceptional excess of drugs, in a case where
the deceased was not dependent on the drug, was usually recorded as non-
dependent abuse of drugs.[96] Sometimes, however, such deaths were recorded (if
appropriate) as accident or misadventure.[97] As the word "drug" was regarded
pejoratively, accidental death caused by deliberate inhalation of solvent fumes could
not be recorded as "acute abuse of a *drug*", though it could be recorded (for
example) as *solvent* abuse.[98]

The new formulation is looser and (perhaps intentionally) less pejorative. It   **13–43**
appears to cover death from both (i) the poisoning effect of the drugs or alcohol in
the drug addict or chronic alcoholic, and (ii) accidental death resulting from abuse
of alcohol or drugs. But these kinds of deaths are quite different, and it is unclear
what advantage is gained by lumping them together. Moreover the role of alcohol
or drugs can be recorded elsewhere, for example in the medical cause of death, and
it may be preferable to employ the conclusion most appropriate to the circumstances (such as natural causes, accident and so on) than to group all such deaths
together.

III *"Industrial disease"*[99]

This expression has no statutorily defined meaning for the purposes of an inquest   **13–44**
determination. Hence it can apply even though the occupation of the deceased is
not one of those prescribed as an industrial disease for the purposes of social
security.[100] In this wider sense it means any disease caused by employment. From
the coroner's point of view, death from such a disease is unnatural.[101] The coroner

---

[94] Form 18 in Sch.3 to the Coroners Rules 1953.
[95] Home Office Circular No. 68 of 1955, App.4, para.3(b).
[96] e.g. *Re Lady Gormanston, The Times*, December 20, 1984, Westminster coroner: aspiration of vomit
   following heroin overdose by non-addict; *Re Jason Fitzsimmons, The Times*, January 30–31, 1986:
   14-year-old boy choked on vomit after overdose of sleeping tablets, heroin and methadone.
[97] *R. v Northampton Coroner Ex p. Tomkinson* (1995) 160 J.P. 69, DC; see, e.g. *Re Michelle Bartlett, The
   Times*, July 17, 1985, Westminster coroner: 14-year-old girl took overdose of paracetamol and
   penicillin without intention to kill herself; *Re Karen Pate, The Times*, July 5, 1985, St Pancras coroner:
   the deceased took five Panadol tablets to relieve back pain, and suffered liver failure; cf. *Re Ian Fuller,
   The Times*, November 16, 1983, Battersea coroner: heroin capsules swallowed by smuggler burst
   inside stomach.
[98] *R. v Southwark Coroner Ex p Kendall* [1988] 1 W.L.R. 1186, DC.
[99] See 15–34—15–35 below.
[100] *R. v South Glamorgan Coroner Ex p. BP Chemicals Ltd* (1987) 151 J.P. 799, DC .
[101] See 5–70 ff above.

(or jury) need only be satisfied on the balance of probabilities that death resulted from a disease caused by work.

13–45   If there were several successive occupations, it is not necessary to be satisfied *which* of them caused the disease, as long as the coroner (or jury) is satisfied that it was one of them. The inquest is not concerned with awarding compensation, but with ascertaining and recording facts.[102] Hence if there are occupational and non-occupational causes available, the coroner (or jury) must be satisfied that it was one of the occupational causes, and the rules of causation in the tort of negligence are irrelevant.[103]

IV *"Lawful/unlawful killing"*[104]

13–46   A lawful killing is one which is deliberate, and which would amount to murder (or voluntary manslaughter) but for the presence of an additional factor which justifies it. This may be, for example, self-defence, or the defence of others or of property.[105] Thus, in one case a conclusion of "justifiable homicide" (the forerunner of lawful killing) was quashed, because the evidence disclosed circumstances either amounting to an accident or to unlawful killing, but there was no basis for saying that the injuries to the deceased were legally justified if deliberately inflicted.[106] For the purpose of returning a conclusion, lawful killing does not include execution of sentence of death or killing by accident or misadventure, which are separate conclusions.

13–47   As to unlawful killing, the law before 1887, as continued by the Coroners Act of that year, required the coroner's inquest, in the case of a finding of murder or manslaughter,[107] to name the person(s) found to have committed the homicide.[108] The inquisition then operated as an indictment of the person(s) so charged, who would be committed for trial on the inquisition at the next assizes.[109] This was never the law in relation to any other offence involving killing.

13–48   But in 1977 the power of the inquest to in effect charge a person with homicide was abolished,[110] and further amendments removed the other surviving distinctions in coroners' law between murder, manslaughter and infanticide, on the one hand, and other homicide offences on the other.[111] So since 1977 the inquisition has played no direct role in the criminal process.

13–49   The conclusion of unlawful killing, which was then introduced, was not intended to indicate even a prima facie case of criminal liability. Instead it was introduced in order to enable the judgment-neutral fact of *how the deceased came by*

---

[102] See 1–22—1–24 above.

[103] cf. *Fairchild v Glenhaven Funeral Services Ltd* [2003] 1 A.C. 32, HL; *Barker v Corus UK Ltd* [2006] 2 A.C. 572, HL; *Sienkewicz v Greif (UK) Ltd* [2011] 2 A.C. 229, SC; *Durham v BAI (Run Off) Ltd* [2012] 1 W.L.R. 867, SC; *International Energy Group Ltd v Zurich Insurance plc UK* [2013] 3 All E.R. 395, CA.

[104] See the Chief Coroner's Law Sheet No. 1, *Unlawful killing*.

[105] As to which see the Criminal Law Act 1967 s.3, and 14–112 ff below.

[106] *R. v Durham Coroner Ex p. Attorney General, The Times*, June 29, 1978, DC.

[107] This included infanticide after the Infanticide Act 1922 s.1(1).

[108] Coroners Act 1887 s.4(3) (repealed); Coroners Rules 1953 r.26(c) (repealed).

[109] Coroners Act 1887 s.5 (repealed); see 1–28 above.

[110] Criminal Law Act 1977 s.56(1). This followed the naming of Lord Lucan in the inquisition on the inquest in June 1975 into the death of his children's nanny, Sandra Rivett.

[111] Criminal Law Act 1977 ss.56(2), 65(5) and Sch.13.

his death[112] to be recorded. By concentrating on the deceased rather than any alleged perpetrator (who in any event could not be named),[113] it was hoped to turn the verdict into a purely factual record.

Yet logically it is difficult to state that a person has been the victim of a crime **13–50** without first being satisfied that a crime has been committed. Public perception has accordingly been that unlawful killing is a judgmental, and not merely a factual, conclusion. Although the establishment in civil proceedings of the fact of a crime is only required to be achieved to the civil standard, i.e. the balance of probabilities,[114] the English courts after 1977 established the rule that the conclusion of unlawful killing could not be reached unless the coroner or jury was satisfied to the *criminal* standard of proof, i.e. beyond reasonable doubt.[115]

Prior to 1977 this would have been nonsense. At most, an express finding by an **13–51** inquest coroner or jury of murder or manslaughter by a named person operated to *charge* a person with the offence, not to *convict* him of it.[116] It was a committal for trial. Yet a grand jury, or (later) examining magistrates, did not have to be satisfied of guilt *beyond reasonable doubt* before committing for trial. A case to answer was sufficient. Other common law jurisdictions have accordingly held that the civil standard is enough, thus avoiding the English error.[117]

The impact of the Human Rights Act 1998 on the conclusion of unlawful **13–52** killing is limited. Where the inquest is or constitutes the United Kingdom's means of compliance with the procedural obligation[118] under art.2 (the right to life),[119] it must investigate the facts relevant to the lawfulness (in the criminal sense) of the force causing death.[120]

But there is no requirement that the inquest itself be a method of apportioning **13–53** guilt. Nor, indeed, is it even necessary that a conclusion such as unlawful killing be available.[121] It is sufficient if the facts brought out

"contribute to the prosecution of the offenders by bringing the offences to the attention of those who are responsible for directing prosecutions."[122]

---

[112] Coroners Act 1988 s.11(5)(b)(ii) (repealed); see *R. (Wilkinson) v Greater Manchester South Coroner* [2012] EWHC 2755 (Admin), and 13–01 above.

[113] Coroners Rules 1984, R. 42 (repealed); see 12–112. *Cf. Perre v Chivell* [2000] SASC 279 (finding that named person sent bomb which killed deceased permissible).

[114] *Hornal v Neuberger Products Ltd* [1957] 1 Q.B. 247; *Re Dellow's WT* [1964] 1 W.L.R. 451; *Post Office v Estuary Radio* [1967] 1 W.L.R. 847; *Nishina Trading v Chiyoda Fire Co* [1969] 2 Q.B. 449; *Miles v Cain, The Times*, December 14, 1989.

[115] *R. v West London Coroner Ex p. Gray* [1988] Q.B. 467, DC; *R. v Wolverhampton Coroner Ex p. AG* (1990) 155 J.P. 190, DC; *R. v Inner North London Coroner Ex p. Diesa Koto* (1993) 157 J.P. 857, DC; *R. (Francis) v Inner South London Deputy Coroner* [2005] EWHC 980 (Admin.); *R. (Cash) v Northamptonshire Coroner* [2007] EWHC 1354 (Admin.).

[116] *Wakley v Cooke* (1849) 4 Exch. 511, 154 E.R. 1316; see 1–28.

[117] *Anderson v Balashki* [1993] 2 V.R. 89; *Secretary to the Department of Health and Community Services v Gurrick* [1995] 2 V.R. 69. See also Matthews, "The Coroner and the Quantum of Proof" (1993) 12 C.J.Q. 279, and (1994) 13 C.J.Q. 309, and the *Shipman Inquiry, First Report*, paras 9–40—9–43 (http://webarchive.nationalarchives.gov.uk/20090808154959/http://www.the-shipman-inquiry.org.uk/report-s.asp).

[118] i.e. to investigate how the death occurred.

[119] See 21–15 ff below.

[120] *Re Jordan's Application* Unreported January 29, 2002, HC (NI), Kerr J.

[121] *Re Jordan's Application* Unreported January 29, 2002, HC (NI), Kerr J.

[122] *Re Jordan's Application* Unreported January 29, 2002, HC (NI), Kerr J.

In other words it is the *fact finding* that matters, *not* any expression of legal judgment that might be made. But in any event it seems that the better view is that a conclusion of unlawful killing does not engage, much less than infringe, art.6.[123]

13–54   Unlawful killing covers all cases of unlawful homicide, but does not include cases where the killing was justified, e.g. by self-defence or the prevention of crime.[124] It clearly covers murder,[125] manslaughter (including corporate manslaughter)[126] and infanticide.[127] The question arises whether it includes any of the offences of causing death by dangerous (or other culpable) driving.[128] Unlawful killing serves to distinguish cases where it would be an abuse of language to describe the events leading to death as simply an accident. In the expression itself there is a connotation of the use of violence in contrast to a more neutral expression such as "causing death".

13–55   Accordingly the verdict of unlawful killing is restricted to murder, manslaughter (including corporate manslaughter) and infanticide. Bad driving cases causing death may, therefore, only be regarded as "unlawful killing" for inquest purposes if they satisfy the ingredients for manslaughter (gross negligence manslaughter). The offences of causing death by dangerous driving, causing death by careless driving and other driving offences where death is caused do not fall within the scope of a verdict of unlawful killing in the coroner jurisdiction.[129] In complex cases it may in any event be too confusing for the jury to consider death by dangerous driving separately from manslaughter.[130]

13–56   Unlawful killing is also the appropriate conclusion where killing abroad would have constituted an unlawful homicide under English law had it taken place in England.[131] Since there was no rule that a corporate body could not be guilty of involuntary manslaughter, and there is now a specific offence of corporate manslaughter,[132] it is possible for an unlawful killing conclusion to be recorded where a corporate body would be so liable.[133] Unlawful killing is not, however, appropriate where the killer is not criminally responsible, e.g. because too young[134]

---

[123] See 13–107 ff above.

[124] See 14–112 ff below.

[125] See 14–37 below.

[126] See 14–42 below.

[127] See 14–69 below.

[128] Burton, Chambers and Gill, *Coroners' Inquiries* (1985) p.86 and Thurston's *Coronership*, 3rd edn (1985), para.22–32. See also note (4)(c) to the prescribed form of inquisition (Form 22) in Sch.4 to the Coroners Rules 1984 (which confines it to murder, manslaughter and infanticide).

[129] *R. (Wilkinson) v Greater Manchester South Coroner* [2012] EWHC 2755 (Admin) at [63]–[71]. See the Chief Coroner's Law Sheet No. 1, *Unlawful killing*.

[130] cf. *R. v Inner South London Coroner Ex p. Douglas-Williams* [1999] 1 All E.R. 344 at 349, CA; 12–115 above.

[131] See, e.g. *Re Winifred Smith, The Times*, October 3, 1985 (Reading coroner) (death by criminal negligence in Vienna). *Re Aimee Stephenson, Daily Telegraph*, April 10, 2002, Wiltshire coroner (criminal negligence in Peru).

[132] See 14–52 below.

[133] *Re Herald of Free Enterprise, The Times*, October 10, 1987; *Re Towy Rail Bridge, The Independent*, July 22, 1988; *Re Gulf War Deaths, The Times*, May 15, 1992.

[134] e.g. *Re Perry Osbourne, Daily Telegraph*, November 19, 1986, St Pancras coroner (open verdict); *Re Karla Granville, Daily Telegraph*, July 12, 2002, Southwark coroner (misadventure)

or insane.[135] In the latter case, where insanity is raised it must be disproved, to the criminal standard, before unlawful killing is appropriate.[136]

Although it is in general prohibited for a verdict to appear to determine criminal **13–57** liability on the part of a named person,[137] there are cases where it will be obvious that a particular person, though not named in the verdict, was responsible for the death,[138] and a conclusion of unlawful killing must be recorded if appropriate.[139] It is unarguable that, wherever the evidence and the circumstances are such that a conclusion of unlawful killing must relate to the conduct of a person who is in fact identifiable, it would infringe ECHR art.8[140] to return such a conclusion, and therefore such a conclusion is not open to the coroner.[141]

As with suicide,[142] and as already stated, the standard of proof in unlawful killing **13–58** cases is the criminal one, i.e. beyond all reasonable doubt,[143] for all the relevant elements of the relevant form of unlawful killing, which must all inhere in the same person.[144] If the jury is not properly directed on this standard, the verdict will be quashed.[145]

Where a coroner or jury has to consider the twin possibilities of unlawful killing **13–59** and accident/misadventure, unlawful killing should be considered first.[146] If the coroner or jury is not satisfied beyond reasonable doubt that the death was the result of unlawful killing, then they must go on to consider whether, *on the balance of probabilities*, the death was the result of accident/misadventure.[147] But if they are not satisfied on the balance of probabilities that it was accident/misadventure, the only conclusion available is an "open verdict".[148]

---

[135] *R. (O'Connor) v Avon Coroner* [2009] EWHC 854 (Admin.).
[136] *R. (O'Connor) v Avon Coroner* [2009] EWHC 854 (Admin.).
[137] Coroners and Justice Act 2009 s.10(2)(a); formerly Coroners Rules 1984 r.42; *Hay v Devon Coroner* (1998) 162 J.P. 96, CA. see also 13–103 ff.
[138] See Home Office Circular No. 187 of 1977, App.C para.11.
[139] Such cases include (a) those of a gunman going on the rampage: *Re Michael Ryan and others*, *The Independent*, September 30, 1987, Berkshire coroner; (b) those where a person has killed his family or friends and then himself; *Re Parry*, *The Times*, April 28, 1984, Rotherham coroner; *Re Fryer*, *The Times*, January 30 1985, Walthamstow coroner; *Re Peter and Laurie Gray*, *The Independent*, November 19, 1988, Wiltshire coroner; and (c) cases where the evidence showed that one of two people must have killed the victim, but not which of them it was: *Re Jenkins*, *The Times*, November 12, 1985, Coventry coroner. For a study of suicide preceded by murder, see Barraclough and Harris (2002) 32 *Psychological Medicine* 577.
[140] See 21–29 ff.
[141] *R. (Evans) v Cardiff and Vale of Glamorgan Coroner* [2010] EWHC 3478 (Admin.); affirmed [2011] EWCA Civ. 719.
[142] See 13–70 above.
[143] *R. v West London Coroner's Court Ex p. Gray* [1988] Q.B. 467, DC; *R. v Wolverhampton Coroner Ex p. McCurbin* [1990] 1 W.L.R. 719, CA; *R. v Hampshire Coroner Ex p. Attorney General* (1990) 155 J.P. 190, DC. See *Matthews*, "The Coroner and the Quantum of Proof" (1993) 12 C.J.Q. 279; also (1994) 13 C.J.Q. 309. See the Chief Coroner's Law Sheet No. 1, *Unlawful killing*.
[144] *R. (Secretary of State for Justice) v West Yorkshire (Eastern District) Deputy Coroner* [2012] EWHC 1634 (Admin) at [48]–[53].
[145] *R. v St Pancras Coroner Ex p. Higgins* (1988) 152 J.P. 637, DC; *R. v South Powys Coroner Ex p. Jones* [1991] C.O.D. 14, DC; *R. v Hampshire Coroner Ex p. Attorney General* (1990) 155 J.P. 190, DC.
[146] See the Chief Coroner's Law Sheet No. 1, *Unlawful killing*.
[147] *R. v Wolverhampton Coroner Ex p. McCurbin* [1990] 1 W.L.R. 719 at 728; *R. (Francis) v Inner South London Deputy Coroner* [2005] EWHC 980 (Admin.) at [35], [37].
[148] *R. (Francis) v Inner South London Deputy Coroner* [2005] EWHC 980 (Admin.) at [37]. Cf. *R. (Lagos) v City of London Coroner* [2013] EWHC 423 (Admin.) at [35] (suicide).

V *"Natural causes"*

13–60   A case which is referred to the coroner because there is reason to suspect it is "unnatural"[149] or "unknown"[150] may still after investigation turn out to be one of "natural causes". In part, this is because a death from natural causes may nonetheless be "unnatural" within the meaning of coroner law, for example because of late diagnosis of disease, poor treatment, or unsuccessful operations. In part it is also because much depends upon current social conventions. And what is socially acceptable behaviour may change over time.

13–61   The distinction between natural causes and accidental death/misadventure, in both medical and non-medical cases, has already been discussed.[151] For the purposes of an inquest determination, a person dependent on alcohol or drugs who dies from a naturally acquired natural disease has died from natural causes, even though a person not so dependent might not have succumbed. On the other hand, a person who dies from an industrial disease does not die from natural causes, even if death from the same disease in a non-industrial context might be so treated. A person who dies from a natural disease whose pathogens were deliberately or recklessly introduced into his or her body may have been unlawfully killed.[152]

VI *"Open verdict"*

13–62   If there is insufficient evidence to record any of the other suggested conclusions, an "open verdict" may be recorded.[153] This includes the case where there *is* evidence for another conclusion, but it fails to reach the required standard of proof.[154] The notes to the prescribed 1984 form of inquisition explained this conclusion as where "the evidence did not fully or further disclose the means whereby the cause of death arose".[155]

13–63   To return this conclusion is not a failure of any kind on the part of the coroner or jury, and does not reflect on them.[156] But coroners should not direct juries that open verdict is some kind of refuge from making a decision.[157] It must be clearly distinguished from a failure by a jury to agree.[158] Open verdict is the *agreed* (or majority) view of the jury that there is insufficient evidence to return any other conclusion.

13–64   Coroners must also guard against the mischievous seeking of open verdict in order to have a death clouded in suspicion,[159] but there will be cases where there

---

[149] See 5–70ff.
[150] See 5–80ff.
[151] See 5–74.
[152] cf. *R. v Clarence* (1888) 22 Q.B.D 23, CCR, as overtaken by *R. v Wilson* [1984] A.C. 242 at 260, and *R. v Burstow* [1997] 4 All E.R. 225, HL.
[153] *R. v Huntbach Ex p. Lockley* [1944] K.B. 606.
[154] See previous paragraph, and also 13–59, 13–71.
[155] Coroners Rules 1984 Sch.4 Form 22 Note (4)(b) (repealed).
[156] *R. v City of London Coroner Ex p. Barber* [1975] 1 W.L.R. 1310, DC; *R. (Francis) v Inner South London Deputy Coroner* [2005] EWHC 980 (Admin) at [40].
[157] *R. v City of London Coroner Ex p. Calvi, The Times*, April 2, 1983, DC.
[158] See 13–13 ff.
[159] *Re Tabarn* Unreported January 20, 1998, DC.

is a real doubt and any other conclusion would be unjust.[160] On the other hand, the fact that there may be uncertainty as to other parts of the inquisition, for example as to the precise medical cause, time or place of death, does not authorise recording an open verdict if there is sufficient evidence to record how the deceased came by his death. In other words, the coroner or jury should not fail to reach a positive conclusion merely because there is doubt on some minor point.

VII *"Road traffic collision"*

This is a completely new conclusion in 2013, on which there is as yet no guidance.   **13–65**
It would appear to cover all cases where a person dies as a result of a collision between two vehicles, or a vehicle and a stationary or fixed object, or even a vehicle and a pedestrian or passer-by, as long as it arises from *road* traffic. So it would not cover collisions not on roads (such as on private land) or collisions not with road traffic (such as railway vehicles). Most of these cases would have been cases of accident or misadventure before 2013. It is not clear what, if any, advantage is achieved by this change, since the fact of the road traffic collision will be apparent from the statement in box 3 ("How, when and where?").

VIII *"Stillbirth"*

A coroner might not be sure in a particular case whether a death is or is not a   **13–66**
stillbirth, and so the matter goes to an inquest. In such a case, If the "death" is found in fact to have been stillbirth,[161] the determination is marked "stillbirth" in para.(4), but the rest of the form is not completed,[162] for the child not having been born had no independent life and cannot properly form the subject of an inquest.[163]

IX *Suicide*[164]

Suicide means self-murder. It should never be presumed, but must always be based   **13–67**
upon some evidence that the deceased intended to take his own life.[165] On the other hand, once there is *sufficient* evidence, it is a matter for the coroner (or jury, if there is one) as to whether or not it *was* suicide, and the High Court will not quash a conclusion (whether of suicide or open verdict) unless no reasonable coroner (or jury) properly directed could have found such a conclusion in such

---

[160] *R. v City of London Coroner Ex p. Barber* [1975] 1 W.L.R. 1310, DC; *R. v Northamptonshire Coroner Ex p. Walker* (1998) 153 J.P. 289, DC; see also *Attorney General v South London Coroner* (1988) 152 J.P. 641.
[161] As to this expression, see 5–04 above.
[162] See Coroners Rules 1984 Sch.4 Form 22, note 4(d) (repealed); the notes to the current form (Coroners (Inquests) Rules 2013 (SI 2013/1616) r.34 Sch. Form 2) are silent on the point.
[163] See 5–04 above.
[164] For a discussion of suicide by statistical analysis, see Henderson, Mellin and Patel, *Journal of Clinical Forensic Medicine*, 12 (2005) 305–309.
[165] *R. v Huntbach Ex p. Lockley* [1944] K.B. 606; *Re Davis* [1968] 1 Q.B. 72; *R. v Cardiff City Coroner Ex p. Thomas* [1970] 1 W.L.R. 1475; *R. v City of London Coroner Ex p. Barber* [1975] 1 W.L.R. 1310; *R. v Northamptonshire Coroner Ex p. Walker* (1988) 151 J.P. 773, DC; *R. (Jenkins) v Bridgend Coroner* [2012] EWHC 3175 (Admin.) at [18]–[20].

circumstances.[166] The test of sufficiency of evidence for suicide has been stated to be "whether other possible explanations were totally ruled out".[167]

13–68   Although suicide ceased to be a crime in 1961,[168] it was the law until 1996 that a death could not be recorded as suicide if it ensued more than a year and a day after the injury was inflicted.[169] Since 1996, the "year and a day" rule has been abolished, and a death caused by suicide is to be so recorded, whenever the causative injury occurred.[170]

13–69   The question of causation can be troublesome in suicide cases. In one civil case, the House of Lords held that, where the claimant's husband was injured in an accident through the defendant's negligence, foreseeably causing depression, which caused him subsequently to commit suicide, the defendant was liable for damages flowing from the death.[171] But it was still suicide. And, in another such case, Blake J held that, where a young offender was subject to restraint a few hours before taking his own life, and his state of mind may have been affected by it, the coroner should have ruled on the lawfulness of the restraint and directed the jury accordingly.[172]

13–70   At least since 1984 it has been consistently held in England that the standard of proof in suicide cases should be the same as in criminal prosecutions, i.e. beyond reasonable doubt,[173] although there is no crime involved and an inquest is not a criminal trial (or any sort of trial[174]). The comparative difficulty in obtaining a conclusion of suicide may well mean that official statistics significantly underestimate the occurrence of suicide.[175]

13–71   All other definite conclusions (except unlawful killing)[176] operate on the civil standard, i.e. the balance of probabilities.[177] This logically means that if the coroner (or jury) is satisfied *on the balance of probabilities* that it was suicide, but is not satisfied

---

[166] *R. v Devon Coroner Ex p. Glover* (1984) 149 J.P. 208; *R. (Lagos) v City of London Coroner* [2013] EWHC 423 (Admin.) at [41].

[167] *R. v Essex Coroner Ex p. Hopper* Unreported May 13, 1988, DC; *R. (Jenkins) v Bridgend Coroner* [2012] EWHC 3175 (Admin.) at [29]; *R. (Lagos) v City of London Coroner* [2013] EWHC 423 (Admin.) at [41].

[168] Suicide Act 1961.

[169] *R. v Inner West London Coroner Ex p. De Luca* [1989] Q.B. 249, DC; see the 9th ed.n of this work (1957), p.229.

[170] See the Law Reform (Year and a Day) Rule 1996.

[171] *Corr v IBC Vehicles Ltd* [2008] UKHL 13.

[172] *R. (Pounder) v Durham and Darlington Coroner* [2009] EWHC 76 (Admin.).

[173] *R. v Dyfed Coroner Ex p. Evans* Unreported May 24, 1984, DC; *R. v North Northumberland Coroner Ex p. Armstrong* (1987) 151 J.P. 773 at 785; *R. v Wolverhampton Coroner Ex p. McCurbin* [1990] 1 W.L.R. 719 at 728; *R. v Newbury Coroner Ex p. John* (1991) 156 J.P. 456 at 457; *R. v Birmingham and Solihull Coroner Ex p. Nutt* [1993] COD 449, DC; *R. (Jenkins) v Bridgend Coroner* [2012] EWHC 3175 (Admin) at [17]; *R. (Lagos) v City of London Coroner* [2013] EWHC 423 (Admin) at [35]; cf. *Re Beckon* (1992) 93 D.L.R. (4th) 161, Ontario CA; *Re Sutherland* [1994] 2 N.Z.L.R. 22, HC (NZ) (balance of probabilities). See Matthews, "The Coroner and the Quantum of Proof" (1993) 12 C.J.Q. 279, and also (1994) 13 C.J.Q. 309.

[174] See 1–19, 10–01 ff, 12–61.

[175] See Chambers (1989) 29 Med. Sci. Law 181. For examples, see *Re David Paulton, Daily Telegraph*, May 23, 2002; *Re Natasha Lake, Daily Telegraph*, May 29, 2002, South Staffs coroner; *Re Morgan Musson, The Daily Telegraph*, February 21, 2002, Nottingham coroner; *Re Jevan Richardson, Daily Telegraph*, June 12, 2001, Southwark coroner.

[176] See 13–47 ff above.

[177] *Re Tabarn* Unreported January 23, 1998, DC.

beyond reasonable doubt, the conclusion must be an open one.[178] The suggested form of conclusion in suicide cases is "suicide"[179] (formerly that the deceased "killed himself [whilst the balance of his mind was disturbed]").[180]

The use of the additional words "the balance of his [or her] mind was disturbed" **13–72** (which do not appear in the current rules) is still possible, but ought to be based upon some evidence to that effect given at the inquest,[181] even though insufficient to negative the intention to take his or her own life. They do not imply any psychopathy, and for this reason it may be better to use a more explanatory phrase such as "whilst suffering extremely anxiety/distress". But if the inquest, on the basis of evidence, finds that the deceased's mind *was* disturbed, then it is a finding that should be recorded. Other forms of words, such as "self-harm",[182] have sometimes been used instead of "suicide" or "killed himself", but this is not recommended.

Other conclusions

That concludes the "official" list of short-form conclusions in the notes to the **13–73** current form of record of inquest. There now follow the remaining conclusions discussed in the notes to the former form of inquisition. As already stated,[183] there is nothing in law to prevent these conclusions being employed where appropriate.

"Want of attention at birth"

Want of attention at birth is an old-fashioned conclusion, but plainly a form of **13–74** neglect. It states the facts, and obviously should not be used where the death was caused by such negligence or intention to cause harm that the conclusion could be one of unlawful killing, or would be better recorded as neglect.[184] As with neglect, there must be a clear causal link between the want of attention and the death. In the period 2004-12 there were 12 such cases reported, the most in any one year being three.

"Attempted/self-induced abortion"

This conclusion is not about the death of the baby. Instead, it applies where the **13–75** *mother* dies as a result of an attempted or self-induced abortion. Until the passing of the Abortion Act 1967 it was a significant conclusion. Nowadays it is very rare. In the period 2004-12 there were two such cases reported, the most in any one year being one.

---

[178] cf. *R. v City of London Coroner Ex p. Barber* [1975] 1 W.L.R. 1310 at 1313; *R. v Northamptonshire Coroner Ex p. Walker* (1988) 151 J.P. 773, DC; *R. (Lagos) v City of London Coroner* [2013] EWHC 423 (Admin.) at [35]. See also *R. (Francis) v Inner South London Deputy Coroner* [2005] EWHC 980 (Admin.) at [37] (unlawful killing).
[179] Coroners (Inquests) Rules 2013 (SI 2013/1616) r.34 Sch. Form 2, Note (i) IX.
[180] Coroners Rules 1984, Sch.4 Form 22, Note (repealed).
[181] *R. v Horner Ex p. Jones* [1956] Crim.L.R. 482, CA.
[182] See, e.g. *Re Hannah Taylerson, Daily Telegraph*, March 6, 2002, Bristol coroner.
[183] See 13–35.
[184] Home Office Circular No. 68 of 1955, App.4 para.3(a).

"Disaster"

13–76   In 1999 the law was changed to require a coroner to adjourn an inquest pending a public inquiry into a disaster in which the deceased died.[185] According to the notes to the 1984 inquisition form (as amended in 1999), where such an inquest is resumed,[186] it will be open to the coroner or jury to conclude that the deceased "died in the [*name*] disaster".[187] But the notes have no legislative force, and hence this conclusion may be used in appropriate circumstances not otherwise falling within the terms of the notes.[188] In the period 2004-12 there were nine such cases reported, the most in any one year being four.

"Execution of sentence of death"

13–77   After the abolition of the death penalty for murder,[189] treason,[190] aggravated piracy,[191] and spying in naval ships and foreign establishments,[192] the death penalty in Britain remained possible in military cases only. But even in these cases it was finally abolished.[193] However, other legal systems retain the death penalty, and hence this will be the appropriate conclusion if the body of a person upon whom sentence of death has been lawfully executed is brought into England or Wales and becomes the subject of an inquest. But the inquest in such a case is not a basis for examining whether the sentence of death was legally or morally justified. There were no such cases in the period 2004–12.[194]

"Death on active service"

13–78   Historically, the bodies of service personnel who had died abroad on active service were rarely brought back to England and Wales, but were buried where they fell.[195] Consequently coroners were not troubled with such cases. Since the Falklands War in 1982, however, increasing numbers of British war dead have been repatriated, and nowadays nearly all are. So (where the bodies are repatriated to England and Wales) coroners are now very much involved. There are even special statutory provisions relating to such deaths.[196] ECHR art.2 may sometimes be engaged.[197]

---

[185] See 10–81 above.

[186] See 10–81 above.

[187] See the Coroners Rules 1984 Sch.4 Form 22 fn.4(b), as amended by SI 1999/3325 r.18. The notes to the 2013 record of inquest do not mention this conclusion at all.

[188] See 13–35 above.

[189] Murder (Abolition of the Death Penalty) Act 1965 s.1.

[190] Crime and Disorder Act 1998 s.36.

[191] Crime and Disorder Act 1998 s.36.

[192] Armed Forces Act 1981 s.17.

[193] See Human Rights Act 1998 s.21(5) and the Armed Forces Act 2001 s.38, Sch.7 Pt 4, repealing the Army Act 1955 s.70(1)(a), the Air Force Act 1955 s.(1)(a), and the Naval Discipline Act 1957 s.43(1)(a), as from May 11, 2001.

[194] The last occasion appears to have been the inquest into the death of the journalist Farzad Bazoft, executed by the then Iraqi regime for spying in March 1990, whose body was returned to Britain.

[195] The case of Lord Nelson, whose body was brought back from Trafalgar (in a barrel of spirits) for burial in St Paul's Cathedral, is a rare exception.

[196] Coroners and Justice Act 2009 ss.12-13; see 4–25—4–27. See also the Armed Forces (Service Inquiries) Regulations 2008 (SI 2008/1651), providing for separate service inquiries.

[197] See 21–15.

The Chief Coroner has created a cadre of coroners with specialist military training for inquests into such deaths.[198]

The question is what, if any, conclusion as to death is appropriate in such cases? **13–79** In considering this question, coroners will take into account the fact that the families of deceased service personnel will commonly wish such conclusion to reflect the active service involved, and also that other consequences may flow from the fact of death being the result of active service.[199] This conclusion will of course depend on the evidence in the particular case, and the standard of proof will be the same as if the events had occurred in England and Wales.

Where the circumstances are such that, if the events took place in England and **13–80** Wales, they would amount to murder or manslaughter, then the appropriate conclusion is unlawful killing. This would apply, for example, to peacekeeping forces killed by terrorist action. On the other hand, the death of a member of such a peacekeeping force by accident (e.g. a road traffic collision), suicide or even natural causes would be just that.

But where the deceased died during a war covered by the Geneva Conven- **13–81** tions[200] the position is different.[201] There can still be cases of unlawful killing (e.g. shooting a prisoner who has surrendered and is not trying to escape), but death from enemy action in accordance with the Convention is not unlawful. It should be recorded as "Death [or killed] on active service". Where the deceased died from some other event than enemy action, but the other event *arises out of* military service, then it should be "Accidental death [or whatever] whilst on active service". Otherwise it is just "Accidental death [or whatever]".

If the deceased was injured abroad whilst on active service, and then died from **13–82** the injuries once back in England and Wales, even some time later, the position is similar. If the causative injuries were from terrorist action, the conclusion should be unlawful killing. If the causative injuries were from enemy action in a war, the conclusion should be "Died from injuries [or wounds] sustained on active service". If the injuries were not from enemy action, but arose out of military service, it should be "Died from injuries [accidentally sustained *or* whatever] whilst on active service".

"Self-neglect or lack of care/neglect"

One of the most troublesome conclusions in recent years has been lack of care (as **13–83** it used to be called) or neglect (as it is now called). There is also a self-induced version, called self-neglect, but that is easier to deal with. The history of lack of care or neglect can be divided into four main periods as follows:

(i) from the Coroners Rules 1953 to the abolition of criminal jurisdiction in 1977;[202]

---

[198] Chief Coroner's Guidance No. 7, *A Cadre of Coroners for Service Deaths*; see 2–151.
[199] For example, inheritance tax: Inheritance Tax Act 1984 s.154.
[200] See the Geneva Conventions Act 1957.
[201] It is beyond the scope of the coroner's inquest to decide whether a war is lawful or not: see 6–11. In practice there is likely to be a ministerial certificate to deal with the point.
[202] See 1–30 above.

    (ii) from the abolition of criminal jurisdiction to the *Jamieson*[203] case in 1994;

    (iii) from the *Jamieson* case to the coming into force of the Human Rights Act 1998;

    (iv) from the coming into force of the Human Rights Act 1998 to the present day.

First period

13–84 Lack of care and self-neglect were first seen as part of the conclusion as to death in the notes to the new prescribed form of inquisition in the Coroners Rules 1953.[204] Self-neglect was created to cover cases where a person dies from failing to look after himself, e.g. from starvation or exposure.[205] Even if the cause of death is natural, it is self-induced. It is not properly an accident, since it occurs over a long period, and it is not suicide, as there is no intention by the deceased to take his own life.

13–85 Lack of care was intended to be "the other side of the coin to self-neglect",[206] i.e. to cover the cases where death occurred from similar causes, but owing to senility, infancy or other incapacity the deceased was unable to look after himself and was hence in the care of others.[207] It did not depend upon the existence of a legal duty of care; a moral obligation would suffice, but in that case the conclusion implied moral censure.[208] If there *were* a legal duty of care, breached sufficiently seriously, it might be a case of manslaughter.[209]

Second period

13–86 Once the criminal jurisdiction of the inquest had been abolished, the conclusion of lack of care lost any pejorative meaning it might have had, and was no longer used to indicate any breach of duty.[210] Instead it referred to the physical, or mental,[211] condition of the deceased which caused the death, in the circumstances immediately surrounding that death.[212]

---

[203] *R. v North Humberside Coroner Ex p. Jamieson* [1995] Q.B. 1, CA.

[204] SI 1953/205 r.42 Sch.3 Form 18 Note (5)(a). There is an early example of neglect in the form of inquisition prescribed by the Coroners Act 1887 Sch.2, but that was in the context of a serious breach of a (civil) duty of care in failing to fence a pond, amounting to gross negligence manslaughter. The form was replaced in 1916 (S.R. & O. 1916 Nos 374, 375), omitting the neglect example altogether, as did the various substituted forms thereafter (S.R. & O. 1918 No. 1016; S.R. & O. 1923 No. 1365; S.R. & O. 1927, No. 344). On the history of these provisions, see generally *R. v North Humberside Coroner Ex p. Jamieson* [1995] Q.B. 1, CA.

[205] See the 9th edn (1957) of this work, at p.178; Home Office Circular No. 68 of 1955, para.7, App.4, para.3(c).

[206] *R. v Southwark Coroner Ex p. Hicks* [1987] 1 W.L.R. 1624, DC.

[207] See the 9th edn (1957) of this work, at p.179; Home Office Circular No. 68 of 1955 para.7 App.4 para.3(c).

[208] See the 9th edn (1957) of this work, at p.179; Home Office Circular No. 68 of 1955 para.7 App.4 para.3(c).

[209] See the 9th edn (1957) of this work, at p.179; Home Office Circular No. 68 of 1955 para.7 App.4 para.3(c).

[210] *R. v Southwark Coroner Ex p. Hicks* [1987] 1 W.L.R. 1624, DC; *R. v East Berkshire Coroner Ex p. Buckley* (1992) 157 J.P. 425, DC.

[211] *R. v Birmingham Coroner Ex p. Home Secretary* (1990) 155 J.P. 107, DC.

[212] *R. v East Berkshire Coroner Ex p. Buckley* (1992) 157 J.P. 425, DC.

The word "care" here meant physical attention, or care "in the narrow sense of   **13–87**
the word",[213] rather than in the wider, more abstract sense of the duty of care.[214]
It became a purely factual statement: here was a person receiving physical attention;
that attention stopped (for whatever reason) and the stoppage directly caused or
contributed to the death. *Inappropriate* (as opposed to *no*) care could in some cases
amount to accident/misadventure, or even unlawful killing, but not lack of
care.[215]

Third period

The decision of the Court of Appeal in *R. v North Humberside Coroner Ex p.*   **13–88**
Jamieson[216] was a watershed. First, it suggested that in future the concept of lack of
care should be referred to as "neglect", in order to lessen the potential for
confusion between this conclusion and the civil law of negligence. Secondly, it
modified the requirements. It did this both by defining neglect as involving a *gross*
failure to provide physical attention, and by introducing a new requirement
that—at least in some cases—the need for such attention had to be objectively
perceptible by the person who failed to provide it.[217]

In other words, it was no longer necessary that attention *was being* provided, and   **13–89**
then stopped; "neglect" could exist if attention was never provided at all, but
objectively it was clearly needed. This in one sense widened the inquiry, but also
made the standard more difficult to attain. Arguably it made the conclusion more
pejorative, and less objectively fact-based.[218] But it was still not negligence, or
negligent lack of care.[219]

Fourth period

The coming into force of the Human Rights Act 1998[220] added an extra layer of   **13–90**
complexity. The European Convention on Human Rights by art.2 imposes a
procedural obligation on states to investigate deaths in state custody or through
state agency.[221] This may have an impact on inquests in such cases, notably deaths
in prison or police custody. These inquests will usually have to meet additional
criteria based on Strasbourg jurisprudence,[222] and their influence may spill over
into non-art.2 cases. So far it seems that the net result is only to require a broader
inquiry, or at least a broader determination, treating "how" the deceased came by
his or her death as meaning not merely "by what means", but also "in what broad
circumstances" he or she did so.[223] In the period 2004-12 it was reported that there

---

[213] *R. v Southwark Coroner Ex p. Hicks* [1987] 1 W.L.R. 1624, DC; *R. v Poplar Coroner Ex p. Thomas* [1993] Q.B. 610, CA.

[214] *R. v East Berkshire Coroner Ex p. Buckley* (1992) 157 J.P. 425, DC; *R. v Poplar Coroner Ex p. Thomas* [1993] Q.B. 610, CA.

[215] *R. v Inner North London Coroner Ex p Diesa Koto* (1993) 157 J.P. 857, DC.

[216] [1995] Q.B. 1, CA.

[217] *R. v North Humberside Coroner Ex p. Jamieson.*[1995] Q.B. 1, CA , at 25.

[218] See Matthews (1994) 110 L.Q.R. 536.

[219] *Re Wright's Application* (1996) 35 B.M.L.R. 57, CA, affirming [1997] Q.B. 786.

[220] See Ch.21 below.

[221] See 21–15.

[222] See 21–10 ff.

[223] See 6–14 above.

were 337 cases of a conclusion "aggravated by neglect or self-neglect", the most in any one year being 51.

What is neglect today?

13–91   The governing view is still that of the Court of Appeal in 1994:

> "Neglect in this context means a gross failure to provide adequate nourishment or liquid, or provide or procure basic medical attention or shelter or warmth for someone in a dependent position (because of youth, age, illness or incarceration) who cannot provide it for himself. Failure to provide medical attention for a dependent person whose physical condition is such as to show that he obviously needs it may amount to neglect. So it may be if it is the dependent person's mental condition which obviously calls for medical attention . . . In both cases the crucial consideration will be what the dependent person's condition, whether physical or mental, appears to be."[224]

13–92   It follows from this view that, in order for there to be neglect, there must be an opportunity to offer or provide the relevant nourishment, liquid, medical attention, shelter or warmth. If the timescale between the (i) moment when the deceased first showed signs of needing attention, and (ii) the moment when he went beyond assistance, is too short for attention to be provided, there is no neglect.[225] The failure to offer or provide must be "gross", that is, serious.[226]

13–93   Neglect unfortunately means different things to different people and in different contexts. In the legal context it does not necessarily imply a finding of common law negligence.[227] Instead it refers to a (factual) gap in the care that was being or, given the objectively perceptible condition of the person concerned, should have been, given. It is "continuous or at least non-transient neglect".[228]

---

[224] *R. v North Humberside Coroner Ex p. Jamieson* [1995] Q.B. 1, CA; see *R. v Southwark Coroner's Court Ex p. Epsom Health Care NHS Trust* (1994) 158 J.P. 973, DC; *R. v Birmingham Coroner Ex p. Cotton* (1955) 160 J.P. 123, DC; *R. v South Yorkshire Coroner Ex p. Tremble* (1995) 159 J.P. 761; *Re Clegg* (1996) 161 J.P. 521, DC; *R. v Surrey Coroner Ex p. Wright* [1997] Q.B. 786; *R. v Swansea and Gower Coroner Ex p. Chief Constable of Wales* (1999) 164 J.P. 191; *R. (Scott) v Inner West London Coroner* [2001] EWHC Admin. 105; *R. (Touche) v Inner North London Coroner* [2001] EWCA Civ. 383; [2001] Q.B. 1206; *R. (Marshall) v Coventry Coroner* [2001] EWHC Admin. 804; *Nicholls v Liverpool Coroner* [2001] EWHC 922 (Admin.); [2001] Inquest L.R. 249; *R. (Khan) v West Hertfordshire Coroner* [2002] EWHC 302 (Admin.); *R. (Mumford) v Berkshire Coroner* [2002] EWHC 2184 (Admin.); *R. (Metropolitan Police Commissioner) v South London Coroner* [2003] EWHC 1829 (Admin.); *Mullholland v Inner North London Coroner* [2003] EWHC 2612 (Admin.); *R. (Davies) v Birmingham Deputy Coroner* [2003] EWCA Civ. 1739; *R. (Sacker) v West Yorkshire Coroner* [2004] UKHL 11; [2004] 1 W.L.R. 796; *R. (Middleton) v West Somerset Coroner* [2004] UKHL 10; [2004] 2 A.C. 182; *R. (Longfield Care Homes Ltd) v Blackburn Coroner* [2004] EWHC 2467; *Bloom v North London ADC* [2004] EWHC 3071 (Admin.); *R. (Pekkelo) v Central & South East Kent Coroner* [2006] EWHC 1265 (Admin.); *R. (Hurst) v Commissioner of Police of the Metropolis* [2007] UKHL 13; [2007] 2 A.C. 189; *R. (Lewis) v Mid & North Shropshire Coroner* [2009] EWHC 661 (Admin.); (2009) 108 B.M.L.R. 87.

[225] *R. v Inner South London Coroner Ex p. Douglas-Williams* [1999] 1 All E.R. 344, 355, CA.

[226] *Smith v Oxfordshire Assistant Deputy Coroner* [2008] EWHC 694 (Admin.) at [40]–[47].

[227] As to negligence leading to the suicide of a detainee, see *Orange v West Yorkshire Police* [2001] EWCA Civ. 611.

[228] *Re Wright* [1997] Q.B. 786; permission to appeal refused (1996) 35 B.M.L.R. 57, CA.

The notes to the prescribed 1984 form of inquisition[229] recommended that   **13–94**
"self-neglect" or "lack of care" be used as a qualification rather than as a separate
conclusion, and then only to qualify conclusions of natural causes, industrial
diseases, dependence on drugs/non-dependent abuse of drugs, or want of attention
at birth. But these notes had no legal force, being no part of the Coroners Rules,[230]
and the forms might be modified as circumstances require.[231]

Accordingly, it had been several times held that the conclusion of "lack of care"   **13–95**
and "self-neglect" could be "free-standing" if circumstances warranted.[232] However, in 1994 the Court of Appeal expressed the view that neglect, like self-neglect,
could "rarely, if ever be an appropriate [conclusion] on its own".[233] The Court of
Appeal preferred the form that the neglect "contributed to" the main cause of
death.[234]

The issue of the free-standing neglect conclusion was revisited in 2002, when   **13–96**
the Court of Appeal indicated that human rights considerations meant that neglect
could be a free-standing conclusion in cases of "system neglect", i.e. defaults in the
system that lead to death (whether by suicide or otherwise).[235] But on appeal to the
House of Lords the distinction between individual and systemic neglect was
criticised, "since the borderline between the two is indistinct and there will often
be some overlap between the two: there are some kinds of individual failing which
a sound system may be expected to detect and remedy before harm is done. There
will, moreover, be individual failings which need to be identified even though an
individual is not to be named."[236] The House confirmed that, despite the Human
Rights Act 1998, "self-neglect" and "neglect" were terms of art in the law of
inquests, and there was no reason to alter their meaning.[237]

As stated above,[238] at an earlier stage in its history the conclusion was concerned   **13–97**
only with an absence of care; death from inappropriate treatment or rough
handling might be an accident/misadventure, or even unlawful killing (as the case
might be), but not neglect/lack of care.[239] Thus, where clinical judgment was badly

---

[229] Coroners Rules 1984 Sch.4 Form 22 note (4)(a) (repealed).
[230] *R. v Turnbull Ex p. Kenyon* Unreported March 15, 1984, DC. See also *R. v Southwark Coroner Ex p. Kendall* [1988] 1 W.L.R. 1186, DC (in relation to the 1984 form), and also *R. (Wilkinson) v Greater Manchester South Coroner* [2012] EWHC 2755 (Admin.) at [65].
[231] *R. v Southwark Coroner Ex p. Hicks* [1987] 1 W.L.R. 1624, DC.
[232] *R. v Surrey Coroner Ex p. Campbell* [1982] Q.B. 661, DC; *R. v Southwark Coroner Ex p. Hicks* [1987] 1 W.L.R. 1624, DC; *R.v Birmingham Coroner Ex p. Home Secretary* (1990) 155 J.P. 107, DC; *R. v East Berkshire Coroner Ex p. Buckley* (1992) 157 J.P. 425, DC.
[233] *R. v North Humberside Coroner Ex p. Jamieson* [1995] Q.B. 1, CA;
[234] *R. v North Humberside Coroner Ex p. Jamieson* [1995] Q.B. 1, CA; *R. v Avon Deputy Coroner Ex p. Lambourne* Unreported July 29, 2002, DC. The old practice was to state a cause of death as having been "aggravated" by lack of care.
[235] *R. (Middleton) v West Somerset Coroner* [2003] Q.B. 581 at [87]–[89]; *R. (Sacker) v Wakefield Coroner* Unreported July 4, 2002, Sir Richard Tucker; *R. (Mumford) v Reading Coroner* [2002] EWHC 2184 (Admin.), and *R. (Metropolitan Police Commissioner) v South London Coroner* [2003] EWHC 1829 Admin. The decision in *Sacker* was reversed by the Court of Appeal [2003] 2 All E.R. 278, and that decision was affirmed by the House of Lords ([2004] UKHL 11; [2004] 2 All E.R. 487), though on different grounds.
[236] *R. (Middleton) v West Somerset Coroner* [2004] UKHL 10; [2004] 2 A.C. 182 at [47].
[237] *R. (Middleton) v West Somerset Coroner* [2004] UKHL 10; [2004] 2 A.C. 182 at [47].
[238] See 13–87.
[239] *R. v Inner North London Coroner Ex p. Diesa Koto* (1993) 157 J.P. 857, DC.

exercised by a doctor, with the result that the wrong medical treatment was given, this was held not to be capable of being neglect.[240]

13–98   Indeed, this may be why neglect was stated to be "a gross failure to . . . procure *basic* medical attention",[241] i.e. excluding complex decision-making, and contrasting basic attention with no attention, rather than the right treatment with the wrong treatment. But subsequently a number of first instance and appellate decisions held or implied that errors by clinicians in diagnosis and treatment were capable of amounting to neglect, and this now represents the current law.[242]

13–99   However, whatever the concept of neglect may consist of, there must be a clear and direct causal connection between that neglect (or self-neglect) and the death.[243] To put it another way, there must be some distinct act or omission closely and directly associated with the death as its cause or as one of its causes.[244] For this reason it will be easier to find neglect contributing in a suicide case where the alleged neglect takes place after the suicide attempt,[245] compared with the case where it takes place before.[246]

13–100   The notion of causation in tort has been re-examined in recent years, concluding that it depends on the scope of the relevant liability rules.[247] But the requirement here for a clear and direct causal connection is not a "liability-based" causation. Instead it is simply "the opportunity of rendering care".[248] If there is no such opportunity, there is no neglect.[249] If there is an opportunity (not taken) but

---

[240] *R. v Birmingham Coroner Ex p. Cotton* (1995) 160 J.P. 123, DC; *R. v Surrey Coroner Ex p. Wright* [1997] Q.B. 786, permission to appeal refused (1996) 35 B.M.L.R. 57, CA; *R. v Lincoln Coroner Ex p. Hay* [2000] Lloyd's Rep. Med. 264, DC; see also *R. v Birmingham and Solihull Coroner Ex p. Benton* (1997) 162 J.P. 807.

[241] *R. v North Humberside Coroner Ex p. Jamieson* [1995] Q.B. 1, at 25; see *Re Harris* Unreported October 5, 2001 at [28], Tomlinson J.

[242] *R. v Northamptonshire Coroner Ex p. Tompkinson* (1995) 160 J.P. 69, DC; *Re Clegg* (1996) 161 J.P. 521 at 528, DC; *R. v Swansea and Gower Coroner Ex p. Chief Constable of Wales* (1999) 164 J.P. 191 at 198–199; *R. (Scott) v Westminster Coroner* (2001) 165 J.P. 417, DC; *Nicholls v Liverpool Coroner* [2001] EWHC Admin. 922, DC; *R. (Marshall) v Coventry Coroner* Unreported October 22, 2001 at [32], Hooper J. (not clinician); *R. (Davies) v Birmingham Deputy Coroner* [2003] EWCA Civ. 1739 at [28]–[29], [72], [74]; *Bloom v North London ADC* [2004] EWHC 3071 (Admin.).

[243] *R. v Southwark Coroner Ex p. Hicks* [1987] 1 W.L.R. 1624, DC; *R. v North Humberside Coroner Ex p. Jamieson* [1995] Q.B. 1, CA; *R. (Scott) v Inner West London Coroner* (2001) 165 J.P. 417, DC; the requirement for "a clear and direct causal connection" is not to be read or applied in an over-literal manner, and the jury is entitled to take a commonsense approach: *Nicholls v Liverpool Coroner* Unreported November 8, 2001 at [56], DC; *R. (Khan) v West Hertfordshire Coroner* [2002] EWHC 302 (Admin.) at [43]; *R. (Metropolitan Police Commissioner) v South London Coroner* [2003] EWHC 1829 (Admin.) at [56]–[57].

[244] *R.v East Berkshire Coroner Ex p. Buckley* (1992) 157 J.P. 425, DC.

[245] *Re Clegg* (1996) 161 J.P. 521.

[246] As in *R. v North Humberside Coroner Ex p. Jamieson* [1995] Q.B. 1, CA.

[247] *Environment Agency v Empress Car Co (Abertillery) Ltd* [1999] 2 A.C. 22, 29–32; *Reeves v Metropolitan Police* Commissioner [2000] 1 A.C. 360, 370; *Kuwait Airways Corporation v Iraqi Airways Co* (Nos 4 & 5) [2002] 2 A.C. 883 at [523]–[524]; *Rahman v Arearose Ltd* [2001] Q.B. 351, 367–368; *Fairchild v Glenhaven Funeral Services Ltd* [2003] 1 A.C. 32, HL at [12]; *Sienkewicz v Greif (UK) Ltd* [2011] 2 A.C. 229, SC; *Durham v BAI (Run Off) Ltd* [2012] 1 W.L.R. 867, SC; *International Energy Group Ltd v Zurich Insurance plc UK* [2013] 3 All E.R. 395, CA.

[248] *R. v Coventry Coroner Ex p. Chief Constable of Staffordshire Police* (2000) 164 J.P. 665; *R. (Scott) v Westminster Coroner* (2001) 165 J.P. 417, DC; *R. (Khan) v West Hertfordshire Coroner* [2002] EWHC 302 (Admin.) at [21], Richards J; *R. (Metropolitan Police Commissioner) v South London Coroner* [2003] EWHC 1829 (Admin.) at [56]–[57]; *cf. R. (Dawson) v East Riding and Hull Coroner* [2001] EWHC Admin. 352 at [77].

[249] *R. v Inner South London Coroner Ex p. Douglas-Williams* [1999] 1 All ER. 344 at 355, CA.

it would not have prevented the death,[250] or other intervening steps broke the chain of causation between that lost opportunity and the death, there is no neglect.[251]

Thus, a person who starves himself to death, or a person who dies through **13–101** refusing medication, may die through self-neglect.[252] Or a person with a medical condition who is deprived of the medication upon which he depends, or a person in custody who is deprived of food or clothing over a period, and thereby dies, may die through neglect, or, in some cases, through natural causes to which neglect contributed.[253] But it may also be appropriate where a person's mental (as opposed to physical) condition is the effective cause of his death, e.g. where a mentally disordered person is left unsupervised and leaps from an upper storey window.[254]

On the other hand, it is not "neglect" if the missing "care" would only have **13–102** ameliorated the pre-existing condition, but its absence did not aggravate it.[255] It is extremely unlikely that an accidental death will have been caused by lack of care.[256] Most cases of lack of care will be cases of omission rather than of commission,[257] although there will be exceptions.[258]

Use of the words "lack of care" or "neglect" does not contravene the **13–103** requirement[259] that the verdict should not appear to determine a question of civil liability, that is, negligence. This is either because it does not state that there was a legal duty of care[260] (which has been broken) or because no one is named in the conclusion.[261] But these reasons have not satisfied every judge.[262]

If that is wrong, there is a potential conflict between the statutory duty imposed **13–104** on the coroner's investigation of finding out *how* the deceased died,[263] and the statutory duty to ensure that the determination does not appear to determine any

---

[250] *R. (Khan) v West Hertfordshire Coroner* [2002] EWHC 302 (Admin.) at [43], Richards J.

[251] cf. *Nicholls v Liverpool Coroner* [2001] EWHC Admin. 922 at [57]–[58], DC.

[252] See, e.g. *Re Eleanor Reekie, The Times*, March 5, 1986 (High Peak coroner); *Re Philip Kitchen, Daily Telegraph*, January 23, 2002 (Worcestershire coroner). Such self-neglect is not unlawful: cf. *B v An NHS Hospital Trust* Unreported March 22, 2002, Fam D.

[253] See, e.g. *An NHS Trust v D, The Times*, July 19, 2002, Fam D. (declaration that lawful for hospital not to resuscitate patient in event of respiratory and/or cardiac failure or arrest).

[254] *R. v Birmingham Coroner Ex p. Home Secretary* (1990) 155 J.P. 107, DC; note that Watkins LJ in that case doubted that there could be the necessary causal connection between lack of supervision and death in the case of a person who was not mentally disordered; see also *R. v East Sussex Coroner Ex p. Homberg* (1994) 158 J.P. 357 at 370.

[255] *R. v Portsmouth Coroner Ex p. Anderson* [1987] 1 W.L.R. 1640, DC; see also *R. v Poplar Coroner Ex p. Thomas* [1993] Q.B. 610, CA; *R. v North Humberside Coroner Ex p. Jamieson* [1995] Q.B. 1, CA.

[256] *R. v Southwark Coroner Ex p. Hicks* [1987] 1 W.L.R. 1624, DC; *R. v Portsmouth Coroner Ex p. Anderson* [1987] 1 W.L.R. 1640, DC. cf. *R. (Davies) v Birmingham and Solihull Deputy Coroner* Unreported February 11, 2003, Moses J (reversed [2003] EWCA Civ. 1739, on different grounds).

[257] *R. v Inner North London Coroner Ex p. Diesa Koto* (1993) 157 J.P. 857, DC.

[258] See *R. v East Berkshire Coroner Ex p. Buckley* (1992) 157 J.P. 425, DC.

[259] Coroners and Justice Act 2009 s.10(2)(a); formerly Coroners Rules 1984 r.42 (repealed).

[260] See the 9th edn of this work (1957), p.179, approved by the court in *R. v Surrey Coroner Ex p. Campbell* [1982] Q.B. 661; and see also *R. v Walthamstow Coroner Ex p. Rubenstein* [1982] Crim. L.R. 509; *R. v Birmingham Coroner Ex p. Home Secretary* (1991) 155 J.P. 107, DC.

[261] *R. v Surrey Coroner Ex p. Campbell* [1982] Q.B. 661; *R. v Walthamstow Coroner Ex p. Rubenstein* [1982] Crim. L.R. 509; *R. v Southwark Coroner Ex p. Hicks* [1987] 1 W.L.R. 1624, 1634, DC.

[262] *R. v Sunderland Coroner Ex p. Sunderland City Council* Unreported October 19, 1994, DC, per Beldam LJ (conclusion of lack of care would "point the finger" and infringe r.42).

[263] Coroners and Justice Act 2009 s.5(2); formerly Coroners Act 1988 s.11(5)(b) (repealed).

question of civil liability, or criminal liability on the part of a named person.[264] In one case in which this point was considered, the court said, obiter:

"such conflict as may in any given circumstance appear to arise between rule 33 [now s.10(2) of the 2009 Act] and the duty to inquire 'how' must be resolved in favour of the statutory duty to inquire whatever the consequences of this may be."[265]

13–105 This view appears to have been implicitly taken more recently by the House of Lords, which held that

"However the jury's factual conclusion is conveyed, rule 42 [now s.10(2) of the 2009 Act] should not be infringed. Thus there must be no finding of criminal liability on the part of a named person. Nor must the verdict appear to determine any question of civil liability. Acts or omissions may be recorded, but expressions suggestive of civil liability, in particular 'neglect' or 'carelessness' and related expressions, should be avoided. Self-neglect and neglect should continue to be treated as terms of art. A verdict such as that suggested in paragraph 45 below ('The deceased took his own life, in part because the risk of his doing so was not recognised and appropriate precautions were not taken to prevent him doing so') embodies a judgmental conclusion of a factual nature, directly relating to the circumstances of the death. It does not identify any individual nor does it address any issue of criminal or civil liability. It does not therefore infringe either rule 36(2) [now s.5(3) of the 2009 Act] or rule 42."[266]

13–106 These views certainly reflect the practice with regard to "unlawful killing" verdicts[267] (where the person who unlawfully killed is not named either), but they were stated at a time when the prohibition on appearing to determine liability was set out in *secondary* rather than primary legislation, and it was thus easier for the court to conclude that the primary legislation should prevail.[268] However, it is difficult to see why the courts should now take a different view, merely because the two statements are both made in the same Act of Parliament. That is not a sufficient basis for assuming that Parliament intended to change the law on this point.

13–107 Since the coming into force of the Human Rights Act 1998,[269] it is also necessary to consider how far a finding by an inquest which did cast an imputation of civil or criminal liability upon a person is consistent with art.6 of the European

---

[264] Coroners and Justice Act 2009 s.10(2). See 13–57.

[265] *R. v Surrey Coroner Ex p. Campbell* [1982] Q.B. 661 at 676; *R. v East Sussex Coroner Ex .p Homberg* (1994) 158 J.P. 357, DC; *R. v North Humberside Coroner Ex p. Jamieson* [1995] Q.B. 1, CA; cf. *R. v Sunderland Coroner Ex p. Sunderland City Council* Unreported October 19, 1994, DC, per Beldam LJ (conclusion of lack of care would "point the finger" and infringe r.42).

[266] *R. (Middleton) v West Somerset Coroner* [2004] UKHL 10; [2004] 2 A.C. 182 at [37]. See also *Perre v Chivell* [2000] SASC 279 (finding that named person sent bomb which killed deceased permissible).

[267] See 13–57 above.

[268] It did not, however, mean that the rule was ultra vires the rule-making power in the Coroners Act: *R. v Surrey Coroner Ex p. Campbell* [1982] Q.B. 661, DC; *R. v Southwark Coroner Ex p. Hicks* [1987] 1 W.L.R. 1624, DC; *R. v West London Coroner Ex p. Gray* [1988] Q.B. 467, DC.

[269] See Ch.21.

Convention on Human Rights.[270] This article is only engaged when a court or tribunal is concerned with "the determination of [a person's] civil rights and obligations or of any criminal charge against him".[271] Under the old coroners' law prior to 1977 a person was not charged with a criminal offence at any time prior to being named in the inquisition as responsible for the murder or manslaughter of the deceased.[272] Under the current law a conclusion of unlawful killing does not even operate as such a charge.

Strasbourg jurisprudence suggests that "charge" for art.6 purposes extends   **13–108** beyond official notification of an allegation of an offence[273] to "other measures which carry the implication of such an allegation".[274] It is just possible that an unlawful killing conclusion, in certain circumstances, could therefore amount to a "charge".[275] But the inquest can only *result* in such a charge; it does not in any way *determine* it. Article 6 does not regulate how charges come to be preferred, only how they are determined. Hence it does not apply to any criminal imputation cast by an inquest. Nor does art.8 assist the person, not mentioned in the determination of unlawful killing but arguably identifiable, from the surrounding circumstances, as having caused the death.[276]

As for civil liability, it is not enough that civil rights and obligations are *in issue*:   **13–109** the question must be whether the inquest, by, for example, finding that the death was caused or contributed to by neglect, is *determining* civil rights and obligations.[277] It is submitted that the answer is No. The inquest is investigating and recording, in the public interest, limited but important facts about the death.[278] If during the investigation statements or findings are made which are detrimental to the interests of a particular person, that does not amount to a determination of rights and obligations. That person is not adjudicated to be civilly liable to any other, or required to pay compensation or provide any other remedy. For that purpose, further, *civil* proceedings are required, in which the findings of the inquest will not only not be conclusive,[279] but may not even be admissible.[280]

This conclusion is consistent with case law on art.6, holding that the investiga-   **13–110** tion and report by an inspector appointed to look into the affairs of a public company,[281] and the request pursuant to statute by a local authority requiring information relevant to the commission of possible offences committed by a

---

270 See 21–22 ff.
271 Article 6 para.1.
272 *Wakley v Cooke* (1847) 4 Ex. 511, 154 E.R. 1316; see 1–28, 12–73 above.
273 See *Eckle v Germany* (1983) E.H.R.R. I, ECtHR.
274 *Foti v Italy* (1983) 5 E.H.R.R. 313; *Corigliano v Italy* (1983) 5 E.H.R.R. 334; see also *X v United Kingdom* (1978) 14 D.R. 26.
275 See 20–03 ff.
276 *R. (Evans) v Cardiff and Vale of Glamorgan Coroner* [2010] EWHC 3478 (Admin.); affirmed [2011] EWCA Civ. 719.
277 Starmer, *European Human Rights Law* (1999), para.12–34.
278 *R. v North Humberside Coroner Ex p. Jamieson* [1995] Q.B. 1, CA; *Jordan v Lord Chancellor* [2007] 2 A.C. 226, HL at [39]; *R. (Middleton) v West Somerset Coroner* [2004] 2 A.C. 182, HL at [37].
279 *Garnett v Ferrand* (1827) 6 B. & C. 611; 108 E.R. 577.
280 See 20–14 ff below.
281 *Fayed v United Kingdom* (1994) 18 E.H.R.R. 393, ECtHR; *Saunders v United Kingdom* (1996) 23 E.H.R.R. 313 at [57].

company,[282] were not "determining" civil rights and obligations within art.6. It also seems that a narrative conclusion of neglect, stating that a medical condition later leading to death had not been recognised by (unidentified) carers, is not even arguably unlawful.[283]

Riders and recommendations

13–111   Although the rules before 1980 forbade the coroner (and jury) from expressing any opinion on any matters, other than the identity of the deceased, how, when and where he came by his death, the person(s) to be charged with his homicide, and the registration particulars,[284] there was an exception for the coroner or jury to make recommendations.[285]

13–112   But this power was abused. Juries used sometimes to add riders to their verdicts, that is, expressions of opinion, often on matters about which nothing (or not enough) had been given in evidence. And, indeed, it is difficult to see how, especially with limited resources, coroners or juries could easily be put in the appropriate position to make decisions about technical feasibility and funding priorities. In 1980, therefore, the power for coroner or jury to add a recommendation to a verdict was simply abolished.[286]

13–113   The power to make recommendations in the 1953 Rules coexisted until 1980 with another power, for the coroner (and not the jury) to record a rider which in his opinion was "designed to prevent the recurrence of fatalities similar to that in respect of which the inquest is being held.'[287] In 1980, when the power for the coroner or jury to make recommendations was abolished, this latter power was recast in the modern form,[288] as a power to refer matters to an appropriate person to enable action to be taken to prevent similar fatalities in future,[289] but not power to make any particular recommendation.[290] In the new coroner system, this power has been turned into a contingent duty,[291] and is dealt with below.[292]

---

[282] *R. v Hertfordshire County Council Ex p. Green Environmental Services Ltd* [2002] 2 A.C. 412, HL. See further 21–22 below.

[283] *My Care (UK) Ltd v Coventry Coroner* [2009] EWHC 3630 (Admin.) ("It explains the cause of death rather than purports to determine civil liability").

[284] Coroners Rules 1953 r.27 (repealed), replaced by Coroners Rules 1984 r.36(2) (repealed), and now by Coroners and Justice Act 2009 s.5(3).

[285] Coroners Rules 1953 r.27, proviso (repealed) ("Provided that nothing in this rule shall preclude the coroner or the jury from making a recommendation designed to prevent the recurrence of fatalities similar to that in respect of which the inquest is being held."). On the like power in New South Wales, see *X v Deputy State Coroner for New South Wales* [2001] NSWSC 46.

[286] Coroners (Amendment) Rules 1980 r.11 (repealed), following the *Report of the Departmental Committee on Coroners* (1936), Cmd. 5070; *R. v Shrewsbury Coroner's Court Ex p. British Parachute Association* (1987) 152 J.P. 123, DC; juries since then do sometimes attempt to add riders, which have to be rejected, often because they are inconsistent with the verdict, e.g. *Re James Davey, The Times*, March 31, 1984 (Coventry coroner) (verdict of accidental death with rider that police used unreasonable force rejected, the final verdict was accidental death).

[287] Coroners Rules 1953 r.34 (repealed).

[288] Becoming r.43 in the Coroners Rules 1984.

[289] Coroners and Justice Act 2009 Sch.5 para.7; formerly Coroners Rules 1984 r.43 (repealed); see the Coroners' Society's *Practice Notes for Coroners* (1998) para.11.

[290] Unlike, say, sheriffs in Scottish fatal accident inquiries.

[291] Coroners and Justice Act 2009 Sch.5 para.7.

[292] See 13–122 ff.

The prohibition on collateral comments is not confined to the determination   **13–114**
and findings themselves, but extends to anything said by the coroner or the jury at
the time or afterwards.[293] Despite this, both coroners and juries still sometimes
make "recommendations"[294] for the avoidance of similar deaths, although these
have no legal significance, and are not part of the determination.[295] And in high-
profile cases senior judges sitting temporarily as coroners sometimes make detailed
recommendations in the form of "reports",[296] even though strictly they go too far.
However, if coroners and juries fulfil their statutory duty to find "how, when and
where the deceased came by his or her death"[297] by finding all the material facts,
the need for such riders or recommendations often disappears. Apart from cases of
illegality or internal inconsistency, a coroner should be careful not to "edit" the
jury's expressed verdict.[298]

Registration particulars

Paragraph (5) of the prescribed form of inquisition makes provision for the   **13–115**
particulars required by the registration legislation to be registered concerning the
death.[299] These particulars consist of the date and place of death, name and
surname of the deceased, the sex of the deceased, the maiden surname of a woman
who has married, the date and place of birth, and the occupation and usual address
of the deceased.[300] Specific instructions for completion in the case of a child are
provided by the Registrar General.

Attestation

When the inquisition is complete, it should be signed by the coroner and, if there   **13–116**
is a jury, such of the jurors as agree with it.[301] Though the contrary has been

---

[293] *R. v Shrewsbury Coroner's Court Ex p. British Parachute Association* (1987) 152 J.P. 123, DC.

[294] See, e.g., the 20 recommendations made by the jury at the Bradford football fire inquest: *The Times*,
July 30, 1985.

[295] Just as a rider was not part of the inquisition: *R. v Harding* (1908) 25 T.L.R. 139, CCA.

[296] See for example the "Report under Rule 43 of The Coroner's Rules 1984" made to the Home
Secretary and other public bodies on 6 May 2011 by Hallett LJ after the "7/7 bombings" inquests,
running to 65 pages, which (i) named the perpetrators of the bombings, (ii) recorded the success of
the security services in preventing other terrorist attacks, (iii) set out (a) a very detailed summary of
the history leading up to the attacks, and (b) detailed summaries of much of the evidence given at
the inquest hearings, including the emergency response, and (iv) included nine detailed recommendations for particular action, each one beginning "I recommend that . . . " No ordinary coroner
could hope to get away with this without being judicially reviewed, and none should attempt to
emulate it. cf *R. v Shrewsbury Coroner's Court Ex p. British Parachute Association* (1987) 152 J.P. 123,
DC; *Re Clegg* (1996) 161 J.P. 521, DC; *R. (Farah) v Southampton and New Forest Coroner* [2009]
EWHC 1605 (Admin); Chief Coroner's Guidance No. 5, *Reports to Prevent Future Deaths* at [31]; and
see 13–122 ff.

[297] Coroners and Justice Act 2009 ss.5(1)(b), 10(1)(a); formerly Coroners Act 1988 s.11(5)(b)(ii)
(repealed); para.13–01 above.

[298] *R. v West London Coroner Ex p. Gray* [1988] Q.B. 467, DC.

[299] Coroners and Justice Act 2009 ss.5(1)(c), 10 (1)(b); formerly Coroners Act 1988 s.11(3)(b), (4)(b)
(repealed).

[300] Registration of Births, Marriages and Deaths Regulations 1968 reg.48(1).

[301] This was explicit under the Coroners Act 1988 s.11(5)(a) (repealed). It is implicit in the Coroners
and Justice Act 2009 ss.5(1), 10(1), and the Coroners (Inquests) Rules 2013 (SI 2013/1616) r.34 Sch.
Form 2.

stated,[302] it is considered that it is not necessary for the jurors to subscribe their names in full. If a deputy or assistant deputy coroner is holding the inquest, he should sign the form of inquisition in his own name.[303]

13–117   Formerly the coroner might, if he thought fit, excuse the jurors from further jury service at a coroner's court for such period as he thought appropriate, and this would provide the jurors concerned with an excusal as of right if summoned to serve on a coroner's jury within that period.[304] But this, together with the form of certificate of attendance (and excusal),[305] have now gone, and it appears that coroners can no longer do this. However, they retain the discretionary power to excuse jurors from service.[306]

Separate judgment

13–118   A coroner may, in addition to delivering the determination and findings of the inquest, give a judgment which refers to matters falling within his jurisdiction,[307] that is (i) who the deceased was, (ii) how, when, and where the deceased came by his death, and (iii) the particulars for the time being required for the registration of the death.[308] Indeed there are matters on which a coroner may well be obliged to give a short judgment, for example why a line of questioning is objectionable and why a particular verdict cannot be left to the jury.[309] Furthermore, the coroner might be justified in explaining in a judgment the procedure he adopted in providing the verdict on the specified issues, such as how he had dealt with a claim by a witness that he need not answer a question because of his privilege against self-incrimination.[310]

13–119   But this judgment must of course not infringe the rules requiring that no opinion be expressed on anything else.[311] In order to police this, the High Court has jurisdiction on judicial review to make a declaration of unlawfulness in relation to, and strike out from any such judgment, comments which (a) do not relate to any of the issues (i) to (iii) above in any way; (b) are matters of opinion; and (c) are sufficiently unfairly critical and offensive of any party as to justify the intervention of the courts.[312] Probably an allegation of criminal conduct or professional misconduct, or behaviour which would be regarded as repugnant by right-thinking members of the community, would fall into that category.

---

[302] *R. v Evett* (1827) 6 B. & C. 247.

[303] Coroners and Justice Act 2009 Sch.3 para.8; formerly Coroners Rules 1984 r.58 (repealed).

[304] Coroners Rules 1984 r.49(c) (repealed).

[305] Coroners Rules 1984 Sch.4 Form 6 App.2 (repealed).

[306] See 10–48.

[307] *R. (Farah) v Southampton and New Forest Coroner* [2009] EWHC 1605 (Admin) at [20(d)], [47].

[308] See 13–115.

[309] See 11–66, 12–63 ff, 12–114.

[310] See 12–95.

[311] Coroners and Justice Act 2009 ss.5(3), 10(2); *R. v Shrewsbury Coroner's Court Ex p. British Parachute Association* (1987) 152 J.P. 123, DC; *R. (Farah) v Southampton and New Forest Coroner* [2009] EWHC 1605 (Admin.) at [20(f)].

[312] *Nichol v Gateshead MBC* (1988) 87 L.G.R. 435, 460; *R. (Mowlem plc) v Avon Assistant Deputy Coroner* [2005] EWHC 1359 (Admin.); *R. (Farah) v Southampton and New Forest Coroner* [2009] EWHC 1605 (Admin.) at [27], [47]. See also *R. v Shrewsbury Coroner's Court Ex p. British Parachute Association* (1987) 152 J.P. 123, DC.

CLOSING THE INQUEST

There is no rule that the coroner must formally discharge the jury in cases where **13–120** they have given a verdict. But it is usual for the coroner at least to thank them for their efforts, before closing the inquest. It would seem that if, before they separate, or see or hear anything which they should not, there is good reason to allow the jury to deliberate further (e.g. to correct a misunderstanding or a mistake), the coroner may allow them to do so.[313] But it must be clear that the jury has not simply changed its mind.[314]

Once all the business of the inquest is finished, it should be formally closed,[315] **13–121** though no particular form is prescribed. Usually the coroner's officer simply calls "Silence" or asks those present in the court to rise as the coroner leaves the bench, though in the past proclamations[316] have been used. Where the coroner does not leave the bench at the conclusion of the inquest, as where he proceeds with another inquest, it is usual for the coroner or his officer to announce the end of the inquest and that all those persons involved in it may now leave.

REPORTS TO PREVENT FUTURE DEATHS[317]

As already stated, the coroner (and not the jury) has a contingent duty (formerly **13–122** a power) to refer matters to an appropriate person to enable action to be taken to prevent similar fatalities in future.[318] The duty arises where:

(a) a coroner has been conducting an investigation under this Part into a person's death;

(b) anything revealed by the investigation gives rise to a concern[319] that circumstances[320] creating a risk of other deaths will occur, or will continue to exist, in the future; and

(c) in the coroner's opinion, action should be taken to prevent the occurrence or continuation of such circumstances, or to eliminate or reduce the risk of death created by such circumstances.

---

[313] cf. *Igwemma v Chief Constable of Greater Manchester Police* [2002] Q.B. 1012, CA (civil case).

[314] *R. v Tantram* [2001] Crim. LR. 824, CA.

[315] Coroners Rules 1984 r.16 (repealed) formerly so provided. But it is sensible so to do even now.

[316] For forms, see App.3, Forms 21 and 22.

[317] See the Chief Coroner's Guidance No. 5, *Reports to Prevent Future Deaths*; *Chief Coroner's Guide to the Coroners and Justice Act 2009* at [172] ff.

[318] Coroners and Justice Act 2009 Sch.5 para.7; formerly Coroners Rules 1984 r.43 (repealed); see the Coroners' Society's *Practice Notes for Coroners* (1998) para.11.

[319] A relatively low threshold: see Hallett LJ as Westminster Assistant Deputy Coroner in the London bombings inquests in a ruling dated May 6, 2011, p.5.

[320] The Chief Coroner's Guidance No. 5, *Reports to Prevent Future Deaths* at [17], says that the failure to use words such as "similar circumstances" means that this rule is not restricted to matters causative or potentially causative of the death in question. But if that were right, it would broaden the scope of the rule too far, and, in the context of an obligation (rather than discretion) to report could lead to a deluge of reports that had nothing to do with the case at hand. That cannot have been Parliament's intention.

There is power to do this even before the inquest is concluded,[321] but the coroner must first consider all relevant matters.[322]

13–123   The function of the coroner under this provision is not to punish anyone for what has happened, nor to advance the interests of the family, nor even to judge whether the evidence in particular cases reaches or does not reach any particular standard required for (say) professional disciplinary proceedings to be commenced. That would not only require in many cases specialist knowledge which the coroner does not possess. It would also duplicate or render otiose any gate-keeping functions built into the processes for such professional disciplinary proceedings.

13–124   Instead, the duty is imposed upon the coroner to respond to a perceived public interest in reducing or eliminating similar fatalities in future, of whatever kind it may be. That perceived public interest, taken with the fact that a report does not in itself have any *direct* impact on the situation, requires that the paragraph be interpreted broadly rather than narrowly, so that matters are reported to those who, having more specialist knowledge than the coroner may decide what, if anything, should be done for the future.

13–125   Condition (b) must be considered in the light of the evidence given at the inquest, but as at the date of making the decision to report, that is, taking into account any changes which have been made or developments which have taken place since the events the subject of the inquest occurred. The point of a report is to enable a risk to be met. If the risk has since gone, it is unnecessary to spend time reporting it.

13–126   Where the three conditions are satisfied, but only after the coroner has considered all the documents, evidence and information that in his or her opinion are relevant to the investigation,[323] the coroner *must* report the matter to a person whom the coroner believes may have power to take such action,[324] copying it (i) to the Chief Coroner[325] and every interested person who in the coroner's opinion should receive it,[326] and (ii) to the Local Safeguarding Children Board where the coroner believes that the deceased was under the age of 18 years.[327] The coroner *may* also send a copy (iii) to any other person whom he or she believes may find it useful or of interest.[328] The Chief Coroner on receipt may publish a copy or a summary of the report,[329] and may send a copy to any other person whom he or she believes may find it useful or of interest.[330]

13–127   The person to whom it is addressed must respond in writing,[331] within 56 days of the date on which it is sent.[332] This period may be extended by the coroner.[333] The response must (a) contain details of action that has been or is proposed to be

---

[321] See the Chief Coroner's Guidance No. 5, *Reports to Prevent Future Deaths* at [13].
[322] Coroners (Investigations) Regulations 2013 (SI 2013/1629) reg.28(3).
[323] Coroners (Investigations) Regulations 2013 (SI 2013/1629) reg.28(3).
[324] Coroners and Justice Act 2009 Sch.5 para.7(1).
[325] Email address: chiefcoronersoffice@judiciary.gsi.gov.uk.
[326] Coroners (Investigations) Regulations 2013 (SI 2013/1629) reg.28(4)(a).
[327] Coroners (Investigations) Regulations 2013 (SI 2013/1629) reg.28(4)(b).
[328] Coroners (Investigations) Regulations 2013 (SI 2013/1629) reg.28(4)(c).
[329] Coroners (Investigations) Regulations 2013 (SI 2013/1629) reg.28(5)(a).
[330] Coroners (Investigations) Regulations 2013 (SI 2013/1629) reg.28(5)(b).
[331] Coroners and Justice Act 2009 Sch.5 para.7(2).
[332] Coroners (Investigations) Regulations 2013 (SI 2013/1629) reg.29(4).
[333] Coroners (Investigations) Regulations 2013 (SI 2013/1629) reg.29(5).

taken and set out a timetable for this, or (b) explain why no action is proposed.[334] A responder may make written representations to the coroner about release or publication of the response,[335] no later than the response itself,[336] and the coroner must pass these on to the Chief Coroner for his or her consideration.[337]

The coroner *must* send a copy of the response to the Chief Coroner[338] and every   **13–128** interested person who in the coroner's opinion should receive it,[339] and *may* send a copy to any other person who he or she believes may find it useful or of interest.[340] The Chief Coroner on receipt may publish a copy or a summary of the response,[341] and may send a copy to any other person who he or she believes may find it useful or of interest.[342]

It was held under the previous coroner system that the coroner's power to report   **13–129** the facts is ancillary to the inquest procedure, not its mainspring, and its existence was not a basis for holding a new inquest if otherwise there would be no sufficient reason to do so.[343] The change from *power* to *duty* may have strengthened the importance of the provision, but the investigation is still the most important aspect of the process, and there is no reason to suppose that Parliament intended thereby to create a new basis for holding a fresh inquest. As stated elsewhere, the critical point is that the Strasbourg caselaw relating to art.2 now require that the state's own art.2-complaint inquiry must inter alia ascertain "any shortcomings in the operation of the regulatory system", even if they were not causative of the death.[344] The coroner's previous power, now duty, to report is the means of compliance with this requirement in England and Wales.[345]

---

[334] Coroners (Investigations) Regulations 2013 (SI 2013/1629) reg.29(3).
[335] Coroners (Investigations) Regulations 2013 (SI 2013/1629) reg.29(8).
[336] Coroners (Investigations) Regulations 2013 (SI 2013/1629) reg.29(9).
[337] Coroners (Investigations) Regulations 2013 (SI 2013/1629) reg.29(10).
[338] Email address: chiefcoronersoffice@judiciary.gsi.gov.uk.
[339] Coroners (Investigations) Regulations 2013 (SI 2013/1629) reg.29(6)(a), (b).
[340] Coroners (Investigations) Regulations 2013 (SI 2013/1629) reg.29(6)(c).
[341] Coroners (Investigations) Regulations 2013 (SI 2013/1629) reg.29(7)(a).
[342] Coroners (Investigations) Regulations 2013 (SI 2013/1629) reg.29(7)(b).
[343] *Re Kelly* (1996) 161 J.P. 417, DC; see also *Re Clegg* (1996) 161 J.P. 521, DC.
[344] *R. (Lewis) v Mid and North Shropshire Coroner* [2009] EWCA Civ. 1403 at [11], [35]. See also *R. (Duffy) v Worcestershire Deputy Coroner* [2013] EWHC 1654 (Admin.) at [41].
[345] *R. (Lewis) v Mid and North Shropshire Coroner* [2009] EWCA Civ. 1403 at [16], [38]. See also *R. (Middleton) v West Somerset Coroner* [2004] UKHL 10; [2004] 2 A.C. 182 at [38] and 6–19.

Part IV

SPECIAL CASES

Chapter 14

HOMICIDE

THE PRACTICE IN HOMICIDE CASES

As has been seen,[1] the coroner has the duty to investigate deaths which he or she   **14–01**
has reason to suspect are violent or unnatural. Some of these will be obvious
homicides; others may not seem so at first, but may later turn out to be homicides.
Although the various procedures have been covered elsewhere, it is convenient to
draw together in summary form the practice in homicide cases, together with a
short exposition of the relevant principles of the criminal law.

Cases which seem to be obvious homicides will fall into a number of different   **14–02**
categories, from the coroner's point of view:

(i) cases where charges are made in connection with a death, and criminal
proceedings follow;

(ii) cases where no charges are made because the suspect is immune from the
criminal law (such as where he has diplomatic immunity[2]) or is dead;

(iii) cases where, whether or not charges are brought, the coroner is otherwise
obliged to cease his investigation (for example because the deceased was a
member of a visiting force,[3] or he had diplomatic immunity);

(iv) cases where the perpetrator has not been found[4];

(v) cases where no charges are made, the inquest is held, *but* unexpected
evidence is given that obliges the coroner to adjourn and notify the Crown
Prosecution Service[5];

(vi) cases where the Crown Prosecution Service considers the matter but does
not consider that the evidence is sufficient to support a charge of unlawful
killing[6];

---

[1] See 5–01.
[2] See 5–109 ff.
[3] See 5–98 ff.
[4] See 14–28.
[5] See 14–30 ff.
[6] See 14–31.

(vii) cases where ultimately the matter turns out not to have been a homicide.

14–03   In addition, there will be cases where a death appears not to be suspicious at first, but evidence subsequently is found to give grounds for suspicion of homicide. Although in each of these cases the procedure for coroners will differ, certain principles are common.

INITIAL INQUIRIES

The incidence of jurisdiction

14–04   A coroner has no jurisdiction until death has taken place. Thus the investigation of potentially unlawful injuries to a person dying in hospital or elsewhere is initially a police matter and the coroner is not involved.

14–05   Once the victim has died, it is the coroner's investigation and the coroner's body, and therefore only the coroner (or, with the coroner's authority, the officer on his or her behalf) can give permission for any interference with the body (including its examination at, or removal from, the place where it was found).[7] In practice the coroner's officer will either attend the scene, or give any necessary permission by telephone. In rare cases, the coroner may attend the scene in person.

14–06   However, it is the police who have the experience and the resources to do much of the work involved, and there will need to be consultation and co-operation between the police and the coroner. In particular, if the police inform the coroner that a person may be charged with a homicide offence in relation to the deceased, the coroner must consult the chief officer of police with regard to who should carry out the post-mortem examination.[8]

Recovery and removal of body

14–07   Where a Home Office or specialist pathologist is available, the scene may be visited before the body is removed.[9] The recovery of the body may be carried out by police scientific support (formerly "scenes of crime") officers, using special techniques to retain trace evidence (nowadays, especially DNA evidence) and to avoid extraneous contamination. The so-called "Murder Manual" should be followed.[10] Photographs may be taken at all stages, and the full spectrum of scientific tests may be utilised. The post-mortem examination may be preceded by radiographic examination for missiles or evidence of bony injury. Continuity of evidence of the finding of the body and of the origin of all specimens and exhibits is essential. Subsequent criminal proceedings may otherwise be prejudiced.

---

[7] See 8–11.
[8] See 8–48 above.
[9] Knight, *Forensic Pathology,* 3rd edn (2004), pp.4–7.
[10] ACPO, *Murder Investigation Manual* (2006); available at *http://www.acpo.police.uk/documents/crime/2006/2006CBAMIM.pdf* [Accessed June 13, 2014].

POST-MORTEM EXAMINATION

The coroner alone has the legal power to order an examination of the body of a   **14–08**
suspected homicide victim, but this is invariably carried out by agreement with the
police. Indeed, in some cases the police ask the coroner to instruct a particular
pathologist. In most cases, the coroner has no reason not to agree.[11]

Fees for examination

The payment of the fees incurred is also a matter of agreement. The special nature   **14–09**
of the post-mortem examination in a homicide case is recognised by provision for
an enhanced fee.[12] In addition, the pathologist may be paid a further fee or a
retainer by the police, to cover parts of the examination beyond the post-mortem
examination. So long as the coroner is satisfied that the pathologist is an
appropriate person for his or her purposes, and is content that the pathologist may
carry out additional services for the police, he or she is not concerned with the
performance of those additional services.

Position of pathologist

The pathologist carrying out an autopsy in a homicide case has two sets of powers   **14–10**
and duties, and two masters. One master is the coroner,[13] from whom is derived
one set of powers and duties, and the other is the local police force, from which
is derived another set, under their responsibility for the detection and prosecution
of crime. In exercising these, the pathologist must also follow the directives of the
Pathology Delivery Board.[14] To the extent that the coroner is responsible at all for
the actions of the pathologist, he or she is only responsible in respect of what is
done on *his or her* instructions, and not for what the pathologist does on the
instructions of the police. The coroner's role is to investigate the death and try to
find answers to the statutory questions. For *these* purposes (but not for others) the
pathologist may remove and retain body material which bears on the cause of death
or the identity of the deceased.[15] But the coroner has no power to investigate or
prosecute possible criminal activity.

The consequence is that the coroner has no power to authorise the pathologist   **14–11**
to remove and retain material from the body which does not bear on the identity
of the deceased or the cause of death, but which may be useful for the purposes of
any criminal investigation or proceedings. That must be authorised, if at all, by the
police under their own powers.[16] The coroner's role in relation to this exercise of
police power is at most limited to consenting to the interference with the body by
the pathologist on behalf of the police for their criminal justice purposes (just as he
may consent to the removal of organs for the purposes of transplantation), on the
basis that this interference is not itself permitted by police powers.[17]

---

[11] See 8–54.
[12] See 18–38 below.
[13] See 8–39 ff above.
[14] See its constitution, at *https://www.gov.uk/government/publications/constitution-of-the-pathology-delivery-board* [Accessed June 13, 2014], and see also 8–55—8–56.
[15] See 8–72, 8–76.
[16] Either under the Police and Criminal Evidence Act 1984 or at common law. See 8–11.
[17] See also the Human Tissue Act 2004 s.39.

The effect of homicide investigation on examination

14–12 There may be pressure on the coroner to have the post-mortem examination performed as quickly as possible, either because the police seek information to enable them to identify or trace a suspect, or because a suspect is or suspects are being held in custody. However, this must not be regarded simply as a police investigation. Two cases out of three investigated in this manner are subsequently shown not to be homicidal deaths, and the coroner must still inquire into a death that once appeared to be suspicious.

14–13 Even if the death continues to appear to be homicidal, the coroner may still have to hold an inquest (for example, if no person is ever charged with causing the death). In either event, the coroner will still need to know (a) who the deceased person was and (b) what was the medical cause of death. Obtaining identification evidence may present problems. These may be due to the circumstances of the death,[18] or it may be that the next of kin (who would normally identify the body) are suspects, or potential suspects.

14–14 In the converse case, it may be discovered in the course of a post-mortem examination of an apparently non-suspicious death that there are grounds for suspicion of homicide. In such a case, the examination should be halted and the evidence preserved until a full homicide investigation can be mounted.

Findings of post-mortem examination

14–15 Following the conclusion of the post-mortem examination, any one of a number of situations may arise:

    (i) it may be certain that the death was not due to homicide;

    (ii) the evidence is inconclusive at this stage;

    (iii) further tests may be required, as for example in poisoning cases;

    (iv) the police enquiries and preparations for inquest continue while a suspect is being traced;

    (v) a person or persons may be charged in connection with the death.

PROCEDURE FOLLOWING POST-MORTEM EXAMINATION

Where death is not homicidal

14–16 If the death is not homicidal and the autopsy discloses a natural cause of death, it may be possible to use the Pink Form B procedure.[19] Whereas under the old law[20] a special examination (e.g. histological) could only be carried out once the coroner had decided to hold an inquest, under the new law the coroner may direct such an

---

[18] For example, where the body is found badly decomposed.
[19] See 8–36—8–37 above.
[20] Coroners Act 1988 ss.19–20 (repealed).

examination once he is under a duty to investigate.[21] This makes it more likely that a natural causes death can be so identified and disposed of quickly.[22]

Where a person is, or may be, charged

In certain cases where criminal proceedings may be or have been begun, the coroner must suspend any investigation into the death. These cases have already been discussed.[23] Where the investigation is suspended, the coroner *must* adjourn any inquest being held as part of the investigation,[24] and *may* discharge any jury summoned.[25] (He may later resume the inquest, in certain circumstances, which also have already been discussed.)[26] Exceptionally, in these cases the death can be registered before the investigation is complete. So the coroner receives the minimum of information required to allow the death to be registered, and issues the relevant certificate.[27] Then he has to deal with the question of the release of the body for the funeral.[28] Where the coroner subsequently notifies the registrar of the result of the criminal proceedings the registrar will record it.[29]

14–17

Release of the body

Obviously the coroner should not consider releasing the body until he has received the pathologist's report, or at any rate a summary of the report to come.[30] If the death appears to be homicidal, but no suspect has been traced and arrested, the coroner is in a difficulty in releasing the body for disposal. If the body is released and subsequently destroyed by cremation, or taken to another country for burial or other disposal, a suspect when finally charged with the killing may claim that his defence has been jeopardised by the impossibility of having an examination on behalf of the defence to substantiate any assertions or challenge the prosecution in evidence.

14–18

Of course, the pathologist should have retained such specimens as are required for further examination or even demonstration at a trial, but realistically this cannot apply to every wound or injury, however slight. The strength of the defendant's argument will however depend on the nature of the case. For example, there may be more value in a further examination where the deceased died in a fight, than where he was shot dead from a considerable distance. Also, the argument weakens over time, as deterioration of the tissues (even when frozen) makes them less likely to yield anything of value on a second or subsequent examination.

14–19

It has been suggested that the coroner in such cases should order a second post-mortem examination by another pathologist, and keep the report on file in case charges are subsequently brought.[31] But that pathologist will not have received any

14–20

---

[21] See 8–18, 8–69.

[22] See 8–36.

[23] See 10–73 ff.

[24] Coroners and Justice Act 2009 s.11 Sch.1 para.6(1).

[25] Coroners and Justice Act 2009 s.11 Sch.1 para.6(2).

[26] See 10–83 ff.

[27] See 10–82. If the body is returned from abroad, however, there is no registration.

[28] See 9–14 ff above.

[29] Births and Deaths Registration Act 1953, s.23(2B).

[30] Home Office Circular No. 45 of 1988.

[31] See 8–40 above.

instructions regarding the defence case, and it seems unlikely that the defence will be satisfied by the second autopsy.

14–21   Accordingly, the coroner may feel that he should retain the body for a reasonable time, if there is a prospect of an arrest, and should in the meantime ensure that the body is maintained in a frozen condition. If there is no provision for such storage within the coroner's district, the body may have to be moved to another district that has the appropriate facility. Official guidelines were issued to minimise the delay in releasing the body.[32] The new law now provides that the coroner must release the body for burial or cremation "as soon as reasonably practicable",[33] and, moreover, that if the coroner cannot release the body within 28 days of being made aware that it is in his area, he must notify the next of kin or personal representative of the reason for the delay.[34]

14–22   It has been suggested that the coroner set a time limit for retaining the body, but if a charge has been made the accused may make an application to the High Court. The need to have the prosecution statements and the delay in obtaining legal aid for counsel's advice and the post-mortem examination may mean in practice that, where there is a serious risk of losing potentially useful defence evidence, the High Court would restrain the coroner from releasing the body until the second examination is carried out.[35] But if no sufficient advantage to the defence can be demonstrated, the court is unlikely to interfere with the coroner's decision.[36]

HOLDING THE INQUEST

General

14–23   Despite the abolition in 1977 of the last vestiges of criminal jurisdiction of the coroner's court,[37] the senior judiciary persist in treating it as if it were still a part of the criminal justice system. This manifests itself in relation to a number of specific areas already mentioned, such as requiring the criminal standard of proof for suicide and unlawful killing conclusions,[38] and treating the coroner's jury as if it were performing the same function as a criminal jury.[39] But it also appears more generally in relation to procedure.

14–24   In one case,[40] after the death of the deceased in a fight at a public house in October 2007, the CPS originally declined to prosecute at all.[41] The coroner

---

[32] See originally Home Office Circular No. 30 of 1999, attaching a Memorandum of Guidance, subsequently reissued by the Ministry of Justice in May 2008. See also *R. (McLeish) v North London Coroner* [2010] EWHC 3624 (Admin.).

[33] Coroners (Investigations) Regulations 2013 reg.20(1). See 8–11 above.

[34] Coroners (Investigations) Regulations 2013 reg.20(2). See 8–12 above.

[35] *R. v Bristol Coroner Ex p. Kerr* [1974] Q.B. 652; *R. v Bristol Coroner Ex p. Atkinson* Unreported May 5, 1983. See also 8–40, 9–11, 9–16, 9–17.

[36] See e.g. *Haydon v Chivell* (1999) 73 A.L.J.R. 1311, HC (Aus), Gaudron J.

[37] Criminal Law Act 1977 ss.56, 65. See 1–28 ff.

[38] See 13–47 ff, 13–67 ff.

[39] See 13–04.

[40] *R. v Davies* [2011] EWCA Civ. 871.

[41] A decision described by the Court of Appeal as "the result of incompetence on the part of the CPS and advising counsel".

having read the papers nevertheless formed the view that an unlawful killing conclusion was a real possibility and so informed the police, who, however, did not contact the CPS. The coroner did not contact the appellant or the lawyers that he had instructed, but proceeded to hold an inquest, resulting in a conclusion of unlawful killing. The CPS then reconsidered the position and charged the appellant with manslaughter. At trial, the appellant was convicted of manslaughter, and appealed. The Court of Appeal said, firstly, that "fairness demanded that [the coroner] should have informed" the appellant's solicitors "of her preliminary view".[42] In substance, this conclusion involves giving back to the coroner the grand jury/examining magistrate function of finding a case to answer, which Parliament expressly took away in 1977.

Secondly, at the trial, a critical eye-witness was cross-examined by the Crown on   **14–25**
the basis of the inconsistency of his evidence at the coroner's inquest, and his credibility was damaged. The Court held that at the inquest, the coroner should have given the witness the opportunity to read his statement before giving evidence, saying that it was "normal practice at a criminal trial, particularly where there is a significant delay between the events and the trial itself as there was in this case", and that they "would have hoped it was normal at an inquest."[43] It is not clear if the court considered that such refreshing of memory should take place at *all* inquests, or only at those where there was a risk of criminal proceedings following.

Taken all together, the Court regarded this as "a very serious irregularity in the   **14–26**
inquest taking place in the circumstances it did".[44] The conviction was quashed. The Court appears to have regarded the functions of the coroner as including that of safeguarding the interests of possible future defendants to criminal proceedings, over and above the specific provisions of the coroner legislation. It is submitted that this is not consistent with the intention of Parliament in abolishing the criminal jurisdiction of coroners.

Homicide with no charge brought

Where the death is obviously a homicide, but no person has been charged and a   **14–27**
request for adjournment is made by the police or the CPS, the coroner must adjourn.[45] But if no request for an adjournment has been made by the police or the CPS, the coroner must proceed to hold the inquest.

Suspect untraced or dead

Whether the reason that no one has been charged is that the suspect has not yet   **14–28**
been traced, or that he or she is already dead, the coroner must take sufficient evidence to find the facts required by the law.[46] These findings must not include

---

[42] *R. v Davies* [2011] EWCA Civ. 871 at [68].
[43] *R. v Davies* [2011] EWCA Civ. 871 at [69]. The Court appears to have been unaware that neither the witness himself, nor the appellant nor his legal representative at the inquest asked that the witness should be permitted to refresh his memory from his statement before giving evidence at the inquest.
[44] *R. v Davies* [2011] EWCA Civ. 871 at [72].
[45] See 10–78 above.
[46] See 13–02 above.

any finding of criminal liability against a named person,[47] and care should be taken to avoid any evidence or comment that might be held to prejudice any subsequent criminal trial.[48] In a case where the suspect is dead, the evidence may make it obvious who this person was, and the coroner has to balance the duty not to name any person who was responsible against the need to allay any suspicion that may have fallen on others.

Where evidence insufficient to identify person responsible for death

14–29   The greatest problems for the coroner arise where neither the post-mortem examination nor the other evidence available is sufficient to enable any person to be identified as responsible for the death. In many cases, the surrounding circumstances may require the coroner to sit with a jury.[49] Even where they do not, allegations may be made, in advance of the evidence being heard by the inquest, which if true would require a jury, and in practice a jury will often have to be summoned. If the coroner refuses to sit with a jury, an application to the High Court for an order compelling the coroner to do so is likely to be heard before the coroner can hear evidence that may refute the allegations, unless a "split" inquest is held, taking only the evidence in question, and adjourning the remainder.[50]

Where inquest to be adjourned

14–30   The coroner is required to adjourn the inquest and to inform the CPS if evidence is given in the course of an inquest from which it appears likely that a person may be charged with murder, manslaughter, infanticide, causing death by dangerous driving or complicity in the suicide of the deceased.[51] This avoids the risk of the inquest prejudicing any subsequent criminal trial. However, the coroner need not adjourn if the CPS has already been made aware of that particular evidence and has informed him or her that the inquest need not be adjourned.

14–31   Where the coroner sits without a jury, there is little difficulty in adjourning the inquest for further reference to the CPS When sitting with a jury in a long inquest, it creates serious logistical difficulties if the case has to be adjourned. A coroner who does *not* adjourn (because not satisfied from evidence given that a charge is likely) will nonetheless have to consider whether there is sufficient evidence to justify leaving an unlawful killing conclusion to the jury.[52] There may be strong evidence of unlawful killing, yet no adjournment, e.g. because the killer is dead, or cannot be found, or immune from prosecution (or conviction), or the CPS has declined to prosecute and/or has told the coroner to continue, or the offence was committed, and is being prosecuted, in Scotland.[53]

14–32   In other cases the evidence may be less strong, but still sufficient for a jury to consider. An additional problem is that the coroner cannot know what weight the jury has attached to the matters given in evidence, until they give their findings. In

---

[47] See 12–112, 13–57 above.
[48] cf. *R. v Home Secretary Ex p. Weatherhead* (1995) 32 BMLR 72.
[49] See 10–34 above.
[50] See 11–36.
[51] See 11–47 above.
[52] See 12–114 above.
[53] As to the "Scottish anomaly", see 10–79.

these cases, the coroner accordingly has to deal with such issues as whether the omission of a person amounted to criminal recklessness, whether it was self-defence, or whether the killing was a reasonable act in the circumstances, and so on. However, in cases of murder, manslaughter or infanticide, the expression "unlawfully killed" covers all three conclusions, and this usually avoids the need to enquire into matters such as provocation or diminished responsibility.

THE LAW OF HOMICIDE IN OUTLINE

There now follows an overview of the law relating to homicide. As with the **14–33** discussion of the law of evidence, it cannot claim to be a substitute for the many textbooks and other sources which bear on this subject.[54] Moreover, the law of homicide is constantly developing. First there is an exposition of the eight substantive offences involving or resulting in death, and then a discussion of certain problem areas common to them all, such as the issue of causation and the various defences that a defendant might put forward. Finally, there is some discussion of the different degrees of criminal responsibility.

It should be noted that the conclusion (or, in lay terms, "verdict") of "unlawful killing" is generally considered to cover three of these substantive offences, namely murder, manslaughter and infanticide.[55] Nevertheless, it is necessary to distinguish between them, for the necessary elements of *one* of them must be proved in order for "unlawful killing" to be properly recorded.

Components of a substantive offence

It is usual to analyse all substantive criminal offences under English law in their **14–34** component parts. The two most important such components are:

(i) the physical acts or omissions of the defendant for which he must be responsible (sometimes called actus reus); and

(ii) the mental attitude he must have towards those physical acts at the time that they occur (usually called the mens rea).

To be guilty of an offence, both component parts must be present in the **14–35** defendant, and generally at the same time.[56] Thus, a person who kills another without the requisite mental element for a particular offence is not guilty of that offence (though he may be guilty of another offence where the mental element *is* satisfied). Similarly, a person who has the requisite mental element but who does not bring about the death of the victim (for example, where the victim is killed by an accident before the defendant can attack him or her)[57] is not guilty of the offence in question.

---

[54] See e.g. Smith and Hogan, *Criminal Law,* 13th edn (2011); Archbold, *Criminal Pleading, Evidence and Procedure* (2013).
[55] See 13–55 above.
[56] Smith and Hogan, *Criminal Law,* 13th edn (2011), pp.47–49; cf. *R. v Le Brun* [1992] 2 Q.B. 61, CA.
[57] cf. *R. v White* [1910] 2 K.B. 124; see 14–81.

14–36   The four most important substantive "death" offences will each be analysed in turn in terms of actus reus and mens rea: murder, manslaughter, infanticide and causing death by dangerous driving. Causing death by careless driving when under the influence of drink or drugs, child destruction, abortion and aiding and abetting suicide will then be briefly considered.

Substantive offences

Murder

14–37   The actus reus of murder is that a human being born alive should die as a result of the defendant's unlawful acts or (in some cases) omissions.[58] Thus, for example, causing the death of a fetus is not murder, because a fetus is not a human being born alive.[59] But "mercy killing" or euthanasia[60] of a human being born alive is unlawful, and can be murder.[61]

14–38   As for being born alive, the legal test is not whether the child has breathed, but whether it was wholly expelled from the mother's body before dying.[62] If it has been wholly expelled, the fact that the umbilical cord has not been severed at the time of death is legally irrelevant as to whether there is a life in being.[63] Further, once the child has been completely born it does not matter if its subsequent death is due to injuries received before birth.[64] Thus if, in an operation to terminate pregnancy, the fetus is alive at any time after being removed from the mother's body, it becomes a human being born alive and so subject to the law of homicide. Whether an offence is actually committed if the fetus then dies will depend on the particular facts of the case, and the willingness of the jury to convict.[65]

14–39   The mental element required for murder (formerly known as "malice afore-thought", but needing to be neither malicious nor premeditated) is as follows. For murder there must be either an intention to kill or an intention to cause really serious injury.[66] For the defendant merely to foresee that death or serious injury is a probable or even highly probable consequence of his voluntary act is insufficient in itself,[67] although it may constitute material (if it was highly likely that the defendant's act would cause death or serious injury),[68] from which the jury,

---

[58] *R. v Dyson* [1908] 2 K.B. 454. It was formerly necessary that death should occur within a year and a day of the injury being inflicted, but that has been abolished: Law Reform (Year and a Day Rule) Act 1996 ss.1, 3(2).

[59] See 5–04.

[60] *R. (Nicklinson) v Ministry of Justice* [2014] UKSC 38.

[61] *R. v Inglis* [2011] 1 W.L.R. 1110, CA

[62] *R. v Poulton* (1832) 5 C. & P. 330; 172 E.R. 997. Hence a child born without lungs may "die". cf. the test for birth and death registration, 5–04 above.

[63] *R. v Reeves* (1839) 8 C. & P. 25.

[64] *R. v Senior* (1832) 1 Mood. C.C. 346: *R. v West* (1848) 2 Car. & Kir. 784; 175 E.R. 329: *McCluskey v HM Advocate* [1989] R.T.R. 182. A person who injures a pregnant woman, wounding the fetus, which is born prematurely as a result but dies because of prematurity, can be charged with manslaughter: *Attorney General's Reference (No. 3 of 1994)* [1998] A.C. 245, HL.

[65] See, e.g. *R. v Hamilton* [1983] Crim.L.R. 805 (charge of attempted murder of fetus born alive after abortion operation dismissed by Luton magistrates on the ground of insufficient evidence: the child had since been adopted).

[66] *R. v Moloney* [1985] A.C. 905, HL.

[67] Criminal Justice Act 1967 s.8.

[68] *R. v Hancock and Shankland* [1986] A.C. 455, HL.

properly directed, might infer the existence of an actual *intention* to kill or cause serious injury.[69]

However, it must be remembered that intention is quite distinct from motive or desire, so that a person may intend a consequence which he does not at all desire to bring about. It should also be noted that there is no necessity that the defendant should have aimed his act at any particular person: intention to kill or cause serious injury in the abstract will suffice.[70] Similarly intention to kill or cause serious injury to A will suffice, even though B is killed and A is unhurt. **14–40**

A British subject can be charged with and convicted of murder committed anywhere in the world.[71] The penalty for murder is fixed by law, i.e. imprisonment for life,[72] and the judge has no discretion in the matter, although he is entitled to specify a period of years which should elapse before the defendant should be considered for release on licence.[73] **14–41**

Manslaughter

Since 2008, the law of manslaughter has been different for (i) individuals and (ii) corporations and organisations. The latter is dealt with later.[74] As for individuals, there are two kinds of manslaughter, commonly known as "voluntary" and "involuntary" manslaughter. The actus reus of both kinds of manslaughter is the same as that for murder[75]: it is the mental element that differs. "Voluntary" manslaughter involves the same mens rea as murder, with the addition of circumstances amounting either: **14–42**

   (i) to loss of control (formerly provocation);[76] or

   (ii) to diminished responsibility;[77] or

   (iii) to a suicide pact.[78]

---

[69] See *R. v Nedrick* [1986] 1 W.L.R. 1025; *R. v Woollin* [1999] A.C. 82; *R. v Mathews* [2002] Cr.App.Rep. 461.

[70] *R. v Moloney* [1985] A.C. 905, HL.

[71] Offences against the Person Act 1861 ss.9, 10.

[72] Murder (Abolition of the Death Penalty) Act 1965 s.1(1).

[73] Murder (Abolition of the Death Penalty) Act 1965 s.1(2). Elements of the licence system have been held to infringe art.5 of the European Convention on Human Rights: *Stafford v United Kingdom* Unreported May 28, 2002, ECtHR.

[74] See 14–52 ff.

[75] As to which see 14–37 above.

[76] Coroners and Justice Act 2009 ss.54, 55, as from October 4, 2010; see *R. v Clinton* [2012] 2 All E.R. 947, CA; *R. v Dawes* [2013] EWCA Crim. 322; *R. v Asmelach* [2013] 1 Cr. App. Rep. 229. As to provocation, see *Mancini v DPP* [1942] A.C. 1; *R. v Duffy* [1949] 1 All E.R. 932, CCA; Homicide Act 1957 s.3 (repealed); *DPP v Camplin* [1978] A.C. 705; *R. v Smith* [2001] 1 A.C. 146; *Attorney General for Jersey v Holley* [2005] 3 All E.R. 371, PC.

[77] Homicide Act 1957 s.2, as amended by the Coroners and Justice Act 2009 s.52; *R. v Dunbar* [1958] 1 Q.B. 1, CCA; *R. v Lloyd* [1967] 1 Q.B. 175, CA; *R. v Dix* (1982) 74 Cr. App. R. 306, CA; *R. v Gittens* [1984] Q.B. 698, CA; *R. v Tandy* [1989] 1 W.L.R. 350, CA; *R. v Egan* [1992] 4 All E.R. 470, CA; *R. v Antoine* [2001] 1 A.C. 340; *R. v Dietschmann* [2003] 1 A.C. 1209, HL; *R. v Stewart* [2010] 1 All E.R. 260, CA; *R. v Brown* [2011] EWCA Crim. 2796; *R. v Foye* [2013] EWCA Crim. 475; *R. v Dowds* [2013] 3 All E.R. 154, CA.

[78] Homicide Act 1957 s.4; see *R. v West Yorkshire Coroner Ex p. Kenyon* Unreported April 9, 1984, DC; *Attorney General's Reference (No. 1 of 2004)* [2004] 4 All E.R. 457.

14–43   In other words, "voluntary" manslaughter is murder, with a special mitigating factor which reduces the crime to manslaughter. From the coroner's point of view these special factors are not of much interest once the elements for murder are otherwise shown to exist, for, whether it is murder or manslaughter, the conclusion of the inquest will be "unlawful killing". It is however important to distinguish diminished responsibility from insanity and automatism, and this is dealt with later.[79]

14–44   The other kind of manslaughter is commonly called "involuntary manslaughter" because, although it involves the same actus reus as voluntary manslaughter, the mental element is quite different. In fact there are two alternative mental elements. There is no need for an intention to kill or to do serious bodily harm. It is sufficient if the defendant *either* deliberately intended any unlawful act of violence[80] ("unlawful act" manslaughter) *or*, having no intention in the matter at all, was grossly negligent towards the victim ("gross negligence" manslaughter), with the result (in either case) that he died. It is necessary to distinguish the two forms, especially in directing a jury.

14–45   As for the first of the two alternative formulations, a defendant is guilty of manslaughter if he intentionally does an act which is unlawful and dangerous and which inadvertently causes death.[81] Of course, two or more defendants may act together in a "joint enterprise".[82] Thus unreasonable force used by police in detaining the deceased which risks causing him some physical harm and in fact causes death is sufficient.[83]

14–46   It is not necessary to prove that the unlawful and dangerous act was aimed at any person, and in particular at the person whose death is caused,[84] or even that any *direct* harm was caused to that person by the accused, and neither is it necessary to prove that the defendant knew that the act was unlawful or dangerous.[85] So a spouse, or partner, or indeed any other individual whose unlawful conduct causes recognisable psychiatric illness, such as, for example, post-traumatic stress disorder, or battered wife syndrome, or reactive depression, with resulting suicide of the deceased, subject always to issues of causation, is not excluded from the ambit of this offence.[86] The act causing death and the necessary mental state do not always need to coincide in time, particularly where the original "unlawful act" and the eventual act causing death are all part of the same sequence of events.[87]

14–47   For an act to be "unlawful" within the meaning of this rule it must be criminally and not merely civilly wrong,[88] and it is not enough if the criminality consists in mere negligence, as in, for example, driving without due care and attention:[89] a

---

[79] See 14–96, 14–100 below.
[80] *R. v Lamb* [1967] 2 Q.B. 981; *R. v Slingsby* [1995] Crim. L.R. 570.
[81] *DPP v Newbury* [1977] A.C. 500, HL; cf. *R. v Slingsby* [1995] Crim. L.R. 570.
[82] cf. *R. v Inner North London Coroner Ex p. Diesa Koto* (1993) 157 J.P. 857, DC.
[83] *R. (Cash) v Northamptonshire Coroner* [2007] EWHC 1354 (Admin.).
[84] *R. v Mitchell* [1983] Q.B. 741, CA; *R. v Goodfellow* (1986) 84 Cr. App. R. 23, CA.
[85] *DPP v Newbury* [1977] A.C. 500, HL; *R. v Watson* [1989] 2 All E.R. 865, CA.
[86] *R. v D* [2006] EWCA Crim. 1139 at [32]. See also *Corr v IBC Vehicles Ltd* [2008] UKHL 12; *R. (Pounder) v Durham and Darlington Coroner* [2009] EWHC 76 (Admin.).
[87] *R. v Le Brun* [1992] Q.B. 61, CA.
[88] *R. v Franklin* (1883) 15 Cox C.C. 163; *R. v Lamb* [1967] 2 Q.B. 981.
[89] *Andrews v DPP* [1937] A.C. 576, HL; cf. *R. v Meeking* [2012] 1 W.L.R. 3349.

very high degree of negligence is required for manslaughter.[90] But it is not an "unlawful" act for a person to assault another, mistakenly believing circumstances to exist which, if they did exist, would mean that there was no assault.[91] However, notwithstanding the general rule, it seems that in certain exceptional cases an act can be unlawful without constituting either a crime or a tort, as for example where the defendant administers heroin to a fellow addict who dies from an over-dose.[92]

As for dangerousness, this is to be determined objectively: the act must be such **14–48** as all sober and reasonable people inevitably recognise must subject the other person to at least the risk of some harm, even if not serious.[93]

By contrast, for a defendant to be guilty of gross negligence manslaughter does **14–49** not require any other criminality. The classic formulation of this form of manslaughter is that of Lord Hewart CJ:

"The prosecution must prove the matters necessary to establish civil liability [i.e. for negligence] . . . and, in addition, must satisfy the jury that the negligence or incompetence of the accused went beyond a mere matter of compensation and showed such disregard for the life and safety of others as to amount to a crime against the State and conduct deserving punishment."[94]

The elements of this form of the offence, of which the coroner or the jury must **14–50** be satisfied, have been set out as follows:

"On this basis in my opinion the ordinary principles of the law of negligence apply to ascertain whether or not the defendant has been in breach of a duty of care towards the victim who has died. If such breach of duty is established[95] the next question is whether that breach of duty caused the death of the victim. If so, the jury must go on to consider whether that breach of duty should be characterised as gross negligence and therefore as a crime. This will depend on the seriousness of the breach of duty committed by the defendant in all the circumstances in which the defendant was placed when it occurred. The jury will have to consider whether the extent to which the defendant's conduct departed from the proper standard of care incumbent upon him, involving as it

---

[90] cf. *R. v Pimm* [1994] R.T.R. 391, CA.
[91] *R. v Williams* [1987] 3 All E.R. 411, CA; *R. v Scarlett* [1993] 4 All E.R. 629, CA.
[92] *R. v Cato* [1976] 1 W.L.R. 110, CA; see also *R. v Rogers* [2003] 1 W.L.R. 1374; cf. *R. v Andrews* [2003] Crim. L.R. 477; *R. v Kennedy* [2008] 1 A.C. 269, HL; *R. v Burgess* [2008] EWCA Crim. 516; *R. v Meeking* [2012] 1 W.L.R. 3349.
[93] *R. v Church* [1966] 1 Q.B. 59, CCA; *DPP v Newbury* [1977] A.C. 500, HL; *R. v Goodfellow* (1986) 83 Cr. App.R. 23, CA. Although the "harm" must be physical, it may be caused by shock or fright: *R. v Dawson* (1985) 81 Cr.App.R. 150, CA; *R. v Watson* [1989] 1 W.L.R. 684, CA. See also *R. v Scarlett* [1993] 4 All E.R. 629.
[94] *R. v Bateman* (1925) 19 Cr.App.R. 8, CCA; *R. (Brown) v Neath and Port Talbot Coroner* [2006] EWHC 2019 (Admin.).
[95] See *R. v Evans* [2009] 1 All E.R. 13.

must have done a risk of death to the patient, was such that it should be judged criminal."[96]

Evidence of a defendant's state of mind is not a prerequisite to a conviction for this form of manslaughter.[97] This form of manslaughter is not incompatible with the ECHR art.7.[98]

14–51   The penalty for manslaughter, of whatever kind, is at the trial judge's discretion, and may range from, say, probation or a fine to a maximum of life imprisonment.[99] The range reflects the infinitely variable fact situations amounting to manslaughter.

Corporate manslaughter

14–52   At common law, a corporate body could be guilty of involuntary manslaughter.[100] But the position was unsatisfactory. Where the question of corporate manslaughter arose, the reference to "duty of care" was a reference to a duty of the company concerned, but the reference to breach of that duty (and therefore gross negligence) was to conduct of an identified individual which could be attributed to the company because he or she was one of the directing minds of the company.[101] It was not possible to aggregate the acts or omissions of a number of directing minds, none of which individually was grossly negligent, at least in the absence of a joint unlawful enterprise.[102] As a result, the law has been recast by statute,[103] though at a considerable cost in terms of additional layers of complexity.

14–53   As is so often the case, the gestation period of the change was lengthy and slow. The Law Commission first published a consultation paper on the subject of involuntary manslaughter generally in 1994,[104] and a Report in 1996.[105] A first set of government reform proposals was published by the then Home Secretary in 2000. In 2003 his successor announced that the law on corporate manslaughter would be reformed by primary legislation to be introduced in the autumn of that year.

14–54   However it was almost two years after that before the Home Office published a draft bill for consultation.[106] This was the subject of an inquiry by the Home

---

[96] *R. v Adomako* [1995] 1 A.C. 171 at 187, per Lord Mackay of Clashfern LC; see also *R. v Inner South London Coroner Ex p. Douglas-Williams* [1999] 1 All E.R. 344, 350, CA; *R. (Brown) v Neath and Port Talbot Coroner* [2006] EWHC 2019 (Admin.).

[97] *Attorney General's Reference (No. 2 of 1999)* [2000] Q.B. 796; see also *R. (Rowley) v DPP* [2003] EWHC 693 (Admin.), DC.

[98] *R. v Misra* [2004] EWCA Crim. 2375.

[99] cf *R. v Pimm* [1994] R.T.R. 391, CA.

[100] *R. v East Kent Coroner Ex p. Spooner* (1987) 152 J.P. 115, DC; *R. v P&O European Ferries (Dover) Ltd* (1990) 93 Cr. App. R. 72; *Re Stacey's Application* Unreported October 20, 1999, Turner J; *Attorney General's Reference (No. 2 of 1999)* [2000] Q.B. 796, CA.

[101] *Attorney General's Reference (No. 2 of 1999)* [2000] Q.B. 796; *R. (Bodycote HIP Ltd) v Herefordshire Coroner* [2008] EWHC 164 (Admin.).

[102] *R. v Inner South London Coroner Ex p. Douglas-Williams* [1999] 1 All E.R. 344, 353, CA; *R. (W) v Northants Deputy Coroner* [2007] EWHC 1649 (Admin.).

[103] Corporate Manslaughter and Corporate Homicide Act 2007.

[104] LCCP No. 135.

[105] LC No. 237.

[106] Cm. 6497.

Affairs and Work and Pensions Committees of the House of Commons, which reported in 2005, making various recommendations for change to the bill. The Government's response was published in 2006,[107] accepting some of those recommendations. The bill was introduced into Parliament and became an Act in 2007.

The Act, most of which came into force on April 6, 2008, created a new **14–55** offence, called "corporate manslaughter" in England and Northern Ireland, and "corporate homicide" in Scotland.[108] The Act does not affect the law of manslaughter for individuals, who cannot even be liable for aiding and abetting, counselling or procuring the new offence.[109]

The new law applies only to certain organisations. These are (a) corporations, **14–56** (b) police forces, (c) partnerships, trade unions and employers' associations that are also employers, and (d) other departments or bodies specifically listed in the legislation.[110] Such organisations accordingly can no longer be guilty of gross negligence manslaughter at common law.[111] There is power to extend the Act to other organisations,[112] and to amend the specific list.[113]

In summary, henceforward such an organisation is guilty of the new offence if **14–57** the way in which its activities are managed or organised causes a death and amounts to a gross breach of a relevant duty of care to the deceased.[114] A substantial part of the breach must have been in the way activities were managed by senior management.[115] "Relevant duty of care", "gross" breach and "senior management" are all defined terms.[116] There is no longer any need to show that a "directing mind" of the organisation was personally liable.

"Relevant duty of care",[117] in relation to an organisation, means any duty under **14–58** the law of negligence[118] or under any statutory provision imposing liability in place of the law of negligence[119] owed (a) to its employees or other workers, or (b) as occupier of premises, or (c) in connection with the supply of goods or services, the carrying on of certain operations[120] or other commercial activities, or the use or keeping of plant, vehicles or other things, or (d) to certain persons[121] being detained,[122] transported or securely accommodated, for whose safety the organisation is responsible.[123]

---

[107] Cm. 6755.

[108] Corporate Manslaughter and Corporate Homicide Act 2007 s.1(5).

[109] Corporate Manslaughter and Corporate Homicide Act 2007 s.18.

[110] Corporate Manslaughter and Corporate Homicide Act 2007 s.1(2) Sch.1. These include government departments and departmental agencies (e.g. CPS, ECGD, General Register Office, HMRC, National Archives, Royal Mint, SFO, etc.).

[111] Corporate Manslaughter and Corporate Homicide Act 2007 s.20.

[112] Corporate Manslaughter and Corporate Homicide Act 2007 s.21.

[113] Corporate Manslaughter and Corporate Homicide Act 2007 s.22.

[114] Corporate Manslaughter and Corporate Homicide Act 2007 s.1(1).

[115] Corporate Manslaughter and Corporate Homicide Act 2007 s.1(3).

[116] Corporate Manslaughter and Corporate Homicide Act 2007 s.1(4)(a)-(c); see below.

[117] Corporate Manslaughter and Corporate Homicide Act 2007 s.1(4)(a).

[118] See also Corporate Manslaughter and Corporate Homicide Act 2007 s.2(7).

[119] Corporate Manslaughter and Corporate Homicide Act 2007 s.2(4).

[120] See also Corporate Manslaughter and Corporate Homicide Act 2007 s.2(7).

[121] Corporate Manslaughter and Corporate Homicide Act 2007 s.2(2).

[122] See also Corporate Manslaughter and Corporate Homicide Act 2007 s.2(7).

[123] Corporate Manslaughter and Corporate Homicide Act 2007 s.2(1).

14–59   But this definition is subject to important exceptions[124] for certain public policy decisions, exclusively public functions and statutory inspections,[125] and to the activities of the military,[126] the police,[127] the emergency services,[128] and child-protection and probation services.[129] Where these exceptions apply, any duty of care owed is not a "relevant duty of care". Whether a particular organisation owes a duty of care to a particular individual is a question of law, in respect of which the judge must make any findings of fact necessary to decide that question.[130] In the context of an inquest, the coroner is that judge. For this purpose neither unlawful joint conduct nor voluntary acceptance of risk prevents one person from owing a duty to another.[131]

14–60   A breach of a duty of care is a "gross breach' if the conduct alleged to amount to a breach falls "far below' what can reasonably be expected of the organisation in the circumstances.[132] A jury considering whether an organisation committed a gross breach of the duty of care (a) *must* consider whether the evidence shows that it failed to comply with relevant health and safety legislation (and if so how serious it was and how much of a risk of death it posed),[133] (b) *may* consider how far attitudes, policies, systems or accepted practices within the organisation were likely to have encouraged, or produced tolerance of, the failure,[134] and (c) *may* have regard to any relevant health and safety guidance,[135] or "any other matters they consider relevant".[136]

14–61   "Senior management" means the persons who play significant roles in (i) the making of decisions about how all or a substantial part of the activities of the organisation are to be managed or organised, or (ii) the actual managing or organising of such activities.[137] These criteria, more complex than those at common law, will make summing up to juries especially difficult. The offence itself cannot be charged except with the consent of the DPP[138] (which can be given by a Crown Prosecutor). It is triable only on indictment, and the penalty on conviction is an unlimited fine.[139]

---

[124] Corporate Manslaughter and Corporate Homicide Act 2007 s.2(3).
[125] Corporate Manslaughter and Corporate Homicide Act 2007 s.3.
[126] Corporate Manslaughter and Corporate Homicide Act 2007 ss.4, 12.
[127] Corporate Manslaughter and Corporate Homicide Act 2007 ss.5, 13.
[128] Corporate Manslaughter and Corporate Homicide Act 2007 s.6.
[129] Corporate Manslaughter and Corporate Homicide Act 2007 s.7.
[130] Corporate Manslaughter and Corporate Homicide Act 2007 s.2(5).
[131] Corporate Manslaughter and Corporate Homicide Act 2007 s.2(6).
[132] Corporate Manslaughter and Corporate Homicide Act 2007 s.1(4)(b).
[133] Corporate Manslaughter and Corporate Homicide Act 2007 s.8(2).
[134] Corporate Manslaughter and Corporate Homicide Act 2007 s.8(3)(a).
[135] Corporate Manslaughter and Corporate Homicide Act 2007 s.8(3)(b). As to "health and safety guidance", see s.8(5).
[136] Corporate Manslaughter and Corporate Homicide Act 2007 s.8(4).
[137] Corporate Manslaughter and Corporate Homicide Act 2007 s.1(4)(c).
[138] Corporate Manslaughter and Corporate Homicide Act 2007 s.17.
[139] Corporate Manslaughter and Corporate Homicide Act 2007 s.1(6). See *R. v Cotswold Geotechnical Holdings Ltd*[2012] 1 Cr. App. R. (S) 26 (£385,000 fine, likely to put the company into liquidation).

Road Traffic Offences

Causing death by dangerous driving. This is an offence originally created by **14–62** statute in 1956 and significantly amended since. The current wording is as follows:

"A person who causes the death of another person by driving a mechanically propelled vehicle dangerously on a road or other public place is guilty of an offence."[140]

The maximum penalty is 10 years' imprisonment.[141]

The actus reus of the offence is narrower than murder or manslaughter, in that **14–63** death must be caused "by driving a mechanically propelled vehicle . . . on a road or other public place". For this purpose "road" means any highway and any other road to which the public has access (including bridges over which a road passes).[142] Subject to this restriction on the means of causing death, the actus reus is otherwise identical to murder and manslaughter.[143]

The mens rea of the offence consists simply in the intention to drive a **14–64** mechanically propelled vehicle on a road or other public place. "Dangerously" is defined by the statute in completely objective terms, so that the driver need not appreciate the danger. There are two forms of driving dangerously:

(1) where the manner of driving falls far below what would be expected of a competent and careful driver, and it would be obvious to such a driver that that manner would be dangerous[144];

(2) where it would be obvious to a competent and careful driver that driving the vehicle in its current state would be dangerous.[145]

For this purpose, "dangerous" refers to danger either of injury to the person or **14–65** of damage to property, and in determining what would be expected of or obvious to a competent and careful driver regard is had, not only to circumstances of which he could be expected to be aware, but also to circumstances shown to have been in the knowledge of the actual driver.[146] The "current state" of the vehicle can include the vehicle together with any attachments to or load on it, and also the manner in which it is attached or carried.[147]

The offence was originally created in 1956 because criminal juries were **14–66** reluctant to convict of manslaughter in motoring cases (so-called "motor manslaughter"). However, it is clear that the statutory offence has not impliedly

---

[140] Road Traffic Act 1988 s.1, as substituted by Road Traffic Act 1991 s.1.
[141] See the Criminal Justice Act 1993 s.67.
[142] Criminal Justice Act 1993 s.192(1).
[143] See 14–37 above.
[144] Road Traffic Act 1988 s.2A(1) (inserted by Road Traffic Act 1991 s.1).
[145] Road Traffic Act 1988 s.2A(2).
[146] Road Traffic Act 1988 s.2A(3).
[147] Road Traffic Act 1988 s.2A(4); see *R. v Crossman* (1986) 82 Cr.App.R.333, CA (insecure load falling off and killing pedestrian).

abolished motor manslaughter, which still exists.[148] The statutory offence does not however justify the conclusion of unlawful killing.[149] The appropriate conclusion will be "road traffic collision",[150] or, if that does not apply, "accident/mis-adventure".[151]

14–67   **Causing death by careless driving when under influence of drink or drugs.** This is a statutory offence created in 1991. It consists of causing the death of a person by driving a mechanically propelled vehicle on a road or other public place without due care and attention, or without reasonable consideration for other persons using the road or place, and *either:*

(a) the driver is unfit to drive (meaning that his ability to drive properly is impaired)[152] through drink or drugs; *or*

(b) the driver has consumed so much alcohol that his breath/blood/urine alcohol level in breath, blood or urine at that time exceeds the prescribed limit; or

(c) without reasonable excuse the driver fails to provide a specimen under s.7 of the Road Traffic Act 1988 being required to do so within 18 hours of that time; or

(d) without reasonable excuse fails to give permission for a laboratory test of a blood specimen taken from him.[153]

14–68   The maximum penalty is 10 years' imprisonment and a fine. In accordance with the views already expressed,[154] the proper conclusion for the inquisition in a case of this kind is "road traffic collision",[155] or, if that does not apply, "accident/misadventure",[156] rather than "unlawful killing".

Infanticide

14–69   This offence was formerly considered as a form of voluntary manslaughter, i.e. where an offence otherwise murder is rendered less serious by the presence of a mitigating factor. But it is now clear that it is a new and separate offence, and there is no requirement that all the ingredients of murder be proved before a defendant can be convicted of infanticide.[157] It is applicable to a mother who by any wilful act or omission causes the death of her own child aged less than 12 months at a time when the balance of her mind is disturbed by reason of her not having fully recovered from the effect of giving birth to that child or by reason of the effect of

---

[148] *Jennings v United States* [1983] A.C. 624, HL.
[149] See 13–55 above.
[150] See 13–65.
[151] See 13–36 ff.
[152] Road Traffic Act 1988 s.3A(2) (inserted by Road Traffic Act 1991 s.3).
[153] Road Traffic Act 1988 s.3A(1).
[154] See 13–54 above.
[155] See 13–65.
[156] See 13–36 ff.
[157] *R. v Gore* [2007] EWCA Crim. 2789 at [33]; see also *R. v Kai-Whitewind* [2005] 2 Cr. App. Rep. 457 (law of infanticide outdated and should be reconsidered).

lactation consequent upon the birth of that child.[158] The offence is punishable in the same way as manslaughter, although in practice a custodial sentence is rare. Where a coroner or jury is satisfied that the death of the deceased occurred as a result of circumstances amounting to infanticide, the appropriate conclusion is one of unlawful killing.[159]

Child destruction

Child destruction is not a true homicide offence, since it concerns the death of a **14–70** fetus, albeit one "capable of being born alive". For the same reason it is unlikely to concern the coroner, since he has jurisdiction to inquire only into deaths of persons born alive.[160] This means that, once he is satisfied that the fetus was not born alive, he has no power to order a post-mortem examination, and it is a matter as between the police and the person having possession of the fetus as to any such examination.

The offence, which is punishable by a maximum sentence of imprisonment for **14–71** life, is committed by any person who, with intent to destroy the life of a child capable of being born alive, by any wilful act causes a child to die before it has an existence independent of its mother.[161] However, the prosecution must also prove that the act causing the death of the child was not done in good faith for the purpose only of preserving the life of the mother,[162] which can include the case where the person causing the death did so reasonably believing that the probable consequences of the continuance of the pregnancy would be to make the woman a physical or mental wreck, rather than actually to kill her outright.[163]

The difficult (and crucial) words in the statute are "capable of being born alive": **14–72** it is clearly not necessary that the child be capable of surviving for a long time after birth. However, it must be sufficiently developed so as to be able to breathe after birth, either naturally or with the aid of a respirator.[164] For the purpose of proving that a child whose life is destroyed was "capable of being born alive" there is a statutory presumption that a fetus aged 28 weeks or more from conception was a child capable of being born alive.[165] But it is open to the prosecution to prove that a less developed fetus was also so capable.[166]

Abortion

As with child destruction, this is a form of killing which does not give the coroner **14–73** jurisdiction to inquire into the circumstances of death, unless there is reason to suspect that the deceased fetus had been born alive.[167] As an offence its importance has been very largely diminished by the reform of the law in 1967. The original offence consisted in the unlawful administration of "any poison or noxious thing"

---

[158] Infanticide Act 1938 s.1(1).
[159] See 13–54 above.
[160] As to "born alive", see 5–04, 14–37 above.
[161] Infant Life (Preservation) Act 1929 s.1(1).
[162] Infant Life (Preservation) Act 1929 s.1(1), proviso.
[163] *R. v Bourne* [1939] 1 K.B. 687.
[164] *C. v S.* [1988] Q.B. 135, CA; *Rance v Mid-Downs Health Authority* [1991] 1 Q.B. 587.
[165] Infant Life (Preservation) Act 1929 s.1(2).
[166] cf. *C v S* [1988] Q.B. 135, CA; *Rance v Mid-Downs Health Authority* [1991] 1 Q.B. 587.
[167] As to which see 5–04, 14–37 above.

or the unlawful use of "any instrument or other means whatsoever" with the intent (in either case) of procuring a woman to miscarry.[168] A woman acting alone to procure her own miscarriage commits the offence only if she actually is pregnant: another person so acting commits the offence whether or not the woman is indeed pregnant.

14–74 Sympathetic judicial construction of the word "unlawful" in the section creating the offence led to a defence, for medical practitioners at least, of honest and reasonable belief that the abortion was necessary to preserve the mental or physical well-being of the woman.[169] But this has been largely if not completely overtaken by the statutory defence set out in the Abortion Act 1967.

14–75 Under this Act, an abortion is not unlawful if carried out by a registered medical practitioner, where two such practitioners are of the bona fide view *either*: (a) that the continuance of the pregnancy (which must not have exceeded its 24th week) would involve risk, greater than if it were terminated of injury to the physical or mental health of the woman or any existing children of her family; *or* (b) that the termination is necessary to prevent grave permanent injury to the physical or mental health of the woman; *or* (c) to the life of the woman, greater than if the pregnancy were terminated; or (d) that there is a substantial risk that the child would be born seriously physically or mentally handicapped.[170] Where this provision applies to an abortion, the offence of child destruction cannot be committed.[171]

Complicity in suicide

14–76 Voluntary euthanasia of a person unwilling or unable to commit suicide can be murder.[172] But since 1957 for one party to a suicide pact deliberately to kill the other party is manslaughter only.[173] It can also be manslaughter where one person unlawfully causes recognisable psychiatric illness, with resulting suicide of the deceased, subject always to issues of causation.[174] Apart from these cases, and despite the fact that suicide itself is no longer a criminal offence,[175] it is also an offence, punishable by a maximum of 14 years' imprisonment, to do an act capable of encouraging or assisting the suicide or attempted suicide of another person, with the intent to encourage or assist suicide or attempted suicide.[176]

14–77 Thus, for example, a person who knowingly provides the means for a person to commit suicide is guilty of an offence under this section. It seems that a person who advises another as to how successfully to commit suicide may in certain

---

[168] Offences against the Person Act 1861 s.58. See *R. (Smeaton) v Secretary of State for Health* [2002] Crim. L.R. ("morning-after" pill does not procure miscarriage).

[169] *R. v Bourne* [1939] 1 K.B. 687.

[170] Abortion Act 1967 s.1(1), as amended by the Human Fertilization and Embryology Act 1990 s.37(1).

[171] Abortion Act 1967 s.5(1), as similarly substituted.

[172] *Pretty v DPP* [2002] 1 A.C. 800 at [111], per Lord Hobhouse; *R. (Nicklinson) v Ministry of Justice* [2014] UKSC 38, [17].

[173] Homicide Act 1957 s.4. cf. *R. v Croft* [1944] 1 K.B. 295.

[174] *R. v D* [2006] EWCA Crim. 1139 at [32]. See also *Corr v IBC Vehicles Ltd* [2008] UKHL 12; *R. (Pounder) v Durham and Darlington Coroner* [2009] EWHC 76 (Admin.).

[175] Suicide Act 1961 s.1.

[176] Suicide Act 1961 s.2(1), as amended; see *Airedale NHS Trust v Bland* [1993] A.C. 789 at 831, per Hoffmann LJ; *Pretty v DPP* [2002] 1 A.C. 800 at [9], per Lord Bingham.

circumstances be guilty of the offence.[177] But it is not unlawful for a doctor to prescribe medical treatment which will necessarily hasten death where the purpose is to relieve pain and suffering.[178]

Proceedings for such an offence may be instituted only with the consent of the **14–78** Director of Public Prosecutions.[179] The Director has no power to undertake in advance of an assisted suicide not to give his consent.[180] This does not infringe the European Convention on Human Rights,[181] though the Director must publish his policy on when he would prosecute such offences, and what factors he would take into account.[182]

Where a coroner is faced with a case of suicide accompanied by circumstances **14–79** amounting to the commission of the statutory offence, but not to manslaughter or (a fortiori) murder, the appropriate verdict must be one of suicide.[183] "Unlawful killing" is not appropriate unless the aiding and abetting of suicide is so causative of the death as to found the greater criminal responsibility of (at least) manslaughter: in all other cases the killing is (after all) suicide and, since 1961, not unlawful. It was formerly necessary, for suicide, that death occur within a year and a day of the act concerned, but this rule was abolished in 1996.[184]

Causation

The question of causation is of vital importance in considering whether a **14–80** substantive homicide offence has been committed. A person is only criminally responsible for the death of another if he can be said to have "caused" it. There are two questions to be discussed: the first is what causative factors are regarded as legally significant, and secondly, what is the law's treatment of omissions to act, as distinct from positive acts themselves. The concept of causation has been subjected to considerable judicial analysis in recent years.[185]

Sine qua non

A simple way of looking at causation is to use the "but-for" (or sine qua non) test: **14–81** but for such and such an act by the defendant, the death would not have occurred. Although there are a few cases where this test can be useful, as where a person administers poison to a person who dies of a heart attack before the poison can take

---

[177] *Attorney General v Able* [1984] Q.B. 795, QBD (explanatory booklet published by EXIT on suicide). *cf. R. v Reed* [1982] Crim.L.R. 819, CA (guilty of offence by putting would-be suicides in touch with co-accused to assist them in committing suicide).
[178] *R. (Nicklinson) v Ministry of Justice* [2014] UKSC 38, [18].
[179] Suicide Act 1961 s.2(4).
[180] *Pretty v DPP* [2002] 1 A.C. 800, HL.
[181] *Pretty v United Kingdom* (2002) 35 E.H.R.R. 1, ECtHR
[182] *R. (Purdy) v DPP* [2010] 1 A.C. 345; *R. (Nicklinson) v Ministry of Justice* [2014] UKSC 38.
[183] *R. v Turnbull Ex p. Kenyon* Unreported, March 15, 1984, DC.
[184] Law Reform (Year and a Day Rule) Act 1996.
[185] See, e.g. *Environmental Agency v Empress Car Co (Abertillery) Ltd* [1997] 2 A.C. 22, HL; *Kuwait Airways Corporation v Iraqi Airways Co (Nos 4 and 5)* [2002] 2 A.C. 883, HL; *Rahman v Arearose Ltd* [2001] Q.B. 351, CA; *Fairchild v Glenhaven Funeral Services Ltd* [2003] 1 A.C. 32, HL; *Barker v Corus UK Ltd* [2006] 2 A.C. 572, HL; *Sienkewicz v Greif (UK) Ltd* [2011] 2 A.C. 229, SC; *Durham v BAI (Run Off) Ltd* [2012] 1 W.L.R. 867, SC; *International Energy Group Ltd v Zurich Insurance plc UK* [2013] 3 All E.R. 395, CA.

effect,[186] for legal purposes it is not generally much use, as it casts its net too wide.

Causa causans

14–82 There are a great many acts but for which an ultimate consequence would not have resulted, and it would be unreasonable to ascribe criminal responsibility to the actors in each case. As a result, lawyers have searched for a closer cause (sometimes called an imputable or legal cause, or *causa causans*) amongst the "but-for" causes.[187] Much legal effort is devoted to attempting to rationalise the test for "legal" causes amongst all the "but-for" causes. Sometimes the question of "legal" causation is affected by a specific legal rule, such as that which formerly conclusively presumed a death not to have been caused by an injury sustained earlier than a year and a day before death occurred.[188]

14–83 In the final analysis, what makes a "legal" cause is a value judgment by the law that in the particular circumstances the actor should bear responsibility for what transpired. In other words, the question of causation is simply a part of the scope of the relevant legal rule: what is the basis and purpose of liability?[189] Thus, for example, the person who hands a prepared syringe full of heroin for immediate self-injection to another did not "cause" the death of the person who took a deliberate decision to inject himself.[190]

14–84 Nonetheless, and looking at the purpose and scope of the criminal law generally, it is possible to discern certain types of fact situation in which the courts are ready to ascribe criminal responsibility. One is where the acts of the defendant, though they do not cause direct physical harm to the victim, nevertheless put the victim in such fear that he, in an effort perhaps to escape, or as a result of fright, takes some step which causes his death (for example jumping from a window,[191] falling down stairs,[192] or jumping out of a car travelling at speed[193]).

The chain of causation

14–85 This anxiety that causation should be directly related to the perceived degree of criminal responsibility which should be borne by the actor demonstrates itself in a second class of case. This is where, although the defendant by his acts has caused harm to the victim, these acts would not or might not have resulted in death had it not been for some intervening acts. Thus, where a person was stabbed, such that without medical attention he would eventually have died, and he subsequently received such poor medical attention that he did die, it was held that the original actor who stabbed the victim "caused" his death,[194] in the sense that the stab

---

[186] *R. v White* [1910] 2 K.B. 124.

[187] *Hay v Devon Coroner* (1998) 162 J.P. 96, CA.

[188] See now the Law Reform (Year and a Day Rule) Act 1996.

[189] *Kuwait Airways Corporation v Iraqi Airways Co (Nos 4 and 5)* [2002] 2 A.C. 883 at [128]; *Rahman v Arearose Ltd* [2001] Q.B. 351 at [33]. *R v Hughes* [2013] 1 WLR 2461, SC.

[190] *R. v Kennedy* [2008] 1 A.C. 269, HL; *R. v Burgess* [2008] EWCA Crim. 516.

[191] *R. v Curley* (1909) 2 Cr.App.R. 109, CCA.

[192] *R. v Mackie* (1973) 57 Cr.App.R. 453, CA.

[193] *R. v Williams* [1992] 1 W.L.R. 380, CA.

[194] *R. v Smith* [1959] 2 Q.B. 35, CMAC; *R. v Cheshire* [1991] 1 W.L.R. 844, CA; cf. *R. v Jordan* (1956) 40 Cr.App.R. 153, CCA.

wound contributed *significantly* to the death.[195] It is not necessary for the prosecution in such a case to show that the supervening event was *not* a significant cause of death.[196] Instead, it must simply show that the original act "more than minimally, negligibly or trivially contributed to the death".[197]

Similarly, the courts, in cases where a patient has suffered "brain death" as a result of serious assault, have refused to investigate the question whether the doctors in discontinuing treatment and switching off the ventilator "caused" the resulting death, on the grounds that the rightness or wrongness of the intervening medical treatment could not be allowed to prevent the defendant's original conduct (in inflicting wounds from which the victim would otherwise have died) from bearing criminal responsibility for the death.[198] Again, a person applying unlawful force to a victim who then accidentally kills him during the same sequence of events has been held rightly convicted of manslaughter, on the basis that the subsequent action (resulting in death) did not break the "chain of causation".[199]

14–86

Take the victim as you find him

Indeed, the courts have gone further, and have held that the defendant must take his victim as he finds him, and if the victim is already so feeble in mind or body as to succumb more easily than a normal person,[200] or if the victim is of such religious or other beliefs as to refuse medical treatment and dies where an ordinary person would have accepted treatment which would have saved him,[201] then the defendant must nevertheless bear the criminal responsibility for having "caused" the death of the victim.

14–87

Omission to act

Finally, we turn to a quite different topic in the area of causation, that of liability for omissions, rather than for positive acts. In general, for a person to be held to have caused another's death by omission, there has to be some *duty* to act which the defendant has failed to perform, such that performance would have prevented the death in question.

14–88

Such duties to act have been held to arise in three main sets of circumstances: (1) where the defendant is under a contractual duty to act[202]; (2) where the defendant is a parent who owes duties at common law or under statute to care for his children[203]; (3) where the defendant has assumed a duty to care for another person.[204] The criminal law is somewhat wary of attaching criminal responsibility

14–89

---

[195] *R. v Pitts* (1842) C. & Mar. 248; *R. v Henningan* [1971] 3 All E.R. 133, CA.

[196] *R. v Mellor* [1996] 2 Cr. App. R. 245, CA.

[197] *R. v Inner South London Coroner Ex p. Douglas-Williams* [1999] 1 All E.R. 344 at 350, CA.

[198] *R. v Malcherek, R. v Steel* [1981] 1 W.L.R. 690, CA; *Airedale NHS Trust v Bland* [1993] A.C. 789, HL.

[199] *R. v Le Brun* [1992] Q.B. 61, CA. Something which does "break the chain of causation" is often referred to as "novus actus interveniens".

[200] *R. v Martin* (1832) 5 C. & P. 128.

[201] *R. v Blaue* [1975] 1 W.L.R. 1411, CA.

[202] *R. v Pittwood* (1902) 19 T.L.R. 37; see also *R. v Dytham* [1979] Q.B. 722, CA.

[203] *R. v Gibbons and Proctor* (1918) 13 Cr.App.R. 134, CCA; cf. *R. v Sheppard* [1981] A.C. 394, HL.

[204] *R. v Instan* [1893] 1 Q.B. 450, CCR; *R. v Stone* [1977] 1 Q.B. 354, CA; *R. v Khan, The Times*, April 7, 1998, CA.

to an omission to act, so it may be thought unlikely that these categories will be extended in the future. Of course, this analysis only shows when an omission causes death for legal purposes. It does not conclude the question whether so causing the death is a criminal offence or not, e.g. manslaughter. For this purpose regard must be had to the earlier discussion of substantive offences.

Defences

14–90 There are a number of "defences" which a defendant may advance in a homicide case, which we must now briefly consider. They are: infancy, insanity, automatism, mistake, intoxication, necessity, duress, self-defence, superior orders and impossibility. Each will be treated in turn.

Infancy

14–91 Persons under the age of 18 can be divided into three categories for the purposes of criminal responsibility.

14–92 **Children under 10.** Children before their 10th birthday are simply incapable of being criminally responsible for their actions,[205] however much they are aware of what they are doing and that it is wrong.

14–93 **Children of 14 and over.** Children of the age of 14 or more are treated as adults in terms of theoretical criminal responsibility, and therefore the prosecution need only prove the elements of the offence in question for a conviction.[206] However, there are considerable differences in the procedure applicable and range of sentencing options available in the case of a person aged 14 to 18.

14–94 **Children from 10 to 14.** Thirdly, the so-called "twilight zone" formerly covered the intervening period from the 10th birthday to the day before the 14th: in such cases a defendant had to be proved not only to have had the mens rea requisite for the offence, but also to have acted with "mischievous discretion",[207] i.e. that he understood the difference between right and wrong, and knew that what he was doing was wrong.[208] In other words there was a "rebuttable presumption" that a child aged over 10 to under 14 years was incapable of committing crime.[209] But this rebuttable presumption was then abolished,[210] though doubts have been expressed as to whether the abolition affects the substantive law, or merely procedure.[211]

14–95 The coroner needs to be aware of these rules, because, unless the person causing the death can be said to be criminally responsible, it is inappropriate to record a conclusion of "unlawful killing".[212] (The age of a person can also be highly

---

[205] Children and Young Persons Act 1933 s.50, as amended.
[206] *R. v Smith* (1845) 1 Cox C.C. 260.
[207] 1 Hale P.C. 630.
[208] *R. v B* [1979] 1 W.L.R. 1185, CA.
[209] See *C v DPP* [1996] A.C. 1, HL.
[210] Crime and Disorder Act 1998 s.34.
[211] Walker (1999) 149 N.L.J. 64.
[212] See 13–47 ff above.

relevant in considering the intent of such a person to kill another or take his own life,[213] though this is a rather different point.)

Insanity

The classic definition of insanity as a defence to criminal responsibility was given **14–96** by the common law judges in 1843:

> "To establish a defence on the ground of insanity, it must be clearly proved that, at the time of the committing of the act, the party accused was labouring under such a defect of reason, from disease of the mind, as not to know the nature and quality of the act he was doing; or, if he did know it, that he did not know he was doing what was wrong."[214]

"Wrong" in the final phrase means "legally wrong", not "morally wrong".[215] It **14–97** is for the defendant to prove, on the balance of probabilities,[216] that he is insane and not for the prosecution to negative insanity. It should be noted that a disease of the mind by itself is not enough: it does not matter whether the cause of the defect is organic or functional, or whether it is permanent or temporary[217]; thus an epileptic could be legally "insane" for this purpose.[218] If the defence is proved, the verdict is "not guilty by reason of insanity" and the judge must make a special hospital order.[219] The abolition of capital punishment and the serious consequences of the hospital order have made this defence signally unpopular in modern times.

Insanity as a complete legal defence must be distinguished from diminished **14–98** responsibility, which is not a defence but a special factor reducing a case of murder to one of manslaughter.[220] Diminished responsibility is simply where the killer was suffering from such abnormality of mind as substantially to impair (but not extinguish) his mental responsibility for the killing.[221]

Where a person who deliberately killed another was insane at the time, the **14–99** appropriate conclusion in a coroner's inquisition is not "unlawful killing" but "accident/misadventure" or "open verdict" as necessary.[222] The case may be complicated by the need to take into account the position of those who allow a mental patient to escape and kill a person, but even in such a case "neglect" will hardly ever be an option.

Automatism

The defence of automatism must be distinguished from that of insanity. Essentially, **14–100** a plea of automatism is a denial of the voluntariness of the actus reus, in that the

---

[213] *R. v Turnbull Ex p. Kenyon* Unreported March 15, 1984, DC; *R. v North Northumberland Coroner Ex p. Armstrong* (1987) 151 J.P. 773, DC.
[214] *M'Naghten's* case (1843) 10 Cl. & F. 200; 8 E.R. 718, per Tindal CJ.
[215] *R. v Windle* [1952] 2 Q.B. 826, CCA; cf. *Stapleton v R.* (1952) 86 C.L.R. 358, HC (Aus.).
[216] *Sodeman v R.* [1936] 2 All E.R. 1138, PC.
[217] *R. v Burgess* [1991] 2 Q.B. 92, CA.
[218] *R. v Sullivan* [1984] A.C. 156, HL.
[219] Criminal Procedure (Insanity) Act 1964 ss.1 and 5(1).
[220] See 14–42 above.
[221] Homicide Act 1957 s.2.
[222] See 13–56, 13–62 above.

defendant, at any rate without fault, has lost the capacity for voluntary control of his actions otherwise than through a disease of the mind.[223] Where the defendant is at fault, for example by taking drink or drugs or by failing to take medicine to control a pre-existing condition such as diabetes, whether the defendant can rely on non-insane automatism depends on whether the crime is one of basic intent or one of specific or ulterior intent.

14–101   In theory, the distinction between these two classes of case is that a basic intent is an intent to do acts comprising the actus reus, whereas a specific intent is an intent to do acts going beyond this.[224] Intellectually, the distinction is illusory, with the result that whether a particular crime is one of specific or basic intent is a question answered by the courts on an entirely unprincipled and ad hoc basis. Murder is apparently a crime of specific intent,[225] as is wounding or causing grievous bodily harm with intent to do so,[226] whereas manslaughter (all forms)[227] and malicious wounding or inflicting grievous bodily harm[228] are crimes of basic intent.

14–102   In relation to crimes of specific intent, automatism, even if self-induced, is a defence because it negatives the necessary specific intent.[229] In crimes of basic intent, where alcohol or other drugs voluntarily taken by the defendant produce the automatic state, it is no defence to charges of such crimes, because the voluntary taking is sufficiently reckless to constitute the necessary mens rea.[230] However, in other cases of self-induced automatism (e.g. failing to take appropriate medication to prevent a hypoglycaemic episode), the question is whether the defendant's fault amounted in fact to recklessness sufficient for the mens rea of the offence in question.[231] Where this defence applies, the appropriate conclusion in an inquisition is likely to be "accident/misadventure" or "open verdict".

Mistake

14–103   Mistake is not itself a defence, but operates in certain cases by denying the existence of all or part of the requisite mens rea of an offence.[232] Thus, for example, a person who shoots a person thinking him to be a dummy does not intend to kill or cause grievous bodily harm, and accordingly does not have the mens rea for murder. Similarly, a person mistakenly believing circumstances to exist justifying the use of excessive force is not guilty of "unlawful and dangerous act" manslaughter.[233]

---

[223] This might be insanity: *R. v Sullivan* [1984] A.C. 156, HL; *R. v Hennessy* [1989] 1 W.L.R. 287, CA.

[224] See, e.g. *DPP v Majewski* [1977] A.C. 443, HL.

[225] *DPP v Beard* [1920] A.C. 479, HL; *R. v Sheehan* [1975] 1 W.L.R. 739, CA.

[226] *Bratty v Attorney General for Northern Ireland* [1963] A.C. 386, HL; *R. v Pordage* [1975] Crim.L.R. 575, CA.

[227] *DPP v Beard* [1920] A.C. 479, HL; *Attorney General for Northern Ireland v Gallagher* [1963] A.C. 349, HL; *Bratty v Attorney General for Northern Ireland* [1963] A.C. 386, HL; *R. v Lipman* [1970] 1 Q.B. 152, CA.

[228] *Bratty v Attorney General for Northern Ireland* [1963] A.C. 386, HL; *DPP v Majewski* [1977] A.C. 443, HL.

[229] *DPP v Majewski* [1977] A.C. 443, HL; *R. v Bailey* [1983] 1 W.L.R. 760, CA.

[230] *DPP v Majewski* [1977] A.C. 443, HL.

[231] *R. v Bailey* [1983] 1 W.L.R. 760, CA.

[232] *DPP v Morgan* [1976] A.C. 182, HL.

[233] *R. v Scarlett* [1993] 4 All E.R. 629, CA. Of course, it might amount to some lesser offence, e.g. manslaughter.

However, it depends entirely on the exact mens rea required to constitute an offence as to whether the mistake made by the defendant will afford a defence in a particular case. If, for example, negligence is sufficient mens rea for the offence in question, then only an honest mistake that is also objectively reasonable can excuse, for an honest but unreasonable mistake is *ex hypothesi* negligent and hence constitutes the necessary mens rea.[234]

It is sometimes said that mistake (or ignorance) of law is no excuse. As a general **14–104** proposition this is in fact untrue,[235] for there are many offences where a particular attitude towards a proposition of law (criminal or civil) is requisite for criminal liability to attach, and in such cases a mistake of law may excuse.[236] How far this principle is applicable to homicide (if at all) is doubtful. For instance, it might be argued that if a medical practitioner carrying out an abortion caused the death of the child mistakenly believing it not in law to constitute a "human being born alive" he should not be guilty of murder, but this cannot reasonably be expected to represent the law.[237]

Intoxication

Intoxication is a defence to criminal liability only in cases where it leads to the **14–105** defendant's making such a mistake as would itself excuse, on the ground of absence of the necessary mens rea for the offence in question, or in cases where it prevents the defendant from having the capacity to form any mental attitude at all.[238] However, for reasons of policy, the courts have restricted the scope of the defence to: (i) cases where the intoxication was not self-induced and the defendant was not otherwise at fault;[239] (ii) all cases where the intoxication *was* self-induced in bona fide pursuance of medical treatment;[240] and (iii) cases of crimes requiring a specific intent[241] where the intoxication was self-induced.[242]

If the defendant became intoxicated through his own actions, he is not **14–106** permitted to rely on that intoxication to deny mens rea for any crime of basic intent.[243] It is not a defence that a person having formed a sufficient intent thereafter becomes intoxicated in order to commit the crime (so-called "Dutch courage").[244] Nor is it a defence that it was only because he (without fault) became intoxicated that he formed the necessary intent to commit the offence.[245]

---

[234] See, e.g. *R. v Tolson* (1889) 23 Q.B.D. 168, CCR.
[235] See Matthews (1983) 3 *Legal Studies* 174.
[236] e.g. *R. v David Smith* [1974] Q.B. 354, CA.
[237] cf. *R. v David Smith* [1974] Q.B. 354, CA: defendant entitled to be acquitted of criminal damage where he mistakenly believed the property which he damaged to belong to himself in law.
[238] *DPP v Majewski* [1977] A.C. 443, HL.
[239] cf. *R. v Kingston* [1995] 2 A.C. 355.
[240] *R. v Quick* [1957] 1 Q.B. 399.
[241] See 14–101 above.
[242] *DPP v Beard* [1920] A.C. 479, HL; *DPP v Majewski* [1977] A.C. 443, HL.
[243] For the specific intent/basic intent distinction, see 14–101.
[244] *Attorney General for Northern Ireland v Gallagher* [1963] A.C. 349, HL.
[245] *R. v Kingston* [1995] 2 A.C. 355, HL.

Necessity

14–107   The commonly held view has been that there is no general defence of "necessity" in English criminal law.[246] However there are extreme circumstances in which the law recognises such a defence. Chief among these are cases of duress, i.e. where a person's will is overborne by wrongful threats or violence from another, and this is considered below.[247] Further cases, amounting to "self-defence", are also discussed below.[248]

14–108   There are other cases where objective (extraneous[249]) dangers threaten the person concerned, or third parties. Sometimes these cases are called "duress of circumstances".[250] Thus a person who drives recklessly to avoid men believed to be assassins bent on killing his passenger,[251] or who drives while disqualified to prevent his wife from carrying out a threat to commit suicide,[252] can rely on "necessity" as a defence. More relevant to our subject is the defence of necessity open to a medical practitioner on a charge of unlawful abortion, i.e. that the operation was carried out in good faith and for the purpose only of saving the life of the mother.[253] Whereas duress by threats is not a defence to murder, it seems that duress of circumstances may be such a defence.[254]

Duress

14–109   "Duress" (sometimes now called "duress by threats") describes a form of necessity in which the compulsion on the actor *to act as he does* proceeds from threats of death or serious personal injury made to him by another person. These threats are characteristically of the form "do this, or else". It is a defence to all offences[255] except murder (whether as a principal in the first or the second degree[256]) and possibly treason.[257] But the law requires a person to have the self-control reasonably expected of an ordinary citizen, and hence the test for whether that person acted through duress is partly objective.[258]

14–110   The defence of duress is excluded when as a result of the accused's voluntary association with others engaged in crime he foresaw or ought reasonably to have foreseen the risk of being subjected to any compulsion by threats of violence.[259]

---

[246] *R. v Dudley and Stephens* (1884) 11 Q.B.D. 273, CCR; *Lynch v DPP for Northern Ireland* [1975] A.C. 653 at 691, per Lord Simon of Glaisdale.
[247] See 14–109 ff below.
[248] See 14–112 ff below.
[249] *R. v Rodger* [1998] 1 Cr.App.R. 143, CA.
[250] See *R. v Pommell* [1995] 2 Cr.App.R. 607, CA; *R. v Abdul-Hussain* [1999] Crim.L.R. 570; *R. v S (DM)* [2001] Crim.L.R. 986.
[251] *R. v Conway* [1989] Q.B. 290, CA; cf. *R. v Willer* (1986) 83 Cr.App.R. 225, CA.
[252] *R. v Martin* (1989) 153 JP 231, CA.
[253] *R. v Bourne* [1939] 1 K.B. 687; see also *Re F (Mental Patient)* [1990] 2 A.C. 1, HL.
[254] *Re A (Children)* [2000] 4 All E.R. 960.
[255] *R. v Hudson* [1971] 2 Q.B. 202, CA.
[256] *R. v Howe* [1987] A.C. 417, HL, overruling *Lynch v DPP for Northern Ireland* [1975] A.C. 653, HL.
[257] *R. v Hudson* [1971] 2 Q.B. 202, CA .
[258] *R. v Howe* [1987] A.C. 417, HL; see also *R. v Bowen* [1996] 2 Cr.App.R. 157, CA (low IQ irrelevant).
[259] *R. v Hasan* [2005] UKHL 22; [2005] 2 A.C. 467.

But it is available to a defendant who reasonably believes there to have been an appropriate threat, even if in fact there was no such threat.[260]

There is a related defence, usually known as "coercion", available only to a wife **14–111** who commits certain crimes in the presence of her husband. Formerly there was a presumption that a wife who committed an offence in her husband's presence did so under his coercion,[261] but this has long been abolished.[262] The law now is that the wife must prove, on the balance of probabilities, that her will was overborne by the wishes of her husband, so that she was forced unwillingly to participate in the offence.[263] It is unclear to what crimes the defence still extends, although it is clear that it does not apply to treason or murder. Some writers exclude manslaughter and robbery as well. It is today of little significance and its abolition has been recommended.[264]

Self-Defence

"Self-defence" is a term often used (and indeed used here) to cover not merely the **14–112** defence of oneself but also the defence of others, the defence of property and the prevention of crime. Sometimes it is called "public and private defence" to reflect this width of scope.[265] Strictly, self-defence in this sense is not a defence to a criminal charge, since the acts of self-defence which might give rise to such a charge are not unlawful at all if committed in the circumstances to be outlined hereafter. Thus the burden is always on the prosecution to prove that the acts with which the defendant is charged do not amount to self-defence.

The common law rules on the prevention of crime have been replaced by **14–113** statute, as follows:

"A person may use such force as is reasonable in the circumstances in the prevention of crime, or in effecting or assisting in the lawful arrest of offenders or suspected offenders or of persons unlawfully at large."[266]

This does not in terms affect the right of defence of self, others or property, but **14–114** it must implicitly do so, as self-defence and defence of others almost invariably involves the prevention of crime, and it has been judicially stated that the degree of force permissible in self-defence is limited in the same way as the statute limits that for the prevention of crime.[267] The same question arises in each case: were the acts done by the person concerned a reasonably necessary response to the particular circumstances?[268] This is not incompatible with the ECHR art.2.[269]

---

[260] *R. v Safi* [2004] 1 Cr .App. R. 14, CA.
[261] The source of Mr. Bumble's comment that "if the law supposes that . . . the law is a ass—a idiot. If that's the eye of the law, the law's a bachelor . . . " (Dickens, *Oliver Twist*, Ch.51).
[262] Criminal Justice Act 1925 s.47.
[263] *R. v Shortland* [1996] 1 Cr.App.R. 116, CA.
[264] Law Commission No. 83 (1977), paras 3.1–3.9.
[265] e.g. Smith and Hogan, *Criminal Law*, 13th edn (2011), p.379.
[266] Criminal Law Act 1967 s.3(1).
[267] *R. v McInnes* [1971] 1 W.L.R. 1600 at 1610, per Edmund Davies L.J.
[268] *Devlin v Armstrong* [1971] N.I. 13, CA (NI).
[269] *R. (Bennett) v Inner South London Coroner* [2006] EWHC 196 (Admin.); affirmed [2007] EWCA Civ. 617.

14–115   In self-defence, there is no rule that a person must, for example, demonstrate an unwillingness to fight, since that is merely a factor to be taken into account in considering whether he was indeed acting in self-defence.[270] Neither is there any rule that self-defence is confined to spontaneous acts in response to actual violence. The question is whether the acts done were intended to protect himself (or others whom he wished to protect) or his property against an apprehended attack and whether they were (and were believed to be) reasonably necessary in the circumstances.[271]

14–116   The question of reasonable force is of great significance. Reasonableness might imply an absolutely objective standard, but there is an element of subjectivity, in that a person's honest belief that action was reasonably necessary is potent evidence that it really was necessary.[272] The question of reasonableness is a question of fact for the jury or other tribunal of fact after considering various factors, including all the circumstances in which the person concerned was obliged to make his decision.[273] For example, in some circumstances a person need not wait for his assailant to strike the first blow, but may launch a pre-emptive strike.[274]

14–117   It is clear that if someone acts on the basis of a mistaken view of the facts at the time, he is entitled to be treated on the basis that the facts were as he perceived them, and there is no requirement that his mistaken belief was a reasonable one in the circumstances.[275] However, a person is not entitled to rely on self-defence if through self-induced intoxication he makes a mistake as to the amount of force reasonably necessary to defend himself, and uses more force than necessary.[276] Where the defence is prima facie available, but more excessive force than was reasonable in all the circumstances is used by the defendant, then the person is outside the scope of the defence, and will be criminally liable if he otherwise has the requisite mens rea.[277]

Superior orders

14–118   Acting in obedience to superior orders cannot generally amount to a defence.[278] Superior orders may lead a person to make a mistake of law, but under English law,

---

[270] *R. v Bird* [1985] 1 W.L.R. 816, CA.

[271] *Attorney General's Reference (No. 2 of 1983)* [1984] A.C. 456, CA. See, e.g., *Re Paul Everitt, The Times,* March 5, 1986 (deceased was stabbed when, having threatened to kill another, he tried to grab a shotgun: in fact the gun was empty, but the other person was unaware of this); *Re Glyn Davies, Daily Telegraph,* November 9, 1988 (gunman killed by police); *Re Nicholas Payne, The Independent,* October 19, 1988 (armed robbers shot by police).

[272] *Palmer v R.* [1971] A.C. 814, PC; *R. v Shannon* (1980) 124 J.P. 374, CA; *R. v Whyte* [1987] 3 All E.R. 416, CA. cf. *Ashley v Sussex Chief Constable* [2008] 1 A.C. 962 (defence to civil action).

[273] *Attorney General for Northern Ireland's Reference* [1978] A.C. 105, HL; *R. v Whyte* [1987] 3 All E.R. 416, CA.

[274] *Beckford v R.* [1988] A.C. 130, PC.

[275] *R. v Williams* [1987] 3 All E.R. 411, CA; *Beckford v R.* [1988] A.C. 130, PC. See, e.g., *Re Harry Stanley, The Independent,* June 22, 2002 (open verdict on unarmed man shot by police who believed he was pointing a shotgun at them; St Pancras coroner).

[276] *R. v O'Grady* [1987] Q.B. 995, CA.

[277] *R. v Clegg* [1995] 1 A.C. 482, HL.

[278] *R. v Yip Chin-Cheung* [1995] 1 A.C. 111, PC.

a mistake of law will not excuse when so caused, unless it would excuse when not so caused.[279]

Impossibility

There are a number of offences where a defendant is able to plead that through no fault of his own it was impossible for him to fulfil the legal requirements. Thus, for example, a driver who is unaware that an accident has occurred is not liable for failing to report it.[280] However, there is no general principle running through those cases, and it is a question of construction and interpretation in each case whether impossibility is a defence. From the coroner's point of view this is not very significant.   **14–119**

PARTICIPATION IN CRIME

Two or more persons may together commit an offence as a "joint enterprise". For example, they may both attack the victim, and injure him so severely that he dies.[281] Exactly the same principles apply as in the case of a single defendant. But it is not merely the persons who actually perpetrate criminal acts who bear criminal responsibility for those offences. The law recognises not only the primary offender (known as the principal in the first degree) but also secondary parties. It has been said that a secondary party is different from a party to a joint enterprise,[282] but this view has been criticised.[283]   **14–120**

Secondary parties are generally divided into two categories: (i) those taking part at the time of the commission of the main offence (known as principals in the second degree): and (ii) those taking part at an earlier stage (known as accessories before the fact). Secondary parties (of both categories) are liable to be tried and punished as if they were primary offenders, if they "aid, abet, counsel or procure" the commission of the principal offence.[284]   **14–121**

The words, "aid, abet, counsel and procure" in the statute should be given their ordinary meaning if possible, and each word has a meaning different from the other three.[285] It appears that the word "procure" requires a causative link between the procuring and the commission of the offence, but no necessary agreement on the part of the principal offender,[286] whereas "abet" and "counsel" imply some kind of agreement, but no causation,[287] and "aid" seems to require neither agreement   **14–122**

---

[279] *R. v Thomas* (1816) MS of Bayley J. (Turner and Armitage, *Cases on Criminal Law,* p. 42); *R. v James* (1837) 8 C. & P. 131 (master's orders convinced servants that he had a right to obstruct airway of mine, i.e. mistake of law, which negatived their mens rea). cf. *R. v Smith* (1900) 17 S.C.R. 561 (South Africa).

[280] *Harding v Price* [1948] 1 K.B. 695, DC.

[281] cf. *R. v Inner North London Coroner Ex p. Diesa Koto* (1993) 157 J.P. 857, DC.

[282] *R. v Stewart and Scholfield* [1995] 1 Cr.App.R. 441, CA.

[283] Smith and Hogan, *Criminal Law,* 13th edn (2011), p.229.

[284] Accessories and Abettors Act 1861 s.8; Magistrates' Courts Act 1980 s.44.

[285] *Attorney General's Reference (No. 1 of 1975)* [1975] Q.B. 773.

[286] *Attorney General's Reference (No. 1 of 1975)* [1975] Q.B. 773; see also *R. v Rook* [1993] 2 All E.R. 955 at 960–961.

[287] *R. v Calhaem* [1985] Q.B. 808, CA.

with the principal offender nor causation of the latter's offence.[288] Counselling requires only that the person counselled went on to commit the offence still acting within the scope of the counselling, rather than (say) accidentally or in some automatic state.[289]

14–123   In order to be guilty as a secondary party a person must either (a) be present when the crime is committed pursuant to an agreement that it be committed, or (b) assist or encourage the commission of the offence, and with intention so to do.[290] Mere presence at the scene of a crime is in itself not enough,[291] unless it amounts in fact to encouragement of the offence and there is intention that it should.[292] If assistance is knowingly given, it makes no difference that (for other reasons) the person assisting would rather that the offence not be committed,[293] or is indifferent as to whether it should be committed.[294]

14–124   The mens rea of secondary participation, even in offences of "strict" liability or negligence, is that the secondary party should know or be wilfully blind to the circumstances constituting the offence.[295] Where the secondary party is alleged to be an accessory before the fact, there is the additional problem that he may not know the exact details of the principal offence to be committed. It is clear that a general criminal intention on the part of the secondary party is not enough. But it will be sufficient if the defendant knows the type of criminal offence intended,[296] or contemplates the commission of a limited number of crimes by the principal, even if he does not know the details of the target and the surrounding circumstances, or indeed which of the limited number of crimes the principal will in fact commit.[297]

14–125   Where a secondary party takes part in an unlawful joint enterprise he will be liable for acts committed by the primary offender if he foresees (even though he does not intend) such acts as a possible incident of the execution of the planned joint enterprise, unless he genuinely dismisses such possibilities as negligible and too remote to be seriously contemplated.[298]

14–126   Finally, it should be mentioned that the much criticised rule that the accessory before the fact can never be convicted of a more serious offence than the principal in the first degree[299] has now been discarded,[300] and the position is the same as for a principal in the second degree, i.e. that if he has the mens rea to justify it, he can be convicted of a more serious offence than the principal in the first degree. This also accords with the position where the principal offender is not liable for any

---

[288] Smith and Hogan, *Criminal Law,* 13th edn (2011), pp.192–193.
[289] *R. v Calhaem* [1985] Q.B. 808, CA .
[290] *R. v Clarkson* [1971] 3 All E.R. 344.
[291] *R. v Atkinson* (1869) 11 Cox C.C. 330.
[292] *R. v Coney* (1882) 8 Q.B.D. 534.
[293] *Lynch v DPP for Northern Ireland* [1975] A.C. 653, HL.
[294] *National Coal Board v Gamble* [1959] 1 Q.B. 11.
[295] *Johnson v Youden* [1950] 1 K.B. 544, DC.
[296] *R. v Bainbridge* [1960] 1 Q.B. 129, CCA.
[297] *DPP for Northern Ireland v Maxwell* [1978] 1 W.L.R. 1350; and see *R. v Rook* [1993] 2 All E.R. 955, CA, dealing with withdrawal from participation.
[298] *Chan Wing-Sui v R.* [1985] A.C. 168, PC; *R. v Hyde* [1991] 1 Q.B. 134, CA; *Hui Chi-Ming v R.* [1992] 1 A.C. 34, PC; *R. v Roberts* [1993] 1 All E.R. 583, CA; *R. v Powell* [1999] 1 A.C. 1, HL; *R. v Uddin* [1998] 2 All E.R. 744 at 752.
[299] *R. v Richards* [1974] Q.B. 776, CA.
[300] *R. v Howe* [1987] A.C. 417, HL.

offence at all because of insufficient mens rea, although a secondary party can be criminally responsible to the extent of his own mens rea.[301]

---

[301] *R. v Bourne* (1952) 36 Cr.App.R. 125, CCA; *R. v Cogan and Leak* [1976] 2 Q.B. 217, CA.

Chapter 15

NOTIFIABLE ACCIDENTS AND PRESCRIBED DISEASES

GENERAL

Certain types of accident and disease (usually, but not invariably, industrial or occupational in origin) are considered to be sufficiently serious for notification of their occurrence to be given to relevant government bodies for the purpose of investigation and research. Additionally, certain serious diseases are prescribed for social security and other purposes. Where deaths occur as a result of such accidents or diseases, the coroner is usually involved, and the interplay between the coroner and the relevant government bodies causes modifications to the coronial procedures otherwise adopted. **15–01**

These modifications were formerly substantial.[1] However, the impact of the modifications made at the present day lies mainly in an extension of the range of persons who must be notified by the coroner of the time and place of the post-mortem examination[2] and the inquest hearing itself,[3] and who have the right to examine witnesses at the inquest hearing[4] and are generally "interested persons".[5] Moreover, any such inquest hearings will almost always be required to be held with a jury.[6] But it should be noted that, although the changes in coronial procedure are parasitic upon the obligation to notify, the question of whether there should be such an obligation has been decided apparently without reference to the effect it would have upon coroners. Sometimes the distinctions involved are very fine, and make no sense at all in the context of coroners' courts.[7] **15–02**

Effect on coroner's inquiry of possible reportable accident, dangerous occurrence or disease

Where there is or may be a duty to report an accident or dangerous occurrence to the relevant enforcing authority, and a death has resulted from such accident or occurrence, the consequences that follow for the coroner having jurisdiction will **15–03**

---

[1] See the 9th edn of this work, Ch.12.
[2] See 8–60.
[3] See 10–22.
[4] See 11–59.
[5] See 8–22.
[6] See 10–34.
[7] See, e.g. 15–10 below.

depend on the exact terms of the particular provision in the coroner legislation, the relevant test being different in each case.

15–04   The various cases are as follows:

(a) if the death *may have been caused* by a reportable accident or disease, notice of any post-mortem examination must be given to such authority or the appropriate inspector or representative of the authority,[8] unless to do so would cause the examination to be unreasonably delayed;[9]

(b) if a government department *has notified the coroner of its desire to be represented* at the examination, notice of any post-mortem examination must be given to that department,[10] unless to do so would cause the examination to be unreasonably delayed;[11]

(c) if the death *may have been caused* by a reportable accident or disease, such authority or inspector is entitled to be represented at the post-mortem examination by a medical practitioner;[12]

(d) if a government department *has notified the coroner of its desire to be represented* at the examination, it is entitled to be represented at the post-mortem examination by a medical practitioner;[13]

(e) where a person appointed by, or representative of, an enforcing authority, or appointed by a government department to attend an inquest into the death, *has made himself known to the coroner*, the coroner must notify him of the date, time and place of the inquest hearing within one week of setting it,[14] and of any alteration to those details within one week of the decision to alter;[15]

(f) where the coroner has *reason to suspect that* the death was caused by a notifiable accident, poisoning or disease (including an accident where there is a duty to report an accident to a government minister or department), the inquest must be held with a jury;[16]

(g) a person appointed by, or representative of, an enforcing authority, or appointed by a government department to attend an inquest into the death, is entitled to request the disclosure of documents held by the coroner;[17]

(h) a person appointed by, or representative of, an enforcing authority, or appointed by a government department to attend an inquest into the death, is entitled to examine witnesses at the inquest.[18]

---

[8] Coroners (Investigations) Regulations (SI 2013/1629) reg.13(1), (3)(d) (emphasis supplied); see 8–60.

[9] Coroners (Investigations) Regulations (SI 2013/1629) reg.13(2); see 8–60.

[10] Coroners (Investigations) Regulations (SI 2013/1629) reg.13(1), (3)(e) (emphasis supplied); see 8–60.

[11] Coroners (Investigations) Regulations (SI 2013/1629) reg.13(2); see 8–60.

[12] Coroners (Investigations) Regulations (SI 2013/1629) reg.13(4) (emphasis supplied); see 8–61.

[13] Coroners (Investigations) Regulations (SI 2013/1629) reg.13(4) (emphasis supplied); see 8–61.

[14] Coroners (Inquests) Rules 2013 (SI 2013/1616) r.9(2) (emphasis supplied); see 10–22 above.

[15] Coroners (Inquests) Rules 2013 (SI 2013/1616) r.10(1).

[16] Coroners and Justice Act 2009 s.7(2)(c), (4) (emphasis supplied); see 10–34 above.

[17] Coroners (Inquests) Rules 2013 (SI 2013/1616) r.13(1); see 7–25, 8–22.

[18] Coroners (Inquests) Rules 2013 (SI 2013/1616) r.19(1); see 7–25, 11–59.

It will be seen that the consequences flow for the coroner not only when there **15–05** *is* a reportable or notifiable event, but in some cases where there *may be* one, or where the coroner has *reason to suspect that* there is one. In this chapter the various accidents or diseases which involve reporting or notification, or are otherwise prescribed, are set out or referred to. But the modifications themselves are dealt with in more detail in other, more appropriate parts of the text dealing with post-mortem examinations and inquest hearings.

NOTIFIABLE ACCIDENTS AND OCCURRENCES

Most accidents which must be officially notified are set out in the Reporting of **15–06** Injuries, Diseases and Dangerous Occurrences Regulations 2013.[19] Under these regulations, and subject to certain exceptions,[20] (i) where any person[21] dies as a result of a "work-related accident"[22] (i.e. one arising out of or in connection with work)[23] or occupational exposure to a biological agent,[24] or (ii) where a reportable injury to any person at work[25] results in death within a year of the accident, this must be notified by the "responsible person"[26] to the "relevant enforcing authority".[27]

The relevant enforcing authority and the responsible person

The "relevant enforcing authority" is usually the Health and Safety Executive, but **15–07** may be another regulator.[28] The "responsible person" is generally the employer of an employee who is injured or dies.[29] But in relation to a person not at work, or self-employed, it is generally the person who has control of the premises at the time of the accident,[30] although, in relation to certain reportable diseases of self-employed persons, it is the self-employed person.[31] There are exceptional rules for

---

[19] SI 2013/1471, hereinafter called the "2013 Regulations", replacing SI 1995/3163: see App. 2.
[20] See 15–08 below.
[21] cf. *Woking BC v BHS plc* (1994) 159 J.P. 427, DC (decided under the Reporting of Injuriries, Diseases and Dangerous Occurences Regulations 1985).
[22] 2013 Regulations reg.6(1).
[23] 2013 Regulations reg.2(1).
[24] 2013 Regulations reg.6(2). "Biological agent" is defined by reg.2(1) as having the meaning given by reg.2(1) of the Control of Substances Hazardous to Health Regulations 2002 (SI 2002/2677), i.e. "a micro-organism, cell culture, or human endoparasite, whether or not genetically modified, which may cause infection, allergy, toxicity or otherwise create a hazard to human health".
[25] 2013 Regulations reg.4(1).
[26] 2013 Regulations reg.2(1), referring to reg.3.
[27] See the Health and Safety at Work etc. Act 1974 s.18(7).
[28] See the Health and Safety at Work etc. Act 1974 s.18(7). The last formal guidance to coroners as to the proper such authority in any particular case was given in a booklet enclosed with Home Office Circular No. 3 of 1981. The National Liaison Committee for the Work-related Deaths Protocol (England and Wales), September 2011, states that the phrase means "the health and safety regulator with responsibility for the activity or workplace involved and includes the Health and Safety Executive (HSE), Office of Rail Regulation (ORR), local authorities, Maritime and Coastguard Agency (MCA) and the Fire and Rescue Services".
[29] 2013 Regulations reg.3(1)(a)(i), (b)(i).
[30] 2013 Regulations reg.3(1)(a)(ii).
[31] 2013 Regulations reg.3(1)(b)(ii).

mines, closed tips, quarries, pipelines, wells, offshore installations and diving projects.[32]

Accidents with no duty to report

15–08   However, not all accidents otherwise satisfying the statutory criteria are subject to a duty to report and consequently affect the coroner. There are three main classes of otherwise "notifiable" accident where there is no duty to report:

(1) accidents to patients undergoing operations, examinations or treatment under the supervision of a doctor or dentist;[33]

(2) accidents to members of the Crown's armed forces or visiting forces whilst on duty;[34]

(3) accidents arising out of or in connection with the movement of a vehicle on a road, *unless* the victim was killed or injured by an accident involving a train, or by exposure to a substance being conveyed by the vehicle, or was engaged in (or was injured or killed by the activities of another person engaged in) either (i) work connected with loading or unloading such vehicle[35] or (ii) work on or alongside a road concerned (broadly) with construction, demolition, alteration, repair or maintenance of the road or its environs.[36]

There being no duty to report such accidents, these cases are consequently unaffected by the modifications to coronial procedure mentioned below. They may of course lead to inquests in the usual way.

Extension of obligation for gas suppliers

15–09   By way of contrast, there is an extension of the obligation to notify the Health and Safety Executive of any case where (not being a case already made notifiable or reportable under the 2013 Regulations) a supplier of flammable gas through a fixed pipe distribution system, or a filler, importer or supplier (except by retail) of a refillable gas container containing liquefied petroleum gas receives notification of the death, loss of consciousness or taking to hospital of any person because of an injury arising in connection with that gas.[37]

15–10   Thus a death resulting from a heating device with a refillable cartridge or cannister may give rise to an obligation to notify (and hence the other consequences referred to below), whereas a death resulting from a similar device with a disposable cartridge or canister will not. This distinction may have some significance so far as the health and safety procedures are concerned. In the context of the resulting differences in coronial procedures, it is inexplicable.

---

[32] 2013 Regulations reg.3(2).
[33] 2013 Regulations reg.14(1).
[34] 2013 Regulations reg.14(5).
[35] cf. *R. (Aineto) v Brighton and Hove Coroner* [2003] EWHC 1896 (Admin.) (decided under the 1995 Regulations).
[36] 2013 Regulations reg.14(3), (4).
[37] 2013 Regulations reg.11(1).

Dangerous occurrences

In addition, there is a duty to notify the enforcing authority of the existence of any **15–11**
"dangerous occurrences".[38] These are defined by the 2013 Regulations,[39] and
cover various situations too complex to summarise here.[40] They need not result
even in personal injury, let alone death, to be notifiable, but *ex hypothesi* the
coroner will only be involved if death results. Some of them are discussed below in
the context of railway and tramway accidents.[41]

Regulations requiring special notification

There are a number of other classes of accident or occurrence in respect of which **15–12**
there is no duty to report under these regulations,[42] but where there is a duty to
notify an official or body under other, more specialised, legislation.[43] These are as
follows:

(a) deaths through the emission of ionising radiations or the release of
radioactive or toxic substances on licensed sites or in carriage, which must
be reported to the Health and Safety Executive;[44]

(b) accidents involving or on board UK ships (other than pleasure vessels) and
other ships in UK ports or carrying passengers to or from such ports, all of
which must be reported to the Secretary of State for Transport;[45]

(c) accidents in or involving civil aircraft in Britain, which must be reported to
the Secretary of State for Transport;[46]

---

[38] 2013 Regulations, reg.7.
[39] 2013 Regulations reg.2(1).
[40] Schedule 2. There are six parts to the Schedule, as follows:
Pt 1: **General** (lifting equipment, pressure systems, overhead electric lines, electrical incidents
causing explosion or fire, explosives, biological agents, radiation generators and radiography,
breathing apparatus, diving operations, collapse of scaffolding, certain train collisions not reportable
elsewhere, wells, and pipelines or pipeline works);
Pt 2: Dangerous occurrences **reportable except in relation to an offshore workplace** (structural
collapses, explosion or fire, release of flammable liquids and gases, and hazardous escapes of substances);
Pt 3: Dangerous occurrences **reportable in relation to a mine** (fires or ignition of gas, escapes of
gas with solid matter, failures of plant or equipment, breathing apparatus, emergency escape
apparatus, inrushes of gas or flowing material, insecure tips, locomotives, falls of ground, accidents
causing specified injuries);
Pt 4: Dangerous occurrences **reportable in relation to a quarry** (collapse of storage bunkers,
sinking of craft, projection of substances outside quarry, misfires, insecure tips, movement of slopes
or faces, explosion or fire in vehicles or mobile plant);
Pt 5: Dangerous occurrences **reportable in respect of a relevant transport system** (see
15–14—15–15 below);
Pt 6: Dangerous occurrences **reportable in respect of an offshore workplace** (release of
petroleum hydrocarbon, fire or explosion, release of escape of dangerous substances, collapses,
equipment, dropping objects, weather damage, collisions, subsidence or collapse of seabed, loss of
stability or buoyancy, evacuation, falls into water).
[41] See 15–15.
[42] 2013 Regulations reg.14(6).
[43] 2013 Regulations Sch.6.
[44] Nuclear Installations (Dangerous Occurrences) Regulations 1965 (SI 1965/1824).
[45] Merchant Shipping (Accident Reporting and Investigation) Regulations 2012 (SI 2012 No.1743).
[46] Civil Aviation (Investigation of Air Accidents and Incidents) Regulations 1996 (SI 1996/2798).

(d) accidents involving the release or spillage of radioactive substances above a certain quantity, which must be reported to the Health and Safety Executive;[47]

(e) any event, involving a consumer's installation which is connected to the distributor's network, attributable to the generating, transforming, control or carrying of energy, which has given rise to (inter alia) the death of any person other than a person engaged by the generator, distributor or meter operator for the purposes of his business, which must be reported to the Secretary of State for Trade and Industry;[48]

(f) accidents on or near a civil aerodrome where a person suffers a fatal or serious injury as a result of being in or in contact with a military aircraft, which must be reported to the Secretary of State for Transport.[49]

Railway, tramway and trolley vehicle accidents

15–13   Deaths on railways were formerly reportable to the Secretary of State for Transport under specific legislation.[50] This has now been repealed[51] and the reporting of railway deaths now takes place, if at all, pursuant to the Reporting of Injuries, Diseases and Dangerous Occurrences Regulations 2013.[52] As already noted, these regulations make reportable (i) deaths "as a result of a work-related accident", i.e. one "arising out of or in connection with work",[53] and (ii) "dangerous occurrences".[54]

15–14   The latter requirement covers a number of accidents, so long as they arise out of or in connection with work, which are specifically related to "relevant transport systems".[55] A "relevant transport system" is defined[56] as one which is not situated at a factory, dock, construction site, mine or quarry, and is not a guided bus system,[57] but otherwise is (a) a railway, (b) a tramway,[58] (c) a trolley vehicle system,[59] or (d) any other system using guided transport.[60]

15–15   These "dangerous occurrences" include (a) collisions between passenger trains and other trains,[61] (b) derailments of passenger trains, in whole or in part,[62] (c)

---

[47] Ionising Radiations Regulations 1999 (SI 1999/3232).

[48] Electricity Safety, Quality and Continuity Regulations 2002 (SI 2002/2665).

[49] Civil Aviation (Investigation of Military Air Accidents at Civil Aerodromes) Regulations 2005 (SI 2005/2693).

[50] Railways (Notice of Accidents) Order 1986 (SI/1986/2187).

[51] Reporting of Injuries, Diseases and Dangerous Occurrences Regulations ("RIDDOR") 1995 reg.14(1).

[52] SI 2013/1471.

[53] Regulation 6(1), as defined by reg.2(1). See 15–16—15–20.

[54] Regulation 7, as defined by reg.2(1).

[55] See reg.2(1), definition of "dangerous occurrence".

[56] 2013 Regulations reg.2(1).

[57] As defined by the Railways and Other Guided Transport Systems (Safety) Regulations 2006 (SI 2006/599) reg.2(1).

[58] As defined by the Railways and Other Guided Transport Systems (Safety) Regulations 2006 (SI 2006/599).

[59] As defined by the Transport and Works act 1992 s.67.

[60] As defined by the Railways and Other Guided Transport Systems (Safety) Regulations 2006 (SI 2006/599) reg.2(1).

[61] 2013 Regulations reg.7 Sch.2 Pt 5 para.54.

[62] 2013 Regulations reg.7 Sch.2 Pt 5 para.55.

certain collisions[63] or derailments[64] of non-passenger trains, (d) certain accidents where trains strike buffer stops[65] or animals,[66] or strike or are struck by other objects[67] or road vehicles,[68] (e) unintentional division of trains,[69] (f) failure of train parts whilst the train is on a running line,[70] (g) certain fires[71] or severe electrical arcing or fusing[72] on trains, (h) accidents and incidents at level crossings,[73] (i) failures (by fractures or detachments) of rails in a running line or of a rack rail,[74] or buckling[75] of or other damage to railway lines caused by vehicles (including aircraft) coming to rest on or cause damage to them,[76] (j) the runaway of an escalator, lift or passenger conveyor,[77] (k) failures of tunnels, bridges or other structures,[78] or the signalling system,[79] the slipping of cuttings or embankments,[80] floods on the permanent way,[81] the striking of bridges by vessels or road vehicles or their loads,[82] and the failure of any other part of the permanent way or works,[83] and (j) cases of signals being passed without authority.[84] This will cover many, perhaps most, cases of deaths on railways and other relevant transport systems.

But none of these categories directly covers the cases of persons (a) jumping **15–16** from trains, trams, trolley vehicles and so on, or (b) falling under such vehicles, or (c) being hit by them (not being in another vehicle), and so on. So whether such deaths are reportable will depend on whether they are deaths arising out of a "work-related accident". The Home Office view under the old regulations was that these cases were exactly that, whether or not the victim himself was at work, because the train driver and his colleagues on the railway invariably were.

However, two matters have changed since the Home Office expressed its view. **15–17** First, the 2013 Regulations differ importantly from the 1995 Regulations, in that the definition of "accident" has been deliberately altered to exclude "an act of suicide which occurs on, or in the course of operation of, a relevant transport system".[85] So a suicide on the railway or tramway is no longer an accident, let alone work-related. But there is a question as to exactly what "suicide" means in this context.

---

[63] 2013 Regulations reg.7 Sch.2 Pt 5 para.56.
[64] 2013 Regulations reg.7 Sch.2 Pt 5 para.57.
[65] 2013 Regulations reg.7 Sch.2 Pt 5 para.58.
[66] 2013 Regulations reg.7 Sch.2 Pt 5 para.59.
[67] 2013 Regulations reg.7 Sch.2 Pt 5 para.60.
[68] 2013 Regulations reg.7 Sch.2 Pt 5 para.61.
[69] 2013 Regulations reg.7 Sch.2 Pt 5 para.62.
[70] 2013 Regulations reg.7 Sch.2 Pt 5 para.63.
[71] 2013 Regulations reg.7 Sch.2 Pt 5 para.64.
[72] 2013 Regulations reg.7 Sch.2 Pt 5 para.65.
[73] 2013 Regulations reg.7 Sch.2 Pt 5 paras 66-68.
[74] 2013 Regulations reg.7 Sch.2 Pt 5 para.69.
[75] 2013 Regulations reg.7 Sch.2 Pt 5 para.70.
[76] 2013 Regulations reg.7 Sch.2 Pt 5 para.71.
[77] 2013 Regulations reg.7 Sch.2 Pt 5 para.72.
[78] 2013 Regulations reg.7 Sch.2 Pt 5 para.73(a).
[79] 2013 Regulations reg.7 Sch.2 Pt 5 para.73(b).
[80] 2013 Regulations reg.7 Sch.2 Pt 5 para.73(c).
[81] 2013 Regulations reg.7 Sch.2 Pt 5 para.73(d).
[82] 2013 Regulations reg.7 Sch.2 Pt 5 para.73(e).
[83] 2013 Regulations reg.7 Sch.2 Pt 5 para.73(f).
[84] 2013 Regulations reg.7 Sch.2 Pt 5 para.74.
[85] 2013 Regulations reg.2(1).

15–18   The concern of the Regulations is with accidents, and (with one exception) not with deliberate acts of violence.[86] So in these Regulations, "suicide" probably means no more than a non-accidental self-inflicted act of violence causing death, e.g. jumping in front of a train. It is not necessary (as it is at an inquest) to be satisfied that the deceased intended beyond reasonable doubt to kill himself, or to exclude all other possible explanations.[87] A person may therefore be a suicide for the purposes of these Regulations (and the death therefore not an "accident", and therefore not reportable), where he or she would not be for coronial purposes.

15–19   Second, the official guidance to the 2013 Regulations makes clear that "the fact that there is an accident at work premises does not, it itself, mean that the accident is work-related".[88] It suggests that it is work-related if the following plays a significant role in the accident: (i) the way the work was carried out; (ii) any machinery, plant, substances or equipment used for the work; or (iii) the condition of the site or premises where the accident happened.[89]

15–20   So if a passenger slips on a defective platform into the path of an oncoming train, or a broken train door swings open as the train enters the station, hitting a passenger, or the driver of the train goes too fast and it jumps the rails, killing a passenger, this is a "work-related accident", and properly notifiable. But if the passenger dashes onto the platform in a hurry and slips onto the track, not as a result of the surface condition, or is taken ill and collapses onto the track, and (in either case) the driver can do nothing to avoid the accident, it is not a "work-related accident".[90] The fact that *the train* hits and kills the passenger is not enough, since the train is by then committed. The accident is the result of the passenger's interaction with the system, and not the other way around. It would be different if the driver could stop in time and did not.

15–21   The coroner who is informed of a death, particularly one "on, or in the course of operation of, a relevant transport system", will have to make decisions in investigating which will be affected by the question whether the death *is or is not* (or may or may not be) reportable or notifiable to an enforcing authority. As already mentioned, if the death is so reportable or notifiable, (i) the arrangements made for any autopsy will be affected, and (ii) the coroner will have to summon a jury for the inquest hearing. So the coroner needs to take a view right at the outset, long before all the evidence is available, let alone before it has been heard in court.

15–22   For post-mortem examinations, the test is whether the death *may have been caused* by a reportable accident or disease.[91] On the question of summoning a jury, the test is whether the coroner has *reason to suspect that* the death was caused by a notifiable

---

[86] An act of non-consensual violence done to a person at work: 2013 Regulations reg.2(1) (definition of "accident").

[87] See 13–67 ff.

[88] Office of Rail Regulation, *Reporting of Injuries, Diseases and Dangerous Occurrences Regulations 2013: Guidance for railways, tramways and other guided transport systems* para.4.3; HSE *Guide to RIDDOR 2013*, p.31.

[89] Office of Rail Regulation, *Reporting of Injuries, Diseases and Dangerous Occurrences Regulations 2013: Guidance for railways, tramways and other guided transport systems* para.1.23; HSE *Guide to RIDDOR 2013*, p 2. The Chief Coroner's Guidance No. 11, *Juries in railway cases: suicides and accidents* at [12], takes the same view.

[90] See also Chief Coroner's Guidance No. 11, *Juries in railway cases: suicides and accidents* at [13].

[91] See 15–04 (a), (c).

accident, poisoning or disease.[92] For notifying inquest arrangements, the test is whether a person appointed by, or representative of, an enforcing authority *has made himself known to the coroner.*[93] There is no requirement that the coroner be first satisfied that the death itself is reportable. For disclosure and examination of witnesses, the test is whether a person appointed by, or representative of, an enforcing authority is asking for disclosure or to examine witnesses,[94] and again there is no requirement that the coroner be first satisfied that the death itself is reportable.

The coroner informed of a death in circumstances (a) pointing to a deliberate act **15–23** of self-violence,[95] or (b) although accidental, not indicating a sufficient "work" connection, will normally *not* consider that the death "may have been caused" by a reportable accident, nor will he or she normally have "reason to suspect" that the death is notifiable. Hence the modifications to the coronial procedure are not engaged at that stage. The inquiry will therefore proceed without the involvement of an enforcing authority or its representative, and without the need to summon a jury.[96]

But this is necessarily a provisional position only, as new facts and matters may **15–24** come to light thereafter, and the position may have to be revisited. Moreover, if an enforcing authority takes the positive step of informing the coroner that it wants to be involved in the process, then as the rules stand the coroner must allow for its involvement, at least in the inquest procedures. On the other hand, if the coroner's view remains that this is not, and there is no reason to suspect, a notifiable death (whatever the authority says), there is no need to involve the authority in the autopsy procedure nor to summon a jury for the inquest hearing.

AGRICULTURAL ACCIDENTS

Whether or not the accident rises out of or in connection with work (and is thus **15–25** notifiable), where the death may have been caused by an accident occurring in the course of agricultural operations, the coroner must adjourn the inquest unless an inspector or other official of the Health and Safety Executive[97] is present to watch the proceedings, and must give to an inspector notice of the time and place of holding of the adjourned inquest hearing.[98] However, the coroner may take evidence of identification and sign the order for "interment"[99] of the body before adjourning the original inquest,[100] and need not adjourn at all if the inquest relates

---

[92] See 15–04 (f).
[93] See 15–04 (e).
[94] See 15–04 (g), (h).
[95] e.g. where there is a suicide note, or there were previous attempts at suicide, or prolonged depression or other suicidal tendencies demonstrated. See also Chief Coroner's Guidance No. 11, *Juries in railway cases: suicides and accidents*, [11], [15].
[96] See also Chief Coroner's Guidance No. 11, *Juries in railway cases: suicides and accidents*, [11].
[97] Agriculture (Safety, Health and Welfare Provisions) Act 1956 s.24(1) (definition of "inspector").
[98] Agriculture (Safety, Health and Welfare Provisions) Act 1956 s.9(1).
[99] This is not defined, but presumable includes cremation or other lawful disposal.
[100] Agriculture (Safety, Health and Welfare Provisions) Act 1956 s.9(1)(a).

to the death of not more than one person and the coroner gave at least 24 hours' notice of the original hearing.[101]

15–26   For these purposes, "agriculture" is widely defined, to include dairy-farming, the production of consumable procedure which is grown, whether for sale, consumption or other business use, and the use of land for grazing or pasture, for orchards, woodlands, market gardens or nurseries.[102]

15–27   If such an inquest proceeds in the absence of an inspector from the Health and Safety Executive, and evidence is given of any "neglect" as having caused or contributed to the accident or of any defect in any building or machine or equipment seeming to require a remedy, the coroner is obliged to inform the inspector of such neglect or defect.[103] But "neglect" in this context does not necessarily mean what it means in coroners' law.[104]

INJURY IN THE COURSE OF EMPLOYMENT

15–28   Even if an accident or occurrence is not "notifiable", it may have other consequences. Thus, where the death touching which the inquest is being held may have been caused by an injury received during the course of employment, and the deceased belonged to a trade union at the time of his death, a person appointed by that trade union may attend the inquest and examine the witnesses,[105] and is an "interested person" for other purposes, such as the supply of copy documents from the coroner.[106]

15–29   What constitutes an injury "received during the course of employment" is normally easy to determine: for example, it clearly covers an injury received from a machine operated by the deceased pursuant to a contract of employment, and clearly does not include the self-employed. However, there are many borderline cases giving rise to difficulty. As Sir John Donaldson MR said in dealing with industrial injuries benefit[107] (where the same words are used):

"These apparently clear and simple words gave rise to endless litigation in the context of the Workmen's Compensation Acts and have provided to be no less prolific in their present context. None of the authorities purports to construe the words other than in their natural meaning. None provides a simple formula which, on application of the facts, provides a ready answer to the question, 'did he suffer the accident in the course of his employment?' and, in the nature of things, none could do so, because the incidents of employment are so varied. All that they can and do attempt is to draw attention to factors which are material

---

[101] Agriculture (Safety, Health and Welfare Provisions) Act 1956 s.9(1)(b).
[102] Agriculture (Safety, Health and Welfare Provisions) Act 1956 s.24(1).
[103] Agriculture (Safety, Health and Welfare Provisions) Act 1956 s.9(2).
[104] See 13–91 ff.
[105] See 8–22, 11–59.
[106] See 7–25, 18–53.
[107] Under the Social Security Contributions and Benefits Act 1992 s.94, formerly the National Insurance (Industrial Injuries) Act 1965 s.5(1).

and should be taken into account and balance one against the other in answering the question."[108]

In that case, the court concluded:

15–30

"We cannot over-emphasise the importance of looking at the factual picture as a whole and rejecting any approach based on the fallacious concept that any one factor is conclusive. The addition or subtraction of one factor in a given situation may well tip the balance. In another, the addition or subtraction of the same factor may well make no difference. We appreciate that it would assist if we could lay down rules or even guidelines. However, there are no rules, other than that which is contained in the statute."[109]

Thus, the coroner must decide the question whether the injury which may have caused the deceased's death was received during the course of the deceased's employment on looking at the totality of the situation and taking all the factors into account. As with industrial injury benefit, it seems that the courts will only interfere

15–31

"if it is clear that there has been a self-misdirection by the [coroner], or if the only reasonable conclusion on the facts found is inconsistent with that decision".[110]

NOTIFIABLE DISEASES

There are a number of diseases which, when encountered, medical practitioners are obliged to notify to the "proper officer[111] of the local authority",[112] formerly the local medical officer of health. This notification in itself has no significance for the procedures to be followed by the coroner, as notification to such proper officer is not notification to the Government or the Health and Safety Executive.

15–32

However, certain diseases must be notified by the proper officer (who will have been informed usually by medical practitioners) to Public Health England, an executive agency of the Department of Health,[113] or Public Health Wales NHS Trust (as the case may be). These diseases are set out in the regulations,[114] and include cholera, measles, mumps, plague, rubella, smallpox, SARS, yellow fever, leprosy, malaria, rabies, tuberculosis and viral haemorrhagic fever, but not AIDS.[115]

15–33

---

[108] *Nancollas v Insurance Office* [1985] 1 All E.R. 833 at 835.

[109] *Nancollas v Insurance Office* [1985] 1 All E.R. 833 at 840.

[110] *Nancollas v Insurance Office* [1985] 1 All E.R. 833 at 836.

[111] See Public Health (Control of Diseases) Act 1984 s.74.

[112] Public Health (Control of Diseases) Act 1984 ss.13, 45C, 45F; Health Protection (Notification) Regulations 2010 (SI 2010/659) regs 2, 3; Health Protection (Notification) (Wales) Regulations 2010 (SI 2010/1546) regs 2, 3.

[113] Health Protection (Notification) Regulations 2010 (SI 2010/659) reg.1(3).

[114] Health Protection (Notification) Regulations 2010 (SI 2010/659) reg.2(7) Sch.1; Health Protection (Notification) (Wales) Regulations 2010 (SI 2010/1546) reg.2(7) Sch.1. The two lists overlap, but are not the same.

[115] The AIDS (Control) Act 1987 was repealed by the Health and Social Care Act 2012 s.59.

Notification to Public Health England is certainly a notification to the government, but it is unclear that notification to Public Health Wales NHS Trust is the same, as an NHS Trust is not itself a government department. Nevertheless, the better view is that the Trust is acting as agent for the government in being so notified. The consequence for the coroner in dealing with a death from any of these notifiable diseases is that any inquest must be held with a jury.[116]

INDUSTRIAL DISEASES

15–34   A coroner must hold an inquest into deaths which he has reason to suspect of being unnatural.[117] This will usually include cases of diseases contracted by reason of work. These are often called "industrial diseases". However, this phrase is also used in a narrower sense, as a statutorily defined term. Where a coroner holds an inquest into the death of a person who may have died as a result of an "industrial disease" as so defined,[118] just the same consequences flow as if the death had been caused through a injury received in the course of employment.[119] That is that. a representative of a trade union of which the deceased was a member at the time of his death (i) may attend the inquest and examine witnesses (either in person or through lawyers),[120] and (ii) may obtain copy documents from the coroner.[121] As with employment injury cases, such an inquest is not automatically a jury inquest.[122]

15–35   An "industrial disease" for this purpose is one prescribed under the Social Security legislation.[123] The current regulations are the Social Security (Industrial Injuries) (Prescribed Diseases) Regulations 1985.[124] Under these regulations, certain diseases are prescribed in relation to persons who satisfy certain occupational criteria.[125] These criteria are complex and will not be summarised here. It should be noted that the conclusion (in lay terms, "verdict") of death through industrial disease is not restricted to cases falling strictly within the scope of the regulations,[126] although of course the procedural consequences referred to in the previous paragraphs are so restricted. The Home Office asked coroners to draw to the attention of dependants of victims of various dust-related diseases the compensation scheme available under the Pneumoconiosis etc. (Workers' Compensation) Act 1979.[127]

---

[116] See 10–34 above.
[117] See 5–72 above.
[118] See 15–35 above.
[119] See 15–28 ff above.
[120] See 11–59 above.
[121] See 7–25 below.
[122] It will be so if the disease is *notifiable*: for this see 15–32—15–33, 15–36—15–37.
[123] Social Security Contributions and Benefits Act 1992 s.108.
[124] SI 1985/967.
[125] Social Security (Industrial Injuries) (Prescribed Diseases) Regulations 1985 reg.2 and Sch.1.
[126] See 13–44—13–45.
[127] See Home Office Newsletter No. 28 (December 18, 1998) para.3.

OTHER REPORTABLE DISEASES

Certain diseases, infections and other conditions are made reportable by the **15–36**
"responsible person" (the employer in relation to an employee, or a self-employed
person)[128] to the enforcing authority[129] by the Reporting of Injuries, Diseases and
Dangerous Occurrences Regulations 2013, once the responsible person has
received a written diagnosis[130] from a registered medical practitioner.[131] However,
this obligation to report does not apply to any condition notifiable by virtue of the
specialised legislation[132] referred to above.[133] Nor does it apply if the person is by
then no longer working. This is important in the case of diseases (such as
mesothelioma) which take many years to manifest themselves. If, as is common,
the person is by then retired, the disease is not reportable. In such cases, although
there will usually be an inquest (because there is reasonable cause to suspect
unnatural death), it will not be a jury inquest.

There is an overlap between the diseases (and occupational criteria) prescribed **15–37**
under the Social Security (Industrial Injuries) (Prescribed Diseases) Regulations
1985[134] and those prescribed under the Reporting of Injuries, Diseases and
Dangerous Occurrences Regulations 2013,[135] but the two lists are by no means the
same. The consequences for coroners of diseases being reportable under the latter
regulations are those set out above,[136] for accidents and dangerous occurrences.

OTHER FORMS OF INQUIRY

The coroner's inquest is not the only form of inquiry into notifiable accidents **15–38**
which cause death. There is specific statutory provision for specialised discretionary
inquiries into (inter alia):

(1) road traffic accidents;[137]

(2) deaths in UK-registered (and some non-UK registered)[138] ships.[139]

In the first case the inquiry may be held even though no death has resulted. There
also used to be provision for discretionary inquiry into railway accidents, but that
has been repealed.[140] Obligatory investigations must be held into civil aviation
accidents and serious incidents.[141]

---

[128] 2013 Regulations, regs 2(1), 3.
[129] As to which see 15–07 above.
[130] 2013 Regulations reg.2(1).
[131] 2013 Regulations, regs 8–10.
[132] See 15–12 above.
[133] 2013 Regulations reg.15.
[134] See 15–35 above.
[135] See 15–06 above.
[136] See 15–03—15–04 above.
[137] Road Traffic Act 1988 ss.181–182.
[138] Merchant Shipping Act 1970 (Unregistered Ships) Regulations 1991 (SI 1991/1366).
[139] Merchant Shipping Act 1995 s.271.
[140] Regulation of Railways Act 1871 s.7, repealed by the Railway Safety (Miscellaneous Provisions)
    Regulations 1997.
[141] Civil Aviation (Investigation of Air Accidents and Incidents) Regulations 1996 (SI 1996/2798). See
    also 1–34.

Chapter 16

TREASURE

Treasure, formerly known as treasure trove, was of considerable importance in **16–01** medieval times as a source of revenue to the Crown.[1] In modern times, however, it has been of importance only from a historical, antiquarian or archaeological point of view.[2] But unfortunately not all that is valuable or of historical importance and found in the earth was treasure trove (or is now treasure). The law in this area survived in its original medieval form until almost the very end of the twentieth century, but was refashioned by the Treasure Act 1996. Unfortunately, the new law still requires an understanding of the old. For this reason, it is necessary to begin with the medieval idea of treasure trove.

MEDIEVAL DEFINITION

English jurists, from medieval times to the nineteenth century, were by no means **16–02** *ad idem* on the meaning of treasure trove.[3] However, the Court of Appeal finally held[4] that the definitions laid down by Coke and Chitty were to be preferred to those of Bracton, Glanvill and Blackstone. Coke said this:

"Treasure trove is when any gold or silver, in coin, plate or bullion hath been of ancient time hidden, wheresoever it be found, whereof no person can prove any

---

[1] See, e.g. Adam Smith, *The Wealth of Nations* (1770) Vol.1, p.232.
[2] The Treasure Trove Reviewing Committee considered 98 finds over the seven years from April 1977 to September 1984, although this figure excluded reported finds in the City of London, Cornwall, and the Duchy of Lancaster. See Cookson, *Archaeological Heritage Law* (2000), esp. at 229–250.
[3] See, e.g. Glanvill, *Tractatus de Legibus et Consuetudinibus Regni Angliae* Bk.14 c.2: Bracton, *De Legibus et Consuetudinibus Angliae* (ed. Woodbine) Vol.ii p.338; Britton, Vol.i c.17; Dalton, *Sheriffs* (1623) 36b; *Fleta*, Bk.I c.xxv (Selden Soc., Vol.72, p.65); 3 Co. Inst. 132; Comyn, Digest, tit. Treasure trove, p.624; 1 Bl.Com. 295; Chitty, *Prerogatives of the Crown* (1820), p.152. The best twentieth-century survey (which compares the laws of different countries) is Hill, *Treasure Trove in Law and Practice* (1936, reprinted 1980), and see also Palmer, "The Protection of Antiquities" (1981) 44 M.L.R. 178, and Palmer, *Bailment*, 2nd edn (1991), pp.1471–1473.
[4] *Attorney General for the Duchy of Lancaster v G. E. Overton (Farms) Ltd* [1982] Ch. 277, CA.

property, it doth belong to the King, or to some Lord or other by the King's grant, or prescription."[5]

Chitty said the same thing in more modern language.[6]

Essential characteristics

16–03 This meant that, in order for property once found to be held treasure trove, it had to have three essential characteristics:

(i) it had to be made of gold or silver;

(ii) it had to have been deliberately concealed by the owner with a view to later recovery; and

(iii) the owner or his present heirs or successors had to be unknown.

16–04 As to the first of these characteristics, it was clear that base or other metal than gold or silver was not treasure trove,[7] and a fortiori neither were gemstones, pottery, cloth or other possibly valuable items, such as might comprise the containers or wrappings for items which themselves might or might not amount to treasure trove.[8] To constitute treasure trove, it was not necessary that the gold or silver of which the item was made should be pure, but the item had to comprise a "substantial" proportion of gold or silver,[9] perhaps 50 per cent or more.[10]

16–05 As to the second characteristic, property was not treasure trove if it was deliberately abandoned or accidentally lost. As Chitty said:

"If the owner, instead of hiding the treasure, casually lost it or purposely parted with it in such a manner that it is evident he intended to abandon the property altogether and did not purpose to resume it on another occasion, as if he threw it on the ground or other public place, or in the sea, the first finder is entitled to the property against everyone but the owner, and the King's prerogative does not in this respect obtain."[11]

---

[5] 3 Co. Inst. 132.

[6] *Prerogatives of the Crown*, p.152. See also Hill, *Treasure Trove in Law and Practice* (1936, reprinted 1980), pp.218–220.

[7] Thus, finds of such objects, such as coins, did not need to be reported to the coroner, although the British Museum, National Museum of Wales or other local museum was always glad to hear of finds and would advise on disposal or may even buy them outright: Home Office Circular No. 10 of 1989 para.10.

[8] See Palmer, "The Protection of Antiquities" (1981) 44 M.L.R. 178, pp.180–181. Although the coroner had no jurisdiction over such things, they might still be of historical or other importance and the British Museum or National Museum of Wales was to be informed: Home Office Circular No. 10 of 1989 para.9.

[9] *Attorney General for the Duchy of Lancaster v G. E. Overton (Farms) Ltd* [1982] Ch. 277, CA.

[10] *Attorney General for the Duchy of Lancaster v G. E. Overton (Farms) Ltd* [1982] Ch. 277, 292.

[11] *Prerogatives of the Crown*, p.152, citing Britton, c.17 and 1 Bl.Comm. 295. It may have been that, to be treasure trove, the object must have been found concealed either underground or "in places affixed to the ground": Hill, *Treasure Trove in Law and Practice* (1936, reprinted 1980), pp.205–208, 220–221.

Thus, for example, objects buried in graves were unlikely to constitute treasure trove.[12]

So far as the third characteristic was concerned, Chitty said: 16–06

"If he that laid [the property in question] be known or afterwards discovered the owner and not the King is entitled to it, this prerogative right only applying in the absence of an owner to claim the property."[13]

Although this was never decided, it is submitted that this correctly represented the old law.

Crown rights to treasure trove

Prima facie, treasure trove belonged to the Crown by prerogative right,[14] except   16–07
that in Lancashire[15] and the liberties of the Duchy of Lancaster outside that county it belonged to the Crown in right of the Duchy of Lancaster,[16] and in Cornwall it belonged to the Duke of Cornwall in right of the Duchy of Cornwall.[17] However, the prerogative right to treasure trove in a particular area or areas might have been granted to a subject by the Crown, the Duchy of Lancaster or the Duchy of Cornwall (as the case might be),[18] when it became a franchise in the grantee.[19] It was not clear whether the grantee of a franchise, or a person claiming under him, might successfully defend its possession of treasure trove against the Crown merely by demonstrating the weakness of the Crown's case, or whether it was necessary for such grantee positively to prove his own title.[20]

Ownership where object not treasure trove

If an object was not treasure trove, then prima facie it belonged to the original   16–08
owner or his heirs.[21] Subject to that, an object buried in or attached to land or a

---

[12] Home Office Circular No. 10 of 1989 para.8(b); Brodrick Report para.13.24, cf. Burton, Chambers and Gill, *Coroners' Inquiries,* p.119. See further Hill, *Treasure Trove in Law and Practice* (1936, reprinted 1980), pp.223–224; Palmer, "The Protection of Antiquities" (1981) 44 M.L.R. 178, pp.182–183.

[13] *Prerogatives of the Crown,* p.152, citing 3 Co. Inst. 132–133; 1 Bl. Comm. 295.

[14] See the jurists cited in fn.3, above, and the general discussion in Hill, *Treasure Trove in Law and Practice* (1936, reprinted 1980), pp.208–218.

[15] That is, historic Lancashire, before the local government reforms introduced in 1974 by the Local Government Act 1972; see s.271(5) of that Act.

[16] See Hill, *Treasure Trove in Law and Practice* (1936, reprinted 1980), pp.208 and 245. An example is *Attorney General for the Duchy of Lancaster v G. E. Overton (Farms) Ltd* [1982] Ch. 277, CA.

[17] See Hill, *Treasure Trove in Law and Practice* (1936, reprinted 1980), pp.213–215.

[18] See the jurists cited in fn.3, above.

[19] *Attorney General v Trustees of the British Museum* [1903] 2 Ch. 598, a case dealing with the construction of grants of franchises. A list of such grants is to be found in Hill, *Treasure Trove in Law and Practice* (1936, reprinted 1980). For example, the Corporation of London is franchisee of treasure trove in the City of London and Southwark, under charters of 1444, 1462, 1608 and 1638. On the assumption that the Crown had property in treasure trove as yet unfound, the Crown had sometimes granted licences to persons to search for it upon terms, e.g. that anything found would be shared with the Crown in stated proportions; see the list of some such licences in Hill, *op. cit.,* pp.221–225, and cf. *Ponsonby v Boone, The Times,* July 19, 24–26, 1934.

[20] *Attorney General v Trustees of the British Museum* [1903] 2 Ch. 598, 614.

[21] According to the 7th to 9th editions of this work (at pp.110, 20 and 32 respectively) the jurist Statham, writing in 1470, mentioned a case to this effect in 22 Hen. 6.

building was in the legal possession of the owner[22] or occupier[23] of that land or building, who thus had property in the object good against the whole world except the true owner or anyone claiming through him. In a similar position was the occupier of land or a building on or in which an object was found (not being attached to or forming part of the land or building) when the occupier, before the object is found, had manifested an intention to exercise control over the land or building and the things which might be found on or in it.[24]

16–09   However, where an object was lying on land not occupied by anyone, or on land occupied by a person not manifesting an intention to exercise control over it, then, unless he was a trespasser on that land,[25] the first finder of the object had a right to possession of it good against the whole world except the true owner and anyone claiming through him.[26]

16–10   If an object was held not to be treasure trove, the coroner had to be careful to deliver it up only to the person properly entitled,[27] or, if there were several rival claimants, to invite the claimants to take proceedings between themselves to determine which (if any) was entitled. If they would not do this, the coroner's only safe course was to issue interpleader proceedings in the appropriate court, to which those claimants would be respondents, in order to allow the question of ownership to be resolved without risk to the coroner's position.[28] The coroner would normally be awarded his costs of such proceedings out of the value of the property.

THE TREASURE ACT 1996

16–11   This old law was reformed by the Treasure Act 1996. This was the first significant statutory amendment in the history of treasure trove. The drafting is unnecessarily complex and user-unfriendly, but broadly speaking, the Act (according to its long title) purports to abolish the medieval law of treasure trove and to replace it with a broader, more modern concept of "treasure". The right to treasure trove under the old law is abolished for the future,[29] and is replaced by the new right to "treasure", which when found vests in the franchisee if there is one, but otherwise

---

[22] *Elwes v Brigg Gas Co* (1866) 33 Ch.D. 562; *Attorney General for the Duchy of Lancaster v G. E. Overton (Farms) Ltd* [1982] Ch. 277, CA; *Waverley BC v Fletcher* [1996] Q.B. 334, CA.

[23] *South Staffordshire Water Co. v Sharman* [1896] 2 Q.B. 44, DC.

[24] *Parker v British Airways Board* [1982] Q.B. 1004, CA.

[25] *Parker v British Airways Board* [1982] Q.B. 1004, 1009, per Donaldson LJ.

[26] *Armory v Delamirie* (1722) 5 Stra. 505; 93 E.R. 664; *Parker v British Airways Board* [1982] Q.B. 1004.

[27] See Home Office Circular No. 10 of 1989, para.11; cf. misdelivery in bailment: *Youl v Harbottle* (1791) 1 Peake 49 (mere mistaken delivery to wrong person is conversion); but cf. *Elvin and Powell v Plummer Roddis Ltd* (1934) 50 T.L.R. 158 (non-negligent misdelivery by *involuntary* bailee held not actionable). In *Waverley BC v Fletcher* [1996] Q.B. 334, CA, the inquest concluded that the find was not treasure, and returned it to the finder. The landowner brought civil proceedings against the finder and succeeded, as having a better title. The coroner was not involved.

[28] RSC Ord.17 (High Court); CCR Ord.33 (county court). See now CPR Pt 86 (stakeholder claims and applications).

[29] Treasure Act 1996 s.4(3).

in the Crown,[30] as part of the hereditary revenues of the Crown, disposable of by the Secretary of State,[31] but subject to disclaimer by him.[32]

There is a complex definition of "treasure" in s.1 of the Act, supplemented by **16–12** s.3. There are now four categories of treasure, one of which (despite the Act's long title) actually preserves the old law of treasure trove, because it comprises "any object which would have been treasure trove if found before the commencement of section 4". This is likely to be significant only in relation to objects less than 300 years old, or less than 200 years old and not designated by the Secretary of State,[33] because objects at least 300 years old, or 200 years old and so designated, will usually fall within other (new) categories of "treasure" (the main exception is a single gold or silver coin).

The most important new such category comprises objects at least 300 years old **16–13** which, not being coins, have metallic content of at least 10 per cent by weight of gold or silver, or which, being coins, are at least two in number with the same percentage of gold or silver or at least 10 in number altogether. Thus, a hoard of at least 10 non-gold or silver coins at least 300 years old would be treasure, although it could not have been treasure trove.

The third category of treasure is an object at least 200 years old when found, **16–14** belonging to a class designated by the Secretary of State[34] which he considers to be of outstanding historical, archaeological, or cultural importance. As from January 1, 2003, this category includes a prehistoric non-coin object, which is (a) part base metal, forming part of a find of at least two such objects, or (b) part gold or silver.[35] There is a fourth category of treasure, which covers objects found as part of the same find as something else which falls within the categories of treasure.

Unlike the old law, it is not necessary for the owner of the find to be unknown **16–15** in order for it to constitute treasure. Instead, as treasure it vests in the Crown or franchisee, subject to all prior interests and rights. So the practical effect is the same. There are certain exclusions from the definition of treasure. In particular, it does not include objects which are unworked natural objects or minerals extracted from a natural deposit, or wreck within the meaning of Part IX of the Merchant Shipping Act 1995. In addition, the Secretary of State has power to designate a class of objects which are thereupon excluded from the definition. But for something to vest in the Crown or a franchisee as treasure, it is generally no longer necessary to show any intention on the part of the last possessor to retrieve the object subsequently.[36] (But this will still be necessary in relation to an object which is within the scope of "treasure" only because it would have been treasure trove under the old law.)

---

[30] Treasure Act 1996 s.4(1).
[31] Treasure Act 1996 s.6(1),(2).
[32] Treasure Act 1996 s.6(3).
[33] Under Treasure Act 1996 s.2(1). See the Treasure (Designation) Order 2002, 16–14 below.
[34] Under Treasure Act 1996 s.2(1).
[35] Treasure (Designation) Order 2002 art.3. "Prehistoric" means dating from the Iron Age or earlier, above art.2. See also Home Office Circular No.1 of 2003, issued on January 9, 2003, which sets out the revised definition of treasure, and also changes to the Code of Practice.
[36] Treasure Act 1996 s.4(4).

CODES OF PRACTICE AND REPORTS

16–16 The Treasure Act 1996 for the first time requires a Code of Practice to be prepared, reviewed when appropriate, and revised, by the Secretary of State.[37] It must set out the principles and practice to be followed by him in carrying out his functions in relation to treasure,[38] and may include guidance for those who search for and find treasure, and museums and others with treasure-related functions.[39] In the preparation or revision, the Secretary of State must consult interested persons.[40] The Code and any revision must be laid before Parliament[41] and approved by each House before coming into force.[42] It must then be published.[43] The first Code for England and Wales was approved in 1997, and after an outside consultant reported on how the Act had been operating in practice,[44] the new Revised Code was approved in 2002.[45] It was updated in certain respects (but not others)[46] in 2007.[47]

16–17 The Code does not have the force of law. In relation to others than the Secretary of State, it only contains "guidance".[48] In relation to the Secretary of State it may be more significant, in that a failure by him to follow its provisions[49] may ground a successful application for judicial review.[50] The 1996 Act also requires the Secretary of State to prepare and lay before Parliament an annual report on the workings of the Act.[51] Once the treasure provisions of the Coroners and Justice Act 2009 come into force, the coroner will thereafter be protected from civil liability if he or she delivers an object in accordance with the Code.[52]

JURISDICTION OF THE CORONER

16–18 The jurisdiction of the coroner in relation to treasure at the present day is derived from statute. The Coroners Act 1887 continued the pre-existing jurisdiction "to inquire of treasure which is found, who were the finders and who were suspected thereof".[53] In the (consolidating) Coroners Act 1988 this became jurisdiction:

---

[37] Treasure Act 1996 s.11(1).
[38] Treasure Act 1996 s.11(2).
[39] Treasure Act 1996 s.11(3). See App.7 below, for the internet URL for the Code of Practice, 2nd Revision (updated March 19, 2007).
[40] Treasure Act 1996 s.11(4).
[41] Treasure Act 1996 s.11(5).
[42] Treasure Act 1996 s.11(6).
[43] Treasure Act 1996 s.11(7).
[44] *Report on the Operation of the Treasure Act 1996*, October 2001. See also *The Times*, August 15, 2002.
[45] See also Home Office Circular No.1 of 2003, issued on January 9, 2003, which sets out the revised definition of treasure, and also changes to the Code of Practice.
[46] For example, the details of coroners and their offices in App.2 of the Code, which are now very out of date.
[47] See App.7 for the internet URL.
[48] Treasure Act 1996 s.11(3).
[49] See Treasure Act 1996 s.11(2): "the principles and practice *to be followed*" (emphasis supplied).
[50] See generally Ch.19.
[51] Treasure Act 1996 s.12.
[52] See Coroners and Justice Act 2009 s.31(2).
[53] Coroners Act 1887 s.36, derived from the statute *De Coronatoribus*, 4 Edw. 1.

"(a) to inquire into any treasure that is found in his district; and

(b)to inquire who were, or are suspected of being, the finders."[54]

After the commencement of s.4 of the Treasure Act 1996,[55] the coroner **16–19**
continued to have jurisdiction under the 1988 Act[56] to hold a "treasure trove"
inquest under the old law in relation to anything found before that commencement.[57] But, in relation to anything found thereafter, the coroner had jurisdiction,
under the same provision,[58] to hold a "treasure" inquest.[59]

The matter is now further complicated by Pt I of the Coroners and Justice Act **16–20**
2009. When this was (mostly) brought into force in July 2013, those provisions
relating to treasure, and in particular to the appointment of a national Coroner for
Treasure, were not commenced, because of lack of resources.[60] In principle, the
2009 Act repeals the 1988 Act. But the lack of a national Coroner for Treasure
meant that local coroners must continue to deal with treasure cases. Accordingly,
and by way of transitory provision, the repeal of the 1988 Act does not have effect
in so far as it relates to the exercise of a coroner's jurisdiction in relation to treasure inquests
as provided by s.30 of the 1988 Act.[61] It will be noted that it does not keep alive
merely s.30 for this limited purpose, but the *whole* Act *and* the Coroners Rules
1984.[62] Only once the treasure investigations provisions in the 2009 Act are
commenced will the repeal of the 1988 Act and the 1984 Rules become complete.[63]

What this means is that there are now two quite separate coroner regimes in **16–21**
England and Wales, one for deaths (under the 2009 Act) and one for treasure
(under the 1988 Act). But the transitory provision deals with two particular
problems that might thereby have been caused. First, it makes clear that any
reference to a "coroner" in the 1988 Act is to be treated as a reference to a coroner

---

[54] Coroners Act 1988 s.30.

[55] i.e. September 24, 1997 (see SI 1997/1977).

[56] Section 30.

[57] See the Treasure Act 1996 s.7(2).

[58] i.e. Coroners Act 1988 s.30.

[59] Treasure Act 1996 s.7(1).

[60] See 1–41.

[61] Coroners and Justice Act 2009 (Commencement No. 15, Consequential and Transitory Provisions)
Order 2013 art.3(a).

[62] The 1984 Rules were in fact made under the Coroners (Amendment) Act 1926 ss.26–27, but treated
as made under the 1988 Act, by virtue of the Interpretation Act 1978 s.17(2)(b). But it is arguable
that that provision does not save the 1984 Rules on the coming into force of the Coroners and Justice
Act 2009 Pt I, because the new rule-making powers are different, and were used immediately to
make new rules and regulations replacing the 1984 Rules, which are therefore impliedly revoked (cf.
Watson v Winch [1916] 1 K.B. 688).

[63] Coroners and Justice Act 2009 (Commencement No. 15, Consequential and Transitory Provisions)
Order 2013 art.3. When that happens, the Coroner for Treasure will (and assistant coroners for
treasure may) be appointed (Sch.4), who will (to the exclusion of all other coroners) conduct all
treasure investigations in England and Wales (s.26), including any inquests (s.27), which will
determine whether the object is treasure and by whom and where it was found (s.28). For the first
time a disclaimer notice will have the effect of preventing a treasure investigation (s.29), and the
coroner will be protected from civil liability in delivering an object in accordance with the Code of
Practice (s.31). Finally, additional reporting requirements will be laid on the acquirers of certain
objects (s.30).

appointed under the 2009 Act s.23 and Sch.3.[64] So there is only one kind of coroner, operating in both systems. And area and assistant coroners under the 2009 Act are clearly within the meaning of coroner where it appears in the 1988 Act, because s.23 of the 2009 Act specifically mentions them.[65] With that point settled, problems about pay, terms, discipline and so on must clearly be dealt with under the new regime only.

16–22   The other matter concerns coroner areas. The 1988 Act allocated coroners to "coroner districts", which were in administrative areas, normally counties. The 2009 Act allocates coroners to "coroner areas", which have no necessary tie to any administrative area. So the transitory provision makes clear that any reference to a "coroner district" in the 1988 Act is to be treated as a reference to a coroner area constituted under the 2009 Act s.22 and Sch.2.[66] This means that in principle any question of territorial jurisdiction is judged by reference to the new system only, and that the old system of districts in administrative areas has gone.

Extent of jurisdiction

16–23   Formerly, the duty of the coroner was expressed to be that he must go to the place where the treasure was said to be found.[67] This would suggest that the coroner's duty to inquire arises when he has reasonable suspicion that treasure has been found within his area, and this would be consistent with the position in relation to inquiries into deaths, i.e. where the coroner honestly believes facts which, if true, would give him jurisdiction.[68] It is the duty of those finding treasure to report it to the coroner,[69] although in practice many such reports reach the coroner via others. It was formerly an offence to conceal treasure trove,[70] but this has long been abolished.[71] Many, if not all, such cases would now constitute theft.[72] For a person to be convicted of theft of treasure, it is not necessary that a coroner's inquest should already have found the object to be treasure, but it must be proved to the satisfaction of the (criminal) jury that the object is in fact treasure.[73]

Requirements as to finding and presence of objects within coroner area

16–24   But one matter which is not quite clear is whether the coroner's jurisdiction is dependent upon the original finding of the objects within his area, the current presence of the objects within his area, or upon both these things. It will be recalled that, in relation to inquests into deaths, it has been held that it is presence of the

---

[64] Coroners and Justice Act 2009 (Commencement No. 15, Consequential and Transitory Provisions) Order 2013 art.3(b).

[65] See also Coroners and Justice Act 2009 Sch.3 para.8; see 2–16.

[66] Coroners and Justice Act 2009 (Commencement No. 15, Consequential and Transitory Provisions) Order 2013 art.3(c).

[67] Britton, Vol.I c.18 para.1; Fitzherbert, *New Boke of Justices of the Peas* (1538) fol.59a.

[68] See para.5–01 above.

[69] Treasure Act 1996 s.8(1); formerly, see Britton, Vol.I c.18 para.1; Staunford P.C., c.42 fol.40a; 3 Co. Inst. 133; 1 Bl.Comm, 296; Chitty, *Prerogatives of the Crown* (1820) p.153. See also Hill, *Treasure Trove in Law and Practice* (1936, reprinted 1980), pp.228–232.

[70] *R. v Thomas & Willett* (1863) 9 Cox C.C. 376; *R. v Toole* (1867) 11 Cox C.C. 75. See also Hill, *Treasure Trove in Law and Practice* (1936, reprinted 1980), pp.225–228.

[71] Theft Act 1968 s.32(1)(a).

[72] Theft Act 1968 s.1. See, e.g. Smith and Hogan, *Criminal Law*, 13th edn (2011) Ch.19. There are also possible offences under the Dealing in Cultural Objects (Offences) Act 2003.

[73] *R. v Hancock* [1990] 2 Q.B. 242, CA.

body alone which nowadays gives the coroner jurisdiction, though formerly it was necessary for both cause of death and death itself to occur within the coroner's jurisdiction.[74]

So far as treasure is concerned, the difficulty with basing jurisdiction on the **16–25** original finding is that the objects may now be in a completely different area, and the coroner of the first area may have difficulty in obtaining possession of them. If, on the other hand, jurisdiction is based upon current presence of the objects within the area, the coroner of that area may have difficulty in securing the attendance of witnesses as to the circumstances and the place in which the objects were found. The third alternative, that is requiring both finding and presence within the coroner's jurisdiction, would mean that in some cases at least there would be no coroner having jurisdiction at all.

Bracton speaks of the coroner's power, indeed duty, to arrest a person suspected **16–26** of concealing treasure trove "wherever it is found", which suggests that presence of the objects within the coroner's jurisdiction was the connecting factor, because the finder might well move from one jurisdiction into another. Similarly, Coke refers to an object "hidden, wheresoever it be found", which again puts less emphasis on the place of finding than on the actual existence of the objects in question.

Section 30 of the Coroners Act 1988,[75] preserved for the moment, refers to "any **16–27** treasure which is found in his district" [for which read "area"].[76] The Treasure Act 1996 refers all questions of jurisdiction to this section. It is not clear whether "found" refers to the original finding or to current presence. But it is submitted that the better view is that the only necessary connecting factor to give a coroner jurisdiction is the *current* presence within the area of objects which are believed to be treasure trove, wherever they have been found in England and Wales.[77] If they were not originally found somewhere in England and Wales, the prerogative rights of the English Crown could not apply in any event.

There are however other problems with the non-repeal of the 1988 Act, besides **16–28** coroners and areas. The rules relating to the provision of accommodation for treasure inquest hearings must be referrable to the 1988 Act. So too must the rules relating to the expenses of witnesses (so the Schedule of the Home Secretary[78] continues to have effect, rather than the new financial regulations)[79] and also the rules about witness summonses,[80] and about juries.[81] Unlike coroners and areas, these points appear not to have been considered.

---

[74] See 5–87 above.
[75] cf. Coroners Act 1887 s.36.
[76] See 16–22.
[77] 3 Co. Inst. 231. Leckey and Greer, *Coroners' Law and Practice in Northern Ireland* (1998), p.277, take the opposite view, partly based on slightly different wording in the Northern Ireland statute.
[78] See 18–33, 18–47.
[79] See 18–34 ff.
[80] See 7–12.
[81] See 10–33 ff.

THE CORONER'S POWERS AND DUTIES

Duty to inquire

16–29   A coroner who becomes aware of the presence of possible treasure within his area comes under a duty forthwith to inquire into the matter.[82]

Power to take possession of objects at issue

16–30   Just as a coroner inquiring into a death has a right to possession of the body of the deceased person until his inquiries are complete,[83] so too a coroner has the power, if not the duty, to take possession of objects believed to be treasure.[84] Just as a coroner has power to interfere with the rights of executors to possession of a body when he honestly believes to be true facts which, if true, would give him jurisdiction, even if the truth ultimately turns out to be otherwise,[85] so too in the case of objects honestly believed to be treasure the coroner may interfere with the otherwise unimpaired rights of the owner or other person entitled to possession of the object in question. But a coroner who has no reasonable grounds for believing an object to be treasure (e.g. because he knows it does not satisfy the definition) acts at his peril if he interferes with the rights of the finder or owner.

Concealment of treasure trove

16–31   All the old authorities are clear that a coroner had the power to arrest any person suspected of having found and concealed treasure trove, or who had otherwise put it to his own use, and also to grant bail to such a person.[86] In addition, it appears that the county sheriffs and bailiffs were under a duty to assist the coroners in the execution of their duties,[87] and this probably included exercising such powers of arrest on their behalf. However, since the abolition of the specific offences of concealment of treasure trove,[88] and indeed the whole criminal jurisdiction of coroners,[89] it seems doubtful that these powers can have survived. In any event, it is clearly preferable that, insofar as any offences may have been committed in relation to treasure, they should be investigated by the police and prosecuted in the usual way.[90]

Duty to notify, and failure to notify

16–32   A person finding an object which he has grounds for believing to be treasure must notify the coroner for the area in which it was found before the end of a 14-day

---

[82] Fitzherbert, *New Boke of Justices of the Peas* (1538) fol.59a; Treasure Act 1996 s.7(1). The Home Office view is that any delay in dealing with the objects (and therefore leading to delay in rewards being paid) will tend to discourage those who find such objects from reporting them at all: Home Office Circular No. 10 of 1989 para.4.

[83] See 8–11 above.

[84] Britton, Vol.I Bk.1 Ch.II para.18; Fitzherbert, *New Boke of Justices of the Peas* (1538), fol. 57a; Treasure Act 1996 s.7(1).

[85] See 5–01, 5–65 above.

[86] Stat. 4 Edw. 1; Britton, Vol.1 Bk.1 Ch.II para.18; Fitzherbert and Crompton, *Justices de Peace* (1584) fol.177a; 1 Bl.Comm. 337; 2 Hawk P.C., c. 9, 536.

[87] Britton, Vol.1 Bk.1 Ch.II para.18; Fitzherbert and Crompton, *Justices de Peace* (1584) fol.177a.

[88] Theft Act 1968 s.32(1)(a).

[89] Criminal Law Act 1977 s.56.

[90] See, e.g. *R. v Hancock* [1990] 2 Q.B. 242, CA.

notice period. This period begins with the day after the find or such later day as
the finder first believes or has reason to believe that the object is treasure.[91] Failure
to notify is a criminal offence.[92] A coroner proposing to conduct a treasure inquest
must notify the British Museum, if his district is in England, or the National
Museums and Galleries of Wales, if it is in Wales.[93]

He must also take reasonable steps to notify the apparent finder of the treasure   **16–33**
and the occupier of the land where it was found, and this is an obligation which
continues during the inquest if not successfully achieved before it.[94] It also gives
rise to an obligation to take reasonable steps to obtain from any person so notified
the names and addresses of other interested persons and to notify them of the
inquest.[95] The coroner must then take reasonable steps to give any interested
person[96] so notified of the inquest the opportunity to examine witnesses at the
inquest.[97]

Advice on nature or composition of objects

A coroner will need advice or assistance in establishing the age, nature and   **16–34**
composition of objects. In some cases he may need archaeological advice tending
to show whether or not objects were hidden as opposed to abandoned. Under the
Revised Code of Practice made (in 2002, but amended in 2007) under the
Treasure Act 1996,[98] it is contemplated that the coroner will seek advice either
from a local or a national museum, or from a local authority archaeological officer
or unit,[99] under pre-agreed arrangements.[100] A report on the find will be prepared
for the coroner,[101] which will give details of the find together with an assessment
(with reasons) as to whether it falls within the definition of treasure, though not a
valuation.[102] It may also be necessary, in non-coin cases, to analyse the objects,[103]
wherever possible without sampling.

Disclaimer

The 1996 Act conferred an express power on the Secretary of State to disclaim the   **16–35**
Crown's title to treasure.[104] The principles on which the minister acts are set out
in the Code,[105] and involve (inter alia) a consideration of whether any museum

---

[91] Treasure Act 1996 s.8(1),(2). A further duty to notify the coroner will be imposed on *acquirers* of
certain objects when s.30 of the Coroners and Justice Act 2009 comes into force.
[92] Treasure Act 1996 s.8(3).
[93] Treasure Act 1996 s.9(2).
[94] Treasure Act 1996 s.9(3), (4).
[95] Treasure Act 1996 s.9(5).
[96] As defined by Treasure Act 1996 s.9(7).
[97] See Treasure Act 1996 s.9(6).
[98] See App.7 for the internet URL.
[99] Revised Code of Practice, para.49.
[100] Revised Code of Practice, para.41.
[101] Revised Code of Practice, para.54. In the case of Welsh finds, this will normally be from the
National Museums and Galleries of Wales.
[102] Revised Code of Practice, para.55.
[103] Revised Code of Practice, para.56.
[104] Treasure Act 1996 s.6(3).
[105] Revised Code of Practice, paras 48–52.

wishes to acquire the find. If none does, the national museum[106] will advise the Secretary of State to disclaim.[107] If treasure is disclaimed, it is deemed not to have vested in the Crown,[108] and (without prejudice to others' rights) may be delivered to the finder under the Code,[109] unless the occupier or landowner objects.[110] In the latter case, the coroner (or his agent) prima facie retains the find pending a resolution of the dispute in the ordinary courts.[111] The coroner has no power himself to resolve that dispute.[112] If the coroner is sued for return of the find in such a case, he should interplead.[113]

16–36 The power to disclaim is to disclaim the Crown's title.[114] If the treasure vests in a franchisee[115] the position is different. The Revised Code notes[116] that the power "does not specifically apply to franchise-holders, but asserts that "they may choose to follow this practice if they so wish". It is hard to see the justification for this statement. The 1996 Act does not permit the Secretary of State to disclaim anyone else's title, and the disclaimer provision must be read as not giving the Secretary of State power, by disclaiming the Crown's title, to affect the title of the franchisee.[117]

16–37 For a disclaimer by the franchisee to be valid at common law, it must be made before the franchisee does anything to accept the property,[118] and must be of the whole, not merely part, of that property.[119] But the property concerned is not the individual find; it is the original grant by charter of the franchise, accepted long ago. And if (as is likely) the franchisee has accepted individual finds in the past under its grant, it is too late to disclaim the whole grant now.

16–38 On the other hand it may be argued that the title of the franchisee now arises under the Act itself,[120] rather than by virtue of the original grant. But in that case the problem would be that the Act is not facultative, creating a framework for voluntary transfer, but mandatory, vesting property in a person without his or her knowledge or consent. A specific exception is given for the Crown to disclaim, and escape the mandatory effect, but none for the franchisee. This is therefore an unlikely construction.

16–39 The final point on disclaimer is the effect of a valid disclaimer on the inquest process. The Revised Code states that "it will not normally be necessary to hold treasure inquests in such cases".[121] The legal basis for this assertion is not disclosed.

---

[106] i.e. the British Museum or the National Museums & Galleries of Wales, as appropriate.
[107] Paragraph 49.
[108] Treasure Act 1996 s.6(4)(a).
[109] Treasure Act 1996 s.6(4)(b).
[110] Revised Code of Practice, para.50.
[111] Revised Code of Practice, para.50.
[112] Revised Code of Practice, para.50.
[113] See 16–10 above.
[114] Treasure Act 1996 s.6(3).
[115] Under Treasure Act 1996 s.4(1)(a); see 16–07 above.
[116] Paragraph 20.
[117] By virtue of the Human Rights Act 1998 s.3(1), Sch.1 Pt II art.1 (protection of property). This will alter when s.29 of the Coroners and Justice Act 2009 comes into force, and the franchisee will for the first time be able to give a disclaimer notice.
[118] *Standing v Bowring* (1885) 31 Ch.D. 282, CA.
[119] *Re Lord and Fullerton's Contract* [1896] 1 Ch. 228, CA.
[120] See Treasure Act 1996 s.4(1)(a).
[121] Paragraph 48.

The duty on the coroner is to hold an inquest into treasure.[122] Disclaimer affects title, not status: an item of treasure, though disclaimed, remains treasure,[123] and hence its status must still be inquired into. If a suspected treasure find is reported to the coroner, he has no discretion, but must proceed to hold an inquest, at which he (or the jury) will publicly inquire into the facts, so as to determine whether the find is or is not treasure.[124] Who has title to it is quite another matter, and one with which the coroner has nothing to do.[125]

But, even if that were wrong, and the inquest dealt with title, the disclaimer **16–40** could not do away with the need for an inquest for a quite separate reason. There is no provision in the treasure legislation for a "fast-track" determination, comparable with "Pink Form B" procedure in sudden death cases, enabling the coroner to dispense with an inquest.[126] If the find is validly disclaimed, that is as much a relevant fact to consider at the inquest as is scientific evidence presented in advance to the coroner that (say) the find contains less than 10 per cent precious metal. If (conclusive) evidence of the former kind were to take away the coroner's jurisdiction to inquire further, why not the latter? Of course, in practice if the coroner ignores his duty, and simply releases the item to the finder (or occupier or landowner, as the case may be), there will be no complaint.[127] But it is profoundly unsatisfactory.

FUNCTION OF AN INQUEST INTO TREASURE

It is not entirely clear at the present day what is the function of an inquest on **16–41** treasure. There seem to have been three views. The first is that such an inquest was a preliminary to criminal proceedings against a person who had concealed treasure.[128] On this view, whilst it might be part of the function of the coroner's inquest to decide whether the object was treasure or not, this would merely be in order to determine whether criminal proceedings should follow in connection with such treasure. The second possible view is that the inquest is effectively to try the title to the object in question. The third view is that the inquest is merely to find the facts upon which it may be decided whether or not the object constitutes treasure, but without trying title to the object.[129]

---

[122] Treasure Act 1996 s.7, referring back to s.30 of the Coroners Act 1988.

[123] See Treasure Act 1996 s.6(4).

[124] See 16–15 above. This will alter when s.29 of the Coroners and Justice Act 2009 comes into force, and the service of a disclaimer notice will for the first time prevent an investigation being conducted.

[125] *Attorney General* v *Moore* [1893] 1 Ch. 676. See below, 16–43.

[126] See 8–36 ff above.

[127] See also 16–39 above.

[128] See *Attorney General v Moore* [1893] 1 Ch. 676 at 679, per Sir J. Rigby QC, *arguendo*; cf. above at 683, per Stirling J.

[129] *Mirror of Justices* Vol.I c.13 (Selden Soc. Vol.7 p.32); Statute of Exeter (probably 14 Edw. 1, i.e. 1286); Fitzherbert, *New Boke* fol.58b; Fleta Bk.I c.xxv (Selden Soc. Vol.72 p.65); Home Office Circular No. 10 of 1989 para.11; Brodrick Report, at para.13–21; Burton, Chambers and Gill, *Coroners' Inquiries*, p.122.

16–42 · If the first view were correct, the abolition of the coroner's criminal jurisdiction in homicide cases,[130] and the rule change prohibiting verdicts suggesting criminal liability of named persons,[131] would leave the coroner's inquest in cases of treasure without any function whatever. The second view is clearly wrong, for it has been held that the coroner's inquest was not there to try title (as between the Crown and a possible franchisee) to the object in question,[132] for the Crown's title did not depend on the verdict of the jury, but was independent.[133]

16–43 Although the third view may involve a prima facie finding as to title to the object, but finding it treasure, it clearly has nothing to do with trying title between the Crown and any person claiming as a franchisee,[134] and in any case (as we shall see), the verdict of the coroner's inquest is not conclusive as between rival claimants.[135] The weight of opinion[136] is in favour of the third view, and this has certainly been assumed in later cases.[137]

EVIDENCE AND PROCEDURE

Application of Coroners Rules

16–44 By and large, an inquest on treasure trove follows the same general pattern as an inquest on death, with due allowance being made for the different subject matter of the proceedings. However, as a general point it should be noted that the bulk of the Coroners Rules probably do not apply, since the definition of "inquest" in those Rules does not include a treasure trove inquest, "unless the context otherwise requires".[138]

16–45 Until the Treasure Act 1996, every treasure trove inquest had to be held with a jury. This is no longer the case, although the coroner has a discretion to hold a treasure inquest with a jury if he so orders.[139] If the jury is ordered, the requirements and procedure for summoning a jury appear to be the same as for juries summoned in other cases,[140] although the jurors' oath must be slightly modified.[141]

---

[130] Criminal Law Act 1977 s.56; see 1–30.
[131] Coroners (Amendment) Rules 1977 r.7; see now Coroners Rules 1984 r.42(a).
[132] *Attorney General v Moore* [1893] 1 Ch. 676.
[133] *Attorney General v Moore* [1893] 1 Ch. 676, at 684.
[134] Which was the substance of the action at *Attorney General v Moore* [1893] 1 Ch. 676, the jury having already declared the objects to be treasure trove.
[135] See 16–52, 16–61 above.
[136] See 16–41 above.
[137] e.g. *Attorney General of the Duchy of Lancaster v G. E. Overton (Farms) Ltd* [1982] Ch. 277.
[138] Coroners Rules 1984 r.2(1).
[139] Treasure Act 1996 s.7(4). See also s.27 of the Coroners and Justice Act 2009 (not yet in force).
[140] See the Coroners Act 1988 s.30, applying s.3 of that Act.
[141] For a form, see App.3, Form 13.

Evidence

Evidence will be taken at the inquest in the usual way,[142] both from experts as to   **16–46**
the nature and other characteristics of the object in question,[143] and from the
witnesses of fact as to the circumstances in which the object was found. So far as
the latter are concerned, under the old law, in order for the object to be declared
treasure trove, there had to be evidence to show a deliberate concealment as
opposed to an abandonment or a simple loss, although such deliberate concealment
might be shown from the circumstances of the find itself.[144] The usual witnesses of
fact are the finder and the landowner (and/or leaseholder). The usual experts are
those dealing with (i) the type of find in question, and (ii) the history of the land
where it was found.

Questions to be put in summing up

Under the old law, in the course of his summing-up to the jury, it was usual for the   **16–47**
coroner to put the following questions to them:

   (1) Where was the object found?

   (2) What did the find consist of?

   (3) Was it intentionally hidden, accidentally lost, or purposely abandoned?

   (4) Is the owner of the find unknown?

   (5) Who was the finder of the object?

It should be noted that the age of the object found was not itself of   **16–48**
importance,[145] although it might have been relevant in considering the question of
intention. The first four questions went to whether or not the object was indeed
treasure trove, and the final question, though originally relevant for the question of
criminal liability, was relevant for the purposes of any reward that may be
paid.[146]

Under the new law the coroner should consider (or direct the jury to consider)   **16–49**
such of the following questions as are relevant to the particular case:

   (1) Where was the object found?

   (2) What did the find consist of?

   (3) Was it part of another find?

   (4) Does it have the characteristics needed to fall within the definition of
       treasure in the 1996 Act?

---

[142] See Ch.12.
[143] Such expert witnesses can be procured through the British Museum or National Museum of Wales:
Home Office Circular No. 10 of 1989 para.8(d).
[144] See, e.g. *Attorney General v Trustees for the British Museum* [1903] 2 Ch. 598 at 609; *Attorney General
of the Duchy of Lancaster v G. E. Overton (Farms) Ltd* [1980] 3 All E.R. 503 at 508, per Dillon J.
[145] See the 9th edn of this work, p.31.
[146] As to which see 16–54 above.

    (5) Does it have any of the characteristics taking it outside the definition of treasure?

    (6) Is there anyone with a prior interest in or right to it?

    (7) Who was the finder?

16–50   The fourth question is the most complex, because it may involve issues of age, metallic content, being part of the same find, and (in rare cases) the characteristics of treasure trove under the old law. If there is a jury, the coroner will need to formulate the precise attributes suitable for the case. The sixth question is relevant because a positive answer in practice will render the whole process futile. The seventh question is again relevant to the question of reward.

VERDICT

16–51   In answering the questions posed to himself, or left to the jury, the coroner finds or the jury find certain facts in relation to the object, as a result of which the object is declared to be either treasure or not, and this is recorded in a modified form of inquisition.[147] Although the verdict as to whether an object is or is not treasure trove may be prima facie evidence of that fact in any later proceedings,[148] it is clear that it is not conclusive, and that the same issue can be relitigated between rival claimants in further proceedings.[149]

Challenge to the verdict of a jury

16–52   However, although it is clear that the jury's verdict is traversable as to matters of law,[150] it is less clear that facts found by the jury are so challengeable, such as whether the object contained sufficient precious metal.[151] Nonetheless, it is submitted that, just as under the old law of deodand[152] a jury's verdict that an object was deodand, and therefore forfeit to the Crown, was traversable by any person affected by such verdict, so too the inquest verdict in matters of fact relating to treasure should equally be open to challenge and to be relitigated in subsequent proceedings.[153]

16–53   It cannot be doubted, either, that the decisions of the coroner and the inquisition resulting from an inquest on treasure can be quashed or otherwise subjected to judicial review in the same way as any other decisions or inquisitions not involving treasure.[154] The statutory power of the Court to order an inquest to

---

[147] For a form, see App.3, Form 20.

[148] It was so argued in *Attorney General v Moore* [1893] 1 Ch. 676.

[149] *Attorney General for Duchy of Lancaster v G. E. Overton (Farms) Ltd* [1982] Ch. 277 at 287, and see 20–02 below.

[150] *Attorney General for Duchy of Lancaster v G. E. Overton (Farms) Ltd* [1982] Ch. 277; *Attorney General v Moore* [1893] 1 Ch. 676.

[151] See *Attorney General for Duchy of Lancaster v G. E. Overton (Farms) Ltd* [1982] Ch. 277, at 530.

[152] See 1–06 above.

[153] See generally 20–02 below.

[154] See Ch.19 below.

be held or to quash an inquisition in certain circumstances[155] applies to treasure cases.[156]

Disposal of objects held to be treasure

If at the conclusion of the inquest, a museum wishes to acquire objects found by **16–54** the verdict to be treasure, they should be sent to the relevant national museum, so that it can be valued by the Treasure Valuation Committee.[157] The Code of Practice sets out the principles upon which the national museum will arrange the acquisition of the find, including the order in which museums should be entitled to acquire.[158] Rewards are paid to finders, occupiers and landowners, in accordance with principles set out in the Code.[159] Obviously, the coroner will take all possible care in preparing the treasure trove for dispatch, and in suitable cases will discuss it with the museum beforehand.[160] The expenses incurred in and for the purpose of the inquest will of course be treated as with the expenses of any other inquest.[161] If the objects are found not to be treasure, then they will be returned in the same way as if they were disclaimed.[162]

MODERN APPLICATION

Use of the coroner's jurisdiction to inquire into treasure

Although the original importance of the coroner's jurisdiction in treasure appears **16–55** to have been to protect the prerogative right (and therefore the financial interests) of the Crown,[163] its importance in modern times is that of preserving artefacts for their archaeological or historical interest. However, this purpose is not well served by the present situation, for two reasons. First, the definition of treasure trove—albeit expanded in 1996 and again in 2002—does not include all things of archaeological or historical interest. Secondly, the verdict of the inquest is not conclusive, and the question whether or not the object is treasure trove can be, and often is, litigated in the ordinary courts.[164]

Defects in the existing definition

So far as the definition of treasure is concerned, there are two main defects from **16–56** the point of view of preserving important or interesting archaeological finds. First, to constitute treasure, an object or objects must either (a) include at least 10 per cent gold or silver, or (b) be a collection of base metal coins, or (c) be two or more *prehistoric* part-base metal objects or (d) be a single *prehistoric* part-precious metal

---

[155] Coroners Act 1988 s.13; see Ch.19 above.
[156] *R. v Wiltshire Coroner, ex p. Chaddock* (1992) 157 J.P. 209, DC.
[157] Revised Code of Practice, para.60. For valuation principles, see paras 65–70.
[158] Revised Code of Practice, para.63.
[159] Revised Code of Practice, paras 71–85.
[160] Home Office Circular No. 10 of 1989 para.8.
[161] Home Office Circular No. 10 of 1989 para 17; see 18–47.
[162] See 16–10 above.
[163] See 1–06 above.
[164] As demonstrated by *Attorney General for the Duchy of Lancaster v G. E. Overton (Farms) Ltd* [1982] Ch. 277, CA.

object. There is doubt as to how far it includes non-prehistoric plated and composite objects, but in most such cases plated objects seem to be excluded. So too, for the most part, is pottery and other non-metallic material, whether prehistoric or not.

16–57 A great deal of interesting and important archaeological material therefore still falls outside the treasure system. The *Report on the Operation of the Treasure Act 1996*[165] declined to recommend any general move to include this further material (save for the subtle extension to certain prehistoric part-base or precious metal objects, now implemented), on the basis of lack of resources to cope with the likely increase in finds.

16–58 The second problem is that the 1996 Act retained the old law of treasure trove, and for an object to be treasure trove it must be decided that it was deliberately concealed with a view to being retrieved, rather than being accidentally lost or deliberately abandoned.[166] The poverty of evidence usually available means that the coroner or jury must simply guess at the truth, and it is in any event absurd that upon such facts (even if they could be accurately found) the question of treasure should depend. But the recent *Report on the Operation of the Treasure Act 1996*[167] declined to recommend that any change be made, on the basis that this might lead to the loss of important finds.

Applicability of coroner's jurisdiction

16–59 Unlike the law relating to inquests into unnatural deaths, where the coroner's powers and duties in connection with such inquests have been largely reduced to statutory form, too many of the coroner's powers and duties in connection with a treasure inquest remain unclear, despite the reforms wrought by the Treasure Act 1996. The *Report into the Operation of the Treasure Act 1996*[168] has recommended that procedures for dealing with treasure inquests be set out in new rules and practice guidance.

16–60 Secondly, historically the coroner has been an expert in one form of inquiry alone, that into deaths,[169] and there appears to be no good reason for wasting his expertise on a form of inquiry involving very different considerations. It is fair to say that coroners themselves mostly are in favour of continuing the jurisdiction, or alternatively have no view. After all, when one considers the distressing nature of most coroners' inquiries, what coroner would not be in favour of something less gloomy? But the fact remains that very few coroners acquire more than minimal experience of treasure.

16–61 Finally, and most absurd of all, the inquest's verdict is by no means conclusive, but may, where valuable objects are concerned, more than in any other, be merely the precursor to litigation in the ordinary courts, in which the verdict may be quite irrelevant.[170] The title of the Crown to treasure, as indeed the title of a finder of

---

[165] October 2001, paras 62–65, 74.
[166] See 16–03 above.
[167] October 2001, paras 71, 75.
[168] October 2001, paras 118–119.
[169] As shown by the fact that before Part I of the Coroners and Justice Act 2009 came into force in 2013, a medical practitioner with no legal experience might be appointed a coroner: see 2–39 above.
[170] See 20–02 below.

objects or the owner of land on which the objects are found (if the objects are not treasure) is completely independent of the verdict of the coroner's inquest.[171]

In these circumstances, there seems no good reason for not leaving the issue of **16–62** treasure trove or not to be resolved by the ordinary courts in the normal way, and simply abolishing the jurisdiction of the coroner to take inquests on treasure. In Scotland, for example, where there are no coroners, finds of treasure trove are reported to the procurators fiscal (public prosecutors) and the Queen's and Lord Treasurer's Remembrancer (the Treasury's representative in Scotland). It is they who, acting on behalf of the Crown, take the advice of an advisory panel as to historical interest and market value, and deal with the property themselves. Admittedly the Crown's prerogative in Scotland is wider than in England and Wales, and is not restricted to gold or silver objects, but the principle is the same.[172]

It is therefore submitted that, for England and Wales, the convenient method of **16–63** proceeding would be to have finds of treasure trove reported to the Treasury Solicitor,[173] who could administer the property in the same way as (for example) *bona vacantia* is administered at present. Alternative claimants to the objects found could be advertised for, as with *bona vacantia*,[174] and if competing claims were not resolved by agreement, proceedings could be brought to determine the issue conclusively.[175] But this view did not commend itself to the author of the recent *Report on the Operation of the Treasure Act 1996*.[176]

---

[171] *Attorney General v Moore* [1893] 1 Ch. 676; *The King's Prerogative in Saltpetre* (1606) 6 Co.Rep. 208.

[172] As to the Republic of Ireland, see *Webb v Ireland and Attorney General* [1988] I.R. 373.

[173] Or the Solicitor to the Duchy of Lancaster, or the Duchy of Cornwall, as appropriate: *cf.* 9–19, fn.88 and 16–07 above.

[174] Trustee Act 1925 s.27; Administration of Estates Act 1925 s.46(1)(vi).

[175] As with bona vacantia; see, e.g. *Re Wells* [1933] Ch. 29, CA.

[176] October 2001 para.113.

Chapter 17

MAJOR DISASTERS

INTRODUCTION

In recent years there has been a number of major disasters, often attended by large **17–01** loss of life. Some are natural, others accidental, and others again deliberate. Terrorist attacks in particular, and especially after the destruction of the Twin Towers in New York in September 2001, and the London bombings of July 2005, have focused attention on the systems in place for reacting to such incidents. A great deal of information and advice, official and unofficial, is now available.[1] There is also earlier literature.[2]

The legal position of the coroner is not altered in any way by the number of **17–02** persons who die in a particular incident, although the law does make provision for the special case of the multiple homicide where the accused is only charged with the death of one or more of the persons killed.[3] This chapter deals with those cases where the coroner is obliged to modify the usual methods of investigation in order to deal with a major incident. In principle, similar considerations will apply to a coronial investigation into deaths in an incident abroad[4] where the bodies are brought back to this country, as to deaths from such an incident in England and Wales.

There is no definition of a major incident or disaster. Examples are aeroplane **17–03** and train crashes, multiple crashes on motorways, sinking ships, bomb explosions, flooding, and gunmen running amok. An incident may attract considerable public concern and involve extensive investigations, with no loss or minimal loss of life. But if at least one person dies, the coroner will be involved.

---

[1] See, e.g. the Home Office, *Dealing with Disaster* (1997) (available online at *http://www.nationalarchives.gov.uk* [Accessed June 16, 2014]), the Cabinet Office, *Emergency Response and Recovery* (2013) (*http://www.gov.uk/emergency-response-and-recovery* [Accessed June 16, 2014]), and *Resilence in society: infrastructure, communities and business* (2013) (*http://www.gov.uk/resilience-in-society-infrastructure-communities-and-businesses* [Accessed June 16, 2014]); *Mass Fatalities: The Chief Coroner's Role*, 23 July 2014. See also e.g. from the International Red Cross: *http://www.icrc.org/eng/assets/files/other/icrc_002_0880.pdf* [Accessed June 16, 2014].

[2] See, e.g. Doyle and Bolster (1992) 32 Med. Sci. & Law 5; Busuttil and Jones (1992) 32 Med. Sci. & Law, 9; Report of the National Working Party, *Dealing with Fatalities during Disasters* (October 1994); Report of the Department of Health Working Party, *Disaster: Planning for a Caring Response* (1991).

[3] See 17–66 below.

[4] e.g. the Indian Ocean tsunami of 2004 or the Sharm El-Sheikh bombings of 2005.

17–04   The coroner's actions will be governed by two factors:

(1) The number of casualties, both dead and injured; even a low death toll with many injured will create difficulties in identification of the deceased.

(2) The extent of the surrounding inquiry into the incident.

However, the coroner must also bear in mind that, in a busy coroner's district, the ordinary business of death continues, and a service needs to be provided, at least during working hours. So some resources must be kept back for this.

CADRE OF DVI CORONERS

17–05   As a belated response to the London bombings of 2005, the Government sought to form a group of coroners with special training for dealing with major disasters. Unfortunately the resources available for this training were modest at the outset, and have been diminishing ever since. Moreover, the Government's view as to what such coroners could achieve when a disaster took place outside their own districts was muddled and incoherent.[5] But the creation of such a group (or cadre) was nevertheless a considerable step forward. There are currently 22 such coroners in England and Wales,[6] and they are known as the Cadre of DVI[7] Coroners.[8] When a disaster occurs, a cadre coroner should be able, and will be expected, to advise and work with the local (sometimes called "incident") coroner, if called upon to do so.

17–06   The advice could cover (amongst other things):

(i) the opening and running of an emergency mortuary;[9]

(ii) interaction with other emergency and contributory services;

(iii) the possibility of the transfer of the coroner's jurisdiction in respect of some or all of the victims to another coroner area;[10]

(iv) guidance on practical aspects of procedures, including CBRN, and legislation such as the Human Tissue Act 2004;[11]

(v) the working of the "identification commission" and the criteria that might be used to establish the identification of individual victims;[12]

---

[5] At the time there was no power for the government (or anyone else) to appoint a coroner to deal with a disaster over the head of the coroner for that district. See now 4–22.

[6] In the nature of things, however, most of them have never been involved in a major disaster. But they have at least been trained.

[7] "Disaster Victim Identification".

[8] See *UK DVI-Cadre of Advisory Coroners, Terms of Reference,* 2008, agreed between the Home Office and the Coroners' Society of England and Wales.

[9] See 17–23ff.

[10] See 17–07 ff.

[11] See 17–19—17–20.

[12] See 17–47.

(vi) liaison with local and regional authorities, government departments, and ministers.

However, unless and until the local coroner and the cadre coroner agree a   **17–07** transfer of jurisdiction,[13] or the Chief Coroner exercises his power to transfer responsibility for the inquiry to a cadre (or indeed, any other) coroner,[14] the local coroner will retain coronial responsibility for what happens. Indeed, only the local coroner may make decisions; the cadre coroner can only *advise*. The local coroner can no more delegate his or her powers to the cadre coroner than to a coroner's officer.[15] If the local coroner wishes the cadre coroner to act directly in respect of the incident, either the relevant authority of the local coroner will need to appoint the cadre coroner as an assistant coroner (and offer terms, including remuneration),[16] or there will need to be a transfer of jurisdiction.

There are important differences between these two possibilities. If the local   **17–08** coroner and the cadre coroner agree a transfer of jurisdiction,[17] or if the Chief Coroner directs that a cadre coroner being a coroner for a different area than the local coroner should conduct the investigations and any inquests,[18] then in the administrative sense they move to the new coroner's own area (even if, nowadays, investigations and inquests physically can still be run from the original area),[19] and the costs fall thereafter entirely on the authorities which finance the cadre coroner so appointed.

If, on the other hand, the relevant authority appoints a cadre coroner as an   **17–09** assistant coroner for this purpose, the investigations and any inquests (and all their costs) remain in the original coroner area. These costs will be very significant.[20] This means that the coroners concerned will not agree a transfer of jurisdiction, and the Chief Coroner is unlikely to exercise his power to transfer jurisdiction, without first consulting all the persons affected.

CONTINGENCY PLANNING

Although the responsibility for ordering the necessary examinations of a body and   **17–10** inquiring into every violent or unnatural death is vested in the coroner, and no other person may interfere with those investigations, there are many agencies who will be involved in the immediate aftermath of a major disaster, such as the police, the fire brigade, the ambulance and hospital services, government departments, the Health and Safety Executive, perhaps the coastguard, and so on. In order therefore to be prepared to deal with major incidents there has to be contingency planning.

---

[13] See 4–19.
[14] See 4–22; see also *Mass Fatalities: The Chief Coroner's Role*
[15] See 2–142.
[16] See 2–18, 2–27.
[17] See 4–19 ff.
[18] See 4–22.
[19] See 4–28—4–30, 10–16.
[20] See 17–58.

17–11   The Civil Contingencies Act 2004 makes fresh provision[21] for (i) planning for and (ii) reactions to emergencies (as defined). Part 1 of the 2004 Act is entitled "Local arrangements for civil protection".[22] It places a complex duty (which may be modified by subordinate legislation) on local authorities and others, including NHS and other medical agencies, police and emergency services, and public utilities, *but not coroners*, (a) to assess the risk of an "emergency" occurring, and (b) to plan for this.[23]

17–12   An "emergency" is defined in detail,[24] but broadly refers to things which threaten "serious damage" to human welfare or the environment in, or the security of, the United Kingdom. The threat may come from inside or outside the United Kingdom.[25] But the notion of "damage to human welfare" is restricted to a number of matters, including loss of human life.[26] There is also a restriction on the meaning of "damage to the environment".[27] In relation to threats to security, these are restricted to those from war or terrorism.

17–13   The persons on whom this duty is placed are divided into two groups: "Category 1 Responders" and "Category 2 Responders".[28] In broad terms, the public utilities and the HSE are Category 2 Responders, and the others are Category 1 Responders. There are special provisions for Scotland and Wales, and for cross-border collaboration with Scotland. The duties cast on Responders have been qualified and fleshed out to some extent by regulations.[29] The coroner is not a Responder, but should nevertheless play a part in such planning.

17–14   There are special rules requiring contingency planning for persons using or transporting radioactive substances, and their relevant local authorities.[30] The coroner must be aware exactly where he stands in relation to all of these. He must keep copies of the plans available in more than one place, in case his only copy is located within the affected zone. The assistant coroners must be sufficiently trained and informed to be able, at a moment's notice, to perform the coroner's role in his absence.

17–15   Because disasters and major incidents vary so much, in size, intensity and location, there is a danger that too detailed or rigid a plan may be thrown into confusion by the impossibility of implementing some elements. On the other hand, a plan that leaves too much to be decided for the first time when the incident occurs is no plan at all, and risks wasting precious time and resources. A good plan ensures that the essential elements are prepared in advance—or at least considered,

---

[21] Replacing the Civil Defence Act 1948, the Civil Protection in Peacetime Act 1986, and regulations made thereunder.

[22] It partly came into force on April 1, 2005 (see SI 2005/772, dealing with the repeal of provisions concerning the civil defence grant), and partly on July 22 and November 14, 2005, and May 15, 2006 (see SI 2005/2040, dealing with the remainder of Pt 1, except provisions dealing with the functions of Scottish Ministers).

[23] Civil Contingencies Act 2004 s.2 and Sch.1.

[24] Civil Contingencies Act 2004 s.1.

[25] Civil Contingencies Act 2004 s.1(5).

[26] Civil Contingencies Act 2004 s.1(2).

[27] Civil Contingencies Act 2004 s.1(3).

[28] Civil Contingencies Act 2004 s.3(4), (5).

[29] See the Civil Contingencies Act 2004 (Contingency Planning) Regulations 2004 (SI 2005/2042), which came into force on November 14, 2005. They do not refer to coroners.

[30] The Radiation (Emergency Preparedness and Public Information) Regulations 2001 (SI 2001/2001) regs 7–13.

so as not to be forgotten in the heat of the moment—whilst retaining the flexibility to adapt to changing circumstances.

From the coroner's point of view, the elements that must be considered, if not decided upon, in advance will include: **17–16**

(a) co-ordination of the various systems;

(b) communications;

(c) recovery and removal of bodies;

(d) continuity of evidence;

(e) mortuary facilities;

(f) pathology services;

(g) identification of the dead;

(h) dealing with relatives;

(i) dealing with the media;

(j) dealing with the Chief Coroner and the Government.

Police co-ordination

Even though there may be no suspicion of crime, most immediate reports of major incidents are received through the police force, which arranges to co-ordinate the other rescue services. In addition to the police, the fire brigade, the health services and rescue services and the local authorities may have to take immediate action. Although the contingency plan and all training should try to ensure that evidence is not lost or destroyed for the subsequent inquiry, for this may save lives in the future, the immediate concern is to save lives now and to contain the disaster. **17–17**

Communication and common strategy

The first problem that will arise for all concerned is likely to be the difficulty of communication. Initial reports may be wildly inaccurate. Telephone lines and radio frequencies can be swamped in a few minutes.[31] There will be no chain of command as yet. Here lies the first importance of everybody following the same contingency plan. In flooding, explosion or earthquake, the roads may be blocked, and travel will be made difficult by the emergency services and sightseers. The scene of the incident will be chaotic, and perhaps inaccessible at first. In appropriate cases, satellite telephony should be considered. The mobile telephones of the coroner, assistant coroners and officers should be registered by the police under the MTPAS procedure to give them transmitter priority.[32] Police will **17–18**

---

[31] The Home Office Large Major Enquiry System 2 ("Holmes 2") is a second-generation computer system with many investigation management systems: see *http://www.holmes2.com/holmes2/whatish2/HOLMES2.pdf* [Accessed June 16, 2014]. One is a casualty bureau function to allow other police forces to assist in the immediate aftermath of a disaster by taking public calls, with the same access to information as the main force dealing.

[32] MTPAS stands for "mobile telecommunications privileged access scheme".

establish a casualty bureau, away from the scene, to deal with relatives and the public.[33]

Recovery and removal of bodies

17–19   The contingency plan will have to deal with the recovery and removal of dead bodies. Thought must be given to the need for personnel to carry out this difficult and often distressing physical task. Usually the police take it on.[34] In some disasters, bodies may be lying in the districts of several coroners.[35] Alternatively, parts of some bodies may be recovered from different places, perhaps scattered over a wide area. A decision may have to be taken at an early stage by each coroner involved as to whether (a) to remove the bodies to his or her own mortuary and then decide whether to transfer jurisdiction to one of the several coroners concerned,[36] or (b) to take all the bodies to one central mortuary. The former involves the potential scattering of information, the diffusion of resources, potential extra distress to relatives, and an overall increase in security risk. But it is sometimes unavoidable.

17–20   The circumstances will usually suggest the correct action. One factor will be whether the deaths occurred separately, in different places, or in a single incident or single place. Widespread flooding from a tidal surge, for instance, would usually suggest that bodies should go to the nearest mortuary that can be used. Bodies recovered from an aeroplane crash would be taken to a single mortuary for identification from the passenger lists. Where (as happens in violent crashes and explosions), limbs and other body parts become disrupted or detached, it is essential that (i) each individual body part is *separately* retrieved, detailed and stored, and (ii) all the body parts (and bodies) go to the same mortuary. Proper labelling is essential.[37] Where survivors die later in hospital, their bodies must go to the temporary mortuary rather than the hospital mortuary, to enable all the victims to be dealt with together.

Continuity of evidence

17–21   The recovery and removal of the bodies will normally be arranged by those working at the scene. Every effort should be made to ensure continuity of evidence. Bodies, parts of bodies and personal effects should be marked with a pre-printed number, to avoid more than one series of labels. The position of the body should be recorded and photographed, if possible. There will be considerable pressure to remove the bodies from the scene. This should not be allowed to prevent the recording of evidence.

17–22   It must be recognised however that bodies may sometimes need to be removed precipitately, to obtain access to wounded who are trapped, and to avoid destruction by fire or other means. Hence, every contingency plan has to be extremely flexible, to cope with every type of disaster and to be able to pick up the

---

[33] See 17–42.
[34] Where CBRN issues arise, specialist advice will be needed first.
[35] In some parts of England and Wales there are memoranda of understanding which deal with agrements to transfer cases so that one coroner deals all the deaths.
[36] See 4–19 ff.
[37] See 17–43.

threads as rescue work progresses. In cases where the coroner's normal staff and premises would be inadequate to deal with the number of fatalities involved, the police will provide teams to assist in running the mortuary and in obtaining information to identify the bodies.[38]

MORTUARY AND OTHER FACILITIES[39]

Basic requirements for temporary mortuaries

A suitable building will be required to act as a temporary (or emergency) mortuary. **17–23** It must be distinguished from any body-holding area established at the site of the incident. Although some cities have capacious public or hospital mortuaries, much of the space may already be in use with the coroner's or hospitals' routine work. Moreover, such mortuaries, by reason of their other work, will be less secure from media and other intrusion. So a dedicated disaster mortuary is preferable, in a location which is capable of being made secure.

A temporary mortuary must: **17–24**

(i) be large enough to accommodate all the bodies, body parts[40] and personal belongings and have additional space for the investigating staff and office staff;

(ii) be available almost instantly for the length of time (sometimes more than a week) needed to complete the investigation and identification of the bodies;

(iii) be accessible to vehicles, preferably with drive-in/drive-out facilities, but not be easily overlooked (e.g. by the media);[41]

(iv) have, or have access to, suitable facilities for personal hygiene (including showers if possible) and refreshment for all the personnel involved;

(v) have some place available where relatives of the deceased may attend to identify the bodies;

(vi) have facilities to provide lighting, power and water.

In addition there will need to be facilities nearby (but preferably in separate **17–25** places from each other) which can be used:

(vii) as a reception centre for relatives;

---

[38] See 17–42 (casualty bureau), 17–47 ff (identification evidence).
[39] See, generally, the Royal College of Pathologists' *Deaths in Major Disasters—the Pathologists' Role,* 2nd edn (2000).
[40] Each body part must be treated as a separate body, and this means that much more space is needed for a given number of bodies which have been disrupted (e.g. by explosion) than for the same number of bodies which have not.
[41] A limited window area is therefore desirable.

(viii) as a reception centre/enquiry office for the media;

(ix) (if the coroner's own offices are distant) as office space for the coroner and his officer(s).

Each of these will need good communications facilities, and the first two will need, or need to have access to, refreshment facilities. It goes without saying that the mortuary, relatives' and media centres and coroner's offices will need unimpeded 24-hour access.

17–26   **Drainage.** The problem of drainage may need special consultation with health and safety inspectors. Effluent could be treated and removed, if necessary. An empty industrial hangar or warehouse usually has all these facilities.

17–27   **Equipment.** The provision of equipment does not normally present a problem. Folding tables covered with thick polythene sheeting have been used. Industrial grade plastic sheeting, though slippery when wet, produces an impermeable floor that can be taken up and disinfected. Heavy lifting equipment, water pumps, emergency lighting and even generators to operate it, must be traced at short notice. Mobile X-ray equipment will be essential in cases of explosion or other penetrating injuries. A photocopier will also be very useful, as many documents will need to be copied.

Reconnaissance and review of available locations

17–28   The need for contingency planning is illustrated by the above requirements. Suitable premises must have been inspected and recorded. The list must be kept up to date, as once-empty industrial premises may subsequently be brought into use and thus not be available when needed. Equipment must be obtainable from a source that is available at all times. There is no need to stockpile equipment that has a regular use. Body bags will deteriorate with time, and the depots may be widely dispersed. Plastic sheeting is used regularly and can be used for a multitude of purposes, including wrapping the bodies, but a ready source must have been identified in advance. Ideally, a list of all such sources of equipment would be held on a national computer, but there is no such facility as yet.

17–29   Essentially there will be up to five different scenes of action which the coroner must plan for: (i) the incident location itself, (ii) the temporary mortuary, (iii) a body holding area, (iv) the family reception centre and (v) the media centre. Failure to prepare for and adequately manage any of these may lead to mistakes being made. The security of the first and second is normally a matter for the police, who may also be involved as "gatekeepers" in relation to the others. The lead pathologist, in conjunction with the coroner, will manage the second. Local authority social services or voluntary organisations may be persuaded to deal with the fourth. The fifth is problematic. If the local authority has a media or public relations department, it may be appropriate for its personnel to set up and run the media centre. The coroner will probably need to be in contact with all five. A reliable mobile telephone or two-way radio will be essential.

Family needs[42]

It is particularly important, for the proper public perception and understanding of **17–30** what is going on, and why, that the families of the deceased and the media be given (separately) all appropriate assistance and information. Official updates at regular intervals will be important. The presence of relatives enables information (e.g. for identification purposes) to be gathered quickly by the so-called "ante-mortem" team, i.e. police of coroner's officers designated to interview relatives and obtain other useful information about the deceased. It will be desirable to draw up (and enforce) guidelines on media activity, especially in respect of contact with families. Where victims came from other countries, the cultural and linguistic needs of their relatives—and the foreign media who will also be interested—must not be forgotten.

Families will be under immense stress before it is confirmed that their relative is **17–31** amongst the dead. They will usually want an authoritative statement (confirmation *or* exclusion) as soon as possible. Once it is confirmed, they will want the body released as soon as possible. In the meantime they will seek information on what is going on, how long it will take, and why. Where families are from abroad, their diplomatic representatives in the UK will also be involved. Some of these are experienced at dealing with coroners' inquests. Others, however, are not. In addition, there are significant cultural differences, and even sometimes a competitive edge between different diplomatic missions.

But, in addition to these general matters, the families may have specific concerns **17–32** about matters such as the following:

(i) why they cannot visit the site of the incident;

(ii) why bodies are not being removed from the scene, or not faster;

(iii) why bodies are taken to the temporary mortuary rather than a public or hospital mortuary;

(iv) whether (and when) they will be able to view the body of their relative, and, if not, why not;

(v) how a positive identification can be made in the absence of their viewing the body;

(vi) why bodies are not being released faster;

(vii) how the incident occurred.

With the exception of the last, which obviously depends on the particular circumstances, it may be possible to prepare in advance material which, in addition to giving general information about the role of the coroner, provides answers to at least some of the other questions above.

---

[42] See ACPO, *Humanitarian assistance in Emergencies Guidance on Establishing Family Assistance Centres*, and London Resilience Team, *London Family Assistance Centre, Provisional Guidance Document* (2006).

The media

17–33 The media will have quite different concerns. They will be looking to obtain regular supplies of relevant, new and interesting information, preferably accurate. They have deadlines to meet, for publication or broadcast (it should of course be borne in mind that foreign media will have different deadlines to domestic). They will be expecting press conferences and interviews. Those expectations need to be managed. Pre-printed information, distributed in "media packs", about the role (and limitations) of the inquiry, the need to respect families' privacy and grief, and so on, is highly desirable. Above all, the media must be treated equally: no one should obtain special treatment. If need be, a "pool" can be established, whereby representatives obtain information or photographs to be made available to all. The coroner must keep firm control of the situation,[43] but it is generally better to see the media as a positive opportunity, rather than as a negative threat.

The Chief Coroner and the Government

17–34 The Chief Coroner has important powers, including that of transferring jurisdiction to another coroner area,[44] and also that of obtaining information about investigations from the coroner concerned.[45] As an experienced judge, the Chief Coroner will know instinctively not to interfere with judicial decision-making by the local coroner, but will be able to give appropriate advice and support where needed.

17–35 The Government however is in the opposite position. Ministers have no power to require the coroner to provide information about current investigations, or to interfere with them. But they are accountable to the electorate, and will be anxiously concerned with the Government's image as it reacts to the emergency, and will seek information and to influence the coroner as the matter progresses. The coroner must resist such pressure, but would do well not to upset the Government unnecessarily, as the relevant authority may wish to invite the Government to fund all or part of the investigations, especially if they are long and protracted and result from a national rather than merely local disaster.[46]

17–36 All these pressures, especially in a large-scale incident, will make it likely that the coroner cannot manage on his own. If the assistant coroners for the area are available, it may be desirable to allocate them specific responsibilities. After all, they have the legal power to make decisions when the senior coroner is absent or unavailable, or when the senior coroner otherwise consents.[47] (But the ordinary work of the area must also be carried on, so someone will need to attend to that.) Alternatively, a cadre coroner or the coroner, or assistant coroner, from a nearby area may be prepared to assist. All the better if such coroner has (or they have) experience of major incidents.

---

[43] Without necessarily giving personal briefings, for example.
[44] See 4–22.
[45] See 2–62; see also *Mass Fatalites: The Chief Coroner's Role*.
[46] See 17–58.
[47] Coroners and Justice Act 2009 s.23, Sch.3 para.8; see 2–16.

THE COURSE OF THE INQUIRY

Although it is tempting to think of a single coronial investigation into a major   **17–37**
disaster, despite the fact that there are many dead, this is wrong. Each death requires
a separate investigation, even though conducted simultaneously with all the others.
Each such investigation follows the normal legal requirements to find out who the
deceased persons were, and how, when and where they came by their deaths.[48]

But the circumstances are at the same time extraordinary. Because the coroner   **17–38**
will need to move around from place to place, dealing with many different aspects
of the disaster inquiry, but will be constantly sought by telephone and email for
discussion and decisions, it is highly desirable that he or she has a reliable personal
assistant or clerk with him or her at all times, so as to be able to field calls and refer
emails, to record decisions and to implement them. Otherwise there is a danger of
mistakes being made and matters being overlooked.

The legal requirements overlap in three phases: **17–39**

(1) the identification of the bodies;

(2) the immediate cause of the individual deaths;

(3) the circumstances and cause of the incident that caused the deaths.

Of these three phases, the coroner's role in (3) is likely to be nil at the outset,   **17–40**
and even later it may be small, as other experts (e.g. railway, shipping or aviation
investigators) will concentrate on this. His role in (2) will only occupy more than
a minimal amount of time where the causes of death are not obvious. Accordingly,
the bulk of his efforts will be directed towards (1). However, since the deaths will
not have been natural, an inquest will have to be opened in respect of each as soon
as is reasonably practicable.[49]

Identification

Identification is of course necessary to enable families to have their dead returned   **17–41**
to them for the purposes of a funeral. But identification of all the bodies will also
be an important part of the investigation. A key operator, such as the pilot of an
aeroplane, may have suffered a heart attack. Some deceased may have missile
injuries. It is essential to know who they were and where they were when the
injury was inflicted. Some victims may escape unhurt, some may be injured and
some killed. It may be important to know where they were placed to receive or
escape injury.

Establishment of a casualty bureau

In the initial stages of the disaster, the police will establish a casualty bureau. This   **17–42**
is usually a telephone exchange, or interconnected exchanges, usually away from
the scene, as the communications facilities there will be unable to cope. This
bureau takes information from the public, asking for particulars of all people who

---

[48] See 13–01 above.
[49] Coroners (Inquests) Rules 2013 (SI 2013/1616) r.5(1); see 10–05.

are known or believed to be missing. As a result of the introduction of the police major incident computer system, HOLMES II,[50] police forces nationwide can establish satellite bureaux to assist the force actually dealing.[51] As survivors make contact with families, the multitude of inquiries will reduce to those concerning persons who are dead or unable to communicate in hospital. But it is not the bureau's purpose to collect the detailed information needed for identification. This is the job of the so-called "ante-mortem" team, which may be based in the family reception centre.

Transportation of bodies

17–43   The bodies are transported, either from the incident site directly, or via the body holding area, to the mortuary. It takes time to collect and move a large number, and they will not all arrive at the same time. They will be received by the "post-mortem" team. If the bodies have not been numbered at the scene, they are numbered at the mortuary. If there are several sequences of numbers, then they are renumbered, starting at a high number such as 1,000. This also avoids the problems of numbers being read upside down (86/98, 19/61, etc.). Property on or with the body is similarly numbered. The clothing, property and external appearance of the body is recorded on a specially designed form.

Examination of bodies

17–44   The body may be X-rayed and photographed. It is then examined by the pathologist and any specimens that are required are taken. The teeth are inspected and the details of the dentition recorded.

Collation of available information on affected parties

17–45   At the same time, details of the possessions, appearance, scars, tattoos, operations and dental records of all the persons known to be missing, or on a passenger list, are recorded by the ante-mortem team on another specially designed form. The object is to match the forms to complete a positive identification.

Evidence of cause of death

17–46   As stated above[52] the pathological examination will be directed to finding the medical cause of the death and to seeking evidence, such as fragments of missiles, to show how the incident was caused. The type of pathologist required will vary according to the circumstances.[53] The examination may show a pattern of injuries that will be of future use in preventing similar injuries.

Identification evidence

17–47   An "identification commission" may be established,[54] consisting of the coroner (or assistant coroner), a senior police officer, a senior pathologist, representatives of the

---

[50] See *http://www.holmes2.com/holmes2/whatish2/HOLMES2.pdf* [Accessed June 16, 2014].
[51] See 17–18.
[52] See 17–39—17–41.
[53] See 17–53 ff.
[54] See the Metropolitan Police document, *Identification of the Deceased Following Mass Disaster* (January 1994). The position with regard to DNA has, of course, moved on considerably since then.

ante-mortem and post-mortem teams, and other experts. It will monitor the progress of identification evidence in relation to each body. But the ultimate decision as to whether sufficient evidence has been obtained formally to identify the body is for the coroner alone, considering the matter at a later stage. Thus it does not matter if the coroner sitting on the commission is not the local coroner or assistant coroner, because the decision at that stage has no legal force.

Fingerprints and odontology were the original failsafes here. Fingerprints from available digits could be matched against police records, but also against prints found at the home of a suspected victim. Teeth tended to survive explosions and fires, and could be matched against dental records. Now they have been joined by DNA profiling,[55] though this takes more time, and is relatively more expensive. Blood groupings, personal effects (especially jewellery) and distinctive clothing are also useful.[56] Information about a missing person will be obtained from the relatives by the ante-mortem team, information about the deceased person from the post-mortem team. Evidence of tattoos, old operations or wounds, or even some medical conditions, may also assist. **17–48**

Direct visual identification of the deceased *may* be possible in some cases. Using information thus acquired, and also photographs, it may be possible to ensure that the family are shown the deceased to confirm the identification. Ideally two or three viewing rooms (e.g. portacabins) should be available next to, but not in, the mortuary. Taking relatives into a large area where many bodies are visible should be avoided. In many cases of disaster victims, visual identification is not reliable, as a result of the combination of (a) sudden distress to relatives and (b) severe trauma to the deceased. Even where there is no trauma, mistakes can still be made. But relatives will probably want to do everything to help, and also to see the deceased—however disfigured—as part of the bereavement process. **17–49**

A sometimes useful technique is to photograph every victim's face and in the first instance show relatives the photograph corresponding to the most likely body, according to the available information, including any photographs supplied by relatives. If the identification is positive, the relatives can be taken to see the body. This renders less likely the possible need for the relatives to view more than one body. In cases of fire, where the bodies look alike, identification from dental records or DNA (inside the teeth) may be the only positive means, teeth being extremely resistant to heat. **17–50**

Release of bodies

There will be pressure upon the coroner for the early release of bodies to the families. The rules for this are the same as in any other case,[57] and the body must be released as soon as reasonably practicable.[58] However, the coroner must not be too precipitate in releasing a body, as examination of a subsequent body may sometimes cast doubt on an earlier identification. The consequences of a mistake, **17–51**

---

[55] There may be a policy question here, as to the minimum size of body part which is separately collected and so identified.

[56] But in some disasters they can become separated from their owner, so care must be taken.

[57] See Ch.9.

[58] Coroners (Investigations) Regulations 2013 (SI 2013/1629) reg.20(1); see 8–11—8–12, 9–14.

particularly when—as is now common—dealing with victims from several countries, can be devastating for the families concerned.[59]

17-52 Where the bodies are not identified, or where further examination is needed, it may be necessary to preserve the body. Embalming is the easiest method, but it destroys any prospect of future toxicology. Some mortuaries have a facility for lowering the temperature and preserving the body. Bodies may be transferred to another mortuary or commercial refrigerators. Containers for transporting frozen meat have been used on occasion. Where inquests have been opened and bodies can be released, but relatives are not yet in a position to take them (e.g. funeral directors not yet instructed or arrived), it may be desirable to move bodies to the public mortuary with their documentation, for collection there. This will reduce congestion at the temporary mortuary.

PATHOLOGY[60]

Availability of experienced pathologists

17-53 The choice of suitable pathologists must have been considered in advance. In many cases (e.g. explosions) forensic pathologists will be needed. In other cases (e.g. a drowning disaster) non-forensic pathologists may be sufficient. Home Office pathologists have been encouraged to enter into contracts with police forces to hold themselves available to examine bodies in cases of major crime and major disasters.

17-54 In cases of aircraft accidents, the Royal Air Force Pathology team from the RAF Institute of Pathology and Tropical Medicine[61] may be able to attend and give advice and assistance. In addition, Army pathologists have had special training and experience in investigating multiple deaths and the interpretation of missile injuries.[62]

17-55 It is not desirable to seek to employ as many pathologists as possible, with a view to reducing the time taken to identify and release bodies, because (i) there is only a limited supply of appropriately qualified pathologists, and the rest of the system has to continue, and (ii) it is better that the pathologists involved should do multiple cases so as to facilitate comparisons.

Availability of mortuary technicians

17-56 In addition to the pathologists, the mortuary team provided by the police should be supplemented by as many experienced mortuary technicians as can be mustered at short notice, although again it must be remembered that the normal work of the hospital and public mortuaries will be continuing.

---

[59] This has happened in reverse, where in a foreign disaster a body has been mis-identified and sent to the UK for funeral purposes.

[60] See generally the Royal College of Pathologists' *Deaths in Major Disasters—The Pathologists' Role,* 2nd edn (2000), also available online at *www.rcpath.org* [Accessed June 16, 2014]

[61] See 8–47.

[62] Contact the Royal Army Medical College, Millbank, London SW1P 4RJ, Tel: 020 7930 4466.

Use of forensic odontologists

Where the identification of the bodies may require comparison of the teeth found   **17-57**
with the body and dental charts kept by the dentist in private practice during life,
specialist forensic odontologists will need to be available to examine the teeth and
to make the comparison.

COSTS

Although the costs of the coronial investigation of a small incident in which one   **17-58**
or two people die may not exceed the usual costs for other inquiries, the costs of
a coronial inquiry for a major disaster, with all the associated pathology, mortuary,
family and media costs, as well as the cost of the inquests themselves, may run into
millions of pounds.[63] Where the disaster is of national proportions, the relevant
authority may consider that funding such an inquiry is something for national
rather than local government, particularly where the causes of the incident or the
lessons to be learned are national rather than local. The law however is clear: the
liability for costs is local.[64] If national government is to fund all or any part of the
investigation's costs, it will be because someone has persuaded it to do so. In the
case of the London bombings of 2005,[65] this took until October 2009 to
achieve.

CO-ORDINATION WITH OTHER INQUIRIES

While the examination of the bodies is the responsibility of the coroner alone, with   **17-59**
consultation with the police in possible homicide cases,[66] the coroner will have to
act in liaison with other investigators, who will be examining the evidence for their
own, specialist, purposes. These include Inspectors of Marine Accidents,[67]
Inspectors of Air Accidents,[68] Health and Safety Inspectors[69] and specially
appointed boards of inquiry.

Some of these inquiries may be held privately. Some may be in public. They   **17-60**
rarely have the scope of the coroner's inquest, and there may be certain classes of
people who would be considered interested persons for the purposes of an
inquest[70] but who would not have a right to be heard at the inquiry. The outcome

---

[63] For example the costs of the inquests (not including the pathology and other immediate services
    provided), held in 2010–11, into the London bombings 2005 amounted to some £4.6 million. The
    costs of the inquests into the deaths of Diana, Princess of Wales, and Dodi Fayed, in 2007–08,
    exceeded £4.7 million.
[64] See 2–90, 10–17, 18–43.
[65] See   *http://webarchive.nationalarchives.gov.uk/20120216072438/http:/7julyinquests.independent.gov.uk/*
    [Accessed June 16, 2014].
[66] Coroners (Investigations) Regulations 2013 (SI 2013/1629) reg.12; see 8–48, 14–06 above.
[67] Merchant Shipping Act 1995 s.267.
[68] Civil Aviation (Investigation of Air Accidents and Incidents) Regulations 1996 (SI 1996/2798)
    reg.8.
[69] Health and Safety at Work etc. Act 1974 s.19.
[70] See 8–22.

of such inquiries will be of considerable assistance to the coroner in conducting the inquest. They may avoid the need to take evidence from all the witnesses on several occasions, thus saving time, resources and distress.

17–61   In the past the main problem for the coroner lay in coordinating the inquest with one of the specially appointed inquiries, usually set up by a government department. The inquiry is usually headed by a judge or senior lawyer, with a panel of persons with special knowledge sitting as a team. There is usually a counsel to the inquiry, who presents the case for the inquiry. Parties are represented by lawyers and question witnesses. The system is still, basically, adversarial. If some line of inquiry is not in the interests of any of the parties, then it may not be pursued. This must be contrasted with the inquest, where no case is presented until after all the evidence has been heard. Now the law is that if the Lord Chancellor informs the coroner that a judicial public inquiry is proceeding into the disaster, the coroner must normally adjourn the inquest.[71] So conflict is minimised.

Holding the Inquest

17–62   There will be one combined hearing for the inquests into the individual deaths of all the victims, much of the evidence being of course common to all. It is not normally possible for the coroner to combine the inquest with any other inquiry, as the inquest will in practice have to be heard before a jury.[72] In any event the personnel and procedure involved in the other inquiry will be different from that of an inquest.

17–63   The standard practice is for the coroner to open the inquest and then adjourn it.[73] In addition to the case where there is a public inquiry, and the inquest is adjourned[74] where a person is charged with an indictable offence relating to the deaths, then the inquest may have to be adjourned pending the charge.[75] If there is no such charge, then the coroner awaits the outcome of the other inquiry, and then summons a jury.

Evidence and procedure

17–64   Much of the evidence may be given by expert witnesses and the inquest can also deal with matters that were not covered by the inquiry. In principle, the procedure at the inquest is the same as at any other inquest,[76] due allowance being made for the special circumstances. The usual court accommodation may be insufficient for the numbers of persons wishing (and entitled) to attend, and other accommodation may need to be obtained.[77] In the biggest and most serious cases, the documents

---

[71] See 10–81.
[72] See 10–34.
[73] See 10–04 ff; see also *Mass Fatalities: The Chief Coroner's Role.*
[74] See 17–61.
[75] See 10–75 ff.
[76] See Chs 10–13.
[77] See 10–16 ff..

relevant to the inquest, and transcripts evidence given at it, have been made publicly available on a special inquest website.[78]

MULTIPLE DEATHS BY HOMICIDE

The relationship between the coroner and the prosecuting authorities is the same   **17–65**
in multiple deaths as in a single death.[79] The requirement for consultation with the chief officer of police on the choice of a suitable pathologist[80] applies, although the connection between the act causing the deaths (such as planting a bomb in an aircraft) and the nature of the injuries may be less direct than that of a homicide by direct confrontation. Therefore the problems of retaining bodies for subsequent examinations on behalf of the defendants may not be so acute as in a direct killing. There may be a very considerable delay in the decision to prosecute, particularly over such charges as corporate manslaughter.

Where a person is charged with causing death by murder, manslaughter, causing   **17–66**
death by dangerous driving, or causing death by careless driving when under the influence of drink or drugs, the inquest is adjourned in the usual way.[81] However, that person may not be charged with causing all the deaths, and only specimen charges may be brought. In order to enable the other deaths to be registered without delay, the coroner must consult with the Crown Prosecution Service to provide all relevant information.[82] This may enable the inquest to be adjourned and the deaths registered in those remaining cases, where a person has been charged with an offence committed in circumstances connected with the death of the deceased.

This modification of the law was introduced in 1977 to avoid the problems that   **17–67**
had been encountered where there had been multiple deaths from terrorist bombs. The inquest is opened, evidence is given to link the multiple deaths with those that are the subject of the charge or charges, the information from the Crown Prosecution Services is produced, usually in written form, and the inquests are adjourned. The deaths are registered and, upon the conclusion of the criminal proceedings, the registrar of death is notified of the outcome.[83]

---

[78] See   e.g.   *http://webarchive.nationalarchives.gov.uk/20090607230252/http:/www.scottbaker-inquests-.gov.uk/*   [Accessed   June   16,   2014]   and   *http://webarchive.nationalarchives.gov.uk/20120216072438/http:/7julyinquests.independent.gov.uk/* [Accessed June 16, 2014].
[79] See 14–27 ff.
[80] See 8–48, 14–06.
[81] See 10–75 ff, 14–17.
[82] See 10–78, 10–80, 10–82.
[83] Births and Deaths Registration Act 1953, s.23 (2B). See 14–17, 18–17.

17–68   The same procedure can be used where a person has been injured and dies subsequently, although there may have to be a separate inquest if there is any evidence that one of the deaths was not a direct consequence of the criminal act. In such a case, the inquest may still have been adjourned[84] in order to avoid the publication of any evidence at an inquest that might prejudice the criminal trial.[85] The inquest would then be resumed after the trial was completed. In such a case the coroner would comply with the relevant provisions.[86]

---

[84] Under Sch.1 para 1(2)(b), (3)(b), 2(4), (5), or 5.
[85] See 11–47 ff, 14–30.
[86] See 10–83 ff.

Part V

AFTER THE INQUEST

Chapter 18

MATTERS AFTER THE INQUIRY

FUNCTUS OFFICIO

A coroner's power to inquire into a particular death is not general, or capable of **18–01** exercise from time to time. Instead, it is limited, and in the absence of statutory or judicial authority can be exercised once only. Investigation into that death having been completed by holding an inquest, the coroner no longer has jurisdiction to inquire further into it: in the old Latin expression, the coroner is functus officio.[1] Although this is a convenient shorthand, it must be borne in mind that it does not necessarily mean that all powers of the coroner have ceased in relation to the particular death; usually it means only that the power to conduct an investigation or hold an inquest has ceased. Other powers (e.g. correction of errors in certificates, exhumation, and so on) are usually still exercisable. But a coroner who attempts to conduct a second investigation or hold a second inquest into a particular death, without first having been ordered to do so by the court,[2] will be restrained from so doing.[3] There is no necessity for the first inquest to have been held by the same coroner, as long as the first coroner had jurisdiction to inquire.[4]

Prior inquest pursuant to English and Welsh coroner legislation

This rule postulates a prior investigation held pursuant to the English and Welsh **18–02** coroner legislation.[5] It is therefore clear that, where a body is brought back to England and Wales from abroad, the coroner in whose area the body lies is not functus officio merely by reason that some official inquiry has taken place in the foreign country where the deceased died.[6] No inquest pursuant to the English and Welsh legislation having yet taken place, the coroner has jurisdiction to, and indeed must, inquire if the statutory criteria are, or are reasonably believed to be, satisfied.[7]

---

[1] *R. v White* (1860) 3 E. & E. 137; 121 E.R. 394; *Terry v East Sussex Coroner* [2002] Q.B. 312 at [4]; see also *X v Deputy State Coroner for New South Wales* [2001] NSWSC 46; *Baxendale-Walker v Law Society* [2006] EWHC 643 (Admin.) (not a coroner's case); *Re McDonnell's Application* [2014] NIQB 66 (no power to revisit procedural rulings after inquest concluded).

[2] See 19–05, 19–65 below.

[3] *R. v White* (1860) 3 E. & E. 137; 121 E.R. 394.

[4] *R. v West Yorkshire Coroner Ex p. Smith* [1983] Q.B. 335, DC.

[5] Now the Coroners and Justice Act 2009; formerly the Coroners Act 1988, and before that the Coroners Act 1887 and the Coroners (Amendment) Act 1926.

[6] In some countries this may be an inquest on the English model: see Ch.21 below.

[7] See 5–01 above.

This must logically apply even in the case of an inquest held by a coroner in Northern Ireland[8] or a fatal accident inquiry in Scotland,[9] where the body of the deceased subsequently comes to lie in England and Wales.

18–03   The Home Office view was that "it is possible to maintain" that in such circumstances the coroner in England and Wales has no jurisdiction to act, the inquest or inquiry in Northern Ireland or Scotland having satisfied the public interest in inquiring into the death for all parts of the United Kingdom.[10] Whatever the merits of this view as a policy, it is not consistent with legal authority. The rule is that "a coroner cannot hold a second inquest while the first is existing"[11] or, as it was expressed more recently:

> "once an inquest has been held pursuant to the statute, no other coroner will have jurisdiction to hold a further inquest in relation to that body unless and until the verdict of the first inquiry has been set aside."[12]

The reference in each case is to a prior English or Welsh inquest, and not a foreign inquiry. Primary legislation will be needed to alter the position. The coroner reforms of 2013 have made no attempt to do so.

18–04   It should also be borne in mind that the body may be released in Scotland or Northern Ireland for disposal in England and Wales *before* the fatal accident inquiry or inquest is concluded in the country of origin. In such a case the coroner in England and Wales will (assuming the relevant criteria to be satisfied) have to conduct an investigation in any event.[13] But, for the criteria to be satisfied, the coroner must be informed. It is to be noted that, where a certificate for disposal is issued in Scotland or Northern Ireland for use in England and Wales, it is much less likely that the English or Welsh coroner will be informed of the presence of the body before it is disposed of.

At what point does a coroner become functus officio?

18–05   There used to be a question mark as to when exactly a coroner becomes functus officio, in the sense of not being able to inquire further into a death. Before 1927, there was no power to dispense with an inquest where the statutory criteria were satisfied. Nowadays, however, there is a procedure whereby the coroner may direct a post-mortem examination to be made and in some cases thereafter must discontinue the investigation (the so-called "Pink Form B" procedure).[14] But utilising that procedure does not render the coroner then functus officio in relation to that particular death. If he or she thereafter discovers further evidence bringing the case within the statutory criteria for holding an inquest the coroner can and

---

[8] Under the Coroners Act 1959 (N.I.); see 22–12 below.
[9] Under the Fatal Accidents and Sudden Deaths Inquiry (Scotland) Act 1976. See 22–51 below.
[10] Home Office Circular No. 79 of 1983 para.5; Home Office Circular No. 94 of 1985.
[11] *R. v White* (1860) 3 E. & E. 137; 121 E.R. 394, at 144, 397.
[12] *R. v West Yorkshire Coroner Ex p. Smith* [1983] Q.B. 335 at 359.
[13] As indeed happened in relation to the soldiers and civil servants killed in Scotland when their Chinook helicopter crashed on the Mull of Kintyre on June 2, 1994.
[14] See 8–37 above.

must so do without an application to the court having to be made,[15] if the body is still in the coroner area.

A fortiori, a coroner who signs "Pink Form A"[16] to inform the registrar of   **18–06** deaths that he or she does not propose to conduct an investigation or hold an inquest, is not functus officio either. "Pink Form A" is an administrative convenience for the registrar of deaths, and not a substitute for a coronial inquiry. There is no authority on the point, but the position is analogous where the coroner, after suspending an investigation because of criminal proceedings or a public inquiry, firstly decides not to resume, but then subsequently becomes aware of facts constituting sufficient reason for doing so.[17] If any of these cases would otherwise satisfy the criteria, except that the body is by then no longer be in the coroner's area,[18] the coroner cannot inquire without first obtaining from the Chief Coroner a direction to conduct an investigation, but must then do so.[19]

No provision for correction of defective record

If an inquest is held, and subsequently evidence comes to light showing that the   **18–07** record of inquest is wrong in some material respect, the coroner may not correct it on his or her own. If the circumstances justify it, there will have to be an application to the court for an order quashing the determination and findings, and for the conducting of a new investigation.[20] This is subject to two qualifications. First, on judicial review the court in appropriate cases has power at common law to amend a record of inquest to remedy formal defects[21] without the need to conduct another investigation. Secondly, there is a statutory power in the coroner to hold an inquiry to receive evidence for the purpose of correcting a limited range of matters recorded in the certificate after inquest sent to the registrar of deaths. This will not alter the record, but the death will at last be correctly registered. This is dealt with later.[22]

Mistaken identification of the body

Where there has been a mistaken identification of the body, the correct action to   **18–08** be taken by the coroner will depend on the facts. If the coroner has conducted an investigation into a death where the body is that of the person who is the subject of the investigation, but it has been wrongly identified by witnesses at the inquest, and he or she is later informed that the body is in fact that of another person, the

---

[15] *Terry v East Sussex Coroner* [2002] Q.B. 312, CA; Coroners and Justice Act 2009 s.4(3), proviso; *Re Miller's Application for Judicial Review* [2005] NIQB 34; cf. *R. v Avon Coroner Ex p. Smith* (1998) 162 J.P. 403.

[16] See 8–15 above.

[17] Coroners and Justice Act 2009 s.11, Sch.1 para.8; see 10–84.

[18] See 4–02, 5–01.

[19] See 4–12, 4–22, 5–17. The same applies where the death does not come to the coroner's notice until after the body has left the area: see 5–02.

[20] See 19–05, 19–65 below.

[21] See 19–66 ff below. The court may even order the coroner to enter a new conclusion as to death. The statutory power of amendment of an inquisition, in Coroners Act 1887 s.20, was repealed by the Criminal Law Act 1977 s.65(5) and Sch.13 (cf. *R. v Surrey Coroner Ex p. Campbell* [1982] Q.B. 661).

[22] See 18–23.

coroner cannot reopen the inquest as there is no longer any jurisdiction to do so.[23] The coroner could apply to the High Court for the record to be amended, or even for the determination and findings to be quashed.[24] Or, if more appropriate, the statutory power to hold an inquiry could be exercised, with a view to certifying to the Registrar of Deaths that there was an error in the certificate after inquest, namely, that the name of the deceased person was wrongly given.[25]

18–09   If, on the other hand, the coroner has conducted an investigation into a death of a particular person but the wrong body is subjected to post-mortem examination or other procedure, the identity of the deceased will be correctly recorded, but other information such as the cause of death may not be. In such a case the statutory power of subsequent inquiry[26] is unlikely to be available, and the only means of amending the register is to apply for the record to be amended or the determination and findings to be quashed.[27] If the determination and findings are quashed, then at the new inquest the coroner will consider the new information, and then forward a new certificate to the registrar, who will make a fresh entry in the register.[28]

Post-Inquiry Duties

18–10   Despite the fact that a coroner who is functus officio may no longer inquire into a particular death as the subject of an investigation, he or she nonetheless has certain specific duties of an administrative nature in connection with that death, and will also continue to have certain duties of a general nature which will take account of the particular death. The specific duties fall into four main categories: (1) completing and sending to the registrar of deaths the certificate after inquest; (2) completing other, specialised returns; (3) paying fees, allowances and expenses to those entitled to them; and (4) allowing access to and supplying copies of documents, exhibits and other information forming part of the record of the particular inquiry. These will be taken in turn.

Certificate after inquest

18–11   Under the old law before July 25, 2013, it was the duty of the coroner, within five days after the verdict at an inquest held in England and Wales had been given, to send to the appropriate registrar of deaths a certificate giving information concerning the death, including: (1) the particulars required for death registration; (2) the cause of death; and (3) the time and place at which the inquest was held.[29] The form of this certificate was not prescribed, but in practice the forms used were

---

[23] See 18–01.
[24] See 19–65 ff below.
[25] See 18–23.
[26] See 18–23.
[27] See 19–66 ff below.
[28] Births and Deaths Registration Act 1953 s.23(2); *Attorney General v Harte* (1987) 151 J.P. 819.
[29] Coroners Act 1988 s.11(7); Births and Deaths Registration Act 1953 s.23(1).

those supplied to coroners by the Registrar-General.[30] Where a death certificate was to be issued in both English and Welsh, coroners were asked to complete Pt 1 of the form in both languages.[31]

Before 1993, the Registrar-General's Form 99 REV did not explicitly ask the coroner to notify the conclusion as to death. This reflected the fact that the coroner's statutory obligation was only to supply the "cause of death", and not the conclusion as to death.[32] Thereafter, however, without any alteration in the law, the form changed, now asking for the conclusion as to death (calling it "verdict"), though as part of the box headed "cause of death".[33] If the coroner supplied this information, it was recorded on the register and would appear on every copy death certificate thereafter produced. **18–12**

In addition to the statutory information, the form provides for other useful information to be provided, such as whether the coroner has issued a burial order or Form E certificate for cremation.[34] This enables the registrar to carry out his duty to inquire into the disposal of the body in some circumstances. Form 99 REV is also used where an inquest is adjourned under the visiting forces provisions.[35] However, there is no point in sending such a certificate where the death which is the subject of the inquest is not required to be registered. This is the case, for example, where the death occurred outside England and Wales,[36] but the body is brought back there and becomes subject to a coroner's inquiry.[37] **18–13**

The new coroner legislation brought into force in 2013 does not however require the coroner to send a certificate after inquest to the registrar at all. This appears to have been overlooked in the drafting.[38] However, the coroner does have an obligation to make a finding as to the registrable particulars concerning a death,[39] and it is convenient to use the Registrar General's form to record this. Coroners will in practice continue to send such forms to the registrar, because otherwise the death cannot be registered. But it means that the registrar has no legal basis for complaining to the coroner that any of the form's expected contents are lacking or organised in a way which is not convenient for the registrar, or that it has been sent late. **18–14**

---

[30] Known as Form 99 REV. It is divided into two sheets, Pts A and B. Part A contains most of the details, but Pt B requests information about accident or misadventure cases. There is no legal requirement to supply details other than those required by the statutes and set out in the text.

[31] Home Office Circular No. 28 of 2003, of April 16, 2003.

[32] Coroners Act 1988 s.11(7); *Fraser v North West Wales Coroner* [2010] EWHC 1165 (Admin,) at [13].

[33] *Fraser v North West Wales Coroner* [2010] EWHC 1165 (Admin.) at [17].

[34] See 9–20 ff (burial), 9–28 ff (cremation) above.

[35] See 10–74 above.

[36] Coroners Act 1988 s.11(7); Births and Deaths Registration Act 1953 ss 15, 23. See also Home Office Circular No. 79 of 1983, para.11.

[37] See 5–90.

[38] cf. Coroners (Investigations) Regulations 2013 (SI 2013/1629) reg.8, and 10–82 (coroner's duty to supply particulars after certain suspensions of investigation). Births and Deaths Registration Act 1953 s.23 (as amended in 2013) imposes a duty on the registrar to register the death on receiving the particulars from the coroner, but none on the coroner to send it.

[39] Coroners and Justice Act 2009 s.10(1)(b). See 13–01 ff, 13–115.

Stillbirths

18–15   Where the "death" turns out to have been a stillbirth,[40] it is the practice for coroners to complete an appropriate certificate[41] and to send this to the registrar,[42] but it is not a legal requirement. In the past, if the coroner directed a post-mortem examination and on the result of that examination decided to discontinue the investigation under the "Pink Form B" procedure,[43] rather than because the death was actually a stillbirth, the coroner had still to send the registrar a certificate stating the cause of death as disclosed in the post-mortem examination.[44] But in 2013 this was amended so that the coroner no longer has any obligation to do so.[45]

Adjournment following criminal proceedings

18–16   Under the old law, where an inquest was adjourned because criminal proceedings had been brought against some person in connection with the death of the subject of the inquest,[46] the coroner's obligation was, within five days of the adjournment, to supply to the registrar a certificate[47] stating the particulars necessary for the registration of the death, so far as ascertained at the date of the certificate.[48] (Where a death certificate was to be issued in both English and Welsh, coroners were asked to complete Pt 1 of the form in both languages.[49]) Then, once the coroner knew the outcome of the criminal proceedings in question, he or she had to send a further certificate[50] to the registrar informing him or her of such outcome.[51] It was irrelevant whether the inquest was ever resumed, as no certificate after inquest (Form 99 REV) was ever required in such a case. The death had already been registered on the basis of the information supplied after the statutory adjournment, and any information available after the criminal proceedings was ignored.[52] Hence it did not refer to the latter at all.

18–17   Under the new system, however, where the coroner suspends an investigation within any of the criminal charge or inquiry cases, he must furnish the registrar with the particulars necessary[53] for the registration of death.[54] This can still be done by way of the certificate[55] supplied by the Registrar General. But there is no longer

---

[40] As to which see 5–04 above.

[41] Known as Form 99A, redesigned in 1995; see Home Office Circular No. 19 of 1995.

[42] Home Office Circular No. 68 of 1955 App.4 No.4.

[43] See 8–37 above.

[44] Births and Deaths Registration Act s.23(3).

[45] Births and Deaths Registration Act 1953 s.23(3).

[46] See 10–75 ff.

[47] Known as Form 120.

[48] See Coroners Act 1988 s.16(4) (repealed); Coroners Rules 1984 r.21 (repealed).

[49] Home Office Circular No. 28 of 2003, of April 16, 2003.

[50] Known as Form 121.

[51] See Coroners Act 1988 s.16(3) (repealed); Coroners Rules 1984 r.21 (repealed).

[52] Cf. *Fraser v North West Wales Coroner* [2010] EWHC 1165 (Admin.).

[53] Where the death occurred outside England and Wales it is not registrable (Births and Deaths Registration Act 1953 s.15) and consequently no certificate need be furnished to the registrar.

[54] Coroners (Investigations) Regulations 2013 (SI 2013/1629) reg.8; formerly Coroners Act 1988 s.16(4).

[55] Form 120. It is divided into two sheets, Pts A and B. Pt A gives most of the information. Pt B requests details of the incident leading to the death. See Home Office Circular, No. 12 of 1993.

a five-day time limit for this, nor any further obligation to send the registrar the outcome of the criminal proceedings once known.[55a]

Adjournment for reasons other than criminal proceedings

Where an investigation is suspended for any other reason than the institution of **18–18** criminal proceedings, the creation of a public inquiry or by reason of the visiting forces provisions[56] the coroner does not send any certificate of registration particulars to the registrar at that stage. On the other hand the coroner must supply a certificate of the fact of death (often called an "interim certificate") to any interested person who asks for one.[57] The investigation so suspended will either be resumed and completed by an inquest hearing, when the usual certificate after inquest can be completed (voluntarily), or it will be further suspended because criminal proceedings are begun against a person in connection with the death, when the procedure set out above will take effect.

Entry in register of deaths

The eventual entry that is made in the register of deaths depends upon the **18–19** information in the certificates given to the registrar. The registrar must register the particulars contained in the certificate without alteration,[58] and no alteration can be made in any register of deaths except as authorised by legislation.[59] The procedure adopted in case of an error in the register or a certificate depends on the circumstances.

Any clerical error which may from time to time be discovered in any such **18–20** register may, in the prescribed manner and subject to the prescribed conditions, be corrected by any person authorised in that behalf by the Registrar General.[60]

Subject to the next paragraph, an error of fact or substance in any such register **18–21** may be corrected by entry in the margin (without any alteration of the original entry) by the officer having the custody of the register, upon production to him or her of a statutory declaration made by two qualified informants of the death stating the nature of the error and the true facts of the case, or in default then by two credible persons having knowledge of the truth of the case.[61] However, where the special procedure for mistakes as to statements of parenthood applies, one qualified informant or credible person is sufficient.[62]

Where the coroner has discontinued an investigation after post-mortem **18–22** examination, his or her approval is required for any correction of an error of fact or substance in the register relating to the cause of death, and any such error may be corrected by entry in the margin (without any alteration of the original entry) by the officer having the custody of the register on being notified by the coroner of the nature of the error and the true facts of the case.[63]

[55a] Cf Births and Deaths Registration Act 1953 s.23(2B); see 14–17, 17–67.
[56] See 10–73 ff.
[57] See 11–42.
[58] Births and Deaths Registration Act 1953 s.23(2).
[59] Births and Deaths Registration Act 1953 s.29(1).
[60] Births and Deaths Registration Act 1953 s.29(2).
[61] Births and Deaths Registration Act 1953 s.29(3).
[62] Births and Deaths Registration Act 1953 s.29A.
[63] Births and Deaths Registration Act 1953 s.29(3B).

18–23   Where an error of fact or substance (other than an error relating to the cause of death)[64] occurs in the information given by a coroner's certificate after inquest, the coroner, if satisfied by evidence on oath[65] or statutory declaration[66] that such error exists, may certify[67] under his or her hand to the officer having the custody of the register the nature of the error and the true facts of the case as ascertained on that evidence, and the error may thereupon be corrected by that officer in the register by entering the facts as so certified in the margin (without any alteration of the original entry).[68]

18–24   There is no prescribed form for this "certificate", which may simply be a letter, signed by the coroner, informing the registrar that he or she has received evidence on oath or by statutory declaration satisfying him or her of the existence of the error in the certificate after inquest and of the true state of affairs. The coroner does not issue a fresh certificate after inquest, since one has already been issued, and the statute by the word "certify" is referring to a document stating very limited facts, *not* one repeating all the information on the certificate after inquest. In some cases it may be possible to correct the certificate after inquest, but if the coroner does this he or she must re-date it as at the date of correction, otherwise the certificate will be telling a lie about itself, i.e. forgery.

18–25   Where an error of fact or substance relating to the cause of death[69] occurs in the information given by a coroner's certificate after inquest, it does not fall within the scope of any of the above procedures. The only means of correcting the register in such a case is to apply to the High Court for the determination and findings to be quashed and a new investigation to be held, following which a fresh certificate will be sent to the registrar.[70] Where the error in the certificate after inquest is not of fact or substance, but is merely clerical, there is no need for a statutory declaration, but the coroner certifies[71] the error to the registrar in a similar way.[72]

18–26   It will be observed that these provisions confer *power*, and do not impose any *duty*, upon the coroner. He or she is not entitled to charge a fee for adopting this procedure,[73] and it would be improper to act as a commissioner for oaths and take the fee allowed under the Statutory Declarations Act 1835, having already acted judicially as coroner in the case. There is no time limit within which the power has to be exercised, except that the wording of the provision suggests that only the coroner having jurisdiction in relation to the death concerned (i.e. the original

---

[64] As in *Attorney General v Harte* (1987) 151 J.P. 819.

[65] The reference to an oath recognises the power of the coroner to take evidence on oath otherwise than at an inquest.

[66] A statutory declaration is made, pursuant to the Statutory Declarations Act 1835, in any case where an oath cannot be administered, e.g. because no proceedings are pending. For a suitable form see App.3, Form 25.

[67] For a form of certificate, see App.3, Form 23.

[68] Births and Deaths Registration Act 1953 s.29(4).

[69] As in *Attorney General v Harte* (1987) 151 JP 819.

[70] *Attorney General v Harte* (1987) 151 JP 819; see also *Fraser v North West Wales Coroner* [2010] EWHC 1165 (Admin.).

[71] For a suitable form see App.3, Form 24.

[72] Births and Deaths Registration Act 1953 s.29(2); Registration of Births and Deaths Regulations 1987 reg.59.

[73] Coroners and Justice Act 2009 s.23, Sch.3 para.18; formerly Coroners Act 1988 s.3(2).

coroner or a successor) may inquire further into errors in the certificates in this way.

OTHER RETURNS

There is an obligation to inform the Chief Coroner that an investigation has been **18–27** completed more than one year after the death was notified,[73a] but no particular from is prescribed. There is now only one other special kind of certificate after inquest, which it is obligatory for coroners to send.

Death in, or following loss from, UK-registered ship

This is where an inquest (or post-mortem examination without inquest) has been **18–28** held concerning the death (a) of a person in a UK-registered ship[74] or its ship's boat,[75] or (b) outside the United Kingdom of a person employed in such a ship,[76] or (c) of a citizen of the United Kingdom and colonies in a non-UK ship (or its ship's boat)[77] which calls at a UK port during or at the end of a voyage.[78] In these (rare) cases the coroner is obliged to send particulars of the deceased in the form of a certificate[79] to the Registrar-General of Shipping and Seamen.[80] No specific time limit is prescribed for so doing. To the extent that such deaths occur within England and Wales (e.g. whilst the ship is in port) the coroner will normaly notify the registrar of deaths in the usual way.[81]

Although there is no requirement to do so, the coroner is also requested to **18–29** inform the Registrar-General of Shipping and Seamen, in the same way, of the particulars of persons who died on non-UK ships (the Registrar-General being able to register such deaths where the deceased was a citizen of the United Kingdom and colonies, and having undertaken to inform the marine authorities in the country of registration) after an inquest (or post-mortem examination without inquest) has been held.[82] The coroner should use the same form with any necessary modifications.[83]

[73a] See 2–62, 10–14.

[74] A "ship" is defined by the Merchant Shipping Act 1995 s.313(1), as every description of vessel used in navigation. A "United Kingdom ship" is one registered in the United Kingdom under Pt II of the 1995 Act.

[75] Merchant Shipping Act 1995 s.108(11).

[76] Merchant Shipping Act 1995 s.108(2).

[77] Merchant Shipping Act 1995 s.108(11).

[78] Merchant Shipping Act 1995 s.307, and Merchant Shipping (Returns of Births and Deaths) Regulations 1979 (SI 1979/1577), extending the scope of s.108(2) for the purposes of s.273.

[79] The contents of this certificate (though not the form) are prescribed by the Merchant Shipping (Returns of Births and Deaths) Regulations 1979 (SI 1979/1577) reg.8, Sch.3. Duplicated forms (ref. RBD 13) can be obtained from the Registry of Shipping and Seamen (see next note).

[80] Merchant Shipping Act 1995 s.273; Merchant Shipping (Returns of Births and Deaths) Regulations 1979 (SI 1979/1577) reg.8. The address of the Registry is PO Box 165, Cardiff CF14 5FU (tel.: 029 2076 8200; direct 029 2076 8227).

[81] See 18–11 ff above.

[82] Home Office Circular No. 174 of 1979, para.9.

[83] Home Office Circular No. 174 of 1979, para.10.

Deaths on a railway

18–30   There was formerly a requirement for a coroner, within seven days after holding an inquest on the death of a person killed on a railway, or who died in consequence of injuries received on a railway, to make a return to the Secretary of State, in such form as he might require, of the death and the cause of it.[84] But this was not carried over from the old legislation to the new, and has therefore now gone.

Notification to government departments

18–31   Although it is not compulsory for a coroner to comply, coroners are requested by various government departments or bodies to notify them of certain kinds of death relevant to their particular field. Thus, for example, the Transport and Road Research Laboratory is interested in receiving information on the blood alcohol level in victims of road traffic accidents,[85] the Department of Health wish to be notified about adverse drug reactions,[86] or faulty medical supplies or equipment resulting in death,[87] and there are other inquiries sponsored from time to time by that department. The Drugs Branch of the Home Office used to collect information from coroners about the deaths of registered drug addicts, in order to keep their files up to date,[88] but this ceased in 1997.

No obligation to notify relatives of deceased of outcome

18–32   There is no obligation on the coroner to notify the relatives of the deceased of the outcome of the inquest, although of course they will have been notified of the holding of the inquest[89] and indeed, in most cases, will have attended it. The Brodrick Committee recommended[90] that the coroner should be obliged to notify the nearest surviving adult relatives whose existence is known to him and who were not present at the inquest. When other recommendations of the Committee were implemented in 1980,[91] it was decided not to implement this recommendation, apparently on the grounds that coroners are usually in contact with some member of the family of the deceased, and it may not always be appropriate to notify the nearest surviving adult relative.[92] Nonetheless, the Home Office recommended that the coroner should normally ensure that such a person (or some other appropriate person) should be made aware of the result of the inquest, and also of which registrar of deaths would issue a death certificate.[93]

---

[84] Coroners Act 1988 s.11(8). The prescribed form was HSE RF1, provided by the Health & Safety Executive.

[85] See Home Office Circular No. 25 of 1984. It may also be interested in other findings, e.g. the injuries sustained by coach passengers in a motorway accident: see *Re M4 Coach Crash, The Times*, February 28, 1988.

[86] Under the "yellow card scheme": see Coroners' Newsletter No. 17 (April 19, 1995). The scheme is run by the Medicines Control Agency, Market Towers, 1 Nine Elms Lane, London SW8 5NQ (Tel: 020 7273 0000).

[87] Reports on supplies and equipment should be sent (or telephoned) to the MDA Adverse Incident Centre, 14 Russell Square, London WC1B 5EP (tel.: 020 7972 8140).

[88] See Home Office Circular No. 24 of 1971.

[89] See 10–22 above.

[90] See 15–14.

[91] See the Coroners (Amendment) Rules 1980 (SI 1980/557).

[92] Home Office Circular No. 53 of 1980, para.6.

[93] Home Office Circular No. 53 of 1980, para.6.

FEES, ALLOWANCES AND EXPENSES

Under the old law before July 25, 2013, a coroner holding an inquest had an   **18–33**
obligation immediately after the termination of the proceedings to pay fees,
allowances and all expenses reasonably incurred in and about the holding of the
inquest (which would include fees and allowances for expert and other witnesses)
not exceeding the fees, allowances and disbursements which might be lawfully paid
or made under the Coroners Act 1988.[94] This regime still applies in relation to
treasure inquests.[95] But in relation to non-treasure investigations the new law is
differently worded in important respects, even though the substantive effect is
much the same.

Non-treasure cases

Jurors

Subject to any conditions prescribed by regulations,[96] a person who attends for   **18–34**
service as a juror (even though not sworn)[97] or who serves as juror at an inquest is
entitled under primary legislation to be paid an allowance (a) for travelling and
subsistence,[98] and (b) for financial loss,[99] but only (in the case of financial loss) if
attending the inquest has caused non-travelling and subsistence expenses to be
incurred which would not otherwise have been incurred,[100] or loss of earnings[101]
or social security benefits[102] to be suffered which would not otherwise have been
suffered. The rates to be paid are prescribed by regulations,[103] though the coroner
may reimburse a juror for any additional expresses, other than those prescribed,
which the coroner believes to have been reasonably incurred.[104]

According to the primary legislation, the coroner must calculate and (whether   **18–35**
personally or by agent)[105] pay the amount due.[106] According to the regulations
themselves, however, it is for the coroner or the coroner's relevant authority[107] to
calculate and pay.[108] As a matter of law the regulation, being secondary legislation,
cannot go beyond the scope of the primary, so the obligation to calculate and pay
is and remains that of the coroner alone. But in practice this inconsistency is
unlikely to cause a problem. The coroner may require the juror to provide written

---

[94] Coroners Act 1988 s.26(1).
[95] See 18–47.
[96] Coroners Allowances, Fees and Expenses Regulations 2013 (SI 2013/1615).
[97] Coroners and Justice Act 2009 s.34 Sch.7 para.10.
[98] Coroners and Justice Act 2009 s.34 Sch.7 para.1(a).
[99] Coroners and Justice Act 2009 s.34 Sch.7 para.1(b).
[100] Coroners and Justice Act 2009 s.34 Sch.7 para.2(a).
[101] Coroners and Justice Act 2009 s.34 Sch.7 para.2(b).
[102] Coroners and Justice Act 2009 s.34 Sch.7 para.2(c).
[103] Coroners and Justice Act 2009 s.34 Sch.7 paras 3, 11; see Coroners Allowances, Fees and Expenses Regulations 2013 (SI 2013,/1615) reg.8 Sch.
[104] Coroners Allowances, Fees and Expenses Regulations 2013 (SI 2013,/1615) reg.11.
[105] The coroner may delegate this administrative function to his officers or other staff: Coroners Allowances, Fees and Expenses Regulations 2013 (SI 2013,/1615) reg.3.
[106] Coroners and Justice Act 2009 s.34 Sch.7 para.4.
[107] That is, the local authority designated as such under the Coroners and Justice Act 2009 for the area concerned: Coroners Allowances, Fees and Expenses Regulations 2013 (SI 2013/1615) reg.2.
[108] Coroners Allowances, Fees and Expenses Regulations 2013 (SI 2013/1615) reg.4.

evidence of the expense before paying,[109] but must also explain on request how the sum has been calculated.[110]

Witnesses, etc.

18–36   There is no similar primary legislation entitlement to allowances for witnesses[111] or persons producing documents or things,[112] or providing evidence in the form of written statements,[113] to coroners. There is however power to make regulations to prescribe allowances for such persons.[114] Regulations have indeed been made,[115] but only for allowances to witnesses who give evidence at an inquest,[116] and not for allowances to the other persons referred to.

18–37   In the regulations, the witnesses concerned are defined as either professional, expert or ordinary.[117] Professional witnesses are those who practise as members of the medical profession or as dentists and who give evidence at an inquest.[118] Expert witnesses are persons of any calling, profession or trade who give evidence at an inquest because of their expertise, other than professional witnesses.[119] Ordinary witnesses are any other persons who give evidence at an inquest.[120] However, the regulations also refer (but only in the Schedule) to "suitable practitioner", a term not defined, or indeed even mentioned, elsewhere in the regulations. The term is used in the section of the primary legislation dealing with post-mortem examinations,[121] where it means a registered medical practitioner or a practitioner of a description designated by the Chief Coroner.[122]

Post-mortem examiners

18–38   There is also a power to make regulations to prescribe the fees and allowances that may be paid by or on behalf of coroners to persons making post-mortem examinations.[123] Regulations have been so made,[124] referring however (in the

---

[109] Coroners Allowances, Fees and Expenses Regulations 2013 (SI 2013/1615) reg.5.

[110] Coroners Allowances, Fees and Expenses Regulations 2013 (SI 2013/1615) reg.6.

[111] Defined by Coroners and Justice Act 2009 s.34 Sch.7 para.5(2), to mean a person (other than a police officer or full-time prison officer attending as such, or a prisoner conveyed in custody) properly attending before a coroner in order to give evidence at an inquest (whether or not that happens).

[112] See 7–13, 7–14.

[113] See 7–13, 7–14.

[114] Coroners and Justice Act 2009 s.34 Sch.7 paras 5(1), 11.

[115] Coroners Allowances, Fees and Expenses Regulations 2013 (SI 2013/1615).

[116] Coroners Allowances, Fees and Expenses Regulations 2013 (SI 2013/1615) reg.2, definitions of "witness", "expert witness", "professional witness" and "ordinary witness".

[117] Coroners Allowances, Fees and Expenses Regulations 2013 (SI 2013/1615) reg.2, definition of "witness".

[118] Coroners Allowances, Fees and Expenses Regulations 2013 (SI 2013/1615) reg.2, definition of "professional witness".

[119] Coroners Allowances, Fees and Expenses Regulations 2013 (SI 2013/1615) reg.2, definition of "expert witness".

[120] Coroners Allowances, Fees and Expenses Regulations 2013 (SI 2013/1615) reg.2, definition of "ordinary witness".

[121] Coroners and Justice Act 2009 s.14. See 8–35, 8–45 ff.

[122] Coroners and Justice Act 2009 s.14(3). At the time of writing no designation had been made by the Chief Coroner under this section.

[123] Coroners and Justice Act 2009 s.34 Sch.7 paras 6, 11.

[124] Coroners Allowances, Fees and Expenses Regulations 2013 (SI 2013/1615).

Schedule only) to a "suitable practitioner",[125] and (both in the Schedule and elsewhere) to a professional witness.[126] In practice, a post-mortem examiner is likely to be both a "suitable practitioner" and a professional witness, but if not both then at least one of these.

Expert witnesses

A coroner may pay an expert witness a fee that he or she considers reasonable (a)   **18–39** for preparatory work directly related to the giving of evidence at an inquest, having regard to the nature and complexity of that preparatory work,[127] and (b) for attending and giving expert evidence at the inquest, having regard to the nature and complexity of the evidence given by that witness.[128]

Relevant authority schedule

In addition, there is power for a relevant authority[129] for a coroner area, having   **18–40** regard to any guidance from the Lord Chancellor[130] to issue (and amend or revoke)[131] a schedule of fees, allowances and expenses (not including any fees or allowances discussed above)[132] that may be lawfully paid or incurred by the coroner in the performance of coronial functions.[133] A copy of the schedule as issued or amended must be given to the senior coroner.[134] Any such schedule will be a local matter, applying only to the coroner concerned. Where a coroner agrees in advance for a particular expense to be incurred in a particular case, the effect will be in substance the same as the making of a schedule within this power, though only for the case in question. The coroner also has an obligation to notify the authority of any unusual allowances, fees or expenses, if possible before they are incurred; otherwise when they are incurred or as soon as possible thereafter.[134a] Costs (and damages) arising from legal proceedings concerning coronial duties are not governed by the schedule system, but by a separate statutory indemnity, which is discussed later.[135]

Determination and payment of witnesses and other expenses

Unlike the position for jurors' allowances (where the primary legislation puts an   **18–41** obligation to calculate and pay such allowances on the coroner alone),[136] in relation to fees and allowances for *witnesses* there is no primary legislation obligation on the coroner. Instead there is a power for the Lord Chancellor to make regulations prescribing the allowances that may be paid by or on behalf of coroners.[137] But the

---

[125] See 8–37, 18–37.
[126] See 18–37.
[127] Coroners Allowances, Fees and Expenses Regulations 2013 (SI 2013/1615) reg.9.
[128] Coroners Allowances, Fees and Expenses Regulations 2013 (SI 2013/1615) reg.10.
[129] See 2–32.
[130] Coroners and Justice Act 2009 s.34 Sch.7 para.7(3). No such guidance has so far been issued.
[131] Coroners and Justice Act 2009 s.34 Sch.7 para.7(2).
[132] Coroners and Justice Act 2009 s.34 Sch.7 para.7(5).
[133] Coroners and Justice Act 2009 s.34 Sch.7 para.7(1).
[134] Coroners and Justice Act 2009 s.34 Sch.7 para.7(4).
[134a] Coroners Allowances, Fees and Expenses Regulations 2013 (SI 2013/1615) reg.7; see 5–65.
[135] See 18–44 below.
[136] See 18–34.
[137] Coroners Allowances, Fees and Expenses Regulations 2013 (SI 2013/1615) reg.5(1).

regulations made go beyond that, and seek to place an obligation on the coroner or the coroner's relevant authority[138] to calculate and pay.[139] In practice the coroner's officer or clerk will deal with this on behalf of the coroner, as the delegate of the coroner.[140]

18–42   The coroner may require the claimant to provide written evidence[141] of the expense before paying,[142] but must also explain on request how the sum has been calculated.[143] The written evidence must be returned to the claimant on request,[144] in which case the coroner will take and keep a copy for the record. The rates to be paid are prescribed by regulations,[145] though the coroner may reimburse a suitable practitioner or witness for any additional expresses, other than those prescribed, which the coroner believes to have been reasonably incurred.[146]

Record-keeping and indemnities

18–43   There is a power to make regulations for meeting or reimbursing coronial expenses,[147] including an indemnity for legal costs and damages arising out of the exercise of the coroner's functions.[148] Under the regulations, a coroner must provide the relevant authority[149] with an account (including original or copy[150] documentary proof of sums incurred)[151] of all payments under the regulations at agreed time intervals,[152] and the authority once satisfied that it is correct must reimburse the coroner for those payments.[153] "Correctness" here means the fact of the payment having been made, not its propriety. The coroner and the relevant authority must each keep a record of payments under the regulations for three years,[154] and must provide the Chief Coroner with a copy on request.[155] The coroner must retain original or copy documentary proof of sums incurred in a format and for a period agreed with the relevant authority.[156]

18–44   Where proceedings are brought against a coroner in respect of the exercise or purported exercise of the coroner's duty, the coroner must be indemnified by the relevant authority[157] in respect of:

---

[138] That is, the local authority designated as such under the Coroners and Justice Act 2009 for the area concerned: Coroners Allowances, Fees and Expenses Regulations 2013 (SI 2013/1615) reg.2.

[139] Coroners Allowances, Fees and Expenses Regulations 2013 (SI 2013/1615) reg.4.

[140] Coroners Allowances, Fees and Expenses Regulations 2013 (SI 2013/1615) reg.3.

[141] Such as receipts, invoice or other documents proving the expense incurred.

[142] Coroners Allowances, Fees and Expenses Regulations 2013 (SI 2013/1615) reg.5.

[143] Coroners Allowances, Fees and Expenses Regulations 2013 (SI 2013/1615) reg.6.

[144] Coroners Allowances, Fees and Expenses Regulations 2013 (SI 2013/1615) reg.15.

[145] Coroners and Justice Act 2009 s.34 Sch.7 paras 3, 11; see Coroners Allowances, Fees and Expenses Regulations 2013 (SI 2013/1615) reg.8 Sch.

[146] Coroners Allowances, Fees and Expenses Regulations 2013 (SI 2013/1615) reg.11.

[147] Coroners and Justice Act 2009 s.34 Sch.7 paras 9(1), 11.

[148] Coroners and Justice Act 2009 s.34 Sch.7 para.9(3).

[149] See 2–32.

[150] See Coroners Allowances, Fees and Expenses Regulations 2013 (SI 2013/1615) regs 15, 16.

[151] Coroners Allowances, Fees and Expenses Regulations 2013 (SI 2013/1615) reg.13(2).

[152] Coroners Allowances, Fees and Expenses Regulations 2013 (SI 2013/1615) reg.13(1).

[153] Coroners Allowances, Fees and Expenses Regulations 2013 (SI 2013/1615) reg.13(3). See also *Forrest v Lord Chancellor* [2011] EWHC 142 (Admin.) at [30].

[154] Coroners Allowances, Fees and Expenses Regulations 2013 (SI 2013/1615) reg.14(1).

[155] Coroners Allowances, Fees and Expenses Regulations 2013 (SI 2013/1615) reg.14(2).

[156] Coroners Allowances, Fees and Expenses Regulations 2013 (SI 2013/1615) reg.16.

[157] See 2–32.

(a) any costs which the coroner reasonably incurs in or in connection with such proceedings;

(b) any costs which the coroner reasonably incurs in disputing any claim which might have been made in such proceedings;

(c) any damages awarded against or to be paid by the coroner in such proceedings;

(d) any sums payable by the coroner in connection with a reasonable settlement of such proceedings or claims.[158]

Where such proceedings are brought by a coroner, the same applies if and to the **18–45** extent that the relevant authority has agreed in advance to indemnify the coroner.[159] If the relevant authority refuses so to agree, the coroner may appeal such refusal to the Lord Chancellor or his appointee for the purpose.[160]

In each case the coroner deals only with the relevant authority,[161] and where the **18–46** coroner area consists only of the district of that authority, that is an end of the matter. But where a coroner's district consists of two or more local government districts,[162] it is potentially more complex. In the latter case, there was formerly provision for apportioning the coroner's expenses,[163] and also any indemnity for legal costs and damages to which he or she might be entitled,[164] between the different authorities for those local government districts, thus enabling the pro rata reimbursement of the relevant authority. But these provisions have not been carried over into the new coroner regime. It is not clear on what basis the relevant authority will obtain such reimbursement for the future.

Treasure cases

In treasure cases the regime under the Coroners Act 1988 continues to apply, as the **18–47** treasure provisions of the new legislation have not been commenced.[165] Omitting material relating to post-mortem examinations, which is not relevant, this is as follows. A coroner holding an inquest must immediately after the termination of the proceedings pay the allowances of every juror and all expenses reasonably incurred in and about the holding of the inquest (which will include fees and allowances for expert and other witnesses) not exceeding the fees, allowances and disbursements which may be lawfully paid or made under the Coroners Act.[166] All fees and allowances to witnesses[167] and jurors[168] are determined by the Secretary of

---

[158] Coroners Allowances, Fees and Expenses Regulations 2013 (SI 2013/1615) reg.17(1).
[159] Coroners Allowances, Fees and Expenses Regulations 2013 (SI 2013/1615) reg.17(2).
[160] Coroners Allowances, Fees and Expenses Regulations 2013 (SI 2013/1615) reg.17(3).
[161] See 2–32.
[162] They might be metropolitan districts, London boroughs, Welsh principal areas, or non-metropolitan counties.
[163] Coroners Act 1988 s.27(4).
[164] Coroners Act 1988 s.27A(5).
[165] See 16–20.
[166] Coroners Act 1988 s.26(1).
[167] Including persons summoned as witnesses but who do not in fact give evidence.
[168] Including persons summoned as jurors but who do not in fact serve as such.

State with Treasury consent,[169] whereas all other expenses and disbursements made are largely regulated by means of a schedule made by the local authority.[170]

Expert witnesses

18–48   An expert witness at an inquest may be paid such sum as the coroner considers reasonable having regard to the nature and difficulty of the case and the work necessarily involved in the preparation of evidence.[171] The coroner should take into consideration not only the evidence actually given but also the preparatory work in connection with the evidence. As with other witnesses, an expert witness may be entitled to allowances for travel expenses incurred[172] and also in some circumstances to an overnight allowance.[173]

Other witnesses

18–49   A witness who is not an expert witness is entitled in some circumstances to allowances for loss of remuneration,[174] for expenses incurred in travelling[175] and for subsistence,[176] or overnight stay,[177] but it is not entitled to be paid a fee merely by reason of giving evidence. Where a witness is abroad and (exceptionally) returns to give evidence, the allowances (particularly for travel) will be inadequate, and prior relevant authority consent should be sought for payment at levels above those determined.[178] There are special professional allowances for lawyers, dentists and veterinary surgeons attending to give professional evidence.[179] None of these allowances, however, applies to police officers, prison officers or coroner's officers attending in such capacity, or to prisoners produced in custody at an inquest.[180]

Jurors

18–50   A person summoned or who serves as a juror in a coroner's court at a treasure inquest is entitled to allowances at prescribed rates[181] for travelling[182] and subsistence[183] and for financial loss.[184] In abnormally long inquests this may be increased to a maximum of twice the prescribed rates after the first 10 days of attendance, suffered in consequence of jury service, such as loss of earnings or social security benefits, and in some cases to an overnight allowance.[185]

---

[169] Coroners Act 1988 ss.24(1). The Schedule of Fees and Allowances in force on July 25, 2013 took effect on April 1, 2004: see Home Office Circular No. 15 of 2004.
[170] See 18–51 above.
[171] Schedule of Fees and Allowances para.3(a).
[172] Schedule of Fees and Allowances para.5.
[173] Schedule of Fees and Allowances para.3(b).
[174] Schedule of Fees and Allowances para.1(c).
[175] Schedule of Fees and Allowances para.5.
[176] Schedule of Fees and Allowances para.1(a).
[177] Schedule of Fees and Allowances para.1(b).
[178] See Home Office Circular No. 79 of 1983 para.7.
[179] Schedule of Fees and Allowances para.2.
[180] Schedule of Fees and Allowances, Preliminary Note.
[181] Coroners Act 1988 s.25(1).
[182] Schedule of Fees and Allowances para.5.
[183] Schedule of Fees and Allowances para.1(a).
[184] Schedule of Fees and Allowances para.1(c). In abnormally long inquests this may be increased to a maximum of twice the prescribed rates after the first 10 days of attendance.
[185] Schedule of Fees and Allowances para.1(b).

Making, and amendment of, schedule of fees by relevant council

A relevant council may, from time to time, make and, once made, alter and vary   **18–51**
a schedule of fees, allowances and disbursements (not being those prescribed by
regulations and set out above) which may lawfully be paid and made by a coroner
in the course of his duties.[186] A copy of the schedule must be delivered to every
coroner concerned.[187] Both the contents of the schedule and the amount
authorised for each item vary from one authority to another, depending in part on
when the schedule was last revised.[188]

If the schedule does not make provision for some expense which is to be   **18–52**
incurred, the coroner should obtain the agreement of the local authority in
advance. The schedule may be varied by rules made by the Secretary of State,[189]
but in fact no such rules have ever been made. As in non-treasure cases, costs (and
damages) arising from legal proceedings concerning coronial duties are governed
by a separate statutory indemnity.[190]

Access to Documents and Information

Individuals may be able to obtain access to personal data about themselves held by   **18–53**
the coroner under the data protection legislation. This was dealt with earlier.[191]
More important here are provisions entitling certain persons access to information
about *others*. In non-treasure cases the rules for post-inquest disclosure are the same
as for pre- and peri-inquest disclosure, and have already been discussed.[192] So far
as concerns treasure cases, probably there were rules in the old system providing for
the supply to any properly interested person a copy of (inter alia) any notes of
evidence or any document put in evidence at an inquest.[193] The preservation of the
Coroners Act 1988 for treasure cases means that the old Coroners Rules are also
retained for the moment, for the same purpose.[194]

---

[186] Coroners Act 1988 s.24(2)(a), (b).
[187] Coroners Act 1988 s.24(2)(c).
[188] Some of the fees were fixed by the Joint Negotiating Committee for Doctors Assisting Local
Authorities. Note that the statutory authority to pay only arises when the relevant council makes a
schedule including these fees; the fact of national agreement by itself is not enough.
[189] Coroners Act 1988 s.24(3)(b), re-enacting Coroners (Amendment) Act 1926 s.29(2)(b).
[190] See Coroners Act 1988, s.27A.
[191] See 7–33 ff.
[192] See 7–24 ff. The rule in *R (Guardian News & Media Ltd) v City of Westminster Magistrate's Court)*
[2013] QB 618 only applies to documents relied on but not read aloud, so it will be of limited
application in the coroner's court.
[193] Coroners Rules 1984 r.57(a).
[194] See 16–20.

GENERAL ADMINISTRATIVE MATTERS

Register of deaths

18–54   A senior coroner must keep a register of all deaths reported in the coroner area.[195] The register must contain particulars of the date on which the death was reported, the full name, address, age and gender of the deceased, and any other information aiding the identification of the deceased, and the place of the death, or (if that is unknown) the place where the body was found.[196] Unlike under the old law, there is no need to record the procedure used for disposing of the case.[197]

Annual return

18–55   Under the old law, on or before the first day of February in every year, every coroner had to make and transmit to the Secretary of State a return in writing, in such form and containing such particulars as the Secretary of State might direct, of all cases in which an inquest has been held by him or by some person acting for him, during the year ending on the immediately preceding December 31.[198] Further, every coroner had to furnish the Secretary of State as and when required by him to do so, with returns in relation to inquests held and deaths inquired into by him in such form and containing such particulars as the Secretary of State might direct.[199]

18–56   However, these provisions have not been carried over into the new law, even though the Chief Coroner's Guide to the new legislation appears to think that they have (without citation of authority).[200] Consequently there is no longer any duty on coroners to make an annual return to the Lord Chancellor. On the other hand, in the new system the Chief Coroner has the right to information about particular investigations.[201]

Retention of exhibits

18–57   Under the old law, an exhibit at an inquest had to be retained by the coroner until he was satisfied that the exhibit was not required for the purposes of any other legal proceedings.[202] Once the coroner was so satisfied, then, if a request for its delivery had been made by a person appearing to the coroner to be entitled to its possession,[203] the coroner had to deliver it to that person. If no request had been made, the coroner might destroy it or dispose of it as he thought fit.[204] These provisions have also not been carried over into the new law.

---

[195] Coroners (Investigations) Rules 2013 (SI 2013/1629) reg.5(1).
[196] Coroners (Investigations) Rules 2013 (SI 2013/1629) reg.5(2).
[197] Coroners Rules 1984 r.54 and Sch.3 (repealed).
[198] Coroners Act 1988 s.28(1).
[199] Coroners Act 1988 s.28(2).
[200] Paragraph 186.
[201] See 2–62.
[202] Coroners Rules 1984 r.55.
[203] i.e. usually the owner, or (if it belonged to the deceased) the deceased's personal representatives or, failing them, his next of kin: cf. 9–02.
[204] Coroners Rules 1984 r.56.

Care should obviously be exercised in dealing with exhibits in suicide cases, such **18–58** as the instrument with which a suicide was committed,[205] but there is no longer any specific legal power for the coroner to withhold these things from persons otherwise entitled to them.[206] Of course, there may be difficulties in establishing exactly who is so entitled, and the coroner is normally justified in waiting until entitlement has been established between two or more competing claimants before handing them over.[207] There are special provisions for body tissues and fluid samples.[208]

Retention of documents

Any document in the possession of the coroner in connection with an investigation **18–59** or post-mortem examination must, unless a court otherwise directs, be retained by the coroner for at least 15 years.[209] This will include notes of evidence taken by the coroner, post-mortem examination or special examination reports, all documents put in evidence at an inquest, and reports of preliminary enquiries which have led to an investigation or to a post-mortem examination. It will not include any documents on any death reported to the coroner which is dealt with without investigation, e.g. by the "Pink Form A" procedure.

However, the coroner may, instead of keeping a document for the prescribed **18–60** period, deliver it to a person who seems to him or her to be a proper person to have possession of it.[210] Delivery by the coroner to the person appearing to be entitled does not determine the question of legal title to the item in question, but the coroner in following the procedure set out will be protected from suit in the event of the property being delivered to a person not legally entitled to it.

Where the coroner hands over a document, in most cases it may be desirable to **18–61** retain a copy. If the coroner does not exercise the power to hand over, then except in special circumstances he or she should on request supply copies of the document to its owner or other person kept out of possession.[211] This is particularly important in the case of documents in evidence at the inquest which belong to persons not otherwise connected with the deceased or who otherwise have a need for the return of the document.

Fees are payable for disclosure given after an inquest is over,[212] unless the **18–62** document is disclosed by email.[213] There is a separate fee for transcription of an inquest hearing,[214] which appears to have been set without reference to what a professional transcriber would charge. This may mean that in cases where an interested person asks for disclosure of the recording of the inquest hearing the

---

[205] Documents, such as suicide notes, are dealt with below: 18–59 ff.
[206] cf. Coroners and Justice Act 2009 s.32 Sch.5 paras 3, 5(4) (not brought into force).
[207] See cf 9–12, 16–10 and CPR Part 86 (stakeholder claims and applications).
[208] See 8–72 ff above.
[209] Coroners (Investigations) Regulations 2013 (SI 2013/1629) reg.27(1); formerly Coroners Rules 1984 r.56.
[210] Coroners (Investigations) Regulations 2013 (SI 2013/1629) reg.27(2).
[211] *Arias v Metropolitan Police Commissioner* (1984) 128 S.J. 784; *The Times*, August 1, 1984, CA (documents lawfully seized by police under search warrant).
[212] Coroners Allowances, Fees and Expenses Regulations 2013 (SI 2013/1615) reg.12.
[213] Coroners Allowances, Fees and Expenses Regulations 2013 (SI 2013/1615) reg.12(2).
[214] Coroners Allowances, Fees and Expenses Regulations 2013 (SI 2013/1615) reg.12(5).

coroner will only allow this by inspecting (i.e. listening to) it or supplying a copy of the recording,[215] rather than by transcribing it.

Coroners' records

18–63 The records of coroner's courts (including photographs and tape recordings) are public records for the purposes of the Public Records Act 1958, and are in the custody of coroners until removed to a place of permanent deposit.[216] It was decided in 1967 that all records later in date than 1875 should be destroyed after 15 years, except for the indexed registers of deaths and papers relating to treasure trove or matters of special historical interest, which (along with records from earlier then 1875) should be permanently preserved.[217] It is for coroners themselves to decide which records post–1875 are of such interest to justify preservation, though the then Public Record Office (now National Archives) produced an operational selection policy for coroners' records from 1970 to 2000.[218] In cases of doubt, the advice of the Keeper of Public Records should be sought.[219]

18–64 Where a coroner does not have sufficient accommodation for storing documents which must be retained, the older documents should be handed over to the country archives, although the coroner will still be responsible for deciding whether they should be destroyed after 15 years, or preserved.[220] Documents which appear to require preservation should be separated, and may be handed over direct to the local record repository for coroners' records appointed by the Lord Chancellor under the 1958 Act. Those coroners' records of a later date than 1874 and not of historical or other special interest should be destroyed after 15 years, unless the coroner wishes to dispose of them in some other way, when application should be made to the Keeper of Public Records.[221]

18–65 Documents to be preserved should be transferred to the appointed repository as soon as possible after the expiry of the 15-year retainer period (assuming that they have not already been deposited there through lack of storage space) and in any event before they are 30 years old, unless the approval of the Lord Chancellor (through the Keeper of Public Records) is obtained for longer retention.[222] Of course, such records may be borrowed back if required by the coroner.[223] Access to coroners' records deposited under the Public Records Act 1958 will not be given to the public until 75 years have elapsed (in the case of records relating to reported deaths) or 30 years (in the case of other records), unless the coroner of the

---

[215] See 7–25.
[216] Home Office Circular No. 250 of 1967, App. paras 1–2.
[217] Home Office Circular No. 250 of 1967, App. para.3.
[218] *Operational Selection Policy OSP 6: Records created by and relating to Coroners, 1970–2000*, available at http://www.nationalarchives.gov.uk/documents/information-management/osp6.pdf [Accessed June 16, 2014] (revised 2005, and amended 2007).
[219] Home Office Circular No. 250 of 1967, App. The Keeper's address is the Public Record Office, Kew, Richmond, Surrey, TW9 4DU (Tel.: 020 8876 3444; website http://www.nationalarchives.gov.uk/).
[220] Home Office Circular No. 250 of 1967, App. para.4.
[221] Home Office Circular No. 250 of 1967, App. para.5.
[222] Home Office Circular No. 250 of 1967, App. para.6.
[223] Home Office Circular No. 250 of 1967, App. para.8.

court from which the records came gives special permission in writing for such access.[224]

Under the old law, where a coroner vacated office, by death or otherwise, all **18–66** documents, exhibits, registers and other things in the custody of the coroner in connection with inquests or post-mortem examinations had to be transferred to the coroner next appointed to that office.[225] This has not been carried over into the new law. But it seems that under the general law a successor to a public office normally has the right, at least in equity, to the predecessor's official property and documents.[226]

---

[224] Home Office Circular No. 250 of 1967, App. para.9, as substituted by Home Office Circular No. 62 of 1971 and amended by Lord Chancellor's Order No. 69 (April 16, 1984).

[225] Coroners Rules 1984 r.59.

[226] *Coulter v Chief Constable of Dorset* [2004] 1 W.L.R. 1425 at [14]–[17] (equitable assignment of debt owed to predecessor of defendant).

Chapter 19

APPEALS

INTRODUCTION

By reason of the inquisitorial nature of a coronial investigation, the conclusions **19–01** reached in it are not binding on those affected, and may be traversed in further proceedings.[1] But those who are dissatisfied with inquest conclusions do not have to wait for those further proceedings; they may challenge them immediately. This chapter is concerned with that challenge. The common law knew no system of appeal against coroners' decisions. The only recourse was to the prerogative writs, which later became judicial review, and also a limited, statutory form of review, introduced in 1926. The Luce[2] and Shipman[3] reports had recommended that a true appeal system be introduced. Accordingly, the Coroners and Justice Act 2009 as originally enacted provided for appeals from coronial decisions to lie to the Chief Coroner.[4]

But before the Act was brought into force the Government changed, and the **19–02** post of Chief Coroner was destined to be abolished, to save money. As it turned out, political pressure saved the Chief Coroner, but the provisions setting up the appeal system were still repealed (before they came into force),[5] on the grounds of lack of resources. In fact, the cumbersome and bifurcated system of judicial and statutory review probably costs more than the new appeal system would have done. But of course the costs of the current patchwork fall on local authorities, whereas the new system would fall on central government. Whatever the reason, the old system has been retained, as explained below.

That system provides for reviews of two kinds of coronial decision: first, **19–03** interlocutory decisions of the coroner, e.g. as to the conduct of the investigation, or as to some aspect of procedure at the inquest, and secondly, the determination and findings in the record of the inquest. From neither kind of decision is there any appeal as such, in the sense of a rehearing on the merits and a fresh decision being come to in substitution for that already reached. But they may be subject, in some cases, to review by the courts.

---

[1] See 20–02 below.
[2] At 21.105 (ch.15).
[3] Third Report, Recommendation 46 (para.19.132).
[4] Section 40.
[5] Public Bodies Act 2011 s.33.

19–04 Broadly, there are two procedures. The first is entirely statutory, and deals with cases where a coroner has declined to hold an investigation or inquest in circumstances where he should do so, and also with quashing a determination or finding and ordering the holding of a new investigation or inquest in some cases.[6] The second procedure is not confined to coroners' proceedings, but extends generally to the actions and decision of inferior courts and other tribunals, and that is judicial review.[7] Unlike the first, statutory procedure, this extends, in principle, to *all* actions and decisions of the coroner, and not merely to ordering investigations or inquests and quashing determinations or findings.

STATUTORY POWER

Ambit of statutory power

19–05 This power is entirely the creature of statute[8] and did not exist before 1887. It is contained in one[9] of the two sections of the Coroners Act 1988 retained (in an amended form) after the coming into force of Pt I of the Coroners and Justice Act 2009.[10] The High Court, upon application made by or under the authority of the Attorney General, must first be satisfied either (a) that a coroner[11] refuses or neglects to hold an inquest or an investigation which ought to be held; or (b) where an inquest or an investigation has been held by a coroner, that (whether by reason of fraud, rejection of evidence, irregularity of proceedings, insufficiency of inquiry, or the discovery of new facts or evidence or otherwise) it is necessary or desirable, in the interests of justice, that another inquest or investigation, or another investigation, should be held. In such cases, the High Court has power (a) to order an investigation to be held, either by the coroner concerned, or by another coroner in the same coroner area,[12] (b) to order the coroner concerned to pay such costs of, and incidental to, the application as to the court may appear just, and also (c) to quash the inquisition on, or determination or finding made at, the previous inquest.[13]

19–06 Notwithstanding the reference in the statute[14] to ordering an inquest or an investigation "into the death", the statutory power has been held to apply equally to cases of treasure,[15] where of course there is no death to be inquired into.[16] The amendments to the section needed to make it compatible with the reforms made by the 2009 Act do not sit well with the treasure jurisdiction continued under the

---

[6] See 19–05 ff.

[7] See 19–25 ff below.

[8] Coroners Act 1988 s.13, re-enacting Coroners Act 1887 s.6, as extended by the Coroners (Amendment) Act 1926 s.19.

[9] Section 13.

[10] Coroners and Justice Act 2009 (Consequential Provisions) Order 2013 (SI 2013/1874).

[11] Meaning a coroner appointed under the Coroners Act 1988 or the Coroners and Justice Act 2009: s.13(4).

[12] That coroner is treated for the purposes of the 1988 Act as if he were the coroner for the coroner *district* concerned: s.13(3).

[13] Coroners Act 1988 s.13(2).

[14] Section 13(2)(a).

[15] See Ch.16.

[16] *R. v Wiltshire Coroner Ex p. Chaddock* (1992) 157 J.P. 209, DC.

1988 Act.[17] For example, there are no "investigations" under the 1988 Act. But it is not considered that these amendments therefore indicate an intention by Parliament that the section should no longer apply to treasure cases.

The statutory procedure can only be used to obtain an order against a coroner, **19–07** and not against any other person or body who may in some way be connected with the matter.[18] Similarly, where there is no coroner who ever had jurisdiction in a case (because the statutory criteria for such jurisdiction[19] were never satisfied in relation to him), the court has no power to order any coroner to hold an inquest.[20] In particular, a coroner cannot acquire jurisdiction to hold an inquest by agreeing or undertaking to do so.[21]

Prerequisites for the quashing of an inquisition

So far as this power relates to ordering an inquest or an investigation to be held, **19–08** which a coroner has neglected or refused to hold, this has already been dealt with.[22] So far as concerns the power to quash an inquisition or determination or finding, it will be seen that there are three prerequisites:

   (i) the authority (still sometimes called *fiat*) of the Attorney General must be obtained;

   (ii) an inquest or an investigation must already have been held and an inquisition or determination or finding produced;

   (iii) in holding the previous inquest or investigation, there must have been (a) such fraud, rejection of evidence, irregularity of proceedings, insufficiency of inquiry, or other reasons; or (b) since then the discovery of such new facts or evidence, as to make it necessary or desirable to hold another inquest or investigation.[23]

The leave of the court is not necessary to make an application under the **19–09** statute,[24] although it will be necessary for any parallel application for judicial review.[25]

If these prerequisites are satisfied, then the court will order another inquest or **19–10** investigation to be held and the whole of the original inquisition or determination or finding to be quashed.[26] In exercising this jurisdiction, the court has no power merely to amend an existing inquisition or determination or finding, e.g. to

---

[17] As to which, see 16–20.
[18] *Connah v Plymouth Hospitals NHS Trust* [2010] EWHC 1727 (Admin.) at [14].
[19] See 5–01.
[20] *Connah v Plymouth Hospitals NHS Trust* [2010] EWHC 1727 (Admin.) at [15]–[21].
[21] *Connah v Plymouth Hospitals NHS Trust* [2010] EWHC 1727 (Admin.) at [16].
[22] See 5–122 above.
[23] Coroners Act 1988 s.13(1)(b).
[24] *Re Rapier* [1988] Q.B. 26, DC; cf. *R. v South London Coroner Ex p. Thompson, The Times*, May 15, 1982, per Comyn J; *R. v City of London Coroner Ex p. Calvi, The Times*, April 2, 1983, DC.
[25] See 19–45 below.
[26] *Re Bithell* (1986) 150 J.P. 273.

remove offending words.[27] This is in stark contrast to the position on judicial review, where the court has power to quash part only of an inquisition or determination or finding, and to remit an inquisition or determination or finding to the coroner with a direction to insert a new verdict, or even sometimes power to amend an inquisition, determination or finding.[28]

19–11 In exercising the statutory power to order another inquest or investigation to be held, the court may order it to be held by another coroner in the same coroner area, and such coroner for that purpose has the same powers and jurisdiction as the original coroner.[29] This means, for example, that he may exercise the power of exhumation which might have been exercised by the original coroner.[30] The court does not normally name the new coroner, but simply orders that the matter be remitted, e.g. "to be heard by a different coroner".[31]

Circumstances held to have satisfied prerequisites

19–12 Thus an inquisition, determination or finding may be quashed if a coroner fraudulently misdirects a jury,[32] or if he refuses to hear material evidence (including expert or medical evidence)[33] that is available,[34] or if there is an irregularity in the proceeding that is material,[35] such as the coroner having a private conversation with the jury foreman to the exclusion of the others,[36] or if he goes on a preliminary private inspection with one of the jury,[37] or if he retires with the jury to discuss the verdict with them,[38] or if he admits documentary evidence in breach of the Coroners Rules,[39] or if he sits late at night to finish the inquest in a single sitting,[40] or if he puts improper pressure on the jury for or against a particular verdict,[41] or refuses to leave to the jury a verdict open to them on the evidence,[42] or where the inquest finds only the terminal cause of death rather than the

---

[27] *R. v Walthamstow Coroner Ex p. Rubenstein* [1982] Crim. L.R. 509; *Re Sheppard* Unreported April 28, 1992, DC. But see 18–23 above for a statutory power to correct errors in certificates after inquest.

[28] See 19–66 ff below.

[29] Coroners Act 1988 s.13(2)(a)(ii), (3).

[30] See 8–03 ff above.

[31] See also 19–66 below.

[32] cf. *R. v Wakefield* (1717) 1 Str. 69.

[33] *R. v Inner North London Coroner Ex p. Linnane (No. 2)* (1990) 155 J.P. 343, DC; *Nicholls v Liverpool Coroner* Unreported November 8, 2001, DC; *Dowler v North London Coroner* [2009] EWHC 3300 (Admin.).

[34] cf. *R. v Carter* (1876) 45 L.J.Q.D. 711; *R v Rothera, The Times,* July 25, 1930; *R. v West Sussex Coroner Ex p. Edwards* (1991) 156 J.P. 186, DC; *R. v Lincoln Coroner Ex p. Hay* [2000] Lloyd's Rep. Med. 264, DC; *R. v Avon Deputy Coroner Ex p. Lambourne* Unreported July 29, 2002, DC.

[35] *R. v South London Coroner Ex p. Thompson, The Times,* July 9, 1982, DC.

[36] *R. v Reynolds* [1945] K.B. 20.

[37] *R. v Divine Ex p. Walton* [1930] 2 K.B. 29.

[38] *R. v Divine Ex p. Walton* [1930] 2 K.B. 29; *R. v Wood Ex p. Anderson* [1928] 1 K.B. 302.

[39] *R. v City of London Coroner Ex p. Calvi, The Times,* April 2, 1983, DC.

[40] *R. v City of London Coroner Ex p. Calvi, The Times,* April 2, 1983, DC.

[41] *R. v Surrey Coroner Ex p. Campbell* [1982] Q.B. 661; *Clayton v South Yorkshire Coroner* [2005] EWHC 1196 (Admin.), DC.

[42] *R. v Inner North London Coroner Ex p. Linnane (No. 2)* (1990) 155 J.P. 343, DC; *R. v Lincoln Coroner Ex p. Hay* [2000] Lloyd's Rep. Med. 264, DC.

underlying cause of death,[43] or if the investigations are inadequate and yield little or no evidence as to the cause and circumstances of death.[44]

Further, an inquisition, determination or finding may be quashed where further **19–13** facts or evidence later come to light, as where a subsequent post-mortem or histological examination reveals important new evidence,[45] or a subsequent pathologist's report contradicts earlier evidence,[46] or the original pathologist revises his opinion,[47] or an internal inquiry results in new evidence becoming available,[48] or an undocumented fall is alleged in a hospital patient shortly before death,[49] or if there is simply insufficient evidence (or that which is available is inadmissible) to justify the particular verdict arrived at.[50]

What constitutes new evidence?

For the purposes of this provision "new" evidence is evidence which was not **19–14** available at the time of the original inquest,[51] would have been admissible had it been available, is credible and relevant to an issue of significance in the inquisition, and might have made a material difference to the verdict recorded at the original inquest.[52] In one case, the written reports of two medical experts, prepared long after the original inquest (and therefore not then available), but on the basis of the relevant pre-existing medical notes, and histology slides and specimens, were held to be new evidence in this sense, though the court emphasised that "not every different opinion subsequently expressed by an expert witness upon materials which are available would necessarily qualify".[53]

---

[43] *Ex p. Minister of Justice* [1965] NSWR 1598.

[44] *R. v Wood Ex p. Atcherley* (1908) 73 J.P. 40; *Attorney General v South London Coroner* (1988) 152 J.P. 641; *Re O'Reilly* (1996) 160 J.P. 749, DC; *R. v Avon Deputy Coroner Ex p. Lambourne* Unreported July 29, 2002, DC; *Howlett v Devon Coroner* [2006] EWHC 2570 (Admin.), and *Jones v South London Coroner* [2010] EWHC 931 (Admin.). As to the phrase "insufficiency of inquiry" in Australian coronial legislation, see *Quinlan v Deputy State Coroner* [2000] NSWSC 434 (failure to call witness not insufficiency of inquiry) and *Plover v McIndoe* [2000] V.S.C. 475 (application to reopen inquest fails).

[45] *R. v Lewes Coroner Ex p. Attorney General* (1913) 48 L.J. 25, DC; *Re Wilby* Unreported October 10, 1991, DC. However, one factor for the court to take into account in deciding whether to exercise the power to quash is the extent to which the applicant is to blame for the new evidence's non-availability at the earliest inquest: *R. v City of London Coroner Ex p. Calvi, The Times*, April 2, 1983, DC. See also *Parkin v North Lincolnshire and Grimsby Coroner* [2005] EWHC 660 (Admin.), DC at [21]–[21].

[46] *Attorney General v Hampshire Coroner* (1990) 155 J.P. 190, DC; *Re Fletcher* (1992) 156 J.P. 522, DC.

[47] *Attorney General v Harte* (1987) 151 J.P. 819; *R. v Maidstone Coroner's Court Ex p. Johnstone* (1994) 158 J.P. 1115, DC.

[48] *Re Farrer* Unreported April 22, 1991 DC.

[49] *Combe v Blackburn Coroner* [2005] EWHC 2843 (Admin.), DC.

[50] *R. v Durham Coroner Ex p. Attorney General, The Times*, June 29, 1978, DC; *R. v Cardiff Coroner Ex p. Thomas* [1970] 1 W.L.R. 1475, DC; *R. v City of London Coroner Ex p. Barber* [1975] 1 W.L.R. 1310, DC; *R. v Walthamstow Coroner Ex p. Rubenstein, The Times*, February 24, 1982.

[51] Though see *Bloom v North London Assistant Deputy Coroner* [2004] EWHC 3071 (Admin.), DC (coroner not provided with family commissioned independent medical expert report, critical of hospital treatment, nor asked to call any independent expert evidence; inquisition quashed under s.13 on grounds of "fresh" evidence, and new inquest ordered; not decisive that family could have raised issues at inquest but failed to do so).

[52] *Re Fletcher* (1992) 156 J.P. 522, DC.

[53] *Re Fletcher* (1992) 156 J.P. 522, DC; *Howlett v Devon Coroner* [2006] EWHC 2570 (Admin.).

Critical test of whether "necessary or desirable in the interests of justice"

19–15 However, it is important to note that the exercise of the power to quash depends on the court's view that it is "necessary or desirable in the interests of justice" to hold a new inquest. The words have been described as

> "the critical words. The court is not to attend to mere formalities, nor to criticise minutely the summing up, or the nature of the evidence or of the procedure. But if the inquest has been so conducted, or the circumstances attending it are such that there is a real risk that justice has not been done, a real impairment of the security which the right procedure provides that justice is done and is seen to be done, the court ought not to allow the inquisition to stand."[54]

19–16 However, in another case, it was said simply that

> "Consideration of the many authorities in this field suggests that there are no longer any absolute principles in play, save only perhaps that the interests of justice must be the cardinal consideration."[55]

And, in another case, it was held that it was in the interests of justice to investigate "material which was not properly and fully investigated at the previous inquiry", even though some 50 years had elapsed since the death.[56] Lapse of time is a factor, but not conclusive.[57]

Likelihood of different verdict

19–17 In cases of new evidence, where the court is unable fully to evaluate the extent and effect of the proposed evidence, it has been held sufficient that there is a *possibility* that the result of the second inquest would be different from the first[58] although in other cases it has been stressed that this in itself is not determinative.[59] It has even been held that a new inquest may be ordered if there is a high probability that the result would be the same.[60] It may be that the test is more stringent (i.e. probability, not possibility, of different verdict) in cases where the court can fully evaluate the

---

[54] *R. v Divine Ex p. Walton* [1930] 2 K.B. 29 at 37, applied in *R. v South London Coroner Ex p. Thompson*, *The Times*, July 9, 1982, DC; *Herron v Attorney General for New South Wales* (1987) 8 NSWLR 601, CA (NSW); *Re Neal* (1995) 37 B.M.L.R. 164, DC; *Re Kelly* (1996) 61 J.P. 417, DC; *Attorney General v South Yorkshire (West) Coroner* [2012] EWHC 3783 (Admin.); *Markham v West London Coroner* [2013] EWHC 253 (Admin.); *Roberts v North and West Cumbria Coroner* [2013] EWHC 925 (Admin.).

[55] *Re Tabarn* Unreported January 20, 1998, DC, per Simon Brown LJ.

[56] *Re Maddison* [2002] EWHC 2567 (Admin.), DC.

[57] *R. (Sutovic) v North London Coroner* [2006] EWHC 1095 (Admin.) at [55].

[58] *R. v Cardiff Coroner Ex p. Thomas* [1970] 1 W.L.R. 1475, DC; *Re Rapier* [1988] Q.B. 26, DC; *Attorney General v Hampshire Coroner* (1990) 155 J.P. 190, DC; *Re Fletcher* (1992) 156 J.P. 522, DC; *Re Christopher Kelly* (1996) 161 J.P. 417, DC; *R. v Lincoln Coroner Ex p. Hay* [2000] Lloyd's Rep. Med. 264, DC; *Mulholland v St Pancras Coroner* [2003] EWHC 2612 (Admin.); *North West Wales Coroner v Hartley* [2005] EWHC 2343 (Admin.); *R. (Sutovic) v North London Coroner* [2006] EWHC 1095 (Admin.) at [54]; *Sparrow v East Somerset Coroner* [2006] EWHC 2718 (Admin.); *Jones v South London Coroner* [2010] EWHC 931 (Admin.); *R. (Halpin) v Attorney General* [2011] EWHC 3759 (Admin.) at [19].

[59] *Re O'Reilly* (1996) 160 J.P. 749, DC; *Re Clegg* (1996) 161 J.P. 521, DC.

[60] *R. v West Sussex Coroner Ex p. Edwards* (1991) 156 J.P. 186, DC; see *R. (Sutovic) v North London Coroner* [2006] EWHC 1095 (Admin.) at [55].

proposed evidence at the hearing,[61] though the less stringent test has been used more recently.[62]

Where there is new evidence the courts in recent times have in substance relied **19–18** on the test of whether there was a "real possibility" of a different verdict.[63] This echoes the approach in earlier cases.[64]

In cases where there is no new evidence, there is authority for saying that, if the **19–19** result of any new inquest would be the same, then it is not "necessary" within the meaning of those "critical words" to hold a new inquest.[65] In another case the test applied was whether there was "a real possibility" of a different result.[66] And in considering whether it is "desirable" to hold a new inquest, economic, social and humanitarian factors may be taken into account.[67] In cases in which the court is satisfied that a different verdict is not possible or doubts that it would be, the fact that the deceased died in custody may be "a compelling additional factor" in concluding that a further inquest is necessary or desirable in the interests of justice.[68] Lapse of time generally points in the opposite direction.[69] The generality and width of this statutory power to quash inquisitions make it preferable to judicial review in cases where an aggrieved person is unable to point to a clear error in the conduct of the inquest.[70]

Application by any person with sufficient interest

Application to the court for an inquisition to be quashed and a new inquest held **19–20** may be made by any person with sufficient interest, such as the family of the deceased,[71] a person whose conduct may be thought to be called into question by the verdict,[72] the Crown,[73] or indeed the coroner himself.[74] In one case a doctor who thought he could contribute to the inquiry into the mysterious death of a

---

[61] *Re Davis* [1968] 1 Q.B. 72, CA (but the precise test was not disputed); *Mulholland v Inner North London Coroner* (2003) 78 B.M.L.R. 75; [2003] Inquest L.R. 60.

[62] *Re Taylor* (1990) 154 J.P. 933, DC; *Re Tabarn* Unreported January 20, 1998, DC.

[63] *Mulholland v St Pancras Coroner* [2003] EWHC 2612 (Admin.); *North West Wales Coroner v Hartley* [2005] EWHC 2343 (Admin.).

[64] *Re Christopher Kelly* (1996) 161 J.P. 417, DC; *R. (Sutovic) v North London Coroner* [2006] EWHC 1095 (Admin.), DC; *Duggan v North London Coroner* [2010] EWHC 1263 (Admin.); *Jones v South London Coroner* [2010] EWHC 931 (Admin.). See also *Sparrow v East Somerset Coroner* [2006] EWHC 2718 (Admin.).

[65] *R. v South London Coroner Ex p. Thompson*, The Times, July 9, 1982, DC; cf. *R. v West Berkshire Coroner Ex p. Thomas* (1991) 155 J.P. 681 at 699; *Clayton v South Yorkshire Coroner* [2005] EWHC 1196 (Admin.), DC at [31]; *Fraser v North West Wales Coroner* [2010] EWHC 1165 (Admin.).

[66] *R. v Ceredigion Coroner Ex p. Wigley* [1993] C.O.D. 364, DC; *Re Christopher Kelly* (1996) 161 J.P. 417, DC.

[67] *R. v Ceredigion Coroner Ex p. Wigley* [1993] C.O.D. 364, DC; *Re Christopher Kelly* (1996) 161 J.P. 417, DC; *R. v West Sussex Coroner Ex p. Walrond* (1988) 153 J.P. 235, DC; see also *Re Sutherland* [1994] 2 N.Z.L.R. 242, HC (NZ).

[68] *R v West Sussex Coroner Ex p. Homberg* (1994) 158 J.P. 357; *R. (Sutovic) v North London Coroner* [2006] EWHC 1095 (Admin.), DC at [55].

[69] *R v West Sussex Coroner Ex p Homberg* (1994) 158 J.P. 357; *Re Tabarn* Unreported January 20, 1998, DC; *R. (Sutovic) v North London Coroner* [2006] EWHC 1095 (Admin.), DC at [55]; cf. *Nicholls v HM Coroner for the City of Liverpool* [2001] EWHC (Admin.) 922 at [49]–[50], [59].

[70] *R. v Central Cleveland Coroner Ex p. Dent* (1986) 150 J.P. 251.

[71] *R. v City of London Coroner Ex p. Calvi*, The Times, April 1983, DC.

[72] *R. v Walthamstow Coroner Ex p. Rubenstein* [1982] Crim. L.R. 509.

[73] cf. *Re Culley* (1833) 5 B. & Ad. 230.

[74] *R. v Lodder*, Manchester Guardian, June 2, 1956; *Re Rapier* [1988] Q.B. 26, DC; *R. v West Sussex Coroner Ex p. Walrond* (1988) 153, DC; see also *Re Maddison* [2002] EWHC 2567 (Admin.), DC.

scientist was held not to have, even arguably, any civil right infringed by the refusal of the Attorney General to give his *fiat* to statutory review proceedings against the Lord Chancellor who appointed a judge to conduct an inquiry into the death.[75]

19–21   The would-be applicant seeks the consent (*fiat*) of the Attorney General[76] in a document (known as a "memorial") verified by statutory declaration.[77] The form of the memorial is not prescribed.[78] It is just a written application. The Attorney General should give the coroner an opportunity to explain the situation (or his conduct) before the application is made to the court.[79] In practice, the Attorney General invites the coroner's comments before deciding whether to give the *fiat*.

19–22   If the Attorney General gives leave, or if he decides himself to make the application, it is made by Pt 8 claim form[80] (formerly originating motion), stating the grounds of the application, to the Divisional Court of the Queen's Bench Division of the High Court.[81] Unless the Attorney General himself makes the application, his *fiat* must accompany the claim form,[82] which itself must be filed in the Administrative Court and served upon all persons directly affected by the application (obviously including the coroner) within six weeks after the grant of the *fiat*.[83]

19–23   When the court issues the claim form it will fix a hearing date and prepare a notice of the hearing date for each party.[84] The claim form must be served at least 21 days before the hearing.[85] Where the claimant serves it, and it does not specify the hearing date, the claimant must serve notice of the hearing date at the same time.[86] The defendant (usually the coroner) does not have to acknowledge service[87] although he may do so, and indeed may file a defence. On the hearing

---

[75] *R. (Halpin) v Attorney General* [2011] EWHC 3759 (Admin.).

[76] The Solicitor-General may act for the Attorney General: Law Officers Act 1997 s.1. If the Attorney General refuses his *fiat*, the court has no power to review his decision: *Gouriet v Union of Post Office Workers* [1978] A.C. 435, HL, followed by Popplewell J in *R. v Attorney General Ex p. Ferrante* [1995] C.O.D. 18 (the Court of Appeal, *The Independent*, April 3, 1995, did not deal with this point), and by the Divisional Court in *R. v Sol.-Gen. Ex p. Taylor* [1996] 1 F.C.R. 206 (not a coroner's case). See also *R. (Duggan) v Attorney General* Unreported 3 November 2009 (permission for judicial review against the Attorney General given by Wyn Williams J), leading to *Duggan v North London Coroner* [2010] EWHC 1095 (Admin.), DC; *R. (Halpin) v Attorney General* [2011] EWHC 3759 (Admin.).

[77] For a form, see App.4, Form 2.

[78] For a form, see App.4, Form 1. Where the application is to quash, this should be accompanied by copies of the inquisition, statements of witnesses to be called at the new inquest and any newspaper reports available.

[79] *R. v Graham* (1905) 93, L.T. 371 at 376.

[80] CPR Practice Direction, Pt 8 paras 3.3 B.1(1), Table 2 B.8(3).

[81] Originally RSC Ord.94 r.14 (added by RSC (Amendment No. 2) 1988, as from October 1, 1988) and now CPR, PD 8 para.19. This regularised the previous procedure, under which originating motions were often used instead of originating summonses (*R. v City of London Coroner Ex p. Barber* [1975] 1 W.L.R. 1310, DC, and cf. RSC Ord.5 r.3 and *Re Rapier* [1988] Q.B. 26, DC).

[82] CPR Practice Direction, Pt 8 para.19(2).

[83] CPR Practice Direction, Pt 8 para.19(3).

[84] CPR Practice Direction, Pt 8 para.B.9.

[85] CPR Practice Direction, Pt 8, para.B.10.

[86] CPR Practice Direction Pt 8 para.B.11.

[87] CPR Practice Direction Pt 8 para.B.12; cf. CPR r.8.3(1).

date the court may either hear and dispose of the case, or give case management directions.[88]

On the actual hearing of the application, evidence is normally given by witness **19–24** statement,[89] though the court has power to require or permit oral evidence,[90] or to require a person who has given written evidence to attend for cross-examination.[91] Whether or not he attends or is represented, the coroner should make and file a witness statement[92] setting out the situation and the basic facts of the inquest, answering any specific points made by the claimant, and exhibiting to the statement copies of the inquisition, determination or findings[93] and any other relevant documents. The general practice and procedure is otherwise similar to that in cases of judicial review.[94] The question of costs is dealt with later.[95]

JUDICIAL REVIEW

Unified procedure

Applications for judicial review have, since 1977, been brought under a unified **19–25** procedure,[96] which has wrought considerable changes in English and Welsh public law.[97] The relief available on judicial review includes quashing orders[98] (formerly known as certiorari), by which a decision of an inferior tribunal is removed into the High Court to be quashed because it is ultra vires or an error of law has been made, and mandatory orders[99] (formerly known as mandamus), by which an inferior tribunal can be ordered to perform some duty already imposed upon it which it is neglecting to perform. These are the most important from the point of view of coronial law.

Other orders available on judicial review are prohibiting orders[100] (formerly **19–26** known as prohibition), by which an inferior tribunal can be prevented from exceeding its powers in some way which it is threatening to do; declarations,[101] by which the rights of the parties can be declared; and also injunctions[102] and damages[103] in appropriate cases.

---

[88] CPR Practice Direction Pt 8 para.B.13.
[89] For form, see App.4 Form 4.
[90] CPR r.8.6(2).
[91] CPR r.8.6(3).
[92] For form, see App.4 Form 6.
[93] *R. v Turnbull Ex p. Kenyon* Unreported March 15, 1984, DC.
[94] See 19–43 ff.
[95] See 19–30 ff.
[96] Originally RSC Ord.53; now CPR Pt 54.
[97] E.g. *O'Reilly v Mackman* [1983] 2 A.C. 237, HL.
[98] Senior Courts Act 1981 ss.29(1), 31(1)(b), (1A).
[99] Senior Courts Act 1981 ss.29(1), 31(1)(b), (1A).
[100] Senior Courts Act 1981 ss.29(1), 31(1)(b), (1A).
[101] Senior Courts Act 1981 s.31(1)(b), (2).
[102] Senior Courts Act 1981 s.31(1)(b),(c), (2). See *R. v Secretary of State for the Home Department Ex p. Herbage* [1987] Q.B. 872.
[103] Senior Courts Act 1981 s.31(4). As to interest on damages, see *R. v Transport Secretary Ex p. Sherriff & Sons, The Independent,* January 12, 1988.

To what extent is the coroner susceptible to review?

19–27   At the outset, however, there is a question as to how far the acts of the coroner and the coroner's court are amenable to judicial review at all. On the old authorities, it was clear that if there was fraud by the coroner,[104] or an error by him going to his jurisdiction,[105] or if an error of law appeared on the face of the record,[106] the High Court could interfere and quash the decision or inquisition, as the case might be. But at least until the decision of the House of Lords in *Anisminic v Foreign Compensation Commission*,[107] there seemed to be no way in which an error of law *within* the coroner's jurisdiction and not going to that jurisdiction (such as misdirection of the jury,[108] or questions of admissibility of evidence)[109] could be reviewed by the courts.

19–28   Since *Anisminic*, it has been possible for the courts to review errors of law committed by inferior tribunals not going to jurisdiction. These errors might fall into any of a number of categories, such as those set out by Lord Reid in *Anisminic*, in a list expressed to be non-exhaustive:

> "But there are many cases where, although the tribunal had jurisdiction to enter on the enquiry, it has done or failed to do something in the course of the enquiry which is of such a nature that its decision is a nullity. It may have given a decision in bad faith. It may have made a decision which it had no power to make. It may have failed in the course of the enquiry to comply with the requirements of natural justice. It may in perfect good faith have misconstrued the provisions giving it the power to act so that it failed to deal with the question remitted to it and decided some question which was not remitted to it. It may also have refused to take into account something which it was required to take into account. Or it may have based its decision on some matter which, under the provisions setting it up, it had no right to take into account."[110]

19–29   *Anisminic* itself concerned a statutory tribunal, not a coroner's court, and accordingly there was room for argument as to whether the *Anisminic* extension applied to an inferior court such as that of the coroner. In one case,[111] the Divisional Court held that it did not, on the basis that *Anisminic* dealt with statutory tribunals, and probably only with those from whose decisions there was no appeal,[112] whereas in the case of coroners the statutory provisions already considered[113] constituted a form of appeal. But in a later case[114] a differently

---

[104] *R. v Wakefield* (1717) 1 Str. 69.
[105] Such as exceeding or refusing jurisdiction: *R. v Surrey Coroner Ex p. Campbell* [1982] Q.B. 661 at 672.
[106] *Foxhall v Barnett* (1853) 2 E. & B. 928; *R. v Evett* (1827) 6 B. & C. 247; *R. v Northumberland Compensation Appeal Tribunal Ex p. Shaw* [1952] 1 K.B. 338, per Denning LJ.
[107] [1969] 2 A.C. 147, HL.
[108] *R. v McIntosh* (1858) 7 W.R. 52; 32 L.T.O.S. 146.
[109] *R. v Ingham* (1864) 5 B. & S. 257.
[110] [1969] 2 A.C. 147 at 171.
[111] *R. v Surrey Coroner Ex p. Campbell* [1982] Q.B. 661.
[112] See 19–35.
[113] See 19–05 ff.
[114] *R. v Greater Manchester Coroner Ex p. Tal* [1985] Q.B. 67.

constituted Divisional Court held that that case was wrongly decided, and decided to follow it, holding instead that, in principle, the *Anisminic* extension of the law covered the case of a coroner's court. This is the accepted view.[115]

What kind of decisions in coroner's court are susceptible to review?

The inquisition, determination or findings. Given that judicial review is **19–30** available at all, the question arises, in relation to what kinds of decision of the coroner's court is it exercisable? Obviously it extends to reviewing the ultimate verdict of the inquest, as recorded in the inquisition, determination or findings, and such inquisitions, determinations or findings may be quashed, for example if it can be shown that the jurors were not sworn,[116] or one juror was sworn after evidence had already been given (which he had not heard),[117] that the coroner had no jurisdiction at all;[118] that the coroner wrongly refused to hear relevant and available evidence,[119] or admitted evidence not on oath,[120] or otherwise inadmissible,[121] which might have influenced the jury and thus caused a miscarriage of justice; that the inquest was not resumed on the date to which it had been adjourned;[122] that the coroner retired with the jury,[123] or had a private discussion with them not in open court,[124] or passed lengthy and complex notes to them to look at in considering their verdict;[125] that the coroner put pressure on the jury to return a particular verdict,[126] or misdirected them[127] (or himself),[128] or made them sit too long without a proper break;[129] that the coroner made excessive use of the power

---

[115] See also *R. (Cart) v The Upper Tribunal* [2012] 1 AC 663, SC (judicial review available against the Upper Tribunal, but only on "second appeal" criteria).

[116] *R. v Ferrand* (1819) 3 B. & Ald. 260.

[117] *R. v Yorkshire Coroner* (1863) 9 L.T. 424.

[118] *Foxall v Barnett* (1863) 2 E. & B. 928; *R. v White* (1860) 3 E. & E. (where the coroner had already held one inquest and accordingly was *functus officio*); similarly where the inquest is in part conducted outside his jurisdiction: *R. v Hinde* (1844) 5 Q.B. 944.

[119] *R. v Carter* (1876) 45 L.J.Q.B. 711; *R. v Rothera Ex p. Chetwin, The Times*, July 25, 1930; *R v Inner North London Coroner Ex p. Linnane (No. 2)* (1990) 155 J.P. 343, DC; *R. v East Sussex Coroner Ex p. Homberg* (1994) 158 J.P. 357; *Re Potter's Application for Judicial Review* Unreported January 24, 1997, Harrison J; *R. v Lincoln Coroner Ex p. Hay* [2000] Lloyd's Rep. Med. 264, DC; *R. v West Yorkshire Coroner Ex p. Schrompf* Unreported June 8, 1998, CA; *Nicholls v Liverpool Coroner* Unreported November 8, 2001, DC; *R. v Avon Deputy Coroner Ex p. Lambourne* Unreported July 29, 2002, DC; *Quinlan v Deputy State Coroner* [2000] NSWSC 434; *R. (Hair) v Staffordshire (South) Coroner* [2010] EWHC 2580 (Admin.).

[120] *R. v Staffordshire Coroner* (1864) 10 L.T. 650; *R. v Graham* (1905) 93 L.T. 371.

[121] cf. *R. v City of London Coroner Ex p. Calvi, The Times*, April 2, 1983, DC; *Re Siberry's Application for Judicial Review* [2008] N.I.Q.B. 147.

[122] *R. v Payn* (1864) 34 L.J.Q.B. 59.

[123] *R. v Fitzgerald Ex p. O'Brien and Bourchier* (1883) 17 Ir.L.T. 34; *Re Mitchelstown Inquisition* (1888) 22 L.R. IR. 279; *R. v Wood Ex p. Anderson* [1928] 1 K.B. 302.

[124] *R. v Reynolds* [1943] K.B. 20; cf. *R. v Greater Manchester Coroner Ex p. Tal* [1985] Q.B. 67.

[125] *R. v West London Coroner Ex p. Gray* [1988] Q.B. 467, DC.

[126] *R. v Anderson* (1701) 12 Mod.Rep. 493; cf. *R. v Surrey Coroner Ex p. Campbell* [1982] Q.B. 661 at 676–677.

[127] *R. v Turnbull Ex p. Kenyon* Unreported March 15, 1984, DC; *R. v West London Coroner Ex p. Gray* [1988] Q.B. 567, DC; *R. v Birmingham Coroner Ex p. Home Secretary* (1990) 155 J.P. 107, DC; *R. v Birmingham and Solihull Coroner Ex p. Nutt* [1993] C.O.D. 409, DC; *R. (Anderson) v Inner North London Coroner* [2004] EWHC 2729 (Admin.); *R. (P) v Avon Coroner* [2009] EWCA Civ. 1367; *R. (Hair) v Staffordshire (South) Coroner* [2010] EWHC 2580 (Admin.).

[128] *R. (Platts) v South Yorkshire Coroner* [2008] EWHC 2502 (Admin.).

[129] *R. v Southwark Coroner Ex p. Hicks* [1987] 1 W.L.R. 1624, DC.

to adjourn;[130] that he failed to sum up the evidence to the jury;[131] that he refused to hear legal submissions on behalf of the "interested person";[132] that the facts in evidence did not justify the verdict;[133] that there was insufficient inquiry;[134] that there were irregularities in the jury[135]or in the inquisition;[136] or that the coroner himself altered the inquisition, being persuaded that the evidence before the jury did not justify the verdict;[137] or that the verdict was perverse. The courts will not, however, quash an inquisition, determination or findings taken before a wholly unauthorised person, for that is simply void.[138]

19–31   **Preliminary and interlocutory decisions.** But judicial review extends wider than the inquisition, determination or findings, and in principle covers all preliminary and interlocutory decisions made by the coroner in connection with or in the course of his or her official duty. Thus applications for judicial review have been entertained by the courts in relation to decisions whether to release a body for burial,[139] whether an inquest must be held at all,[140] whether a first post-mortem examination should be prohibited[141] or a second post-mortem examination should be permitted,[142] whether a coroner should enter premises and search for evidence,[143] where an inquest should be held,[144] whether it should be held in public or in camera,[145] whether it ought to be held with a jury,[146] whether a

---

[130] *R. v Northern Ireland Secretary Ex p. Devine* Unreported September 9, 1988, HC (NI).

[131] *R. v Antrim Coroner* [1980] N.I. 123; *R. (Bodycote HIP Ltd) v Herefordshire Coroner* [2008] EWHC 164 (Admin.).

[132] *R. v East Berkshire Coroner Ex p. Buckley* (1992) 157 J.P. 425, DC.

[133] *R. v Huntbach Ex p. Lockley* [1944] K.B. 606; *Re Williams*, 118 New L.J. 1174; *R. v Durham Coroner Ex p. Attorney General, The Times*, June 29, 1978, DC; *R. v Devon Coroner Ex p. Glover* (1984) 149 J.P. 208; see also *Khan v West* [2002] V.S.C. 227.

[134] *R. v Lewes Coroner Ex p. Attorney General* (1913) 29 T.L.R. 199, DC; *R. v Rothera Ex p. Chetwin, The Times*, July 25, 1930, DC; *R. v Cave Ex p. Horwill, The Times*, June 9, 1956, DC; *R. v Avon Deputy Coroner Ex p. Lambourne*, July 29, 2002 Unreported DC.

[135] *R v Thompson* [2010] EWCA Crim. 1623.

[136] *Foxall v Barnett* (1853) 2 E. & B. 928 (inquisition did not show coroner to have jurisdiction); *Anon.* (1696) 123 Mod. Rep. 112 (jury's finding uncertain); *R. v Parker* (1675) 2 Lev. 140 (inquisition did not adequately describe manner of death); *R. v Evett* (1827) 6 B. & C. 247 (inquisition did not state where death occurred or the body was found). In *R. v Surrey Coroner Ex p. Campbell* [1982] Q.B. 661, the Divisional Court purported to exercise the statutory power to amend an inquisition contained in s.20 of the Coroners Act 1887, but this section was applicable only to criminal trials upon the inquisition, and in any event was repealed by the Criminal Law Act 1977 Sch.13. As to the common law powers to *amend* an inquisition, rather than quash it, see 19–66.

[137] *R. v Howe Ex p. Powell, The Times*, July 20, 1954, DC.

[138] *Re Daws* (1838) 8 Ad. & El. 936.

[139] *R. v Bristol Coroner Ex p. Atkinson* Unreported May 5, 1983, QBD; *R. v Hampshire Coroner Ex p. Horscroft, The Times*, October 3, 1985.

[140] *R. v West Yorkshire Coroner Ex p. Smith* [1983] Q.B. 335, CA. There is no doubt that, conversely, the courts would hear an application for review of a decision to hold or resume an inquest when there was no power in the coroner to do so: *R. v White* (1860) 3 E. & E. 137; *R. v Bristol Coroner Ex p. Atkinson* Unreported May 5, 1983, QBD.

[141] *R. v Westminster City Coroner Ex p. Rainer*, 112 S.J. 882. See also *R. v Greater Manchester Coroner Ex p. Worch* [1988] Q.B. 513, CA.

[142] *R. v South London Coroner Ex p. Ridley* [1985] 1 W.L.R. 1347.

[143] *Ex p. Zinc Corporation* (1969) 90 W.N. (N.S.W.) 654.

[144] *R. v Inner North London Coroner Ex p. Greater London Council, The Times*, April 30, 1983.

[145] *R. v McHugh Ex p. Trelford* Unreported March 22, 1984, DC.

[146] *R. v West Yorkshire Coroner Ex p. National Union of Mineworkers (Yorkshire Area)* (1985) 150 J.P. 58, DC; *R. v Inner North London Coroner Ex p. Linnane* [1989] 1 W.L.R. 395, DC.

coroner should adjourn,[147] whether a coroner should call an inquest to be held by
a different coroner than himself, for example on grounds of possible bias,[148]
whether the coroner should resume an inquest after the disposal of criminal
charges,[149] whether the coroner should put additional questions to the jury,[150] and
the question whether the coroner possessed any power at all to punish for contempt.[151]

Some of these decisions may have been purely oral and never reduced into   **19–32**
writing, yet no point appears ever to have been taken that certiorari originally lay
only in respect of written decisions (being part of the record).[152] That point should
now be regarded as obsolete since *Anisminic*. In principle, the court has power to
review the coroner's handling of an inquest even whilst that inquest is in progress,
but it will be reluctant to intervene in such a case,[153] and in the ordinary case will
not entertain such a challenge.[154] If it does intervene, it may prohibit any
publication of the report of its decision until after the jury has reached a verdict.[155]

Distinction between review and appeal

The list of types of decision subject to judicial review is obviously not exhaustive,   **19–33**
but, as with judicial review inquisitions, it must not be forgotten that judicial
review is not a process of appeal. The reviewing court does not quash a decision
just because the court might have decided it differently, and a fortiori it does not
substitute its own decision for that of the coroner. The coroner's decision is
reviewed on the basis of the evidence available to him or her then, not that available
since.[156] It is a question of error in the decision-making process, rather than in the
decision itself, with which the court is concerned. If no clear error can be pointed
to, but the decision is unsatisfactory overall, the applicant should proceed under the
statutory power to quash, and not by way of judicial review.[157]

---

[147] *R. v East Sussex Coroner Ex p. Homberg* (1994) 158 J.P 357, DC; *Re Doyle's Application* Unreported
April 18, 2005, Sullivan J (coroner had no duty in circumstances to adjourn until partner of deceased
was well enough to attend).
[148] *R. v West Yorkshire Coroner Ex p. Smith*, *The Times*, November 6, 1982; *R. v Inner West London
Coroner Ex p. Dallaglio* [1994] 4 All E.R. 139, CA.
[149] *R. (Moss) v Durham and Darlington Coroner* [2008] EWHC 2940 (Admin.); *R. (Palmer) v Worcestershire
Coroner* [2011] EWHC 1453 (Admin.).
[150] *R. (D) v Inner South London Assistant Deputy Coroner* [2008] EWHC 3356 (Admin.).
[151] *R. v West Yorkshire Coroner Ex p. Smith (No. 2)* [1985] Q.B. 1096, DC.
[152] See 19–29 above.
[153] *R. v East Kent Coroner Ex p. Spooner* (1987) 152 J.P. 115, DC; *R. v Inner North London Coroner Ex
p Diesa Koto* (1993) 157 J.P. 857, DC; *Re Palmer's Application* Unreported December 10, 1997, CA;
R. (Khan) v West Hertfordshire Coroner [2002] EWHC 302; *R. (Craik) v Wiltshire & Swindon Coroner*
[2004] EWHC 2653 (Admin.); see 11–40 above.
[154] *R. (Cooper) v North East Kent Coroner* [2014] EWHC 586 (Admin.). See also *Re Application by Officers
C, D, H & R* [2012] NICA 47, and *Re McDonnell's Application* [2014] NIQB 66.
[155] Contempt of Court Act 1981 s.4(2); see *The Times*, October 10, 1987; *R. v Inner North London
Coroner Ex p Diesa Koto* (1993) 157 J.P. 857, DC; *Re Palmer's Application* Unreported December 10,
1997, CA; *R. v Worcester Coroner Ex p. UK Detention Services Ltd.*, February 18, 1998 Unreported
Ognall J.
[156] *R. v Poplar Coroner Ex p. Chaudhry* Unreported December 15, 1993, DC; *R. (Sutovic) v North London
Coroner* [2006] EWHC 1095 (Admin.) at [41], [44]–[47], [52]; *R. (Lagos) v City of London Coroner*
[2013] EWHC 423 (Admin.) at [7].
[157] *R. v Central Cleveland Coroner Ex p. Dent* (1986) 150 J.P. 251.

19–34 However, it is true to say that the question of error in reaching a decision is sometimes dealt with by asking whether any reasonable tribunal, directing itself correctly as to both law and fact, could have reached the conclusion to which it in fact came.[158]

Judicial review is a discretionary remedy

19–35 Even though defects may be shown to have existed in the decision–making process, nonetheless the court retains a discretion as to whether it should grant the relief sought. This is because judicial review is a discretionary remedy: it does not follow that an order will be made merely because some error of law has been committed.[159] Apart from other considerations, the court will generally only interfere if the decision or verdict under review would be different if the decision were to be taken or the inquest held afresh.[160] If the outcome would be the same, the error has not caused injustice, and there is no need to make any order.[161]

19–36 Where the court considers that there has been undue delay in making an application for judicial review, it may refuse to grant the relief sought if it considers that this would cause substantial hardship to, or substantially prejudice the rights of, any person, or would be detrimental to good administration.[162] This is without prejudice to any other rule limiting time for making such an application.[163]

Locus standi

19–37 In order for the courts to entertain an application for judicial review, the applicant must show that he has a sufficient interest in the matter or decision to be subjected to review, that is that he has locus standi. In judicial review cases, the court will not give permission to make the application at all unless the would-be applicant passes a preliminary threshold of "sufficient interest"[164]; but the threshold is designed only to exclude clearly unmeritorious, "busybody" cases, since locus standi can only properly be gone into at the full hearing.[165]

19–38 The question appears to be one of mixed law and fact, involving a considerable measure of discretion, but the following are said to be factors which will be taken into account[166]:

---

[158] *R. v City of London Coroner Ex p. Barber* [1975] 1 W.L.R. 1310, DC; *R. v Devon Coroner Ex p. Glover* (1984) 149 J.P. 208.

[159] *R. v Greater Manchester Coroner Ex p. Tal* [1985] Q.B. 67 at 83; *R. v Inner North London Coroner Ex p. Linnane (No. 2)* (1990) 155 J.P. 343, DC.

[160] *Re Davis* [1968] 1 Q.B. 72; *Re Williams, The Times,* December 10, 1968, DC; *R. v Portsmouth Coroner Ex p. Keane* (1989) 153 J.P. 658, DC.

[161] *R. v Wolverhampton Coroner Ex p. McCurbin* [1990] 1 W.L.R. 719, CA; *Re Potter's Application,* January 24, 1997, Harrison J; *R. v Inner South London Coroner Ex p. Douglas-Williams* [1998] 1 All E.R. 344, CA; *R. (Anderson) v Inner North London Coroner* [2004] EWHC 2729 (Admin.); *R. (Bennett) v Inner South London Coroner* [2006] EWHC 196 (Admin.) at [61]; *R. (P) v Avon Coroner* [2009] EWCA Civ. 1367.

[162] Senior Courts Act 1981 s.31(6).

[163] Senior Courts Act 1981 s.31(7). See also 19–47 (three months).

[164] Senior Courts Act 1981 s.31(3); CPR r.54.4.

[165] *IRC v National Federation of Self-Employed and Small Businesses Ltd* [1982] A.C. 617 at 630, 643–644, 649, 659, HL. See also *R. (Halpin) v Attorney General* [2011] EWHC 3759 (Admin.).

[166] Aldous and Alder, *Applications for Judicial Review,* 2nd edn (1993), pp.103–104; see also *Halsbury's Laws of England,* 4th edn reissue, Vol.1(1) para.66.

(1) the scope and purpose of the particular power or duty under consideration, and whether it recognises the applicant's interest;

(2) the gravity of the allegations made;

(3) the strength of the applicant's case;

(4) the degree of public interest in the decision or matter under review;

(5) the nature of the remedy sought, certiorari being more liberally allowed than mandamus;

(6) how seriously the applicant has been injured;

(7) the degree of previous connection with the decision or matter in question.

It should be noted that the parties to an application for judicial review cannot **19–39** *agree* to treat one of them as having locus standi, since this goes to the jurisdiction of the court.[167]

Thus, where a coroner's inquest is concerned, it seems clear that persons having **19–40** a right to be represented at a post-mortem examination[168] or at an inquest[169] shall have locus standi to complain of matters forming part of such proceedings[170]; more specifically, both the family[171] of a deceased and a person who may be charged with causing his death are very much interested (though for different reasons) in a decision whether or not to release a body for disposal or removal out of the country,[172] and a person, whether witness or spectator, punished by a coroner for contempt clearly has locus standi to challenge the decision to impose such punishment,[173] as also a person whose conduct may be thought to be brought into question by an inquest verdict has to challenge that verdict.[174] The coroner has also been held to have standing to challenge a decision, whether his own[175] or that of a predecessor.[176]

A less obvious case (but nonetheless correct, it is submitted) is the locus standi **19–41** of a national newspaper editor and reporter to challenge a decision to hold an

---

[167] *Re Aylmer Ex p Bischoffheim* (1887) 20 Q.B.D. 258, 262; *R. v Social Services Secretary Ex p. Child Poverty Action Group* [1990] 2 Q.B. 540, CA; *Connah v Plymouth Hospitals NHS Trust* [2010] EWHC 1727 (Admin.) at [16].

[168] As to which see 8–60, 8–61 above.

[169] As to which see 11–59 above.

[170] *R. v South London Coroner Ex p. Ridley* [1985] 1 W.L.R. 1347.

[171] Where the family are divided on whether judicial review should be sought, the court should be told: *Re Tabarn* Unreported January 20, 1998, DC.

[172] *R. v Bristol Coroner Ex p. Kerr* [1974] Q.B. 652, DC; *R. v Bristol Coroner Ex p. Atkinson* Unreported May 5, 1983.

[173] *R. v West Yorkshire Coroner Ex p. Smith (No. 2)* [1985] Q.B. 1096, DC.

[174] *R. v Walthamstow Coroner Ex p. Rubenstein* [1982] Crim. L.R. 509.

[175] *R. v Inner North London Coroner Ex p. Chambers, The Times,* April 30, 1983; *R. v West Suffolk Coroner Ex p Walrond* (1989) 153 J.P. 235, DC.

[176] *Re Maddison* [2002] EWHC 2567 (Admin.) DC at [5]. But the lapse of time would normally be fatal to the judicial review application: see 19–47.

inquest in camera or grant anonymity to a witness.[177] The appropriate government department may doubtless challenge a decision not to hold a particular inquest in camera, even though it involved important national security considerations.[178] Similarly, a trades union may have locus standi to challenge coronial decisions made in relation to a death which occurred during picketing in the course of an industrial dispute.[179] But an unrelated correspondent of a prisoner (who had never met him) was held not to have locus standi to bring judicial review proceedings in respect of that prisoner's death.[180]

19–42   A more difficult case is where a person or body wishes to challenge the decision of the coroner that he or it is not an "interested person" for the purposes of the investigation and therefore entitled to be represented at the inquest.[181] In one case, the coroner himself applied for judicial review, by way of declaration, that a particular organisation was *not* a "properly interested person".[182] No doubt, where the person or body claiming to be such person could show a strong case, he or it would be treated as having locus standi to challenge the coroner's decision in the matter.

Procedure for application for judicial review

19–43   Under the RSC, there was no legal requirement for a would-be applicant to engage in any dialogue with the respondent before launching legal proceedings. The applicant was merely expected to complain to the decision-maker about the decision, and give him an opportunity to respond, before embarking upon a judicial review application.[183] Under the CPR, however, a system of pre-action protocols has been devised, including one for judicial review. This sets out the two distinct steps that the parties should follow before the claim for judicial review is made, except in urgent cases (although even then it is good practice to email or fax the draft claim form to the proposed defendant). A failure to follow the protocol may result in sanctions being imposed by the court.

---

[177] *R. v McHugh Ex p. Trelford* Unreported March 22, 1984, DC; see also *R. v Felixstowe Justices Ex p. Leigh* [1987] Q.B. 582, DC; *R. v Bedfordshire Coroner Ex p. Local Sunday Newspapers Ltd* (1999) 164 J.P. 283.

[178] *Cf Foreign Secretary v Inner North London Assistant Deputy Coroner* [2013] EWHC 3724 (Admin.); para.11–09 above.

[179] *R. v West Yorkshire Coroner Ex p. National Union of Mineworkers (Yorkshire Area)* (1985) 150 J.P. 58, DC; see also *Re Medical Defence Union Ltd. v Sinclair* [1990] 1 Med.L.R. 359, HK (MDU has locus standi where doctor's conduct in question).

[180] *R. v North Cambridgeshire Coroner Ex p. Chaney* Unreported May 19, 1995, CA.

[181] See 8–22.

[182] *R. v Inner North London Coroner Ex p. Chambers, The Times,* April 30, 1983: the court did not grant the declaration sought as the coroner indicated that he would hear further submissions by the organisation in question; the coroner did so and held that the organisation was not a "properly interested person" within r.20(2)(h). See also *R. (Southall Black Sisters) v West Yorkshire Coroner* [2002] EWHC 1914 (Admin.), Jackson J.

[183] *R. v Horsham District Council Ex p. Wenman* [1995] 1 W.L.R. 680 (not a coroner's case).

The first step is a letter before action, containing all the essential details,   **19–44**
information, and names of interested parties.[184] The second step is that proposed
defendant should normally respond within 14 days,[185] or failing that should send
an interim reply and propose a reasonable extension. But this will not extend the
time limit for making the claim.[186] The reply should make clear what is conceded
and what is not, and should be sent to all interested parties.

Under the RSC, a would-be applicant for judicial review had to obtain leave ex   **19–45**
parte from the court *before* commencing the proceedings.[187] Under the CPR,
however, the claimant actually starts the proceedings first, by filing a claim form
making the coroner defendant,[188] serving it on the defendant coroner,[189] and then
seeking permission from the court to carry on the proceedings.[190] This different
approach makes the coroner a party from the outset, and has significant costs
implications.[191] Moreover, under the 2013 reforms, each area or assistant coroner
is a separate officeholder,[192] and not merely the deputy of the coroner, the sole
officeholder under the old system. Thus, in respect of the acts of an area or assistant
coroner, proceedings are no longer against the coroner of a particular area, but
against the officeholder in question, senior, area or assistant coroner, as the case
may be. Each of them has an indemnity[193] and is entitled to direct his or her own
defence. It makes no difference if the occupant of the office retires.

Claims for judicial review against coroners can be filed at any of (i) the   **19–46**
Administrative Court at the Royal Courts of Justice, and (ii) the District Registries
of Birmingham, Cardiff, Leeds and Manchester.[194] The expectation is that the
claim will be administered and determined in the region with which the claimant
has the closest connection, having regard however to certain other considerations,
including where the defendant is based.[195] A claim may be transferred from one
venue to another.[196]

The claim form (N 461)[197] is headed "The Queen on the application of [name]   **19–47**
Claimant, versus [coroner or other public body] Defendant".[198] It must be filed
promptly and in any event within three months after the grounds for the claim first
arose.[199] Time for challenging a decision to carry out a post-mortem examination
runs from the date of the decision, not the date of any inquest held thereafter.[200]

---

[184] See Annex A to the Protocol.
[185] See Annex B to the Protocol.
[186] CPR r.54.5(1).
[187] Senior Courts Act 1981 s.31(3); RSC Ord.53 r.4(1).
[188] CPR Pt 54.
[189] CPR r.54.7.
[190] CPR r.54.4.
[191] See 19–70 ff below.
[192] See 2–94, 2–95.
[193] See 18–44.
[194] PD 54D para.2.1.
[195] PD 54D para.5.2.
[196] PD 54D, paras 5.1, 5.4.
[197] See App.4. If the matter is exceptionally urgent, Form N 463 should *also* be completed.
[198] *Practice Direction: The Administrative Court* [2000] 1 W.L.R. 1654.
[199] CPR r.54.5(1). See also Senior Courts Act 1981 s.31(6), (7), 19–36.
[200] *Re Jacobs' Application for Judicial Review* (1999) 53 B.M.L.R. 21, CA; PD 54D, para.4.1.

The time limit may not be extended by agreement.[201] The court, however, has power to extend the period, for "good reason".[202]

19–48 The claim form must state the remedy sought and the basis for it, any enactment under which the claim is brought, any representative capacity in which it is made, and any representative capacity of the defendant.[203] In addition it must state that the claimant is seeking permission to proceed with a claim for judicial review and any interim remedy claimed, as well the name and address of any person whom he or she considers to be an "interested party".[204] This expression means any person (other than the claimant and defendant) who is directly affected by the claim.[205] It will include persons who are parties to court proceedings which become subject to judicial review,[206] but "interested persons" at an inquest are not *parties* to that inquest,[207] and so are not automatically "interested parties" on judicial review.[208] Nonetheless, in practice the interested persons at an inquest are frequently considered interested parties on judicial review of a coronial decision affecting them. Where a human rights issue is raised, further information must also be included.[209] The form must be served (by the claimant)[210] on the defendant and any person considered to be an interested party within seven days of issue.[211] There is a special expedited procedure for urgent applications.[212]

19–49 The claim form must include or be accompanied by a detailed statement of the claimant's grounds, a statement of the facts relied on, any application to extend time for filing, any directions application, and a time estimate for the hearing.[213] It must also be accompanied by any written evidence in support, a copy of any order sought to be quashed, an approved copy of any reasons given, copies of any documents to be relied on and any relevant statutory material, and a list of essential court reading.[214] If some of these are not filed, this fact (and the reasons for it) must be stated.[215] In addition to the original documents, two further copies of an indexed bundle of all these documents must also be supplied.[216] In principle, therefore, the claimant has to have his or her case ready from the outset, though the

---

[201] CPR r.54.5(2).
[202] *Re Jacobs' Application for Judicial Review* (1999) 53 B.M.L.R. 21, CA; and see *R. v Stratford-upon-Avon DC Ex p. Jackson* [1985] 1 W.L.R. 1319, CA (difficulty in obtaining legal aid good reason for extending period), and *Caswell v Dairy Produce Quota Tribunal for England and Wales* [1990] 2 A.C. 738, HL; *Re Berry's Application* Unreported May 30, 2002, Burton J; *R. (Lawrance) v West Somerset Coroner* [2008] EWHC 1293 (Admin.); *R. (Pritchard) v Oxfordshire Coroner* [2008[EWHC 3246 (Admin.); *Allman v West Sussex ADC* [2012] EWHC 534 (Admin.) at [27]; *Re McDonnell's Application* [2014] NIQB 66, [23] ff.
[203] CPR rr.8.2, 54.6(1).
[204] CPR r.54.6(1).
[205] CPR r.54.1(2)(f).
[206] PD 54A, para.5.1.
[207] See 1–19, 10–03.
[208] *Foreign Secretary v Inner North London ADC* [2013] EWHC 1786 (Admin.).
[209] PD 54A para.5.3, and see also para.8.2.
[210] PD 54A, para.6.1 (service is generally effected by the parties, not by the court; as to service on the Crown, see para.6.2).
[211] CPR r.54.7.
[212] *Practice Statement (Administrative Courts: Listing and Urgent Cases)* [2002] 1 W.L.R. 810.
[213] CPR r.54.6(2); PD 54A para.5.6.
[214] PD 54A para.5.7.
[215] PD 54A para.5.8.
[216] PD 54A para.5.9.

court can give permission later for additional grounds,[217] or for other evidence to be adduced.[218]

If the coroner or anyone else served with the claim form wishes to take part in **19–50** the proceedings, he or she must file an acknowledgement of service[219] within 21 days of service, and serve a copy on the claimant and any interested party within seven days thereafter.[220] Again, these limits may not be extended by agreement.[221] The acknowledgement must state whether the claim is contested, and if so on what grounds (in summary form), and the details of any other person considered to be an interested party.[222] It must be signed by the coroner concerned (who may not be the senior coroner, but an area or assistant coroner) or his or her lawyer, and give an address for service.[223]

If the coroner (or anyone else) fails to file an acknowledgement of service, he or **19–51** she may not take part in the "permission" hearing, unless the court specifically so allows.[224] But as long as detailed grounds for contesting the claim (or supporting it on other grounds), and any written evidence, are served and filed within the time limit,[225] the coroner will still be able to appear on the substantive hearing.[226]

The judge will normally consider the question of permission without a **19–52** hearing,[227] i.e. on the documents alone. At the end of 2013 the average waiting time for this to be decided in London was 14.7 weeks. In 2001 it was eight weeks. If the judge gives permission, he or she may also give directions.[228] The order giving or refusing permission will be served on all parties, including interested parties who acknowledge service.[229] The grant of permission cannot be challenged.[230] The refusal (or grant on terms) will be accompanied by reasons.[231]

Unless the court records that the application is totally without merit,[232] in the **19–53** case of a refusal the claimant may within seven days request a hearing to reconsider the matter.[233] This happens in about 50 per cent of refusals. Only the claimant need attend such a hearing.[234] The costs implications are considered later.[235] If permission is refused again, the claimant may within seven days make a paper application for permission to appeal from the Court of Appeal,[236] though that

---

[217] CPR r.54.15.
[218] CPR r.54.16(2).
[219] CPR r.54.8(1).
[220] CPR r.54.8(2).
[221] CPR r.54.8(3).
[222] CPR r.54.8(4).
[223] CPR r.10.5.
[224] CPR r.54.9(1)(a).
[225] CPR r.54.14.
[226] CPR r.54.9(1)(b).
[227] PD 54A para.8.4.
[228] CPR r.54.10; PD 54A, paras 8.1, 8.2.
[229] CPR r.54.11.
[230] CPR r.54.13.
[231] CPR r.54.12(1), (2); PD 54A, para.9.1.
[232] CPR r.54.12(7).
[233] CPR r.54.12(3), (4).
[234] PD 54A para.8.5. A coroner who fears that the court may lack the complete picture should however attend or be represented: cf. *R. (Gracey) v Cheshire Coroner* [2008] EWHC 957 (Admin.).
[235] See 19–70 ff.
[236] CPR r.52.15 (1), (2).

court may then, if it thinks fit, give permission *to apply for judicial review* rather than give *permission to appeal*,[237] and in that case the matter will return directly to the High Court.[238]

19–54   If the High Court refused permission, and recorded that the application was totally without merit, the appeal to the Court of Appeal is restricted to a paper application, the result of which is final.[239] Otherwise, if permission is refused on the papers by the single judge of the Court of Appeal, then, unless, that judge has certified that the decision is final, on the basis that the application is totally without merit,[240] the claimant can apply within seven days for an oral hearing before a Court of Appeal judge.[241] Where the Attorney General has given his *fiat* for a parallel application under the statutory review jurisdiction, the court will rarely refuse permission for judicial review.[242]

19–55   The defendant or other person served with the claim form who wishes to contest the claim (or support it on other grounds) must file and serve detailed grounds for his or her stance, and any written evidence, within 35 days after service of the order giving permission.[243] If the person so filing intends to rely on documents not already filed, he must file a paginated bundle of those documents at the same time.[244] If the claimant seeks to rely on other grounds than those permitted, he must obtain the court's further permission,[245] and he must notify the court and all other persons served with the claim form not less than seven days prior to the hearing (or warned date).[246]

19–56   The court has power to permit any other person (i.e. who is not already involved) to file evidence or make representations at the hearing, but an application for permission should be made promptly.[247] Permission may be given on terms.[248] If everyone consents, the court may deal with the application without a hearing.[249] Disclosure of documents, although possible in theory,[250] is not normally ordered.[251] This is because (i) judicial review proceedings are usually confined to

---

[237] CPR r.52.15 (3).
[238] CPR r.52.15(4).
[239] CPR r.52.15 (1A).
[240] CPR r.52.3(4A).
[241] CPR r.52.16(6), (6A).
[242] *Re Sheppard* Unreported April 22, 1992, DC.
[243] CPR r.54.14.
[244] PD 54A para.10.1
[245] CPR r.54.15.
[246] PD 54A para.11.1.
[247] CPR r.54.17.
[248] PD 54A para.13.2.
[249] PD 54A para.13.1.
[250] CPR rr.31.5, 31.12.
[251] PD 54A para.12.1. See also *R. (Armani da Silva) v DPP* [2006] EWHC 3204 (Admin.) (claimant not entitled to disclosure of the underlying evidence on which the IPCC Report was based, as not necessary to have this in order for judicial review claim to be decided); cf. *R. (Ministry of Defence) v Wiltshire Coroner* [2005] EWHC 889 (Admin.) (tapes of coroner's summing up to jury ordered to be disclosed to MoD counsel to consider whether to plead allegation that coroner's tone of voice indicated attitude dismissive of MoD witness's evidence; in fact counsel did not so plead, and the case was ultimately settled: *Ministry of Defence v Wiltshire Coroner* [2006] EWHC 309 (Admin.)).

the material that was before the decision-maker,[252] and (ii) there is very limited scope for the introduction of fresh evidence.[253]

Evidence at the hearing of the judicial review application will normally be in **19–57** writing, either by way of affidavit or (more likely) witness statement.[254] No such evidence may be relied on unless it has been served in accordance with the rules, or the court's direction, or the court gives permission.[255] There is no express provision for cross-examination on written evidence in judicial review, but it is available in appropriate cases.[256]

Admissibility of fresh evidence

Fresh evidence is admissible at the hearing of judicial review proceedings only if it **19–58** is (a) evidence showing the material before the decision-maker (i.e. the coroner); (b) evidence needed for the court to be able to determine whether a jurisdictional or procedural error occurred; or (c) evidence of misconduct by a party or the decision-maker.[257]

Adjournment

An application for judicial review of a coroner's interlocutory decision will only be **19–59** adjourned for very good reason. Thus in one case[258] the judge refused an application, by the applicant for judicial review of the coroner's refusal to call a named person as witness, to adjourn the hearing of the application for judicial review pending the hearing of the inquest, when it would be known if the coroner in fact did or did not call the named person. The judge said:

> "I am quite satisfied that leave having been granted, and the hearing [ordered to be] expedited, it is in the interests of justice that the matter be determined as quickly as possible. It should not go into limbo until the conclusion of the inquest, or until such time as the application chooses to re-activate the application."

On the other hand, the court may adjourn judicial review proceedings to enable **19–60** them to be heard together with a statutory review application by a Divisional Court,[259] may stay a judicial review of an inquest until the termination of pending criminal proceedings against the applicant arising out of the same facts,[260] and may

---

[252] *R. v Poplar Coroner Ex p. Chaudhry* Unreported December 15, 1993, DC; *R. (Sutovic) v North London Coroner* [2006] EWHC 1095 (Admin.) at [41], [44]–[47], [52]; *R. (Lagos) v City of London Coroner* [2013] EWHC 423 (Admin.) at [7].
[253] See *Civil Procedure*, 2014, para.54. 16.6.
[254] CPR r.32.2(1)(b).
[255] CPR r.54.16(2).
[256] CPR r.32.7(1); *R. (G) v Ealing London Borough Council, The Times*, March 18, 2002, Munby J; *R. (Wilkinson) v Broadmoor Hospital Responsible Medical Officer* [2002] UKHRR 390, CA.
[257] *R. v Environment Secretary Ex p. Powis* [1981] 1 W.L.R. 584, CA; *R. v East Berkshire Coroner Ex p. Buckley* (1992) 157 J.P. 425, DC; *R. (Dwr Cymru Cyfyngedig) v Environment Agency of Wales, The Times*, April 29, 2003, Harrison J (dangerous to admit in judicial review proceedings fresh evidence that was not before the decision-maker).
[258] *R. v Inner North London Coroner Ex p. Keogh* Unreported February 1, 1994, Potts J.
[259] *R. (Mulholland) v St Pancras Deputy Coroner* [2003] EWHC 96 (Admin.).
[260] *R. v Birmingham Coroner Ex p. Najada* (1995) 160 J.P. 210.

stay judicial review proceedings relating to a prosecution decision until after the inquest.[261]

Agreement on disposal prior to hearing

19–61 It may be that, or before the time of the hearing, the parties are agreed as to the terms on which the application can be disposed of. In that case, to avoid the necessity of the parties attending court, the claimant should file a document and two copies) signed by all parties[262] setting out the terms of the proposed order together with material relied on as justifying it.[263] The court will consider the material and make the order if satisfied.[264] If not satisfied, a hearing date will be set.[265] If the agreement relates only to a costs order, it is sufficient to file a signed document setting out the terms.[266] But the court's powers go further, and enable the judge to decide on any application which is still disputed on the papers alone, if the parties so agree.[267]

19–62 The policy for listing hearings in the Administrative Court is the subject of a Practice Statement.[268] The claimant must file and serve a skeleton argument not less than 21 working days before the date of the hearing (or warned date).[269] Any other parties wishing to make representations at the hearing must file and serve a skeleton argument not less than 14 working days before the same date.[270] These skeletons must contain time estimates, issue lists, legal points, a chronology, essential reading lists, and lists of persons referred to.[271] In 2013 the average waiting time from lodging the application to a decision in London was just over 30 weeks. In 2001 it was 20 weeks.

The finding of the court

19–63 Assuming that the application proceeds to a contested hearing, the claimant may succeed in establishing some defect in the decision-making process which makes the decision reviewable by the court. However, as has already been made clear,[272] the courts retain a large discretion as to whether or not they should grant any relief by way of judicial review.[273] A remedy may be refused on various grounds when

---

[261] *R. (Sylvester) v DPP* Unreported May 21, 2001, DC; *R. (Stanley) v Inner North London Coroner* [2003] EWHC 1180 (Admin.) at [32].

[262] That is, the claimant, the defendant, and any persons properly "interested parties": see CPR r.54.1(2)(f) (definition of "interested party").

[263] PD 54A para.17.1.

[264] PD 54A para.17.2. See *Ministry of Defence v Wiltshire and Swindon Coroner* [2006] EWHC 309 (Admin.), DC, where the court gave reasons for approving a compromise between the parties which involved adding words to the verdict returned to the inquest.

[265] PD 54A para.17.3.

[266] PD 54A para.17.4.

[267] CPR r.54.18.

[268] *Practice Statement (Administrative Court: Listing & Urgent Cases)* [2000] 1 W.L.R. 810.

[269] PD 54A para.15.1.

[270] PD 54A para.15.2.

[271] PD 54A para.15.3.

[272] See 19–35.

[273] *R. v Inner West London Coroner Ex p. Dallaglio* [1994] 4 All E.R. 139, CA; *R. (Aineto) v Brighton and Hove Coroner* [2003] EWHC 1896 (Admin.).

it might otherwise have been granted, such as the applicant's delay,[274] waiver of the defect,[275] bad faith (e.g. non-disclosure of material information)[276] or other misconduct,[277] or where the complaint is trivial.[278]

In some cases it may be refused where an equally convenient remedy is open to   **19–64** the applicant,[279] and in the coronial context this might refer to the statutory powers of quashing an inquisition and ordering a new inquest which have already been discussed.[280] However, there is no reported case of judicial review of a coroner's inquest being refused because of the existence of those alternative powers.[281] Other factors that may weigh with the court in deciding whether the order sought should be made are whether the relief would serve any useful purpose, as where even if errors were corrected the result would be the same[282] and whether it would cause considerable administrative or public inconvenience.[283]

Remedies

Where the court considers that relief should be given, the primary remedy is an   **19–65** order quashing the inquisition, with a further order that a fresh inquest be held.[284] But the flexibility of judicial review, as compared with the statutory remedy already considered,[285] means that the court may grant relief which falls short of quashing the whole inquisition and ordering a new inquest.[286]

Thus, in earlier cases, the courts have ordered inaccuracies in the inquisition   **19–66** (e.g. date of death of deceased) to be amended,[287] deleted para.4 (the conclusion as to death, or "verdict," in popular language) and remitted the inquisition to the coroner for him to enter such conclusion as he thinks appropriate in light of the court's judgment,[288] deleted para.4 *without* remitting the matter to the coroner or

---

[274] Senior Courts Act 1981 s.31(6), (7); see 19–36, and *R. v Stratford-on-Avon DC Ex p. Jackson* [1985] 1 W.L.R. 1319 at 1325, *Caswell v Dairy Produce Quota Tribunal for England and Wales* [1990] 2 A.C. 738, HL, *R. v South Yorkshire Coroner Ex p. Stringer* (1993) 158 J.P. 453, DC.

[275] *R. v Williams Ex p. Phillips* [1914] 1 K.B. 608.

[276] *R. v Kensington Income Tax Commissioners Ex p. De Polignac* [1917] 1 K.B. 486, CA.

[277] *Ward v Bradford Corporation* (1971) 70 L.G.R. 27, CA.

[278] *R. v Tower Hamlets LBC Ex p. Kayne-Levenson* [1975] Q.B. 431, CA.

[279] *R. v Huntingdon DC Ex p. Cowan* [1984] 1 W.L.R. 501; *R. v Merseyside Chief Constable Ex p. Calveley* [1986] Q.B. 424, CA; *R. (Sutovic) v North London Coroner* [2006] EWHC 1095 (Admin.).

[280] See 19–05 ff above. Indeed, sometimes those powers are more suitable: *R. v Central Cleveland Coroner Ex p. Dent* (1986) 150 J.P. 251; and see *R. v West Berkshire Coroner Ex p. Thomas* (1991) 155 J.P. 681 at 698.

[281] Though see *R. (Sutovic) v North London Coroner* [2006] EWHC 1095 (Admin.) at [52].

[282] *Re Williams, The Times,* December 10, 1968, DC; *R. v South London Coroner Ex p. Thompson* (1982) 126 S.J. 625, DC; *R. v Portsmouth Coroner Ex p. Keane* (1989) 153 J.P. 658, DC; *R. v Wolverhampton Coroner Ex p. McCurbin* [1990] 1 W.L.R. 719, CA; *R. v South Yorkshire Coroner Ex p. Stringer* (1993) 158 J.P. 453, DC; *R. v East Sussex Coroner Ex p. Homberg* Unreported June 14, 1993, DC and (further hearing) (1994) 158 J.P. 357, DC; *R. v South London Coroner Ex p. Weeks* Unreported December 6, 1996, Scott Baker J; *Re Potter's Application* Unreported January 24, 1997, Harrison J.

[283] *Coney v Choyce* [1975] 1 W.L.R. 422; *Meade v Haringey LBC* [1975] 1 W.L.R. 637.

[284] *R. (Aineto) v Brighton Hove Coroner* [2003] EWHC 1896 (Admin.), DC at [12].

[285] See 19–05 ff above.

[286] The only remedy under s.13 of the 1988 Act.

[287] *R. v Inner North London Coroner Ex p. Linnane (No. 2)* (1990) 155 J.P. 343, DC.

[288] *R. v Southwark Coroners Court Ex p. Kendall* [1988] 1 W.L.R. 1186, DC; *R. v West London Coroner Ex p. De Luca* [1989] Q.B. 249, DC. See now Senior Courts Act 1981 s.31(5)(a).

ordering a new inquest,[289] and quashed the decision not to hold an inquest and remitted the question for him to decide again in light of the judgment.[290]

19–67   In more recent times, the courts have gone further, substituting an accident conclusion for an unlawful killing one,[291] even adding a short narrative,[292] quashing unlawful killing and adding a narrative constructed from the jury findings,[293] and could even add words to an unlawful killing conclusion so as to approve a compromise between the parties which would make clear the basis for that finding and to exclude another possibility for that finding, in a case where the court considered that there was "a strongly arguable case that there was insufficient evidence" for one basis, but that unlawful killing on the other basis was the only one open to the jury on the evidence.[294]

19–68   Finally, in another case,[295] the court held that there was power on judicial review to substitute words in the inquisition (i) where the words used do not accurately convey the inquest's determination, but other words do, and even (ii) where, even though the court cannot be sure which of the rival theories the jury would have preferred, there are words which cover all of them and to which the decision-maker could not object.

19–69   Since April 6, 2008, the relevant procedural law has been amended[296] to provide that where the High Court quashes the decision to which the application relates, it may in addition substitute its own decision for the decision in question, if (a) the decision in question was made by a court or tribunal, (b) the decision is quashed on the ground that there has been an error of law, and (c) without the error, there would have been only one decision which the court or tribunal could have reached.[297] Unless the High Court otherwise directs, a decision substituted by it in this way has effect as if it were a decision of the relevant court or tribunal.[298]

COSTS

19–70   The question of costs in proceedings under the statutory review procedure and in judicial review proceedings is more complex than it need be. Subject to one point, there is no real ground for applying different rules to the two different forms of procedure. It is true that under the statutory power jurisdiction the Act confers

---

[289] *R. v St Pancras Coroner's Court Ex p. Jones* [1991] C.O.D. 14, DC; see also *R. v Southwark Coroner Ex p. Epsom Hospital NHS Trust* (1994) 158 J.P. 973, DC; *R. v Reading Coroner Ex p. West Berkshire Housing* Unreported August 7, 1995, Popplewell J; *R. v Birmingham and Solihull Coroner Ex p. Benton* (1997) 162 J.P. 807.

[290] *R. v Avon Coroner Ex p. Smith* (1998) 162 J.P. 403.

[291] *R. (Wilkinson) v Greater Manchester South Coroner* [2012] EWHC 2755 (Admin.).

[292] *R. (Brown) v Neath and Port Talbot Coroner* [2006] EWHC 2019 (Admin.).

[293] *R. (Anderson) v Inner North London Coroner* [2004] EWHC 2729 (Admin.).

[294] *Ministry of Defence v Wiltshire and Swindon Coroner* [2006] EWHC 309 (Admin.), DC.

[295] *R. (Mowlem plc) v Avon Deputy Assistant Coroner* [2005] EWHC 1359 (Admin.).

[296] Tribunals, Courts and Enforcement Act 2007 s.141.

[297] Senior Courts Act 1981 s.31(5), (5A).

[298] Senior Courts Act 1981 s.31(5B).

express power to make a costs order against the coroner,[299] but the same is true of judicial review generally.[300]

The one point of real difference is that the statutory power to award costs against **19–71**
the coroner is stated *only* to apply where the High Court is satisfied that a coroner ought to hold an investigation or inquest, or another inquest or investigation (as the case may be).[301] So the jurisdiction to order costs against the coroner only exists if the application is successful. Yet in one case the Divisional Court held that, although there was no point in a further inquest, and therefore a s.13 application should fail, it should nevertheless order the coroner to pay the costs, holding that for an award of costs it was not necessary that the application should have been successful.[302] This not only contravenes the express words of the statute, but is out of line with both earlier and later authority.

Where the coroner succeeds

Secondly, the general rule in civil litigation in that costs should follow the event, **19–72**
though the court has power to make a different order.[303] Thus if a challenge to the coroner's decision or to the inquisition, determination or findings fails, then prima facie an order should be made for the claimant to pay the coroner's costs.[304] But if, as often happens, the coroner is not present or represented, the court may not make an order, because no one asks for it.[305] Or the coroner may be present, but not think it appropriate to ask for an order.[306] Or the applicant may be funded by the Legal Services Commission, and therefore it is in practice impossible to obtain a useful order.[307] In principle, the same is true, and the loser pays, if the coroner makes an application which fails.[308]

In one (non-coroner) case[309] the Court of Appeal held that, on the conclusion **19–73**
of full judicial review proceedings where the claim had failed, the nature and purpose of the proceedings was relevant to the exercise of the court's discretion as to costs. If the court awarded costs against the claimant, it must consider whether to award costs of pre-permission preparation as well as costs relating to the

---

[299] Coroners Act 1988 s.13(2)(b); *R. v Turnbull Ex p. Kenyon, The Times*, April 11, 1984, DC; *R. (Touche) v Inner North London Coroner* [2001] Q.B. 1206 at [57], CA.
[300] Senior Courts Act 1981 s.51; CPR r.44.2(1),(2).
[301] Section 13(1).
[302] *Re Clegg* (1997) 161 J.P. 521.
[303] CPR r.44.2(2)(a).
[304] *R. v Inner North London Coroner Ex p. GLC, The Times*, April 30, 1983; *R. v South Glamorgan Coroner Ex p. BP Chemicals Ltd* (1987) 151 J.P. 799, DC; *R. v Greater Manchester Coroner Ex p. Worch* [1988] Q.B. 513, CA; *R. v Portsmouth Coroner Ex p. Keane* (1989) J.P. 658, DC; *Re Taylor* (1990) 154 J.P. 933, DC; *R. v Inner North London Coroner Ex p. Keogh* (1995) 159 J.P. 739, DC; *R. v Birmingham Coroner Ex p. Cotton* (1995) 160 J.P. 123, DC; *R. v Worcester Coroner Ex p. UK Detention Services Ltd.* Unreported February 18, 1998, Ognall J; *R. (Dawson) v East Riding and Hull Coroner* Unreported April 9, 2001, Jackson J. cf. *R. v Ceredigion Coroner Ex p. Wigley* Unreported February 8, 1993, DC.
[305] The coroner may still have incurred costs, e.g. in preparing filing and serving a witness statement to assist the court.
[306] *R. v Portsmouth Coroner Ex p. Anderson* [1987] 1 W.L.R. 1640, DC.
[307] See the Community Legal Service (Cost Protection) Regulations 2000 reg.5. But a so-called "football pools" order (i.e. not to be enforced without the leave of the court) is sometimes made: *R. v West Yorkshire Coroner Ex p. Clements* Unreported July 7, 1993, DC.
[308] *Re Kelly* (1996) 161 J.P. 467, DC.
[309] *Davey v Aylesbury Vale DC* [2007] EWCA Civ. 1166.

acknowledgment of service. It would be for the defendant to justify such pre-permission preparation costs.

19-74   As to pre-permission costs in the coroner context, in one case[310] where the applicant's father died a natural death and the coroner after procuring a pathologist's report to deal with the applicant's concerns refused to hold an inquest, there were held to be "no merits . . . whatsoever" in the application for judicial review, the applicant (who did not comply with the pre-action protocol and was not publicly funded) was ordered to pay the coroner's costs of the acknowledgment of service, and indeed the costs of his representation at the hearing.

19-75   There are two other important situations to consider where the coroner succeeds. One is where a judicial review challenge fails at the permission stage. Under the RSC, the application for leave to move for judicial review was ex parte, that is, without notice. So the respondent (i.e. the coroner) was not necessarily notified, and did not always attend. The proceedings proper did not begin until leave was given. If the application for leave failed, the coroner could not claim to be a party to the proceedings, and hence, even if he had attended the hearing and played a significant part in successfully resisting the application, was not normally in a position to ask for his costs.[311]

19-76   But, under the CPR, the position is otherwise. The coroner is a defendant to judicial review proceedings from the outset. He or she is served with the proceedings, must prepare and serve an acknowledgement of service, and may well attend at the permission stage, though this is not necessary in most cases. If the claimant's application for permission fails, the coroner is in principle entitled to his or her costs of the acknowledgement of service.[312] This is consistent with the position where a respondent to an application for permission to appeal is successful, and he or she too is held entitled to the costs.[313]

19-77   The second point to consider relates to the case where there is more than one defendant to the application for judicial review. The general rule is that the unsuccessful claimant is normally not liable for more than one set of costs in total, no matter how many defendants there were.[314] This means that, if the coroner is a defendant, he usually gets his costs, and the other defendants do not. In order to entitle another defendant to a separate set of costs, it is necessary to show that there were separate interests to be represented.[315] Where the coroner makes no

---

[310] *R. (Gracey) v Cheshire Coroner* [2008] EWHC 957 (Admin.).

[311] Though the court had *discretion* to do so: *R. v Camden LBC Ex p. Martin* [1997] 1 W.L.R. 359.

[312] *R. (Leach) v Commissioner for Local Administration, The Times,* August 2, 2001, Collins J; *Civil Procedure,* Spring 2002 para.54.12.6; cf. PD 54A para.8.6, and *R. (Southall Black Sisters) v West Yorkshire Coroner*[2002] EWHC 1914 (Admin.), Jackson J; *Mount Cook Land Ltd v Westminster City Council, The Times,* October 16, 2003; *R. (Payne) v Caerphilly CBC* [2004] EWCA Civ. 433; *R. (Leeds Teaching Hospitals NHS Trust) v West Yorkshire Coroner* [2004] EWHC 1458 (Admin.).

[313] *Jolly v Jay, The Times,* March 15, 2002, CA.

[314] *Bolton MDC v Secretary of State for the Environment (No. 2)* [1995] 1 W.L.R. 1176, HL; *R. (Mowlem plc) v Avon Deputy Assistant Coroner* [2005] EWHC 1359 (Admin.).

[315] *Bolton MDC v Secretary of State for the Environment (No. 2)* [1995] 1 W.L.R. 1176, HL. In *R. (Leeds Teaching Hospitals NHS Trust) v West Yorkshire Coroner* [2004] EWHC 1458 (Admin.), it was exceptionally held that the claimant should pay not only the defendant coroner's costs of attending the oral renewal of the application for permission, but *also* those of the interested party.

submissions on an issue, which is left to another interested party to deal with successfully, that party should normally have the costs of dealing with that issue.[316]

Where the coroner loses

Cases where the coroner loses have a more complicated history to them. The basic **19–78** rule, derived from cases involving magistrates' courts and other inferior tribunals,[317] used to be that if a coroner did not appear at the hearing, and (although he had been found to be in the wrong) he had done nothing calling for strong disapproval, then the court would not make an order for costs against him.[318] But if he had done something calling for strong disapproval, then the court *might* make a costs order against him.[319]

If the coroner did appear at the hearing, and lost, then the court had a discretion **19–79** whether to order the coroner to pay the successful applicant's costs, even though he had acted reasonably. But such an order was only rarely made[320]; usually no order was made unless the coroner's behaviour called for strong disapproval.[321]

One additional factor against making a costs order was where the applicant was **19–80** legally aided,[322] and therefore it would only be the public paying the public. There were also two unusual cases dating from the period before the statutory indemnity for coroners was introduced in 1999, where the applicant succeeded, and was not legally aided, and the court was persuaded, both times in the absence of the coroner, to make an order that the coroner pay the applicant's costs, such order not to be enforced failing an indemnity of the coroner by the relevant council.[323]

But the old practice has changed, and statute now plays an important role. In **19–81** two significant cases in the 1990s the courts ignored the old case law, and held that coroners, whether they attended court or not, could be ordered to pay a successful

---

[316] R. (Dawson) v East Riding and Hull Coroner Unreported April 9, 2001, Jackson J.

[317] R. v Coventry Rent Tribunal Ex p. Whitcombe Unreported December 1, 1948, DC; R. v Liverpool Justices Ex p. Roberts [1960] 1 W.L.R. 585, DC; R. v Huntingdon Magistrates' Court Ex p. Percy, The Times, March 4, 1994.

[318] R. v West Yorkshire Coroner Ex p. Smith, The Times, November 6, 1982; R. v Turnbull Ex p. Kenyon, The Times, April 11, 1984, DC; R. v Essex Coroner Ex p. Hopper Unreported May 13, 1988; DC; R. v Southwark Coroner Ex p. Epsom Hospital NHS Trust (1994) 158 J.P. 973, DC.

[319] R. v McHugh Ex p. Trelford Unreported March 22, 1984, DC; R. v Dyfed Coroner Ex p. Evans Unreported May 24, 1984, DC.

[320] R. v Inner North London Coroner Ex p. Chambers, The Times, April 30, 1983; R. v South London Coroner Ex p. Driscoll (1993) 159 J.P. 45, DC.

[321] R. v Surrey Coroner Ex p. Ager Unreported July 3, 1974, DC; R. v West Yorkshire Coroner Ex p. Smith, The Times, November 6, 1982; R. v West London Coroner Ex p. Gray (1986) 151 J.P. 209 (rather than [1988] Q.B. 467); R. v Southwark Coroner Ex p. Hicks [1987] 1 W.L.R. 1624, DC; R. v Shrewsbury Coroners Court Ex p. British Parachute Association (1987) 152 J.P. 123, DC; R. v St Pancras Coroner's Court Ex p. Higgins (1988) 152 J.P. 637, DC; R. v Inner North London Coroner Ex p. Diesa Koto (1993) 157 J.P. 857, DC; R. v Merseyside Coroner Ex p. Carr [1993] 4 All E.R. 65, DC; R. v Reading Coroner Ex p. West Berkshire Housing Consortium Ltd. Unreported July 11, 1995; Re Cohen (1993) 158 J.P. 644, DC; R. v Avon Coroner Ex p. Smith (1998) 162 J.P. 403.

[322] R. v Inner North London Coroner Ex p. Linnane (1989) Casebook on Coroners (rather than [1989] 1 W.L.R. 395); R. v Inner North London Coroner Ex p. Diesa Koto, (1993) 157 J.P. 857, DC.

[323] R. v Dyfed Coroner Ex p. Evans Unreported May 24, 1984, DC; Re Bithell (1986) 150 J.P. 273.

applicant's costs, even though their behaviour did not call for strong disapproval.[324] Non-coroners' cases, however, continued to follow the old line: inferior tribunals were to pay costs only in rare and well-defined circumstances.[325]

19–82   In 1999, the Divisional Court re-examined the issue in the coronial context, and concluded that an unsuccessful coroner who appeared in court more as an amicus curiae than in an adversarial mode, and whose conduct did not otherwise excite strong disapproval in the court, should not be ordered to pay the costs of the successful applicant.[326] The court added that central, rather than local, funds should be found for this latter purpose.[327] Shortly afterwards, the statute law was changed, to provide that a coroner's "relevant council" should indemnify him against liability to costs and damages in proceedings relating to the performance of his coronial duties.[328]

19–83   Subsequent to that, the Court of Appeal for the first time considered the costs issue, and held that, if the coroner chose to appear at the hearing, he was at risk as to costs, whether his conduct merited strong disapproval or not.[329] But if he did not appear then, assuming he did nothing calling for specific disapproval, he could "exempt himself from any costs liability".[330] If the court was minded to make such an order, then the court should give the absent coroner the opportunity to attend to make representations.[331]

19–84   However, the new regime did not last long. In 2004 the Court of Appeal comprehensively revisited the question of costs against coroners.[332] Departing from its earlier decision, it held[333] that the established practice of the High Court on judicial review was:

1.   to make no order for costs against an inferior court (like the coroner) which did not appear at all (but might make a witness statement setting out relevant facts and neutrally responding to specific points made by the claimant),

---

[324] *R. v Kent Coroner Ex p. Johnstone* [1995] 6 Med. L.R. 116; *Re Clegg* (1997) 161 J.P. 521, DC (indeed, in this case the substantive application was actually unsuccessful); see also Matthews [1995] *Public Law* 526.

[325] *Seifert v Pensions Ombudsman* [1997] 4 All E.R. 947, 956, CA; *R. v Merthyr Tydfil Crown Court Ex p. Chief Constable of Dyfed-Powys Police*, The Times, December 17, 1998; *R. v Doncaster Justices Ex p. Jack*, The Times, May 26, 1999.

[326] *R. v Lincoln Coroner Ex p. Hay* [2000] Lloyd's Rep. Med. 264, 278, DC; cf. *R. (Scott) v Inner West London Coroner* (2001) 165 J.P. 417 (coroner appeared in adversarial mode; ordered to pay costs).

[327] *R. v Lincoln Coroner Ex p. Hay* [2000] Lloyd's Rep. Med. 264, 279 col.2.

[328] Coroners and Justice At 2009 s.34, Sch.7 para.9; Coroners Allowances, Fees and Expenses Regulations, 2013 (SI 2013/1615) reg.17; formerly Coroners Act 1988 s.27A, inserted by the Access to Justice Act 1999 s.104(1); see now 18–44.

[329] *R. (Touche) v Inner North London Coroner* [2001] Q.B. 1206 at [57]–[59], CA, impliedly overruling *Re Clegg*, where the coroner did not appear, and the court did not allude to any behaviour calling for specific disapproval; *R. (Hurst) v North London Coroner* [2003] EWHC 1721 (Admin.); cf. *R. (Metropolitan Police Commissioner) v South London Coroner* [2003] EWHC 1829 (Admin.) (no order as to costs).

[330] *R. (Touche) v Inner North London Coroner* [2001] Q.B. 1206 at [56]; *R. v Avon Deputy Coroner Ex p. Lambourne* Unreported July 29, 2002, DC.

[331] *R. v Turnbull Ex p. Kenyon* Unreported March 15, 1984, DC. The coroner should expressly make this point in his witness statement if he intends not to be represented at the hearing.

[332] *R. (Davies) v Birmingham Deputy Coroner (No. 2)* [2004] EWCA Civ. 207.

[333] *R. (Davies) v Birmingham Deputy Coroner (No. 2)* [2004] EWCA Civ. 207 at [47], [49].

except for cases of flagrantly improper behaviour or unreasonable refusal to consent to a suitable disposal of the proceedings;

2. where an inferior court actively resisted an application like a party to litigation, to allow costs to follow the event; but

3. where an inferior court appeared merely to assist neutrally on questions of jurisdiction, procedure, specialist case law, and so on, to treat it as a neutral party and make no costs order either in its favour or against it, whatever the outcome;[334] although there were other considerations nowadays in this category, such as the need for a claimant who has no claim on public funds to be compensated for irrecoverable legal expense when a coroner had gone wrong in law.

These principles have been followed since then.[335]

There are three other costs matters to be mentioned. One is that, at least in theory, an applicant for an order under s.13 of the Coroners Act 1988 or for judicial review may seek an order at the outset that the applicant should not in any event bear any part of the respondent's costs. This is a so-called "pre-emptive" costs order, occasionally met with in private law litigation.[336] But it is only proper in the public law context in the most exceptional circumstances, where the court is satisfied that the issues raised are truly of general public importance, and the court has a sufficient appreciation of the merits of the claim to conclude that it was in the public interest to make the order.[337] The court must also have regard to the financial resources of the parties, and to the amount of costs likely to be in issue.[338]   **19–85**

---

[334] On the question whether the coroner is at risk as to costs in any given case, and should make a pre-hearing application to the court for directions, see *R. (Davies) v Birmingham Deputy Coroner (No. 2)* [2004] EWCA (Civ.) 207 at [50].

[335] *R. (Anderson) v Inner North London Coroner* [2004] EWHC 2729 (Admin.); *R. (Longfield Care Homes Ltd) v Blackburn Coroner* [2004] EWHC 2467 (Admin.); *R. (Parkin) v North Lincolnshire and Grimsby Coroner* [2005] EWHC 660 (Admin.), DC; *R. (Sharman) v Inner North London Coroner* [2005] EWHC 857 (Admin.); *R. (Plymouth City Council) v Devon Coroner* [2005] EWHC 1014 (Admin.); *R. (Mowlem plc) v Avon Deputy Assistant Coroner* [2005] EWHC 1359 (Admin.) (coroner not neutral); *Combe v Blackburn Coroner* [2005] EWHC 2843 (Admin.), DC; *R. (Pounder) v North and South Durham and Darlington (No. 2)* [2010] EWHC 328 (Admin.); *R. (Medihani) v Inner South London Coroner* [2012] EWHC 1104 (Admin.); *Jenkins v Bridgend and Glamorgan Valleys Coroner* [2012] EWHC 3175 (Admin.); see also *R. (Mack) v Birmingham Coroner* [2011] EWCA Civ 712; *R. (Cooper) v North East Kent Coroner* [2014] EWHC 586 (Admin.).

[336] See, e.g. *Wallersteiner v Moir (No. 2)* [1975] 1 All E.R. 849; *McDonald v Horn* [1995] 1 All ER 961, CA; *National Grid Co. plc v Laws* [2001] WTLR 741.

[337] *R. v Lord Chancellor Ex p. Child Poverty Action Group* [1999] 1 W.L.R. 347; *Re Campaign for Nuclear Disarmament, The Times*, December 27, 2002, DC; *R. (Corner House Research) v Trade and Industry Secretary* [2005] EWCA Civ. 192 at [74]–[81] (not coroners' cases); *R. (Ministry of Defence) v Wiltshire Coroner* [2005] EWHC 889 (Admin.) (PCO refused); *Goodson v Bedfordshire and Luton Coroner* [2005] EWCA Civ. 1172 (PCO refused).

[338] *R. v Lord Chancellor Ex p. Child Poverty Action Group* [1999] 1 W.L.R. 347; *Re Campaign for Nuclear Disarmament, The Times*, December 27, 2002, DC; *R. (Corner House Research) v Trade and Industry Secretary* [2005] EWCA Civ. 192 at [74]–[81] (not coroners' cases); *R. (Ministry of Defence) v Wiltshire Coroner* [2005] EWHC 889 (Admin.) (PCO refused); *Goodson v Bedfordshire and Luton Coroner* [2005] EWCA Civ. 1172 (PCO refused).

19–86   The second point is that if the coroner is served with proceedings and only then takes (or corrects) the step required or in respect of which complaint is made by the proceedings, the claimant may well be entitled to the costs to that stage.[339] The last matter relates to costs against the legal aid authorities where a legally aided applicant has failed. Under the old law it was possible for the court dealing with the substantive litigation to make an order against the Legal Aid Board,[340] but under the new law it is not. Instead, the court has power to give an indication (by a statement in the court order) that in the circumstances it would be just and equitable for the Legal Services Commission to bear the coroner's costs.[341] It is then for the costs judge to decide.[342]

Appeals to the Court of Appeal

19–87   Where the High Court makes an order in a statutory or a judicial review case, the losing party may appeal to the Court of Appeal, with the permission either of the High Court or of the Court of Appeal.[343] If permission is given, the normal appeals procedure is followed.[344]

Residual Common Law Powers

19–88   Although formerly there was some suggestion that the Queen's Bench Division of the High Court possessed some residual power at common law, not covered by the procedure for judicial review now contained in CPR Pt 54,[345] it is now clear that this is not so. The common law powers are exercisable only on application for judicial review.[346]

Funding of Legal Services

19–89   For proceedings at the inquest themselves, public funding for legal services is extremely limited.[347] However, in applications to the High Court, whether under the statutory power or in judicial review (or other proceedings), public funding for representation is available for parties of modest means, subject to a means test and a possible contribution.[348] Where such funding is obtained, then whatever the

---

[339] See *R. v Kensington and Chelsea LBC Ex p. Ghebregiogis* (1994) 27 HLR 602 (not a coroner's case).

[340] Legal Aid Act 1988 s.18(4); see *Re Palmer's Application* Unreported December 10, 1997, CA.

[341] *R. (Gunn) v Home Secretary* [2001] 1 W.L.R. 1634, CA.

[342] Community Legal Service (Costs Protection) Regulations 2000 reg.5; *Legal Services Commission v F* [2011] EWHC 899 (QB).

[343] CPR r.52.3(1).

[344] CPR Pt 52; *Practice Direction—Appeals*.

[345] *R. v South London Coroner Ex p. Thompson, The Times*, May 15, 1982, per Comyn J. See the 10th edn of this work at para.21–24.

[346] *Re Rapier* [1988] Q.B. 26, DC.

[347] See 10–55 ff.

[348] See 10–53, 10–54.

outcome of the proceedings, and whether or not any other order regarding costs is made, an order for legal aid assessment of the costs of the assisted person should be sought from the court at the hearing.

CONSEQUENCES

As has been seen, the court on a judicial review application may grant relief falling **19–90** short of quashing the inquisition, and may, for example, amend or delete part of it if appropriate.[349] In such a case there is no need for a new inquest. But where an inquisition is quashed, whether under the statutory or the common law powers already discussed, the usual consequence is that a fresh inquest is ordered: under the statutory power this can be done directly; under judicial review this is done by seeking, in addition to the order of certiorari to quash the first inquisition, an order of mandamus to hold the new inquest. In both cases[350] the order may (but need not) be that the new inquest be held before a different coroner.

However, the quashing of the inquest leaves the case in the jurisdiction of the **19–91** senior coroner for the coroner area where it was held, and so prima facie it is a coroner for that area that must hold the fresh investigation and any inquest. The High Court has no power, whether under the statutory or the judicial review system, to transfer jurisdiction elsewhere.[351] Only the Chief Coroner can direct a coroner for a different coroner area to conduct the investigation.[352] If no such direction is given, it will be necessary to find a different coroner from among those available in that area.[353] Prima facie this is the responsibility of the senior coroner. In some cases it has been appropriate to appoint a serving or retired judge, or some other qualified person, to act temporarily for this purpose.

Formerly, in cases whether the inquisition was quashed by a reason of **19–92** misconduct on the part of the coroner, the court under its common law powers ordered a further inquiry, or "*melius inquirendum*" before the sheriff, justices of the peace, or special commissioners,[354] but this power has not been exercised for very many years, and is now obsolete.[355]

---

[349] See 19–66 ff.

[350] e.g. *R. v City of London Coroner Ex p. Calvi*, *The Times*, April 2, 1983, DC; *R. v South Powys Coroner's Court Ex p. Jones* [1991] C.O.D. 14, DC (Coroners Act); *R. v Turnbull Ex p. Kenyon* Unreported March 15, 1984, DC; *R. v Southwark Coroner Ex p. Hicks Walker* (1988) 151 J.P. 773, DC (both); *R. (Cash) v Northamptonshire Coroner* [2007] EWHC 1354 (Admin.); *R. (Mack) v Birmingham Coroner* [2011] EWCA Civ 712; *Jenkins v Bridgend Coroner* [2012] EWHC 3175 (Admin.) (Coroners Act).

[351] Coroners Act 1988 s.13(2)(a)(ii), as amended, expressly refers to a coroner "in the same coroner area".

[352] See 4–22.

[353] For the difficulties that could arise under the old system, see *R. v Inner West London Coroner Ex p. Dallaglio and Lockwood Croft* [1994] 4 All E.R. 139, where the original coroner was unable to act, and the coroner for another district (but in the same administrative area) volunteered to act, if ordered to do so: the court so ordered at a further hearing on July 20, 1994. Because coroners are now appointed to coroner areas, and not districts within administrative areas, that solution is no longer possible.

[354] *R. v Bunney* (1689) 1 Salk. 190; *R. v Parker* (1675) 2 Lev. 140; Short and Mellor, *Practice of the Crown Office,* 1st edn (1890), p.443.

[355] See 5–126 ff above.

Chapter 20

FURTHER PROCEEDINGS

Introduction

In most cases, the conclusion of the inquest is the end of legal proceedings **20–01** concerning the death. But in other cases the inquest is followed by further proceedings. These may include High Court proceedings to quash the determination and findings and to order a new inquest to be held. Such proceedings have already been discussed.[1]

However, our concern in this chapter lies, not so much with further inquiries **20–02** *into* the same death, but with other proceedings, civil or criminal, *arising out of* that death. Because the coroner's court is inquisitorial and not accusatorial in nature, its findings do not bind any person affected by them. As Lord Tenterden CJ once said, "Nothing that is done will be conclusive upon the person to be affected by it. All is traversable."[2] Thus in former times even a conclusion by a coroner's jury of murder by a named individual did not *convict* him of murder—it operated merely to *charge* him with the offence, for which he could thereafter be tried at a full criminal trial in which he could deny his guilt.[3]

Criminal proceedings

Conclusions imputing criminal responsibility to named persons have now dis- **20–03** appeared from coroner's courts,[4] but the principle remains the same, both for criminal and civil cases. As already stated, the inquest conclusion may not be framed in such a way as to appear to determine any question of criminal responsibility on the part of a named person or any question of civil liability.[5] This will reduce substantially the number of cases in which an inquisition would be even relevant for the purposes of establishing legal liability in relation to the death. Nowadays, only in a small minority of cases will the conclusion indicate any legal responsibility on the part of other persons than the deceased.[6]

The chief examples of such cases are conclusions of unlawful killing. It does not **20–04** follow, however, that criminal proceedings will necessarily be instituted thereafter. The chief suspect may be dead, or immune from prosecution, or lack criminal responsibility. In other cases the matter will usually be referred to (or referred back

---

[1] See Ch.19.
[2] *Garnett v Ferrand* (1827) 6 B. & C. 611 at 627; 108 E.R. 577 at 582; see also the discussion at 578, 615–616. In *Re Sheppard* Unreported April 28, 1992, DC, Beldam LJ said: "The opinion of the coroner, as to the cause of death, is in my opinion irrelevant as between the parties to a claim under a policy of insurance."
[3] *R. v Davies, The Times*, March 18, 1890, per Wills J, reprinted in the 7th edn (1927), of this work, at pp.254–256, in the 8th edn (1946), at pp.296–298, and in the 9th edn (1957), at pp.508–510.
[4] See 1–30 above, and *R. v Crown Prosecution Service Ex p. Hitchens* Unreported June 13, 1997, DC.
[5] See 13–57, 13–103 ff above.
[6] See 13–57, 13–103 ff above.

to) the Crown Prosecution Service for consideration. However, the inquest may have received evidence unavailable to a criminal jury, and the test for prosecuting may involve a high threshold. The CPS may decide to prosecute or it may not.[7]

20–05   But the DPP will generally be required to give reasons for not prosecuting in respect of the death.[8] Even then the DPP's decision will only be quashed on proper judicial review grounds.[9] The Attorney General in May 2002 issued a consultation paper on, and then in July 2003 a Review of, the role of the CPS in cases of death in custody, one aspect of which being the significance attached to inquest verdicts of unlawful killing.[10]

20–06   The Attorney General concluded that, where an unlawful killing conclusion was reached at an inquest, there could be a number of reasons why the CPS might decide not to prosecute, but that, if that were the decision, a full explanation would have to be given for the decision. And in reaching the decision it would be important for the reviewing officer to attend the inquest and observe crucial parts of the evidence on which any prosecution might rely.[11]

20–07   Moreover, the present law requires the coroner to adjourn an inquest in most cases when a person has been charged with an offence arising out of the death of the deceased,[12] or when an arrest or charge for such offence is likely to occur in the near future.[13] Consequently, it is unlikely that a modern inquest would have proceeded far enough to provide much useful material for subsequent criminal proceedings.

Depositions

20–08   The old law required depositions (written statements signed by the maker) to be made of witnesses' evidence in murder and manslaughter cases.[14] That requirement has long been abolished. Nevertheless, it is theoretically still possible that a witness might make a deposition before the coroner.[15] In such a case it was formerly held that a deposition might be admitted at a criminal trial if signed by the deponent and the coroner, and if the accused was present when the deposition was made and had

---

[7] See, e.g. *Re Eugene Swaine*, *The Times*, September 26, 1985, Hornsey coroner (conclusion of unlawful killing; DPP declined to prosecute); *R. v Crown Prosecution Service Ex p. Hitchins* Unreported June 13, 1997, DC, Bodmin coroner (unlawful killing; CPS declined to prosecute).

[8] *R. v DPP Ex p. Manning* [2001] Q.B. 330, DC; cf. *Re Adams' Application* [2001] N.I.C.A. 2. See also *Re Jordan's Application* [2003] N.I.Q.B. 1.

[9] *R. v DPP Ex p. C* [1995] 1 Cr. App. R. 136; *R. v DPP Ex p. Duckenfield* [2002] 1 W.L.R. 55, DC; *R. v DPP Ex p. Stephens* Unreported January 28, 2000, Potts J; *R. v DPP Ex p. Jones* Unreported March 22, 2000, DC; *R. (Sylvester) v DPP,* unreported, May 21, 2001, DC. See also *R. (Rowley) v DPP* [2003] EWHC 693 (Admin.), DC; *R. (Armani da Silva) v DPP* [2006] EWHC 3204 (Admin.) (pre-HRA test for reviewing decisions of the DPP not to prosecute following an unlawful killing conclusion by a coroner's jury, i.e. that the court should interfere only if the decision was arrived at (i) because of some unlawful policy, (ii) because of a failure to act in accordance with settled policy, or (iii) because the decision was perverse, is not altered by the advent of the HRA; on the facts, the DPP's decision not to prosecute was lawful and not open to challenge).

[10] *A Review of the Role and Practices of the Crown Prosecution Service in Cases arising from a Death in Custody,* available at *http://www.cps.gov.uk* [Accessed June 17, 2014].

[11] See at paras 8.154–8.160.

[12] See 10–79—10–80 above.

[13] See 10–78 above.

[14] Coroners Act 1887 s.4(2) (repealed).

[15] See *Morris v Dublin City Coroner* [2000] 3 I.R. 603 at [17], Ir. Sup. Ct.

full opportunity to cross-examine the deponent.[16] In order for the deposition to be admitted, the coroner (or some other person who could give evidence of the circumstances in which the deposition was taken) had to be called to prove the document.[17]

However, the law relating to the admissibility of depositions and other written **20–09** statements in criminal proceedings today is considerably more relaxed. For example, a provision in 1967 rendered statements made in a certain form and served on all other parties capable of admission as evidence if there was no objection.[18] And subsequent provisions in 1980 and 1996 have rendered such written statements admissible in committal proceedings,[19] and at trial,[20] even if objected to.

Civil proceedings

Not only the evidence, but also the determination and findings at an inquest may **20–10** be helpful in civil proceedings. For example, a conclusion of suicide may be material where an insurance company otherwise liable to pay out on a life assurance policy desires to rely on a "suicide" clause as a justification for non-payment. Again, a conclusion that certain valuable items found do or do not constitute treasure trove will in practice affect both the Crown (or any franchisee of treasure trove of the Crown) and the person who would otherwise be entitled to the property if it were not treasure trove[21] and the person out of possession may wish to take action against the person having possession in order to recover it.[22]

Determination and transcript of evidence

First of all, there has never been anything (and still is nothing) to prevent the **20–11** determination or transcript of evidence at an inquest being used as the basis for further inquiry by interested persons before trial, or indeed as the basis of cross-examination at trial.[23] Despite the fact that, as Dillon LJ once observed, "it is not the function of a coroner's inquest to provide a forum for attempts to gather evidence for pending or future criminal or civil proceedings",[24] this has historically been the reason why insurance companies, employees and employees' representatives, and relatives attend inquests and exercise their respective rights to cross-

---

[16] *R. v Cowley* (1907) 71 J.P. 152; *R. v Black* (1910) 74 J.P. 71.
[17] *R. v Marriott* (1911) 75 J.P. 288.
[18] Criminal Justice Act 1967 s.9.
[19] Magistrates' Courts Act 1980 ss.5A–5F.
[20] Criminal Procedure and Investigations Act 1996 s.68, Sch.2.
[21] See 16–08 above.
[22] See, e.g. *Attorney General for Duchy of Lancaster v G.E. Overton (Farms) Ltd* [1982] Ch.277, CA; cf. *R. v Hancock* [1990] 2 Q.B. 242, CA.
[23] Criminal Procedure Act 1865 s.4; *Calmenson v Merchants' Warehousing Co* (1921) 90 LJPC 134.
[24] *R. v Inner North London Coroner Ex p. Thomas* [1993] Q.B. 610 at 629, CA. For examples of detailed assessments of costs of clinical negligence proceedings where it was held that the costs of attending the inquest into the death of the deceased were in principle recoverable under the usual costs order in the civil proceedings, see *Stewart v The Medway NHS Trust* [2004] EWHC 9013 (Costs) and *King v Milton Keynes General NHS Trust* [2004] EWHC 9007 (Costs) (in para.17 of which the dictum of Dillon LJ in *Ex p. Thomas* was cited).

examine witnesses[25] and obtain copies of the record of the inquest and of the documents admitted in evidence at the inquest.[26]

Procedure for proving transcript of evidence

20–12 However, even for the purpose of being used for cross-examination in court the transcript of evidence should be duly proved. In order to avoid the need to call the coroner (or similar person) able to prove the transcript, it was formerly the practice in civil litigation under the Rules of the Supreme Court 1965 to seek an order on the summons for directions in the following terms:

> "That a copy of the notes of evidence (or depositions) taken at the coroner's inquest upon the deceased [duly certified by the coroner or his officer or agreed between the parties] be admissible at the trial for the same purposes and to the same extent as the contents of the original would have been if duly provided by the coroner (or the person who took down the same) without calling the coroner (or such person) and without providing the original or copy."[27]

20–13 The Rules of the Supreme Court 1965 were replaced by the Civil Procedure Rules 1998.[28] These provide (inter alia) that the court has power to control the evidence placed before it.[29] They also provide that, although the general rule is that facts should be proved at trial by oral evidence, this is subject to any order of the court.[30] The court may therefore make a similar order to the old order under the RSC at the case management conference[31] or at the pre-trial review,[32] as appropriate. Or the parties may simply agree the order, and the court can approve and make it without the necessity of a hearing.[33]

Admissibility in evidence

20–14 But in modern times, the question arises as to the admissibility in evidence of (a) the determination (formerly inquisition) itself, and (b) the transcript of evidence taken by the coroner. There were indeed old cases in which an inquisition was received at common law as evidence (though not conclusive evidence) of facts found.[34] However, all the more modern cases held the opposite: neither inquisition (now determination) nor record of evidence was admissible evidence of the facts

---

[25] cf. Burton, Chambers and Gill, *Coroners' Inquiries*, pp.4–7. For the right to cross-examine witnesses, see 11–59, 12–58 above.

[26] See 18–53 above.

[27] See RSC Ord.25 r.3 and *The Supreme Court Practice 1997*, note 25/3/3; the final edition (1999) does not mention the point.

[28] SI 1998/3132.

[29] CPR r.32.1.

[30] CPR r.32.2(1), (2)(b).

[31] CPR r.29.2–29.3.

[32] CPR r.29.7.

[33] CPR r.29.4; *Lavelle v Noble* [2011] EWCA Civ. 441 at [55]–[59].

[34] *R. v Gregory* (1846) 8 Q.B. 508; *Prince of Wales' Association v Palmer* (1858) 25 Beav. 605; *Walpole v Colonial Bank of Australasia* (1884) 10 V.L.R. (E) 315; See also *Hill v Clifford* [1907] 2 Ch. 236, CA.

stated.[35] A rider to the conclusion is no longer possible,[36] but even when it was possible it formed no part of the conclusion, and was similarly inadmissible in subsequent proceedings.[37]

In the cases, the basis of the exclusion of the determination has sometimes been **20–15** put on the rule that opinion evidence is inadmissible[38] and sometimes as that the inquiry is *res inter alios acta*.[39] For the moment, at least, these objections survive.

However, the common law objection to the admissibility at trial of evidence **20–16** given at the inquest was always put on the basis of infringement of the hearsay rule. The objection must therefore have been removed by the statutory relaxation of that rule.[40] Thus, the evidence given at the inquest may be admitted in subsequent civil proceedings as hearsay evidence,[41] though various safeguards must first be satisfied.[42] To prove the evidence, it is sufficient to produce the transcript.[43] Indeed, in an appropriate case it may be that the recording itself would be admissible. But these provisions do not apply to criminal proceedings.[44]

---

[35] *Grime v Fletcher* [1915] 1 K.B. 634; *Bird v Keep* [1918] 2 K.B. 692; *Calmenson v Merchants' Warehousing Co* (1921) 90 L.J.P.C. 134, HL; *Barnett v Cohen* [1921] 2 K.B. 461; *Re Sigsworth* [1935] Ch. 89; *Re Pollock* [1941] Ch. 219. For an earlier case to the same effect, see *The Mangerton* (1856) Swab. 120.

[36] See 12–110, 13–111 ff above.

[37] *R. v Harding* (1908) 1 Cr. App. R. 219, CCA.

[38] e.g. *Bird v Keep* [1918] 2 K.B. 692 at 701.

[39] e.g. *Calmenson v Merchants' Warehousing Co* (1921) 90 L.J.P.C. 134.

[40] By the Civil Evidence Act 1968, and now the Civil Evidence Act 1995; see s.14(1) of the 1995 Act.

[41] Civil Evidence Act 1995 s.1(1); Civil Procedure Rules 1998 r.33.1–33.5.

[42] Civil Evidence Act 1995 ss.2–7.

[43] Civil Evidence Act 1995 s.8.

[44] cf. the Criminal Procedure and Investigations Act 1996, s.68 Sch.2.

Part VI

THE INTERNATIONAL DIMENSION

Chapter 21

CORONERS AND HUMAN RIGHTS

INTRODUCTION

This chapter is about certain aspects of international law, that is, rights and **21–01** obligations between states. These are commonly, but not always, the product of international agreement called treaties or conventions. Those aspects of international law relate to the European Convention on Human Rights 1950 ("the Convention").[1] The coroner needs to know about the Convention, because it can have a significant impact on death investigation, particularly when the death concerned is of a person in state custody or detention, or who died as a result of state action. However, as will be seen, the scope of the Convention is wider than that, and it can affect aspects of other death investigations too.

Unlike the position in some other states, international law affects English (and **21–02** other UK) domestic law only to the extent that statute law so permits. The relevant domestic law, applying throughout the United Kingdom, is contained in the Human Rights Act 1998, which came fully into effect on October 2, 2000.[2] This has given more direct effect than hitherto in domestic UK law to a number of rights guaranteed by the Convention (the so called "Convention rights").[3] Before the Act, the scope for UK judges to have regard to the Convention was limited.[4] A person complaining that UK law infringed the Convention had first to exhaust domestic remedies before applying to the Convention institutions to determine whether there had been a violation. But the scheme of the 1998 Act now empowers those judges to consider the compatibility of legislation with Convention rights, whilst maintaining the principle of parliamentary sovereignty.[5]

The Act works at a number of levels. First, it requires a domestic court or **21–03** tribunal (of whatever level) in determining questions concerning Convention rights to take into account various sources of relevant information, including jurisprudence of the European Court of Human Rights, and opinions and decisions of the European Commission on Human Rights.[6] This is more difficult

---

[1] ETS No. 5, signed at Rome on November 4, 1950.
[2] SI 2000/1851 art.2.
[3] 1998 Act s.1(1); they are set out in Sch.1 to the 1998 Act.
[4] See Hunt, *Using Human Rights Law in English Courts* (1997).
[5] See Bingham (1998) 2 J.L.Rev. 257 at 262–263.
[6] 1998 Act s.2(1); *R. v Davis* [2001] 1 Cr. App. R. 8, CA; the Commission and the Court were merged into a single institution (the Court) by the 11th Protocol, as from November 1, 1998.

than it sounds. The broad statements of principle in the Strasbourg jurisprudence are "hard to interpret, and even harder to follow".[7] Moreover, the meaning of "take into account" is itself controversial. The duty of national courts is to "keep pace" with the Strasbourg Court as the Convention evolves.[8] Thus the weight of the case law is in favour of the view that in practice the United Kingdom courts *normally* will follow Strasbourg decisions.[9] But some serving and former senior judges are unhappy about this.[10]

21–04 Domestically, the position is simpler. Where English courts have considered the provisions of the ECHR and decisions of the European Court of Human Rights, and have decided on their interpretation and effect in English law under the Human Rights Act, the English courts are bound by those decisions (or not) in accordance with the ordinary English rules of precedent. They may offer their opinion of decisions of higher courts as to whether they are compatible with the treaty or international tribunal's own decisions, and if appropriate give permission to appeal, but pending any appeal should consider those higher decisions binding.[11]

21–05 Secondly, it is unlawful for a public authority to act in a way which is incompatible with a Convention right.[12] A claim for damages may be made against a public authority which so acts.[13] So courts and tribunals, including coroners' inquiries (as "public authorities"),[14] must not apply the common law, or award remedies, in a way which is incompatible with a Convention right.[15] Indeed, there may be a positive obligation on the courts to develop the common law in ways compatible with such rights.[16] Thirdly, primary and subordinate legislation must, so far as is possible, be read and given effect to in a way compatible with the

---

[7] *Rabone v Pennine Care NHS Trust* [2012] 2 A.C. 72 at [97].

[8] *R. (Ullah) v Special Adjudicator* [2004] 2 A.C. 323; *Huang v Secretary of State for the Home Department* [2007] 2 A.C. 167 at [18]; *R. (Al-Skeini) v Secretary of State for Defence* [2008] 1 A.C. 153 at [90], [105]; *Re G (adoption: unmarried couple)* [2008] UKHL 38; [2008] 3 W.L.R. 76 at [30], [50], [79], [120], [127]; *Kennedy v Charity Commission* [2014] UKSC 20 at [100], [212]. See also *Smith v Ministry of Defence* [2014] A.C. 52.

[9] *Kay v Lambeth LBC* [2006] 2 A.C. 465 at [28]; *R. v Horncastle* [2010] 2 A.C. 373 at [11]; *Osborn v Parole Board* [2013] UKSC 61; *R. (Chester) v Secretary of State for Justice* [2014] 1 A.C. 271. Cf. *Doherty v Birmingham City Council* [2009] A.C. 367 at [126]; *Manchester City Council v Pinnock* [2011] 2 A.C. 104 at [48].

[10] Laws, Hamlyn Lecture III, "The Common Law and Europe", 27 November 2013 at [23] ff.; Judge, *Constitutional Change: Unfinished Business*, December 4, 2013 at [40]–[47]; cf. Moses, "Hitting the balls out of court", Creaney Memorial Lecture, February 26, 2014; Arden, "An English judge in Europe", Neill Lecture, February 28, 2014.

[11] *Kay v Lambeth LBC* [2006] 2 A.C. 465 at [40]–[45].

[12] Human Rights Act 1998 s.6(1).

[13] Human Rights Act 1998 s.6(1). *R (Greenfield) v Home Secretary* [2005] 1 WLR 673, [19]. No claim against a coroner under this provision has yet succeeded (though see *R. (McLeish) v North London Coroner* [2010] EWHC 3624 (Admin.) for an unsuccessful attempt). Claims against a police force and a hospital trust for breaches of the substantive art.2 obligation have however succeeded: *Van Colle v Chief Constable of Hertfordshire Police* [2007] 1 W.L.R. 1821; *Savage v South Essex Partnership NHS Foundation Trust* [2010] EWHC 865 (QB); see also *Rabone v Pennine Care NHS Trust* [2012] 2 A.C. 72 at [88], and see also *Re Jordan's Application* [2014] NIQB 71.

[14] Human Rights Act 1998 ss.6(3)(a), 21(1); see *R. (A and others) v Partnerships in Care Ltd* [2002] 1 W.L.R. 2610; *Aston Cantlow and Wilmcote with Billesley Parochial Church Council v Wallbank* [2004] 1 A.C. 546.

[15] Human Rights Act 1998 s.6(1); Starmer, *European Human Rights Law* (2000), para.1.42. See also *R. (N) v Home Secretary, The Times*, March 7, 2003, Silber J.

[16] Lester, Pannick and Herberg, *Human Rights Law and Practice*, 3rd edn (2009), para.2.6.3, fn.3.

Convention rights.[17] The phrase "the Convention rights" here means the same as "a Convention right" earlier.[18]

However, there may be cases where the legislation concerned cannot be read **21–06** and given effect to compatibly with the Convention rights. The approach to be taken then differs for primary and subordinate legislation. Incompatible subordinate legislation will be one of two kinds: (i) that where the relevant primary legislation does not prevent removal of the incompatibility, and (ii) that where it does. In the former case the action of making (or perhaps of failing to exercise a power to revoke)[19] the subordinate legislation will, if occurring after the commencement of the 1998 Act, have been unlawful,[20] with limited exceptions.[21]

One of these exceptions is where there is a failure to lay before Parliament a **21–07** "proposal for legislation".[22] In the context of coroners' investigations, the Lord Chancellor and the Lord Chief Justice each has power, with the concurrence of the other, to make rules for (i) coronial investigations and (ii) inquests. These powers are exercisable by statutory instrument,[23] but such instrument does not have even to be laid before Parliament before coming into effect.[24] So this exception does not apply. Hence in such a case the subordinate legislation will be invalid or unenforceable,[25] apparently "on vires grounds in the ordinary way".[26] The coroner as a public authority will be acting unlawfully if he gives effect to such incompatible subordinate legislation,[27] so he must ignore it, to the extent of the incompatibility.

Incompatible primary legislation, or incompatible subordinate legislation where **21–08** the primary legislation prevents removal of the incompatibility, remains in full force and effect: the courts may not strike it down, but the higher courts (including in England the High Court, the Court of Appeal and the Supreme Court)[28] may make a "declaration of incompatibility".[29] However, lower courts and tribunals (including the coroner) may not do this. Such a declaration does not affect the validity of the legislation, or the rights of the parties,[30] but may lead to "fast-track" amendment of the legislation to remove the incompatibility.[31]

---

[17] Human Rights Act 1998 s.3; see e.g. *Haig v Aitken* [2001] Ch. 110.
[18] *Metropolitan Police Commissioner v Hurst* [2007] 2 A.C. 189.
[19] cf. Human Rights Act 1998 s.3(2)(b).
[20] Human Rights Act 1998 s.6(1).
[21] Human Rights Act 1998 s.6(2).
[22] Human Rights Act 1998 s.6(6)(a)
[23] Coroners and Justice Act 2009 ss.43, 45, 176; Constitutional Reform Act 2005 s.12, Sch.1 Pt I.
[24] See Statutory Instruments Act 1946 s.4(1).
[25] Lester, Pannick and Herberg, *Human Rights Law and Practice,* 3rd edn (2009), para.2.3.6; Starmer, *European Human Rights Law* (2000), para.1.36; Grosz, Beatson, Duffy, *Human Rights* (2000), para.3–42; the Act does not say this expressly (cf. s.10(4)), and the point is regrettably obscure.
[26] Per the Lord Chancellor, *Hansard*, HL Debs, col. 544 (November 18, 1997). See Squires [2000] E.H.R.R. 116, esp. at 123–125; Allen and Sales [2000] *Public Law* 361 at 364–65; Hansard, HC Debs, cols. 426ff (June 3, 1998)..
[27] Human Rights Act 1998 s.6(1).
[28] Human Rights Act 1998 s.4(5).
[29] Human Rights Act 1998 s.4(1)–(4); the Crown may intervene in the proceedings: s.5.
[30] Human Rights Act 1998 s.4(6).
[31] Human Rights Act 1998 s.10.

21–09   The Coroners and Justice Act 2009 is primary legislation, and hence falls within the latter rules. On the other hand, the rules and regulations made under it are subordinate legislation which were not required by the terms of the rule-making power to be in the particular form which they are. Hence they are subject to the former rules above. If they cannot be "read down" and interpreted consistently with the Convention rights,[32] they must not be given effect to, so far as they are incompatible with such rights.

21–10   It is necessary to say a few words about both the temporal and the territorial application of the Convention and the Human Rights Act 1998. Both have spawned considerable litigation since the Act came into force. As to the former, suppose a death before the coming into force of the Act on October 2, 2000, where the circumstances were otherwise such that art.2 of the Convention would be engaged, so that any coroner's investigation and inquest would be of the *Middleton* kind rather than the *Jamieson* kind.[33] After a number of early cases,[34] it was held that the Human Rights Act did not render the art.2 rights and obligations arising in such a case justiciable before United Kingdom courts.[35]

21–11   But a subsequent decision of the European Court of Human Rights[36] on the temporal scope of *the Convention* concluded that the procedural obligation arising under art.2 was a detachable or freestanding duty, instead of being merely secondary or ancillary to the death itself. This decision led the United Kingdom courts to reconsider, and ultimately change their mind, in respect of the application of the Human Rights Act.[37] Henceforward, where a coroner has a duty after the coming into force of the Act to hold an investigation which would otherwise be a *Middleton* investigation, it does not fail to be so merely because the death itself occurred before that coming into force.

21–12   As for the territorial scope of the Convention and the Human Rights Act, it was held that the Act applied outside the United Kingdom's national territory only in places which United Kingdom forces controlled.[38] But the European Court of Human Rights subsequently held that the Convention extended to places outside such territory for which the United Kingdom assumed authority and responsibility for the maintenance of security, whether or not the United Kingdom actually controlled them.[39]

21–13   Convention rights may be relevant to coroners' law in a number of areas, and reference has been made throughout this work to Convention jurisprudence at

---

[32] i.e. under s.3 of the 1998 Act.

[33] As to these terms, see 6–14.

[34] *R. (Wright) v Home Secretary* [2001] Lloyd's Rep. Med. 478, *R. (Hurst) v North London Coroner* [2003] EWHC 1721 (Admin.); *R. (Khan) v Secretary of State for Health* [2003] EWCA Civ. 1129; *R. (Challender) v Legal Services Commission* [2004] EWHC 925 (Admin.), *Police Service of Northern Ireland v McCaughey and Grew* [2005] N.I.C.A. 1; *R. (Pearson) v Inner North London Coroner* [2005] EWHC 833 (Admin.).

[35] *Re McKerr* [2004] 1 W.L.R. 807; *Metropolitan Police Commissioner v Hurst* [2007] 2 A.C. 189; *Re Jordan* [2007] 2 A.C. 226.

[36] *Šilih v Slovenia* (2009) 49 E.H.R.R. 996.

[37] *Re McCaughey's Application* [2012] 1 A.C. 725.

[38] *R. (Smith) v Secretary of State for Defence* [2011] 1 A.C. 1. See also *R. (Al Skeini) v Secretary of State for Defence* [2008] A.C. 153; *R. (Gentle) v Prime Minister* [2008] A.C. 1356.

[39] *Al-Skeini v UK* (2011) 53 E.H.R.R. 18, ECtHR; *Smith v Ministry of Defence* [2014] A.C. 52.

appropriate points. In summary, however, the rights most likely to be raised in this context are:

(1) the right to life (art.2);

(2) the right to a fair hearing (art.6(1));

(3) the right to respect for private and family life (art.8(1));

(4) the right to freedom of religion (art.9);

(5) the right to freedom of expression (art.10(1));

(6) the prohibition on discrimination (art.14).

The most important of these, by far, is art.2, the right to life. But the others need **21–14** also to be kept in mind. The text of these rights is set out in Appendix 1, as a Schedule to the Human Rights Act 1998. Because the United Kingdom and Ireland are the only states parties to the Convention with fully developed coroner systems, there have been very few cases before the Convention institutions dealing with the subject, but amongst these the response to terrorism plays a disproportionately large part. Nonetheless, a brief discussion of some of the available jurisprudence follows.[40]

The Right to Life

Scope

Article 2 is one of the most fundamental provisions in the Convention,[41] imposing **21–15** at least three separate duties on Member States,[42] as explained below. It was originally considered to cover cases where the state's agents killed the deceased.[43] It has also been applied to cases where it was not clear if the state's agents had killed the deceased,[44] and to cases where the state has failed to protect the deceased against a human threat,[45] or a suicide[46] or other risk.[47] More relevantly for the coroner's inquiry, it has been applied to cases where the deceased has died in the

---

[40] For full treatments of the subject, see Lester, Pannick and Herberg, *Human Rights Law and Practice,* 3rd edn (2009); Starmer, *European Human Rights Law* (2000); Grosz, Beatson, Duffy, *Human Rights* (2000); Clayton and Tomlinson, *The Law of Human Rights.* Most of the case law is available on the ECtHR website, at *http://www.echr.coe.int* [Accessed June 17, 2014].

[41] *McCann v UK* (1996) 21 E.H.R.R. 97 at [147]; *Andronicon v Cyprus* (1997) 25 E.H.R.R. 491 at [171].

[42] See *R. (P) v Avon Coroner* [2009] EWCA Civ. 1367 at [33].

[43] *McCann v UK* (1996) 21 E.H.R.R. 97; *Jordan v UK* (2001) 11 BHRC 1, ECtHR; *McShane v UK* (2002) 35 E.H.R.R. 593, ECtHR.

[44] *Ergi v Turkey* Unreported July 28, 1998, ECtHR.

[45] e.g. *Osman v UK* [1999] 1 F.L.R. 193, 29 E.H.R.R. 245, ECtHR (mentally disturbed stalker); *Re A's Application for Judicial Review* Unreported October 10, 2001, HC (NI), Kerr J.

[46] *Kiliç v Turkey* (2001) 33 E.H.R.R. 1357 at [41] (army conscripts).

[47] e.g. *LCB v UK* (1998) 27 E.H.R.R. 212, ECtHR at [36] (radiation from nuclear tests); *Barrett v UK* (1997) 23 E.H.R.R.CD 185, ECtHR (excess alcohol consumption). cf. *R. (Southall Black Sisters) v West Yorkshire Coroner* [2002] EWHC 1914 (Admin.), Jackson J (death in mysterious circumstances not through state agency).

custody of the state,[48] i.e. in prison or police custody, and, more latterly, as a detained mental patient.[49] It can also apply, in some aspects at least, to non-violent deaths which occur under the care and responsibility of the state's healthcare professionals, even though the deceased was not in hospital or otherwise unable to make choices for himself (or, being a child, have them made for him by his parents).[50] It is unclear whether a fetus *in utero* has a protectable "life" for the purposes of this article.[51]

Relevant rights

21-16   There are at least three separate duties imposed on Member states by this article. First, a state has a positive obligation to protect the right to life by law. This breaks down into (i) a general or systemic duty, and (ii) an operational duty. As to (i), this involves both enacting legislation and other rule-based systems (e.g. for professional discipline) to protect life,[52] and also putting in place effective criminal law and other provisions to deter offences and to enforce the law.[53] As to (ii), there is a duty to take preventative operational measures to protect an individual at risk,[54] where the state knows, or ought to know, of a real and immediate risk to life,[55] whether it arises in relation to a public or a private activity.[56] Here, "real" means objectively well-founded,[57] and "immediate" means present and continuing, not remote,

---

[48] *Keenan v UK* (2001) 33 E.H.R.R. 38, 10 BHRC 319 at [90], ECtHR; *R. (Wright) v Home Secretary* [2001] Lloyd's Rep. Med. 478, 62 BMLR 16; [2001] UKHRR 1399; *Edwards v UK* (2002) 35 E.H.R.R. 19, ECtHR.

[49] *Savage v South Essex Partnership NHS Foundation Trust* [2009] 1 A.C. 681.

[50] *Powell v UK* Unreported May 4, 2000, ECtHR; *Calvelli v Italy* Unreported January 17, 2002, ECtHR; *R. (Khan) v Secretary of State for Health* [2003] EWCA Civ. 1129; *R. (Goodson) v Bedfordshire Coroner* [2006] 1 W.L.R. 432; *R. (Takoushis) v Inner North London Coroner* [2006] 1 W.L.R. 461, CA; *R. (Canning) v Northampton Coroner* [2006] EWCA Civ. 1225; *R. (Mack) v Birmingham and Solihull Coroner* [2011] EWCA Civ. 712; *R. (Antoniou) v Central and North West London NHS Foundation Trust* [2013] EWHC 3055 (Admin.), DC; *Gray v Germany*, App. no. 49278/09 (ECtHR, May 22, 2014).

[51] *Vo v France* [2005] 40 E.H.R.R. 12 at [85]–[86].

[52] *Osman v UK* [1999] 1 F.L.R. 193; 29 E.H.R.R. 245 at [115], ECtHR; *Öneryildiz v Turkey* (2005) 41 E.H.R.R. 20 at [89]–[90]; *Savage v South Essex NHS Trust* [2009] A.C. 681 at [19]; *Smith v Ministry of Defence* [2014] 1 A.C. 52 at [67].

[53] *Osman v UK* [1999] 1 F.L.R. 193, 29 E.H.R.R. 245 at [115], ECtHR; *Keenan v United Kingdom* (2001) 33 E.H.R.R. 38; *Öneryildiz v Turkey* (2005) 41 E.H.R.R. 20 at [89]–[90]; *Smith v Ministry of Defence* [2014] 1 A.C. 52 at [68].

[54] *Osman v UK* [1999] 1 F.L.R. 193; 29 E.H.R.R. 245 at [115], ECtHR; *Edwards v UK* (2002) 35 E.H.R.R. 19; *Öneryildiz v Turkey* (2005) 41 E.H.R.R. 20 at [91].

[55] *Osman v UK* [1999] 1 F.L.R. 193; 29 E.H.R.R. 245 at [116], ECtHR; *Edwards v UK* (2002) 35 E.H.R.R. 19; *Scavuzzo-Hager v Switzerland*, App. no. 417773/98 (ECtHR, February 7, 2006); *Van Colle v Chief Constable of Hertfordshire Police* [2009] 1 A.C. 225 at [32]; *Watts v United Kingdom* (2010) 51 E.H.R.R. 66 at [83]. See *R. (DF) v Norfolk Chief Constable* [2002] EWHC 1738 (Admin.); *R. (Kent County Council) v Kent Coroner* [2012] EWHC 2768 (Admin.), DC; *Re Applications by C, D, H and R* [2012] NICA 47; *R. (Rowe) v Bedfordshire and Luton Coroner* [2012] EWCA Civ. 1597.

[56] *Öneryildiz v Turkey* (2005) 41 E.H.R.R. 20 at [71]; *Watts v United Kingdom* (2010) 51 E.H.R.R. SE5 at [82].

[57] *Re Officer L* [2007] 1 W.L.R. 2135 at [20]; *Re W's Application* [2004] N.I.Q.B. 67 at [17].

fanciful or negligible.[58] But the threshold is high.[59] Moreover, it is necessary to attain the threshold in relation to a public authority who has the operational duty concerned (usually the police), rather than, say, a public sector landlord.[60] The content of the duty is to take reasonable steps to prevent the risk materialising.[61]

Secondly, a state has a negative duty to refrain from intentionally and unlawfully taking life.[62] This can also be separated out into a general or systemic duty, and an operational duty. The general or systemic duty has already been covered in the discussion in relation to the positive duty, above, and nothing need be added here. As to the operational duty, there is no breach of art.2 where death results from the use of force no more than absolutely necessary (a) in defence of any person from unlawful violence, (b) in order to effect a lawful arrest or prevent the escape of a detainee, (c) in lawful action to quell a disturbance.[63] These exceptions are largely but not exclusively concerned with intentional killing.[64] The words "absolutely necessary" indicate a higher test than the words "necessary in a democratic society", found elsewhere in the Convention.[65] But they are consistent with the English law of self-defence,[66] i.e. such force as is reasonably necessary in the circumstances.[67]   **21–17**

But, thirdly, the article also includes a procedural obligation to investigate deaths which may arguably amount to a breach of the positive or negative obligations imposed by the article,[68] including suspicious deaths.[69] This is particularly relevant to coroners, as in England and Wales the coroner's investigation is the normal way to satisfy the state's obligation.[70] The investigation must begin promptly and proceed with reasonable expedition,[71] and possess the necessary expertise.[72] The minimum content of the investigation obligation will be to provide a mechanism for public and independent scrutiny of the circumstances of the death.[73] A public   **21–18**

---

[58] *Rabone v Pennine Care NHS Trust* [2012] 2 A.C. 72 at [39]; *Re Officers C, D H & R.* [2012] NICA 47 at [26]; *Re Officer L* [2007] 1 W.L.R. 2135 at [20]; *Re W's Application* [2004] N.I.Q.B. 67 at [17].

[59] *Re Officer L* [2007] 1 W.L.R. 2135 at [20]; *Van Colle v Chief Constable of Hertfordshire Police* [2009] 1 A.C. 225 at [32]; *Savage v South Essex Partnership NHS Foundation Trust* [2009] 1 A.C. 681 at [41], [66]; *Mitchell v City of Glasgow* [2009] 1 A.C. 874 at [31].

[60] *Mitchell v City of Glasgow* [2009] 1 A.C. 874 at [67]–[71], [85].

[61] *Osman v UK* [1999] 1 F.L.R. 193, 29 E.H.R.R. 245 at [116], ECtHR; *Keenan v United Kingdom* (2001) 33 E.H.R.R. 38 at [89]; *Edwards v UK* (2002) 35 E.H.R.R. 19 at [55]; *Watts v United Kingdom* (2010) 51 E.H.R.R. 66 at [83].

[62] *LCB v UK* (1998) 27 E.H.R.R. 212 at [36], ECtHR

[63] Convention, art.2(2).

[64] *McCann v UK* (1996) 21 E.H.R.R. 97 at [148].

[65] e.g. arts 8–11; see *McCann v UK* (1996) 21 E.H.R.R. 97 at [149].

[66] Criminal Law Act 1967 s.3; see 14–112 above.

[67] *McCann v UK* (1996) 21 E.H.R.R. 97 at [155]; *Bubbins v UK* (2005) 41 E.H.R.R. 24; *R. (Bennett) v Inner South London Coroner* [2006] EWCA Civ. 617 at [14]–[15].

[68] *McCann v UK* (1995) 21 E.H.R.R. 97 at [161]; *R. (Middleton) v West Somerset Coroner* [2004] 2 A.C. 182 at [2]; *R. (Hurst) v North London Coroner* [2007] 2 A.C. 189 at [28].

[69] *Aksoy v Turkey* (1997) 23 E.H.R.R. 553; *Aydin v Turkey* (1998) 25 E.H.R.R. 251; *Kurt v Turkey* (1999) 27 E.H.R.R. 373; *R. (Southall Black Sisters) v West Yorkshire Coroner* [2002] EWHC 1914 (Admin.), Jackson J at [41]–[44].

[70] *R. (Middleton) v West Somerset Coroner* [2004] 2 A.C. 182 at [20]; *R. (Antoniou) v Central and North West London NHS Foundation Trust* [2013] EWHC 3055 (Admin.) at [24], DC.

[71] *McCaughey v UK* (2013) 58 E.H.R.R. 13 at [130]–[140].

[72] *Stoyanovi v Bulgaria*, App. no 42980/04 (November 9, 2010) at [64].

[73] *Taylor v UK* (1994) 79–A D.R. 127, 136, ECtHR; *Scavuzzo-Hager v Switzerland*, App no. 417773/98 (ECtHR, February 7, 2006); *Ramsahai v The Netherlands* (2008) 46 E.H.R.R. 43.

prosecutor's investigation will not be independent if he relies too heavily on the information provided by the state agents involved.[74] The degree of public scrutiny required may vary from case to case,[75] but the next of kin must be involved in the procedure sufficiently to safeguard their legitimate interests.[76] It is not necessary that there be a public hearing.[77] If there is one, however, it may be necessary in some cases, but not all, for legal aid to be provided to the family.[78]

21–19   The investigation must be effective in the sense that it is capable of leading to a determination of whether the force used was justifiable, and to the identification and punishment of those responsible.[79] It is not necessary that the investigation itself should make such a determination, much less punish wrongdoers. On the contrary, it is expressly accepted by the European organs that the common law model coroner's inquest is a fact-finding exercise, rather than a method of apportioning guilt.[80] So it is sufficient that the factual findings of the inquest could, for example, lead to the referral of the case to the prosecuting authorities, or cause the prosecuting authority to reconsider an earlier decision not to prosecute.[81] Or there may be disciplinary proceedings against the person concerned.[82] For this purpose it is fact-finding that counts, and, not, for instance, the availability of a conclusion such as "unlawful killing".[83]

21–20   The essential principle is that the key facts should be exposed and that the procedures provide for effective accountability. It is not necessary that there should be one unified procedure satisfying all requirements. The aims of fact-finding and accountability may be carried out by or shared between several authorities, as long as the various procedures provide for the necessary safeguards in an accessible and

---

[74] *Ergi v Turkey* Unreported July 28, 1998 at [83]–[84], ECtHR. See also *Re Kelly's Application* [2004] N.I.Q.B. 72 at [27]–[32].

[75] *Jordan v UK* (2001) 37 E.H.R.R. 54, 11 BHRC 1 at [109].

[76] *Öğur v Turkey* Unreported October 30, 1997, ECtHR; *Jordan v UK* (2001) 37 E.H.R.R. 54; 11 BHRC 1 at [109]; *Edwards v UK* (2002) 35 E.H.R.R. 19; *Bubbins v United Kingdom* (2005) 41 E.H.R.R. 24 at [15]; *Gray v Germany*, App no. 49278/09 (ECtHR, 22 May 2014). cf. *Re Doyle's Application* Unreported April 18, 2005, Sullivan J (coroner has no obligation to adjourn inquest until deceased's partner well enough to attend); *R. (Hair) v Staffordshire Coroner* [2010] EWHC 2580 (Admin.) (inability to address coroner on facts at inquest does not make inquiry incompatible with ECHR).

[77] *Gray v Germany*, App no. 49278/09 (ECtHR, 22 May 2014).

[78] *Jordan v United Kingdom* (2003) 37 E.H.R.R. 2 at [132], [137], [142]; *R. (Khan) v Health Secretary* [2003] EWCA Civ. 1129; *Re Hemsworth (No. 2)* [2004] N.I.Q.B. 26; *R. (Challender) v Legal Services Commission* [2004] EWHC 925 (Admin.); *R. (Wright) v Home Secretary* [2006] HRLR 1 at [60]; *R. (Main) v Minister for Legal Aid* [2007] EWCA Civ. 1147 at [50], [51]; *R. (Patel) v Lord Chancellor* [2010] EWHC 2220 (Admin.); *R. (Humberstone) v Legal Service Commission* [2010] EWCA Civ. 1479.

[79] *Jordan v UK* (2001) 37 E.H.R.R. 54; 11 BHRC 1 at [107]; *Edwards v UK* (2002) 35 E.H.R.R. 19 at [71]; *Ramsahai v The Netherlands* (2008) 46 E.H.R.R. 43.

[80] *McCann v UK* (1995) 21 E.H.R.R. 97 at [162]; *Jordan v UK* (2001) 37 E.H.R.R. 54; 11 BHRC 1 at [128]. See also *R. (Amin) v Home Secretary* [2004] 1 A.C. 653 at [31]; *R. (JL) v Secretary of State for Justice* [2009] 1 A.C. 588 at [18]–[19]; *R. (Smith) v Oxfordshire Assistant Deputy Coroner* [2011] 1 A.C. 1 at [72]; *R. (Antoniou) v Central and North West London NHS Foundation Trust* [2013] EWHC 3055 (Admin.), DC.

[81] *Jordan v UK* (2001) 37 E.H.R.R. 54; 11 BHRC 1 at [129]; *McShane v UK* Unreported May 28, 2002 at [121], ECtHR; *Bubbins v United Kingdom* (2005) 41 E.H.R.R. 24 at [7].

[82] *Calvelli v Italy*, App no. 32967/96 (ECtHR, 17 January 2002). See e.g. *Gosai v General Medical Council* [2003] UKPC 31.

[83] *Re Jordan's Application* Unreported January 29, 2002, HC (NI), Kerr J; *Re Jordan's Application* Unreported March 8, 2002, HC (NI), Kerr J.

effective manner.[84] Where an inquest is held it will not normally be necessary to hold a public inquiry as well.[85] But where there is no death (e.g. an attempted suicide in the custody of the state) and hence no inquest,[86] or a death in circumstances involving matters of state policy, which an inquest cannot properly investigate,[87] there may have to be an ad hoc inquiry instead or as well. However, this does not apply to deaths of persons detained on mental health grounds,[88] or indeed in state custody otherwise. In such cases, the inquest is sufficient.

Thus, if the infringement of the right to life is not caused intentionally, the 21–21 obligation to set up an effective judicial system does not necessarily require the provision of a criminal law remedy. In the case of deaths through alleged medical negligence (whether in the public or private sector), the Strasbourg Court has found that that obligation may be satisfied if the legal system affords victims a remedy in the civil courts, either alone or in conjunction with a remedy in the criminal courts,[89] enabling any civil liability to be established and appropriate civil redress to be obtained, such as an order for damages and for the publication of the decision, to be obtained, together with the additional possibility of disciplinary measures.[90]

THE RIGHT TO A FAIR HEARING

Scope

Article 6(1) confers upon a person the right "to a fair and public hearing" in the 21–22 "determination of his civil rights and obligations or of any criminal charge against him".[91] Here, "civil rights and obligations" is used in a narrow sense, unfamiliar to an English lawyer.[92] It has been said that art.6 does no more than reflect the approach of the common law, and there is no difference between the right to a fair hearing and the overriding objective of the CPR.[93] It is not engaged until there are proceedings to determine those rights and obligations,[94] and so cannot apply (for

---

[84] *Rowley v United Kingdom*, App. no. 31914/03 (ECtHR, February 22, 2005); *Pearson v United Kingdom*, App. no. 40957/07 (ECtHR, 13 December 2011) at [71]. See also *R. (Rowley) v DPP* [2003] EWHC 693 (Admin.), DC; *R. (Khan) v Health Secretary* [2003] EWCA Civ. 1129.

[85] *R. (Scholes) v Home Secretary* [2006] EWCA Civ. 2043; *R. (Lin) v Secretary of State for Transport* [2006] EWHC 2575 (Admin.); *R. (Antoniou) v Central and North West London NHS Foundation Trust* [2013] EWHC 3055 (Admin.), DC.

[86] *R. (L) v Secretary of State for Justice* [2009] 1 A.C. 588.

[87] *R. (Smith) v Oxfordshire Assistant Deputy Coroner* [2011] 1 A.C. 1.

[88] *R. (Antoniou) v Central and North West London NHS Foundation Trust* [2013] EWHC 3055 (Admin.), DC.

[89] e.g. a charge of manslaughter in a medical setting: see 14–42—14–51.

[90] *Erikson v Italy*, App no. 37900/97 (ECtHR, October 26, 1999); *Powell v UK*, App no 45305/99 (ECtHR, May 4, 2000); *Calvelli v Italy*, App. no. 32967/96 (ECtHR, January 17, 2002). See also *R. (Takoushis) v Inner North London Coroner* [2006] 1 W.L.R. 461, CA at [99]–[107].

[91] The French version uses the word *contestation* (dispute), which is not replicated in the English version.

[92] *R. (Alconbury Developments Ltd) v Secretary of State for the Environment and the Regions* [2003] 2 A.C. 295 at [78]–[79]; *Meerabux v AG of Belize* [2005] UKPC 12 at [38].

[93] *Ebert v Venvil* [2000] Ch. 484. Cf *Meerabux v AG of Belize* [2005] UKPC 12 at [39]–[40].

[94] *Powell v UK* (1990) 12 E.H.R.R. 355 at [36]; *Masson v Netherlands* (1995) 22 E.H.R.R. 491 at [50]–[52]; *R. v Secretary of State for Health, ex.p C* [2000] 1 F.L.R. 627 C.A;. cf. *Osman v UK* [1999] 1 F.L.R. 193, 5 BHRC 293, ECtHR at [133]–[140].

example) to the collection of information for tax purposes,[95] or in order to consider whether and whom to prosecute for a road traffic offence,[96] to the investigative functions of company inspectors under the Companies Act 1985 s.432(2),[97] to adjudication proceedings under the Housing, Grants, Construction and Regeneration Act 1996,[98] to those of local authorities under the Environmental Protection Act 1990 s.71(2),[99] and to the question whether the court should issue a bench warrant to bring a person before the court.[100]

21–23   Accordingly it cannot apply, for the most part at least, to coroners holding an inquest, because this is, at most, a preliminary inquiry or investigation of the same kind.[101] This is the position in relation to the functionally equivalent inquiry of the *juge d'instruction* in civil law systems, and plainly art.6 must apply the same standard across Europe. Nor can it apply in favour of a person who has no civil rights to be determined in the proceedings, or where, if he has, those rights cannot be determined in them.[102] It is true that the coroner may decide whether a person has certain rights, e.g. to be represented and ask questions. But these are rights of a public law nature, and hence not "civil rights" within the essentially private law meaning of that phrase in the Convention.[103] On the other hand the article is engaged where proceedings are taken in another, specialist tribunal whose decision may influence the outcome of other proceedings in the ordinary (i.e. generalist) courts.[104] But the findings in coroners' courts are certainly not determinative of other proceedings in the ordinary courts.[105] Nor is the record of the inquest (formerly inquisition) even admissible evidence.[106] There is no direct influence at all. Accordingly, it is submitted that art.6(1) is not engaged by an inquest as such.[107]

21–24   In the criminal context it has been held not to apply to preliminary hearings concerning matters of procedure,[108] or hearings under the Criminal Procedure (Insanity) Act 1964 s.4A, to determine whether an insane person (who had no criminal responsibility) committed the act in question.[109] Article 6(2) and (3) only apply where there is a criminal charge, to be determined by Convention rather

---

[95] *Abas v Netherlands* (1997) 88B D.R. 120, ECtHR

[96] *Stott (Procurator Fiscal) v Brown* [2001] 2 W.L.R. 817, PC; *Tolmas v Spain*, App. no. 23816/94 (ECtHR, May 17, 1995) (penalty imposed for failure by car's registered owner to reveal identity of driver on particular occasion: no violation).

[97] *Fayed v UK* (1994) 18 E.H.R.R. 393; *Saunders v UK* (1997) 23 E.H.R.R. 313 at [67].

[98] *Elanay Contract Ltd v Vestry* [2001] B.L.R. 33; 3 T.C.L.R. 6.

[99] *R. v Hertfordshire CC Ex p. Green Environmental Industries Ltd* [2000] 2 A.C. 412.

[100] *Zakarov v White* [2003] EWHC 2463 (Ch).

[101] cf. de Mello (ed.), *Human Rights Act 1998, A Practical Guide* (2000), para.3.13 (mistaking the nature and lack of admissibility of inquest findings).

[102] *McMichael v UK* (1995) 20 E.H.R.R. 205 at [76]–[77]; *Hamer v France* (1996) 23 E.H.R.R. 313 at [73]–[78].

[103] *Ferrazzini v Italy* [2001] S.T.C. 1314; 34 E.H.R.R. 45, ECtHR

[104] *Ruiz-Mateos v Spain* (1993) 16 E.H.R.R. 505 at [31]–[32]; *Sussmann v Germany* (1996) 25 E.H.R.R. 64 at [43]–[45]; *Probstmeier v Germany* Unreported July 1, 1997 at [48]–[53]; *Pammel v Germany* (1997) 26 E.H.R.R. 100 at [53]–[57] (Constitutional Court ruling on validity of legislation).

[105] See 20–02.

[106] See 20–14.

[107] Criminal offences committed in the context of the inquest process itself are dealt with in the next paragraph.

[108] *X v UK* (1982) 5 E.H.R.R. 273 (appointment of new solicitor to represent defendant).

[109] *R. v M* [2002] 1 W.L.R. 824, CA; *R. v Grant, The Times*, December 10, 1991, CA.

than local law, and depend on (a) the classification of the proceedings in local law, (b) the nature of the offence, and (c) the severity of the penalty imposed.[110] For this purpose it has been held that company director disqualification proceedings do not involve a criminal charge,[111] whereas prison disciplinary proceedings,[112] proceedings for penalties for tax evasion,[113] and committal for non-payment of community charge[114] or for contempt of court[115] have all been held to do so. The coroner may, of course, be involved in contempt proceedings, and for fining persons who do not comply with notices[116] and summonses,[117] and in such cases art.6 will be engaged.

Relevant rights

The principle of "equality of arms" underlying art.6(1)[118] requires that, in cases where that provision is engaged, the parties[119] must have the same access to records and documents of a case which play a part in the Court's opinion,[120] and must have the opportunity to present their case under conditions not putting them at a disadvantage[121] and to know of and comment on the documents[122] or other evidence produced or observations or arguments made by others (whether opponents,[123] independent counsel,[124] a legal assessor,[125] or a lower court),[126] or even obtained by the court of its own motion and not disclosed to anyone.[127] Being informed of the material orally during the hearing is not enough.[128]

21–25

---

[110] *Engel v Netherlands (No. 1)* (A/22) (1980) 1 E.H.R.R. 647 at [82]; *AP v Switzerland* (1997) 26 E.H.R.R. 541, ECtHR

[111] *EDC v UK* [1998] B.C.C. 370, ECtHR; *DC v UK* [2000] B.C.C. 710, ECtHR; *Official Receiver v Stern* [2000] 1 W.L.R. 2230, CA.

[112] *Campbell v UK* (1984) 7 E.H.R.R. 165; cf. *R. v Board of Visitors of Hull Prison Ex p. St Germain (No. 1)* [1979] Q.B. 425.

[113] *Bendenoun v France* (1994) 18 E.H.R.R. 54; *Han v Customs and Excise Commissioners* [2001] 1 W.L.R. 2253, CA.

[114] *Benham v UK* (1996) 22 E.H.R.R. 293.

[115] *Harman v UK* (1984) 38 D.R. 53.

[116] See 7–17.

[117] See 10–29 (witnesses), and 11–09 (jurors).

[118] *Borgers v Belgium* Unreported October 30, 1999, ECtHR

[119] Or at any rate their lawyers: *Kamasinski v Austria* (1989) 13 E.H.R.R. 36.

[120] *McMichael v UK* (1995) 20 E.H.R.R. 205 at [80]; *Vermeulen v Belgium*, February 20, 1996, ECtHR

[121] *Dombo Beheer v Netherlands* (1993) 18 E.H.R.R. 188 at [33] (rule prohibiting party from giving evidence held violation); *Bulut v Austria* (1996) 24 E.H.R.R. 84; *Ankerl v Switzerland* Unreported 1996, ECtHR at [38]; *Helle v Finland* (1997) 26 E.H.R.R. 159.

[122] *Mantovanelli v France* (1997) 24 E.H.R.R. 370 at [33]–[36] (court expert's report).

[123] *Feldbrugge v Netherlands* (1986) 8 E.H.R.R. 425; *Ruiz-Mateos v Spain* (1993) 16 E.H.R.R. 505; *Kuopila v Finland* (2000) 33 E.H.R.R. 25, ECtHR

[124] *Lobo Machado v Portugal* (1996) 23 E.H.R.R. 79; *Van Orhoven v Belgium* (1998) 26 E.H.R.R. 55 at [39].

[125] *Nwabueze v The General Medical Council* [2000] 1 W.L.R. 1769, 1775, PC.

[126] *Niderost-Huber v Switzerland* (1998) 25 E.H.R.R. 709.

[127] *Kerojavi v Finland* [1996] E.H.R.L.R. 66; *Krcmar v Czech Republic,* (2000) 31 E.H.R.R. 41 at [40].

[128] *Krcmar v Czech Republic* (2000) 31 E.H.R.R. 41 at [42]–[43].

21–26   In some cases the principle requires that a party should be able to obtain legal aid,[129] and that parties be able to cross-examine witnesses.[130] It may also require communications with lawyers to be protected.[131] In civil (as opposed to criminal[132]) cases, art.6(1) appears to confer no right to obtain disclosure from an opponent of relevant material in the opponent's possession not being produced to the court,[133] unless the opponent is the state itself (or an equivalent public authority).[134] Were it otherwise, the civilian systems of Europe would nearly all be in constant violation of art.6(1). Where a party chooses not to use a system of disclosure provided by the rules, he cannot complain of lack of disclosure as a breach of art.6.[135]

21–27   The court must be independent and impartial. As stated elsewhere,[136] the test for bias at common law[137] has been modified in the light of Convention jurisprudence.[138] The test is now to ascertain all the circumstances which have a bearing on the suggestion that that tribunal was biased, and then ask whether those circumstances would lead a fair-minded and informed observer to conclude that there was a real possibility (or real danger) that the tribunal was biased.[139] Although this modified test is strictly speaking applicable only when art.6 is engaged, it has been applied to a non-art.6 coroner's case on at least one occasion.[140]

21–28   The rules of evidence are for each state to determine, and the Court's only role in relation to them is to see if the proceedings as a whole were fair.[141] So for example the burden or standard of proof is not regulated, except that it must not create an imbalance between the parties[142] (but in criminal cases, the jurisprudence has developed specific rules, like the right of an accused to remain silent[143]). The court must give reasons for its judgment,[144] though the degree of detail may vary

---

[129] *Steel and Morris v United Kingdom*, App. no. 68416/01 (ECtHR, February 15, 2005).

[130] *X v Austria* (1972) 42 C.D. 145, ECtHR; see also *Unterpetinger v Austria* (1986) 13 E.H.R.R. 175 (criminal case), and *R. (Wilkinson) v Broadmoor Hospital Responsible Medical Officer* [2002] UKHRR 390, CA.

[131] *General Mediterranean Holdings Ltd v Patel* [2000] 1 W.L.R. 272; cf. *Re L (A Minor)* [1997] A.C. 16, HL.

[132] *Jespers v Belgium* (1981) 27 D.R. 61; *Bonisch v Austria* (1985) 9 E.H.R.R. 191; *Edwards v UK* (1992) 15 E.H.R.R. 417; *Foucher v France* (1997) 25 E.H.R.R. 234; *Cannon v UK* Unreported January 17, 1997, ECtHR; *Rowe & Davis v UK* (2000) 30 E.H.R.R. 1.

[133] cf. *McMichael v UK* (1995) 20 E.H.R.R. 205 at [80] ("vital documents" undisclosed to the other parties, but produced to the court).

[134] *McGinley and Egan v UK* (1998) 27 E.H.R.R. 1; 4 EHRC 421 at [86].

[135] *McGinley and Egan v UK* (1998) 27 E.H.R.R. 1; 4 EHRC 421.

[136] See 5–67 above.

[137] *R. v Gough* [1993] A.C. 646, HL; *Locabail (UK) Ltd v Bayfield Properties Ltd* [2000] Q.B. 451, CA.

[138] Including *Delcourt v Belgium* (1970) 1 E.H.R.R. 355; *Piersack v Belgium* (1982) 5 E.H.R.R. 169; *De Cubber v Belgium* (1984) 7 E.H.R.R. 236; *Hauschildt v Denmark* (1989) 12 E.H.R.R. 266; *Borgers v Belgium* (1993) 15 E.H.R.R. 92; *Gregory v UK* (1977) 25 E.H.R.R. 577.

[139] *Director General of Fair Trading v Proprietary Association of Great Britain* [2001] 1 W.L.R. 700, CA.

[140] *R. v East Riding and Kingston-upon-Hull Coroner Ex p. Dawson* [2001] A.C.D. 68, Jackson J.

[141] *Miailhe v France (No. 2)* (1996) 23 E.H.R.R. 491 at [43].

[142] *G v France* (1988) 57 D.R. 100, 106.

[143] *Funke v France* (1993) 16 E.H.R.R. 297; *Saunders v UK* (1996) 23 E.H.R.R. 313; cf. *Murray v UK* (1996) 22 E.H.R.R. 29 (adequate safeguards; no violation).

[144] *Van de Hurk v Netherlands* (1994) 18 E.H.R.R. 481 at [61]; *Hiro Balani v Spain* (1995) 19 E.H.R.R. 566 at [27].

according to the nature of the decision.[145] In criminal cases, the use of screens[146] or other methods to preserve the anonymity of witnesses is justified in some cases,[147] provided (i) such methods are restricted to what is strictly necessary,[148] and (ii) there are "counterbalancing procedures" to enable the reliability of the evidence to be tested.[149] But it is harder to justify anonymity for police officer witnesses.[150]

THE RIGHT TO RESPECT FOR PRIVATE AND FAMILY LIFE

Scope

Article 8 confers the right to respect[151] for a person's private and family life, home   **21–29** and correspondence,[152] subject to important exceptions, in the form of justification for prima facie infringements.[153] There is some doubt as to whether this right attaches to legal persons,[154] such as companies, but they can have rights of confidence in law, the law of privilege protects their communications, and the Convention elsewhere extends to legal persons, so the better view is that art.8 can do so to at least some extent (e.g. privacy of communications). States' obligations under this article are both negative[155] and positive.[156] But inaction cannot be a breach of a positive duty in the absence of culpability.[157] A person claiming a violation of this article needs to show that he is a "victim",[158] although sometimes the threat of a violation has been sufficient for this.[159] The article does not, however, protect against the effects of a person's own conduct.[160] In the context of coroner law, the most important aspects of the right are those concerning respect

---

[145] *Ruiz Torija v Spain* (1994) 19 E.H.R.R. 553 at [29]; *Georgiadis v Greece* (1997) 24 E.H.R.R. 606 at [42]–[43]; *Helle v Finland* (1997) 26 E.H.R.R. 159 at [55]–[60]; *Stefan v General Medical Council* [2000] 1 W.L.R. 1299, PC.

[146] *X v UK* (1993) 15 E.H.R.R. CD 113.

[147] *Doorson v Netherlands* (1996) 22 E.H.R.R. 330.

[148] *Van Mechelen v Netherlands* (1998) 25 E.H.R.R. 647.

[149] *Kostovski v Netherlands* (1990) 12 E.H.R.R. 434.

[150] *Van Mechelen v Netherlands* (1998) 25 E.H.R.R. 647.

[151] Thus an interference is not automatically a violation: see further *Abdulaziz, Cabales, and Balkandali v UK* (1985) 7 E.H.R.R. 471 at [67], and *Sheffield and Horsham v UK* (1998) 27 E.H.R.R. 163 at [52].

[152] Article 8(1).

[153] Article 8(2) (accordance with the law, *and* necessity in a democratic society in certain national interests, or to protect others' rights: see 21–36).

[154] *R. v Broadcasting Standards Commission Ex p. BBC* [2000] UKHRR 158, 169 (no); cf. on appeal at [2000] 3 All E.R. 989, 999, 1001 (point left open); *Cantabrica Coach Holdings Ltd v Vehicle Inspectorate* (2000) 164 J.P. 593, DC (point left open).

[155] *Belgian Linguistics Case (No. 2)* (1968) 1 E.H.R.R. 252; *Lingens v Austria* (1986) 8 E.H.R.R. 407.

[156] *Marckx v Belgium* (1979) 2 E.H.R.R. 330; *X and Y v Netherlands* (1985) 8 E.H.R.R. 235 at [23]; *Johnstone v Ireland* (1986) 9 E.H.R.R. 203 at [55]; *Gaskill v UK* (1989) 12 E.H.R.R. 36 at [38]; *Kroon v Netherlands* (1994) 19 E.H.R.R. 263 at [31]; *Sheffield and Horsham v UK* (1998) 27 E.H.R.R. 163 at [52]; *MC v Bulgaria* (2005) 40 E.H.R.R. 459 at [150].

[157] *Anufrijeva v Southwark LBC* [2004] Q.B. 1124, CA at [45], [48].

[158] *Campbell v UK* (1992) 15 E.H.R.R. 137 at [32]–[33].

[159] *Klass v Germany* (1978) 2 E.H.R.R. 214; *Dudgeon v UK* (1981) 4 E.H.R.R. 149; *Leander v Sweden* (1987) 9 E.H.R.R. 433; *Norris v Ireland* (1988) 13 E.H.R.R. 186; *Modinos v Cyprus* (1993) 16 E.H.R.R. 485.

[160] *McFeely v UK* (1980) 20 D.R. 44, ECtHR (prisoners' "dirty protest").

for the physical integrity of the individual, in relation to funerals, and for private communications and information. Other aspects include respect for private life and family life.

Integrity of the individual

21–30   A decision by hospital doctors to overrule a mother's objections to their proposed treatment of her disabled son in the absence of court authorisation has been held a breach of the article.[161] A failure to comply with the art.2 obligation to protect life may well also involve a breach of art.8.[162] But where there is no violation of art.2, it is unlikely that the same facts could amount to a breach of art.8.[163] Positive obligations on the state are inherent in the right to effective respect for private life under art.8; these obligations may involve the adoption of measures even in the sphere of the relations of individuals between themselves.[164] The article is also enagaged by the desire to end life.[164a]

Funerals and memorials

21–31   A failure by state authorities to return a dead body to the family for funeral purposes once all technical and scientific examinations have been completed and there is no need to retain it further is a breach.[165] It is also a breach not to permit a prisoner to leave prison to attend his parents' funerals without compelling reasons.[166] The article is engaged in that, while choice of place and determination of the modalities of burial are made for a time after life has come to an end, individuals may feel the need to express their personality by the way they arrange how they are to be buried,[167] and therefore their views are to be taken into account.[168] In Scotland this has been held, obiter, to extend to other near relatives' expressions of views.[169]

21–32   In some circumstances the respect accorded to private life in art.8 can extend to aspects of funeral arrangements, although a requirement that the cremation of human remains takes place in a building, and a corresponding prohibition on an open-air pyres, do not amount to an interference with the right of respect for privacy and family life accorded by art.8.[170] And it is not a breach for a parent not

---

[161] *Glass v UK*, App. no.61827/00 (ECtHR, March 9, 2004). See also *R (Tracey) v Cambridge University Hospital NHS Foundation Trust* [2014] EWCA Civ 822.
[162] *Van Colle v Hertfordshire Chief Constable* [2007] 1 W.L.R. 1821, CA, reversed [2009] 1 A.C. 225, HL, on different grounds.
[163] *Van Colle v United Kingdom* (2012) 56 E.H.R.R. 23 at [107]–[108].
[164] *MC v Bulgaria* (2005) 40 E.H.R.R. 459 at [150].
[164a] *Pretty v UK* (2002) 35 EHRR 1, [67]; *Haas v Switzerland* (2011) 53 EHRR 33, [51]; *Koch v Germany* [2013] 56 EHRR 6, [46], [51]; *Gray v Switzerland* (2014) 58 EHRR 7, [60]; *R v (Nicklinson) v Ministry of Justice* [2014] UKSC 38.
[165] *Pannullo v France* (2003) 36 E.H.R.R. 757, ECtHR.
[166] *Ploski v Poland*, App. no. 26761 (ECtHR, November 12, 2002).
[167] *X v Federal Republic of Germany*, App. no. 8741/79 (March 10, 1981); D.R. 24, 137.
[168] *Borrows v Preston Coroner* [2008] EWHC 1387 (QB); *Ibuna v Arroyo* [2012] EWHC 428 (Ch); *R. (The Plantagenet Alliance Ltd) v Secretary of State for Justice* Unreported August 15, 2013, Haddon-Cave J. cf. *R. (Plantagenet Alliance Ltd) v Secretary of State for Justice* [2014] EWHC 1662 at [134].
[169] *C v Advocate General of Scotland* 2012 S.L.T. 103 at [36].
[170] *R. (Ghai) v Newcastle City Council* [2009] EWHC 978 (Admin.) at [138], [141] (not pursued on appeal). See also *Esfandieri v Secretary of State for Work and Pensions* [2006] EWCA Civ. 282 at [23].

to be able to have a monument of his choice on the grave of his dead child.[171] Nor is it a breach to refuse a request to move ashes from a cemetery where they have been placed in an urn to another resting place.[172]

Private communications and information

Article 8 refers to "correspondence",[173] but this includes telephone calls,[174] and no **21–33** doubt other means of communication. Hence state telephone tapping,[175] mail interception[176] and even secret filming in a public place[177] are all prima facie an infringement of art.8(1). But in principle, so is requiring a person, whether a party to proceedings or a third party (or witness), to reveal confidential information to a court[178] or other state agency.[179] The communications intercepted may be from the person's business premises,[180] and need not be domestic in nature.[181] Indeed, they may even be criminal.[182] Similarly, the information required to be revealed may be of a commercial rather than domestic nature. The respect for private correspondence may involve positive obligations on the state.[183] But a suicide note intended for or addressed to the coroner or "To whom it may concern" is not private in this sense.

Private and family life

The state may be obliged under this article to adopt measures to protect the public **21–34** against media intrusion into private life, e.g. by photography, even in public places, particularly where such intrusion conveys information without contributing to public debate.[184] This may be relevant, for example, to the photographing of persons arriving at the coroner's court. Late supply of a post-mortem examination

---

[171] *Jones v United Kingdom*, App. no. 42639/04 (ECtHR, September 13, 2005).

[172] *Dödsbo v Sweden* (2006) 45 E.H.R.R. 22, ECtHR.

[173] This includes the medium as well as the message: *Haig v Aitken* [2000] Ch. 110 (trustee in bankruptcy has no right to sell personal letters).

[174] *Klass v Germany* (1978) 2 E.H.R.R. 214.

[175] *Klass v Germany* (1978) 2 E.H.R.R. 214; *Malone v UK* (1984) 7 E.H.R.R. 14; *Huvig v France* (1990) 12 E.H.R.R. 528; *Kruslin v France* (1990) 12 E.H.R.R. 547; *A v France* (1994) 17 E.H.R.R. 462; *Halford v UK* (1997) 24 E.H.R.R. 523; *Kopp v Switzerland* (1998) 27 E.H.R.R. 91.

[176] *Silver v UK* (1983) 5 E.H.R.R. 347; *Campbell v UK* (1993) 15 E.H.R.R. 137; *Herczegfalvy v Austria* (1993) 15 E.H.R.R. 437; *Foxley v UK* Unreported June 20, 2000, ECtHR.

[177] *R. v Loveridge* Unreported April 11, 2001, CA. See also *Peck v UK* (ECtHR, February 3, 2003).

[178] *Z v Finland* (1998) 25 E.H.R.R. 371; 45 B.M.L.R. 107 (doctor required to give evidence of patient's medical condition); see also *R. v Home Secretary Ex p. Belgium* Unreported February 15, 2000, DC (disclosure to other parties of medical reports relied on by Home Secretary).

[179] *X v Belgium* (1982) 31 D.R. 231, ECtHR (taxpayer required to explain personal expenditure in detail); *Visser v Netherlands* Unreported May 2, 1989, ECtHR (disclosure by telephone service to tax authorities of telephone number); *MS v Sweden* (1997) 28 E.H.R.R. 313; 3 B.H.R.C.; 45 B.M.L.R. 133 (disclosure of medical records to Social Insurance Office); *Cantabrica Coach Holdings Ltd v Vehicle Inspectorate* [2001] 1 W.L.R. 2288, HL (transport business required to hand over tachograph records).

[180] *Halford v UK* (1997) 24 E.H.R.R. 523; *Cantabrica Coach Holdings Ltd v Vehicle Inspectorate* [2001] 1 W.L.R. 2288, HL.

[181] *Huvig v France* (1990) 12 E.H.R.R. 538 at [8], [25]; *Kopp v Switzerland* (1998) 27 E.H.R.R. 91; *Cantabrica Coach Holdings Ltd v Vehicle Inspectorate* [2001] 1 W.L.R. 2288, HL.

[182] *A v France* (1993) 17 E.H.R.R. 462 at [34]–[37].

[183] *Boyle v UK* (1985) 41 D.R. 90, ECtHR; *Grace v UK* (1988) 62 D.R. 22, ECtHR; cf. *X v Germany* (1979) 17 D.R. 227, ECtHR (no positive obligation to ensure perfectly functioning postal service).

[184] *Von Hannover v Germany* (2005) 40 E.H.R.R. 1 at [56]–[60], ECtHR.

report to the deceased's mother, so in effect preventing further inquiry by her into the cause of death, is not a breach of the article.[185] Nor is it a breach for the coroner to return unlawful killing in circumstances where the killer although not named in the conclusion is nonetheless readily identifiable.[186]

21–35   Police files[187] and local authority social services case files[188] relating to an individual relate to private and family life, and hence access to those files falls under art.8. But although art.8 may give rise to positive duties,[189] there is no requirement for a general right of access. On the other hand, a system giving access to the person concerned conditionally on the consent of the various contributors to the files (given a confidentiality undertaking) must provide for an independent authority to decide whether access should be given in cases where a contributor fails to answer or improperly refuses consent.[190] In the last resort, however, judicial review meets this need.[191]

Exceptions

21–36   Article 8(2) allows significant exceptions to the basic rights in art.8(1), where (i) the law permits it on a sufficiently precise basis to foresee when it will be applied,[192] and (ii) it is necessary in a democratic society in the interests of national security, public safety or the economic well-being of the country, for the prevention of disorder or crime, for the protection of health or morals, or the protection of the rights or freedoms of others. The phrase "necessary in a democratic society" has been interpreted as implying the existence of a "pressing social need".[193] So, for example, it has been held that requiring a doctor to reveal his patient's medical history in criminal proceedings against her husband was proportionate measure taken in the interests of investigating and prosecuting crime, and hence justifiable,[194] and a search (*Anton Piller*) order was not a violation of art.8, because the relevant law was accessible and sufficiently precise as to be foreseeable, and there were sufficient safeguards against abuse.[195] Similar conclusions have been reached in relation to out of court disclosure.[196]

---

[185] *R. (McLeish) v North London Coroner* [2010] EWHC 3624 (Admin) at [64].

[186] *R. (Evans) v Cardiff Coroner* [2011] EWCA Civ. 719.

[187] *Leander v Sweden* (1987) 9 E.H.R.R. 433.

[188] *Gaskin v UK* (1989) 12 E.H.R.R. 36 at [36]–[37].

[189] See 21–29 above.

[190] *Gaskin v UK* (1989) 12 E.H.R.R. 36 at [49].

[191] *Gunn-Russo v Nugent Care Society* [2001] UKHRR 1320.

[192] *Silver v UK* (1983) 5 E.H.R.R. 347; *Huvig v France* (1990) 12 E.H.R.R. 538; *Amann v Switzerland* Unreported February 16, 2000, ECtHR at [56]; *Foxley v UK* (2000) 31 E.H.R.R. 25; 8 B.H.R.C. 571, ECtHR at [34].

[193] *Handyside v UK* (1976) 1 E.H.R.R. 737 at [48]; *Dudgeon v UK* (1982) 4 E.H.R.R. 149.

[194] *Z v Finland* (1998) 25 E.H.R.R. 371, 45 B.M.L.R. 107.

[195] *Chappell v UK* (1990) 12 E.H.R.R. 1; cf. *Niemietz v Germany* (1992) 16 E.H.R.R. 97 (violation, where no safeguards, and interference with professional secrecy disproportionate), *Funke v France* (1993) 16 E.H.R.R. 97 (violation, where no judicial authorisation).

[196] *MS v Sweden* (1997) 28 E.H.R.R. 313; 3 B.H.R.C.; 45 B.M.L.R. 133 (disclosure of medical records to Social Insurance Office to resolve claim made by patient held justifiable), *Cantabrica Coach Holdings Ltd v Vehicle Inspectorate* [2001] 1 W.L.R. 2288, HL (disclosure of tachograph records necessary in interests of public safety), *R. v Banque Internationale à Luxembourg* [2000] S.T.C. 708 (disclosure of client banking records to Inland Revenue held justifiable), and *A Health Authority v X* [2001] UKHRR 1213 (patients' health records disclosable in investigation of GP's practice). See also *R. (Marper) v Chief Constable of South Yorkshire, The Independent*, October 1, 2002, CA (retention of fingerprints and DNA samples).

Witness summonses or court questioning seeking the production of highly   **21–37** confidential documents or information may be justified, as in the interests of protecting the rights of others,[197] as where the expert report obtained by a mother in care proceedings relating to her child was compulsorily disclosed to the police in the interests of protecting the child.[198] As to anonymity orders, in one particular case it was held that, where a claimant was appealing against an order by the Treasury designating him as suspected of involvement in terrorism, there was a powerful general public interest in identifying him in any report of the legal proceedings which justified curtailment to that extent of his and his family's art.8 rights to respect for their private and family life.[199]

Privilege

Communications protected by legal privilege[200] must be specially mentioned.   **21–38** There is no specific regime for them in the Convention, but they are protected by art.8 on the same basis as other confidential information. However, lawyer-client privilege may be given a higher degree of protection than other confidential information cases.[201] In the context of criminal proceedings the question of privilege overlaps with the right to a fair hearing under art.6,[202] and is hence doubly protected. There are special considerations where the correspondence of convicted prisoners is concerned, but in particular their privileged communications should not be interfered with unless there is some basis for suspecting the integrity of the lawyer.[203]

The Right to Freedom of Religion and Belief

Scope

The right to freedom of religion and belief is absolute,[204] but the *manifestation* of   **21–39** religion may be subject to limitations prescribed by law as necessary for public safety, the protection of public order, health or morals, or of the rights or freedoms of others.[205] The right is confined to individuals,[206] but may extend to groups of individuals.[207] Religion and belief includes non-religious belief,[208] such as humanism.[209]

---

[197] This was argued, but not decided, in *Z v Finland* (1998) 25 E.H.R.R. 371; 45 B.M.L.R. 107.
[198] *L. v UK* [2000] 2 F.L.R. 322, ECtHR; see also *Re L (A Minor)* [1997] A.C. 16, HL.
[199] *Treasury v Ahmed* [2010] 2 A.C. 697.
[200] The privilege against self-incrimination falls under art.6: see 21–28 above.
[201] *Niemietz v Germany* (1993) 16 E.H.R.R. 97 at [37].
[202] *S v Switzerland* (1992) 14 E.H.R.R. 670 at [48]; see 21–27 above.
[203] *Campbell v UK* (1993) 15 E.H.R.R. 137; see also *Silver v UK* (1984) 5 E.H.R.R. 347; *R. v Home Secretary Ex p. Leach* [1994] Q.B. 198; *R. v Home Secretary Ex p. Simms* [1999] Q.B. 349.
[204] *Kokkinakis v Greece* (1994) 17 E.H.R.R. 397 at [33], ECtHR.
[205] Article 9(2).
[206] *Church of X v UK* (1969) 12 Y.B. 306, ECtHR; *Company X v Switzerland* (1981) 16 D.R. 85, ECtHR; *Vereniging Rechtswinkels Utrecht v Netherlands* (1986) 46 D.R. 200, ECtHR.
[207] *Chappell v UK* (1987) 53 D.R. 241, ECtHR.
[208] *Kokkinakis v Greece* (1994) 17 E.H.R.R. 397.
[209] *Re Crawley Green Road Cemetery, Luton* [2001] W.T.L.R. 1269, Con. Ct.

Relevant rights

21–40   Manifestation of religion or belief does not generally justify refusal to comply with domestic law of general application, e.g. paying taxes which are partly spent on defence,[210] or contributing to compulsory pensions,[211] or complying with planning rules.[212] It is not a violation of the article for a school with a majority of Muslim pupils to forbid a Muslim student to attend wearing a *jilbab*, in breach of a dress code agreed with local imams.[213] Nor was it a violation for HM Treasury not to establish a special fund for taxes collected from pacifists, from which payments out could be made only for non-military uses.[214] A claim to total exemption from the law authorising invasive post-mortem examination of the dead would likewise fail. An invasive post-mortem will be justified even against religious belief or other objection where it contributes to the inquest's purpose in promoting and protecting public safety, public health and the rights and freedom of others, and is not disproportionate in effects.[214a]

21–41   But on the other hand a law banning all proselytism has been held not justified.[215] The blasphemy law was held an acceptable protection of Christian religious rights,[216] but the United Kingdom was not required to extend it to protect Muslims.[217] Failing to secure the interment (or reinterment) in an appropriate time, place or way of the body of a deceased believer where such interment is of religious significance may infringe the rights of co-religionists to manifest their religion,[218] unless subject to a legal limitation of the permissible type set out above.

THE RIGHT TO FREEDOM OF EXPRESSION

Scope

21–42   Article 10(1) confers the right to freedom of expression, to hold opinions, and to receive and impart information without public interference. But it is subject to the limitations in art.10(2), being those prescribed by law,[219] necessary in a democratic society, and in one of various public interests, or the protection of others' rights or

---

[210] *C. v UK* (1983) 37 D.R. 142, ECtHR; *Bouessel del Bourg v France* (1993) 16 E.H.R.R. CD 49.
[211] *V. v Netherlands* (1984) 39 D.R. 267.
[212] *Iskcon v UK* (1994) 76A D.R. 90.
[213] *R. (Begum) v Denbigh High School* [2007] 1 A.C. 100, HL. See also *R. (X) v Y School* [2007] EWHC 298 (Admin.) (*niqab* forbidden after change of policy: no violation), and *SAS v France*, ECtHR, Grand Chamber, July 1, 2014 (law forbidding wearing burqa/niqab in public places: no violation).
[214] *R. (Boughton) v HM Treasury* [2006] EWCA Civ. 504.
[214a] Cf *R (Goldstein) v Inner North London Coroner*, unreported, July 16, 2014, QBDivCt (interim injunction varied to permit staged autopsy from CT scan, through "needle" autopsy to "full" autopsy).
[215] *Kokkinakis v Greece* (1994) 17 E.H.R.R. 397.
[216] *Lemon v UK* (1982) 28 D.R. 77.
[217] *Choudhury v UK*, App. no. 17439/90 (ECtHR, March 5, 1991). .
[218] *Re Durrington Cemetery* [2001] Fam. 33; *Re Crawley Green Road Cemetery, Luton* [2001] W.T.L.R. 1269.
[219] This includes common law: *Tolstoy Miloslavsky v UK* (1995) 20 E.H.R.R. 442 at [37].

preventing the disclosure of confidential information.[220] Moreover, it does not impose any duty on states to collect, disseminate or supply information.[221] A statutory or other inquiry is not required by art.10 to be held in public,[222] and even if it is held in public, art.10 does not confer a right to film it.[223] But art.10 covers nearly all[224] kinds of expression, including artistic[225] and commercial and professional,[226] and legal as well as natural persons may take advantage of it.[227] However, the margin of appreciation accorded to states has been greater in commercial than political matters.[228] The right not to be restricted in receiving information does not depend on what use will be made of it.[229] Article 10 can sometimes give rise to positive obligations on the part of states.[230]

Relevant rights

An order that a journalist disclose sources must be justified, if at all, under art.10(2).   **21–43** Sometimes the public interest in protection of a journalist's source has been held to outweigh an employer's need for disclosure in order to identify a disloyal employee,[231] sometimes not.[232] Although reporting of court proceedings contributes to the achievement of a fair hearing,[233] by exposing judges to public scrutiny,[234] it is legitimate to restrict reporting which may prejudice pending proceedings, especially criminal proceedings.[235] But the restriction must be proportionate to the aim, whether of achieving a fair hearing,[236] or of protecting national security.[237] A complaint under art.10 following the conviction of a journalist for reporting the confidential deliberations of a criminal jury has been dismissed.[238] On the other hand, a conviction for breaching confidentiality of

---

[220] cf. *Attorney General v Punch Ltd* [2001] Q.B. 1028, CA.

[221] *Leander v Sweden* (1987) 9 E.H.R.R. 433; *Guerra v Italy* (1998) 26 E.H.R.R. 357 at [53].

[222] *R. (Persey) v Secretary of State for Environment, Food and Rural Affairs, The Times*, March 28, 2002, DC; *R. (Howard) v Secretary of State for Health, The Times*, March 28, 2002.

[223] Decision dated October 25, 2001, of Dame Janet Smith, Chairman of the Shipman Inquiry (see *http://webarchive.nationalarchives.gov.uk/20090808154959/http://www.the-shipman-inquiry.ord.uk/reports.asp*) at [60].

[224] It does not cover physical expressions of feelings: *Case of X* (1977) 19 D.R. 66, ECtHR.

[225] *Muller v Switzerland* (1988) 13 E.H.R.R. 212; *Chorherr v Austria* (1993) 17 E.H.R.R. 358.

[226] *Markt Intern Verlag v Germany* (1989) 12 E.H.R.R. 161; *Open Door Counselling v Ireland* (1992) 15 E.H.R.R. 244; *Casado Coca v Spain* (1994) 18 E.H.R.R. 1; *Jacubowski v Germany* (1994) 19 E.H.R.R. 64.

[227] *Autronic A.G. v Switzerland* (1990) 12 E.H.R.R. 485; *The Observer Ltd v UK* (1991) 14 E.H.R.R. 153; *Open Door Counselling v Ireland* (1992) 15 E.H.R.R. 244.

[228] *Markt Intern Verlag v Germany* (1989) 12 E.H.R.R. 161; *Casado Coca v Spain* (1994) 18 E.H.R.R. 1.

[229] *Autronic A.G. v Switzerland* (1990) 12 E.H.R.R. 485.

[230] e.g. *Plattform Artze fur das Leben v Austria* (1988) 13 E.H.R.R. 204 (state's duty to take steps to prevent disruption of demonstration by mob).

[231] *Goodwin v UK* (1997) 22 E.H.R.R. 123.

[232] *Camelot Group Ltd v Centaur Communications Ltd* [1999] Q.B. 124, CA; and see *Fressoz and Roire v France* [1999] E.H.R.L.R. 339.

[233] *Axen v Germany* (1984) 6 E.H.R.R. 195 at [25]; *Worm v Austria* (1997) 25 E.H.R.R. 454 at [50].

[234] *Scott v Scott* [1913] A.C. 417, HL.

[235] *Hodgson v UK* (1987) 51 D.R. 136; *C Ltd v UK* (1989) 61 D.R. 285; cf. *Worm v Austria* (1997) 25 E.H.R.R. 454 at [50].

[236] *Sunday Times v UK* (1979) 2 E.H.R.R. 245 at [56].

[237] *The Observer Ltd v UK* (1991) 14 E.H.R.R. 153.

[238] *Associated Newspapers Ltd v UK* Unreported November 30, 1994, ECtHR.

court proceedings was not justifiable where the material concerned was already public.[239] As to anonymity orders, in one particular case, where a claimant appealed an order by the Treasury designating him as suspected of involvement in terrorism, there was a powerful general public interest in identifying him in any report of the legal proceedings which justified curtailment to that extent of his and his family's art.8 rights to respect for their private and family life.[240]

Other Miscellaneous Rights

Forced labour

21–44 Article 4 prohibits slavery (art.4(1)) and forced labour (art.4(2)), subject to exceptions (art.4(3)). But the obligation imposed on employers to calculate and deduct tax from employees' salaries, and to account to the tax authorities for it, does not infringe art.4(2), as it does not go beyond "normal civic obligations" (one of the exceptions in art.4(3)).[241] Similarly, compulsory fire service[242] and participation by gun licensees in anti-rabies activity[243] have been held within the same exception. Accordingly there is no real scope for arguing that complying with a witness summons or other court order, and producing documents or other information, infringes this article.

Right to liberty

21–45 Article 5(1) confers the right to liberty, subject to six enumerated cases, and in all cases in accordance with a legally prescribed procedure.[244] The second case is that of lawful arrest or detention of a person (i) for non-compliance with a lawful order of the court or (ii) in order to secure the fulfilment of any obligation prescribed by law.[245] As to (i), this has been held to justify detention for (inter alia) failure to pay a fine,[246] or refusal to undergo a court-ordered blood test[247] or medical examination.[248] The alternative limb (ii) only justifies detention to secure the fulfilment of the obligation, not to punish the offender.[249] It has been held in particular to justify detention to secure the provision of information and documentation at border controls.[250]

---

[239] *Weber v Switzerland* (1990) 12 E.H.R.R. 508.
[240] *Treasury v Ahmed* [2010] 2 A.C. 697.
[241] *Companies W, X, Y, Z v Austria* (1976) 7 D.R. 148, ECtHR; *Borghini v Italy* Unreported November 29, 1995, ECtHR.
[242] *Schmidt v Germany* (1994) 18 E.H.R.R. 513 at [22].
[243] *X v Germany* (1984) 39 D.R. 90, ECtHR.
[244] See also art.5(2)–(4), setting out procedural safeguards.
[245] Article 5(1)(b).
[246] *Airey v Ireland* (1977) 8 D.R. 42.
[247] *X v Austria* (1979) 18 D.R. 154.
[248] *X v Germany* (1975) 3 D.R. 92.
[249] *Engel v Netherlands* (1979) 1 E.H.R.R. 647; *Johansen v Norway* (1985) 44 D.R. 155; see also *Benham v UK* (1996) 22 E.H.R.R. 293.
[250] *McVeigh, O'Neill and Evans v UK* (1981) 25 D.R. 15.

Prohibition of discrimination

Article 14 prohibits discrimination, but only "in the enjoyment of the rights and   **21–46**
freedoms" set out in the Convention (and Protocols). So it is not a "free-standing"
guarantee of equal treatment. A claim cannot be made unless the case falls within
one of the articles conferring substantive rights.[251] So a breach of the art.2
procedural obligation would not also breach art.14 unless the state failed to take
steps to investigate whether discrimination played a part in the events leading to an
unjustified killing by state agents.[252] Article 14 refers to "property", but it is not
clear whether discrimination on financial grounds is covered.[253] The article does
not convert what would otherwise be a lawful investigation into an unlawful one
by reason of the disability of a detained psychiatric patient.[254]

A difference in treatment is discriminatory unless it has an "objective and   **21–47**
reasonable justification",[255] which means showing the pursuit of a "legitimate aim"
and proportionality.[256] In one case, brought by Muslim residents of the UK who
wished to bury their dead in their country of origin (Iran, Bangladesh and
Pakistan), it was held that there was no discrimination within the article where
social security regulations provided for funeral expenses to be paid in certain cases
where the funeral was to take place in the UK (where facilities for Muslim burial
were available), but not where it was to take place elsewhere (with certain
exceptions for the EU).[257]

---

[251] *Botta v Italy* (1998) 26 E.H.R.R. 241 at [39]–[40].
[252] *Nachova v Bulgaria* , App. nos 43577/98 and 43579/98 (ECtHR, July 6, 2005).
[253] See *Airey v Ireland* (1979) 2 E.H.R.R. 305 at [30]; *Johnstone v Ireland* (1987) 9 E.H.R.R. 203.
[254] *R. (Antoniou) v Central and North West London NHS Foundation Trust* [2013] EWHC 3055 (Admin.)
at [105], DC.
[255] *Belgian Linguistic Case (No. 2)* (1979) 1 E.H.R.R. 252 at [32].
[256] *Darby v Sweden* (1991) 13 E.H.R.R. 774 at [31]; *Petrovic v Austria* (1998) 5 B.H.R.C. 232 at
[30].
[257] *Esfandieri v Secretary of State for Work and Pensions* [2006] EWCA Civ. 282.

Chapter 22

COMPARATIVE DEATH INQUIRY LAW

INTRODUCTION

It has been said, of the legal institution of the trust, that half the world (the   **22–01**
common law part) considers it essential for everyday life, while the other half is
unaware of its existence. In the same way, the coroner is peculiarly a product of the
common law. Most countries in the common law tradition have a coroner system,
or something resembling it, investigating many (or all) kinds of unnatural death,
even if no crime is involved. However those in the civil law tradition do not, and
death inquiries are carried out (if at all) largely as a part of the investigation of
crime. Secondly, the coroner's inquiry is, in principle, a public affair, in that the
evidence is presented before a public court. But as a rule in the civil law systems
the inquiry is private, although the *conclusions* may be published.

The purpose of this chapter is to provide a broad review of death inquiry systems   **22–02**
in some common law and civil law systems. Not every important country is
represented, and it is not exhaustive in its treatment of those that are. It is designed
to show that, even within the common law group or the civil law group, there are
significant differences from one to another, in addition to the more obvious
differences between the two groups. It is hoped that the survey will assist those in
England and Wales (coroners and others) who have to deal with the results of death
inquiries that have taken place abroad, particularly when an inquest thereafter
follows in this country.[1]

COMMON LAW SYSTEMS

The Republic of Ireland[2]

The coroner system was introduced into Ireland from England at an early date   **22–03**
(probably the thirteenth century), and was adapted and modified over the
following countries in a similar (though not identical) way to England.[3] The office
was a local one, elected locally. The legislation basis was similar to that in England.[4]

---

[1] See 5–87 ff.
[2] Farrell, *Coroners: Practice and Procedure* (2000; new edition expected December 2014); see also
O'Connor, *Handbook for Coroners in the Republic of Ireland* (1997).
[3] Farrell, *Coroners: Practice and Procedure* (2000), Ch.1.
[4] Coroners (Ireland) Act 1846.

But no professional qualifications were required, until specific legislation for Dublin so required in 1876, stipulating for a doctor or lawyer. The same rule for the rest of the country followed suit five years later.[5] Election to office became appointment by local authorities in 1898,[6] and deputies possible nationwide in 1908.[7] Further reforms were made in 1927,[8] including the introduction of an equivalent procedure to "Form B", and compulsory adjournment in homicide cases, as in England.

22–04 The whole system was reformed and consolidated in 1962, in a law which is still in force today.[9] There are coroners' rules dealing with fees and with forms, but none regulating practice and procedure more generally. Inquests are required where the coroner is of the opinion that a deceased may have died violently or unnaturally, or suddenly and from unknown causes, or in a place or circumstances requiring an inquest under another legislative provision.[10] Inquests may also be held in cases where a medical certificate of the cause of death is not procurable.[11] The Attorney General may direct a coroner to hold an inquest in certain circumstances.[12]

22–05 A coroner has power to direct a post-mortem examination to be carried out, and may request a special examination of parts or contents of the body.[13] An inquest may be dispensed with in the case of sudden death from unknown causes, if a post-mortem examination shows it is unnecessary.[14] Questions of civil or criminal liability are not to be investigated at an inquest,[15] and neither are verdicts or riders to verdicts to censure or exonerate anyone,[16] but general recommendations to prevent further fatalities are possible.[17] A jury is compulsory in cases of homicide, death in prison, notifiable accident, poisoning or disease, and death in circumstances prejudicial to public health or safety, but is otherwise optional.[18]

22–06 In some cases fairness will require that the family be provided with advance disclosure of depositions of intended witnesses,[19] though not copies of other unused material.[20] The coroner may conduct the inquest in the manner which he best thinks appropriate to serve the public interest, provided he complies with the statute and the rules of natural justice.[21] Coroners enjoy privilege in respect of what

---

[5] Coroners (Dublin) Act 1876 s.2.
[6] Local Government (Ireland) 1898 s.14(1).
[7] Coroners Act 1908 (1876 in Dublin).
[8] Coroners (Amendment) Act 1927.
[9] Coroners Act 1962, as amended by the Coroners (Amendment) Act 2005 and the Courts and Civil Law (Miscellaneous Provisions) Act 2013.
[10] Coroners Act 1962 s.17; this last phrase will cover (inter alia) prison deaths.
[11] Coroners Act 1962 s.18.
[12] Coroners Act 1962 s.24; *Farrell v Attorney General* [1997] I.E.H.C. 20.
[13] Coroners Act 1962 s.33; see *Hanley v Cusack* [1999] I.E.H.C. 6; *Bingham v Farrell* [2010] I.E.H.C. 74, and cf. *Callanan v Geraghty* [2007] I.E.H.C. 419.
[14] Coroners Act 1962 s.19.
[15] Coroners Act 1962 s.30; *Northern Area Health Board v Geraghty* [2001] I.E.H.C. 109; *Eastern Health Board v Farrell* [2001] I.E.S.C. 96; *Grant v Roche Products (Ireland) Ltd* [2008] I.E.S.C. 35.
[16] Coroners Act 1962 s.31(1).
[17] Coroners Act 1962 s.31(2)
[18] Coroners Act 1962 s.40(1)
[19] *Ramseyer v Mahon* [2005] I.E.S.C. 82; cf. *Northern Area Health Board v Geraghty* [2001] I.E.H.C. 109.
[20] *Morris v Farrell* [2004] I.E.H.C. 127.
[21] *Morris v Dublin City Coroner* [2000] I.E.S.C. 24.

they may say at the inquest.[22] There is no prescribed list of "verdicts" (i.e. conclusions as to death). But it is suggested that the verdicts available are similar to those in England and Wales,[23] with the notable exception of lack of care/neglect.[24]

Judicial review is available in relation to all coronial decisions.[25] Decisions   **22–07**
quashed include a refusal to adjourn to obtain medical records from abroad.[26] Decisions challenged unsuccessfully include a refusal to call other witnesses,[27] and a conclusion of death from misadventure where there was evidence of cannabis use.[28] The European Convention on Human Rights applies as much to the Republic of Ireland as to the other Council of Europe Member States, and the Convention rights are justiciable before the local courts by virtue of Irish legislation.[29] In addition, the Irish constitution guarantees the right to life.[30]

In late 2000 the report of a government Working Group, *Review of the Coroner*   **22–08**
Service, was published.[31] It recommended a number of important changes, including central government appointment of coroners, the production of a set of coroners' rules,[32] and making a jury no longer compulsory in road traffic cases. A bill to reform the system completely, introducing a national coroner service headed by a Chief Coroner, was introduced in April 2007, and progressed to committee stage in October 2007 before lapsing. The 1962 system therefore continues in force although, by a reform in 2013, legal aid has now been provided for certain inquests, where the deceased died in the custody or care of the state.[33]

Northern Ireland[34]

Ireland, north and south, was a single jurisdiction until partition in 1922. Hence   **22–09**
the 1926 reforms in England, largely mirrored in the Republic in 1927, were not taken up in the north, although in 1955 a limitation on the need for a jury was introduced.[35] Henceforward jury cases were the same four as in the Republic, *plus* the case of death from a road traffic accident (i.e. the same five compulsory cases as in England and Wales at the time).[36] A significant overhaul of the system took

---

[22] *Desmond v Riordan* [1999] I.E.H.C. 237.

[23] Farrell, *Coroners: Practice and Procedure,* 347–357.

[24] Farrell, *Coroners: Practice and Procedure*, 358 (where it is suggested that such a verdict is not available in Ireland).

[25] Farrell, *Coroners: Practice and Procedure*, Ch.18.

[26] *Lawlor v Geraghty* [2010] I.E.H.C. 168.

[27] *Bingham v Farrell* [2010] I.E.H.C. 74.

[28] *Byrne v Geraghty* [2010] I.E.H.C. 154.

[29] European Convention on Human Rights Act 2003; see Ch.21.

[30] Irish Constitution 1937 art.40. See *Morris v Farrell* [2004] I.E.H.C. 127; *Magee v Farrell* [2009] I.E.S.C. 60; *Grant v Roche Products (Ireland) Ltd* [2008] I.E.S.C. 35.

[31] See *http://www.justice.ie/en/JELR/ReviewCoronerService.pdf/Files/ReviewCoronerService.pdf* [Accessed June 17, 2014].

[32] See the Report of the Coroners Rules Committee, 2003, at *http://www.justice.ie/en/JELR/coronersfulljob.pdf/Files/coronersfulljob.pdf* [Accessed June 17, 2014].

[33] Courts and Civil Law (Miscellaneous Provisions) Act 2013 ss.24–25. cf. *Magee v Farrell* [2009] I.E.S.C. 60 (no constitutional or ECHR right to legal aid at inquest into death in custody).

[34] Leckey and Greer, *Coroners' Law and Practice in Northern Ireland* (1998).

[35] Coroners (Amendment) Act (Northern Ireland) 1955 s.1.

[36] A sixth case, suicide, was added by the Criminal Justice Act (N.I.) 1966 s.13(4).

place in 1959, when the principal law still in force today was enacted.[37] A curiosity
is that this law implemented a number of recommendations of the Report of the
(English) Departmental Committee on Coroners, chaired by Lord Wright, in
1936,[38] which had not up to then been implemented for England and Wales. The
European Convention on Human Rights applies as much to Northern Ireland as
to the rest of the United Kingdom, and the Convention rights are justiciable before
the local courts by virtue of the same United Kingdom legislation.[39]

22–10   Coroners since 1959 have been required to have a *legal* qualification for
appointment: doctors are not as such qualified.[40] The coroner service ceased to be
run locally, by local authorities, and became a service of central government,
initially under the Ministry of Home Affairs and later the Lord Chancellor's
Department. In 2006 the seven districts (six part-time, and one full-time) were
amalgamated into one,[41] centred on Belfast, and the system was reorganised. The
Coroners Service for Northern Ireland now comprises a High Court judge,
appointed as Presiding Judge and Coroner,[42] a senior coroner and two further (full-
time) coroners, a solicitor and a medical adviser, as well as administrative staff. Since
2010 it is the Northern Ireland Judicial Appointments Commission that makes
appointments, rather than the Lord Chancellor.[43] Northern Irish coroners do not
have coroners' officers, unlike in England and Wales, though there are now
"coroners' liaison officers", to deal directly with the bereaved family.

22–11   A duty to inform the coroner of reason to believe that a person died as a result
of violence, misadventure, unfair means, negligence, misconduct, malpractice, or
any non-natural cause is imposed on doctors, registrars, undertakers, occupiers of
homes and persons in charge of any institution where the deceased was residing.[44]
A further duty is imposed on the police to inform the coroner of a dead body, of
an unexpected or unexplained death or one attended by suspicious circumstances.[45]

22–12   In principle the presence of the body founds jurisdiction to inquire,[46] and the
coroner *may* if he thinks fit hold an inquest,[47] notifying the family[48] and persons
whose conduct may be called into question at the inquest.[49] But the coroner may
decide that there is no need to hold an inquest, and simply issue authority to

---

[37] Coroners Act (Northern Ireland) 1959, supplemented by the Coroners (Practice and Procedure) Rules (Northern Ireland) 1963.

[38] Cmd. 5070.

[39] Human Rights Act 1998; see Ch.21.

[40] Coroners Act (Northern Ireland) 1959 s.2(3).

[41] Under Coroners Act (Northern Ireland) 1959 s.3.

[42] The Legal Aid and Coroners Bill (expected to become law later in 2014) provides for the Lord Chief Justice to become titular President of coroners' courts.

[43] Coroners Act (Northern Ireland) 1959 s.2(1), as amended by the Northern Ireland Act 2009 Sch.4 para.2(2).

[44] Coroners Act (Northern Ireland) 1959 s.7. The governor of a prison is obliged under separate legislation to notify the coroner of a death in the prison and give certain other information.

[45] Coroners Act (Northern Ireland) 1959 s.8.

[46] This is subject to ss.15 (inquest without exhuming body) and 16 (inquest where body cannot be found). As to s.15, see *Re Howard's Application* [2011] N.I.Q.B. 125.

[47] Coroners Act (Northern Ireland) 1959 s.13. As to the need for promptness, see the Coroners (Practice and Procedure) Rules (Northern Ireland) 1963 r.3.

[48] *Re Price's Application* [1986] N.I. 390.

[49] Coroners (Practice and Procedure) Rules (Northern Ireland) 1963 r.10.

bury.[50] On the other hand, in order to be able to decide whether an inquest is necessary, the coroner may take possession of the body[51] and deposit it in a convenient mortuary or other suitable place.[52] He may direct a post-mortem examination,[53] but if as a result he is satisfied that it is unnecessary to hold an inquest, he certifies the cause of death, and the inquiry comes to an end.[54] But the coroner *must* hold an inquest into the death of a prisoner.[55]

If the coroner does not hold an inquest, the Attorney General for Northern **22–13** Ireland may direct a coroner to do so, if he has reason to believe that the deceased died in circumstances which in his opinion make it advisable to do so.[56] But in certain circumstances involving national security, the function of the Attorney General is carried out by (in effect) the Attorney General for England and Wales.[57] Unlike the position in England and Wales, in the Northern Irish legislation the definition of "deceased person" includes a fetus *in utero* then capable of being born alive.[58] However, there is no jurisdiction to inquire, and the Attorney General may not direct an inquest, where the deceased dies abroad and the body is returned to Northern Ireland.[59]

The proceedings and evidence at an inquest are directed solely to ascertaining **22–14** who the deceased was, how, when and where he came by his death, and the registration particulars.[60] The expression of any opinion on any other matter or on questions of criminal or civil liability is forbidden.[61] The coroner has the power to summon witnesses to give evidence.[62] "Properly interested persons" (not defined) may examine witnesses.[63] Juries are required in only three cases: death in prison, death caused by accident, poisoning or disease notifiable to the government or health and safety inspector, and death in circumstances prejudicial to public health and safety.[64] Juries in homicide and road traffic cases were made non-mandatory in 1980.[65]

There has never been statutory provision for "conclusions as to death" in **22–15** Northern Ireland inquests, but a short list of possible conclusions was included in

---

[50] Coroners Act (Northern Ireland) 1959 s.24.
[51] Coroners Act (Northern Ireland) 1959 s.11; *Re Millar's Application* [2005] N.I.Q.B. 34 (power of investigation may be exercised again if new material arises). The coroner may order exhumation for this purpose: s.11(4).
[52] Coroners Act (Northern Ireland) 1959 s.12.
[53] Usually one of the pathologists on the staff of the State Pathologist's Department. As to procedure, see the Coroners (Practice and Procedure) Rules (Northern Ireland) 1963 rr.25-31, and, as to the report of the examination, see rr.37-38.
[54] Coroners Act (Northern Ireland) 1959 s.28.
[55] Prisons Act (NI) 1953 s.39(2).
[56] Coroners Act (Northern Ireland) 1959 s.14.
[57] Coroners Act (Northern Ireland) 1959 s.14(2), (3) (as amended in 2010).
[58] *Attorney General for Northern Ireland v Senior Coroner for Northern Ireland* [2013] N.I.C.A. 68.
[59] *Re Forde's Application* [2008] N.I.Q.B. 40.
[60] Coroners (Practice and Procedure) Rules (Northern Ireland) 1963 r.15. See *Re Ramsbottom's Application* [2009] N.I.Q.B. 55; *Re JR 29's Application* [2009] N.I.Q.B. 97.
[61] Coroners (Practice and Procedure) Rules (Northern Ireland) 1963 r.16.
[62] Coroners Act (Northern Ireland) 1959 s.17. See also Coroners (Practice and Procedure) Rules (Northern Ireland) 1963 r.8. Witnesses are entitled to the privilege against self-incrimination: r.9. The Coroners and Justice Act 2009 s.49 and Sch.11, contains prospective changes to the rules governing the summoning of witnesses.
[63] Coroners (Practice and Procedure) Rules (Northern Ireland) 1963 r.7.
[64] Coroners Act (Northern Ireland) 1959 s.18(1).
[65] Criminal Justice (N.I.) Order 1980 art.13 and Sch.1.

a note to the prescribed form of inquisition,[66] and these were generally followed. However, in 1980 a recommendation of the Brodrick Report[67] (never implemented in England and Wales),[68] to the effect that "conclusions as to death" suggested attribution of responsibility and should be replaced by "Findings",[69] was implemented,[70] apparently without much discussion.[71] Since then inquests have had to produce factual "findings" only.[72] The consequent absence of an opportunity for the jury to return "unlawful killing"—particularly in the context of the sectarian strife there—has been vigorously attacked, but has so far survived a human rights challenge.[73] The coroner may report matters to a person who may have the power to take action to prevent future deaths,[74] but there is no power to make recommendations.

New Zealand

22–16   The coroner system was brought to New Zealand in about 1840. Historical material relating to coroner's inquests is held by Archives New Zealand.[75] The first coroners' legislation was enacted in 1846, giving coroners the same powers and duties as they had under English law.[76] From 1858[77] until 1951[78] coroners had jurisdiction to inquire into non-fatal fires. But the primary role was to investigate homicide, drowning, sudden death, and death in prison or lunatic asylum.[79] Inquests had to be held with a jury.[80] In 1908 the rule that the inquest verdict of homicide had the effect of an indictment for the offence was abolished,[81] as also was the requirement to hold inquests with a jury.[82]

22–17   The whole law of coroners was reformed and consolidated in 1951,[83] and it was reformed again in 1988.[84] However, a completely new system was put in place in 2006 to apply to all deaths from July 1, 2007.[85] Instead of over 70 coroners (nearly

---

[66] Coroners (Practice and Procedure) Rules (Northern Ireland) 1963 Sch.3, Form 22 (original version).

[67] See para.1–04, fn.9.

[68] The Coroners and Justice Act 2009 refers to "determination and findings", but the findings are only as to the particulars required for the registration of the death: s.10(1)(b); see 13–01.

[69] Brodrick Report, paras 16.40, 16.43.

[70] Coroners (Practice and Procedure) (Amendment) Rules (N.I.) 1980 (SI 1980/444).

[71] See Leckey and Greer, *Coroners' Law and Practice in Northern Ireland*, para.11–04.

[72] *Re Bradley and Larkin's Application* Unreported April 7, 1995, HC (NI), Carswell LJ; see also *R. v North Humberside Coroner Ex p. Jamieson* [1995] Q.B. 1 at 24 (Conclusion (6)), CA.

[73] *Re Jordan's Application* [2002] N.I.Q.B. 7; *Re Jordan's Application* [2002] N.I.Q.B. 19; see 21–19 above.

[74] Coroners (Practice and Procedure) Rules (Northern Ireland) 1963 r.23.

[75] See *http://archives.govt.nz/*

[76] Coroners Ordinance 1846 s.4.

[77] Coroners Act 1858 s.7.

[78] Coroners Act 1951.

[79] Coroners Act 1867 s.8.

[80] Coroners Act 1867 s.10.

[81] Coroners Act 1908.

[82] Coroners Amendment Act 1908 s.2.

[83] Coroners Act 1951.

[84] Coroners Act 1988.

[85] Coroners Act 2006, supplemented by various secondary legislation, including the Coroners (Forms) Regulations 2008.

all part-time, and mainly lawyers), there are now 16,[86] all full-time[87] and all lawyers,[88] and headed for the first time by a Chief Coroner, a serving judge.[89]

The purpose of the new legislation is expressly stated as being to help prevent **22–18** deaths and to promote justice, through carrying out investigations and making recommendations.[90] The coroner's role is to receive death reports, to direct autopsies and release the body where and when appropriate, to decide whether to open an inquiry (for the purposes of (i) establishing a death, the identity of the deceased and the causes and circumstances of the death, (ii) making recommendations or comments to prevent future deaths, and (iii) determining whether other agencies should investigate the death),[91] opening and conducting such inquiries, giving family members and others notice of significant matters in relation to the processes required to be performed.[92]

Reports of certain deaths must be made by anyone becoming aware of them to **22–19** the police,[93] who will report them to the coroner.[94] In practice the report is to the National Initial Investigation Office, supporting the National Duty Coroner (designated under a rota system). The deaths to be reported are those apparently without known cause, or which are suicides or otherwise violent and unnatural, or for which no doctor has given a certificate, or occurring during medical, surgical or dental treatment, or apparently as a result of pregnancy or giving birth, or in official custody or care (including police, corrective, mental health or social services, and whether in the institution concerned or not).[95]

The exclusive right to custody of the body is first in the police,[96] and then in the **22–20** designated coroner,[97] who can give directions for removal.[98] The National Duty Coroner makes initial decisions, including those on autopsy. The coroner must give notice to the family[99] of certain significant matters,[100] and must supply them with a copy of any autopsy report.[101] Certain documents in a case are in effect publicly available,[102] although sometimes with appropriate consent.[103] A coroner may direct (and the High Court may order)[104] a post-mortem examination,[105] in accordance with certain criteria,[106] although in some circumstances the immediate

---

[86] Coroners Act 2006 s.109(1) (maximum 20).
[87] Coroners Act 2006 s.108.
[88] Coroners Act 2006 s.103(2).
[89] Coroners Act 2006 s.105.
[90] Coroners Act 2006 s.3(1).
[91] Coroners Act 2006 s.4(2).
[92] Coroners Act 2006 s.4(1).
[93] Coroners Act 2006 s.14.
[94] Coroners Act 2006 s.15.
[95] Coroners Act 2006 s.13.
[96] Coroners Act 2006 s.18.
[97] Coroners Act 2006 s.19.
[98] Coroners Act 2006 s.20. See also ss.128-130 (District Court warrant to back up coroner's direction).
[99] Coroners Act 2006 s.23.
[100] Coroners Act 2006 s.24.
[101] Coroners Act 2006 s.27.
[102] Coroners Act 2006 s.28.
[103] Coroners Act 2006 s.29.
[104] Coroners Act 2006 s.41.
[105] Coroners Act 2006 ss.31, 36-39.
[106] Coroners Act 2006 s.32.

family may object,[107] with a procedure in the High Court for dealing with such objections.[108] Subject to certain restrictions on the release of bodies[109] or body parts,[110] the coroner must release the body once satisfied that it is no longer necessary to be withheld from the family.[111] If the case is taken, it is then allocated for investigation to a coroner under the oversight of the Chief Coroner.

22–21   As now in England and Wales, there is a difference between an inquiry and an inquest. The coroner may open an inquiry into a reported death as long as the body is in New Zealand, or was so but is now destroyed, irrecoverable or lost, or (but in this case only with the Solicitor-General's authority) the death occurred on a ship or aeroplane.[112] The coroner must do so in cases of apparent suicide or death in official custody or care,[113] but may decide not to do so in other cases.[114] The inquiry may be postponed or adjourned in certain cases of criminal proceedings[115] or other investigation,[116] and need not be opened or resumed in some circumstances.[117] The coroner has various powers to obtain information for the inquiry,[118] which can be supported by a District Court warrant to enter and search premises in some cases.[119] Information so obtained may only be used for the purposes of the inquiry.[120]

22–22   The inquiry may in some cases be held on the papers.[121] If there is a hearing, choice of witnesses (including experts) at the inquiry is for the coroner,[122] and the ordinary rules of evidence do not apply,[123] although witnesses and counsel have the same privileges and immunities as in courts of law.[124] As part of the inquiry, there must be an inquest if the death appears to be one in official custody or care, and may be an inquest in any other case.[125] The coroner must give notice of the inquest.[126] He or she may sit with advisers,[127] but usually sits alone.[128] Inquests into deaths arising out of the same incident may be held jointly. Inquests are generally held in public,[129] and witnesses who give evidence (whether orally[130] or by written

---

[107] Coroners Act 2006 ss.33-34.
[108] Coroners Act 2006 s.35.
[109] Coroners Act 2006 s.43.
[110] Coroners Act 2006 ss.44, 48-56.
[111] Coroners Act 2006 s.42.
[112] Coroners Act 2006 s.59.
[113] Coroners Act 2006 s.60.
[114] Coroners Act 2006 ss.61-63. The decision may be changed later to open an inquiry: s.65.
[115] Coroners Act 2006 s.68.
[116] Coroners Act 2006 s.69.
[117] Coroners Act 2006 s.70.
[118] Coroners Act 2006 ss.120-121. See also s.131 (police power to seize relevant evidence).
[119] Coroners Act 2006 ss.122-126.
[120] Coroners Act 2006 s.127.
[121] Coroners Act 2006 s.77.
[122] Coroners Act 2006 s.76.
[123] Coroners Act 2006 s.79.
[124] Coroners Act 2006 s.78.
[125] Coroners Act 2006 s.80.
[126] Coroners Act 2006 s.81.
[127] Coroners Act 2006 s.83.
[128] Coroners Act 2006 s.82.
[129] Coroners Act 2006 s.85, but see ss.74 (power to prohibit publication of evidence) and 86-87 (power to exclude certain persons).
[130] Coroners Act 2006 s.88(a).

statement)[131] may be cross-examined.[132] Evidence may be taken at a distance where necessary.[133] A coroner must prepare interim findings and reasons for them, and make them publicly available,[134] before completing the certificate of findings[135] (which supersedes the interim findings).[136] These too are publicly available.[137]

The Solicitor-General and the High Court have various powers to order[138]   **22–23**
inquiries and further inquiries in certain cases, for example in case of failure to inquire,[139] or where an inquiry was defective[140] or new facts are discovered,[141] and the coroner must inquire accordingly.[142] The New Zealand Law Commission has recently produced a paper dealing with burial and cremation.[143]

Australia[144]

Each Australian state and territory has its own coroner system, or (in the case of   **22–24**
smaller territories) is linked to another state's coroner system.[145] Although every system is slightly different from the others, the common functions are to determine the identity of the deceased, when and where he died, the cause of death and how it occurred.[146] In all systems there is provision for recommendations to be made to avoid future fatalities.[147] Almost all jurisdictions provide for investigation of non-fatal fires, and some for other non-fatal accidents.[148] There are important differences between the systems in relation to criminal procedure. Some stop the coronial inquiry altogether once criminal charges relating to the death have been made. Others postpone the inquiry, but still proceed to an ultimate conclusion.

Nearly all states now have a "State Coroner" (or Chief Coroner) system, in   **22–25**
which a senior coroner co-ordinates and oversees the activities of several local

---

[131] Coroners Act 2006 s.90(1).
[132] Coroners Act 2006 ss.88–90.
[133] Coroners Act 2006 s.91.
[134] Coroners Act 2006 s.93(3), referring back to s.28(1)(c).
[135] Coroners Act 2006 s.94.
[136] Coroners Act 2006 s.94(3).
[137] Coroners Act 2006 s.94(4), referring back to s.28(1)(c).
[138] See Coroners Act 2006 ss.98–100.
[139] Coroners Act 2006 s.95.
[140] Coroners Act 2006 s.97.
[141] Coroners Act 2006 s.96.
[142] Coroners Act 2006 s.101; see also s.102 (procedure at ordered inquiries).
[143] *The Legal Framework for Burial and Cremation in New Zealand,* Issues Paper, October 2013.
[144] *Waller's Coronial Law in New South Wales,* 4th edn (2010); Malbon, *Review of Queensland Coronial Laws* (1997); Selby (ed.), *The Inquest Handbook* (1998); Freckleton and Ranson, *Death Investigation and the Coroner's Inquest* (2006).
[145] The main legislation includes: Coroners Act 1993 (NT), Coroners Act 1995 (TAS), Coroners Act 1996 (WA), Coroners Act 1997 (ACT), Coroners Act 2003 (QLD), Coroners Act 2003 (SA), Coroners Act 2008 (VIC), Coroners Act 2009 (NSW).
[146] Coroners Act 1993 (NT) ss.3, 34(1)(a); Coroners Act 1995 (TAS) ss.3, 28(1); Coroners Act 1996 (WA) ss.3, 25(1); Coroners Act 1997 (ACT) s.52(1); Coroners Act 2003 (QLD) s.45(2); Coroners Act 2003 (SA) s.25(1); Coroners Act 2008 (VIC) s.67; Coroners Act 2009 (NSW) s.81(1).
[147] Coroners Act 1993 (NT) ss.26, 34(2), 35(2); Coroners Act 1995 (TAS) ss.28(2), (3), 30(2); Coroners Act 1996 (WA) ss.25(2), (3), 27(3); Coroners Act 1997 (ACT) s.52(4), 57(3); Coroners Act 2003 (QLD) ss.46–47; Coroners Act 2003 (SA) s.25(2), (4); Coroners Act 2008 (VIC) ss.67(3), 72; Coroners Act 2009 (NSW) s.82.
[148] Coroners Act 1993 (NT) s.34(1)(b), Coroners Act 1995 (TAS) s.45(1), Coroners Act 1997 (ACT) s.52(2), Coroners Act 2003 (SA) s.25(1), Coroners Act 2008 (VIC) ss.30-31, Coroners Act 2009 (NSW) ss.30-32.

coroners. There is a national computer database, called the National Coroners Information system (NCIS), which has transformed the way in which information on deaths in Australia is managed. Generally speaking, the coroner will investigate all violent deaths, sudden deaths of unknown cause, and deaths in prison or residential institutions. Some states' systems require the coroner to state the identity of any person who contributed to the death. All of them except one, however, prohibit findings of criminal liability,[149] and some prohibit findings of civil liability too.[150] Coronial decisions are subject to review by the superior courts, though the powers vary from state to state.

The United States of America[151]

22–26   Coroners and their inquests were exported to America with the rest of the common law by the original British colonists. It is said that William Penn appointed the first coroner in the American colonies. Coroners still exist in many parts of the USA, including areas which were never colonised by the British at all, but only became part of the Union after independence. These include Ohio (introduced 1788) and even Louisiana, for example, where the legal system is not based on the English common law, but is largely civilian (based on French law). The range of deaths investigated was similar to that in England.

22–27   But in some areas the coroner system fell into disrepute, partly because it was an elective office, and partly because coroners did not need any qualifications, legal or medical (and in some places this is still the case). So in Massachusetts in 1877 it was abolished, to be replaced by a system of medical examiners (usually known by the initials "ME"). Unlike coroners, they were medically qualified, though not necessarily pathologists. Other populated areas followed, such as New York (where the coroner system was reckoned to be corrupt) from 1918.[152]

22–28   Each state has its own system, some more than one. So today the USA operates a range of different systems, operating from 2,342 offices in 2004.[153] These include (i) coroners appointed or (more often) elected on a county basis, (ii) medical examiners appointed in a statewide system, (iii) medical examiners appointed on a county basis, and (iv) mixed coroner and medical examiner systems. The county coroner systems (about 80 per cent of the total number of jurisdictions in 2004) are usually found in more rural and smaller population areas, and the medical examiners in more urban and larger population areas. At least since 1928 there have

---

[149] Coroners Act 1993 (NT) s.34(3), Coroners Act 1995 (TAS) s.28(4), Coroners Act 1996 (WA) s.25(5), Coroners Act 2003 (QLD) s.45(5), Coroners Act 2003 (SA) s.25(3), Coroners Act 2008 (VIC) s.69, Coroners Act 2009 (NSW) ss.81(3), 82(3). The exception is the Coroners Act 1997 (ACT), though s.55 of the Act requires the coroner to give advance notice to a person identifiable in the draft findings of a finding adverse to that person (there is a similar provision in Coroners Act 1996 (WA) s.44(2). See *Lucas-Smith v Coroner's Court of the ACT* [2009] ACTSC 40.

[150] Coroners Act 1996 (WA) s.25(5), Coroners Act 2003 (QLD) ss.45(5), 46(3), Coroners Act 2003 (SA) s.25(3).

[151] Jentzen, *Death Investigation in America* (2009).

[152] See, e.g. Milton Helpern, *Autopsy*, Ch.1, and Michael Baden, *Unnatural Death* (1989), Ch.4; "Medical Examiner and Coroner Systems: Current and Future Needs", Ch.9 in National Research Council of the National Academies, *Strengthening Forensic Science in the United States: A Path Forward* (August 2009), 241–242.

[153] "Medical Examiner and Coroner Systems: Current and Future Needs", Ch.9 in National Research Council of the National Academies, *Strengthening Forensic Science in the United States: A Path Forward* (August 2009), 243, 245.

been proposals to move towards a universal system of publicly funded medical examiners.[154]

Coroners (where they still exist) are not necessarily lawyers or doctors; there is   **22–29** usually no professional requirement.[155] Very often they oversee the service, but appoint professional deputies to carry out their functions. Medical examiners, on the other hand, are invariably medical practitioners, usually specialists in forensic pathology.[156] They carry out similar functions to coroners, except that they are competent to (and often do) carry out post-mortem examinations themselves, but they do not hold or preside over public inquests. There is usually a file on a deceased, which contains the findings of the medical examiner and the results of his various inquiries. There is a National Association of Medical Examiners ("NAME"), and also in states which still have coroners there are coroners' associations, such as in California, in Washington and in Ohio. Many individual coroners have their own websites.

Canada[157]

Each of the Canadian provinces and territories has its own death investigation   **22–30** system. Some (including Quebec, a civil law system)[158] are coroner systems. On the other hand, Alberta, Manitoba, Prince Edward Island and Nova Scotia have medical examiners. Newfoundland has a system of judicial inquiry, a little like Scotland. Taking the Ontario system as typical of the coroners' systems, the office of coroner has been established since at least 1780. The inquisition ceased to have the effect of an indictment in 1892. Ontario operates a "Chief Coroner" system, in which the Chief Coroner supervises, directs and controls the other coroners in the performance of their duties.[159] There is a pyramidic structure, with regional coroners[160] below the Chief Coroner and above the investigating coroners.[161] All coroners must be medical practitioners.[162]

Deaths must be notified where the deceased is believed to have died as a result   **22–31** of violence, misadventure, negligence and the like, by "unfair means", during or as a result of pregnancy, suddenly and unexpectedly, from untreated disease, non-disease causes, or under other circumstances which may require investigation,[163] or

---

[154] "Medical Examiner and Coroner Systems: Current and Future Needs", Ch.9 in National Research Council of the National Academies, *Strengthening Forensic Science in the United States: A Path Forward* (August 2009), 242-243, 251-256.

[155] "Medical Examiner and Coroner Systems: Current and Future Needs", Ch.9 in National Research Council of the National Academies, *Strengthening Forensic Science in the United States: A Path Forward* (August 2009), 247.

[156] "Medical Examiner and Coroner Systems: Current and Future Needs", Ch.9 in National Research Council of the National Academies, *Strengthening Forensic Science in the United States: A Path Forward* (August 2009), 248-249.

[157] Granger, *Canadian Coroner Law* (1984); Ontario Law Reform Commission, *Report on the Law of Coroners* (1995); Marshall, *Canadian Law of Inquests*, 3rd edn (2009).

[158] See the *Loi sur la recherche des causes et des circonstances des décès*, chapitre R-0.2, and the *Code de déontologie des coroners*, made thereunder.

[159] RSO 1990 c.37 s.4; see the Chief Coroner's website at *http://www.mcscs.jus.gov.on.ca/english/DeathInvestigations/office coroner/coroner.html*.

[160] RSO 1990 c.37 s.5.

[161] RSO 1990 c.37 s.3.

[162] RSO 1990 c.37 s.3. This is not necessarily true of other provinces.

[163] RSO 1990 c.37 s.10(1).

died "in care"[164] or in custody,[165] or died as a result of an accident at work.[166] The coroner must take possession of the body, examine it and decide whether to hold an inquest.[167] There are a number of factors to consider,[168] including whether the five "facts" about the death are already known: who the deceased was, how, when, where and by what means the deceased came to his death.[169] In practice, coroners hold inquests in only a small percentage of cases referred to them, where the public interest makes this desirable. In investigating the matter, the coroner enjoys a number of powers, including entry, search and seizure,[170] and also directing a post-mortem examination.[171]

22–32   Only one case is mandatory for an inquest: where a child dies in specified statutory circumstances.[172] In other cases the coroner may decide that an inquest is unnecessary,[173] or (giving the Chief Coroner a summary of grounds for the decision) that it is.[174] A refusal to hold an inquest is subject to review by the Chief Coroner at the request of the family.[175] Every person who is substantially and directly interested in the inquest can on application be designated as having standing at the inquest, and may call and examine witnesses, present arguments and submissions, and cross-examine other witnesses at the inquest.[176] The strict rules of evidence do not apply at an inquest.[177] Every inquest is held with a jury of five persons,[178] deciding by a majority.[179] The jury may make recommendations directed to the avoidance of death in similar circumstances,[180] but may not make any finding of legal responsibility.[181] Witnesses may refuse to answer on the grounds of self-incrimination.[182]

Isle of Man

22–33   The English coroner system has also been transplanted to the Isle of Man. The Isle of Man (like the Channel Islands) has a curious constitutional relationship with the United Kingdom. The Queen is the head of state, and the UK government is responsible for external affairs, but the island has a separate legal system (the final court of appeal being the Judicial Committee of the Privy Council), and is self-

---

[164] RSO 1990 c.37 s.10(2), (2.1), (3).

[165] RSO 1990 c.37 s.10(4)-(4.8).

[166] RSO 1990 c.37 s.10(5).

[167] RSO 1990 c.37 s.15. In exceptional circumstances the coroner can continue to investigate without the body: s.15(5). But he cannot hold an inquest without the direction of the Chief Coroner: s.21.

[168] RSO 1990 c.37 s.20.

[169] RSO 1990 c.37 s.31(1).

[170] RSO 1990 c.37 s.16.

[171] RSO 1990 c.37 ss.28-29.

[172] RSO 1990 c.37 s.22.1

[173] RSO 1990 c.37 s.18.

[174] RSO 1990 c.37 s.19.

[175] RSO 1990 c.37 s.26.

[176] RSO 1990 c.37 s.41, though see s.50(2) (limitation on cross-examination).

[177] RSO 1990 c.37 s.44.

[178] RSO 1990 c.37 s.33(1). There are no juries in Quebec, but they remain in New Brunswick, Saskatchewan and British Columbia.

[179] RSO 1990 c.37 s.38.

[180] RSO 1990 c.37 s.31(3).

[181] RSO 1990 c.37 s.31(2).

[182] RSO 1990 c.37 s.42.

governing, with its own legislature, Tynwald. Under Manx law the term coroner is used to refer to an executive officer of the High Court (like "sheriff" or "bailiff", formerly used in England and Wales).[183] The official responsible for the investigation of death is called the "coroner of inquests". The current legislation on the subject dates from 1987.[184] Under this law the coroner of inquests is nominally the High Bailiff,[185] but the Governor may appoint deputy or acting coroners to carry out his statutory functions.[186]

Coroners of inquests must be notified of deaths believed to be the result of **22–34** violence, misadventure, unfair means, negligence and similar causes, non-natural causes, and other circumstances requiring investigation,[187] as well as deaths in public places, unexpected deaths of unknown cause, deaths in suspicious circumstances, in prison or police custody or as a result of police action.[188] The coroner investigates to decide whether to hold an inquest. An inquest must be held if the death is believed to have occurred as a result of violence, misadventure, unfair means, negligence, etc., or in prison or police custody or as a result of police action, or the Attorney General directs an inquest.[189] There is discretion to hold an inquest in the other cases.[190] Inquests into deaths in prison or police custody, or as a result of police action, must be held with a jury[191] of seven persons.[192] A jury may be summoned in any other case if the coroner considers it desirable to do so.[193]

The provisions of the law dealing with the proceedings at inquest[194] (including **22–35** the need for an inquisition to be completed, and what it must contain) and with adjournment and resumption because of criminal charges,[195] are based on, and virtually identical to, the equivalent former English provisions. Coroners also have jurisdiction to inquire into the finding of treasure trove.[196] The European Convention on Human Rights applies as much to the Isle of Man as to the United Kingdom, and the Convention rights are justiciable before the local courts by virtue of local legislation, modelled on that of the United Kingdom.[197]

Gibraltar

Captured from the Spanish in 1704, and ceded by Spain to Britain in 1713,[198] **22–36** Gibraltar is a British Overseas Territory, measuring about 6 square kilometres, and jutting out into the Mediterranean Sea where it meets the Atlantic Ocean. It has a local legislature and government, but its law and legal system are based heavily on

---

[183] See 2–;114.
[184] Coroners of Inquests Act 1987, supplemented by the Coroners of Inquests Rules 1998 (as amended), made under s.21.
[185] Coroners of Inquests Act 1987 s.1(1).
[186] Coroners of Inquests Act 1987 s.1(2).
[187] Coroners of Inquests Act 1987 s.2(1).
[188] Coroners of Inquests Act 1987 s.2(4).
[189] Coroners of Inquests Act 1987 s.6(1).
[190] Coroners of Inquests Act 1987 s.5(1).
[191] Coroners of Inquests Act 1987 s.8(1).
[192] Coroners of Inquests Act 1987 s.10(1).
[193] Coroners of Inquests Act 1987 s.8(1).
[194] Coroners of Inquests Act 1987 s.12 corresponding to s.11 of the (English) Coroners Act 1988.
[195] Coroners of Inquests Act 1987 s.13, corresponding to ss.16 and 17 of the 1988 Act.
[196] Coroners of Inquests Act 1987 s.18; see the Treasure Trove Act 1586.
[197] Human Rights Act 2001 (IOM); see Ch.21.
[198] Treaty of Utrecht, 1713.

English models. The Gibraltar Supreme Court has jurisdiction similar to that of the English High Court, there is a Court of Appeal, and further appeals lie to the Judicial Committee of the Privy Council. The law relating to death investigations is drawn from the legislation in force in England and Wales before 1988,[199] with some updating since. The Governor, on the advice of the Judicial Service Commission,[200] must appoint a "fit and proper person"[201] as coroner, and may appoint a deputy coroner,[202] who can act in his place in the event of the coroner's death, resignation, absence or incapacity from whatever cause.[203]

22–37 The coroner must inquire into the death of any person whose body is found in Gibraltar and there is reasonable cause to suspect a violent or unnatural death, or a sudden death of unknown cause or in prison or in such circumstances as to require one under another enactment.[204] The coroner also has jurisdiction to inquire into treasure trove.[205] If the coroner refuses to hold an inquest which ought to be held, the Supreme Court may order him to do so.[206] Where the body has been destroyed or is irrecoverable, out of Gibraltar, but the coroner has reason to believe that an inquest ought to be held, he can report the case to the minister for justice, who may direct him to hold an inquest.[207]

22–38 In the case of a suspected sudden death of unknown cause the coroner may direct a medical practitioner to carry out an autopsy,[208] and if the result shows that an inquest is unnecessary he can dispense with one.[209] In other cases, he has powers to direct an autopsy or special examination to be made and the medical practitioner or other person performing it to give evidence at the inquest.[210] The coroner has power to move bodies for the purposes of autopsies.[211]

22–39 Where a person has been charged with any of certain homicide offences involving the deceased, or with any of certain other offences committed in circumstances connected with the death of the deceased (but in this case only at the request of the Attorney General), the coroner must adjourn the inquest until after the conclusion of the criminal proceedings, in the absence of reason to the contrary.[212] After such conclusion, he may resume the inquest if there is sufficient

---

[199] Coroners Act 1887, as amended, in particular by the Coroners (Amendment) Act 1926, supplemented by the Coroner Rules LN 1980/027, which provide for the (English) Coroners Rules 1953 (except for r.26(c)) to apply so far as applicable, and with any necessary modifications. See the 9th edn (1957) and the 10th edn (1986) of this work.

[200] Judicial Service Act 2007 s.21, referring to s.2 and Sch.

[201] No other qualification is required.

[202] Coroner Act No. 1889-11 s.3(1). In practice the stipendiary magistrate is usually also appointed coroner.

[203] Coroner Act No. 1889-11 s.3(2).

[204] Coroner Act No. 1889-11 s.4(1). There is an exception for British naval personnel who die on board a Royal Navy ship in Gibraltar: s.13.

[205] Coroner Act No. 1889-11 s.24.

[206] Coroner Act No. 1889-11 s.12(1)(a).

[207] Coroner Act No. 1889-11 s.10.

[208] Coroner Act No. 1889-11 s.5(1).

[209] Coroner Act No. 1889-11 s.5(2).

[210] Coroner Act No. 1889-11 ss.17, 18. See also Coroner Rules, LN 1980/027 r.2, referring to Coroners Rules 1953 rr.2-10.

[211] Coroner Act No. 1889-11 s.20.

[212] Coroner Act No. 1889-11 s.11(1). There are further provisions for adjournment at police request in Coroner Rules, LN 1980/027 r.2, referring to Coroners Rules 1953 r.22.

cause to do so,[213] but the finding of the inquest as to the cause of death must not be inconsistent with that conclusion.[214]

The coroner must view the body, and the jury (if there is one) may do so.[215] **22–40**
Once the coroner has decided to hold an inquest,[216] and has viewed the body,[217] he may authorise the burial of the body. At the inquest (which must be held in public)[218] the proceedings and evidence are directed solely at ascertaining who the deceased was, how, when and where the deceased came by his death, and the registration particulars,[219] and neither coroner nor jury must express any opinion on any other matter.[220] The coroner examines the witnesses he thinks expedient to call,[221] and "properly interested persons" may also examine them.[222] There is specific provision for the privilege against self-incrimination.[223]

A jury (of 7 to 11 persons) must be summoned[224] where there is reason to **22–41**
suspect that the death occurred in prison, or in circumstances the continuance or recurrence of which is prejudicial to public health or safety, or was caused by a notifiable accident, poisoning or disease.[225] After hearing the evidence the jury gives its verdict, and finds the registration particulars.[226] The verdict cannot be framed so as to appear to determine any question of civil liability.[227] The jury may add a rider if the coroner is of opinion that it is designed to prevent the recurrence of similar fatalities.[228] The jury may decide by majority, so long as the minority is not greater than two.[229] If the jury cannot otherwise agree it is discharged and there is a further inquest with a fresh jury.[230]

The Supreme Court can quash an inquisition and order a fresh inquest where it **22–42**
is necessary or desirable in the interest of justice to so because of fraud, rejection of evidence, insufficiency of inquiry, the discovery of new facts or evidence, or otherwise.[231] Because the United Kingdom is responsible for the government of Gibraltar and its international relations, the ECHR applies, and a death investigation and inquest there can be the subject of proceedings before the Strasbourg

---

[213] Coroner Act No. 1889–11 s.11(3).
[214] Coroner Act No. 1889–11 s.11(6)(a).
[215] Coroner Act No. 1889–11 s.7(1).
[216] Coroner Rules, LN 1980/027 r.2, referring to Coroners Rules 1953 r.11.
[217] Coroner Act No. 1889–11 s.7(2).
[218] Coroner Rules, LN 1980/027 r.2, referring to Coroners Rules 1953 r.14. This is subject to an exception for national security.
[219] Coroner Rules, LN 1980/027 r.2, referring to Coroners Rules 1953 r.26(a), (b) and (d).
[220] Coroner Rules, LN 1980/027 r.2, referring to Coroners Rules 1953 r.27.
[221] Coroner Act No. 1889–11 s.8(1).
[222] Coroner Rules, LN 1980/027 r.2, referring to Coroners Rules 1953 r.16.
[223] Coroner Rules, LN 1980/027 r.2, referring to Coroners Rules 1953 r.18.
[224] As to failure to attend, see s.16. The jurors' oath is prescribed: Coroner Rules, LN 1980/027 r.3, Sch.1.
[225] Coroner Act No. 1889–11 s.5(1).
[226] Coroner Act No. 1889–11 s.8(2).
[227] Coroner Rules, LN 1980/027 r.2, referring to Coroners Rules 1953 r.33.
[228] Coroner Rules, LN 1980/027 r.2, referring to Coroners Rules 1953 r.34, and see also r.27.
[229] Coroner Act No. 1889–11 s.9(1).
[230] Coroner Act No. 1889–11 s.9(2).
[231] Coroner Act No. 1889–11 s.12(1)(b).

Court.[232] The Gibraltar Constitution guarantees various human rights, including the right to life.[233] These rights are justiciable in the local courts.[234]

Hong Kong

22–43   Hong Kong is now part of China. But, as a former British colony, it has retained its common law, including its coroner system.[235] The English legislation is the basis for the local law,[236] and English case law is much relied on.[237] One or more of the local stipendiary magistrates is appointed to act as coroner. A long list of categories of death is made reportable to the coroner,[238] and he may investigate them.[239] He may hold an inquest into a death which is sudden, or accidental or violence, or suspicious, or where a dead body is found in or brought into Hong Kong.[240] Such inquests may, but need not, be held with a jury.[241] He must hold an inquest into a death in custody (which must be a jury inquest),[242] and if the Secretary of Justice so requires (which need not).[243] There are also powers to hold inquests where a body has been destroyed or is irrecoverable[244] and in the case of certain air or marine accidents outside Hong Kong.[245] In certain cases the Court of First Instance may order an inquest, or another inquest, to be held.[246]

22–44   The purpose of the inquest is to inquire into the cause and circumstances of the death, and to ascertain the identity of the deceased, how, when and where he came by his death, the registration particulars, and the conclusion as to death.[247] As in England, there are special rules for the admission of documentary evidence,[248] and "properly interested persons" (as defined)[249] may examine witnesses at the hearing by counsel or a solicitor.[250] The inquest findings are recorded in a prescribed form, signed by the jury if there is one.[251] These findings must not appear to determine any question of civil liability, or express opinions on other matters,[252] though the

---

[232] See *McCann v United Kingdom* (1996) 21 E.H.R.R. 97.
[233] Gibraltar Constitution Order 2006 para.2 Annex 1 s.3.
[234] Gibraltar Constitution Order 2006 para.2 Annex 1 s.16.
[235] See generally *China Light & Power Company Ltd v Banks* [1995] H.K.C.A. 5.
[236] Coroners Ordinance, No. 27 of 1997 c.504.
[237] e.g. *Chen Yuk Lun v Banks* [1994] HKCFI 126; *Police Commissioner v Hong Kong Coroner* [1997] HKCFI 173; *Tien v Lam* [2004] 2 HKLRD 719.
[238] Coroners Ordinance s.4 Sch.1.
[239] Coroners Ordinance s.9.
[240] Coroners Ordinance s.14(1).
[241] Coroners Ordinance s.14(2). A jury may decide by a majority: s.42.
[242] Coroners Ordinance s.15.
[243] Coroners Ordinance s.16.
[244] Coroners Ordinance s.17.
[245] Coroners Ordinance s.18.
[246] Coroners Ordinance s.20; see *Pearce v Lam and Chan* [2007] HKCA 386; *Secretary for Justice v Ng* [2009] HKCFI 936; [2010] 1 HKLRD 283; *Rai v Ng* [2011] HKCFI 42; [2011] 2 HKLRD 245.
[247] Coroners Ordinance s.27; see *Secretary for Justice v Ng* [2009] HKCFI 936; [2010] 1 HKLRD 283; *Rai v Ng* [2011] HKCFI 42; [2011] 2 HKLRD 245.
[248] Coroners Ordinance s.40.
[249] Coroners Ordinance s.2 Sch.2; see *Pearce v Lam and Chan* [2007] HKCA 386.
[250] Coroners Ordinance s.32.
[251] Coroners Ordinance s.43.
[252] Coroners Ordinance s.44; see *Secretary for Justice v Ng* [2009] HKCFI 936; [2010] 1 HKLRD 283.

coroner or jury may make recommendations,[253] just as in England before 1980.[254] The Hong Kong Basic Law[255] protects the right to life.[256]

MIXED JURISDICTIONS

The Channel Islands

The Bailiwicks of Jersey and Guernsey have independent legal systems originally **22–45** derived from customary Norman law. They are dependencies of the British Crown, and not part of the United Kingdom, enjoying local autonomy. Although not part of France since 1204, their law was in the past subject to considerable French influence. In modern times the English language has supplanted both the French language and the local dialects, *jèrriais* and *guernésiais*, and English law ideas have been considerably introduced. Thus the islands' Norman roots are tempered by common law modernity. That makes them "mixed" jurisdictions, a kind of bridge between the common law and civil law worlds.

Both Jersey and Guernsey have, nonetheless, inquest systems similar to that of **22–46** England and Wales. In Jersey the current law dates from 1995,[257] though earlier legislation on the subject goes back to the nineteenth century.[258] The key figure in the modern system is the Viscount, who is the executive officer of the Royal Court. In practice it is the Deputy Viscount who takes responsibility for conducting inquests. The legislation is based to some extent on the Manx law, but with some features borrowed from elsewhere (notably England). The European Convention on Human Rights applies as much to the Channel Islands as to the United Kingdom (which is responsible for their external relations), and the Convention rights are justiciable before the local courts by virtue of local legislation, modelled on that of the United Kingdom.[259]

The police must be notified of deaths believed to be from violence, mis- **22–47** adventure, negligence and so on, from non-natural cause or untreated natural causes, or in circumstances requiring investigation.[260] The police must then notify the Viscount.[261] Deaths in custody must be reported directly to the Viscount,[262] as must deaths in mental hospitals and nursing homes and in children's homes.[263] The Viscount *must* hold an inquest (a) where the body is in Jersey and the death is believed to have been from violence, misadventure, negligence, etc., or occurred in custody, or (b) where there is reason to believe the death took place "in care" and

---

[253] Coroners Ordinance s.44(2); see *Rai v Ng* [2011] HKCFI 42; [2011] 2 HKLRD 245.
[254] See 13–111—13–112.
[255] Adopted April 4, 1990.
[256] Articles 28 (Hong Kong residents), 41 (others).
[257] See the Inquests and Post-Mortem Examination (Jersey) Law 1995.
[258] Inquests and Post-Mortem Examination (Jersey) Law 1995, Third Schedule.
[259] Human Rights (Jersey) Law 2000; Human Rights (Guernsey) Law 2000; see Ch.21.
[260] Inquests and Post-Mortem Examination (Jersey) Law 1995 art.2(1).
[261] Inquests and Post-Mortem Examination (Jersey) Law 1995 art.2(1).
[262] Inquests and Post-Mortem Examination (Jersey) Law 1995 art.2(3).
[263] Inquests and Post-Mortem Examination (Jersey) Law 1995 art.2(4).

there is no adequate medical certificate.[264] In other cases the Viscount *may* hold an inquest.[265] The Viscount may summon a jury (of 12 persons) for any inquest: there are no cases where a jury is obligatory. The test is whether the Viscount considers it to be in the public interest.[266] The Viscount has power to summon witnesses to the hearing.[267]

22–48   The jury gives a finding in writing, stating who the deceased was, and how when and where he came by his death, and also the registration particulars,[268] but may not make any finding of legal responsibility.[269] The inquest proceedings are subject to review by the Royal Court, which may quash its findings and order a new inquest to be held.[270] The Court also has power to order an inquest to be held where the Viscount fails to do so.[271] There are provisions for post-mortem examinations to be authorised,[272] and a similar procedure to the English "Form B" for dispensing with an inquest which shows the death to have been natural.[273] There are also procedural rules for both post-mortem examinations and inquests,[274] based in large part on the equivalent English ones in force at the time.[275]

22–49   By contrast with Jersey, Guernsey has no specific inquest legislation. The Magistrate's Court has jurisdiction to hold inquests into the cause of death, wherever occurring,[276] and the local legislature (the States of Deliberation) may make further provision for the holding of inquests,[277] but has not so far done so. On the comparatively rare occasions when it has been necessary, the Magistrate's Court has held the inquest, the judge acting as coroner, and following the (English) Coroners Rules 1984, subject to necessary local modifications.[278] A few local laws make reference to inquests,[279] so acknowledging their existence and role, but contribute nothing to the substance of inquest law in Guernsey.

---

[264] Inquests and Post-Mortem Examination (Jersey) Law 1995 art.5 (but there is a "let-out" under para.(b)).

[265] Inquests and Post-Mortem Examination (Jersey) Law 1995 art.4.

[266] Inquests and Post-Mortem Examination (Jersey) Law 1995 art.7(1); see *Re Cotter* 1997 J.L.R. 12, CA.

[267] Inquests and Post-Mortem Examination (Jersey) Law 1995 art.6; his failure to call witnesses may be challenged: see *Re Cassin* 1997 J.L.R. 187, R. Ct.

[268] Inquests and Post-Mortem Examination (Jersey) Law 1995 art.14(1), based on the (English) Coroners Act 1988 s.11(5)(b).

[269] Inquests and Post-Mortem Examination (Jersey) Law 1995 art.14(3).

[270] Inquests and Post-Mortem Examination (Jersey) Law 1995 art.16, based on the 1988 Act s.13(1)(b).

[271] Inquests and Post-Mortem Examination (Jersey) Law 1995 art.15, based on the 1988 Act s.13(1)(a).

[272] Inquests and Post-Mortem Examination (Jersey) Law 1995 art.17.

[273] Inquests and Post-Mortem Examination (Jersey) Law 1995 art.18.

[274] Inquests and Post-Mortem Examinations (Jersey) Rules 1995.

[275] i.e. the Coroners Rules 1984.

[276] Magistrate's Court (Guernsey) Law 2008 s.21.

[277] Magistrate's Court (Guernsey) Law 2008 s.22.

[278] *Re Inquest on Schofield* 2009-10 G.L.R. 33. But the 1984 Rules did not deal with the question in which cases there must be an inquest (these were in the Coroners Act 1988 s.8(1)), which leaves the matter rather in limbo. Moreover, the English law has of course significantly changed since July 2013, and it is not clear whether Guernsey law will change with it.

[279] See Cremation Ordinance 1972 s.8(3), (6)-(8) Sch.1 Forms C, D1, D2 and E; Registration of Births and Deaths (Supplementary Provisions) (Guernsey) Law 1978 Sch. Form E; Registration of Births, Deaths and Marriages (Miscellaneous Provisions) (Bailiwick of Guernsey) Law 1979 Sch. Form E; Human Tissue (Bailiwick of Guernsey) Law 1981 s.1(5).

Scotland[280]

Scotland is another "mixed" jurisdiction, a civilian foundation, but influenced by   **22–50**
England. Its death investigation system leans more towards the civilian ideas than
the common law. There are essentially two stages, but the second does not happen
in every case. Deaths falling within a wide range[281] are reported to the procurator
fiscal, who is essentially the local public prosecutor (a lawyer). He or she will be
advised by the police (including the police surgeon) as to whether further inquiry
is needed. If so, the procurator fiscal may authorise a post-mortem examination, in
suspicious cases carried out by two doctors. He or she may also interview
witnesses. So far, the inquiry is private. Some deaths must be reported by the
procurator fiscal to the Crown Office in Edinburgh. In some cases, of course,
criminal proceedings follow. This is, after all, the main point of the procurator fiscal
being involved at all.

But, if there are no criminal proceedings, and either the death appears to have   **22–51**
resulted from an accident at work, or the deceased was in legal custody, the
procurator fiscal must apply to the local sheriff (criminal and civil judge for the
district concerned) to hold a statutory inquiry, in public.[282] And in any event the
Lord Advocate can direct the procurator fiscal to apply for such an inquiry if the
Lord Advocate thinks it is expedient to hold one on the ground that the death was
sudden, suspicious or unexplained, or occurred in circumstances giving rise to
serious public concern.[283]

The sheriff sits without a jury (though sometimes with an assessor). He or she   **22–52**
determines when and where the accident—and the death—occurred, what caused
them, what might have prevented them, and similar relevant matters.[284] But none
of this will be admissible in any subsequent proceedings.[285] The sheriff's inquiry is
a factual one, and thus to that extent resembles an English inquest. But the reports
and determinations resulting from them can be much longer and more detailed
than anything produced by an English coronial investigation.[286]

In 2009 a review was carried out of the statutory inquiry system by a retired   **22–53**
senior judge, which recommended a number of relatively modest changes.[287] The
European Convention on Human Rights applies as much to Scotland as to the rest
of the United Kingdom, and the Convention rights are justiciable before the local
courts by virtue of the same United Kingdom legislation.[288]

---

[280] See generally Carmichael, *Sudden Deaths and Fatal Accident Inquiries,* 3rd edn (2005); *R. (Amin) v
Home Secretary* [2004] 1 A.C. 653 at [55]–[59].

[281] See Carmichael, *Sudden Deaths and Fatal Accident Inquiries,* para.1.07.

[282] Under the Fatal Accidents and Sudden Deaths Inquiry (Scotland) Act 1976 s.1(1)(a).

[283] Fatal Accidents and Sudden Deaths Inquiry (Scotland) Act 1976 s.1(1)(b); see *Niven v Lord Advocate*
[2009] CSOH 110 (failed murder prosecution; art.2 not engaged); *Emms v Lord Advocate* [2011]
CSIH 7 (hospital death; art.2 not engaged).

[284] Fatal Accidents and Sudden Deaths Inquiry (Scotland) Act 1976 s.6(1).

[285] Fatal Accidents and Sudden Deaths Inquiry (Scotland) Act 1976 s.6(3).

[286] See e.g. that for the case of *John Willock* 2013 FAI 15 (available, as with other such inquiries, on the
BAILII website).

[287] Lord Cullen, *Review of Fatal Accident Inquiry Legislation, The Report,* 2009.

[288] Human Rights Act 1998; see Ch.21.

Malta

22–54   Malta is even more of a civil-law jurisdiction than Scotland. But because of its long association with Britain, and its use of English as a second language (first for business), its law contains many common law institutions, including that of the inquest into death. The police have a duty to report sudden, violent, or suspicious deaths, or those of unknown cause, to a magistrate.[289] They may do so verbally, but in such a case it needs to be confirmed in writing within two weeks.[290] Upon receiving such report the magistrate will transmit a copy of the report to the Attorney General within a period of three working days from when the report was received.[291]

22–55   The magistrate will hold an inquest on the body to ascertain the cause of death, taking all the evidence available and drawing up and signing a *procès-verbal* stating the findings as to that cause.[292] If this is not done within 60 days from the report, the magistrate must report to the Attorney General not later than three working days after the expiry of the 60-day period stating the reasons for the delay.[293] This same procedure applies whenever a person dies in prison, while detained in any place of confinement contemplated by the Prisons Act,[294] while in police custody[295] or whilst kept at a mental hospital under a court order.[296]

22–56   The magistrate holding the inquest has the same powers as a magistrate presiding in the Court of Magistrates as a court of criminal enquiry.[297] However, where the death is sudden or of unknown cause, the magistrate may, instead of himself holding an inquest on the body, appoint a senior police officer (assisted by a photographer or other expert) to establish the facts and to give evidence on the facts, by producing all photographs taken and other articles or documents relevant to the investigation.[298] In the case of sudden, violent, or suspicious deaths, or those of unknown cause, the magistrate also has power to order an autopsy and order medical experts to hear evidence to establish the identity of the body and to ascertain the cause of death.[299] If the body has been buried, the magistrate may also order its exhumation with all due precautions, if this can be effected without prejudicing public health.[300]

22–57   A magistrate who at an inquest considers that there is sufficient circumstantial evidence against a person for a charge in connection with the death, or even that the person is guilty of that offence, may order his or her arrest, the seizure of material thought necessary for the discovery of the truth, or the search of any property, where from the evidence collected the magistrate is led to believe that

---

[289] Criminal Code c.9 of the Laws of Malta art.551(1).
[290] The magistrate may, if it is considered appropriate proceed in accordance with his or her powers even though the report was not confirmed in writing within the required period of time. Criminal Code art.546(4).
[291] Criminal Code art.546(5).
[292] Criminal Code art.551(1).
[293] Criminal Code art.550A(1).
[294] Chapter 260 of the Laws of Malta.
[295] Criminal Code art.551(2).
[296] Criminal Code art.551(3).
[297] Criminal Code art.554(3).
[298] Criminal Code art.551(4), referring to art.546(3).
[299] Criminal Code art.552.
[300] Criminal Code art.553.

any material necessary for the discovery of the truth may be found there.[301] The magistrate may also order the fingerprinting, measuring or photographing of the suspect and the examination of any part of his or her body or clothing by appointed experts.[302] Where the magistrate is of the opinion that the photographs, finger-print impressions, records of measurements or any other thing obtained from the body or clothing of the suspect, is or are no longer required for the purposes of the inquiry, the magistrate is to order their destruction or that they be handed over to the suspect.

The European Convention on Human Rights applies as much to Malta as to the   **22–58** other Council of Europe Member States. The Maltese Constitution guarantees various human rights, including the right to life.[303] These rights are justiciable in the local courts.[304]

Civilian Systems

France

In some ways the French system is a model of the civilian approach. Certain deaths,   **22–59** including those involving violence (but *not* suicide), those in custody, or arising out of police action, and those arising out of large-scale disasters, are reportable to the *Procureur de la République* (public prosecutor), and may give rise to an *enquête judiciaire* (judicial inquiry) by the *juge d'instruction* (investigating magistrate).[305] Formerly it was not possible for the family to be constituted *partie civile* to such an inquiry,[306] and to be involved in the investigation. However, following an adverse report by the European Committee for the Prevention of Torture in relation to certain French prisons, at a time when a case was pending before the European Court of Human Rights involving a death in such a prison where the wife was entirely excluded from the investigation,[307] the law was changed to allow this.[308]

An alternative is for the family of the deceased to lodge a criminal complaint for   **22–60** homicide with the *juge d'instruction* and seek leave to join the proceedings as a *partie civile*.[309] Even if the facts are unclear, they can make a *plainte contre X*—a criminal complaint against an unknown person.[310] The investigating judge investigates in the same way as if an application to open an investigation had been lodged by the public prosecutor. Where the case is then brought before the criminal courts, they can also rule on the civil claims in the action.

---

[301] Criminal Code art.554(1).

[302] Criminal Code art.554(2).

[303] Malta Constitution 1964 s.33.

[304] Malta Constitution 1964 s.46; see Ch.21.

[305] *Code de Procédure Pénale* art.74.

[306] Cass Crim, 26 juill 1966.

[307] *Slimani v France*, App. no. 57671/00 (ECtHR, Second Section, Judgment July 27, 2004). She unsuccessfully requested access to the autopsy and toxicology reports, and was never interviewed by the investigating judge.

[308] See now *Code de Procédure Pénale* art.80-4.

[309] *Code de Procédure Pénale* art.85.

[310] As in *Bone v France*, App. no. 69869/01 (ECtHR, Judgment May 1, 2005) (railway passenger who got out of the train on the wrong side and was killed by a passing train),.

22–61   The *juge d'instruction* may delegate some of his information-gathering functions to a police officer, who will question witnesses.[311] An external or internal post-mortem examination may be ordered, as may a special examination of tissues or samples.[312] A full autopsy only happens in more serious cases. The *juge d'instruction* may in effect also delegate the decision-making function, for example by appointing experts to decide what was the cause of death, whether any medical treatment was in accordance with current medical knowledge, whether there are any deficiencies in the institutions which had care of the deceased, with power to question witnesses and request documents.[313]

22–62   If the investigating judge dealing with a complaint lodged by the family of a person who died in suspicious circumstances considers, at the end of the investigation, that the death was not caused by acts or omissions capable of being classified as criminal, he or she issues an order discontinuing the proceedings, which terminates the prosecution.[314] Such discontinuance may be the subject of an appeal.[315] If it appears to the victim's family that the death is likely to have been caused by errors or shortcomings on the part of the state and its administration, they can still sue the state for damages in the administrative courts.

22–63   Thereafter a death certificate is prepared, in two parts. The *open* part of the certificate states personal particulars, and also whether there is any obstacle to burial. The *closed* part, which is not seen by relatives (but *is* seen by government officials),[316] contains the cause of death, including an opinion whether the death occurred through violence, crime or accident.

22–64   There is no public hearing, unless a criminal trial takes place, or unless a refusal to prosecute is challenged.[317] Essentially, the whole exercise is directed not, as in England, to establishing the circumstances of death, but instead to whether any criminality was involved. Apart from the fact that prison and other custody deaths are initially reportable, there is no special regime attaching to such deaths, which are otherwise treated in the same way.

Spain

22–65   Sudden and unexplained violent (including suicide) or industrial deaths, deaths in custody or involving the police, potential medical negligence deaths and deaths from disasters are all reportable to authority. The body must first be identified.[318] As in France, the investigation may be instituted by the police, who may involve the *Juez de Instruccion* (investigating magistrate). If he is involved, he will direct the inquiry, ordering any necessary post-mortem examination (more likely in non-

---

[311] As happened in *Slimani v France*, App. no. 57671/00 (ECtHR, Second Section, Judgment July 27, 2004).

[312] See e.g. *Pannullo v France*, App. no. 37794/97 (ECtHR Third Section, Judgment October 30, 2001).

[313] As also happened in *Slimani v France*, App. no. 57671/00 (ECtHR, Second Section, Judgment July 27, 2004).

[314] As happened in *Bone v France*, App. no. 69869/01 (Judgment May 1, 2005).

[315] As happened in *Hamouda-Lahari v France*, App. no. 21296/05 (Second Section, Judgment July 3, 2007).

[316] This gives an idea of the relative values informing the system.

[317] As in the case of the death of Diana, Princess of Wales: see the decision of the Criminal Chamber of the *Cour de Cassation* dated April 2002.

[318] Spanish Code of Criminal Procedure of September 14, 1882 arts 340-342.

natural or criminal cases),[319] which he or the judicial police attend.[320] There is no public inquiry equivalent to the English inquest.

Italy

All non-natural deaths, sudden and unexpected deaths, and deaths in custody or through state agency or medical negligence must be reported to the *Procuratore della Repubblica* (public prosecutor)[321] where there is a suspicion of crime, and to other public bodies (e.g. the Italian health service) where other criteria are satisfied. In cases of suspected crime the police or the public prosecutor will investigate and ascertain the cause of death,[322] instructing medical and other experts as needed.[323] An *autopsia* (autopsy) may be ordered by the public prosecutor or a judge,[324] informing the suspect and the victim's family.[325] A judge may also order the exhumation of the body if there is serious evidence of crime.[326] The body cannot be buried without the public prosecutor's consent,[327] or cremated without the judge's.[328] Where there is no suspicion of crime but it is impossible to ascertain the cause of death (e.g. there are no witnesses), the local health authority instructs a doctor to carry out an *esame diagnostico* (non-forensic autopsy), and a death certificate is given.

22–66

The Netherlands

If a medical practitioner will not sign a certificate of natural death, the public prosecutor must be informed, and he may order an autopsy. In practice he will instruct an expert to examine the body. If external examination of the body, and other inquiries, satisfy him that the death was natural, an autopsy is unlikely. However, an autopsy is inevitable if there is suspicion of criminal activity. In addition, family members (and other interested parties) may also seek an autopsy. Both pathologist and public prosecutor will retain copies of the autopsy report. These preliminary investigations are private. The expert's view as to whether a non-natural death was accidental, suicidal or homicidal is usually accepted by the public prosecutor. But ultimately the public prosecutor will decide whether criminal charges should be brought and, if so, will undertake their prosecution, which will of course normally be in public. There is no special regime for deaths in custody or through state agents, though of course ECHR art.2 will have a role to play.[329]

22–67

---

[319] Spanish Code of Criminal Procedure of September 14, 1882 art.343.

[320] Spanish Code of Criminal Procedure of September 14, 1882 art.353.

[321] Responsible, with the judicial police, for carrying out all necessary enquiries in connection with criminal procedure (*Codice di Procedura Penale* arts 326, 358).

[322] *Norme di attuazione del codice di procedura penale* art.116(1).

[323] *Codice di Procedura Penale* art.359.

[324] *Norme di attuazione del codice di procedura penale* art.116(1).

[325] *Codice di Procedura Penale* art.360. See *Giuliano and Gaggio v Italy*, App. no. 23458/02 (ECtHR, March 24, 2011).

[326] *Norme di attuazione del codice di procedura penale* art.116(2).

[327] *Norme di attuazione del codice di procedura penale* art.116(2).

[328] Presidential Decree no. 285 of September 10, 1990 art.79.

[329] See *Ramsahai v The Netherlands*, App. no. 52391/99 (ECtHR (Grand Chamber), judgment May 15, 2007).

Switzerland

22–68   Since 2007, procedure has been governed by federal rather than cantonal law.[330] Only a doctor who examines a dead body externally may issue a certificate of the cause of death. Where the body is unidentified, or there are indications of unnatural death, the public prosecutor must order the inspection of the body by a specialist, to identify it or to establish a cause of death.[331] If the inspection reveals no evidence of crime, the body is released.[332] If there is any such evidence, further tests and if necessary an autopsy will be carried out by a forensic medicine institute. The body and its parts may be retained for as long as needed.[333] The police investigate the circumstances where crime is suspected, and also report to the magistrate. If no criminal proceedings ensue, the matter stops there.

Germany

22–69   Death apparently from an unnatural cause, or the discovery the dead body of an unknown person, must be reported by the police and the local authority to the state prosecutor or the local court immediately.[334] They determine whether an external examination or internal examination (i.e. autopsy) is necessary. Where there is only an external examination, the state prosecutor carries it out, or in special circumstances an investigating magistrate does so. The state prosecutor prepares a report. If the cause of death is beyond doubt, there is no autopsy. If there is one, it is conducted by two doctors, one of whom at least will be a forensic pathologist,[335] and (after identifying the deceased)[336] involves opening the three major body cavities.[337] Sometimes the investigating magistrate is present.[338] A written report is made to the state prosecutor. In addition, every death is reported to the local *Standesbeamter* (civil status registry officer), and there will be a file referring to any investigation that was carried out by the state prosecutor. The investigating magistrate (or in urgent cases the public prosecutor)[339] has power to exhume a body for the purposes of conducting an autopsy.[340]

Austria

22–70   Each province has its own rules. But in principle the position is as follows. Every dead body *must* be externally examined by a medical practitioner. If there is good reason to suppose that the death was not natural, an autopsy is mandatory, unless there is no doubt of the (non-natural) cause (e.g. accident, suicide, crime). If crime is suspected, the federal police must be informed. The record of a mandatory

---

[330] Swiss Criminal Procedure Code of October 5, 2007.
[331] Swiss Criminal Procedure Code art.253 para.1.
[332] Swiss Criminal Procedure Code art.253 para.2.
[333] Swiss Criminal Procedure Code art.253 para.3.
[334] *Strafprozessordnung* (Criminal Procedure Code) s.159.
[335] *Strafprozessordnung* (Criminal Procedure Code) s.87(2).
[336] *Strafprozessordnung* (Criminal Procedure Code) s.88.
[337] *Strafprozessordnung* (Criminal Procedure Code) s.89. As to autopsies on newborn children, see s.90, and, in cases of suspected poisoning s.91.
[338] *Strafprozessordnung* (Criminal Procedure Code) s.87(2).
[339] *Strafprozessordnung* (Criminal Procedure Code) s.87(4).
[340] *Strafprozessordnung* (Criminal Procedure Code) s.87(3).

autopsy will be sent to the municipality or (in the case of suspected crime) the police. There is no special regime for deaths in custody.

Liechtenstein

Deaths occurring in a non-natural way must be investigated, by the public **22–71** prosecutor, acting with a local medical practitioner (on call according to a rota system). If there is a suspicion of crime an investigating magistrate may become involved. An autopsy must be carried out if crime cannot be excluded, or if it is necessary in order to determine the cause of death (e.g. if a contagious disease is suspected). Deaths in custody, or caused by state agents, would usually be non-natural, and so subject to investigation as stated.

Denmark

A doctor attending a death must report unnatural deaths and (most) deaths in **22–72** custody to the police. They then investigate together with the district public health officer. The police decide whether an autopsy should be undertaken, usually because the death is suspected to be the result of a crime, or where no cause of death has been established. The Minister of Justice can also direct an autopsy. Again the investigation is private, unless there are criminal proceedings, which are normally public.

Czech Republic

An autopsy is compulsory (a) where death is suspected to be the result of a crime, **22–73** (b) in order to establish the cause of death in the case of children and pregnant women who die in hospital, (c) where there is sudden or violent death (including suicide) of unknown cause, in state custody, from industrial injuries, or from medical negligence. Two doctors appointed by the prosecuting authority carry out the autopsy. In addition, if there is a suspicion that death is the result of a crime, the police will commence an inquiry, and this may lead to prosecution. Apart from the compulsory autopsy in the case of sudden or violent death, there are no special rules applicable to deaths in custody.

Poland

An external examination and an autopsy of a dead body are ordered if it is **22–74** suspected that death has been caused by criminal means.[341] If necessary for these purposes, exhumation of the body may be ordered by the state prosecutor or a judge.[342] The external examination is carried out, at the place where the body was found, and without so far as possible moving it,[343] by a state prosecutor (or in some cases a judge) with the assistance of a medical practitioner, preferably a specialist in forensic medicine, though in urgent cases the police carry it out, and notify the state prosecutor accordingly.[344] The autopsy is carried out by an expert, with the state prosecutor or judge present.[345] A medical practitioner who has recently

---

[341] Polish Criminal Procedure Code of 6 June 1997 art.209(1).
[342] Polish Criminal Procedure Code of 6 June 1997 art.210.
[343] Polish Criminal Procedure Code of 6 June 1997 art.209(3).
[344] Polish Criminal Procedure Code of 6 June 1997 art.209(2).
[345] Polish Criminal Procedure Code of 6 June 1997 art.209(4).

treated the deceased may also be summoned to be present. The expert will make a written report about both examination and autopsy.[346]

Greece

22–75   Where a doctor does not issue a death certificate showing a natural cause of death, the police or public prosecutor will be informed (either by the attending doctor, or by the relative seeking to deal with deceased's affairs).[347] The police may initiate an inquiry of their own motion, or because others have asked them to, or when directed to do so by the public prosecutor.[348] As part of that inquiry an autopsy will usually be ordered, and a report sent back to the police or public prosecutor.[349] When the inquiry is complete, the prosecutor will decide whether to initiate criminal proceedings, or whether to archive the file.[350] Deaths in prison or in the army are always investigated, and an autopsy carried out, even if apparently natural.

Brazil

22–76   If a death occurs in a non-natural way, whether of obvious cause (e.g. crime, accident, suicide) or of apparently unknown cause, there must be an autopsy, carried out by a doctor affiliated to the Security State Department. The report is filed with that department. If crime is suspected, an investigation is carried out by the public prosecutor, who may initiate criminal proceedings in respect of the death. There is no special regime for deaths in custody.

Conclusion

22–77   The descriptions of the civil law systems given in this chapter are limited in scope, and there is much more of a comparative nature that could be said, e.g. in relation to legal tests for death, the rules for organ transplants, and the formalities for the repatriation of dead bodies. But it is hoped that the details that have been given show how the civilian approach is to see death investigation merely as part of the investigation of possible criminal activity, rather than (as in the common law world) as a worthy object of investigation in its own right. There is no sense that the civilian systems are trying to discover causes of death for public health or policy purposes, only for those of criminal justice. It is also reasonably clear that, with a very few exceptions, death in custody or through state agency is not given special attention, again unlike the common law system, which treats such a death as justifying a full inquiry even though on the face of it the death was perfectly natural. On the other hand, it seems likely that the common law system involves a greater use of the invasive autopsy to explain unnatural death than the civilian systems, which tend to rely on the external examination of the body, coupled with the other evidence available, to reach a conclusion as to the likelihood of criminal

---

[346] Polish Criminal Procedure Code of 6 June 1997 art.209(5).
[347] Greek Penal Procedure Code arts 37, 40.
[348] Greek Penal Procedure Code arts 42, 43.
[349] Greek Penal Procedure Code arts 180-182, 251.
[350] Greek Penal Procedure Code art.43.

involvement in the death in many such cases. There are important social, cultural and historical factors in play here, but this is not the place to deal with them.

Part VII

APPENDICES

Appendix 1

STATUTES AND STATUTORY EXTRACTS

Administration of Justice Act 1960 c. 65

Right of appeal

1.—(1) Subject to the provisions of this section, an appeal shall lie to the [Supreme **A1–001** Court],[1] at the instance of the defendant or the prosecutor—

(a) from any decision of [the High Court][2] in a criminal cause or matter;

[. . .][3]

---

[1] Words substituted by Constitutional Reform Act 2005 c. 4 Sch.9(1) para.13(2)(a) (October 1, 2009).

[2] Words substituted by Access to Justice Act 1999 c. 22 Pt IV s.63(1) (September 27, 1999).

[3] S. 1(1)(b) repealed by Criminal Appeal Act 1968 (c. 19), Sch. 7 and Criminal Appeal (Northern Ireland) Act 1968 (c. 21), Sch. 5.

(2) No appeal shall lie under this section except with the leave of the court below or of [the Supreme Court];[4] and such leave shall not be granted unless it is certified by the court below that a point of law of general public importance is involved in the decision and it appears to that court or to [the Supreme Court],[4] as the case may be, that the point is one which ought to be considered by [the Supreme Court].[4]

[. . .][5]

(4) For the purpose of disposing of an appeal under this section the [Supreme Court][6] may exercise any powers of the court below or may remit the case to that court.

(5) In this Act, unless the context otherwise requires, "leave to appeal" means leave to appeal to the [Supreme Court][6] under this section.

Application for leave to appeal

A1–002   **2.**—(1) Subject to the provisions of this section, an application to the court below for leave to appeal shall be made within the period of [28][7] days beginning with the [relevant date];[8] and an application to the [Supreme Court][9] for such leave shall be made within the period of [28][7] days beginning with the date on which the application is refused by the court below.

[(1A) In subsection (1), "the relevant date" means—

(a) the date of the decision of the court below, or

(b) if later, the date on which that court gives reasons for its decision.][10]

[. . .][11]

(3) [The][12] [Supreme Court][9] or the court below may, upon application made at any time by the defendant, extend the time within which an application may be made by him to [the Supreme Court or the court below][13] under subsection (1) of this section.

Appeal in cases of contempt of court

A1–003   **13.**—(1) Subject to the provisions of this section, an appeal shall lie under this section from any order or decision of a court in the exercise of jurisdiction to punish for contempt of court (including criminal contempt); and in relation to any such order or decision the provisions of this section shall have effect in substitution for any other enactment relating to appeals in civil or criminal proceedings.

(2) An appeal under this section shall lie in any case at the instance of the defendant and, in the case of an application for committal or attachment, at the instance of the applicant; and the appeal shall lie—

---

[4] Words substituted by Constitutional Reform Act 2005 c. 4 Sch.9(1) para.13(2)(b) (October 1, 2009).

[5] Repealed by Constitutional Reform Act 2005 c. 4 Sch.18(5) para.1 (October 1, 2009).

[6] Words substituted by Constitutional Reform Act 2005 c. 4 Sch.9(1) para.13(2)(d) (October 1, 2009).

[7] Word substituted by Courts Act 2003 c. 39 Pt 8 s.88(2)(a) (April 1, 2005).

[8] Words substituted by Courts Act 2003 c. 39 Pt 8 s.88(2)(b) (April 1, 2005).

[9] Words substituted by Constitutional Reform Act 2005 c. 4 Sch.9(1) para.13(3)(a) (October 1, 2009).

[10] Added by Courts Act 2003 c. 39 Pt 8 s.88(3) (April 1, 2005).

[11] Repealed by Criminal Appeal Act 1968 (c. 19), s. 55(3), Sch. 7.

[12] Words repealed by Courts Act 2003 c. 39 Sch.10 para.1 (April 1, 2005 as SI 2005/910).

[13] Words substituted by Constitutional Reform Act 2005 c. 4 Sch.9(1) para.13(3)(b) (October 1, 2009).

(a) from an order or decision of any inferior court not referred to in the next following paragraph, to [. . .]¹⁴ the High Court;

(b) from an order or decision of [the county court]¹⁵ or any other inferior court from which appeals generally lie to the Court of Appeal, and from an order or [decision (other than a decision on an appeal under this section) of a single]¹⁶ judge of the High Court, or of any court having the powers of the High Court or of a judge of that court, to the Court of Appeal;

[(bb) from an order or decision of the Crown Court to the Court of Appeal]¹⁷

(c) [from a decision of a single judge of the High Court on an appeal under this section,]¹⁸ from an order or decision of a Divisional Court or the Court of Appeal (including a decision of either of those courts on an appeal under this section), [and from an order or decision (except one made in Scotland or Northern Ireland) of the Court Martial Appeal Court],¹⁹ to the [Supreme Court].²⁰

[(2A) Paragraphs (a) to (c) of subsection (2) of this section do not apply in relation to appeals under this section from an order or decision of the family court, but (subject to any provision made under section 56 of the Access of Justice Act 1999 or by or under any other enactment) such an appeal shall lie to the Court of Appeal.]²¹

(3) The court to which an appeal is brought under this section may reverse or vary the order or decision of the court below, and make such other order as may be just; and without prejudice to the inherent powers of any court referred to in subsection (2) of this section, provision may be made by [rules of court]²² [rules made under section seven of the Northern Ireland Act 1962]²³ for authorising the release on bail of an appellant under this section.

(4) Subsections (2) to (4) of section one and section two of this Act shall apply to an appeal to [the Supreme Court]²⁴ under this section as they apply to an appeal to [the Supreme Court]²⁴ under the said section one, except that so much of the said subsection (2) as restricts the grant of leave to appeal shall apply only where the decision of the court below is a decision on appeal to that court under this section.

(5) In this section "court" includes any tribunal or person having power to punish for contempt; and references in this section to an order or decision of a court in the exercise of jurisdiction to punish for contempt of court include references—

---

¹⁴ Words repealed by Access to Justice Act 1999 c. 22 Sch.15(III) para.1 (September 27, 1999).

¹⁵ Words substituted by Crime and Courts Act 2013 c. 22 Sch.9(3) para.52(1)(b) (April 22, 2014: substitution has effect as SI 2014/954 subject to savings and transitional provisions specified in 2013 c.22 s.15 and Sch.8 and transitional provision specified in SI 2014/954 arts 2(c) and 3).

¹⁶ Words substituted by Access to Justice Act 1999 c. 22 Pt IV s.64(3) (September 27, 1999).

¹⁷ S. 13(2)(bb) inserted by Courts Act 1971 (c. 23), Sch. 8 Pt. II para. 40(1).

¹⁸ Words added by Access to Justice Act 1999 c. 22 Pt IV s.64(4) (September 27, 1999).

¹⁹ Words substituted by Armed Forces Act 2006 c. 52 Sch.16 para.45(2) (October 31, 2009).

²⁰ Words substituted by Constitutional Reform Act 2005 c. 4 Sch.9(1) para.13(7)(a) (October 1, 2009).

²¹ Added by Crime and Courts Act 2013 c. 22 Sch.10(2) para.15(2) (April 22, 2014: insertion has effect as SI 2014/954 subject to savings and transitional provisions specified in 2013 c.22 s.15 and Sch.8 and transitional provision specified in SI 2014/954 arts 2(d) and 3).

²² Words "rules" to "1962" substituted for words "rules of court" in application of s. 13 to N.I. by Northern Ireland Act 1962 (c.30), Sch. 1 Pt. I.

²³ Words "rules" to "1962" substituted for words "rules of court" in application of s. 13 to N.I. by Northern Ireland Act 1962 (c.30), Sch. 1 Pt. I.

²⁴ Words substituted by Constitutional Reform Act 2005 c. 4 Sch.9(1) para.13(7)(b) (October 1, 2009).

(a) to an order or decision of the High Court [, the family court,][25] [the Crown Court][26] or [the county court][15] under any enactment enabling that court to deal with an offence as if it were contempt of court;

(b) to an order or decision of [the county court][15], or of any court having the powers of [the county court][15], under [section 14, 92 or 118 of the County Courts Act 1984];[27]

(c) to an order or decision of a magistrates' court under [subsection (3) of section 63 of the Magistrates' Courts Act 1980][28] [;][29]

[(d) to an order or decision (except one made in Scotland or Northern Ireland) of the Court Martial, the Summary Appeal Court or the Service Civilian Court under section 309 of the Armed Forces Act 2006,][29]

but do not include references to order under section five of the Debtors Act 1869, or under any provision of the [Magistrates' Courts Act 1980][28], or the County Courts Act [1984][30], except those referred to in paragraphs (b) and (c) of this subsection and except [sections 38 and 142][31] of the last mentioned Act so far as those sections confer jurisdiction in respect of contempt of court.

(6) This section does not apply to a conviction or sentence in respect of which an appeal lies under [Part I of the Criminal Appeal Act 1968,or to a decision of the criminal division of the Court of Appeal under that Part of that Act;][32] [. . .][33]

Agriculture (Safety, Health and Welfare Provisions) Act 1956 c. 49

Inquest in case of death by accident

A1–004   **9.**—(1) Where a coroner holds an inquest on the body of a person whose death may have been caused by an accident occurring in the course of agricultural operations, the coroner, shall adjourn the inquest unless an inspector or some other person on behalf of the appropriate Minister is present to watch the proceedings, and shall, at least four days before holding the adjourned inquest, give to an inspector notice of the time and place of holding the adjourned inquest:

Provided that—

(a) the coroner, before the adjournment, may take evidence to identify the body and may order the interment thereof; and

(b) if the inquest relates to the death of not more than one person, the coroner shall not be bound to adjourn the inquest in pursuance of this section if, not less than twenty-four hours before it is held, he informed an inspector of the time and place of the holding thereof.

---

[25] Words inserted by Crime and Courts Act 2013 c. 22 Sch.10(2) para.15(3) (April 22, 2014: insertion has effect as SI 2014/954 subject to savings and transitional provisions specified in 2013 c.22 s.15 and Sch.8 and transitional provision specified in SI 2014/954 arts 2(d) and 3).

[26] Words inserted by Courts Act 1971 (c. 23), Sch. 8 Pt. II para. 40(2).

[27] Words substituted by County Courts Act 1984 (c.28), s.148(1), Sch.2 Pt.V para.25(a).

[28] Words substituted by Magistrates' Court Act 1980 (c.43), s.154(1), Sch.7 para.36.

[29] Added by Armed Forces Act 2006 c. 52 Sch.16 para.45(3) (October 31, 2009).

[30] Word substituted by County Courts Act 1984 (c.28), s.148(1), Sch.2 Pt.V para.25(b).

[31] Words substituted by County Courts Act 1984 (c.28), s.148(1), Sch.2 Pt.V para.25(c).

[32] Words substituted by Criminal Appeal Act 1968 (c. 19), Sch. 5.

[33] Words repealed by Supreme Court Act 1981 (c.54), s.152(4), Sch.7.

(2) Where evidence is given at any such inquest at which an inspector is not present of any neglect as having caused or contributed to the accident, or of any defect in any building, structure, machinery, plant, equipment or appliance appearing to the coroner or jury to require a remedy, the coroner shall give to an inspector notice of the neglect or defect.

Interpretation

24.—(1) In this Act, unless the context otherwise requires, the following expressions have the meanings hereby assigned to them respectively, that is to say–   A1–005

"agriculture" includes dairy-farming, the production of any consumable produce which is grown for sale or for consumption or other use for the purposes of a trade or business or of any other undertaking (whether carried on for profit or not), and the use of land as grazing, meadow or pasture land or orchard or osier land or woodland or for market gardens or nursery grounds, and "agricultural" shall be construed accordingly;

"agricultural holding", "fixed equipment" and "landlord" have the same meanings as in the [Agricultural Holdings Act 1986];[34]

"agricultural unit" means land which is occupied as a unit for agricultural purposes; [. . .][35]

"consumable produce" means produce grown for consumption or for other use after severance from the land on which it is grown;

["inspector" means an inspector appointed by the Health and Safety Executive under section 19 of the Health and Safety at Work etc. Act 1974][36]

[. . .][37]

"worker" means a person employed under a contract of service or apprenticeship and "employer" and "employed" have corresponding meanings;

"young person" means a person who is over compulsory school age for the purposes of the [(construed in accordance with section 8 of the Education Act 1996)][38], but has not attained the age of eighteen.

(2) Any reference in this Act to a contravention of any provision shall include a reference to a failure to comply with that provision.

[. . .][39]

(4) Any reference in this Act to any other enactment shall be construed as a reference to that enactment as amended by any subsequent enactment.

Births and Deaths Registration Act 1926 c. 48

Prohibition of disposal except on registrar's certificate or coroner's order

1.—(1) Subject as hereinafter provided, the body of a deceased person shall not be disposed of before a certificate of the registrar given [under subsection (2) or (3) of section eleven or under section twenty-four of the Births and Deaths Registration Act 1953][40] or an order of the coroner has been delivered to the person effecting the disposal: A1–006

---

[34] Words substituted by Agricultural Holdings Act 1986 (c.5), ss. 99, 100, Sch. 13 para. 3, Sch. 14 para. 23.

[35] Definition of the appropriate Minister repealed by SI 1976/1247, Sch. 2.

[36] Definition substituted by SI 1976/1247, Sch. 2.

[37] Definition of sanitary authority repealed by SI 1977/746, Sch. 2.

[38] Words substituted in definition by Education Act 1996 c. 56 Sch.37(II) para.134 (September 1, 1997).

[39] Repealed by SI 1977/746, Sch. 2.

[40] Words substituted by virtue of Births and Deaths Registration Act 1953 (c. 20), Sch. 1.

Provided that it shall be lawful for the person effecting the disposal by burial of the body of any deceased person, if satisfied by a written declaration in the prescribed form by the person procuring the disposal that a certificate of the registrar or order of the coroner has been issued in respect of the deceased, to proceed with the burial notwithstanding that the certificate or order has not been previously delivered to him.

(2) Any person contravening the provisions of this section shall be liable on summary conviction to a fine not exceeding [level 1 on the standard scale][41]

Notification of disposal to registrar

A1–007

3.—(1) The person effecting the disposal of the body of any deceased person shall, within ninety-six hours of the disposal, deliver to the registrar in the prescribed manner a notification as to the date, place and means of disposal of the body.
[. . .][42]

Prohibition of removal of body out of England without notice

A1–008

4. The body of a deceased person shall not be removed out of England until the expiration of the prescribed period after notice of the removal has been given to [the senior coroner in whose area the body is situated,][43] or otherwise than in accordance with such procedure as may be prescribed, and any person contravening the provisions of this section shall be liable on summary conviction to a fine not exceeding [level 3 on the standard scale][44]

Burial of still-born children

A1–009

5. It shall not be lawful for a person who has control over or who ordinarily buries bodies in any burial ground to permit to be buried or to bury in such burial ground a still-born child before there is delivered to him [either—][45]

[(a) a certificate given by the registrar under section 11(2) or (3) of the Births and Deaths Registration Act 1953, or

(b) in a case in relation to which a senior coroner has made enquiries under section 1(7) of the Coroners and Justice Act 2009 (or has purported to conduct an investigation under Part 1 of that Act), an order of the coroner.][45]

Regulations

A1–010

9. The [Secretary of State][46] [. . .][47] may make regulations—

(a) prescribing the period and form of notice to be given to the coroner of an intention to remove a body out of England; and as to the procedure upon removal and the notification of the registrar as to the date and place of such removal;

[. . .][48]

---

[41] Words substituted by Criminal Justice Act 1982 (c.48), ss. 38, 46.
[42] Repealed by Births and Deaths Registration Act 1953 (c. 20), Sch. 2.
[43] Words substituted by Coroners and Justice Act 2009 c. 25 Sch.21(1) para.3 (July 25, 2013).
[44] Words substituted by Criminal Justice Act 1982 (c.48), ss. 38, 46.
[45] S.5(a) and (b) and word substituted for words by Coroners and Justice Act 2009 c. 25 Sch.21(1) para.4 (July 25, 2013).
[46] Words substituted by Transfer of Functions (Registration) Order 2008/678 Sch.2 para.3(2)(a) (April 3, 2008).
[47] Words repealed by Transfer of Functions (Registration) Order 2008/678 Sch.2 para.3(2)(b) (April 3, 2008).
[48] Repealed by Public Health Act 1936 (c. 49), s. 346, Sch. 3 and Public Health (London) Act 1936 (c. 50), Sch. 7.

Application to cremation

10. The power to make regulations under section seven of the Cremation Act 1902 shall **A1–011**
include a power to make regulations for the purpose of applying the provisions of this Act
to cases where human remains are disposed of by cremation, and except as may be provided
by any such regulations this Act shall not apply to cremation.

Penalties

11. Any person contravening any of the provisions of this Act in respect of which no **A1–012**
penalty is expressly imposed shall be liable on summary conviction to a fine not exceeding
[level 1 on the standard scale].[49]

Definitions

12. In this Act, unless the context otherwise requires— **A1–013**

"Prescribed" means prescribed by the Registrar-General with the concurrence of [the
Secretary of State];[50]
"Registrar" means, with respect to any death or birth the registrar who is the registrar for
the sub-district in which the death or birth takes place;
"disposal" means disposal by burial, cremation or any other means, and "disposed of" has
a corresponding meaning;
"person effecting the disposal" means the person by whom or whose officer the register
of burials in which the disposal is to be registered is kept, except that in the case of
a burial under the Burial Laws Amendment Act 1880 in the churchyard or graveyard
of a parish or ecclesiastical district the expression "person effecting the disposal" shall
be construed as referring to the relative, friend, or legal representative having charge
of or being responsible for the burial of the deceased person;
"still-born" and "still-birth" shall apply to any child which has issued forth from its
mother after the [twenty-fourth week][51] of pregnancy and which did not at any time
after being completely expelled from its mother, breathe or show any other signs of
life.

Repeals, extent, short title and commencement

13.—[. . .][52] **A1–014**
(2) This Act shall not apply to Scotland or Northern Ireland.
(3) This Act may be cited as the Births and Deaths Registration Act 1926 [. . .][53]
[. . .][52]

---

[49] Words substituted by Criminal Justice Act 1982 (c.48), ss. 38, 46.
[50] Words substituted by Transfer of Functions (Registration) Order 2008/678 Sch.2 para.3(3) (April 3, 2008).
[51] Words substituted in both places where they occur by Still-Birth (Definition) Act 1992 c. 29 s.1(1) (October 1, 1992).
[52] Repealed by Statute Law Revision Act 1950 (c. 6).
[53] Words repealed by Births and Deaths Registration Act 1953 (c. 20), Sch. 2.

Births and Deaths Registration Act 1953 c. 20

Particulars of deaths to be registered

A1–015   **15.** Subject to the provisions of this Part of this Act, the death of every person dying in England or Wales and the cause thereof shall be registered by the registrar of births and deaths for the sub-district in which the death occurred by entering in a register kept for that sub-district such particulars concerning the death as may be prescribed:

Provided that where a dead body is found and no information as to the place of death is available, the death shall be registered by the registrar of births and deaths for the sub-district in which the body is found.

Information concerning death in a house

A1–016   **16.**—(1) The following provisions of this section shall have effect where a person dies in a house.

(2) The following persons shall be qualified to give information concerning the death, that is to say—

(a) any relative of the deceased person present at the death or in attendance during his last illness;

(b) any other relative of the deceased residing or being in the sub-district where the death occurred;

(c) any person present at the death;

(d) the occupier of the house if he knew of the happening of the death;

(e) any inmate of the house who knew of the happening of the death;

(f) the person causing the disposal of the body.

(3) It shall be the duty—

(a) of the nearest relative such as is mentioned in paragraph (a) of the last foregoing subsection; or

(b) if there is no such relative, of each such relative as is mentioned in paragraph (b) of that subsection; or

(c) if there are no such relatives, of each such person as is mentioned in paragraph (c) or (d) of that subsection; or

(d) if there are no such relatives or persons as aforesaid, of each such person as is mentioned in paragraph (e) or (f) of that subsection,

to give to the registrar, before the expiration of five days from the date of the death, information to the best of his knowledge and belief of the particulars required to be registered concerning the death, and in the presence of the registrar to sign the register;

Provided that—

(i) the giving of information and the signing of the register by any one qualified informant shall act as a discharge of any duty under this subsection of every other qualified informant;

[(ii) this subsection shall not have effect if an investigation is conducted under Part 1 of the 2009 Act into the death of the deceased person and has not been discontinued under section 4 of that Act (cause of death revealed by post-mortem examination).][54]

Information concerning other deaths

17.—(1) The following provisions of this section shall have effect where a person dies elsewhere than in a house or where a dead body is found and no information as to the place of death is available.

(2) The following persons shall be qualified to give information concerning the death, that is to say—

    (a) any relative of the deceased who has knowledge of any of the particulars required to be registered concerning the death;

    (b) any person present at the death;

    (c) any person finding or taking charge of the body;

    (d) any person causing the disposal of the body.

(3) It shall be the duty—

    (a) of each such relative as is mentioned in paragraph (a) of the last foregoing subsection; or

    (b) if there are no such relatives, of each other qualified informant,

to give to the registrar, before the expiration of five days from the date of the death or of the finding of the body, such information of the particulars required to be registered concerning the death as the informant possesses, and in the presence of the registrar to sign the register:

Provided that—

    (i) the giving of information and the signing of the register by any one qualified informant shall act as a discharge of any duty under this subsection of every other qualified informant:

    [(ii) this subsection shall not have effect if an investigation is conducted under Part 1 of the 2009 Act into the death of the deceased person and has not been discontinued under section 4 of that Act (cause of death revealed by postmortem examination).][55]

A1–017

Notice preliminary to information of death

18. If, before the expiration of five days from the date of the death or of the finding of the dead body of any person, a qualified informant of that person's death sends to the registrar a written notice of the occurrence of the death or of the finding of the body accompanied by a notice given under subsection (2) of section twenty-two of this Act of the signing of a certificate of the cause of death, the information of the particulars required to be registered concerning the death need not be given before the expiration of the said five days, but shall, notwithstanding the notice, be given before the expiration of fourteen days from the date aforesaid by the person giving the notice or by some other qualified informant.

A1–018

---

[54] Substituted by Coroners and Justice Act 2009 c. 25 Sch.21(1) para.8(4) (July 25, 2013).
[55] Substituted by Coroners and Justice Act 2009 c. 25 Sch.21(1) para.9(3)(d) (July 25, 2013).

Registrar's power to require information concerning death

A1–019   **19.**—(1) Where, after the expiration of the relevant period from the date of the death or finding of the dead body of any person, the death of that person has, owing to the default of the persons required to give information concerning it, not been registered, the registrar may by notice in writing require any qualified informant—

(a) to attend personally at the registrar's office, or at some other place appointed by the registrar within his sub-district, before such date (being not less than seven days after the receipt of the notice nor more than twelve months from the date of the death or of the finding of the body) as may be specified in the notice; and

(b) to give information to the best of the informant's knowledge and belief of the particulars required to be registered concerning the death; and

(c) to sign the register in the presence of the registrar:

Provided that any such requirement shall cease to have effect if, before the date specified in the notice and before the person to whom the notice is given complies with it, either—

(i) the death is duly registered; or

[(ii) an investigation under Part 1 of the 2009 Act is conducted into the death of the deceased person and has not been discontinued under section 4 of that Act.][56]

(2) In this section, the expression "the relevant period" means—

(a) where notice has been duly given to the registrar in accordance with the last foregoing section, fourteen days;

(b) in any other case, five days.

Registration of death free of charge

A1–020   **20.** Where the registrar receives personally from any qualified informant, at any time before the expiration of twelve months from the date of the death or finding of the dead body of any person, information of the particulars required to be registered concerning that person's death, then, so soon as he has received any particulars required to be registered concerning the cause of death which are required to be given by any person other than the informant, he shall forthwith register the death and the particulars, if not previously registered, in the prescribed form and manner without any fee or reward from the informant:

[. . .][57]

Registration of death after twelve months

A1–021   **21.**—(1) After the expiration of twelve months from the date of the death or finding of the dead body of any person, the death of that person shall not be registered except with the written authority of the Registrar General and in such manner and subject to such conditions as may be prescribed, and the fact that the authority of the Registrar General has been obtained shall be entered in the register.

[. . .][58]

---

[56] Substituted by Coroners and Justice Act 2009 c. 25 Sch.21(1) para.11(3) (July 25, 2013).
[57] ???.
[58] Repealed by SI 1968/1242, Sch. 2.

(3) Any person who registers any death, or causes any death to be registered, in contravention of this section shall be liable on summary conviction to a fine not exceeding [level 1 on the standard scale].[59]

Certificates of cause of death

22.—(1) In the case of the death of any person who has been attended during his last illness by a registered medical practitioner, that practitioner shall sign a certificate in the prescribed form stating to the best of his knowledge and belief the cause of death and shall forthwith deliver that certificate to the registrar.

A1–022

(2) On signing a certificate of the cause of death under the foregoing subsection the medical practitioner shall give in the prescribed form to some qualified informant of the death notice in writing of the signing of the certificate, and that person shall, except where an inquest is held [. . .][60] touching the death of the deceased person, deliver the said notice to the registrar.

(3) [Except where an inquest is held into the death of the deceased person or a post-mortem examination of his body is made under section 19 of the Coroners Act 1988][61], a registrar to whom a certificate of case of death is delivered under subsection (1) of this section shall enter in the register the cause of death as stated in the certificate, together with the name of the certifying medical practitioner.

(4) The Registrar General shall from time to time furnish to every registrar printed forms of the certificates required to be signed by registered medical practitioners under subsection (1) of this section, and every registrar shall furnish such forms free of charge to any registered medical practitioner residing or practicing in that registrar's sub-district.

Furnishing of information by coroner

23.—[. . .][62]

A1–023

[(2) Where there has been an investigation under Part 1 of the 2009 Act into a death and the senior coroner sends to the registrar a certificate giving information concerning the death, including the particulars found under section 10(1)(b) of that Act, the registrar shall in the prescribed form and manner register the death and those particulars; and, if the death has been previously registered, those particulars shall be entered in the prescribed manner without any alteration of the original entry.][63]

[(2A) Where—

(a) an investigation under Part 1 of the 2009 Act into a death is suspended under Schedule 1 to that Act, and

(b) the senior coroner sends to the registrar a certificate stating the particulars required by this Act to be registered concerning the death (so far as they have been ascertained at the date of the certificate),

the registrar shall in the prescribed form and manner register the death and those particulars.

(2B) Where—

(a) an investigation under Part 1 of the 2009 Act into a death is suspended under paragraph 2 of Schedule 1 to that Act (suspension where certain criminal proceedings brought), and

---

[59] Words substituted by Criminal Justice Act 1982 (c.48), s. 46.
[60] Words repealed by Coroners Act 1980 (c.38), Sch. 2.
[61] Words substituted by Coroners Act 1988 (c.13), s. 36(1), Sch. 3 para. 3.
[62] Repealed by Coroners Act 1988 (c.13), s. 36(1), (2), Sch. 3 para. 4(1), Sch. 4.
[63] Substituted by Coroners and Justice Act 2009 c. 25 Sch.21(1) para.15(2) (July 25, 2013 as SI 2013/1869 art.2(o)(vi)).

(b) the senior coroner sends to the registrar a certificate—

    (i) stating the result of the proceedings in respect of the charge or charges by reason of which the investigation was suspended, or of any proceedings that had to be concluded before the investigation could be resumed, or

    (ii) setting out any changes or additions to the particulars mentioned in subsection (2A) of this section,

the registrar shall in the prescribed form and manner register the result of those proceedings, or the changes or additions, without any alteration of the original entry.

(2C) Where—

(a) an investigation under Part 1 of the 2009 Act into a death is suspended under paragraph 3 of Schedule 1 to that Act (suspension pending inquiry), and

(b) the senior coroner sends to the registrar a certificate—

    (i) stating the findings of the inquiry by reason of which the investigation was suspended,

    (ii) stating the result of any proceedings that had to be concluded before the investigation could be resumed, or

    (iii) setting out any changes or additions to the particulars mentioned in subsection (2A) of this section,

the registrar shall in the prescribed form and manner register the findings of that inquiry, or the result of those proceedings, or the changes or additions, without any alteration of the original entry.][64]

(3) [[Where an investigation is discontinued under section 4 of the 2009 Act by reason of an examination under section 14 of that Act (post-mortem examinations) and the senior coroner sends to the registrar a certificate stating][65] the cause of death as disclosed by the report of the person making the examination,][66] the registrar shall in the prescribed form and manner make an entry thereof in the register accordingly.

[Giving of information concerning a death to a person other than the registrar

A1–024   23A.—(1) Subject to subsection (2) of this section, any person required by or under this Act to give information to the registrar of the particulars required to be registered concerning a death may give that information by making and signing in the presence of and delivering to such officer as may be prescribed a declaration in writing.

(2) A declaration shall not be made under this section unless the officer in whose presence the declaration is to be made has in his possession-

(a) if no post-mortem examination of the deceased person's body is made by virtue of section 19 of the Coroners Act 1988, a copy of the certificate delivered to the registrar under subsection (1) of section 22 of this Act; or

(b) if a post-mortem examination of the deceased person's body is so made, a copy of the certificate delivered to the registrar under subsection (3) of section 23 of this Act;

---

[64] S.23(2A) to 2(2C) substituted for s.(2A) by Coroners and Justice Act 2009 c. 25 Sch.21(1) para.15(3) (July 25, 2013).

[65] Words substituted by Coroners and Justice Act 2009 c. 25 Sch.21(1) para.15(4) (July 25, 2013).

[66] Words substituted by Coroners Act 1988 (c.13), s. 36(1), Sch. 3 para. 4(4).

and the registrar shall, if so requested by the officer in whose presence the declaration is to be made, supply to that officer a copy of the certificate mentioned in paragraph (a) or, as the case may be, paragraph (b) of this subsection.

(3) The officer in whose presence a declaration is made under this section shall send the declaration to the registrar who shall in the prescribed manner enter the death in the register.

(4) An entry made under the last foregoing subsection shall be deemed for the purposes of this Act to have been signed by the person who signed the declaration and a person making a declaration under this section shall be deemed to have given information concerning the death to the registrar and to have complied with any requirement of the registrar made under this Act to attend and give that information.

(5) Where the person by whom a declaration under this section is made is a relative of the deceased person, he shall be deemed, for the purposes of determining his qualification to give the information given by making the declaration, to be in the sub-district where the death occurred.

(6) A person who, upon making a declaration under this section, delivers to the officer in whose presence the declaration is made the notice to be delivered to the registrar under subsection (2) of section 22 of this Act shall be deemed to have delivered that notice to the registrar.][67]

Certificates as to registration of death

24.—(1) The registrar, upon registering any death, shall forthwith give to the person giving information concerning the death a certificate under this hand that he has registered the death; but may, before registering the death and subject to such conditions as may be prescribed, upon receiving written notice of the occurrence of a death in respect of which he has received a certificate under section twenty-two of this Act, give to the person sending the notice, if required to do so, a certificate under his hand that he has received notice of the death; and any certificate given under this subsection shall be given without fee: **A1–025**

Provided that the registrar shall not issue any such certificate in any case in which he is satisfied that a coroner's order has been issued authorising the disposal of the body.

(2) Where the body of a deceased person has been removed into England or Wales from some place outside both those countries for disposal, and no order has been given by a coroner in respect thereof, the registrar of the sub-district in which it is intended to dispose of the body, if it appears that the death is not required by law to be registered in England or Wales, shall, upon application by the person procuring the disposal [. . .][68] give a certificate to that effect in the prescribed form.

(3) A person to whom any certificate issued by the registrar under this section is delivered shall transmit it to the person effecting the disposal of the body of the deceased person.

(4) A registrar by whom a certificate has been given under this section may, upon receiving a satisfactory explanation of any circumstances by reason of which the certificate is not available for the purposes of the enactments relating to the disposal of the bodies of dead persons, issue [. . .][68] a duplicate thereof either to the person to whom the original certificate was given or to the person effecting the disposal of the body; and any such duplicate certificate shall be in a distinctive form.

(5) Where, on the expiration of the prescribed period after the issue in respect of any deceased person of a certificate under this section or of a coroner's order authorising the disposal of the body, no notification as to the date, place and means of disposal of the body has been received by the registrar from the person effecting its disposal, the registrar shall make enquiry of the person to whom the certificate or order was issued and it shall be the duty of that person to give information to the best of his knowledge and belief as to the

---

[67] Added by Deregulation (Still-Birth and Death Registration) Order 1996/2395 art.3 (April 1, 1997).
[68] Words repealed by SI 1968/1242, Sch. 2.

person having the custody of the certificate or order, the place in which the body is lying, or, if the body has been disposed of, the person effecting the disposal.

(6) In this section, the expression "person effecting the disposal" means the person by whom or whose officer the register in which the disposal is to be recorded is kept, except that, in the case of a burial under the Burial Laws Amendment Act 1880, or section four of the Welsh Church (Burial Grounds) Act 1945, in the churchyard or graveyard of a parish or ecclesiastical district, it shall be construed as referring to the relative, friend or legal personal representative having charge of or being responsible for the burial of the deceased person.

PART III

GENERAL

Registers, certified copies, etc.

Provision of registers, etc., by Registrar General

A1–026   **25.** Registers of live-births, still-births and deaths shall be in such form as may be respectively prescribed, and the Registrar General shall provide any such registers, and any of the forms hereafter mentioned for making certified copies of entries in registers, which may be required for the purposes of this Act.

Correction of errors in registers

A1–027   **29.**—(1) No alteration shall be made in any register of live-births, still-births or deaths except as authorised by this or any other Act.

(2) Any clerical error which may from time to time be discovered in any such register may, in the prescribed manner and subject to the prescribed conditions, be corrected by any person authorised in that behalf by the Registrar General.

(3) An error of fact or substance in any such register may be corrected by entry in the margin (without any alteration of the original entry) by the officer having the custody of the register, [. . .][69] and upon production to him by that person of a statutory declaration setting forth the nature of the error and the true facts of the case made by two qualified informants of the birth or death with reference to which the error has been made, or in default of two qualified informants then [either][70] by two credible persons having knowledge of the truth of the case [or, where it applies, in accordance with section 29A of this Act.][71]

[(3B) In the case of a death in relation to which an investigation under Part 1 of the 2009 Act has been discontinued under section 4 of that Act (cause of death revealed by post-mortem examination)—

(a)   no correction under subsection (3) of this section relating to the cause of death may be made without the approval of the senior coroner concerned;

(b)   any error of fact or substance relating to the cause of death in a register of deaths may be corrected by entry in the margin (without any alteration of the original entry) by the officer having the custody of the register on being notified by the senior coroner of the nature of the error and the true facts of the case.][72]

---

[69] Words repealed by SI 1968/1242, Sch. 2.

[70] Word inserted by Deregulation (Correction of Birth and Death Entries in Registers or Other Records) Order 2002/1419 art.2(1)(a) (July 23, 2002).

[71] Words inserted by Deregulation (Correction of Birth and Death Entries in Registers or Other Records) Order 2002/1419 art.2(1)(b) (July 23, 2002).

[72] Added by Coroners and Justice Act 2009 c. 25 Sch.21(1) para.18(2) (July 25, 2013 as SI 2013/1869 art.2(o)(vii)).

[(4) Where—

(a) an error of fact or substance (other than an error relating to the cause of death) occurs in the information given by a coroner's certificate concerning [. . .][73] a death [into which he has conducted an investigation under Part 1 of the 2009 Act (other than one that has been discontinued under section 4 of that Act)];[74]
[. . .][75]
[. . .][74][76]

the coroner, if satisfied by evidence on oath or statutory declaration that such an error exists, may certify under his hand to the officer having the custody of the register in which the information is entered the nature of the error and the true facts of the case as ascertained by him on that evidence, and the error may thereupon be corrected by that officer in the register by entering in the margin (without any alteration of the original entry) the facts as the certified by the coroner.

[Alternative procedure for certain corrections

29A.—(1) [This section applies where, in an entry in a register of live-births, still-births or deaths, a person is wrongly shown as—   **A1–028**

(a) the father of the person to whose birth or death the entry relates; or

(b) a parent of that person (having been so registered on the basis of being such a parent by virtue of 42, 43 or 46(1) or (2) of the Human Fertilisation and Embryology Act 2008).][77]

(2) Where this section applies, the statutory declaration required by section 29(3) of this Act may be made—

(a) in default of two qualified informants, by one qualified informant of the birth or death to which the entry relates;

(b) in default of any qualified informant, by one credible person having knowledge of the truth of the case.

(3) Such a statutory declaration must be accompanied by documentary evidence of a finding that the person shown as the father was not the father [or, as the case may be, that the person shown as a parent was not such a parent by virtue of 42, 43 or 46(1) or (2) of the Human Fertilisation and Embryology Act 2008].[78]

(4) But subsection (5) applies if it appears to the officer having custody of the register that the only evidence on which the finding was made was that of the person making the statutory declaration.

(5) In that case, the officer may correct the error only if satisfied that another person, who is either a qualified informant or a credible person having knowledge of the truth of the case, has (whether before or since the making of the declaration) confirmed the material facts stated in the declaration.

---

[73] Words repealed by Coroners Act 1980 (c.38), Sch. 2.
[74] Words substituted by Coroners and Justice Act 2009 c. 25 Sch.21(1) para.18(3) (July 25, 2013).
[75] Repealed by Coroners and Justice Act 2009 c. 25 Sch.21(1) para.18(4) (July 25, 2013).
[76] Words substituted by Criminal Law Act 1977 (c. 45), Sch. 12.
[77] S.29A(1)(a) and (b) substituted for words by Human Fertilisation and Embryology Act 2008 c. 22 Sch.6(1) para.10(2) (April 6, 2009 for the purpose of enabling the exercise of any power to make orders, regulations or other instruments or other documents; September 1, 2009 otherwise).
[78] Words inserted by Human Fertilisation and Embryology Act 2008 c. 22 Sch.6(1) para.10(3) (April 6, 2009 for the purpose of enabling the exercise of any power to make orders, regulations or other instruments or other documents; September 1, 2009 otherwise).

(6) "Finding" means a finding made expressly in judicial proceedings in the United Kingdom or elsewhere.][79]

Offences relating to registers

A1–029   **35.** If any person commits any of the following offences, that is to say—

(a) if, being a registrar, he refuses or without reasonable cause omits to register any birth or death or particulars concerning which information has been tendered to him by a qualified informant and which he is required by or under this Act to register; or

(b) if, being a person having the custody of any register of births or register of deaths, he carelessly loses or injures the register or allows the register to be injured,

he shall be liable on summary conviction to a fine not exceeding [level 3 on the standard scale].[80]

Penalties for failure to given information, etc.

A1–030   **36.** If any person commits any of the following offences, that is to say—

(a) if, being required by or under this Act to give information concerning any birth or death [. . .][81] or any dead body, he wilfully refuses to answer any question put to him by the registrar relating to the particulars required to be registered concerning the birth or death, or save as provided in this Act, fails to comply with any requirement of the registrar made thereunder;

(b) if he refuses or fails without reasonable excuse to give, deliver or send any certificate which he is required by this Act to give, deliver or send;

(c) if, being a parent and save as provided in this Act, he fails to give information concerning the birth of his child as required by this Act; or

(d) if, being a parent of a legitimate person [. . .][82] he fails to comply with any requirement of the Registrar General made under or by virtue of section fourteen of this Act; or

(e) if, being a person upon whom a duty to give information concerning a death is imposed by paragraph (a) of subsection (3) of section sixteen or seventeen of this Act, he fails to give that information and that information is not given,

he shall be liable on summary conviction to a fine not exceeding [level 1 on the standard scale][83] for each offence.

Penalty for forging certificate, etc.

A1–031   **37.** If any person [. . .][84] falsifies any certificate, declaration or order under this Act, or knowingly uses, or gives or sends to any person, as genuine any false [. . .][84] certificate,

---

[79] Added by Deregulation (Correction of Birth and Death Entries in Registers or Other Records) Order 2002/1419 art.2(2) (July 23, 2002).

[80] Words substituted by Criminal Justice Act 1982 (c.48), ss. 38, 46.

[81] Words repealed by Children Act 1975 (c. 72), Sch. 4 Pt. VI.

[82] Words repealed by Legitimation (Re-registration of Birth) Act 1957 (c. 39), s. 1(2).

[83] Words substituted by virtue of Criminal Justice Act 1967 (c. 80), s. 92, Sch. 3 Pt. I.

[84] Words repealed by Forgery and Counterfeiting Act 1981 (c.45), s. 30, Sch. Pt. I.

declaration in order for the purposes of this Act, he shall be liable on summary conviction to a fine not exceeding [level 1 on the standard scale][85]

Prosecution of offences and application of fines

38.—(1) Subject as may be prescribed, a superintendent registrar may prosecute any person for an offence under this Act committed within his district, and any costs incurred by him in any such prosecution, being costs which are not otherwise provided for, shall be defrayed out of moneys provided by Parliament.

[. . .][86]

A1–032

Regulations

39. The Registrar General may, with the approval of the Minister, by statutory instrument make regulations—

A1–033

(a) prescribing anything which by this Act is required to be prescribed;

(b) providing that any provisions of this Act specified in the regulations, being a provision relating to the registration or entry of births, shall cease to apply in relation to still-births or, in the case of a provisions expressed by this Act not to apply in relation to still-births, shall apply in relation to still-births with such modifications, if any, as may be prescribed:

Provided that paragraph (b) of this section shall not apply in relation to section nine or eleven of this Act.

Sending documents by post

40. Any notice, information, declaration, certificate, requisition, return or other document required by or under this Act may be sent by post.

A1–034

Interpretation

41. [(1) In this Act, except where the context otherwise requires, the following expressions have the meanings hereby respectively assigned to them, that is to say—

A1–035

["the 2009 Act" means the Coroners and Justice Act 2009;][87]
"birth" includes a live-birth and a still-birth;
"disposal", in relation to a dead body, means disposal by burial, cremation or any other means, and cognate expressions shall be construed accordingly;
"father", in relation to an adopted child, means the child's natural father;
"general search" means a search conducted during any number of successive hours not exceeding six, without the object of the search being specified;
"house" includes a public institution;
"live-birth" means the birth of a child born alive;
"the Minister" means the Secretary of State;
"mother", in relation to an adopted child, means the child's natural mother;
"occupier" in relation to a public institution, includes the governor, keeper, master, matron, superintendent, or other chief resident officer, and, in relation to a house let in separate apartments or lodgings, includes any person residing in the house who is the person under whom the lodgings or separate apartments are immediately held, or his agent;

---

[85] Words substituted by Criminal Justice Act 1982 (c.48), s. 46.
[86] Repealed by Criminal Justice Act 1972 (c. 71), Sch. 6 Pt. II.
[87] Definition inserted by Coroners and Justice Act 2009 c. 25 Sch.21(1) para.21(1) (July 25, 2013 as SI 2013/1869 art.2(o)(ix)).

"particular search" means a search of the indexes covering a period not exceeding five years for a specified entry;

"public institution" means a prison, lock-up or hospital, and such other public or charitable institution as may be prescribed;

"prescribed" means prescribed by regulations made under section thirty-nine of this Act;

"qualified informant", in relation to any birth or death, means a person who is by this Act or, in the case of a birth or death occurring before the commencement of this Act, by any enactment repealed by this Act required, or stated to be qualified, to give information concerning that birth or death;

"registrar" in relation to any birth or death, means the registrar of births and deaths for the sub-district in which the birth or death takes place, or where any still-born child is found exposed or any dead body is found and no information as to the place of birth or death is available, for the sub-district in which the child or the dead body is found;

"relative" includes a relative by marriage or civil partnership;

"still-born child" means a child which has issued forth from its mother after the twenty-fourth week of pregnancy and which did not at any time after being completely expelled from its mother breathe or show any other signs of life, and the expression "still-birth" shall be construed accordingly;

"superintendent registrar" in relation to any registrar, means the superintendent registrar of births, deaths, and marriages for the district in which that registrar's sub-district is situate.

(3) A reference in this Act to an investigation under Part 1 of the 2009 Act being conducted includes a reference to the case where such an investigation has begun and—

(a) has not yet finished,

(b) is suspended under Schedule 1 to that Act (whether temporarily or otherwise), or

(c) is discontinued under section 4 of that Act.][88]

Burial Act 1857 c. 81

Bodies not to be removed from burial grounds, save under faculty, without licence of Secretary of State

A1–036   25. Except in the cases where a body is removed from one consecrated place of burial to another by faculty granted by the ordinary for that purpose, it shall not be lawful to remove any body, or the remains of any body, which may have been interred in any place of burial, without licence under the hand of one of Her Majesty's Principal Secretaries of State, and with such precautions as such Secretary of State may prescribe as the condition of such licence; and any person who shall remove any such body or remains, contrary to this enactment, or who shall neglect to observe the precautions prescribed as the condition of the licence for removal, shall, on summary conviction before any two justices of the peace, forfeit and pay for every such offence a sum not exceeding [level 1 on the standard scale].[89]

---

[88] Existing text renumbered as s.41(1) and (3) inserted by Coroners and Justice Act 2009 c. 25 Sch.21(1) para.21(2) (July 25, 2013 as SI 2013/1869 art.2(o)(x)).
[89] Words substituted by Criminal Justice Act 1982 (c.48), s. 46.

Children and Young Persons Act 1933 c. 12

PART III

PROTECTION OF CHILDREN AND YOUNG PERSONS IN RELATION TO
CRIMINAL AND SUMMARY PROCEEDINGS

General Provisions as to Proceedings in Court

Power to prohibit publication of certain matter in newspapers

39.—(1) In relation to any proceedings in any court [. . .][90], the court may direct   **A1–037**
that—

(a) no newspaper report of the proceedings shall reveal the name, address or school, or
include any particulars calculated to lead to the identification, of any child or young
person concerned in the proceedings, either as being the person [by or against][91] or
in respect of whom the proceedings are taken, or as being a witness therein:

(b) no picture shall be published in any newspaper as being or including a picture of any
child or young person so concerned in the proceedings as aforesaid;

except in so far (if at all) as may be permitted by the direction of the court.

(2) Any person who publishes any matter in contravention of any such direction shall on
summary conviction be liable in respect of each offence to a fine not exceeding [level 5 on
the standard scale][92].

Age of criminal responsibility

50. It shall be conclusively presumed that no child under the age of [ten][93] years can be   **A1–038**
guilty of any offence.

Civil Evidence Act 1968 c. 64

PART II

MISCELLANEOUS AND GENERAL

Privilege

Privilege against incrimination of self or spouse [or civil partner][94]

14.—(1) The right of a person in any legal proceedings other than criminal proceedings   **A1–039**
to refuse to answer any question or produce any document or thing if to do so would tend
to expose that person to proceedings for an offence or for the recovery of a penalty—

(a) shall apply only as regards criminal offence under the law of any part of the United
Kingdom and penalties provided for by such law; and

---

[90] Words repealed by Children and Young Persons Act 1963 (c. 37), s. 64, Sch. 5.
[91] Words substituted by Children and Young Persons Act 1963 (c. 37), s. 57(1).
[92] Words substituted by Criminal Justice Act 1982 (c. 48), s. 46.
[93] Word substituted by Children and Young Persons Act 1963 (c. 37), s. 16(1).
[94] Words inserted by Civil Partnership Act 2004 c. 33 Sch.27 para.30(b) (December 5, 2005).

(b) shall include a like right to refuse to answer any question or produce any document or thing if to do so would tend to expose the [spouse or civil partner][95] of that person to proceedings for any such criminal offence or for the recovery of any such penalty.

(2) In so far as any existing enactment conferring (in whatever words) powers of inspection or investigation confers on a person (in whatever words) any right otherwise than in criminal proceedings to refuse to answer any question or give any evidence tending to incriminate that person, subsection (1) above shall apply to that right as it applies to the right described in that subsection; and every such existing enactment shall be construed accordingly.

(3) In so far as any existing enactment provides (in whatever words) that in any proceedings other than criminal proceedings a person shall not be excused from answering any question or giving any evidence on the ground that to do so may incriminate that person, that enactment shall be construed as providing also that in such proceedings a person shall not be excused from answering any question or giving any evidence on the ground that to do so may incriminate the husband or wife of that person.

(4) Where any existing enactment (however worded) that—

(a) confers powers of inspection or investigation; or

(b) provides as mentioned in subsection (3) above,

further provides (in whatever words) that any answer or evidence given by a person shall not be admissible in evidence against that person in any proceedings or class of proceedings (however described, and whether criminal or not), that enactment shall be construed as providing also that any answer or evidence given by that person shall not be admissible in evidence against the husband or wife of that person in the proceedings or class of proceedings in question.

(5) In this section "existing enactment" means any enactment passed before this Act; and the references to giving evidence are references to giving evidence in any manner, whether by furnishing information, making discovery, producing documents or otherwise.

Constitutional Reform Act 2005 c. 4

PART 4

JUDICIAL APPOINTMENTS AND DISCIPLINE

Chapter 3 Discipline

Disciplinary powers

Disciplinary powers

A1–040   108.—(1) Any power of the Lord Chancellor to remove a person from an office listed in Schedule 14 is exercisable only after the Lord Chancellor has complied with prescribed procedures (as well as any other requirements to which the power is subject).

(2) The Lord Chief Justice may exercise any of the following powers but only with the agreement of the Lord Chancellor and only after complying with prescribed procedures.

(3) The Lord Chief Justice may give a judicial office holder formal advice, or a formal warning or reprimand, for disciplinary purposes (but this section does not restrict what he

---

[95] Words substituted by Civil Partnership Act 2004 c. 33 Sch.27 para.30(a) (December 5, 2005).

may do informally or for other purposes or where any advice or warning is not addressed to a particular office holder).

(4) He may suspend a person from a judicial office for any period during which any of the following applies—

(a) the person is subject to criminal proceedings;

(b) the person is serving a sentence imposed in criminal proceedings;

(c) the person has been convicted of an offence and is subject to prescribed procedures in relation to the conduct constituting the offence.

(5) He may suspend a person from a judicial office for any period if—

(a) the person has been convicted of a criminal offence,

(b) it has been determined under prescribed procedures that the person should not be removed from office, and

(c) it appears to the Lord Chief Justice with the agreement of the Lord Chancellor that the suspension is necessary for maintaining confidence in the judiciary.

(6) He may suspend a person from office as a senior judge for any period during which the person is subject to proceedings for an Address.

(7) He may suspend the holder of an office listed in Schedule 14 for any period during which the person—

(a) is under investigation for an offence, or

(b) is subject to prescribed procedures.

(8) While a person is suspended under this section from any office he may not perform any of the functions of the office (but his other rights as holder of the office are not affected).

Disciplinary powers: interpretation

109.—(1) This section has effect for the purposes of section 108.   **A1–041**

(2) A person is subject to criminal proceedings if in any part of the United Kingdom proceedings against him for an offence have been begun and have not come to an end, and the times when proceedings are begun and come to an end for the purposes of this subsection are such as may be prescribed.

(3) A person is subject to proceedings for an Address from the time when notice of a motion is given in each House of Parliament for an Address for the removal of the person from office, until the earliest of the following events—

(a) either notice is withdrawn;

(b) either motion is amended so that it is no longer a motion for an address for removal of the person from office;

(c) either motion is withdrawn, lapses or is disagreed to;

(d) where an Address is presented by each House, a message is brought to each House from Her Majesty in answer to the Address.

(4) "Judicial office" means—

(a) office as a senior judge, or

(b) an office listed in Schedule 14;

and "judicial office holder" means the holder of a judicial office.

(5) "Senior judge" means any of these—

  (a) Master of the Rolls;

  (b) President of the Queen's Bench Division;

  (c) President of the Family Division;

  (d) Chancellor of the High Court;

  [(da) Senior President of Tribunals;][96]

  (e) Lord Justice of Appeal;

  (f) puisne judge of the High Court.

(6) "Sentence" includes any sentence other than a fine (and "serving" is to be read accordingly).

(7) The times when a person becomes and ceases to be subject to prescribed procedures for the purposes of section 108(4) or (7) are such as may be prescribed.

(8) "Under investigation for an offence" has such meaning as may be prescribed.

Applications for review and references

Applications to the Ombudsman

A1–042   **110.**—(1) This section applies if an interested party makes an application to the Ombudsman for the review of the exercise by any person of a regulated disciplinary function, on the grounds that there has been—

  (a) a failure to comply with prescribed procedures, or

  (b) some other maladministration.

(2) The Ombudsman must carry out a review if the following three conditions are met.

(3) The first condition is that the Ombudsman considers that a review is necessary.

(4) The second condition is that—

  (a) the application is made within the permitted period,

  (b) the application is made within such longer period as the Ombudsman considers appropriate in the circumstances, or

  (c) the application is made on grounds alleging undue delay and the Ombudsman considers that the application has been made within a reasonable time.

(5) The third condition is that the application is made in a form approved by the Ombudsman.

(6) But the Ombudsman may not review the merits of a decision made by any person.

(7) If any of the conditions in subsections (3) to (5) is not met, or if the grounds of the application relate only to the merits of a decision, the Ombudsman—

  (a) may not carry out a review, and

  (b) must inform the applicant accordingly.

---

[96] Added by Tribunals, Courts and Enforcement Act 2007 c. 15 Sch.8 para.63 (September 19, 2007).

(8) In this section and sections 111 to 113, "regulated disciplinary function" means any of the following—

(a) any function of the Lord Chancellor that falls within section 108(1);

(b) any function conferred on the Lord Chief Justice by section 108(3) to (7);

(c) any function exercised under prescribed procedures in connection with a function falling within paragraph (a) or (b).

(9) In this section, in relation to an application under this section for a review of the exercise of a regulated disciplinary function—

"interested party" means—

(a) the judicial office holder in relation to whose conduct the function is exercised, or

(b) any person who has made a complaint about that conduct in accordance with prescribed procedures;

"permitted period" means the period of 28 days beginning with the latest of—

(a) the failure or other maladministration alleged by the applicant;

(b) where that failure or maladministration occurred in the course of an investigation, the applicant being notified of the conclusion or other termination of that investigation;

(c) where that failure or maladministration occurred in the course of making a determination, the applicant being notified of that determination.

(10) References in this section and section 111 to the exercise of a function include references to a decision whether or not to exercise the function.

Review by the Ombudsman

111.—(1) Where the Ombudsman is under a duty to carry out a review on an application under section 110, he must—　　**A1–043**

(a) on the basis of any findings he makes about the grounds for the application, decide to what extent the grounds are established;

(b) decide what if any action to take under subsections (2) to (7).

(2) If he decides that the grounds are established to any extent, he may make recommendations to the Lord Chancellor and Lord Chief Justice.

(3) A recommendation under subsection (2) may be for the payment of compensation.

(4) Such a recommendation must relate to loss which appears to the Ombudsman to have been suffered by the applicant as a result of any failure or maladministration to which the application relates.

(5) If the Ombudsman decides that a determination made in the exercise of a function under review is unreliable because of any failure or maladministration to which the application relates, he may set aside the determination.

(6) If a determination is set aside under subsection (5)—

(a) the prescribed procedures apply, subject to any prescribed modifications, as if the determination had not been made, and

(b) for the purposes of those procedures, any investigation or review leading to the determination is to be disregarded.

(7) Subsection (6) is subject to any direction given by the Ombudsman under this sub-section—

(a) for a previous investigation or review to be taken into account to any extent, or

(b) for any investigation or review which may form part of the prescribed procedures to be undertaken, or undertaken again.

(8) This section is subject to section 112.

Reports on reviews

A1–044   **112.**—(1) In this section references to the Ombudsman's response to an application are references to the findings and decisions referred to in section 111(1).

(2) Before determining his response to an application the Ombudsman must prepare a draft of a report of the review carried out on the application.

(3) The draft report must state the Ombudsman's proposed response.

(4) The Ombudsman must submit the draft report to the Lord Chancellor and the Lord Chief Justice.

(5) If the Lord Chancellor or the Lord Chief Justice makes a proposal that the Ombudsman's response to the application should be changed, the Ombudsman must consider whether or not to change it to give effect to that proposal.

(6) The Ombudsman must produce a final report that sets out—

(a) the Ombudsman's response to the application, including any changes made to it to give effect to a proposal under subsection (5);

(b) a statement of any proposal under subsection (5) that is not given effect to.

(7) The Ombudsman must send a copy of the final report to each of the Lord Chancellor and the Lord Chief Justice.

(8) The Ombudsman must also send a copy of the final report to the applicant, but that copy must not include information—

(a) which relates to an identified or identifiable individual other than the applicant, and

(b) whose disclosure by the Ombudsman to the applicant would (apart from this subsection) be contrary to section 139.

(9) Each copy must be signed by the Ombudsman.

(10) No part of the Ombudsman's response to an application has effect until he has complied with subsections (2) to (9).

References to the Ombudsman relating to conduct

A1–045   **113.**—(1) The Ombudsman must investigate any matter referred to him by the Lord Chancellor or the Lord Chief Justice that relates to the exercise of one or more regulated disciplinary functions.

(2) A matter referred to the Ombudsman under subsection (1) may relate to the particular exercise of a regulated disciplinary function or to specified descriptions of the exercise of such functions.

Reports on references

A1–046   **114.**—(1) Where the Ombudsman carries out an investigation under section 113 he must prepare a draft of a report of the investigation.

(2) If the investigation relates to a matter which is the subject of a review on an application under section 110, subsection (1) applies only when the Ombudsman has sent a copy of the final report on that review to the Lord Chancellor, the Lord Chief Justice and the applicant.

(3) The draft report must state the Ombudsman's proposals as to—

    (a) the findings he will make;

    (b) any recommendations he will make for action to be taken by any person in relation to the matter subject to investigation.

(4) Those findings and recommendations are referred to in this section as the Ombudsman's response on the investigation.

(5) The Ombudsman must submit the draft report to the Lord Chancellor and the Lord Chief Justice.

(6) If the Lord Chancellor or the Lord Chief Justice makes a proposal that the Ombudsman's response on the investigation should be changed, the Ombudsman must consider whether or not to change it to give effect to that proposal.

(7) The Ombudsman must produce a final report that sets out—

    (a) the Ombudsman's response on the investigation, including any changes made to it to give effect to a proposal under subsection (6);

    (b) a statement of any proposal under subsection (6) that is not given effect to.

(8) The Ombudsman must send a copy of the final report to each of the Lord Chancellor and the Lord Chief Justice.

(9) Each copy must be signed by the Ombudsman.

General

Regulations about procedures

115. The Lord Chief Justice may, with the agreement of the Lord Chancellor, make   **A1–047**
regulations providing for the procedures that are to be followed in—

    (a) the investigation and determination of allegations by any person of misconduct by judicial office holders;

    (b) reviews and investigations (including the making of applications or references) under sections 110 to 112.

Contents of regulations

116.—(1) Regulations under section 115(a) may include provision as to any of the   **A1–048**
following—

    (a) circumstances in which an investigation must or may be undertaken (on the making of a complaint or otherwise);

    (b) steps to be taken by a complainant before a complaint is to be investigated;

    (c) the conduct of an investigation, including steps to be taken by the office holder under investigation or by a complainant or other person;

    (d) time limits for taking any step and procedures for extending time limits;

    (e) persons by whom an investigation or part of an investigation is to be conducted;

    (f) matters to be determined by the Lord Chief Justice, the Lord Chancellor, the office holder under investigation or any other person;

    (g) requirements as to records of investigations;

    (h) requirements as to confidentiality of communications or proceedings;

(i) requirements as to the publication of information or its provision to any person.

(2) The regulations—

(a) may require a decision as to the exercise of functions under section 108, or functions mentioned in subsection (1) of that section, to be taken in accordance with findings made pursuant to prescribed procedures;

(b) may require that prescribed steps be taken by the Lord Chief Justice or the Lord Chancellor in exercising those functions or before exercising them.

(3) Where regulations under section 115(a) impose any requirement on the office holder under investigation or on a complainant, a person contravening the requirement does not incur liability other than liability to such procedural penalty if any (which may include the suspension or dismissal of a complaint)—

(a) as may be prescribed by the regulations, or

(b) as may be determined by the Lord Chief Justice and the Lord Chancellor or either of them in accordance with provisions so prescribed.

(4) Regulations under section 115 may—

(a) provide for any prescribed requirement not to apply if the Lord Chief Justice and the Lord Chancellor so agree;

(b) make different provision for different purposes.

(5) Nothing in this section limits the generality of section 115.

Procedural rules

A1–049   **117.**—(1) Regulations under section 115 may provide for provision of a prescribed description that may be included in the regulations to be made instead by rules made by the Lord Chief Justice with the agreement of the Lord Chancellor.

(2) But the provision that may be made by rules does not include—

(a) provision within section 116(2);

(b) provision made for the purposes of section 108(7) or (8) or 116(3).

(3) The rules are to be published in such manner as the Lord Chief Justice may determine with the agreement of the Lord Chancellor.

Extension of discipline provisions to other offices

A1–050   **118.**—(1) This Chapter applies in relation to an office designated by the Lord Chancellor under this section as it would apply if the office were listed in Schedule 14.

(2) The Lord Chancellor may by order designate any office, not listed in Schedule 14, the holder of which he has power to remove from office.

(3) An order under this section may be made only with the agreement of the Lord Chief Justice.

Delegation of functions

A1–051   **119.**—(1) The Lord Chief Justice may nominate a judicial office holder (as defined in section 109(4)) to exercise any of his functions under the relevant sections.

(2) The relevant sections are—

(a) section 108(3) to (7);

(b) section 111(2);

(c) section 112;

(d) section 116(3)(b).

Chapter 4 Interpretation Of Part 4

Interpretation of Part 4

122. In this Part—   A1–052

"appoint" includes nominate or designate (and "appointment" is to be read accordingly);

the "Commission" means the Judicial Appointments Commission;

"Head of Division" means any of these—

    (a) the Master of the Rolls;
    (b) the President of the Queen's Bench Division;
    (c) the President of the Family Division;
    (d) the Chancellor of the High Court;

"High Court" means the High Court in England and Wales;

"high judicial office" has the meaning given by section 60;

["lay member", in relation to the Commission, has such meaning as may be given by regulations under paragraph 3C(a) of Schedule 12;][97]

"Lord Chief Justice", unless otherwise stated, means the Lord Chief Justice of England and Wales;

"Lord Justice of Appeal" means a Lord Justice of Appeal in England and Wales;

"office" includes a position of any description;

the "Ombudsman" means the Judicial Appointments and Conduct Ombudsman;

"prescribed" means prescribed by regulations under section 115 or, subject to section 117(2), by rules under section 117;

"vacancy" in relation to an office to which one of sections 68, 77 and 86 applies, means a vacancy arising on a holder of the office vacating it at any time after the commencement of that section.

SCHEDULE 1

POWERS TO MAKE RULES

PART 1

THE PROCESS

Interpretation

1 In this Part "designated rules" means rules under another Act which are, by virtue of provision in   A1–053
that Act, to be made in accordance with this Part.

2 (1) It is for the Lord Chief Justice, or a judicial office holder nominated by the Lord Chief Justice
with the agreement of the Lord Chancellor, to make designated rules.

(2) The Lord Chief Justice may nominate a judicial office holder in accordance with sub-paragraph
(1)—

---

[97] Definition substituted by Crime and Courts Act 2013 c. 22 Sch.13(3) para.26 (September 4, 2013:
substitution has effect as SI 2013/2200 subject to savings and transitional provisions specified in 2013
c.22 s.15 and Sch.8).

(a) to make designated rules generally, or

(b) to make designated rules under a particular enactment.

(3) In this Part—

(a) "judicial office holder" has the same meaning as in section 109(4);

(b) references to the Lord Chief Justice's nominee, in relation to designated rules, mean a judicial office holder nominated by the Lord Chief Justice under sub-paragraph (1) to make those rules.

3 (1) The Lord Chief Justice, or his nominee, may make designated rules only with the agreement of the Lord Chancellor.

(2) If the Lord Chancellor does not agree designated rules made by the Lord Chief Justice, or by his nominee, the Lord Chancellor must give that person written reasons why he does not agree the rules.

4 (1) Designated rules made by the Lord Chief Justice, or by his nominee, and agreed by the Lord Chancellor—

(a) come into force on such day as the Lord Chancellor directs, and

(b) are to be contained in a statutory instrument to which the Statutory Instruments Act 1946 (c. 36) applies as if the instrument contained rules made by a Minister of the Crown.

(2) A statutory instrument containing designated rules is subject to annulment in pursuance of a resolution of either House of Parliament.

5 (1) This paragraph applies if the Lord Chancellor gives the Lord Chief Justice, or his nominee, written notice that he thinks it is expedient for designated rules to include provision that would achieve a purpose specified in the notice.

(2) The Lord Chief Justice, or his nominee, must make such designated rules as he considers necessary to achieve the specified purpose.

(3) Those rules must be—

(a) made within a reasonable period after the Lord Chancellor gives notice under sub-paragraph (1);

(b) made in accordance with the provisions of this Part.

Contempt of Court Act 1981 c. 49

Strict liability

The strict liability rule

1. In this Act "the strict liability rule" means the rule of law whereby conduct may be treated as a contempt of court as tending to interfere with the course of justice in particular legal proceedings regardless of intent to do so.

Limitation of scope of strict liability

2.—(1) The strict liability rule applies only in relation to publications, and for this purpose "publication" includes any speech, writing, [programme included in a cable programme service][98] or other communication in whatever form, which is addressed to the public at large or any section of the public.

(2) The strict liability rule applies only to a publication which creates a substantial risk that the course of justice in the proceedings in question will be seriously impeded or prejudiced.

---

[98] Words substituted by Broadcasting Act 1990 (c.42), s. 203(1), Sch. 20 para. 31(1)(a).

(3) The strict liability rule applies to a publication only if the proceedings in question are active within the meaning of this section at the time of the publication.

(4) Schedule 1 applies for determining the times at which proceedings are to be treated as active within the meaning of this section.

[(5) In this section "programme service" has the same meaning as in the Broadcasting Act 1990.][99]

Defence of innocent publication or distribution

3.—(1) A person is not guilty of contempt of court under the strict liability rule as the publisher of any matter to which that rule applies if at the time of publication (having taken all reasonable care) he does not know and has no reason to suspect that relevant proceedings are active.   **A1–056**

(2) A person is not guilty of contempt of court under the strict liability rule as the distributor of a publication containing any such matter if at the time of distribution (having taken all reasonable care) he does not know that it contains such matter and has no reason to suspect that it is likely to do so.

(3) The burden of proof of any fact tending to establish a defence afforded by this section to any person lies upon that person.

[. . .][100]

Contemporary reports of proceedings

4.—(1) Subject to this section a person is not guilty of contempt of court under the strict liability rule in respect of a fair and accurate report of legal proceedings held in public, published contemporaneously and in good faith.   **A1–057**

(2) In any such proceedings the court may, where it appears to be necessary for avoiding a substantial risk of prejudice to the administration of justice in those proceedings, or in any other proceedings pending or imminent, order that the publication of any report of the proceedings, or any part of the proceedings, be postponed for such period as the court thinks necessary for that purpose.

[(2A) Where in proceedings for any offence which is an administration of justice offence for the purposes of section 54 of the Criminal Procedure and Investigations Act 1996 (acquittal tainted by an administration of justice offence) it appears to the court that there is a possibility that (by virtue of that section) proceedings may be taken against a person for an offence of which he has been acquitted, subsection (2) of this section shall apply as if those proceedings were pending or imminent.][101]

(3) For the purposes of subsection (1) of this section [. . .][102] a report of proceedings shall be treated as published contemporaneously—

(a) in the case of a report of which publication is postponed pursuant to an order under subsection (2) of this section, if published as soon as practicable after that order expires;

[(b) in the case of a report of allocation or sending proceedings of which publication is permitted by virtue only of subsection (6) of section 52A of the Crime and Disorder Act 1998 ("the 1998 Act"), if published as soon as practicable after publication is so permitted;

---

[99] S. 2(5) inserted by Broadcasting Act 1990 (c.42), s. 203(1), Sch. 20, para. 31(1)(b).
[100] Repeals Administration of Justice Act 1960 (c. 65), s. 11.
[101] Added by Criminal Procedure and Investigations Act 1996 c. 25 Pt VII s.57(3) (July 4, 1996).
[102] Words repealed by Defamation Act 1996 c. 31 Sch.2 para.1 (April 1, 1999 as SI 1999/817).

(c) in the case of a report of an application of which publication is permitted by virtue only of sub-paragraph (5) or (7) of paragraph 3 of Schedule 3 to the 1998 Act, if published as soon as practicable after publication is so permitted.][103]
[. . .][104]

Discussion of public affairs

A1–058   **5.** A publication made as or as part of a discussion in good faith of public affairs or other matters of general public interest is not to be treated as a contempt of court under the strict liability rule if the risk of impediment or prejudice to particular legal proceedings is merely incidental to the discussion.

Savings

A1–059   **6.** Nothing in the foregoing provisions of this Act—

(a) prejudices any defence available at common law to a charge of contempt of court under the strict liability rule;

(b) implies that any publication is punishable as contempt of court under that rule which would not be so punishable apart from those provisions;

(c) restricts liability for contempt of court in respect of conduct intended to impede or prejudice the administration of justice.

Consent required for institution of proceedings

A1–060   **7.** Proceedings for a contempt of court under the strict liability rule (other than Scottish proceedings) shall not be instituted except by or with the consent of the Attorney General or on the motion of a court having jurisdiction to deal with it.

Other aspects of law and procedure

Confidentiality of jury's deliberations

A1–061   **8.**—(1) Subject to subsection (2) below, it is a contempt of court to obtain, disclose or solicit any particulars of statements made, opinions expressed, arguments advanced or votes cast by members of a jury in the course of their deliberations in any legal proceedings.

(2) This section does not apply to any disclosure of any particulars—

(a) in the proceedings in question for the purpose of enabling the jury to arrive at their verdict, or in connection with the delivery of that verdict, or

(b) in evidence in any subsequent proceedings for an offence alleged to have been committed in relation to the jury in the first mentioned proceedings,

or to the publication of any particulars so disclosed.

---

[103] S.4(3)(b)–(c) substituted for s.4(3)(b) by Criminal Justice Act 2003 c. 44 Sch.3(2) para.53 (June 18, 2012: substitution has effect as SI 2012/1320 subject to savings as specified in SI 2012/1320 art.6(2)).

[104] Repeals Magistrates' Courts Act 1980 (c. 43), s. 8(9) and subsequently repealed on June 18, 2012 by Criminal Justice Act 2003 (c. 44), s. 332, Sch. 37 Pt. 4 in relation to the relevant local justice areas as specified in SI 2012/1320 art.4(1)(d) subject to savings as specified in SI 2012/1320 art.5; June 18, 2012 for purposes specified in SI 2012/1320 art.4(3) subject to savings as specified in SI 2012/1320 art.5; not yet in force otherwise.

(3) Proceedings for a contempt of court under this section (other than Scottish proceedings) shall not be instituted except by or with the consent of the Attorney General or on the motion of a court having jurisdiction to deal with it.

Use of tape recorders

9.—(1) Subject to subsection (4) below, it is a contempt of court—   **A1–062**

    (a) to use in court, or bring into court for use, any tape recorder or other instrument for recording sound, except with the leave of the court;

    (b) to publish a recording of legal proceedings made by means of any such instrument, or any recording derived directly or indirectly from it, by playing it in the hearing of the public or any section of the public, or to dispose of it or any recording so derived, with a view to such publication;

    (c) to use any such recording in contravention of any conditions of leave granted under paragraph (a).

    [(d) to publish or dispose of any recording in contravention of any conditions of leave granted under subsection (1A).][105]

[(1A) In the case of a recording of Supreme Court proceedings, subsection (1)(b) does not apply to its publication or disposal with the leave of the Court.][106]

(2) Leave under paragraph (a) of subsection (1), [or under subsection (1A),][107] may be granted or refused at the discretion of the court, and [if granted—

    (a) may, in the case of leave under subsection (1)(a), and be granted subject to such conditions as the court thinks proper with respect to the use of any recording made pursuant to the leave; and

    (b) may, in the case of leave under subsection (1A), be granted subject to such conditions as the Supreme Court thinks proper with respect to publication or disposal of any recording to which the leave relates;

and][107] where leave has been granted the court may at the like discretion withdraw or amend it either generally or in relation to any particular part of the proceedings.

(3) Without prejudice to any other power to deal with an act of contempt under paragraph (a) of subsection (1), the court may order the instrument, or any recording made with it, or both, to be forfeited; and any object so forfeited shall (unless the court otherwise determines on application by a person appearing to be the owner) be sold or otherwise disposed of in such manner as the court may direct.

(4) This section does not apply to the making or use of sound recordings for purposes of official transcripts of proceedings.

[(5) See section 32 of the Crime and Courts Act 2013 for power to provide for further exceptions.][108]

---

[105] Added by Crime and Courts Act 2013 c. 22 Pt 2 s.31(4) (June 25, 2013: insertion has effect subject to savings and transitional provisions specified in 2013 c.22 s.15 and Sch.8).

[106] Added by Crime and Courts Act 2013 c. 22 Pt 2 s.31(2) (June 25, 2013: insertion has effect subject to savings and transitional provisions specified in 2013 c.22 s.15 and Sch.8).

[107] Words and s.9(2)(a) and (b) inserted for words by Crime and Courts Act 2013 c. 22 Pt 2 s.31(3) (June 25, 2013: substitution has effect subject to savings and transitional provisions specified in 2013 c.22 s.15 and Sch.8).

[108] Added by Crime and Courts Act 2013 c. 22 Pt 2 s.32(8) (July 15, 2013: insertion has effect as SI 2013/1725 subject to savings and transitional provisions specified in 2013 c.22 s.15 and Sch.8).

Sources of information

A1–063 **10.** No court may require a person to disclose, nor is any person guilty of contempt of court for refusing to disclose, the source of information contained in a publication for which he is responsible, unless it be established to the satisfaction of the court that disclosure is necessary in the interests of justice or national security or for the prevention of disorder or crime.

Publication of matters exempted from disclosure in court

A1–064 **11.** In any case where a court (having power to do so) allows a name or other matter to be withheld from the public in proceedings before the court, the court may give such directions prohibiting the publication of that name or matter in connection with the proceedings as appear to the court to be necessary for the purpose for which it was so withheld.

Offences of contempt of magistrates' courts

A1–065 **12.**—(1) A magistrates' court has jurisdiction under this section to deal with any person who—

   (a) wilfully insults the justice or justices, any witness before or officer of the court or any solicitor or counsel having business in the court, during his or their sitting or attendance in court or in going to or returning from the court; or

   (b) wilfully interrupts the proceedings of the court or otherwise misbehaves in court.

(2) In any such case the court may order any officer of the court, or any constable, to take the offender into custody and detain him until the rising of the court; and the court may, if it thinks fit, commit the offender to custody for a specified period not exceeding one month or impose on him a fine not exceeding [£2,500][109], or both.

[(2A) A fine imposed under subsection (2) above shall be deemed, for the purposes of any enactment, to be a sum adjudged to be paid by a conviction..][110]

[. . .][111]

(4) A magistrates' court may at any time revoke an order of committal made under subsection (2) and, if the offender is in custody, order his discharge.

(5) [Section 135 of the Powers of Criminal Courts (Sentencing) Act 2000 (limit on fines in respect of young persons) and the][112] following provisions of the Magistrates' Courts Act 1980 apply in relation to an order under this section as they apply in relation to a sentence on conviction or finding of guilty of an offence [; and those provisions of the Magistrates' Courts Act 1980 are][113] section 36 (restriction on fines in respect of young persons); sections 75 to 91 (enforcement); section 108 (appeal to Crown Court); section 136 (overnight detention in default of payment); and section 142(1) (power to rectify mistakes).

---

[109] Amount substituted by Criminal Justice Act 1991 c. 53 Sch.4(I) para.1 (October 1, 1992: represents law in force as at date shown).

[110] Substituted by Criminal Justice Act 1993 c. 36 Sch.3 para.6(4) (September 20, 1993).

[111] Repealed by Criminal Justice Act 1982 (c.48), s. 78, Sch. 16.

[112] Words inserted by Powers of Criminal Courts (Sentencing) Act 2000 c. 6 Sch.9 para.83(a) (August 25, 2000).

[113] Words substituted by Powers of Criminal Courts (Sentencing) Act 2000 c. 6 Sch.9 para.83(b) (August 25, 2000).

Penalties for contempt and kindred offences

Proceedings in England and Wales

14.—(1) In any case where a court has power to commit a person to prison for contempt of court and (apart from this provision) no limitation applies to the period of committal, the committal shall (without prejudice to the power of the court to order his earlier discharge) be for a fixed term, and that term shall not on any occasion exceed two years in the case of committal by a superior court, or one month in the case of committal by an inferior court.

(2) In any case where an inferior court has power to fine a person for contempt of court and (apart from this provision) no limit applies to the amount of the fine, the fine shall not on any occasion exceed [£2,500][114].

[(2A) In the exercise of jurisdiction to commit for contempt of court or any kindred offence the court shall not deal with the offender by making an order under [section 60 of the Powers of Criminal Courts (Sentencing) Act 2000][115] (an attendance centre order) if it appears to the court, after considering any available evidence, that he is under 17 years of age.][116]

[(2A) A fine imposed under subsection (2) above shall be deemed, for the purposes of any enactment, to be a sum adjudged to be paid by a conviction.][117]

[. . .][118]

(4) Each of the superior courts shall have the like power to make a hospital order or guardianship order under [section 37 of the Mental Health Act 1983][119] [or an interim hospital order under][120] [section 38 of that Act][119] in the case of a person suffering from [mental disorder within the meaning of that Act][121] who could otherwise be committed to prison for contempt of court as the Crown Court has under that section in the case of a person convicted of an offence.

[(4A) Each of the superior courts shall have the like power to make an order under [section 35 of the said Act of 1983][122] (remand for report on accused's mental condition) where there is reason to suspect that a person who could be committed to prison for contempt of court is suffering from [mental disorder within the meaning of that Act][121] as the Crown Court has under that section in the case of an accused person within the meaning of that section.][123]

[(4A) For the purposes of the preceding provisions of this section [the county court][124] shall be treated as a superior court and not as an inferior court.][125]

[(4B) The preceding provisions of this section do not apply to the family court, but—

(a) this is without prejudice to the operation of section 31E(1)(a) of the Matrimonial and Family Proceedings Act 1984 (family court has High Court's powers) in relation

---

[114] Amount substituted by Criminal Justice Act 1991 c. 53 Sch.4(I) para.1 (October 1, 1992: represents law in force as at date shown).

[115] Words substituted by Powers of Criminal Courts (Sentencing) Act 2000 c. 6 Sch.9 para.84 (August 25, 2000).

[116] Inserted by CriminalJustice Act 1982 (c.48), Sch. 14 para.60.

[117] Substituted by Criminal Justice Act 1993 c. 36 Sch.3 para.6(5) (September 20, 1993).

[118] Repealed by Criminal Justice Act 1982 (c.48), Sch. 16.

[119] Words substituted by Mental Health Act 1983 (c.20), Sch. 4 para. 57(a).

[120] Words inserted by Mental Health (Amendment) Act 1982 (c.51), Sch. 3 para. 59(a).

[121] Words substituted subject to savings/transitional provisions specified in 2007 c.12 Sch.10 para.2 by Mental Health Act 2007 c. 12 Sch.1(2) para.19 (November 3, 2008: substitution has effect subject to savings/transitional provisions specified in 2007 c.12 Sch.10 para.2).

[122] Words substituted by Mental Health Act 1983 (c. 20), Sch. 4 para. 57(b).

[123] Inserted by Mental Health (Amendment) Act 1982 (c. 51), Sch.3 para. 60.

[124] Words substituted by Crime and Courts Act 2013 c. 22 Sch.9(3) para.52(1)(b) (April 22, 2014: substitution has effect as SI 2014/954 subject to savings and transitional provisions specified in 2013 c.22 s.15 and Sch.8 and transitional provision specified in SI 2014/954 arts 2(c) and 3).

[125] Inserted by County Courts (Penalties for Contempt) Act 1983 (c. 45), ss 1, 2.

to the powers of the High Court that are limited or conferred by those provisions of this section, and

(b) section 31E(1)(b) of that Act (family court has county court's powers) does not apply in relation to the powers of the county court that are limited or conferred by those provisions of this section.][126]
    [. . .][127]

Penalties for contempt of court in Scottish proceedings

A1–067   **15.**—[Applies to Scotland]

Enforcement of fines imposed by certain superior courts

A1–068   **16.**—(1) Payment of a fine for contempt of court imposed by a superior court, other than the Crown Court or one of the courts specified in subsection (4) below, may be enforced upon the order of the court—

(a) in like manner as a judgment of the High Court for the payment of money; or

(b) in like manner as a fine imposed by the Crown Court.

(2) Where payment of a fine imposed by any court falls to be enforced as mentioned in paragraph (a) of subsection (1)—

(a) the court shall, if the fine is not paid in full forthwith or within such time as the court may allow, certify to Her Majesty's Remembrancer the sum payable;

(b) Her Majesty's Remembrancer shall thereupon proceed to enforce payment of that sum as if it were due to him as a judgment debt;
    [. . .][128]

(3) Where payment of a fine imposed by any court falls to be enforced as mentioned in paragraph (b) of subsection (1), the provisions of [sections 139 and 140 of the Powers of Criminal Courts (Sentencing) Act 2000][129] shall apply as they apply to a fine imposed by the Crown Court.

(4) Subsection (1) of this section does not apply to fines imposed by the criminal division of the Court of Appeal or by the [Supreme Court][130] on appeal from that division.

(5) The Fines Act 1833 shall not apply to a fine to which subsection (1) of this section applies.
    [. . .][131]

---

[126] Added by Crime and Courts Act 2013 c. 22 Sch.10(2) para.53 (April 22, 2014: insertion has effect as SI 2014/954 subject to savings and transitional provisions specified in 2013 c.22 s.15 and Sch.8 and transitional provision specified in SI 2014/954 arts 2(d) and 3).

[127] Provides for amendments of enactments specified in Sch. 2 Pt. III.

[128] Para.(c) and the word preceding it repealed by Supreme Court Act 1981 (c. 54), Sch. 7.

[129] Words substituted by Powers of Criminal Courts (Sentencing) Act 2000 c. 6 Sch.9 para.85 (August 25, 2000).

[130] Words substituted by Constitutional Reform Act 2005 c. 4 Sch.9(1) para.35(2) (October 1, 2009).

[131] Repealed by Employment Tribunals Act 1996 c. 17 Sch.3(I) para.1 (August 22, 1996).

Interpretation

19. In this Act—   **A1–069**

"court" includes any tribunal or body exercising the judicial power of the State, and "legal proceedings" shall be construed accordingly;

"publication" has the meaning assigned by subsection (1) of section 2, and "publish" (except in section 9) shall be construed accordingly;

"Scottish proceedings" means proceedings before any court, including the [Court Martial Appeal Court][132] [. . .][133] and the Employment Appeal Tribunal, sitting in Scotland, and includes proceedings before the [Supreme Court][134] in the exercise of any appellate jurisdiction over proceedings in such a court;

"the strict liability rule" has the meaning assigned by section 1;

"superior court" means [the Supreme Court,][135] the Court of Appeal, the High Court, the Crown Court, the [Court Martial Appeal Court][132], [. . .][133] the Employment Appeal Tribunal and any other court exercising in relation to its proceedings powers equivalent to those of the High Court [. . .][136].

Supplemental

Tribunals of Inquiry

20.—(1) In relation to any tribunal to which the Tribunals of Inquiry (Evidence) Act   **A1–070** 1921 applies, and the proceedings of such a tribunal, the provisions of this Act (except subsection (3) of section 9) apply as they apply in relation to courts and legal proceedings; and references to the course of justice or the administration of justice in legal proceedings shall be construed accordingly.

(2) The proceedings of a tribunal established under the said Act shall be treated as active within the meaning of section 2 from the time when the tribunal is appointed until its report is presented to Parliament.

Short title, commencement and extent

21.—(1) This Act may be cited as the Contempt of Court Act 1981.   **A1–071**

(2) The provisions of this Act relating to legal aid in England and Wales shall come into force on such day as the Lord Chancellor may appoint by order made by statutory instrument; and the provisions of this Act relating to legal aid in Scotland and Northern Ireland shall come into force on such day or days as the Secretary of State may so appoint.

Different days may be appointed under this subsection in relation to different courts.

(3) Subject to subsection (2), this Act shall come into force at the expiration of the period of one month beginning with the day on which it is passed.

(4) Sections 7, 8(3), 12, 13(1) to (3), 14, 16, 17 and 18, Parts I and III of Schedule 2 and Schedules 3 and 4 of this Act do not extend to Scotland.

(5) This Act, except sections 15 and 17 and Schedules 2 and 3, extends to Northern Ireland.

---

[132] Words substituted by Armed Forces Act 2006 c. 52 Sch.16 para.91 (October 31, 2009).

[133] Words repealed by Competition Act 1998 (Consequential Provisions) Order 2013/294 Sch.1 para.1 (March 10, 2013).

[134] Words substituted by Constitutional Reform Act 2005 c. 4 Sch.9(1) para.35(3) (October 1, 2009).

[135] Words inserted by Constitutional Reform Act 2005 c. 4 Sch.9(1) para.35(3) (October 1, 2009).

[136] Words repealed by Constitutional Reform Act 2005 c. 4 Sch.18(5) para.1 (October 1, 2009).

SCHEDULE 1

TIMES WHEN PROCEEDINGS ARE ACTIVE FOR PURPOSES OF SECTION 2

PRELIMINARY

A1–072   1. In this Schedule "criminal proceedings" means proceedings against a person in respect of an offence, not being appellate proceedings or proceedings commenced by motion for committal or attachment in England and Wales or Northern Ireland; and "appellate proceedings" means proceedings on appeal from or for the review of the decision of a court in any proceedings.

[**1ZA.** Proceedings under the Double Jeopardy (Scotland) Act 2011 (asp 16) are criminal proceedings for the purposes of this Schedule.][137]

[**1A** In paragraph 1 the reference to an offence includes a service offence within the meaning of the Armed Forces Act 2006.][138]

2. Criminal, appellate and other proceedings are active within the meaning of section 2 at the times respectively prescribed by the following paragraphs of this Schedule; and in relation to proceedings in which more than one of the steps described in any of those paragraphs is taken, the reference in that paragraph is a reference to the first of those steps.

CRIMINAL PROCEEDINGS

A1–073   [3. Subject to the following provisions of this Schedule, criminal proceedings are active from the relevant initial step specified in paragraph 4 or 4A until concluded as described in paragraph 5.][139]

4. The initial steps of criminal proceedings are–

(a) arrest without warrant;

(b) the issue, or in Scotland the grant, of a warrant for arrest;

(c) the issue of a summons to appear, or in Scotland the grant of a warrant to cite;

(d) the service of an indictment or other document specifying the charge;

(e) except in Scotland, oral charge [;][140]

[(f) the making of an application under section 2(2) (tainted acquittals), 3(3)(b) (admission made or becoming known after acquittal), 4(3)(b) (new evidence), 11(3) (eventual death of injured person) or 12(3) (nullity of previous proceedings) of the Double Jeopardy (Scotland) Act 2011 (asp 16).][140]

[**4A.** Where as a result of an order under section 54 of the Criminal Procedure and Investigations Act 1996 (acquittal tainted by an administration of justice offence) proceedings are brought against a person for an offence of which he has previously been acquitted, the initial step of the proceedings is a certification under subsection (2) of that section; and paragraph 4 has effect subject to this.][141]

5. Criminal proceedings are concluded—

(a) by acquittal or, as the case may be, by sentence;

(b) by any other verdict, finding, order or decision which puts an end to the proceedings;

(c) by discontinuance or by operation of law [;][141]

[(d) where the initial steps of the proceedings are as mentioned in paragraph 4(f)—

(i) by refusal of the application;

---

[137] Added by Double Jeopardy (Scotland) Act 2011 asp 16 (Scottish Act) Sch.1 para.2 (November 28, 2011).

[138] Added by Armed Forces Act 2006 c. 52 Sch.16 para.92 (October 31, 2009).

[139] Words added by Criminal Procedure and Investigations Act 1996 c. 25 Pt VII s.57(4) (July 4, 1996).

[140] Added by Double Jeopardy (Scotland) Act 2011 asp 16 (Scottish Act) Sch.1 para.3 (November 28, 2011).

[141] Para. 7(aa) inserted by Prosecution of Offences Act 1985 (c.23), s. 31(5), Sch. 1 Pt. I para. 4.

(ii) if the application is granted and within the period of 2 months mentioned in section 6(3) of the Double Jeopardy (Scotland) Act 2011 (asp 16) a new prosecution is brought, by acquittal or, as the case may be, by sentence in the new prosecution.][141]

6. The reference in paragraph 5(a) to sentence includes any order or decision consequent on conviction or finding of guilt which disposes of the case, either absolutely or subject to future events, and a deferment of sentence under [section 1 of the Powers of Criminal Courts (Sentencing) Act 2000][141], section 219 or 432 of the Criminal Procedure (Scotland) Act 1975 or Article 14 of the Treatment of Offenders (Northern Ireland) Order 1976.

7. Proceedings are discontinued within the meaning of paragraph 5(c)—

(a) in England and Wales or Northern Ireland, if the charge or summons is withdrawn or a nolle prosequi entered;

[(aa) in England and Wales, if they are discontinued by Virtue of section 23 of the Prosecution of Offences Act 1985;][141]

[(ab) in England and Wales, if they are discontinued by virtue of paragraph 11 of Schedule 17 to the Crime and Courts Act 2013 (deferred prosecution agreements);][142]

(b) in Scotland, if the proceedings are expressly abandoned by the prosecutor or are deserted simpliciter;

(c) in the case of proceedings in England and Wales or Northern Ireland commenced by arrest without warrant, if the person arrested is released, otherwise than on bail, without having been charged [;][143]

[(d) where the initial steps of the proceedings are as mentioned in paragraph 4(f) and the application is granted, if no new prosecution is brought within the period of 2 months mentioned in section 6(3) of the Double Jeopardy (Scotland) Act 2011 (asp 16).][143]

9. Criminal proceedings in England and Wales or Northern Ireland cease to be active if an order is made for the charge to lie on the file, but become active again if leave is later given for the proceedings to continue.

[**9A.** Where proceedings in England and Wales have been discontinued by virtue of section 23 of the Prosecution of Offences Act 1985, but notice is given by the accused under subsection (7) of that section to the effect that he wants the proceedings to continue, they become active again with the giving of that notice.][144]

10. Without prejudice to paragraph 5(b) above, criminal proceedings against a person cease to be active—

(a) if the accused is found to be under a disability such as to render him unfit to be tried or unfit to plead or, in Scotland, is found to be insane in bar of trial; or

(b) if a hospital order is made in his case under [section 51(5) of the Mental Health Act 1983][145] or paragraph (b) of subsection (2) of section 62 of the Mental Health Act (Northern Ireland) 1961 or, in Scotland, where [an assessment order or a treatment order ceases to have effect by virtue of sections 52H or 52R respectively of the Criminal Procedure (Scotland) Act 1995][146],

but become active again if they are later resumed.

11. Criminal proceedings against a person which become active on the issue or the grant of a warrant for his arrest cease to be active at the end of the period of twelve months beginning with the date of the warrant unless he has been arrested within that period, but become active again if he is subsequently arrested.

---

[142] Added by Crime and Courts Act 2013 c. 22 Sch.17(3) para.34 (February 24, 2014: insertion has effect subject to transitional provisions and savings specified in 2013 c.22 s.15, Sch.8 and Sch.17 para.39).

[143] Added by Double Jeopardy (Scotland) Act 2011 asp 16 (Scottish Act) Sch.1 para.5 (November 28, 2011).

[144] Para. 9A inserted by Prosecution of Offences Act 1985 (c.23), s. 31(5), Sch. 1 Pt. I para. 5.

[145] Words substituted by Mental Health Act 1983 (c.20), Sch. 4 para. 57(c).

[146] Words substituted by Mental Health (Care and Treatment) (Scotland) Act 2003 (Modification of Enactments) Order 2005/465 (Scottish SI) Sch.1 para.11(2) (September 27, 2005).

OTHER PROCEEDINGS AT FIRST INSTANCE

A1–074   **12.** Proceedings other than criminal proceedings and appellate proceedings are active from the time when arrangements for the hearing are made or, if no such arrangements are previously made, from the time the hearing begins, until the proceedings are disposed of or discontinued or withdrawn; and for the purposes of this paragraph any motion or application made in or for the purposes of any proceedings, and any pre-trial review in the county court, is to be treated as a distinct proceeding.

13. In England and Wales or Northern Ireland arrangements for the hearing of proceedings to which paragraph 12 applies are made within the meaning of that paragraph—

(a) in the case of proceedings in the High Court for which provision is made by rules of court for setting down for trial, when the case is set down;

(b) in the case of any proceedings, when a date for the trial or hearing is fixed.

14. [Applies to Scotland]

15. Appellate proceedings are active from the time when they are commenced—

(a) by application for leave to appeal or apply for review, or by notice of such an application;

(b) by notice of appeal or of application for review;

(c) by other originating process,

until disposed of or abandoned, discontinued or withdrawn.

16. Where, in appellate proceedings relating to criminal proceedings, the court—

(a) remits the case to the court below; or

(b) orders a new trial or a venire de novo, or in Scotland grants authority to bring a new prosecution,

any further or new proceedings which result shall be treated as active from the conclusion of the appellate proceedings.

Coroners Act 1988 c. 13

[[Coroner areas]^{147} : Wales

A1–075   **4A.**—[. . .]^{148}

(8) [A senior coroner]^{149} appointed for any [coroner area]^{150} in Wales—

(a) shall for all purposes be regarded as a [senior coroner]^{151} for the whole of Wales; and

---

^{147} Words substituted by Coroners and Justice Act 2009 (Consequential Provisions) Order 2013/1874 art.2(2) (July 25, 2013).

^{148} Repealed by Coroners and Justice Act 2009 c. 25 Sch.23(1) para.1 (July 25, 2013 as SI 2013/1869 art.2(p) subject to transitory modifications specified in SI 2013/1869 art.3).

^{149} Words substituted by Coroners and Justice Act 2009 (Consequential Provisions) Order 2013/1874 art.2(3)(a) (July 25, 2013).

^{150} Words substituted by Coroners and Justice Act 2009 (Consequential Provisions) Order 2013/1874 art.2(3)(b) (July 25, 2013).

^{151} Word substituted by Coroners and Justice Act 2009 (Consequential Provisions) Order 2013/1874 art.2(3)(c) (July 25, 2013).

(b) shall have the same jurisdiction, rights, powers and authorities throughout Wales as if he had been appointed as [a senior coroner][152] for the whole of Wales. [. . .][148][153]

Order to hold [investigation][154]

13.—(1) This section applies where, on an application by or under the authority of the Attorney-General, the High Court is satisfied as respects a coroner ("the coroner concerned") either—   **A1–076**

   (a) that he refuses or neglects to hold an inquest [or an investigation][155] which ought to be held; or

   (b) where an inquest [or an investigation][156] has been held by him, that (whether by reason of fraud, rejection of evidence, irregularity of proceedings, insufficiency of inquiry, the discovery of new facts or evidence or otherwise) it is necessary or desirable in the interests of justice that [an investigation (or as the case may by, another investigation)][157] should be held.

(2) The High Court may—

   (a) order an [investigation under Part 1 of the Coroners and Justice Act 2009][158] to be held into the death either—

      (i) by the coroner concerned; or

      (ii) by [a senior coroner, area coroner or assistant coroner in the same coroner area][159];

   (b) order the coroner concerned to pay such costs of and incidental to the application as to the court may appear just; and

   (c) where an inquest has been held, quash [any inquisition on, or determination or finding made at][160] that inquest.

[. . .][161]

---

[152] Word substituted by Coroners and Justice Act 2009 (Consequential Provisions) Order 2013/1874 art.2(3)(d) (July 25, 2013).

[153] Added by Local Government (Wales) Act 1994 c. 19 Sch.16 para.82(5) (April 3, 1995 for purposes specified in SI 12995/852 Sch.5; April 1, 1996 otherwise).

[154] Word substituted by Coroners and Justice Act 2009 (Consequential Provisions) Order 2013/1874 art.2(4) (July 25, 2013).

[155] Words inserted by Coroners and Justice Act 2009 (Consequential Provisions) Order 2013/1874 art.2(5)(a) (July 25, 2013).

[156] Words inserted by Coroners and Justice Act 2009 (Consequential Provisions) Order 2013/1874 art.2(5)(b)(i) (July 25, 2013).

[157] Words substituted by Coroners and Justice Act 2009 (Consequential Provisions) Order 2013/1874 art.2(5)(b)(ii) (July 25, 2013).

[158] Words substituted by Coroners and Justice Act 2009 (Consequential Provisions) Order 2013/1874 art.2(5)(c) (July 25, 2013).

[159] Words substituted by Coroners and Justice Act 2009 (Consequential Provisions) Order 2013/1874 art.2(5)(d) (July 25, 2013).

[160] Words substituted by Coroners and Justice Act 2009 (Consequential Provisions) Order 2013/1874 art.2(5)(e) (July 25, 2013).

[161] Repealed by Coroners and Justice Act 2009 c. 25 Sch.23(1) para.1 (July 25, 2013 as SI 2013/1869 art.2(p) subject to transitory modifications specified in SI 2013/1869 art.3).

[(4) For the purposes of this section, "coroner" means a coroner appointed under section 1 of this Act, or a senior coroner, area coroner or assistant coroner appointed under the Coroners and Justice Act 2009.][162]

Coroners and Justice Act 2009 c. 25

Part 1

Coroners Etc

Chapter 1 Investigations Into Deaths

Duty to investigate

Duty to investigate certain deaths

A1–077   **1.**—(1) A senior coroner who is made aware that the body of a deceased person is within that coroner's area must as soon as practicable conduct an investigation into the person's death if subsection (2) applies.

(2) This subsection applies if the coroner has reason to suspect that—

(a) the deceased died a violent or unnatural death,

(b) the cause of death is unknown, or

(c) the deceased died while in custody or otherwise in state detention.

(3) Subsection (1) is subject to sections 2 to 4.

(4) A senior coroner who has reason to believe that—

(a) a death has occurred in or near the coroner's area,

(b) the circumstances of the death are such that there should be an investigation into it, and

(c) the duty to conduct an investigation into the death under subsection (1) does not arise because of the destruction, loss or absence of the body,

may report the matter to the Chief Coroner.

(5) On receiving a report under subsection (4) the Chief Coroner may direct a senior coroner (who does not have to be the one who made the report) to conduct an investigation into the death.

(6) The coroner to whom a direction is given under subsection (5) must conduct an investigation into the death as soon as practicable.

This is subject to section 3.

(7) A senior coroner may make whatever enquiries seem necessary in order to decide—

(a) whether the duty under subsection (1) arises;

(b) whether the power under subsection (4) arises.

(8) This Chapter is subject to Schedule 10.

---

[162] Added by Coroners and Justice Act 2009 (Consequential Provisions) Order 2013/1874 art.2(5)(f) (July 25, 2013).

Investigation by other coroner

Request for other coroner to conduct investigation

2.—(1) A senior coroner (coroner A) who is under a duty under section 1(1) to conduct   **A1–078**
an investigation into a person's death may request a senior coroner for another area (coroner
B) to conduct the investigation.

(2) If coroner B agrees to conduct the investigation, that coroner (and not coroner A)
must conduct the investigation, and must do so as soon as practicable.

(3) Subsection (2) does not apply if a direction concerning the investigation is given under
section 3 before coroner B agrees to conduct the investigation.

(4) Subsection (2) is subject to—

(a) any direction concerning the investigation that is given under section 3 after the
agreement, and

(b) section 4.

(5) A senior coroner must give to the Chief Coroner notice in writing of any request
made by him or her under subsection (1), stating whether or not the other coroner agreed
to it.

Direction for other coroner to conduct investigation

3.—(1) The Chief Coroner may direct a senior coroner (coroner B) to conduct an   **A1–079**
investigation under this Part into a person's death even though, apart from the direction, a
different senior coroner (coroner A) would be under a duty to conduct it.

(2) Where a direction is given under this section, coroner B (and not coroner A) must
conduct the investigation, and must do so as soon as practicable.

(3) Subsection (2) is subject to—

(a) any subsequent direction concerning the investigation that is given under this
section, and

(b) section 4.

(4) The Chief Coroner must give notice in writing of a direction under this section to
coroner A.

(5) A reference in this section to conducting an investigation, in the case of an
investigation that has already begun, is to be read as a reference to continuing to conduct the
investigation.

Discontinuance of investigation

Discontinuance where cause of death revealed by post-mortem examination

4.—(1) A senior coroner who is responsible for conducting an investigation under this   **A1–080**
Part into a person's death must discontinue the investigation if—

(a) an examination under section 14 reveals the cause of death before the coroner has
begun holding an inquest into the death, and

(b) the coroner thinks that it is not necessary to continue the investigation.

(2) Subsection (1) does not apply if the coroner has reason to suspect that the
deceased—

(a) died a violent or unnatural death, or

(b) died while in custody or otherwise in state detention.

(3) Where a senior coroner discontinues an investigation into a death under this section—

(a) the coroner may not hold an inquest into the death;

(b) no determination or finding under section 10(1) may be made in respect of the death.

This subsection does not prevent a fresh investigation under this Part from being conducted into the death.

(4) A senior coroner who discontinues an investigation into a death under this section must, if requested to do so in writing by an interested person, give to that person as soon as practicable a written explanation as to why the investigation was discontinued.

Purpose of investigation

Matters to be ascertained

A1–081   5.—(1) The purpose of an investigation under this Part into a person's death is to ascertain—

(a) who the deceased was;

(b) how, when and where the deceased came by his or her death;

(c) the particulars (if any) required by the 1953 Act to be registered concerning the death.

(2) Where necessary in order to avoid a breach of any Convention rights (within the meaning of the Human Rights Act 1998 (c. 42)), the purpose mentioned in subsection (1)(b) is to be read as including the purpose of ascertaining in what circumstances the deceased came by his or her death.

(3) Neither the senior coroner conducting an investigation under this Part into a person's death nor the jury (if there is one) may express any opinion on any matter other than—

(a) the questions mentioned in subsection (1)(a) and (b) (read with subsection (2) where applicable);

(b) the particulars mentioned in subsection (1)(c).

This is subject to paragraph 7 of Schedule 5.

Inquests

Duty to hold inquest

A1–082   6. A senior coroner who conducts an investigation under this Part into a person's death must (as part of the investigation) hold an inquest into the death. This is subject to section 4(3)(a).

Whether jury required

A1–083   7.—(1) An inquest into a death must be held without a jury unless subsection (2) or (3) applies.

(2) An inquest into a death must be held with a jury if the senior coroner has reason to suspect—

(a) that the deceased died while in custody or otherwise in state detention, and that either—

    (i) the death was a violent or unnatural one, or

    (ii) the cause of death is unknown,

(b) that the death resulted from an act or omission of—

    (i) a police officer, or

    (ii) a member of a service police force,

    in the purported execution of the officer's or member's duty as such, or

(c) that the death was caused by a notifiable accident, poisoning or disease.

(3) An inquest into a death may be held with a jury if the senior coroner thinks that there is sufficient reason for doing so.

(4) For the purposes of subsection (2)(c) an accident, poisoning or disease is "notifiable" if notice of it is required under any Act to be given—

(a) to a government department,

(b) to an inspector or other officer of a government department, or

(c) to an inspector appointed under section 19 of the Health and Safety at Work etc. Act 1974 (c. 37).

Assembling a jury

8.—(1) The jury at an inquest (where there is a jury) is to consist of seven, eight, nine, ten or eleven persons.   **A1–084**

(2) For the purpose of summoning a jury, a senior coroner may summon persons (whether within or without the coroner area for which that coroner is appointed) to attend at the time and place stated in the summons.

(3) Once assembled, the members of a jury are to be sworn by or before the coroner to inquire into the death of the deceased and to give a true determination according to the evidence.

(4) Only a person who is qualified to serve as a juror in the Crown Court, the High Court and the [county court],[163] under section 1 of the Juries Act 1974 (c. 23), is qualified to serve as a juror at an inquest.

(5) The senior coroner may put to a person summoned under this section any questions that appear necessary to establish whether or not the person is qualified to serve as a juror at an inquest.

Determinations and findings by jury

9.—(1) Subject to subsection (2), a determination or finding that a jury is required to make under section 10(1) must be unanimous.   **A1–085**

(2) A determination or finding need not be unanimous if—

(a) only one or two of the jury do not agree on it, and

(b) the jury has deliberated for a period of time that the senior coroner thinks reasonable in view of the nature and complexity of the case.

---

[163] Words substituted by Crime and Courts Act 2013 c. 22 Sch.9(3) para.73 (April 22, 2014: substitution has effect as SI 2014/954 subject to savings and transitional provisions specified in 2013 c.22 s.15 and Sch.8 and transitional provision specified in SI 2014/954 arts 2(c) and 3).

Before accepting a determination or finding not agreed on by all the members of the jury, the coroner must require one of them to announce publicly how many agreed and how many did not.

(3) If the members of the jury, or the number of members required by subsection (2)(a), do not agree on a determination or finding, the coroner may discharge the jury and another one may be summoned in its place.

Determinations and findings to be made

A1–086   **10.**—(1) After hearing the evidence at an inquest into a death, the senior coroner (if there is no jury) or the jury (if there is one) must—

    (a) make a determination as to the questions mentioned in section 5(1)(a) and (b) (read with section 5(2) where applicable), and

    (b) if particulars are required by the 1953 Act to be registered concerning the death, make a finding as to those particulars.

(2) A determination under subsection (1)(a) may not be framed in such a way as to appear to determine any question of—

    (a) criminal liability on the part of a named person, or

    (b) civil liability.

(3) In subsection (2) "criminal liability" includes liability in respect of a service offence.

Suspension

Duty or power to suspend or resume investigations

A1–087   **11.** Schedule 1 makes provision about suspension and resumption of investigations.

Death of service personnel abroad

Investigation in Scotland

A1–088   **12.**—(1) This section applies to the death outside the United Kingdom of a person within subsection (2) or (3).

(2) A person is within this subsection if at the time of the death the person was subject to service law by virtue of section 367 of the Armed Forces Act 2006 (c. 52) and was engaged in—

    (a) active service,

    (b) activities carried on in preparation for, or directly in support of, active service, or

    (c) training carried out in order to improve or maintain the effectiveness of those engaged in active service.

(3) A person is within this subsection if at the time of the death the person was not subject to service law but—

    (a) by virtue of paragraph 7 of Schedule 15 to the Armed Forces Act 2006 was a civilian subject to service discipline, and

    (b) was accompanying persons subject to service law who were engaged in active service.

(4) If—

(a) the person's body is within Scotland or is expected to be brought to the United Kingdom, and

(b) the Secretary of State thinks that it may be appropriate for the circumstances of the death to be investigated under the Fatal Accidents and Sudden Deaths Inquiry (Scotland) Act 1976 (c. 14),

the Secretary of State may notify the Lord Advocate accordingly.

(5) If—

(a) the person's body is within England and Wales, and

(b) the Chief Coroner thinks that it may be appropriate for the circumstances of the death to be investigated under that Act,

the Chief Coroner may notify the Lord Advocate accordingly.

Investigation in England and Wales despite body being brought to Scotland

13.—(1) The Chief Coroner may direct a senior coroner to conduct an investigation into **A1–089** a person's death if—

(a) the deceased is a person within subsection (2) or (3) of section 12,

(b) the Lord Advocate has been notified under subsection (4) or (5) of that section in relation to the death,

(c) the body of the deceased has been brought to Scotland,

(d) no inquiry into the circumstances of the death under the Fatal Accidents and Sudden Deaths Inquiry (Scotland) Act 1976 (c. 14) has been held (or any such inquiry that has been started has not been concluded),

(e) the Lord Advocate notifies the Chief Coroner that, in the Lord Advocate's view, it may be appropriate for an investigation under this Part into the death to be conducted, and

(f) the Chief Coroner has reason to suspect that—

(i) the deceased died a violent or unnatural death,
(ii) the cause of death is unknown, or
(iii) the deceased died while in custody or otherwise in state detention.

(2) The coroner to whom a direction is given under subsection (1) must conduct an investigation into the death as soon as practicable.
This is subject to section 3.

Ancillary powers of coroners in relation to deaths

Post-mortem examinations

14.—(1) A senior coroner may request a suitable practitioner to make a post-mortem **A1–090** examination of a body if—

(a) the coroner is responsible for conducting an investigation under this Part into the death of the person in question, or

(b) a post-mortem examination is necessary to enable the coroner to decide whether the death is one into which the coroner has a duty under section 1(1) to conduct an investigation.

(2) A request under subsection (1) may specify the kind of examination to be made.

(3) For the purposes of subsection (1) a person is a suitable practitioner if he or she—

(a) is a registered medical practitioner, or

(b) in a case where a particular kind of examination is requested, a practitioner of a description designated by the Chief Coroner as suitable to make examinations of that kind.

(4) Where a person informs the senior coroner that, in the informant's opinion, death was caused wholly or partly by the improper or negligent treatment of a registered medical practitioner or other person, that practitioner or other person—

(a) must not make, or assist at, an examination under this section of the body, but

(b) is entitled to be represented at such an examination.

This subsection has no effect as regards a post-mortem examination already made.

(5) A person who makes a post-mortem examination under this section must as soon as practicable report the result of the examination to the senior coroner in whatever form the coroner requires.

Power to remove body

A1–091   15.—(1) A senior coroner who—

(a) is responsible for conducting an investigation under this Part into a person's death, or

(b) needs to request a post-mortem examination under section 14 in order to decide whether the death is one into which the coroner has a duty under section 1(1) to conduct an investigation,

may order the body to be removed to any suitable place.

(2) That place may be within the coroner's area or elsewhere.

(3) The senior coroner may not order the removal of a body under this section to a place provided by a person who has not consented to its being removed there.

This does not apply to a place within the coroner's area that is provided by a district council, a county council, a county borough council, a London borough council or the Common Council.

Miscellaneous

Investigations lasting more than a year

A1–092   16.—(1) A senior coroner who is conducting an investigation under this Part into a person's death that has not been completed or discontinued within a year—

(a) must notify the Chief Coroner of that fact;

(b) must notify the Chief Coroner of the date on which the investigation is completed or discontinued.

(2) In subsection (1) "within a year" means within the period of 12 months beginning with the day on which the coroner was made aware that the person's body was within the coroner's area.

(3) The Chief Coroner must keep a register of notifications given under subsection (1).

Monitoring of and training for investigations into deaths of service personnel

17.—(1) The Chief Coroner must—

(a) monitor investigations under this Part into service deaths;

(b) secure that coroners conducting such investigations are suitably trained to do so.

(2) In this section "service death" means the death of a person who at the time of the death was subject to service law by virtue of section 367 of the Armed Forces Act 2006 (c. 52) and was engaged in—

(a) active service,

(b) activities carried on in preparation for, or directly in support of, active service, or

(c) training carried out in order to improve or maintain the effectiveness of those engaged in active service.

Chapter 2

Notification, Certification And Registration Of Deaths

Notification by medical practitioner to senior coroner

18.—(1) The Lord Chancellor may make regulations requiring a registered medical
practitioner, in prescribed cases or circumstances, to notify a senior coroner of a death of which the practitioner is aware.

(2) Before making regulations under this section the Lord Chancellor must consult—

(a) the Secretary of State for Health, and

(b) the Chief Coroner.

Medical examiners

19.—(1) [Local authorities][163a] (in England) and Local Health Boards (in Wales) must
appoint persons as medical examiners to discharge the functions conferred on medical examiners by or under this Chapter.

(2) Each [local authority][163a] or Board must—

(a) appoint enough medical examiners, and make available enough funds and other resources, to enable those functions to be discharged in its area;

(b) monitor the performance of medical examiners appointed by the [local authority][163a] or Board by reference to any standards or levels of performance that those examiners are expected to attain.

(3) A person may be appointed as a medical examiner only if, at the time of the appointment, he or she—

(a) is a registered medical practitioner and has been throughout the previous 5 years, and

(b) practises as such or has done within the previous 5 years.

[163a] Words substituted by the Health and Social Care Act 2012, s.54(2).

(4) The appropriate Minister may by regulations make—

(a) provision about the terms of appointment of medical examiners and about termination of appointment;

(b) provision for the payment to medical examiners of remuneration, expenses, fees, compensation for termination of appointment, pensions, allowances or gratuities;

(c) provision as to training—

(i) to be undertaken as a precondition for appointment as a medical examiner;
(ii) to be undertaken by medical examiners;

(d) provision about the procedure to be followed in connection with the exercise of functions by medical examiners;

(e) provision conferring functions on medical examiners;

(f) provision for functions of medical examiners to be exercised, during a period of emergency, by persons not meeting the criteria in subsection (3).

(5) Nothing in this section, or in regulations under this section, gives a [local authority][163a] or a Local Health Board any role in relation to the way in which medical examiners exercise their professional judgment as medical practitioners.

(6) In this section "the appropriate Minister" means—

(a) in relation to England, the Secretary of State;

(b) in relation to Wales, the Welsh Ministers.

(7) For the purposes of this section a "period of emergency" is a period certified as such by the Secretary of State on the basis that there is or has been, or is about to be, an event or situation involving or causing, or having the potential to cause, a substantial loss of human life throughout, or in any part of, England and Wales.

(8) A certification under subsection (7) must specify—

(a) the date when the period of emergency begins, and

(b) the date when it is to end.

(9) Subsection (8)(b) does not prevent the Secretary of State certifying a new period of emergency in respect of the same event or situation.

Medical certificate of cause of death

A1–096   20.—(1) The Secretary of State may by regulations make the following provision in relation to a death that is required to be registered under Part 2 of the 1953 Act—

(a) provision requiring a registered medical practitioner who attended the deceased before his or her death (an "attending practitioner")—

(i) to prepare a certificate stating the cause of death to the best of the practitioner's knowledge and belief (an "attending practitioner's certificate"), or
(ii) where the practitioner is unable to establish the cause of death, to refer the case to a senior coroner;

(b) provision requiring a copy of an attending practitioner's certificate to be given to a medical examiner;

(c) provision allowing an attending practitioner, if invited to do so by the medical examiner or a registrar, to issue a fresh attending practitioner's certificate superseding the existing one;

(d) provision requiring a senior coroner to refer a case to a medical examiner;

(e) provision requiring a medical examiner to make whatever enquiries appear to be necessary in order to confirm or establish the cause of death;

(f) provision requiring a medical examiner to whom a copy of an attending practitioner's certificate has been given—

    (i) to confirm the cause of death stated on the certificate and to notify a registrar that the cause of death has been confirmed, or

    (ii) where the examiner is unable to confirm the cause of death, to refer the case to a senior coroner;

(g) provision for an attending practitioner's certificate, once the cause of death has been confirmed as mentioned in paragraph (f), to be given to a registrar;

(h) provision requiring a medical examiner to whom a case has been referred by a senior coroner—

    (i) to issue a certificate stating the cause of death to the best of the examiner's knowledge and belief (a "medical examiner's certificate") and to notify a registrar that the certificate has been issued, or

    (ii) where the examiner is unable to establish the cause of the death, to refer the case back to the coroner;

(i) provision for a medical examiner's certificate to be given to a registrar;

(j) provision allowing a medical examiner, if invited to do so by the registrar, to issue a fresh medical examiner's certificate superseding the existing one;

(k) provision requiring a medical examiner or someone acting on behalf of a medical examiner—

    (i) to discuss the cause of death with the informant or with some other person whom the examiner considers appropriate, and

    (ii) to give him or her the opportunity to mention any matter that might cause a senior coroner to think that the death should be investigated under section 1;

(l) provision for confirmation to be given in writing, either by the informant or by a person of a prescribed description, that the requirement referred to in paragraph (k) has been complied with;

(m) provision prescribing forms (including the form of an attending practitioner's certificate and of a medical examiner's certificate) for use by persons exercising functions under the regulations, and requiring the forms to be made available to those persons;

(n) provision requiring the Chief Medical Officer of the Department of Health, after consulting—

    (i) the Officer with corresponding functions in relation to Wales,

    (ii) the Registrar General, and

    (iii) the Statistics Board,

to issue guidance as to how certificates and other forms under the regulations are to be completed;

(o) provision for certificates or other forms under the regulations to be signed or otherwise authenticated.

(2) Regulations under subsection (1) imposing a requirement—

(a) may prescribe a period within which the requirement is to be complied with;

(b) may prescribe cases or circumstances in which the requirement does, or does not, apply (and may, in particular, provide for the requirement not to apply during a period of emergency).

(3) The power under subsection (1)(m) to prescribe forms is exercisable only after consultation with—

(a) the Welsh Ministers,

(b) the Registrar General, and

(c) the Statistics Board.

(4) Regulations under subsection (1) may provide for functions that would otherwise be exercisable by a registered medical practitioner who attended the deceased before his or her death to be exercisable, during a period of emergency, by a registered medical practitioner who did not do so.

(5) The appropriate Minister may by regulations provide for a fee to be payable to a [local authority][163b] or Local Health Board in respect of—

(a) a medical examiner's confirmation of the cause of death stated on an attending practitioner's certificate, or

(b) the issue of a medical examiner's certificate.

(6) Section 7 of the Cremation Act 1902 (c. 8) (regulations as to burning) does not require the Secretary of State to make regulations, or to include any provision in regulations, if or to the extent that he or she thinks it unnecessary to do so in consequence of—

(a) provision made by regulations under this Chapter or by Coroners regulations, or

(b) provision contained in, or made by regulations under, Part 2 of the 1953 Act as amended by Part 1 of Schedule 21 to this Act.

(7) In this section—

"the appropriate Minister" has the same meaning as in section 19;
"informant", in relation to a death, means the person who gave particulars concerning the death to the registrar under section 16 or 17 of the 1953 Act;
"period of emergency" has the same meaning as in section 19;
"the Statistics Board" means the body corporate established by section 1 of the Statistics and Registration Service Act 2007 (c. 18).

National Medical Examiner

A1–097   21.—(1) The Secretary of State may appoint a person as National Medical Examiner.
(2) The National Medical Examiner is to have—

(a) the function of issuing guidance to medical examiners with a view to securing that they carry out their functions in an effective and proportionate manner;

(b) any further functions conferred by regulations made by the Secretary of State.

(3) Before appointing a person as National Medical Examiner or making regulations under subsection (2)(b), the Secretary of State must consult the Welsh Ministers.
(4) A person may be appointed as National Medical Examiner only if, at the time of the appointment, he or she—

[163b] Words substituted by the Health and Social Care Act 2012, s.54(3).

(a) is a registered medical practitioner and has been throughout the previous 5 years, and

(b) practises as such or has done within the previous 5 years.

(5) The appointment of a person as National Medical Examiner is to be on whatever terms and conditions the Secretary of State thinks appropriate.

(6) The Secretary of State may pay to the National Medical Examiner—

(a) amounts determined by the Secretary of State by way of remuneration or allowances;

(b) amounts determined by the Secretary of State towards expenses incurred in performing functions as such.

(7) The National Medical Examiner may amend or revoke any guidance issued under subsection (2)(a).

(8) The National Medical Examiner must consult the Welsh Ministers before issuing, amending or revoking any such guidance.

(9) Medical examiners must have regard to any such guidance in carrying out their functions.

Chapter 3

Coroner Areas, Appointments Etc

Coroner areas

22. Schedule 2 makes provision about coroner areas.   A1–098

Appointment etc of senior coroners, area coroners and assistant coroners

23. Schedule 3 makes provision about the appointment etc of senior coroners, area   A1–099
coroners and assistant coroners.

Provision of staff and accommodation

24.—(1) The relevant authority for a coroner area—   A1–100

(a) must secure the provision of whatever officers and other staff are needed by the coroners for that area to carry out their functions;

(b) must provide, or secure the provision of, accommodation that is appropriate to the needs of those coroners in carrying out their functions;

(c) must maintain, or secure the maintenance of, accommodation provided under paragraph (b).

(2) Subsection (1)(a) applies to a particular coroner area only if, or to the extent that, the necessary officers and other staff for that area are not provided by a [local policing body].[164]

(3) Subsection (1)(c) does not apply in relation to accommodation the maintenance of which is the responsibility of a person other than the relevant authority in question.

---

[164] Words substituted by Police Reform and Social Responsibility Act 2011 c. 13 Sch.16(3) para.372 (July 25, 2013: substitution came into force on January 16, 2012 but could not take effect until the commencement of 2009 c.25 s.24 on July 25, 2013).

(4) In deciding how to discharge its duties under subsection (1)(b) and (c), the relevant authority for a coroner area must take into account the views of the senior coroner for that area.

(5) A reference in subsection (1) to the coroners for an area is to the senior coroner, and any area coroners or assistant coroners, for that area.

Chapter 4

Investigations Concerning Treasure

Coroner for Treasure and Assistant Coroners for Treasure

A1–101   **25.** Schedule 4 makes provision about the appointment etc of the Coroner for Treasure and Assistant Coroners for Treasure.

Investigations concerning treasure

A1–102   **26.**—(1) The Coroner for Treasure must conduct an investigation concerning an object in respect of which notification is given under section 8(1) of the Treasure Act 1996 (c. 24).

(2) The Coroner for Treasure may conduct an investigation concerning an object in respect of which notification has not been given under that section if he or she has reason to suspect that the object is treasure.

(3) The Coroner for Treasure may conduct an investigation concerning an object if he or she has reason to suspect that the object is treasure trove.

(4) Subsections (1) to (3) are subject to section 29.

(5) The purpose of an investigation under this section is to ascertain—

(a) whether or not the object in question is treasure or treasure trove;

(b) if it is treasure or treasure trove, who found it, where it was found and when it was found.

(6) Senior coroners, area coroners and assistant coroners have no functions in relation to objects that are or may be treasure or treasure trove. This is subject to paragraph 11 of Schedule 4 (which enables an assistant coroner acting as an Assistant Coroner for Treasure to perform functions of the Coroner for Treasure).

Inquests concerning treasure

A1–103   **27.**—(1) The Coroner for Treasure may, as part of an investigation under section 26, hold an inquest concerning the object in question (a "treasure inquest").

(2) A treasure inquest must be held without a jury, unless the Coroner for Treasure thinks there is sufficient reason for it to be held with a jury.

(3) In relation to a treasure inquest held with a jury, sections 8 and 9 apply with the following modifications—

(a) a reference to a senior coroner is to be read as a reference to the Coroner for Treasure;

(b) the reference in section 8(3) to the death of the deceased is to be read as a reference to the matters mentioned in section 26(5).

Outcome of investigations concerning treasure

A1–104   **28.** Where the Coroner for Treasure has conducted an investigation under section 26, a determination as to the question mentioned in subsection (5)(a) of that section, and (where applicable) the questions mentioned in subsection (5)(b) of that section, must be made—

(a) by the Coroner for Treasure after considering the evidence (where an inquest is not held),

(b) by the Coroner for Treasure after hearing the evidence (where an inquest is held without a jury), or

(c) by the jury after hearing the evidence (where an inquest is held with a jury).

Exception to duty to investigate

29.—(1) Where the Coroner for Treasure is conducting, or proposes to conduct, an   **A1–105**
investigation under section 26 concerning—

(a) an object that would vest in the Crown under the Treasure Act 1996 (c. 24) if the object was in fact treasure and there were no prior interests or rights, or

(b) an object that would belong to the Crown under the law relating to treasure trove if the object was in fact treasure trove,

the Secretary of State may give notice to the Coroner for Treasure disclaiming, on behalf of the Crown, any title that the Crown may have to the object.

(2) Where the Coroner for Treasure is conducting, or proposes to conduct, an investigation under section 26 concerning—

(a) an object that would vest in the franchisee under the Treasure Act 1996 if the object was in fact treasure and there were no prior interests or rights, or

(b) an object that would belong to the franchisee under the law relating to treasure trove if the object was in fact treasure trove,

the franchisee may give notice to the Coroner for Treasure disclaiming any title that the franchisee may have to the object.

(3) A notice under subsection (1) or (2) may be given only before the making of a determination under section 28.

(4) Where a notice is given under subsection (1) or (2)—

(a) the object is to be treated as not vesting in or belonging to the Crown, or (as the case may be) the franchisee, under the Treasure Act 1996, or the law relating to treasure trove;

(b) the Coroner for Treasure may not conduct an investigation concerning the object under section 26 or, if an investigation has already begun, may not continue with it;

(c) without prejudice to the interests or rights of others, the object may be delivered to a person in accordance with a code of practice published under section 11 of the Treasure Act 1996.

(5) For the purposes of this section the franchisee, in relation to an object, is the person who—

(a) was, immediately before the commencement of section 4 of the Treasure Act 1996, or

(b) apart from that Act, as successor in title, would have been,

the franchisee of the Crown in right of treasure trove for the place where the object was found.

Duty to notify Coroner for Treasure etc of acquisition of certain objects

A1–106   **30.**—(1) After section 8 of the Treasure Act 1996 (c. 24) there is inserted—

"8A Duty to notify coroner of acquisition of certain objects

(1) A person who—

(a) acquires property in an object, and
(b) believes or has reasonable grounds for believing—

(i) that the object is treasure, and
(ii) that notification in respect of the object has not been given under section 8(1) or this subsection,

must notify the Coroner for Treasure before the end of the notice period.

(2) The notice period is fourteen days beginning with—

(a) the day after the person acquires property in the object; or
(b) if later, the day on which the person first believes or has reason to believe—

(i) that the object is treasure; and
(ii) that notification in respect of the object has not been given under section 8(1) or subsection (1) of this section.

(3) Any person who fails to comply with subsection (1) is guilty of an offence if—

(a) notification in respect of the object has not been given under section 8(1) or subsection (1) of this section; and
(b) there has been no investigation in relation to the object.

(4) Any person guilty of an offence under this section is liable on summary conviction to—

(a) imprisonment for a term not exceeding 51 weeks;
(b) a fine of an amount not exceeding level 5 on the standard scale; or
(c) both.

(5) In proceedings for an offence under this section, it is a defence for the defendant to show that he had, and has continued to have, a reasonable excuse for failing to notify the Coroner for Treasure.

(6) If the office of Coroner for Treasure is vacant, notification under subsection (1) must be given to an Assistant Coroner for Treasure.

(7) In determining for the purposes of this section whether a person has acquired property in an object, section 4 is to be disregarded.

(8) For the purposes of an investigation in relation to an object in respect of which notification has been given under subsection (1), the object is to be presumed, in the absence of evidence to the contrary, to have been found in England and Wales after the commencement of section 4.

(9) This section has effect subject to section 8B.

(10) In this section "investigation" means an investigation under section 26 of the Coroners and Justice Act 2009.

(11) In its application to Northern Ireland this section has effect as if—

(a) in subsection (1), for "Coroner for Treasure" there were substituted "coroner for the district in which the object is located";
(b) in subsection (3)(b), for "investigation" there were substituted "inquest";
(c) in subsection (4)(a), for "51 weeks" there were substituted "three months";
(d) in subsection (5), for "Coroner for Treasure" there were substituted "coroner";
(e) in subsection (6), for the words from "Coroner for Treasure" to "Assistant Coroner for Treasure" there were substituted "coroner for a district is vacant, the person acting as coroner for that district is the coroner for the purposes of subsection (1)";

(f) in subsection (8), for "investigation" there were substituted "inquest" and for "England and Wales" there were substituted "Northern Ireland";

(g) in subsection (10), for ""investigation" means an investigation under section 26 of the Coroners and Justice Act 2009" there were substituted ""inquest" means an inquest held under section 7"."

(2) In section 10 of that Act (rewards), in subsection (5) (persons to whom reward may be paid), at the end insert—

"(d) any person who gave notice under section 8A in respect of the treasure."

(3) In relation to an offence under section 8A of that Act (inserted by subsection (1) above) committed before the commencement of section 280(2) of the Criminal Justice Act 2003 (c. 44), a reference in the inserted section to 51 weeks is to be read as a reference to three months.

Code of practice under the Treasure Act 1996

31.—(1) A code of practice under section 11 of the Treasure Act 1996 (c. 24) may make provision to do with objects in respect of which notice is given under section 29(1) or (2). **A1–107**

(2) No civil liability on the part of the Coroner for Treasure arises where he or she delivers an object, or takes any other action, in accordance with a code of practice under section 11 of the Treasure Act 1996.

Chapter 5

Further Provision To Do With Investigations And Deaths

Powers of coroners

32. Schedule 5 makes provision about powers of senior coroners and the Coroner for Treasure. **A1–108**

Offences

33. Schedule 6 makes provision about offences relating to jurors, witnesses and evidence. **A1–109**

Allowances, fees and expenses

34. Schedule 7 makes provision about allowances, fees and expenses. **A1–110**

Chapter 6

Governance Etc

Chief Coroner and Deputy Chief Coroners

35.—(1) Schedule 8 makes provision about the appointment etc of the Chief Coroner and Deputy Chief Coroners. **A1–111**

(2) The Lord Chief Justice may nominate a judicial office holder (as defined in section 109(4) of the Constitutional Reform Act 2005 (c. 4)) to exercise any of the functions of the Lord Chief Justice under Schedule 8.

Reports and advice to the Lord Chancellor from the Chief Coroner

36.—(1) The Chief Coroner must give the Lord Chancellor a report for each calendar year. **A1–112**

(2) The report must cover—

(a) matters that the Chief Coroner wishes to bring to the attention of the Lord Chancellor;

(b) matters that the Lord Chancellor has asked the Chief Coroner to cover in the report.

(3) The report must contain an assessment for the year of the consistency of standards between coroners areas.

(4) The report must also contain a summary for the year of—

(a) the number and length of—

(i) investigations in respect of which notification was given under subsection (1)(a) or (b) of section 16, and

(ii) investigations that were not concluded or discontinued by the end of the year and in respect of which notification was given under subsection (1)(a) of that section in a previous year,

as well as the reasons for the length of those investigations and the measures taken with a view to keeping them from being unnecessarily lengthy;

[. . .]¹⁶⁵

(c) the matters recorded under paragraph 4 of Schedule 5;

(d) the matters reported under paragraph 7 of that Schedule and the responses given under sub-paragraph (2) of that paragraph.

(5) A report for a year under this section must be given to the Lord Chancellor by 1 July in the following year.

(6) The Lord Chancellor must publish each report given under this section and must lay a copy of it before each House of Parliament.

(7) If requested to do so by the Lord Chancellor, the Chief Coroner must give advice to the Lord Chancellor about particular matters relating to the operation of the coroner system.

Regulations about training

A1–113   37.—(1) The Chief Coroner may, with the agreement of the Lord Chancellor, make regulations about the training of—

(a) senior coroners, area coroners and assistant coroners;

(b) the Coroner for Treasure and Assistant Coroners for Treasure;

(c) coroners' officers and other staff assisting persons within paragraph (a) or (b).

(2) The regulations may (in particular) make provision as to—

(a) the kind of training to be undertaken;

(b) the amount of training to be undertaken;

(c) the frequency with which it is to be undertaken.

---

¹⁶⁵ Repealed by Public Bodies Act 2011 c. 24 Pt 2 s.33(2) (July 25, 2013: repeal came into force on February 14, 2012 but could not take effect until the commencement of 2009 c.25 s.36(4)(b) on July 25, 2013).

Medical Adviser and Deputy Medical Advisers to the Chief Coroner

38. Schedule 9 makes provision about the appointment etc of the Medical Adviser to the   **A1–114**
Chief Coroner and Deputy Medical Advisers to the Chief Coroner.
   39. [. . .]¹⁶⁶
   40. [. . .]¹⁶⁷

Investigation by Chief Coroner or Coroner for Treasure or by judge, former judge or former coroner

41. Schedule 10 makes provision for an investigation into a person's death to be carried   **A1–115**
out by the Chief Coroner or the Coroner for Treasure or by a judge, former judge or former
coroner.

Guidance by the Lord Chancellor

42.—(1) The Lord Chancellor may issue guidance about the way in which the coroner   **A1–116**
system is expected to operate in relation to interested persons within section 47(2)(a).
   (2) Guidance issued under this section may include provision—

   (a) about the way in which such persons are able to participate in investigations under
       this Part into deaths;
       [. . .]¹⁶⁸

   (c) about the role of coroners' officers and other staff in helping such persons to
       participate in investigations [. . .]¹⁶⁹.

This subsection is not to be read as limiting the power in subsection (1).
   (3) The Lord Chancellor may amend or revoke any guidance issued under this section.
   (4) The Lord Chancellor must consult the Chief Coroner before issuing, amending or
revoking any guidance under this section.

Chapter 7

Supplementary Regulations And Rules

Coroners regulations

43.—(1) The Lord Chancellor may make regulations—   **A1–117**

   (a) for regulating the practice and procedure at or in connection with investigations
       under this Part (other than the practice and procedure at or in connection with
       inquests);

   (b) for regulating the practice and procedure at or in connection with examinations
       under section 14;

---

¹⁶⁶ Repealed, never in force, by Public Bodies (Abolition of Her Majesty's Inspectorate of Courts
   Administration and the Public Guardian Board) Order 2012/2401 Sch.1 para.34 (September 18,
   2012).
¹⁶⁷ Repealed, never in force, by Public Bodies Act 2011 c. 24 Pt 2 s.33(1) (February 14, 2012).
¹⁶⁸ Repealed by Public Bodies Act 2011 c. 24 Pt 2 s.33(2) (July 25, 2013: repeal came into force on
   February 14, 2012 but could not take effect until the commencement of 2009 c.25 s.42(2)(b) on July
   25, 2013).
¹⁶⁹ Words repealed by Public Bodies Act 2011 c. 24 Pt 2 s.33(2) (July 25, 2013: repeal came into force
   on February 14, 2012 but could not take effect until the commencement of 2009 c.25 s.42(2)(c) on
   July 25, 2013).

(c) for regulating the practice and procedure at or in connection with exhumations under paragraph 6 of Schedule 5.

Regulations under this section are referred to in this Part as "Coroners regulations".
(2) Coroners regulations may be made only if—

(a) the Lord Chief Justice, or

(b) a judicial office holder (as defined in section 109(4) of the Constitutional Reform Act 2005 (c. 4)) nominated for the purposes of this subsection by the Lord Chief Justice,

agrees to the making of the regulations.
(3) Coroners regulations may make—

(a) provision for the discharge of an investigation (including provision as to fresh investigations following discharge);

(b) provision for or in connection with the suspension or resumption of investigations;

(c) provision for the delegation by a senior coroner, area coroner or assistant coroner of any of his or her functions;

(d) provision allowing information to be disclosed or requiring information to be given;

(e) provision giving to the Lord Chancellor or the Chief Coroner power to require information from senior coroners;

(f) provision requiring a summary of specified information given to the Chief Coroner by virtue of paragraph (e) to be included in reports under section 36;

(g) provision with respect to the preservation, retention, release or disposal of bodies (including provision with respect to reinterment and with respect to the issue of orders authorising burial);

(h) provision, in relation to authorisations under paragraph 3 of Schedule 5 or entry and search under such authorisations, equivalent to that made by any provision of sections 15 and 16 of the Police and Criminal Evidence Act 1984 (c. 60), subject to any modifications the Lord Chancellor thinks appropriate;

(i) provision, in relation to the power of seizure conferred by paragraph 3(4)(a) of that Schedule, equivalent to that made by any provision of section 21 of that Act, subject to any modifications the Lord Chancellor thinks appropriate;

(j) provision about reports under paragraph 7 of that Schedule.

This subsection is not to be read as limiting the power in subsection (1).
(4) Coroners regulations may apply any provisions of Coroners rules.
(5) Where Coroners regulations apply any provisions of Coroners rules, those provisions—

(a) may be applied to any extent;

(b) may be applied with or without modifications;

(c) may be applied as amended from time to time.

Treasure regulations

A1–118   **44.**—(1) The Lord Chancellor may make regulations for regulating the practice and procedure at or in connection with investigations under this Part concerning objects that are or may be treasure or treasure trove (other than the practice and procedure at or in connection with inquests concerning such objects). Regulations under this section are referred to in this Part as "Treasure regulations" .

(2) Treasure regulations may be made only if—

(a) the Lord Chief Justice, or

(b) a judicial office holder (as defined in section 109(4) of the Constitutional Reform Act 2005 (c. 4)) nominated for the purposes of this subsection by the Lord Chief Justice,

agrees to the making of the regulations.

(3) Treasure regulations may make—

(a) provision for the discharge of an investigation (including provision as to fresh investigations following discharge);

(b) provision for or in connection with the suspension or resumption of investigations;

(c) provision for the delegation by the Coroner for Treasure (or an Assistant Coroner for Treasure) of any of his or her functions;

(d) provision allowing information to be disclosed or requiring information to be given;

(e) provision giving to the Lord Chancellor or the Chief Coroner power to require information from the Coroner for Treasure;

(f) provision requiring a summary of specified information given to the Chief Coroner by virtue of paragraph (e) to be included in reports under section 36;

(g) provision of the kind mentioned in paragraph (h) or (i) of section 43(3).

This subsection is not to be read as limiting the power in subsection (1).

(4) Treasure regulations may apply any provisions of Coroners rules.

(5) Where Treasure regulations apply any provisions of Coroners rules, those provisions—

(a) may be applied to any extent;

(b) may be applied with or without modifications;

(c) may be applied as amended from time to time.

Coroners rules

45.—(1) Rules may be made in accordance with Part 1 of Schedule 1 to the   **A1–119** Constitutional Reform Act 2005 (c. 4)—

(a) for regulating the practice and procedure at or in connection with inquests [.][170]
  [. . .][170]

Rules under this section are referred to in this Part as "Coroners rules" .

(2) Coroners rules may make—

---

[170] Repealed by Public Bodies Act 2011 c. 24 Pt 2 s.33(2) (July 3, 2013: repeal came into force on February 14, 2012 but could not take effect until the commencement of 2009 c.25 s.45(1)(b) and (c) on July 3, 2013).

(a) provision about evidence (including provision requiring evidence to be given on oath except in prescribed cases);

(b) provision for the discharge of a jury (including provision as to the summoning of new juries following discharge);

(c) provision for the discharge of an inquest (including provision as to fresh inquests following discharge);

(d) provision for or in connection with the adjournment or resumption of inquests;

(e) provision for a senior coroner to have power to give a direction, in proceedings at an inquest, allowing or requiring a name or other matter not to be disclosed except to persons specified in the direction;

(f) provision for the delegation by—

    (i) a senior coroner, area coroner or assistant coroner, or
    (ii) the Coroner for Treasure (or an Assistant Coroner for Treasure),

of any of his or her functions, except for functions that involve making judicial decisions or exercising any judicial discretion;

(g) provision with respect to the disclosure of information;

(h) provision for persons to be excused from service as jurors at inquests in cases specified in the rules;

(i) provision as to the matters to be taken into account by the Coroner for Treasure in deciding whether to hold an inquest concerning an object that is or may be treasure or treasure trove [.][171]
    [. . .][171]

(3) Coroners rules may make provision conferring power on a senior coroner or the Coroner for Treasure—

(a) to give a direction excluding specified persons from an inquest, or part of an inquest, if the coroner is of the opinion that the interests of national security so require;

(b) to give a direction excluding specified persons from an inquest during the giving of evidence by a witness under the age of 18, if the coroner is of the opinion that doing so would be likely to improve the quality of the witness's evidence.

In this subsection "specified persons" means persons of a description specified in the direction, or all persons except those of a description specified in the direction.
(4) Subsections (2) and (3) are not to be read as limiting the power in subsection (1).
(5) Coroners rules may apply—

(a) any provisions of Coroners regulations;

(b) any provisions of Treasure regulations;

(c) any rules of court that relate to proceedings other than inquests.

(6) Where any provisions or rules are applied by virtue of subsection (5), they may be applied—

(a) to any extent;

---

[171] Repealed by Public Bodies Act 2011 c. 24 Pt 2 s.33(2) (July 3, 2013: repeal came into force on February 14, 2012 but could not take effect until the commencement of 2009 c.25 s.45(2)(j) on July 3, 2013).

(b) with or without modifications;

(c) as amended from time to time.

(7) Practice directions may be given in accordance with Part 1 of Schedule 2 to the Constitutional Reform Act 2005 (c. 4) on any matter that could otherwise be included in Coroners rules.

(8) Coroners rules may, instead of providing for a matter, refer to provision made or to be made by practice directions under subsection (7).

(9) In this section "rules of court" include any provision governing the practice and procedure of a court that is made by or under an enactment.

Coroner of the Queen's household

Abolition of the office of coroner of the Queen's household

46. The office of coroner of the Queen's household is abolished.   A1–120

Interpretation

"Interested person"

47.—(1) This section applies for the purposes of this Part.   A1–121

(2) "Interested person", in relation to a deceased person or an investigation or inquest under this Part into a person's death, means—

(a) a spouse, civil partner, partner, parent, child, brother, sister, grandparent, grandchild, child of a brother or sister, stepfather, stepmother, half-brother or half-sister;

(b) a personal representative of the deceased;

(c) a medical examiner exercising functions in relation to the death of the deceased;

(d) a beneficiary under a policy of insurance issued on the life of the deceased;

(e) the insurer who issued such a policy of insurance;

(f) a person who may by any act or omission have caused or contributed to the death of the deceased, or whose employee or agent may have done so;

(g) in a case where the death may have been caused by—

    (i) an injury received in the course of an employment, or

    (ii) a disease prescribed under section 108 of the Social Security Contributions and Benefits Act 1992 (c. 4) (benefit in respect of prescribed industrial diseases, etc),

a representative of a trade union of which the deceased was a member at the time of death;

(h) a person appointed by, or representative of, an enforcing authority;

(i) where subsection (3) applies, a chief constable;

(j) where subsection (4) applies, a Provost Marshal;

(k) where subsection (5) applies, the Independent Police Complaints Commission;

(l) a person appointed by a Government department to attend an inquest into the death or to assist in, or provide evidence for the purposes of, an investigation into the death under this Part;

(m) any other person who the senior coroner thinks has a sufficient interest.

(3) This subsection applies where it appears that a person has or may have committed—

(a) a homicide offence involving the death of the deceased, or

(b) a related offence (other than a service offence).

(4) This subsection applies where it appears that a person has or may have committed—

(a) the service equivalent of a homicide offence involving the death of the deceased, or

(b) a service offence that is a related offence.

(5) This subsection applies where the death of the deceased is or has been the subject of an investigation managed or carried out by the Independent Police Complaints Commission in accordance with Part 3 of Schedule 3 to the Police Reform Act 2002 (c. 30), including that Part as extended or applied by or under any statutory provision (whenever made).

(6) "Interested person", in relation to an object that is or may be treasure or treasure trove, or an investigation or inquest under Chapter 4 concerning such an object, means—

(a) the British Museum, if the object was found or is believed to have been found in England;

(b) the National Museum of Wales, if the object was found or is believed to have been found in Wales;

(c) the finder of the object or any person otherwise involved in the find;

(d) the occupier, at the time the object was found, of the land where it was found or is believed to have been found;

(e) a person who had an interest in that land at that time or who has had such an interest since;

(f) any other person who the Coroner for Treasure thinks has a sufficient interest.

(7) For the purposes of this section, a person is the partner of a deceased person if the two of them (whether of different sexes or the same sex) were living as partners in an enduring relationship at the time of the deceased person's death.

Interpretation: general

A1–122 48.—(1) In this Part, unless the context otherwise requires—

"the 1953 Act" means the Births and Deaths Registration Act 1953 (c. 20);
"the 1988 Act" means the Coroners Act 1988 (c. 13);
"active service" means service in—

(a) an action or operation against an enemy (within the meaning given by section 374 of the Armed Forces Act 2006 (c. 52)),

(b) an operation outside the British Islands for the protection of life or property, or

(c) the military occupation of a foreign country or territory;

"area", in relation to a senior coroner, area coroner or assistant coroner, means the coroner area for which that coroner is appointed;
"area coroner" means a person appointed under paragraph 2(3) of Schedule 3;
"assistant coroner" means a person appointed under paragraph 2(4) of Schedule 3;
"Assistant Coroner for Treasure" means an assistant coroner, designated under paragraph 7 of Schedule 4, acting in the capacity of Assistant Coroner for Treasure;
"body" includes body parts;
"chief constable" means—

(a) a chief officer of police (within the meaning given in section 101(1) of the Police Act 1996 (c. 16));

(b) the Chief Constable of the Ministry of Defence Police;

(c) the Chief Constable of the Civil Nuclear Constabulary;

(d) the Chief Constable of the British Transport Police;

"the Chief Coroner" means a person appointed under paragraph 1 of Schedule 8;

"the Common Council" means the Common Council of the City of London, and "common councillor" is to be read accordingly;

"coroner area" is to be read in accordance with paragraph 1 of Schedule 2;

"the Coroner for Treasure" means a person appointed under paragraph 1 of Schedule 4;

"Coroners regulations" means regulations under section 43;

"Coroners rules" means rules under section 45;

"the coroner system" means the system of law and administration relating to investigations and inquests under this Part;

"the court of trial" means—

(a) in relation to an offence (other than a service offence) that is tried summarily, the magistrates' court by which the offence is tried;

(b) in relation to an offence tried on indictment, the Crown Court;

(c) in relation to a service offence, a commanding officer, a Court Martial or the Service Civilian Court (depending on the person before whom, or court before which, it is tried);

"Deputy Chief Coroner" means a person appointed under paragraph 2 of Schedule 8;

"document" includes information stored in an electronic form;

"enforcing authority" has the meaning given by section 18(7) of the Health and Safety at Work etc. Act 1974 (c. 37);

"functions" includes powers and duties;

"homicide offence" has the meaning given in paragraph 1(6) of Schedule 1;

"interested person" is to be read in accordance with section 47;

"land" includes premises within the meaning of the Police and Criminal Evidence Act 1984 (c. 60);

"local authority" means—

(a) in relation to England, a county council, the council of any district comprised in an area for which there is no county council, a London borough council, the Common Council or the Council of the Isles of Scilly;

(b) in relation to Wales, a county council or a county borough council;

"medical examiner" means a person appointed under section 19;

"person", in relation to an offence of corporate manslaughter, includes an organisation;

"prosecuting authority" means—

(a) the Director of Public Prosecutions, or

(b) a person of a description prescribed by an order made by the Lord Chancellor;

"related offence" has the meaning given in paragraph 1(6) of Schedule 1;

"relevant authority", in relation to a coroner area, has the meaning given by paragraph 3 of Schedule 2 (and see paragraph 2 of Schedule 22);

"senior coroner" means a person appointed under paragraph 1 of Schedule 3;

"the service equivalent of a homicide offence" has the meaning given in paragraph 1(6) of Schedule 1;

"service offence" has the meaning given by section 50(2) of the Armed Forces Act 2006 (c. 52) (read without regard to any order under section 380 of that Act) and also includes an offence under—

(a) Part 2 of the Army Act 1955 (3 & 4 Eliz. 2 c. 18) or paragraph 4(6) of Schedule 5A to that Act,

(b) Part 2 of the Air Force Act 1955 (3 & 4 Eliz. 2 c. 19) or paragraph 4(6) of Schedule 5A to that Act, or

(c) Part 1 or section 47K of the Naval Discipline Act 1957 (c. 53) or paragraph 4(6) of Schedule 4A to that Act;

"service police force" means—

(a) the Royal Navy Police,

(b) the Royal Military Police, or

(c) the Royal Air Force Police;

"state detention" has the meaning given by subsection (2);

"statutory provision" means provision contained in, or in an instrument made under, any Act (including this Act);

"treasure" means anything that is treasure for the purposes of the Treasure Act 1996 (c. 24) (and accordingly does not include anything found before 24 September 1997);

"Treasure regulations" means regulations under section 44;

"treasure trove" does not include anything found on or after 24 September 1997.

(2) A person is in state detention if he or she is compulsorily detained by a public authority within the meaning of section 6 of the Human Rights Act 1998 (c. 42).

(3) For the purposes of this Part, the area of the Common Council is to be treated as including the Inner Temple and the Middle Temple.

(4) A reference in this Part to a coroner who is responsible for conducting an investigation under this Part into a person's death is to be read as a reference to the coroner who is under a duty to conduct the investigation, or who would be under such a duty but for the suspension of the investigation under this Part.

(5) A reference in this Part to producing or providing a document, in relation to information stored in an electronic form, is to be read as a reference to producing or providing a copy of the information in a legible form.

Northern Ireland and Scotland amendments

Amendments to the Coroners Act (Northern Ireland) 1959

A1–123   **49.** [Applies to Northern Ireland]

Amendments to the Fatal Accidents and Sudden Deaths Inquiry (Scotland) Act 1976

A1–124   **50.** [Applies to Scotland]

Part 9

General

Orders, regulations and rules

A1–125   **176.**—(1) Orders or regulations made by the Secretary of State, the Lord Chancellor, the Welsh Ministers or the Chief Coroner under this Act are to be made by statutory instrument.

(2) The Statutory Instruments Act 1946 (c. 36) applies in relation to the power of the Chief Coroner under section 37 to make regulations as if the Chief Coroner were a Minister of the Crown.

[(2A) Any power of the Department of Justice in Northern Ireland to make an order under this Act is exercisable by statutory rule for the purposes of the Statutory Rules (Northern Ireland) Order 1979[172].][173]

(3) Any power conferred by this Act to make orders, regulations or rules includes power—

(a) to make provision generally or only for specified purposes, cases, circumstances or areas;

(b) to make different provision for different purposes, cases, circumstances or areas;

(c) to make incidental, supplementary, consequential, transitional, transitory or saving provision.

(4) A statutory instrument containing an order or regulations under this Act is subject to negative resolution procedure unless it is—

(a) an instrument within subsection (5), or

(b) an instrument containing an order under section 182 only.

(5) A statutory instrument containing (whether alone or with other provision)—

(a) regulations under section 20(5) setting a fee for the first time or increasing the fee by more than is necessary to reflect changes in the value of money,

(b) an order under section 40(6),

(c) an order under section 74, 75, 77 or 78,

(d) an order under section 148(1) or (3),

(e) an order under section 161(2)(a)(ii) or (4),

(f) an order under section 177 which contains provision amending or repealing any provision of an Act, or

(g) an order under paragraph 34 or 35 of Schedule 22. is subject to affirmative resolution procedure.

(6) In this section—

"affirmative resolution procedure" means—

(a) in relation to any statutory instrument made by the Secretary of State or the Lord Chancellor, a requirement that a draft of the instrument be laid before, and approved by a resolution of, each House of Parliament;

(b) in relation to any statutory instrument made by the Welsh Ministers, a requirement that a draft of the instrument be laid before, and approved by a resolution of, the National Assembly for Wales;

"negative resolution procedure" means—

(a) in relation to any statutory instrument made by the Secretary of State, Lord Chancellor or Chief Coroner, annulment in pursuance of a resolution of either House of Parliament;

---

[172] SI 1979/1573 (N.I. 12).

[173] Added by Northern Ireland Act 1998 (Devolution of Policing and Justice Functions) Order 2010/976 Sch.14 para.101(2) (April 12, 2010: insertion has effect subject to transitional provision specified in SI 2010/976 art.28).

(b) in relation to any statutory instrument made by the Welsh Ministers, annulment in pursuance of a resolution of the National Assembly for Wales.

[(7) No order may be made under this Act by the Department of Justice in Northern Ireland unless a draft of the order has been laid before, and approved by a resolution of, the Northern Ireland Assembly.

(8) Section 41(3) of the Interpretation Act (Northern Ireland) 1954 applies for the purposes of subsection (7) in relation to the laying of a draft as it applies in relation to the laying of a statutory document under an enactment.

(9) Subsection (7) does not apply to the making by the Department of Justice of—

(a) an order under section 177 which does not contain any provision amending or repealing any provision of an Act;

(b) an order under section 182;

and an order within paragraph (a) above made by the Department of Justice is subject to negative resolution (within the meaning of section 41(6) of the Interpretation Act (Northern Ireland) 1954[174]).][175]

Consequential etc amendments and transitional and saving provisions

A1–126   **177.**—(1) Schedule 21 contains minor and consequential amendments.

(2) Schedule 22 contains transitional, transitory and saving provisions.

(3) An appropriate minister may by order make—

(a) such supplementary, incidental or consequential provision, or

(b) such transitory, transitional or saving provision,

as the appropriate minister considers appropriate for the general purposes, or any particular purposes, of this Act, or in consequence of, or for giving full effect to, any provision made by this Act.

[(3A) In relation to the making of provision that could be made by an Act of the Northern Ireland Assembly without the consent of the Secretary of State (see sections 6 to 8 of the Northern Ireland Act 1998), in subsection (3) references to the appropriate minister are to be read as references to the Department of Justice in Northern Ireland.][176]

(4) An order under subsection (3) may, in particular—

(a) provide for any amendment or other provision made by this Act which comes into force before any other provision (whether made by this or any other Act or by any subordinate legislation) has come into force to have effect, until that other provision has come into force, with specified modifications, and

(b) modify any provision of—

(i) any Act (including this Act and any Act passed in the same session as this Act);

(ii) subordinate legislation made before the passing of this Act;

(iii) Northern Ireland legislation passed, or made, before the passing of this Act;

---

[174] Section 41(6) was amended by SI 1999/663.

[175] Added by Northern Ireland Act 1998 (Devolution of Policing and Justice Functions) Order 2010/976 Sch.14 para.101(3) (April 12, 2010: insertion has effect subject to transitional provision specified in SI 2010/976 art.28).

[176] Added by Northern Ireland Act 1998 (Devolution of Policing and Justice Functions) Order 2010/976 Sch.14 para.102(2) (April 12, 2010: insertion has effect subject to transitional provision specified in SI 2010/976 art.28).

(iv) any instrument made, before the passing of this Act, under Northern Ireland legislation.

(5) Nothing in this section limits the power, by virtue of section 176(3), to include incidental, supplementary, consequential, transitional, transitory or saving provision in an order under section 182 (commencement).

(6) The modifications that may be made by virtue of subsection (4)(b) are in addition to those made by, or which may be made under, any other provision of this Act.

(7) Her Majesty may by Order in Council extend any provision made by virtue of subsection (4)(b), with such modifications as may appear to Her Majesty to be appropriate, to the Isle of Man or any British overseas territory.

(8) The power under subsection (7) includes power to make supplementary, incidental, consequential, transitory, transitional or saving provision.

(9) Subsection (7) does not apply in relation to amendments of the Armed Forces Act 2006 (c. 52).

(10) In this section—

"appropriate minister" means the Secretary of State or the Lord Chancellor;
"modify" includes amend, repeal and revoke, and modification is to be construed accordingly;
"subordinate legislation" has the same meaning as in the Interpretation Act 1978 (c. 30).

Repeals

178. Schedule 23 contains repeals (including repeals of spent provisions).   A1–127

Financial provision

179. The following are to be paid out of money provided by Parliament—   A1–128

(a) any expenditure incurred by a Minister of the Crown under or by virtue of this Act;

(b) any increase attributable to this Act in the sums payable out of money so provided under any other Act.

Effect of amendments to provisions applied for purposes of service law

180.—(1) In this section "relevant criminal justice provisions" means provisions of, or   A1–129
made under, an Act which—

(a) relate to criminal justice, and

(b) are applied (with or without modifications) for any purposes of service law by any provision of, or made under, any Act.

(2) Unless the contrary intention appears, any amendment by this Act of relevant criminal justice provisions also amends those provisions as so applied.

(3) In this section "service law" means—

(a) the system of service law established by the Armed Forces Act 2006, or

(b) any of the systems of service law superseded by that Act (namely, military law, air force law and the Naval Discipline Act 1957 (c. 53)).

Extent

181.—(1) Subject to the following provisions of this section and any other provision of   A1–130
this Act, this Act extends to England and Wales only.

(2) The following provisions extend to England and Wales, Scotland and Northern Ireland—

(a) section 84;

(b) the service courts provisions of Chapter 2 of Part 3;

(c) section 143;

(d) Part 7 (except sections 158(1) and (2), 170(2) and 171 and Schedule 19);

(e) sections 176 to 183;

(f) paragraph 4 of Schedule 1;

(g) paragraphs 8, 15, 29, 42 and 45 of Schedule 22.

(3) The following provisions extend to England and Wales and Northern Ireland—

(a) sections 54, 55 and 56(1);

(b) section 61 and Schedule 12;

(c) sections 62 to 66;

(d) section 67(3);

(e) section 68 and Schedule 13;

(f) section 71;

(g) section 73;

(h) Chapter 1 of Part 3 (except section 84);

(i) Chapter 2 of that Part, and paragraphs 16 and 17 of Schedule 22, (subject to subsection (2)(b));

(j) paragraphs 7, 12(2), 39, 40 and 41 of Schedule 22.

(4) The following provisions extend to Northern Ireland only—

(a) section 49 and Schedule 11;

(b) section 67(2);

(c) paragraphs 11, 38 and 44(2) of Schedule 22.

(5) Paragraphs 34 and 35 of Schedule 22 extend to England and Wales and Scotland, and paragraph 36 of that Schedule extends to Scotland only.

(6) Except as otherwise provided by this Act, an amendment, repeal or revocation of any enactment by any provision of this Act extends to the part or parts of the United Kingdom to which the enactment extends.

(7) In section 338(1) of the Criminal Justice Act 2003 (c. 44) (power to extend the provisions of that Act to the Channel Islands etc) the reference to that Act includes a reference to that Act as amended by any provision of this Act.

(8) In section 384 of the Armed Forces Act 2006 (c. 52) (extent to Channel Islands, Isle of Man etc) any reference to that Act includes a reference to—

(a) that Act as amended by or under any provision of this Act;

(b) section 84;

(c) the service courts provisions of Chapter 2 of Part 3;

(d) section 180.

(9) In section 79(3) of the International Criminal Court Act 2001 (c. 17) (power to extend provisions of that Act to Channel Islands, Isle of Man etc) the reference to that Act includes a reference to that Act as amended by section 70.

(10) In this section "the service courts provisions of Chapter 2 of Part 3" means the provisions of Chapter 2 of Part 3, and paragraph 70 of Schedule 21 and paragraphs 16 to 22 of Schedule 22, so far as having effect in relation to service courts.

Commencement

182.—(1) The following provisions come into force on the day on which this Act is passed—

(a) sections 47 and 48;

(b) section 116;

(c) section 143;

(d) sections 151 and 152;

(e) section 154;

(f) this section and sections 176, 177(3) to (10), 179, 181 and 183;

(g) Schedule 18;

(h) paragraphs 62(3) and 94 to 98 of Schedule 21 (and section 177(1) so far as relating to those provisions);

(i) Part 1 and paragraphs 26 and 47 of Schedule 22 (and section 177(2) so far as relating to those provisions);

(j) in Schedule 23—

    (i) in Part 3, the repeals relating to the Administration of Justice (Miscellaneous Provisions) Act 1933 (c. 36) and the Supreme Court Act 1981 (c. 54),

    (ii) in Part 4, the repeals in the Criminal Justice and Immigration Act 2008 (c. 4),

    (iii) in Part 5, the repeal of section 8(6) of the Animal Welfare Act 2006 (c. 45),

    (iv) in Part 6, the repeals in sections 17 and 17A of, and Schedule 3 to, the Access to Justice Act 1999 (c. 22), and

    (v) Part 9,

and section 178 so far as relating to those repeals.

(2) The following provisions come into force at the end of the period of 2 months beginning with the day on which this Act is passed—

(a) section 73;

(b) section 138;

(c) Part 4 of Schedule 21 (and section 177(1) so far as relating to that Part);

(d) paragraph 37 of Schedule 22 (and section 177(2) so far as relating to that provision);

(e) in Part 2 of Schedule 23, the repeals relating to the following Acts—

    (i) Libel Act 1792 (c. 60),

    (ii) Criminal Libel Act 1819 (60 Geo. 3 & 1 Geo. 4 c. 8),

    (iii) Libel Act 1843 (c. 96),

    (iv) Newspaper Libel and Registration Act 1881 (c. 60),

    (v) Law of Libel Amendment Act 1888 (c. 64),

    (vi) Defamation Act 1952 (c. 66),

    (vii) Theatres Act 1968 (c. 54),

    (viii) Broadcasting Act 1990 (c. 42),

    (ix) Criminal Procedure and Investigations Act 1996 (c. 25),

  (x) Defamation Act 1996 (c. 31), and

  (xi) Legal Deposit Libraries Act 2003 (c. 28),

and section 178 so far as relating to those repeals.

(3) The following provisions come into force on 1 January 2010—

(a) Chapter 2 of Part 3;

(b) paragraphs 69 to 71 of Schedule 21 (and section 177(1) so far as relating to those provisions);

(c) paragraphs 16 to 22 of Schedule 22 (and section 177(2) so far as relating to those provisions);

(d) in Part 3 of Schedule 23, the repeals relating to the Criminal Evidence (Witness Anonymity) Act 2008 (c. 15) (and section 178 so far as relating to those repeals).

(4) The following provisions come into force on such day as the Lord Chancellor may by order appoint—

(a) Part 1 (other than sections 19, 20, 21, 47 and 48);

(b) Chapter 1 of Part 4;

(c) sections 146 to 148;

(d) sections 149, 150 and 153;

(e) Parts 1 and 8 of Schedule 21 (and section 177(1) so far as relating to those provisions);

(f) paragraphs 27, 28 and 44 of Schedule 22 (and section 177(2) so far as relating to those provisions);

(g) in Schedule 23—

  (i) the repeals in Part 1,

  (ii) the repeals in Part 4 (other than those relating to the Criminal Procedure (Scotland) Act 1995 (c. 46) and the Criminal Justice and Immigration Act 2008 (c. 4)), and

  (iii) in Part 6, the repeals of section 2(2) of, and paragraph 1(h) of Schedule 2 to, the Access to Justice Act 1999 (c. 22), and section 178 so far as relating to those repeals.

(5) The other provisions of this Act come into force on such day as the Secretary of State may by order appoint.

[(6) The power to make provision by order under subsection (4) or (5) is exercisable by the Department of Justice in Northern Ireland (and not by the Lord Chancellor or the Secretary of State) so far as it may be used to make provision which could be made by an Act of the Northern Ireland Assembly without the consent of the Secretary of State (see sections 6 to 8 of the Northern Ireland Act 1998).

(7) Before making an order under subsection (4) or (5) bringing into force any provision for the purposes of the law of Northern Ireland, the Lord Chancellor or the Secretary of State must consult the Department of Justice.][177]

---

[177] Added by Northern Ireland Act 1998 (Devolution of Policing and Justice Functions) Order 2010/976 Sch.14 para.103(2) (April 12, 2010: insertion has effect subject to transitional provision specified in SI 2010/976 art.28).

Short title

183. This Act may be cited as the Coroners and Justice Act 2009.

SCHEDULE 1

DUTY OR POWER TO SUSPEND OR RESUME INVESTIGATIONS

PART 1

SUSPENSION OF INVESTIGATIONS

Suspension where certain criminal charges may be brought

1.—(1) A senior coroner must suspend an investigation under this Part of this Act into a person's
death in the following cases.

(2) The first case is where a prosecuting authority requests the coroner to suspend the investigation on the ground that a person may be charged with—

(a) a homicide offence involving the death of the deceased, or

(b) an offence (other than a service offence) that is alleged to be a related offence.

(3) The second case is where a Provost Marshal or the Director of Service Prosecutions requests the coroner to suspend the investigation on the ground that a person may be charged with—

(a) the service equivalent of a homicide offence involving the death of the deceased, or

(b) a service offence that is alleged to be a related offence.

(4) Subject to paragraphs 2 and 3, a suspension of an investigation under this paragraph must be for—

(a) a period of 28 days beginning with the day on which the suspension first takes effect, or

(b) whatever longer period (beginning with that day) the coroner specifies.

(5) The period referred to in sub-paragraph (4) may be extended or further extended—

(a) in the first case, at the request of the authority by which the suspension was originally requested;

(b) in the second case, at the request of—

    (i) the Provost Marshal by whom the suspension was originally requested, or
    (ii) the Director of Service Prosecutions.

(6) In this Act—

"homicide offence" means—

    (a) murder, manslaughter, corporate manslaughter or infanticide;
    (b) an offence under any of the following provisions of the Road Traffic Act 1988 (c. 52)—

        (i) section 1 (causing death by dangerous driving);
        (ii) section 2B (causing death by careless, or inconsiderate, driving);
        (iii) section 3ZB (causing death by driving: unlicensed, disqualified or uninsured drivers);
        (iv) section 3A (causing death by careless driving when under the influence of drink or drugs);

    (c) an offence under section 2(1) of the Suicide Act 1961 (c. 60) (encouraging or assisting suicide);

(d) an offence under section 5 of the Domestic Violence, Crime and Victims Act 2004 (c. 28) [of causing or allowing the death of a child or vulnerable adult][178];

"related offence" means an offence (including a service offence) that—

(a) involves the death of the deceased, but is not a homicide offence or the service equivalent of a homicide offence, or

(b) involves the death of a person other than the deceased (whether or not it is a homicide offence or the service equivalent of a homicide offence) and is committed in circumstances connected with the death of the deceased;

"the service equivalent of a homicide offence" means an offence under section 42 of the Armed Forces Act 2006 (c. 52) (or section 70 of the Army Act 1955 (3 & 4 Eliz. 2. c. 18), section 70 of the Air Force Act 1955 (3 & 4 Eliz. 2 c. 19) or section 42 of the Naval Discipline Act 1957 (c. 53)) corresponding to a homicide offence.

Suspension where certain criminal proceedings are brought

A1–134   **2.**—(1) Subject to sub-paragraph (6), a senior coroner must suspend an investigation under this Part of this Act into a person's death in the following cases.

(2) The first case is where the coroner—

(a) becomes aware that a person has appeared or been brought before a magistrates' court charged with a homicide offence involving the death of the deceased, or

(b) becomes aware that a person has been charged on an indictment with such an offence without having appeared or been brought before a magistrates' court charged with it.

(3) The second case is where the coroner becomes aware that a person has been charged with the service equivalent of a homicide offence involving the death of the deceased.

(4) The third case is where a prosecuting authority informs the coroner that a person—

(a) has appeared or been brought before a magistrates' court charged with an offence (other than a service offence) that is alleged to be a related offence, or

(b) has been charged on an indictment with such an offence without having been sent for trial for it,

and the prosecuting authority requests the coroner to suspend the investigation.

(5) The fourth case is where the Director of Service Prosecutions informs the coroner that a person has been charged with a service offence that is alleged to be a related offence, and the Director requests the coroner to suspend the investigation.

(6) The coroner need not suspend the investigation—

(a) in the first case, if a prosecuting authority informs the coroner that it has no objection to the investigation continuing;

(b) in the second case, if the Director of Service Prosecutions informs the coroner that he or she has no objection to the investigation continuing;

(c) in any case, if the coroner thinks that there is an exceptional reason for not suspending the investigation.

(7) In the case of an investigation that is already suspended under paragraph 1—

(a) a suspension imposed by virtue of sub-paragraph (2) of that paragraph comes to an end if, in reliance of sub-paragraph (6)(a) above, the coroner decides not to suspend the investigation;

(b) a suspension imposed by virtue of sub-paragraph (3) of that paragraph comes to an end if, in reliance on sub-paragraph (6)(b) above, the coroner decides not to suspend the investigation;

---

[178] Words substituted by Domestic Violence, Crime and Victims (Amendment) Act 2012 c. 4 Sch.1 para.12 (July 25, 2013: substitution came into force on July 2, 2012 but could not take effect until the commencement of 2009 c.25 Sch.1 para.1 on July 25, 2013).

(c) a reference above in this paragraph to suspending an investigation is to be read as a reference to continuing the suspension of an investigation;

(d) if the suspension of the investigation is continued under this paragraph, the investigation is to be treated for the purposes of paragraphs 1(4), 7 and 8 of this Schedule as suspended under this paragraph (and not as suspended under paragraph 1).

Suspension pending inquiry under Inquiries Act 2005

3.—(1) Subject to sub-paragraph (2), a senior coroner must suspend an investigation under this Part   **A1–135** of this Act into a person's death if—

(a) the Lord Chancellor requests the coroner to do so on the ground that the cause of death is likely to be adequately investigated by an inquiry under the Inquiries Act 2005 (c. 12) that is being or is to be held,

(b) a senior judge has been appointed under that Act as chairman of the inquiry, and

(c) the Lord Chief Justice has indicated approval to the Lord Chancellor, for the purposes of this paragraph, of the appointment of that judge.

In paragraph (b) "senior judge" means a judge of the High Court or the Court of Appeal or a Justice of the Supreme Court.

(2) The coroner need not suspend the investigation if there appears to be an exceptional reason for not doing so.

(3) In the case of an investigation that is already suspended under paragraph 1—

(a) a reference above in this paragraph to suspending the investigation is to be read as a reference to continuing the suspension of the investigation;

(b) if the suspension of the investigation is continued under this paragraph, the investigation is to be treated for the purposes of paragraphs 1(4), 7 and 9 of this Schedule as suspended under this paragraph (and not as suspended under paragraph 1).

4.—(1) This paragraph applies where an investigation is suspended under paragraph 3 on the basis that the cause of death is likely to be adequately investigated by an inquiry under the Inquiries Act 2005 (c. 12).

(2) The terms of reference of the inquiry must be such that it has as its purpose, or among its purposes, the purpose set out in section 5(1) above (read with section 5(2) where applicable); and section 5 of the Inquiries Act 2005 has effect accordingly.

General power to suspend

5. A senior coroner may suspend an investigation under this Part of this Act into a person's death in   **A1–136** any case if it appears to the coroner that it would be appropriate to do so.

Effect of suspension

6.—(1) Where an investigation is suspended under this Schedule, the senior coroner must adjourn   **A1–137** any inquest that is being held as part of the investigation.

(2) Where an inquest held with a jury is adjourned under this paragraph, the senior coroner may discharge the jury.

PART 2

RESUMPTION OF INVESTIGATIONS

Resumption of investigation suspended under paragraph 1

7. An investigation that is suspended under paragraph 1 must be resumed once the period under sub-   **A1–138** paragraph (4) of that paragraph, or as the case may be the extended period under sub-paragraph (5) of that paragraph, has ended.

(But see paragraphs 2(7)(d) and 3(3)(b).)

Resumption of investigation suspended under paragraph 2

A1–139   **8.**—(1) An investigation that is suspended under paragraph 2 may not be resumed unless, but must be resumed if, the senior coroner thinks that there is sufficient reason for resuming it.
(2) Subject to sub-paragraph (3)—

(a) an investigation that is suspended under paragraph 2 may not be resumed while proceedings are continuing before the court of trial in respect of a homicide offence, or the service equivalent of a homicide offence, involving the death of the deceased;

(b) an investigation that is suspended by virtue of sub-paragraph (4) or (5) of that paragraph may not be resumed while proceedings are continuing before the court of trial in respect of the offence referred to in that sub-paragraph.

(3) The investigation may be resumed while the proceedings in question are continuing if—

(a) in the case of an investigation suspended by virtue of sub-paragraph (2) or (4) of paragraph 2, the relevant prosecuting authority informs the coroner that it has no objection to the investigation being resumed;

(b) in the case of an investigation suspended by virtue of sub-paragraph (3) or (5) of that paragraph, the Director of Service Prosecutions informs the coroner that he or she has no objection to the investigation being resumed.

(4) For the purposes of sub-paragraph (3)(a), the relevant prosecuting authority—

(a) in the case of an investigation suspended by virtue of sub-paragraph (2) of paragraph 2, is the prosecuting authority responsible for the prosecution in question;

(b) in the case of an investigation suspended by virtue of sub-paragraph (4) of that paragraph, is the prosecuting authority that made the request under that sub-paragraph.

(5) In the case of an investigation resumed under this paragraph, a determination under section 10(1)(a) may not be inconsistent with the outcome of—

(a) the proceedings in respect of the charge (or each charge) by reason of which the investigation was suspended;

(b) any proceedings that, by reason of sub-paragraph (2), had to be concluded before the investigation could be resumed.

Resumption of investigation suspended under paragraph 3

A1–140   **9.**—(1) Where an investigation is suspended under paragraph 3—

(a) it may not be resumed unless, but must be resumed if, the senior coroner thinks that there is sufficient reason for resuming it;

(b) it may not be resumed before the end of the period of 28 days beginning with the relevant day;

(c) where sub-paragraph (4), (6), (8) or (10) applies, it may be resumed only in accordance with that sub-paragraph (and not before the end of the 28-day period mentioned in paragraph (b)).

(2) In sub-paragraph (1)(b) "the relevant day" means—

(a) if the Lord Chancellor gives the coroner notification under this paragraph, the day on which the inquiry concerned is concluded;

(b) otherwise, the day on which the findings of that inquiry are published.

(3) Sub-paragraph (4) applies where, during the suspension of the investigation, the coroner—

(a) becomes aware that a person has appeared or been brought before a magistrates' court charged with a homicide offence involving the death of the deceased, or

(b) becomes aware that a person has been charged on an indictment with such an offence without having appeared or been brought before a magistrates' court charged with it.

(4) The coroner must not resume the investigation until after the conclusion of proceedings before the court of trial in respect of the offence in question, unless a prosecuting authority informs the coroner that it has no objection to the investigation being resumed before then.

(5) Sub-paragraph (6) applies where, during the suspension of the investigation, the coroner becomes aware that a person has been charged with the service equivalent of a homicide offence involving the death of the deceased.

(6) The coroner must not resume the investigation until after the conclusion of proceedings before the court of trial in respect of the offence in question, unless the Director of Service Prosecutions informs the coroner that he or she has no objection to the investigation being resumed before then.

(7) Sub-paragraph (8) applies where, during the suspension of the investigation, a prosecuting authority informs the senior coroner that a person—

(a) has appeared or been brought before a magistrates' court charged with an offence (other than a service offence) that is alleged to be a related offence, or

(b) has been charged on an indictment with such an offence without having been sent for trial for it.

(8) If the prosecuting authority requests the coroner not to resume the investigation until after the conclusion of proceedings before the court of trial in respect of the offence in question, the coroner must not do so. But the coroner may resume the investigation before the conclusion of those proceedings if the prosecuting authority subsequently informs the coroner that it has no objection to the investigation being resumed before then.

(9) Sub-paragraph (10) applies where the Director of Service Prosecutions informs the coroner that a person has been charged with a service offence that is alleged to be a related offence.

(10) If the Director of Service Prosecutions requests the coroner not to resume the investigation until after the conclusion of proceedings before the court of trial in respect of the offence in question, the coroner must not do so. But the coroner may resume the investigation before the conclusion of those proceedings if the Director subsequently informs the coroner that he or she has no objection to the investigation being resumed before then.

(11) In the case of an investigation resumed under this paragraph, a determination under section 10(1)(a) may not be inconsistent with the outcome of—

(a) the inquiry under the Inquiries Act 2005 (c. 12) by reason of which the investigation was suspended;

(b) any proceedings that, by reason of sub-paragraph (4), (6), (8) or (10), had to be concluded before the investigation could be resumed.

Resumption of investigation suspended under paragraph 5

10. An investigation that is suspended under paragraph 5 may be resumed at any time if the senior coroner thinks that there is sufficient reason for resuming it.   **A1-141**

Supplemental

11.—(1) Where an investigation is resumed under this Schedule, the senior coroner must resume any inquest that was adjourned under paragraph 6.   **A1-142**

(2) The following provisions apply, in place of section 7, to an inquest that is resumed under this paragraph.

(3) The resumed inquest may be held with a jury if the senior coroner thinks that there is sufficient reason for it to be held with one.

(4) Where the adjourned inquest was held with a jury and the senior coroner decides to hold the resumed inquest with a jury—

(a) if at least seven persons who were members of the original jury are available to serve at the resumed inquest, the resumed inquest must be held with a jury consisting of those persons;

(b) if not, or if the original jury was discharged under paragraph 6(2), a new jury must be summoned.

Schedule 2

Coroner Areas

Coroner areas

A1–143
1.—(1) England and Wales is to be divided into areas to be known as coroner areas.

(2) Each coroner area is to consist of the area of a local authority or the combined areas of two or more local authorities.

(3) Subject to paragraph 2—

(a) the coroner areas are to be those specified in an order made by the Lord Chancellor;

(b) each coroner area is to be known by whatever name is specified in the order.

(4) Before making an order under this paragraph, the Lord Chancellor must consult—

(a) every local authority,

(b) the Welsh Ministers, and

(c) any other persons the Lord Chancellor thinks appropriate.

Alteration of coroner areas

A1–144
2.—(1) The Lord Chancellor may make orders altering coroner areas.

(2) Before making an order under this paragraph the Lord Chancellor must consult—

(a) whichever local authorities the Lord Chancellor thinks appropriate,

(b) in the case of a coroner area in Wales, the Welsh Ministers, and

(c) any other persons the Lord Chancellor thinks appropriate.

(3) "Altering", in relation to a coroner area, includes (as well as changing its boundaries)—

(a) combining it with one or more other coroner areas;

(b) dividing it between two or more other coroner areas;

(c) changing its name.

Relevant authorities

A1–145
3.—(1) This paragraph sets out for the purposes of this Part what is the "relevant authority" for a given coroner area.

(2) In the case of a coroner area consisting of the area of a single local authority, that authority is the relevant authority for the coroner area.

(3) In the case of a coroner area consisting of the areas of two or more local authorities, the relevant authority for the coroner area is—

(a) whichever one of those authorities they jointly nominate;

(b) if they cannot agree on a nomination, whichever one of them the Lord Chancellor determines.

(4) Before making a determination under sub-paragraph (3)(b) the Lord Chancellor must consult—

(a) the Secretary of State, in a case involving local authorities in England;

(b) the Welsh Ministers, in a case involving local authorities in Wales.

(5) This paragraph has effect subject to paragraph 2 of Schedule 22.

Effect of body being outside coroner area etc.

4.—(1) This paragraph applies where—   **A1–146**

(a) a senior coroner is responsible for conducting an investigation under this Part into a person's death, and

(b) the body is outside the coroner's area (whether because of its removal or otherwise).

(2) The coroner has the same functions in relation to the body and the investigation as would be the case if the body were within the coroner's area.

(3) The presence of the body at a place outside the coroner's area does not confer any functions on any other coroner.

SCHEDULE 3

APPOINTMENT ETC OF SENIOR CORONERS, AREA CORONERS AND ASSISTANT CORONERS

PART 1

APPOINTMENT OF SENIOR, AREA AND ASSISTANT CORONERS

Appointment of senior coroners

1.—(1) The relevant authority for each coroner area must appoint a coroner (the "senior coroner")   **A1–147**
for that area.

(2) In the case of a coroner area that consists of the areas of two or more local authorities, the relevant authority for the area must consult the other authorities before making an appointment under this paragraph.

(3) A person may not be appointed as a senior coroner unless the Lord Chancellor and the Chief Coroner consent to the appointment of that person.

Appointment of area and assistant coroners

2.—(1) The Lord Chancellor may by order require the appointment, for any coroner area, of—   **A1–148**

(a) an area coroner, or a specified number of area coroners;

(b) a minimum number of assistant coroners.

(2) Before making an order under this paragraph in relation to a particular coroner area, the Lord Chancellor must consult—

(a) the Chief Coroner, and

(b) every local authority whose area falls within the coroner area (or, as the case may be, the local authority whose area is the same as the coroner area).

(3) The relevant authority for a coroner area in relation to which provision is made under sub-paragraph (1)(a) must appoint an area coroner or, as the case may be, the number of area coroners specified for the area in the order.

(4) The relevant authority for a coroner area in relation to which provision is made under sub-paragraph (1)(b) must appoint at least the number of assistant coroners specified for the area in the order.

(5) A person may not be appointed as an area coroner or assistant coroner unless the Lord Chancellor and the Chief Coroner consent to the appointment of that person.

PART 2

QUALIFICATIONS OF SENIOR, AREA AND ASSISTANT CORONERS

3. To be eligible for appointment as a senior coroner, area coroner or assistant coroner, a person   **A1–149**
must—

(a) be under the age of 70, and

(b) satisfy the judicial-appointment eligibility condition on a 5-year basis.

4.—(1) A person who is a councillor for a local authority, or has been during the previous 6 months, may not be appointed as the senior coroner, or as an area coroner or assistant coroner, for a coroner area that is the same as or includes the area of that local authority.

(2) In the application of this paragraph to the Common Council, the reference to a councillor is to be read as a reference to an alderman of the City of London or a common councillor.

PART 3

VACANCIES; FUNCTIONS OF AREA AND ASSISTANT CORONERS

A1–150   **5.**—(1) This paragraph applies where a vacancy occurs—

(a) in the office of senior coroner for an area, or

(b) in an office of area coroner for an area.

(2) The relevant authority for the area must—

(a) give notice in writing of the vacancy to the Lord Chancellor and the Chief Coroner as soon as practicable after the vacancy occurs;

(b) appoint a person to fill the vacancy under paragraph 1 or 2 (as the case may be) within 3 months of the vacancy occurring, or within whatever further period the Lord Chancellor allows;

(c) give notice in writing of the appointment of a person to fill the vacancy to the Lord Chancellor and the Chief Coroner as soon as practicable after it is filled.

Filling of vacancies

A1–151   **6.**—(1) This paragraph applies where—

(a) a vacancy occurs in an office of assistant coroner for an area, and

(b) the vacancy causes the number of assistant coroners for the area to fall below (or further below) the minimum number specified under paragraph 2(1)(b).

(2) Within 3 months of the vacancy occurring, or within whatever further period the Lord Chancellor allows, the relevant authority for the area must appoint a person to fill the vacancy.

Person to act as senior coroner in case of vacancy

A1–152   **7.**—(1) This paragraph applies where a vacancy occurs in the office of senior coroner for an area.
(2) Subject to sub-paragraph (3), the area coroner for the area (or, if there is more than one such area coroner, whichever of them is nominated by the relevant authority for the area) is to act as senior coroner for the area while the office remains vacant.
(3) Where there is no area coroner for the area, whichever assistant coroner for the area is nominated by the relevant authority for the area is to act as senior coroner for the area while the office remains vacant.
(4) In the case of a coroner area that consists of the area of two or more local authorities, the relevant authority for the area must consult the other authority or authorities before making a nomination under this paragraph.
(5) A person who acts as senior coroner for an area by virtue of this paragraph is to be treated for all purposes of this Part of this Act (except those of this paragraph and paragraphs 1 to 5 and 9 to 19 of this Schedule) as being the senior coroner for the area.

Functions of area and assistant coroners

A1–153   **8.**—(1) An area coroner or assistant coroner for an area may perform any functions of the senior coroner for the area (including functions which that senior coroner has by virtue of section 2 or 3)—

(a) during a period when that senior coroner is absent or unavailable;

(b) at any other time, with the consent of that senior coroner.

(2) Accordingly a reference in a statutory provision (whenever made) to a senior coroner is to be read, where appropriate, as including an area coroner or assistant coroner.

Part 4

Terms Of Office Of Senior, Area And Assistant Coroners

Status of office

9. The offices of senior coroner, area coroner and assistant coroner are not to be regarded as freehold **A1–154** offices.

Vacation or termination of office

10. A senior coroner, area coroner or assistant coroner must vacate office on reaching the age of **A1–155** 70.

11.—(1) The senior coroner or an area coroner or assistant coroner for an area ("the relevant coroner area") must vacate office immediately if—

(a) he or she becomes a councillor for a local authority, and

(b) the area of that local authority is the same as or falls within the relevant coroner area.

(2) In the application of this paragraph to the Common Council, the reference to a councillor is to be read as a reference to an alderman of the City of London or a common councillor.

12. The senior coroner or an area coroner or assistant coroner for an area may resign office by giving notice in writing to the relevant authority for the area. But the resignation does not take effect unless and until it is accepted by the authority.

13.—(1) The Lord Chancellor may, with the agreement of the Lord Chief Justice, remove a senior coroner, area coroner or assistant coroner from office for incapacity or misbehaviour.

(2) The Lord Chief Justice may nominate a judicial office holder (as defined in section 109(4) of the Constitutional Reform Act 2005 (c. 4)) to exercise the functions of the Lord Chief Justice under sub-paragraph (1).

Discipline

14. Chapter 3 of Part 4 of the Constitutional Reform Act 2005 (c. 4) (discipline) applies in relation **A1–156** to the offices of senior coroner, area coroner and assistant coroner as it would apply if those offices were listed in Schedule 14 to that Act.

Salary of senior and area coroners

15.—(1) The senior coroner for an area is entitled to a salary. **A1–157**

(2) The amount of the salary is to be whatever is from time to time agreed by the senior coroner and the relevant authority for the area.

(3) If the senior coroner and the relevant authority cannot agree about an alteration in the amount of the salary—

(a) either of them may refer the matter to the Lord Chancellor;

(b) the Lord Chancellor may determine the amount of the salary and the date on which it is to become payable.

Any alteration in the amount of salary is to take effect in accordance with the Lord Chancellor's determination.

(4) In making a determination under sub-paragraph (3), the Lord Chancellor must have regard—

(a) to the nature and extent of the coroner's functions, and

(b) to all the circumstances of the case.

(5) The salary to which the senior coroner for an area is entitled under this paragraph is payable by the relevant authority for the area.

(6) This paragraph applies in relation to an area coroner for an area as it applies in relation to the senior coroner for an area (references to the senior coroner being read as references to an area coroner).

Fees payable to assistants

A1–158   **16.**—(1) An assistant coroner for an area is entitled to fees.

(2) The amount of the fees is to be whatever is agreed from time to time by the assistant coroner and the relevant authority for the area.

(3) The fees to which an assistant coroner for an area is entitled under this paragraph are payable by the relevant authority for the area.

Pensions for senior and area coroners

A1–159   **17.** A relevant authority for a coroner area must make provision for the payment of pensions, allowances or gratuities to or in respect of persons who are or have been senior coroners or area coroners for the area.

Prohibition on receipt of fees etc

A1–160   **18.** Except as permitted by or under this or any other Act, a senior coroner, area coroner or assistant coroner may not accept any remuneration or fee in respect of anything done by that coroner in the performance of his or her functions.

Other terms of office

A1–161   **19.** Subject to the preceding provisions of this Part, the senior coroner or an area coroner or assistant coroner for an area holds office on whatever terms are from time to time agreed by that coroner and the relevant authority for the area.

Schedule 4

Coroner For Treasure And Assistant Coroners For Treasure

Part 1

Appointment, Qualifications And Terms Of Office Of Coroner For Treasure

Appointment

A1–162   **1.** The Lord Chancellor may appoint a person as the Coroner for Treasure.

Qualifications

A1–163   **2.** To be eligible for appointment as the Coroner for Treasure, a person must—

(a) be under the age of 70, and

(b) satisfy the judicial-appointment eligibility condition on a 5-year basis.

Vacation or termination of office

A1–164   **3.** The Coroner for Treasure must vacate office on reaching the age of 70.

4. The Coroner for Treasure may resign office by giving notice to the Lord Chancellor.
But the resignation does not take effect unless and until it is accepted by the Lord Chancellor.

5.—(1) The Lord Chancellor may, with the agreement of the Lord Chief Justice, remove the Coroner for Treasure from office for incapacity or misbehaviour.

(2) The Lord Chief Justice may nominate a judicial office holder (as defined in section 109(4) of the Constitutional Reform Act 2005 (c. 4)) to exercise the functions of the Lord Chief Justice under sub-paragraph (1).

Remuneration, allowances and expenses

6.—(1) The Lord Chancellor may pay to the Coroner for Treasure amounts determined by the Lord Chancellor by way of remuneration or allowances.   **A1–165**

(2) The Lord Chancellor may pay to the Coroner for Treasure amounts determined by the Lord Chancellor towards expenses incurred by the Coroner for Treasure in performing functions as such.

PART 2

DESIGNATION AND REMUNERATION OF ASSISTANT CORONERS FOR TREASURE

Designation

7. The Chief Coroner may designate one or more assistant coroners to act as Assistant Coroners for Treasure.   **A1–166**

8. A person who is designated under paragraph 7 to act as an Assistant Coroner for Treasure may act as such for so long as the designation continues to have effect.

9. A person's designation under that paragraph ceases to have effect—

(a) when the person ceases to be an assistant coroner;

(b) if earlier, when the designation is terminated by notice given—

(i) by the person to the Chief Coroner, or

(ii) by the Chief Coroner to the person.

Remuneration, allowances and expenses

10.—(1) The Lord Chancellor may pay to an Assistant Coroner for Treasure amounts determined by the Lord Chancellor by way of remuneration or allowances.   **A1–167**

(2) The Lord Chancellor may pay to an Assistant Coroner for Treasure amounts determined by the Lord Chancellor towards expenses incurred by the Assistant Coroner for Treasure in performing functions as such.

PART 3

MISCELLANEOUS

Functions of Assistant Coroners for Treasure

11.—(1) An Assistant Coroner for Treasure may perform any functions of the Coroner for Treasure—   **A1–168**

(a) during a period when the Coroner for Treasure is absent or unavailable;

(b) during a vacancy in the office of Coroner for Treasure;

(c) at any other time, with the consent of the Coroner for Treasure.

(2) Accordingly a reference in this Part of this Act to the Coroner for Treasure is to be read, where appropriate, as including an Assistant Coroner for Treasure.

Staff

12.—(1) The Lord Chancellor may appoint staff to assist the Coroner for Treasure and any Assistant Coroners for Treasure in the performance of their functions.   **A1–169**

(2) Such staff are to be appointed on whatever terms and conditions the Lord Chancellor thinks appropriate.

SCHEDULE 5

POWERS OF CORONERS

Power to require evidence to be given or produced

A1–170   **1.**—(1) A senior coroner may by notice require a person to attend at a time and place stated in the notice and—

(a) to give evidence at an inquest,

(b) to produce any documents in the custody or under the control of the person which relate to a matter that is relevant to an inquest, or

(c) to produce for inspection, examination or testing any other thing in the custody or under the control of the person which relates to a matter that is relevant to an inquest.

(2) A senior coroner who is conducting an investigation under this Part may by notice require a person, within such period as the senior coroner thinks reasonable—

(a) to provide evidence to the senior coroner, about any matters specified in the notice, in the form of a written statement,

(b) to produce any documents in the custody or under the control of the person which relate to a matter that is relevant to the investigation, or

(c) to produce for inspection, examination or testing any other thing in the custody or under the control of the person which relates to a matter that is relevant to the investigation.

(3) A notice under sub-paragraph (1) or (2) must—

(a) explain the possible consequences, under paragraphs 6 and 7 of Schedule 6, of not complying with the notice;

(b) indicate what the recipient of the notice should do if he or she wishes to make a claim under sub-paragraph (4).

(4) A claim by a person that—

(a) he or she is unable to comply with a notice under this paragraph, or

(b) it is not reasonable in all the circumstances to require him or her to comply with such a notice,

is to be determined by the senior coroner, who may revoke or vary the notice on that ground.

(5) In deciding whether to revoke or vary a notice on the ground mentioned in sub-paragraph (4)(b), the senior coroner must consider the public interest in the information in question being obtained for the purposes of the inquest or investigation, having regard to the likely importance of the information.

(6) For the purposes of this paragraph a document or thing is under a person's control if it is in the person's possession or if he or she has a right to possession of it.

(7) The validity of a notice under sub-paragraph (1) or (2) is not limited to the coroner area for which the senior coroner issuing the notice is appointed.

(8) A reference in this paragraph to a senior coroner is to be read as including the Coroner for Treasure.

As it applies in relation to the Coroner for Treasure, this paragraph has effect with the omission of sub-paragraph (7).

2.—(1) A person may not be required to give, produce or provide any evidence or document under paragraph 1 if—

(a) he or she could not be required to do so in civil proceedings in a court in England and Wales, or

(b) the requirement would be incompatible with a [EU][179] obligation.

(2) The rules of law under which evidence or documents are permitted or required to be withheld on grounds of public interest immunity apply in relation to an investigation or inquest under this Part as they apply in relation to civil proceedings in a court in England and Wales.

Power of entry, search and seizure

3.—(1) A senior coroner conducting an investigation under this Part, if authorised—

(a) by the Chief Coroner, or

(b) by another senior coroner nominated by the Chief Coroner to give authorisation,

may enter and search any land specified in the authorisation.

(2) An authorisation may be given only if—

(a) the senior coroner conducting the investigation has reason to suspect that there may be anything on the land which relates to a matter that is relevant to the investigation, and

(b) any of the conditions in sub-paragraph (3) are met.

(3) Those conditions are—

(a) that it is not practicable to communicate with a person entitled to grant permission to enter and search the land;

(b) that permission to enter and search the land has been refused;

(c) that the senior coroner has reason to believe that such permission would be refused if requested;

(d) that the purpose of a search may be frustrated or seriously prejudiced unless the senior coroner can secure immediate entry to the land on arrival.

(4) A senior coroner conducting an investigation under this Part who is lawfully on any land—

(a) may seize anything that is on the land;

(b) may inspect and take copies of any documents.

(5) A reference in this paragraph to land is not limited to land within the coroner area for which the senior coroner in question is appointed.

(6) A reference in this paragraph to a senior coroner is to be read as including the Coroner for Treasure. As it applies in relation to the Coroner for Treasure, this paragraph has effect with the omission of sub-paragraphs (1)(b) and (5).

4.—(1) The person by whom an authorisation under paragraph 3(1) is given must make a record—

(a) setting out the reasons for the suspicion referred to in paragraph 3(2)(a);

(b) specifying which of the conditions in paragraph 3(3) is met.

(2) Where the authorisation is given by a senior coroner nominated under paragraph 3(1)(b), that coroner must give the record made under this paragraph to the Chief Coroner.

(3) The Chief Coroner must retain a record made this paragraph until the Chief Coroner has given to the Lord Chancellor the report under section 36 for the calendar year in which the authorisation in question was given.

5.—(1) A power under paragraph 3(4) is not exercisable unless the person exercising the power has reasonable grounds for believing—

---

[179] Words substituted by Treaty of Lisbon (Changes in Terminology) Order 2011/1043 Pt 2 art.6(1)(e) (July 25, 2013: substitution came into on April 22, 2011 but could not take effect until the commencement of 2009 c.25 Sch.5, para.2(1)(a) on July 25, 2013).

(a) that its exercise may assist the investigation, and

(b) in the case of the seizure of anything, that the seizure is necessary to prevent the thing being concealed, lost, damaged, altered or destroyed.

(2) The power under paragraph 3(4)(b) includes power to require any information that is stored in an electronic form and is on, or accessible from, the land to be produced in a form—

(a) in which it can be taken away, and

(b) in which it is legible or from which it can readily be produced in a legible form.

(3) A power under paragraph 3(4) does not apply to any item that the person by whom the power is exercisable has reasonable grounds for believing to be subject to legal privilege.

(4) Anything that has been seized or taken away under paragraph 3 may be retained for so long as is necessary in all the circumstances.

(5) A person on whom a power is conferred by virtue of paragraph 3 may use reasonable force, if necessary, in the exercise of the power.

(6) In this paragraph "subject to legal privilege", in relation to an item, has the meaning given by section 10 of the Police and Criminal Evidence Act 1984 (c. 60).

Exhumation of body for examination

A1–172   **6.**—(1) A senior coroner may order the exhumation of a person's body if subparagraph (2) or (3) applies.

(2) This sub-paragraph applies if—

(a) the body is buried in England and Wales (whether or not within the coroner area for which the coroner is appointed), and

(b) the coroner thinks it necessary for the body to be examined under section 14.

(3) This sub-paragraph applies if—

(a) the body is buried within the coroner area for which the coroner is appointed, and

(b) the coroner thinks it necessary for the body to be examined for the purpose of any criminal proceedings that have been instituted or are contemplated in respect of—

   (i) the death of the person whose body it is, or
   (ii) the death of another person who died in circumstances connected with the death of that person.

(4) In sub-paragraph (3) "criminal proceedings" includes proceedings in respect of an offence under section 42 of the Armed Forces Act 2006 (c. 52) (or section 70 of the Army Act 1955 (3 & 4 Eliz. 2 c. 18), section 70 of the Air Force Act 1955 (3 & 4 Eliz. 2 c. 19) or section 42 of the Naval Discipline Act 1957 (c. 53)).

Action to prevent other deaths

A1–173   **7.**—(1) Where—

(a) a senior coroner has been conducting an investigation under this Part into a person's death,

(b) anything revealed by the investigation gives rise to a concern that circumstances creating a risk of other deaths will occur, or will continue to exist, in the future, and

(c) in the coroner's opinion, action should be taken to prevent the occurrence or continuation of such circumstances, or to eliminate or reduce the risk of death created by such circumstances,

the coroner must report the matter to a person who the coroner believes may have power to take such action.

(2) A person to whom a senior coroner makes a report under this paragraph must give the senior coroner a written response to it.

(3) A copy of a report under this paragraph, and of the response to it, must be sent to the Chief Coroner.

Schedule 6

Offences

Part 1

Offences Relating To Jurors

1.—(1) It is an offence for a person to serve on a jury at an inquest if the person—　　

(a) is disqualified from jury service (by reason of being a person listed in Part 2 of Schedule 1 to the Juries Act 1974 (c. 23)), and

(b) knows that he or she is disqualified from jury service.

(2) A person guilty of an offence under this paragraph is liable on summary conviction to a fine not exceeding level 5 on the standard scale.

2.—(1) It is an offence for a person—

(a) to refuse without reasonable excuse to answer any question put under section 8(5),

(b) to give an answer to such a question knowing the answer to be false in a material particular, or
(c) recklessly to give an answer to such a question that is false in a material particular.

(2) A person guilty of an offence under this paragraph is liable on summary conviction to a fine not exceeding level 3 on the standard scale.

3.—(1) It is an offence for a person who is duly summoned as a juror at an inquest—

(a) to make any false representation, or

(b) to cause or permit to be made any false representation on his or her behalf,

with the intention of evading service as a juror at an inquest.

(2) A person guilty of an offence under this paragraph is liable on summary conviction to a fine not exceeding level 3 on the standard scale.

4.—(1) It is an offence for a person to make or cause to be made, on behalf of a person who has been duly summoned as a juror at an inquest, any false representation with the intention of enabling the other person to evade service as a juror at an inquest.

(2) A person guilty of an offence under this paragraph is liable on summary conviction to a fine not exceeding level 3 on the standard scale.

5.—(1) A senior coroner, or (as the case may be) the Coroner for Treasure, may impose a fine not exceeding £–100 on a person duly summoned as a juror at an inquest who—

(a) fails without reasonable excuse to attend in accordance with the summons, or

(b) attends in accordance with the summons but refuses without reasonable excuse to serve as a juror.

(2) But a fine may not be imposed under this paragraph unless the summons was duly served on the person in question not later than 14 days before the day on which he or she was required to attend.

Part 2

Offences Relating To Witnesses And Evidence

6. A senior coroner, or (as the case may be) the Coroner for Treasure, may impose a fine not　　
exceeding £–100 on a person who fails without reasonable excuse to do anything required by a notice under paragraph 1 of Schedule 5.

7.—(1) It is an offence for a person to do anything that is intended to have the effect of—

(a) distorting or otherwise altering any evidence, document or other thing that is given, produced or provided for the purposes of an investigation under this Part of this Act, or

(b) preventing any evidence, document or other thing from being given, produced or provided for the purposes of such an investigation, or to do anything that the person knows or believes is likely to have that effect.

(2) It is an offence for a person—

(a) intentionally to suppress or conceal a document that is, and that the person knows or believes to be, a relevant document, or

(b) intentionally to alter or destroy such a document.

(3) For the purposes of sub-paragraph (2) a document is a "relevant document" if it is likely that a person conducting an investigation under this Part of this Act would (if aware of its existence) wish to be provided with it.

(4) A person does not commit an offence under sub-paragraph (1) or (2) by doing anything that is authorised or required—

(a) by a senior coroner or the Coroner for Treasure, or

(b) by virtue of paragraph 2 of Schedule 5 or any privilege that applies.

(5) Proceedings for an offence under sub-paragraph (1) or (2) may be instituted only by or with the consent of the Director of Public Prosecutions.

(6) A person guilty of an offence under sub-paragraph (1) or (2) is liable on summary conviction to a fine not exceeding level 3 on the standard scale, or to imprisonment for a term not exceeding 51 weeks, or to both.

8.—(1) It is an offence for a person, in giving unsworn evidence at an inquest by virtue of section 45(2)(a), to give false evidence in such circumstances that, had the evidence been given on oath, he or she would have been guilty of perjury.

(2) A person guilty of an offence under this paragraph is liable on summary conviction to a fine not exceeding £–100, or to imprisonment for a term not exceeding 51 weeks, or to both.

(3) In relation to a person under the age of 14, sub-paragraph (2) has effect as if for the words following "summary conviction" there were substituted "to a fine not exceeding £250".

(4) For the purposes of sub-paragraph (3), a person's age is to be taken to be that which it appears to the court to be after considering any available evidence.

PART 3

MISCELLANEOUS

A1–176   **9.**—(1) The powers of a senior coroner or the Coroner for Treasure under paragraph 5 or 6 are additional to, and do not affect, any other power the coroner may have—

(a) to compel a person to appear before him or her;

(b) to compel a person to give evidence or produce any document or other thing;

(c) to punish a person for contempt of court for failure to appear or to give evidence or to produce any document or other thing.

(2) But a person may not be fined under paragraph 5 or 6 and also be punished under any such other power.

10. In relation to an offence committed before the commencement of section 281(5) of the Criminal Justice Act 2003 (c. 44), a reference in this Schedule to 51 weeks is to be read as a reference to 6 months.

SCHEDULE 7

ALLOWANCES, FEES AND EXPENSES

PART 1

ALLOWANCES PAYABLE TO JURORS

A1–177   **1.** A person who serves as a juror at an inquest is entitled, in respect of attending the inquest, to receive payments by way of allowance—

(a) for travelling and subsistence;

(b) for financial loss.

This is subject to any conditions prescribed by regulations.

2. But a person is entitled to receive payments by way of allowance for financial loss only if, in consequence of attending the inquest, the person has—

(a) incurred expenses (other than on travelling and subsistence) that he or she would otherwise not have incurred,

(b) suffered a loss of earnings that he or she would otherwise not have suffered, or

(c) suffered a loss of benefit under the enactments relating to social security that he or she would otherwise not have suffered.

3. Regulations may prescribe the rates of any allowances payable under paragraph 1.

4. The amount due to a person under paragraph 1 is to be calculated by the senior coroner and paid by (or on behalf of) the senior coroner or, where appropriate, the Coroner for Treasure.

PART 2

ALLOWANCES PAYABLE TO WITNESSES

5.—(1) Regulations may prescribe the allowances that may be paid by (or on behalf of) senior **A1–178** coroners or the Coroner for Treasure—

(a) to witnesses;

(b) to persons who produce documents or things by virtue of paragraph 1(1) or (2) of Schedule 5;

(c) to persons who provide evidence in the form of a written statement by virtue of paragraph 1(2)(a) of that Schedule.

(2) In this paragraph "witness" means a person properly attending before a senior coroner to give evidence at an inquest or in connection with the possibility of doing so (whether or not the person actually gives evidence), but does not include—

(a) a police officer, or a member of a service police force, attending in his or her capacity as such;

(b) a full-time officer of an institution to which the Prison Act 1952 (c. 52) applies in his or her capacity as such;

(c) a prisoner in respect of an occasion on which he or she is conveyed in custody to appear before a senior coroner.

PART 3

MISCELLANEOUS FEES, ALLOWANCES AND EXPENSES

6. Regulations may prescribe the fees and allowances that may be paid by (or on behalf of) senior **A1–179** coroners to persons who make examinations under section 14.

7.—(1) A relevant authority for a coroner area may issue a schedule of the fees, allowances and expenses that may be lawfully paid or incurred by the senior coroner for the area in the performance of the coroner's functions.

(2) The power under sub-paragraph (1) includes power to amend or revoke any schedule issued.

(3) In exercising the power under sub-paragraph (1) a relevant authority must have regard to any guidance from time to time issued by the Lord Chancellor.

(4) A copy of any schedule that is issued or amended must be given to the senior coroner.

(5) The reference in sub-paragraph (1) to fees and allowances does not include fees or allowances within any of the preceding paragraphs of this Schedule.

8. Regulations may prescribe the fees payable to coroners for supplying copies of documents in their custody relating to investigations or inquests under this Part of this Act that they are conducting or have conducted.

PART 4

MEETING OR REIMBURSING EXPENSES

A1–180   **9.**—(1) Regulations may make provision for or in connection with meeting or reimbursing—

(a) expenses incurred by senior coroners (including expenses incurred under or by virtue of paragraph 4, 5 or 6);

(b) expenses incurred by area coroners and assistant coroners;

(c) expenses incurred by virtue of Schedule 10 in the conduct of an investigation by the Chief Coroner or the Coroner for Treasure or by a judge, former judge or former coroner.

(2) The regulations may make provision—

(a) for accounts or evidence relating to expenses to be provided to relevant authorities;

(b) for or in connection with the meeting or reimbursement by relevant authorities of expenses of a description specified in the regulations;

(c) for or in connection with appeals relating to decisions with respect to meeting or reimbursing expenses.

This sub-paragraph is not to be read as limiting the power in sub-paragraph (1).

(3) A reference in this paragraph to meeting or reimbursing expenses incurred by a person ("P") includes a reference to indemnifying P in respect of—

(a) costs that P reasonably incurs in or in connection with proceedings in respect of things done or omitted in the exercise (or purported exercise) by P of duties under this Part of this Act;

(b) costs that P reasonably incurs in taking steps to dispute claims that might be made in such proceedings;

(c) damages awarded against P, or costs ordered to be paid by P, in such proceedings;

(d) sums payable by P in connection with a reasonable settlement of such proceedings or of claims that might be made in such proceedings.

PART 5

SUPPLEMENTAL

A1–181   **10.** For the purposes of paragraph 1, a person who attends for service as a juror in accordance with a summons is to be treated as serving as a juror even if he or she is not sworn.

11.—(1) The power to make regulations under this Schedule is exercisable by the Lord Chancellor.

(2) Regulations under this Schedule may be made only if—

(a) the Lord Chief Justice, or

(b) a judicial office holder (as defined in section 109(4) of the Constitutional Reform Act 2005 (c. 4)) nominated for the purposes of this sub-paragraph by the Lord Chief Justice,

agrees to the making of the regulations.

SCHEDULE 8

CHIEF CORONER AND DEPUTY CHIEF CORONERS

Appointment of Chief Coroner

A1–182   **1.**—(1) The Lord Chief Justice may appoint a person as the Chief Coroner.

(2) To be eligible for appointment as the Chief Coroner a person must be—

(a) a judge of the High Court or a Circuit judge, and

(b) under the age of 70.

(3) The Lord Chief Justice must consult the Lord Chancellor before making an appointment under this paragraph.

(4) The appointment of a person as the Chief Coroner is to be for a term decided by the Lord Chief Justice after consulting the Lord Chancellor. The term must be one that expires before the person's 70th birthday.

(5) In this paragraph "appointment" includes re-appointment.

Appointment of Deputy Chief Coroners

2.—(1) The Lord Chief Justice may secure the appointment as Deputy Chief Coroners of however many persons the Lord Chief Justice thinks appropriate.   **A1–183**

(2) To be eligible for appointment as a Deputy Chief Coroner a person must be—

(a) a judge of the High Court, a Circuit judge, the Coroner for Treasure or a senior coroner, and

(b) under the age of 70.

(3) The Lord Chief Justice must consult the Lord Chancellor as to—

(a) the appropriate number of persons to be appointed as Deputy Chief Coroners;

(b) how many of them are to be persons eligible for appointment by virtue of being judges and how many are to be persons eligible for appointment by virtue of being senior coroners or the Coroner for Treasure.

(4) The function of appointing a person as a Deputy Chief Coroner is exercisable, in the case of a judge of the High Court or a Circuit judge, by the Lord Chief Justice after consulting the Lord Chancellor.

(5) The appointment by the Lord Chief Justice of a person as a Deputy Chief Coroner is to be for a term decided by the Lord Chief Justice after consulting the Lord Chancellor.
The term must be one that expires before the person's 70th birthday.

(6) The function of appointing a person as a Deputy Chief Coroner is exercisable, in the case of a senior coroner or the Coroner for Treasure, by the Lord Chancellor at the invitation of the Lord Chief Justice.

(7) The appointment by the Lord Chancellor of a person as a Deputy Chief Coroner is to be for a term decided by the Lord Chancellor after consulting the Lord Chief Justice. The term must be one that expires before the person's 70th birthday.

(8) In this paragraph "appointment" includes re-appointment.

Resignation or removal

3.—(1) The Chief Coroner, or a Deputy Chief Coroner appointed by the Lord Chief Justice, may resign from office by giving notice in writing to the Lord Chief Justice.   **A1–184**

(2) But the resignation does not take effect unless and until it is accepted by the Lord Chief Justice, who must consult the Lord Chancellor before accepting it.

(3) A Deputy Chief Coroner appointed by the Lord Chancellor may resign from office by giving notice in writing to the Lord Chancellor.

(4) But the resignation does not take effect unless and until it is accepted by the Lord Chancellor, who must consult the Lord Chief Justice before accepting it.

4.—(1) The Lord Chief Justice may, after consulting the Lord Chancellor, remove the Chief Coroner, or a Deputy Chief Coroner appointed by the Lord Chief Justice, from office for incapacity or misbehaviour.

(2) The Lord Chancellor may, after consulting the Lord Chief Justice, remove a Deputy Chief Coroner appointed by the Lord Chancellor from office for incapacity or misbehaviour.

Remuneration, allowances and expenses

5. The Lord Chancellor may pay to the Chief Coroner—   **A1–185**

(a) amounts determined by the Lord Chancellor by way of remuneration or allowances;

(b) amounts determined by the Lord Chancellor towards expenses incurred by the Chief Coroner in performing functions as such.

6. The Lord Chancellor may pay to a Deputy Chief Coroner—

(a) amounts determined by the Lord Chancellor by way of remuneration or allowances;

(b) amounts determined by the Lord Chancellor towards expenses incurred by that Deputy Chief Coroner in performing functions as such.

7. A reference in paragraph 5 or 6 to paying expenses incurred by a person ("P") includes a reference to indemnifying P in respect of—

(a) costs that P reasonably incurs in or in connection with proceedings in respect of things done or omitted in the exercise (or purported exercise) by P of duties under this Part;

(b) costs that P reasonably incurs in taking steps to dispute claims that might be made in such proceedings;

(c) damages awarded against P, or costs ordered to be paid by P, in such proceedings;

(d) sums payable by P in connection with a reasonable settlement of such proceedings or of claims that might be made in such proceedings.

Exercise of Chief Coroner's functions by Deputy Chief coroner

A1–186   **8.**—(1) A Deputy Chief Coroner may perform any functions of the Chief Coroner—

(a) during a period when the Chief Coroner is absent or unavailable;

(b) during a vacancy in the office of Chief Coroner;

(c) at any other time, with the consent of the Chief Coroner.

(2) Accordingly a reference in this Part to the Chief Coroner is to be read, where appropriate, as including a Deputy Chief Coroner.

Staff

A1–187   **9.**—(1) The Lord Chancellor must appoint staff to assist the Chief Coroner and any Deputy Chief Coroners in the performance of their functions.
(2) Such staff are to be appointed on whatever terms and conditions the Lord Chancellor thinks appropriate.

SCHEDULE 9

MEDICAL ADVISER AND DEPUTY MEDICAL ADVISERS TO THE CHIEF CORONER

Appointment and functions of Medical Adviser to the Chief Coroner

A1–188   **1.** The Lord Chancellor may appoint a person as Medical Adviser to the Chief Coroner ("the Medical Adviser") to provide advice and assistance to the Chief Coroner as to medical matters in relation to the coroner system.

Appointment and functions of Deputy Medical Advisers to the Chief Coroner

A1–189   **2.**—(1) The Lord Chancellor may appoint however many Deputy Medical Advisers to the Chief Coroner ("Deputy Medical Advisers") the Lord Chancellor thinks appropriate.
(2) A Deputy Medical Adviser may perform any functions of the Medical Adviser—

(a) during a period when the Medical Adviser is absent or unavailable;

(b) during a vacancy in the office of Medical Adviser;

(c) at any other time, with the consent of the Medical Adviser.

Qualification for appointment

3. A person may be appointed as the Medical Adviser or as a Deputy Medical Adviser only if, at the time of the appointment, he or she—

    (a) is a registered medical practitioner and has been throughout the previous 5 years, and

    (b) practises as such or has done within the previous 5 years.

A1–190

Consultation before making appointment

4. Before appointing a person as the Medical Adviser or as a Deputy Medical Adviser, the Lord Chancellor must consult—

    (a) the Chief Coroner, and

    (b) the Welsh Ministers.

A1–191

Terms and conditions of appointment

5. The appointment of a person as the Medical Adviser or as a Deputy Medical Adviser is to be on whatever terms and conditions the Lord Chancellor thinks appropriate.

A1–192

Remuneration, allowances and expenses

6.—(1) The Lord Chancellor may pay to the Medical Adviser—

    (a) amounts determined by the Lord Chancellor by way of remuneration or allowances;

    (b) amounts determined by the Lord Chancellor towards expenses incurred in performing functions as such.

(2) The Lord Chancellor may pay to a Deputy Medical Adviser—

    (a) amounts determined by the Lord Chancellor by way of remuneration or allowances;

    (b) amounts determined by the Lord Chancellor towards expenses incurred by that Deputy Medical Adviser in performing functions as such.

A1–193

Schedule 10

Investigation By Chief Coroner Or Coroner For Treasure Or By Judge, Former Judge Or Former Coroner

Investigation by Chief Coroner

1.—(1) The Chief Coroner may conduct an investigation into a person's death.

(2) Where the Chief Coroner is responsible for conducting an investigation by virtue of this paragraph—

    (a) the Chief Coroner has the same functions in relation to the body and the investigation as would be the case if he or she were a senior coroner in whose area the body was situated;

    (b) no senior coroner, area coroner or assistant coroner has any functions in relation to the body or the investigation.

(3) Accordingly a reference in a statutory provision (whenever made) to a senior coroner is to be read, where appropriate, as including the Chief Coroner exercising functions by virtue of this paragraph.

A1–194

Investigation by Coroner for Treasure

2.—(1) The Chief Coroner may direct the Coroner for Treasure to conduct an investigation into a person's death.

A1–195

(2) Where a direction is given under this paragraph—

(a) the Coroner for Treasure must conduct the investigation;

(b) the Coroner for Treasure has the same functions in relation to the body and the investigation as would be the case if he or she were a senior coroner in whose area the body was situated;

(c) no senior coroner, area coroner or assistant coroner has any functions in relation to the body or the investigation.

(3) Accordingly, a reference in a statutory provision (whenever made) to a senior coroner is to be read, where appropriate, as including the Coroner for Treasure exercising functions by virtue of this paragraph.

Investigation by judge, former judge or former coroner

A1–196   **3.**—(1) If requested to do so by the Chief Coroner, the Lord Chief Justice may nominate a person within sub-paragraph (2) to conduct an investigation into a person's death.
(2) A person is within this sub-paragraph if at the time of the nomination he or she is—

(a) a judge of the High Court,

(b) a Circuit judge, or

(c) a person who has held office as a judge of the Court of Appeal or of the High Court (but no longer does so),

and is under the age of 75.
(3) The Chief Coroner may request a person who at the time of the request—

(a) has held office as a senior coroner (but no longer does so), and

(b) is under the age of 75,

to conduct an investigation into a person's death.
(4) If a person nominated or requested under this paragraph agrees to conduct the investigation—

(a) that person is under a duty to do so;

(b) that person has the same functions in relation to the body and the investigation as would be the case if he or she were a senior coroner in whose area the body was situated;

(c) no senior coroner, area coroner or assistant coroner has any functions in relation to the body or the investigation.

(5) Accordingly a reference in a statutory provision (whenever made) to a coroner is to be read, where appropriate, as including a person who has been nominated or requested under this paragraph to conduct an investigation and has agreed to do so.
(6) The Lord Chief Justice must consult the Lord Chancellor before making a nomination under this paragraph.
    4. [. . .][180]

Investigations already begun

A1–197   **5.** A reference in this Schedule to conducting an investigation, in the case of an investigation that has already begun, is to be read as a reference to continuing to conduct the investigation.

---

[180] Repealed, never in force by Public Bodies Act 2011 c. 24 Pt 2 s.33(2) (February 14, 2012).

Corporate Manslaughter and Corporate Homicide Act 2007
c. 19

Corporate manslaughter and corporate homicide

The offence

1.—(1) An organisation to which this section applies is guilty of an offence if the way in   **A1–198**
which its activities are managed or organised—

  (a) causes a person's death, and

  (b) amounts to a gross breach of a relevant duty of care owed by the organisation to the
deceased.

(2) The organisations to which this section applies are—

  (a) a corporation;

  (b) a department or other body listed in Schedule 1;

  (c) a police force;

  (d) a partnership, or a trade union or employers' association, that is an employer.

(3) An organisation is guilty of an offence under this section only if the way in which its
activities are managed or organised by its senior management is a substantial element in the
breach referred to in subsection (1).

(4) For the purposes of this Act—

  (a) "relevant duty of care" has the meaning given by section 2, read with sections 3 to
7;

  (b) a breach of a duty of care by an organisation is a "gross" breach if the conduct
alleged to amount to a breach of that duty falls far below what can reasonably be
expected of the organisation in the circumstances;

  (c) "senior management", in relation to an organisation, means the persons who play
significant roles in—

    (i) the making of decisions about how the whole or a substantial part of its
activities are to be managed or organised, or

    (ii) the actual managing or organising of the whole or a substantial part of those
activities.

(5) The offence under this section is called—

  (a) corporate manslaughter, in so far as it is an offence under the law of England and
Wales or Northern Ireland;

  (b) corporate homicide, in so far as it is an offence under the law of Scotland.

(6) An organisation that is guilty of corporate manslaughter or corporate homicide is
liable on conviction on indictment to a fine.

(7) The offence of corporate homicide is indictable only in the High Court of Justiciary.

Relevant duty of care

Meaning of "relevant duty of care"

2.—(1) A "relevant duty of care", in relation to an organisation, means any of the   **A1–199**
following duties owed by it under the law of negligence—

(a) a duty owed to its employees or to other persons working for the organisation or performing services for it;

(b) a duty owed as occupier of premises;

(c) a duty owed in connection with—

(i) the supply by the organisation of goods or services (whether for consideration or not),

(ii) the carrying on by the organisation of any construction or maintenance operations,

(iii) the carrying on by the organisation of any other activity on a commercial basis, or

(iv) the use or keeping by the organisation of any plant, vehicle or other thing;

(d) a duty owed to a person who, by reason of being a person within subsection (2), is someone for whose safety the organisation is responsible.

(2) A person is within this subsection if—

(a) he is detained at a custodial institution or in a custody area at a court [, a police station or customs premises]¹⁸¹;

[(aa) he is detained in service custody premises;]¹⁸²

(b) he is detained at a removal centre or short–term holding facility;

(c) he is being transported in a vehicle, or being held in any premises, in pursuance of prison escort arrangements or immigration escort arrangements;

(d) he is living in secure accommodation in which he has been placed;

(e) he is a detained patient.

(3) Subsection (1) is subject to sections 3 to 7.

(4) A reference in subsection (1) to a duty owed under the law of negligence includes a reference to a duty that would be owed under the law of negligence but for any statutory provision under which liability is imposed in place of liability under that law.

(5) For the purposes of this Act, whether a particular organisation owes a duty of care to a particular individual is a question of law.

The judge must make any findings of fact necessary to decide that question.

(6) For the purposes of this Act there is to be disregarded—

(a) any rule of the common law that has the effect of preventing a duty of care from being owed by one person to another by reason of the fact that they are jointly engaged in unlawful conduct;

(b) any such rule that has the effect of preventing a duty of care from being owed to a person by reason of his acceptance of a risk of harm.

(7) In this section—

"construction or maintenance operations" means operations of any of the following descriptions—

(a) construction, installation, alteration, extension, improvement, repair, maintenance, decoration, cleaning, demolition or dismantling of—

---

¹⁸¹ Words substituted by Corporate Manslaughter and Corporate Homicide Act 2007 (Amendment) Order 2011/1868 art.2(2) (September 1, 2011).

¹⁸² Added by Corporate Manslaughter and Corporate Homicide Act 2007 (Amendment) Order 2011/1868 art.2(3) (September 1, 2011).

(i) any building or structure,

(ii) anything else that forms, or is to form, part of the land, or

(iii) any plant, vehicle or other thing;

(b) operations that form an integral part of, or are preparatory to, or are for rendering complete, any operations within paragraph (a);

"custodial institution" means a prison, a young offender institution, a secure training centre, a young offenders institution, a young offenders centre, a juvenile justice centre or a remand centre;

["customs premises" means premises wholly or partly occupied by persons designated under section 3 (general customs officials) or 11 (customs revenue officials) of the Borders, Citizenship and Immigration Act 2009;][183]

"detained patient" means—

(a) a person who is detained in any premises under—

(i) Part 2 or 3 of the Mental Health Act 1983 (c. 20) ("the 1983 Act"), or

(ii) Part 2 or 3 of the Mental Health (Northern Ireland) Order 1986 (SI 1986/595 (N.I. 4)) ("the 1986 Order");

(b) a person who (otherwise than by reason of being detained as mentioned in paragraph (a)) is deemed to be in legal custody by—

(i) section 137 of the 1983 Act,

(ii) Article 131 of the 1986 Order, or

(iii) article 11 of the Mental Health (Care and Treatment) (Scotland) Act 2003 (Consequential Provisions) Order 2005 (SI 2005/2078);

(c) a person who is detained in any premises, or is otherwise in custody, under the Mental Health (Care and Treatment) (Scotland) Act 2003 (asp 13) or Part 6 of the Criminal Procedure (Scotland) Act 1995 (c. 46) or who is detained in a hospital under section 200 of that Act of 1995;

"immigration escort arrangements" means arrangements made under section 156 of the Immigration and Asylum Act 1999 (c. 33);

"the law of negligence" includes—

(a) in relation to England and Wales, the Occupiers' Liability Act 1957 (c. 31), the Defective Premises Act 1972 (c. 35) and the Occupiers' Liability Act 1984 (c. 3);

(b) in relation to Scotland, the Occupiers' Liability (Scotland) Act 1960 (c. 30);

(c) in relation to Northern Ireland, the Occupiers' Liability Act (Northern Ireland) 1957 (c. 25), the Defective Premises (Northern Ireland) Order 1975 (SI 1975/1039 (N.I. 9)), the Occupiers' Liability (Northern Ireland) Order 1987 (SI 1987/1280 (N.I. 15)) and the Defective Premises (Land-lord's Liability) Act (Northern Ireland) 2001 (c. 10);

"prison escort arrangements" means arrangements made under section 80 of the Criminal Justice Act 1991 (c. 53) or under section 102 or 118 of the Criminal Justice and Public Order Act 1994 (c. 33);

"removal centre" and "short-term holding facility" have the meaning given by section 147 of the Immigration and Asylum Act 1999;

---

[183] Definition inserted by Corporate Manslaughter and Corporate Homicide Act 2007 (Amendment) Order 2011/1868 art.2(4)(a) (September 1, 2011).

"secure accommodation" means accommodation, not consisting of or forming part of a custodial institution, provided for the purpose of restricting the liberty of persons under the age of 18 [;][184]

["service custody premises" has the meaning given by section 300(7) of the Armed Forces Act 2006.][4]

Public policy decisions, exclusively public functions and statutory inspections

A1–200   **3.**—(1) Any duty of care owed by a public authority in respect of a decision as to matters of public policy (including in particular the allocation of public resources or the weighing of competing public interests) is not a "relevant duty of care" .

(2) Any duty of care owed in respect of things done in the exercise of an exclusively public function is not a "relevant duty of care" unless it falls within section 2(1)(a), (b) or (d).

(3) Any duty of care owed by a public authority in respect of inspections carried out in the exercise of a statutory function is not a "relevant duty of care" unless it falls within section 2(1)(a) or (b).

(4) In this section—

"exclusively public function" means a function that falls within the prerogative of the Crown or is, by its nature, exercisable only with authority conferred—

(a) by the exercise of that prerogative, or

(b) by or under a statutory provision;

"statutory function" means a function conferred by or under a statutory provision.

Military activities

A1–201   **4.**—(1) Any duty of care owed by the Ministry of Defence in respect of—

(a) operations within subsection (2),

(b) activities carried on in preparation for, or directly in support of, such operations, or

(c) training of a hazardous nature, or training carried out in a hazardous way, which it is considered needs to be carried out, or carried out in that way, in order to improve or maintain the effectiveness of the armed forces with respect to such operations,

is not a "relevant duty of care" .

(2) The operations within this subsection are operations, including peacekeeping operations and operations for dealing with terrorism, civil unrest or serious public disorder, in the course of which members of the armed forces come under attack or face the threat of attack or violent resistance.

(3) Any duty of care owed by the Ministry of Defence in respect of activities carried on by members of the special forces is not a "relevant duty of care" .

(4) In this section "the special forces" means those units of the armed forces the maintenance of whose capabilities is the responsibility of the Director of Special Forces or which are for the time being subject to the operational command of that Director.

---

[184] Definition inserted by Corporate Manslaughter and Corporate Homicide Act 2007 (Amendment) Order 2011/1868 art.2(4)(b) (September 1, 2011).

Policing and law enforcement

5.—(1) Any duty of care owed by a public authority in respect of—   **A1–202**

(a) operations within subsection (2),

(b) activities carried on in preparation for, or directly in support of, such operations, or

(c) training of a hazardous nature, or training carried out in a hazardous way, which it is considered needs to be carried out, or carried out in that way, in order to improve or maintain the effectiveness of officers or employees of the public authority with respect to such operations,

is not a "relevant duty of care" .
(2) Operations are within this subsection if—

(a) they are operations for dealing with terrorism, civil unrest or serious disorder,

(b) they involve the carrying on of policing or law–enforcement activities, and

(c) officers or employees of the public authority in question come under attack, or face the threat of attack or violent resistance, in the course of the operations.

(3) Any duty of care owed by a public authority in respect of other policing or law–enforcement activities is not a "relevant duty of care" unless it falls within section 2(1)(a), (b) or (d).
(4) In this section "policing or law–enforcement activities" includes—

(a) activities carried on in the exercise of functions that are—

(i) functions of police forces, or
(ii) functions of the same or a similar nature exercisable by public authorities other than police forces;

(b) activities carried on in the exercise of functions of constables employed by a public authority;

(c) activities carried on in the exercise of functions exercisable under Chapter 4 of Part 2 of the Serious Organised Crime and Police Act 2005 (c. 15) (protection of witnesses and other persons);

(d) activities carried on to enforce any provision contained in or made under the Immigration Acts.

Emergencies

6.—(1) Any duty of care owed by an organisation within subsection (2) in respect of the   **A1–203**
way in which it responds to emergency circumstances is not a "relevant duty of care" unless
it falls within section 2(1)(a) or (b).
(2) The organisations within this subsection are—

(a) a fire and rescue authority in England and Wales;

[(b) the Scottish Fire and Rescue Service;][185]

(c) the Northern Ireland Fire and Rescue Service Board;

---

[185] Substituted by Police and Fire Reform (Scotland) Act 2012 (Consequential Provisions and Modifications) Order 2013/602 Sch.1 para.9 (April 1, 2013).

(d) any other organisation providing a service of responding to emergency circumstances either—

    (i) in pursuance of arrangements made with an organisation within paragraph (a), (b) or (c), or

    (ii) (if not in pursuance of such arrangements) otherwise than on a commercial basis;

(e) a relevant NHS body;

(f) an organisation providing ambulance services in pursuance of arrangements—

    (i) made by, or at the request of, a relevant NHS body, or

    (ii) made with the Secretary of State or with the Welsh Ministers;

(g) an organisation providing services for the transport of organs, blood, equipment or personnel in pursuance of arrangements of the kind mentioned in paragraph (f);

(h) an organisation providing a rescue service;

(i) the armed forces.

(3) For the purposes of subsection (1), the way in which an organisation responds to emergency circumstances does not include the way in which—

(a) medical treatment is carried out, or

(b) decisions within subsection (4) are made.

(4) The decisions within this subsection are decisions as to the carrying out of medical treatment, other than decisions as to the order in which persons are to be given such treatment.

(5) Any duty of care owed in respect of the carrying out, or attempted carrying out, of a rescue operation at sea in emergency circumstances is not a "relevant duty of care" unless it falls within section 2(1)(a) or (b).

(6) Any duty of care owed in respect of action taken—

(a) in order to comply with a direction under Schedule 3A to the Merchant Shipping Act 1995 (c. 21) (safety directions), or

(b) by virtue of paragraph 4 of that Schedule (action in lieu of direction),

is not a "relevant duty of care" unless it falls within section 2(1)(a) or (b).

(7) In this section—

"emergency circumstances" means circumstances that are present or imminent and—

    (a) are causing, or are likely to cause, serious harm or a worsening of such harm, or

    (b) are likely to cause the death of a person;

"medical treatment" includes any treatment or procedure of a medical or similar nature;

"relevant NHS body" means—

    [(za) the National Health Service Commissioning Board;][186]

---

[186] Added by Health and Social Care Act 2012 c. 7 Sch.5 para.147(a) (October 1, 2012).

(a) [a clinical commissioning group,]¹⁸⁷ [. . .]¹⁸⁸ [. . .]¹⁸⁹ NHS trust, Special Health Authority or NHS foundation trust in England;

(b) a Local Health Board, NHS trust or Special Health Authority in Wales;

(c) a Health Board or Special Health Board in Scotland, or the Common Services Agency for the Scottish Health Service;

(d) a Health and Social Services trust or Health and Social Services Board in Northern Ireland;

"serious harm" means—

(a) serious injury to or the serious illness (including mental illness) of a person;

(b) serious harm to the environment (including the life and health of plants and animals);

(c) serious harm to any building or other property.

(8) A reference in this section to emergency circumstances includes a reference to circumstances that are believed to be emergency circumstances.

Child-protection and probation functions

7.—(1) A duty of care to which this section applies is not a "relevant duty of care" unless it falls within section 2(1)(a), (b) or (d). **A1–204**

(2) This section applies to any duty of care that a local authority or other public authority owes in respect of the exercise by it of functions conferred by or under—

(a) Parts 4 and 5 of the Children Act 1989 (c. 41),

(b) Part 2 of the Children (Scotland) Act 1995 (c. 36) , [. . .]¹⁹⁰

[(ba) the Children's Hearings (Scotland) Act 2011, or]¹

(c) Parts 5 and 6 of the Children (Northern Ireland) Order 1995 (SI 1995/755 (N.I. 2)).

(3) This section also applies to any duty of care that a local probation board [, a provider of probation services]¹⁹¹ or other public authority owes in respect of the exercise by it of functions conferred by or under—

(a) Chapter 1 of Part 1 of the Criminal Justice and Court Services Act **2000** (c. 43),

[(aa) section 13 of the Offender Management Act 2007 (c. 21),]¹⁹²

(b) section 27 of the Social Work (Scotland) Act 1968 (c. 49), or

---

¹⁸⁷ Words inserted by Health and Social Care Act 2012 c. 7 Sch.5 para.147(b)(i) (October 1, 2012).

¹⁸⁸ Words repealed by Health and Social Care Act 2012 c. 7 Sch.5 para.147(b)(ii) (April 1, 2013 subject to savings and transitional provisons specified in SI 2013/160 arts 5-9).

¹⁸⁹ Words repealed by Health and Social Care Act 2012 c. 7 Sch.5 para.147(b)(iii) (April 1, 2013 subject to savings and transitional provisons specified in SI 2013/160 arts 5-9).

¹⁹⁰ Added by Children's Hearings (Scotland) Act 2011 (Consequential and Transitional Provisions and Savings) Order 2013/1465 Sch.1(1) para.11 (June 24, 2013 being the date on which 2011 asp 1 s.7 comes into force).

¹⁹¹ Words inserted by Offender Management Act 2007 (Consequential Amendments) Order 2008/912 Sch.1(1) para.25(2)(a)(i) (April 6, 2008: insertion came into force on April 1, 2008 but could not take effect until the commencement of s.7(3) on April 6, 2008).

¹⁹² Added by Offender Management Act 2007 (Consequential Amendments) Order 2008/912 Sch.1(1) para.25(2)(a)(ii) (April 6, 2008: insertion came into force on April 1, 2008 but could not take effect until the commencement of s.7(3) on April 6, 2008).

(c) Article 4 of the Probation Board (Northern Ireland) Order 1982 (SI 1982/713 (N.I. 10)).

[(4) This section also applies to any duty of care that a provider of probation services owes in respect of the carrying out by it of activities in pursuance of arrangements under section 3 of the Offender Management Act 2007.][193]

Gross breach

Factors for jury

A1–205   8.—(1) This section applies where—

(a) it is established that an organisation owed a relevant duty of care to a person, and

(b) it falls to the jury to decide whether there was a gross breach of that duty.

(2) The jury must consider whether the evidence shows that the organisation failed to comply with any health and safety legislation that relates to the alleged breach, and if so—

(a) how serious that failure was;

(b) how much of a risk of death it posed.

(3) The jury may also—

(a) consider the extent to which the evidence shows that there were attitudes, policies, systems or accepted practices within the organisation that were likely to have encouraged any such failure as is mentioned in subsection (2), or to have produced tolerance of it;

(b) have regard to any health and safety guidance that relates to the alleged breach.

(4) This section does not prevent the jury from having regard to any other matters they consider relevant.

(5) In this section "health and safety guidance" means any code, guidance, manual or similar publication that is concerned with health and safety matters and is made or issued (under a statutory provision or otherwise) by an authority responsible for the enforcement of any health and safety legislation.

Remedial orders and publicity orders

Power to order breach etc to be remedied

A1–206   9.—(1) A court before which an organisation is convicted of corporate manslaughter or corporate homicide may make an order (a "remedial order") requiring the organisation to take specified steps to remedy—

(a) the breach mentioned in section 1(1) ("the relevant breach");

(b) any matter that appears to the court to have resulted from the relevant breach and to have been a cause of the death;

---

[193] Added by Offender Management Act 2007 (Consequential Amendments) Order 2008/912 Sch.1(1) para.25(2)(b) (April 6, 2008: insertion came into force on April 1, 2008 but could not take effect until the commencement of s.7 on April 6, 2008).

(c) any deficiency, as regards health and safety matters, in the organisation's policies, systems or practices of which the relevant breach appears to the court to be an indication.

(2) A remedial order may be made only on an application by the prosecution specifying the terms of the proposed order.

Any such order must be on such terms (whether those proposed or others) as the court considers appropriate having regard to any representations made, and any evidence adduced, in relation to that matter by the prosecution or on behalf of the organisation.

(3) Before making an application for a remedial order the prosecution must consult such enforcement authority or authorities as it considers appropriate having regard to the nature of the relevant breach.

(4) A remedial order—

(a) must specify a period within which the steps referred to in subsection (1) are to be taken;

(b) may require the organisation to supply to an enforcement authority consulted under subsection (3), within a specified period, evidence that those steps have been taken.

A period specified under this subsection may be extended or further extended by order of the court on an application made before the end of that period or extended period.

(5) An organisation that fails to comply with a remedial order is guilty of an offence, and liable on conviction on indictment to a fine.

Power to order conviction etc to be publicised

10.—(1) A court before which an organisation is convicted of corporate manslaughter or corporate homicide may make an order (a "publicity order") requiring the organisation to publicise in a specified manner— **A1–207**

(a) the fact that it has been convicted of the offence;

(b) specified particulars of the offence;

(c) the amount of any fine imposed;

(d) the terms of any remedial order made.

(2) In deciding on the terms of a publicity order that it is proposing to make, the court must—

(a) ascertain the views of such enforcement authority or authorities (if any) as it considers appropriate, and

(b) have regard to any representations made by the prosecution or on behalf of the organisation.

(3) A publicity order—

(a) must specify a period within which the requirements referred to in subsection (1) are to be complied with;

(b) may require the organisation to supply to any enforcement authority whose views have been ascertained under subsection (2), within a specified period, evidence that those requirements have been complied with.

(4) An organisation that fails to comply with a publicity order is guilty of an offence, and liable on conviction on indictment to a fine.

Application to particular categories of organisation

Application to Crown bodies

A1–208   **11.**—(1) An organisation that is a servant or agent of the Crown is not immune from prosecution under this Act for that reason.

(2) For the purposes of this Act—

(a) a department or other body listed in Schedule 1, or

(b) a corporation that is a servant or agent of the Crown,

is to be treated as owing whatever duties of care it would owe if it were a corporation that was not a servant or agent of the Crown.

(3) For the purposes of section 2—

(a) a person who is—

(i) employed by or under the Crown for the purposes of a department or other body listed in Schedule 1, or

(ii) employed by a person whose staff constitute a body listed in that Schedule,

is to be treated as employed by that department or body;

(b) any premises occupied for the purposes of—

(i) a department or other body listed in Schedule 1, or

(ii) a person whose staff constitute a body listed in that Schedule,

are to be treated as occupied by that department or body.

(4) For the purposes of sections 2 to 7 anything done purportedly by a department or other body listed in Schedule 1, although in law by the Crown or by the holder of a particular office, is to be treated as done by the department or other body itself.

(5) Subsections (3)(a)(i), (3)(b)(i) and (4) apply in relation to a Northern Ireland department as they apply in relation to a department or other body listed in Schedule 1.

Application to armed forces

A1–209   **12.**—(1) In this Act "the armed forces" means any of the naval, military or air forces of the Crown raised under the law of the United Kingdom.

(2) For the purposes of section 2 a person who is a member of the armed forces is to be treated as employed by the Ministry of Defence.

(3) A reference in this Act to members of the armed forces includes a reference to—

(a) members of the reserve forces (within the meaning given by section 1(2) of the Reserve Forces Act 1996 (c. 14)) when in service or undertaking training or duties;

(b) persons serving on Her Majesty's vessels (within the meaning given by section 132(1) of the Naval Discipline Act 1957 (c. 53)).

Application to police forces

A1–210   **13.**—(1) In this Act "police force" means—

(a) a police force within the meaning of—

(i) the Police Act 1996 (c. 16) , [. . .]¹⁹⁴

[. . .]¹⁹⁵

---

¹⁹⁴ Word repealed by Police and Fire Reform (Scotland) Act 2012 (Consequential Provisions and Modifications) Order 2013/602 Sch.2(1) para.57(2)(a) (April 1, 2013).
¹⁹⁵ Repealed by Police and Fire Reform (Scotland) Act 2012 (Consequential Provisions and Modifications) Order 2013/602 Sch.2(1) para.57(2)(b) (April 1, 2013).

[(aa) the Police Service of Scotland;][196]

  (b) the Police Service of Northern Ireland;

  (c) the Police Service of Northern Ireland Reserve;

  (d) the British Transport Police Force;

  (e) the Civil Nuclear Constabulary;

  (f) the Ministry of Defence Police.

(2) For the purposes of this Act a police force is to be treated as owing whatever duties of care it would owe if it were a body corporate.

(3) For the purposes of section 2—

  (a) a member of a police force is to be treated as employed by that force;

  (b) a special constable appointed for a police area in England and Wales is to be treated as employed by the police force maintained by the [local policing body][197] for that area;

  (c) a special constable appointed for a police force mentioned in paragraph (d) or (f) of subsection (1) is to be treated as employed by that force;

  (d) a police cadet undergoing training with a view to becoming a member of a police force mentioned in paragraph (a) [, (aa)][198] or (d) of subsection (1) is to be treated as employed by that force;

  (e) a police trainee appointed under section 39 of the Police (Northern Ireland) Act 2000 (c. 32) or a police cadet appointed under section 42 of that Act is to be treated as employed by the Police Service of Northern Ireland;

  (f) a police reserve trainee appointed under section 40 of that Act is to be treated as employed by the Police Service of Northern Ireland Reserve;

  (g) a member of a police force [seconded to the National Crime Agency to serve as a National Crime Agency officer is to be treated][199] as employed by that Agency.

(4) A reference in subsection (3) to a member of a police force is to be read, in the case of [the Police Service of Scotland, as a reference to a constable of that Service.][200]

(5) For the purposes of section 2 any premises occupied for the purposes of a police force are to be treated as occupied by that force.

(6) For the purposes of sections 2 to 7 anything that would be regarded as done by a police force if the force were a body corporate is to be so regarded.

(7) Where—

  (a) by virtue of subsection (3) a person is treated for the purposes of section 2 as employed by a police force, and

---

[196] Added by Police and Fire Reform (Scotland) Act 2012 (Consequential Provisions and Modifications) Order 2013/602 Sch.2(1) para.57(2)(c) (April 1, 2013).

[197] Words substituted by Police Reform and Social Responsibility Act 2011 c. 13 Sch.16(3) para.365 (January 16, 2012).

[198] Word inserted by Police and Fire Reform (Scotland) Act 2012 (Consequential Provisions and Modifications) Order 2013/602 Sch.2(1) para.57(2)(d) (April 1, 2013).

[199] Words substituted by Crime and Courts Act 2013 c. 22 Sch.8(2) para.174 (October 7, 2013: substitution has effect as SI 2013/1682 subject to savings and transitional provisions specified in 2013 c.22 s.15 and Sch.8).

[200] Words substituted by Police and Fire Reform (Scotland) Act 2012 (Consequential Provisions and Modifications) Order 2013/602 Sch.2(1) para.57(2)(e) (April 1, 2013).

(b) by virtue of any other statutory provision (whenever made) he is, or is treated as, employed by another organisation,

the person is to be treated for those purposes as employed by both the force and the other organisation.

Application to partnerships

A1–211   **14.**—(1) For the purposes of this Act a partnership is to be treated as owing whatever duties of care it would owe if it were a body corporate.

(2) Proceedings for an offence under this Act alleged to have been committed by a partnership are to be brought in the name of the partnership (and not in that of any of its members).

(3) A fine imposed on a partnership on its conviction of an offence under this Act is to be paid out of the funds of the partnership.

(4) This section does not apply to a partnership that is a legal person under the law by which it is governed.

Miscellaneous

Procedure, evidence and sentencing

A1–212   **15.**—(1) Any statutory provision (whenever made) about criminal proceedings applies, subject to any prescribed adaptations or modifications, in relation to proceedings under this Act against—

(a) a department or other body listed in Schedule 1,

(b) a police force,

(c) a partnership,

(d) a trade union, or

(e) an employers' association that is not a corporation,

as it applies in relation to proceedings against a corporation.

(2) In this section—

"prescribed" means [—

(a) in relation to proceedings under this Act in England and Wales, prescribed by an order made by the Secretary of State;

(b) in relation to proceedings under this Act in Northern Ireland, prescribed by an order made by the Department of Justice in Northern Ireland;][201]

"provision about criminal proceedings" includes—

(a) provision about procedure in or in connection with criminal proceedings;

(b) provision about evidence in such proceedings;

(c) provision about sentencing, or otherwise dealing with, persons convicted of offences;

"statutory" means contained in, or in an instrument made under, any Act or any Northern Ireland legislation.

---

[201] S.15(2)(a) and (b) substituted for words by Northern Ireland Act 1998 (Devolution of Policing and Justice Functions) Order 2010/976 Sch.9 para.2(2) (April 12, 2010: substitution has effect subject to transitional provision specified in SI 2010/976 art.28).

(3) A reference in this section to proceedings [(except in the definition of "prescribed" in subsection (2))]²⁰² is to proceedings in England and Wales or Northern Ireland.

(4) An order [of the Secretary of State]²⁰³ under this section is subject to negative resolution procedure.

Transfer of functions

16.—(1) This section applies where—   **A1–213**

(a) a person's death has occurred, or is alleged to have occurred, in connection with the carrying out of functions by a relevant public organisation, and

(b) subsequently there is a transfer of those functions, with the result that they are still carried out but no longer by that organisation.

(2) In this section "relevant public organisation" means—

(a) a department or other body listed in Schedule 1;

(b) a corporation that is a servant or agent of the Crown;

(c) a police force.

(3) Any proceedings instituted against a relevant public organisation after the transfer for an offence under this Act in respect of the person's death are to be instituted against—

(a) the relevant public organisation, if any, by which the functions mentioned in subsection (1) are currently carried out;

(b) if no such organisation currently carries out the functions, the relevant public organisation by which the functions were last carried out.

This is subject to subsection (4).

(4) If an order made by the Secretary of State so provides in relation to a particular transfer of functions, the proceedings referred to in subsection (3) may be instituted, or (if they have already been instituted) may be continued, against—

(a) the organisation mentioned in subsection (1), or

(b) such relevant public organisation (other than the one mentioned in subsection (1) or the one mentioned in subsection (3)(a) or (b)) as may be specified in the order.

(5) If the transfer occurs while proceedings for an offence under this Act in respect of the person's death are in progress against a relevant public organisation, the proceedings are to be continued against—

(a) the relevant public organisation, if any, by which the functions mentioned in subsection (1) are carried out as a result of the transfer;

(b) if as a result of the transfer no such organisation carries out the functions, the same organisation as before.

This is subject to subsection (6).

---

²⁰² Words inserted by Northern Ireland Act 1998 (Devolution of Policing and Justice Functions) Order 2010/976 Sch.9 para.2(3) (April 12, 2010: insertion has effect subject to transitional provision specified in SI 2010/976 art.28).

²⁰³ Words inserted by Northern Ireland Act 1998 (Devolution of Policing and Justice Functions) Order 2010/976 Sch.9 para.2(4) (April 12, 2010: insertion has effect subject to transitional provision specified in SI 2010/976 art.28).

(6) If an order made by the Secretary of State so provides in relation to a particular transfer of functions, the proceedings referred to in subsection (5) may be continued against—

(a) the organisation mentioned in subsection (1), or

(b) such relevant public organisation (other than the one mentioned in subsection (1) or the one mentioned in subsection (5)(a) or (b)) as may be specified in the order.

(7) An order under subsection (4) or (6) is subject to negative resolution procedure.

DPP's consent required for proceedings

A1–214   **17.** Proceedings for an offence of corporate manslaughter—

(a) may not be instituted in England and Wales without the consent of the Director of Public Prosecutions;

(b) may not be instituted in Northern Ireland without the consent of the Director of Public Prosecutions for Northern Ireland.

[No individual liability

A1–215   **18.**—(1) An individual cannot be guilty of aiding, abetting, counselling or procuring the commission of an offence of corporate manslaughter.

(1A) An individual cannot be guilty of an offence under Part 2 of the Serious Crime Act 2007 (encouraging or assisting crime) by reference to an offence of corporate manslaughter.

(2) An individual cannot be guilty of aiding, abetting, counselling or procuring, or being art and part in, the commission of an offence of corporate homicide.][204]

Convictions under this Act and under health and safety legislation

A1–216   **19.**—(1) Where in the same proceedings there is—

(a) a charge of corporate manslaughter or corporate homicide arising out of a particular set of circumstances, and

(b) a charge against the same defendant of a health and safety offence arising out of some or all of those circumstances,

the jury may, if the interests of justice so require, be invited to return a verdict on each charge.

(2) An organisation that has been convicted of corporate manslaughter or corporate homicide arising out of a particular set of circumstances may, if the interests of justice so require, be charged with a health and safety offence arising out of some or all of those circumstances.

(3) In this section "health and safety offence" means an offence under any health and safety legislation.

Abolition of liability of corporations for manslaughter at common law

A1–217   **20.** The common law offence of manslaughter by gross negligence is abolished in its application to corporations, and in any application it has to other organisations to which section 1 applies.

---

[204] Added by Serious Crime Act 2007 c. 27 Pt 2 s.62 (October 1, 2008).

General and supplemental

Power to extend section 1 to other organisations

21.—(1) The Secretary of State may by order amend section 1 so as to extend the **A1–218** categories of organisation to which that section applies.

(2) An order under this section may make any amendment to this Act that is incidental or supplemental to, or consequential on, an amendment made by virtue of subsection (1).

(3) An order under this section is subject to affirmative resolution procedure.

Power to amend Schedule 1

22.—(1) The Secretary of State may amend Schedule 1 by order. **A1–219**

(2) A statutory instrument containing an order under this section is subject to affirmative resolution procedure, unless the only amendments to Schedule 1 that it makes are amendments within subsection (3).

In that case the instrument is subject to negative resolution procedure.

(3) An amendment is within this subsection if—

(a) it is consequential on a department or other body listed in Schedule 1 changing its name,

(b) in the case of an amendment adding a department or other body to Schedule 1, it is consequential on the transfer to the department or other body of functions all of which were previously exercisable by one or more organisations to which section 1 applies, or

(c) in the case of an amendment removing a department or other body from Schedule 1, it is consequential on—

(i) the abolition of the department or other body, or

(ii) the transfer of all the functions of the department or other body to one or more organisations to which section 1 applies.

Power to extend section 2(2)

23.—(1) The Secretary of State may by order amend section 2(2) to make it include any **A1–220** category of person (not already included) who—

(a) is required by virtue of a statutory provision to remain or reside on particular premises, or

(b) is otherwise subject to a restriction of his liberty.

(2) An order under this section may make any amendment to this Act that is incidental or supplemental to, or consequential on, an amendment made by virtue of subsection (1).

(3) An order under this section is subject to affirmative resolution procedure.

[Powers of Department of Justice in Northern Ireland

23A. [Applies to Northern Ireland]][205] **A1–221**

---

[205] Added by Northern Ireland Act 1998 (Devolution of Policing and Justice Functions) Order 2010/976 Sch.9 para.3 (April 12, 2010: insertion has effect subject to transitional provision specified in SI 2010/976 art.28).

Orders

A1–222   **24.**—(1) A power of the Secretary of State to make an order under this Act is exercisable by statutory instrument.

(2) Where an order under this Act is subject to "negative resolution procedure" the statutory instrument containing the order is subject to annulment in pursuance of a resolution of either House of Parliament.

(3) Where an order under this Act is subject to "affirmative resolution procedure" the order may not be made unless a draft has been laid before, and approved by a resolution of, each House of Parliament.

(4) An order under this Act—

(a) may make different provision for different purposes;

(b) may make transitional or saving provision.

[(5) A power of the Department of Justice in Northern Ireland to make an order under this Act is exercisable by statutory rule for the purposes of the Statutory Rules (Northern Ireland) Order 1979.[206]

(6) An order made by the Department of Justice under section 15 or 16 is subject to negative resolution (within the meaning of section 41(6) of the Interpretation Act (Northern Ireland) 1954[207]).

(7) No order shall be made by the Department of Justice under section 21 or 23 or (subject to subsection (8)) section 22, unless a draft of it has been laid before, and approved by a resolution of, the Northern Ireland Assembly.

(8) If the only amendments to Schedule 1 made by an order of the Department of Justice under section 22 are amendments within subsection (3) of that section—

(a) subsection (7) of this section does not apply to the making of the order, and

(b) the order is subject to negative resolution (within the meaning of section 41(6) of the Interpretation Act (Northern Ireland) 1954).

(9) No order shall be made by the Department of Justice under section 27 bringing into force paragraph (d) of section 2(1) unless a draft of the order has been laid before, and approved by a resolution of, the Northern Ireland Assembly.

(10) Section 41(3) of the Interpretation Act (Northern Ireland) 1954[208] applies for the purposes of subsections (7) and (9) in relation to the laying of a draft as it applies in relation to the laying of a statutory document under an enactment.][209]

Interpretation

A1–223   **25.** In this Act—

"armed forces" has the meaning given by section 12(1);
"corporation" does not include a corporation sole but includes any body corporate wherever incorporated;
"employee" means an individual who works under a contract of employment or apprenticeship (whether express or implied and, if express, whether oral or in writing), and related expressions are to be construed accordingly; see also sections 11(3)(a), 12(2) and 13(3) (which apply for the purposes of section 2);

---

[206] SI 1979/1573 (N.I. 12).
[207] 1954 c. 33 (N.I.). Section 41(6) was amended by SI 1999/663.
[208] Section 41(3) was substituted by SI 1999/663.
[209] Added by Northern Ireland Act 1998 (Devolution of Policing and Justice Functions) Order 2010/976 Sch.9 para.4(2) (April 12, 2010: insertion has effect subject to transitional provision specified in SI 2010/976 art.28).

"employers' association" has the meaning given by section 122 of the Trade Union and Labour Relations (Consolidation) Act 1992 (c. 52) or Article 4 of the Industrial Relations (Northern Ireland) Order 1992 (SI 1992/807 (N.I. 5));

"enforcement authority" means an authority responsible for the enforcement of any health and safety legislation;

["health and safety legislation" means any statutory provision dealing with health and safety matters, including in particular provision contained in the Health and Safety at Work etc. Act 1974 (c. 37) or the Health and Safety at Work (Northern Ireland) Order 1978 (SI 1978/1039 (N.I. 9)) and provision dealing with health and safety matters contained in Part 3 of the Energy Act 2013 (nuclear regulation);][210]

"member", in relation to the armed forces, is to be read in accordance with section 12(3);

"partnership" means—

(a) a partnership within the Partnership Act 1890 (c. 39), or

(b) a limited partnership registered under the Limited Partnerships Act 1907 (c. 24),

or a firm or entity of a similar character formed under the law of a country or territory outside the United Kingdom;

"police force" has the meaning given by section 13(1);

"premises" includes land, buildings and moveable structures;

"public authority" has the same meaning as in section 6 of the Human Rights Act 1998 (c. 42) (disregarding subsections (3)(a) and (4) of that section);

"publicity order" means an order under section 10(1);

"remedial order" means an order under section 9(1);

"statutory provision", except in section 15, means provision contained in, or in an instrument made under, any Act, any Act of the Scottish Parliament or any Northern Ireland legislation;

"trade union" has the meaning given by section 1 of the Trade Union and Labour Relations (Consolidation) Act 1992 (c. 52) or Article 3 of the Industrial Relations (Northern Ireland) Order 1992 (SI 1992/807 (N.I. 5)).

Minor and consequential amendments

26. Schedule 2 (minor and consequential amendments) has effect.   **A1–224**

Commencement and savings

27.—(1) The preceding provisions of this Act come into force in accordance with   **A1–225**
provision made by order by the Secretary of State [(subject to subsection (1A))].[211]

[(1A) The power in subsection (1) is exercisable by the Department of Justice in Northern Ireland (and not by the Secretary of State) for the purposes of the law of Northern Ireland.][212]

(2) An order [of the Secretary of State][213] bringing into force paragraph (d) of section 2(1) is subject to affirmative resolution procedure.

---

[210] Words inserted by Energy Act 2013 c. 32 Sch.12(5) para.93 (April 1, 2014).

[211] Words inserted by Northern Ireland Act 1998 (Devolution of Policing and Justice Functions) Order 2010/976 Sch.9 para.5(2) (April 12, 2010: insertion has effect subject to transitional provision specified in SI 2010/976 art.28).

[212] Added by Northern Ireland Act 1998 (Devolution of Policing and Justice Functions) Order 2010/976 Sch.9 para.5(3) (April 12, 2010: insertion has effect subject to transitional provision specified in SI 2010/976 art.28).

[213] Words inserted by Northern Ireland Act 1998 (Devolution of Policing and Justice Functions) Order 2010/976 Sch.9 para.5(4) (April 12, 2010: insertion has effect subject to transitional provision specified in SI 2010/976 art.28).

(3) Section 1 does not apply in relation to anything done or omitted before the commencement of that section.

(4) Section 20 does not affect any liability, investigation, legal proceeding or penalty for or in respect of an offence committed wholly or partly before the commencement of that section.

(5) For the purposes of subsection (4) an offence is committed wholly or partly before the commencement of section 20 if any of the conduct or events alleged to constitute the offence occurred before that commencement.

Extent and territorial application

A1–226   **28.**—(1) Subject to subsection (2), this Act extends to England and Wales, Scotland and Northern Ireland.

(2) An amendment made by this Act extends to the same part or parts of the United Kingdom as the provision to which it relates.

(3) Section 1 applies if the harm resulting in death is sustained in the United Kingdom or—

(a) within the seaward limits of the territorial sea adjacent to the United Kingdom;

(b) on a ship registered under Part 2 of the Merchant Shipping Act 1995 (c. 21);

(c) on a British-controlled aircraft as defined in section 92 of the Civil Aviation Act 1982 (c. 16);

(d) on a British-controlled hovercraft within the meaning of that section as applied in relation to hovercraft by virtue of provision made under the Hovercraft Act 1968 (c. 59);

(e) in any place to which an Order in Council under section 10(1) of the Petroleum Act 1998 (c. 17) applies (criminal jurisdiction in relation to offshore activities).

(4) For the purposes of subsection (3)(b) to (d) harm sustained on a ship, aircraft or hovercraft includes harm sustained by a person who—

(a) is then no longer on board the ship, aircraft or hovercraft in consequence of the wrecking of it or of some other mishap affecting it or occurring on it, and

(b) sustains the harm in consequence of that event.

Short title

A1–227   **29.** This Act may be cited as the Corporate Manslaughter and Corporate Homicide Act 2007.

SCHEDULE 1

List Of Government Departments Etc

A1–228   [. . .]²¹⁴
Attorney General's Office
Cabinet Office
Central Office of Information
Crown Office and Procurator Fiscal Service

---

²¹⁴ Words repealed subject to transitional and transitory provisions and savings as specified in SI 2008/755 arts 3–14 by Serious Crime Act 2007 c. 27 Sch.14 para.1 (April 6, 2008: repeal comes into force on April 1, 2008 as specified in SI 2008/755 art.2(1)(d)(xviii) subject to transitional and transitory provisions and savings as specified in arts 3–14, but cannot take effect until the coming into force of 2007 c.19 Sch.1 on April 6, 2008).

Crown Prosecution Service
[. . .]²¹⁵
[Department for Business, Innovation and Skills]²¹⁶
[. . .]²¹⁷
Department for Communities and Local Government
[. . .]²¹⁸
[. . .]²¹⁸
Department for Culture, Media and Sport
[Department for Education]²¹⁹
[. . .]²¹⁸
[. . .]²¹⁸
Department for Environment, Food and Rural Affairs
[. . .]²²⁰
Department for International Development
Department for Transport
Department for Work and Pensions
[Department of Energy and Climate Change]²²¹
Department of Health
[. . .]²¹⁸
[. . .]²¹⁸
Export Credits Guarantee Department
Foreign and Commonwealth Office
Forestry Commission
General Register Office for Scotland
Government Actuary's Department
Her Majesty's Land Registry
Her Majesty's Revenue and Customs
Her Majesty's Treasury
Home Office
Ministry of Defence
[Ministry of Justice (including the Scotland Office and the Wales Office)]²²²
National Archives
National Archives of Scotland
[National Crime Agency]²²³
[. . .]²²⁴
National Savings and Investments
National School of Government
Northern Ireland Audit Office

---

²¹⁵ Entry repealed by Secretary of State for Business, Innovation and Skills Order 2009/2748 Sch.1(1) para.8(b) (November 13, 2009).
²¹⁶ Words inserted by Secretary of State for Business, Innovation and Skills Order 2009/2748 Sch.1(1) para.8(a) (November 13, 2009).
²¹⁷ Entry repealed by Secretary of State for Education Order 2010/1836 Sch.1(1) para.4(a) (August 18, 2010: repeal has effect subject to transitional provisions specified in SI 2010/1836 art.5).
²¹⁸ Items repealed by Corporate Manslaughter and Corporate Homicide Act 2007 (Amendment of Schedule 1) Order 2008/396 art.2(3) (April 6, 2008).
²¹⁹ Entry inserted by Secretary of State for Education Order 2010/1836 Sch.1(1) para.4(b) (August 18, 2010: insertion has effect subject to transitional provisions specified in SI 2010/1836 art.5).
²²⁰ Entry repealed by Secretary of State for Business, Innovation and Skills Order 2009/2748 Sch.1(1) para.8(c) (November 13, 2009).
²²¹ Item inserted by Secretary of State for Energy and Climate Change Order 2009/229 Sch.2(1) para.5 (March 5, 2009).
²²² Items inserted by Corporate Manslaughter and Corporate Homicide Act 2007 (Amendment of Schedule 1) Order 2008/396 art.2(2) (April 6, 2008).
²²³ Entry inserted by Crime and Courts Act 2013 c. 22 Sch.8(2) para.175 (October 7, 2013: insertion has effect as SI 2013/1682 subject to savings and transitional provisions specified in 2013 c.22 s.15 and Sch.8).
²²⁴ Entry repealed by Budget Responsibility and National Audit Act 2011 c. 4 Sch.5(2) para.32(1) (April 1, 2012: insertion has effect subject to savings specified in 2011 c.4 Sch.5 para.32(2)).

[. . .]²²⁵
Northern Ireland Office
Office for National Statistics
[. . .]²¹⁸
[. . .]²¹⁸
Office of Her Majesty's Chief Inspector of Education and Training in Wales
Ordnance Survey
[. . .]²¹⁸
Public Prosecution Service for Northern Ireland
Registers of Scotland Executive Agency
[. . .]²²⁶
Royal Mint
Scottish Executive
Serious Fraud Office
Treasury Solicitor's Department
UK Trade and Investment
Welsh Assembly Government

Courts and Legal Services Act 1990 c. 41

PART III

JUDICIAL AND OTHER OFFICES AND JUDICIAL PENSIONS

Judicial appointments

Qualification for judicial and certain other appointments

A1–229   **71.**—(1) [Outside the scope of this work]²²⁷

(2) Schedule 10 shall have effect for the purpose of making amendments to other enactments, measures and statutory instruments which relate to qualification for judicial and certain other appointments.

(3) For the purposes of this section, a person has—

(a) a ["Senior Courts qualification" if he has a right of audience in relation to all proceedings in the Senior Courts]²²⁸;

(b) a "High Court qualification" if he has a right of audience in relation to all proceedings in the High Court;

(c) a "general qualification" if he has a right of audience in relation to any class of proceedings in any part of the [Senior Courts]², or all proceedings in county courts or magistrates' courts;

(d) a "Crown Court qualification" if he has a right of audience in relation to all proceedings in the Crown Court;

---

²²⁵ Entry repealed by Northern Ireland Court Service (Abolition and Transfer of Functions) Order (Northern Ireland) 2010/133 Sch.1(1) para.11 (April 12, 2010: repeal has effect subject to transitional provisions specified in SR 2010/133 arts 5-7).

²²⁶ Entry repealed by Public Bodies (Merger of the Director of Public Prosecutions and the Director of Revenue and Customs Prosecutions) Order 2014/834 Sch.2 para.44 (March 27, 2014).

²²⁷ Words substituted by Constitutional Reform Act 2005 c. 4 Sch.11(1) para.1(2) (October 1, 2009).

²²⁸ Words substituted by Constitutional Reform Act 2005 c. 4 Sch.11(2) para.4(1) (October 1, 2009).

(e) a "county court qualification" if he has a right of audience in relation to all proceedings in [the county court][229];

(f) a "magistrates' court qualification" if he has a right of audience in relation to all proceedings in magistrates' courts.

(4) References in subsection (3) to a right of audience are references to a right of audience [exercisable by virtue of an authorisation given by a relevant approved regulator].[230]

(5) Any reference in any enactment, measure or statutory instrument to a person having such a qualification of a particular number of years' length shall be construed as a reference to a person who—

(a) for the time being has that qualification, and

(b) has had it for a period (which need not be continuous) of at least that number of years.

[(6) Any period during which a person had a right of audience but was, as a result of disciplinary proceedings, prevented by [the relevant approved regulator][231] from exercising it shall not count towards the period mentioned in subsection (5)(b).][232]

[(6A) In this section "relevant approved regulator" is to be construed in accordance with section 20(3) of the Legal Services Act 2007.][233]

[. . .][234]

[. . .][234]

Judges

Judges etc. barred from legal practice

75. No person holding as a full-time appointment any of the offices listed in Schedule 11   **A1–230**
shall—

(a) provide any advocacy or litigation services (in any jurisdiction);

(b) provide any conveyancing or probate services;

[(ba) carry on any notarial activities (within the meaning of the Legal Services Act 2007);][235]

(c) practise as a barrister, solicitor, public notary or licensed conveyancer, or be indirectly concerned in any such practice;

(d) practise as an advocate or solicitor in Scotland, or be indirectly concerned in any such practice; or

(e) act for any remuneration to himself as an arbitrator or umpire.

---

[229] Words substituted by Crime and Courts Act 2013 c. 22 Sch.9(2) para.35 (April 22, 2014: substitution has effect as SI 2014/954 subject to savings and transitional provisions specified in 2013 c.22 s.15 and Sch.8 and transitional provision specified in SI 2014/954 arts 2(c) and 3).

[230] Words substituted by Legal Services Act 2007 c. 29 Sch.21 para.94(a) (January 1, 2010).

[231] Words substituted by Legal Services Act 2007 c. 29 Sch.21 para.94(b) (January 1, 2010).

[232] Substituted by Access to Justice Act 1999 c. 22 Sch.6 para.9 (September 27, 1999: brought into force by comm order).

[233] Added by Legal Services Act 2007 c. 29 Sch.21 para.94(c) (January 1, 2010).

[234] Repealed by Access to Justice Act 1999 c. 22 Sch.15(II) para.1 (September 27, 1999: commencement order SI).

[235] Added by Legal Services Act 2007 c. 29 Sch.21 para.95 (January 1, 2010).

SCHEDULE 11

JUDGES ETC BARRED FROM LEGAL PRACTICE

A1–231   The following are the offices for the purposes of section 75—

[Judge of the Supreme Court]²³⁶
Lord Justice of Appeal
Puisne judge of the High Court
Circuit judge
District judge, including district judge of the principal registry of the Family Division
Master of the Queen's Bench Division
Queen's Coroner and Attorney and Master of the Crown Office and Registrar of Criminal Appeals
Admiralty Registrar
Master of the Chancery Division
Registrar in Bankruptcy of the High Court
Taxing Master of the [Senior Courts]²³⁷
Registrar of Civil Appeals
[Senior Judge of the Court of Protection
President of the Court of Protection
Vice-President of the Court of Protection]²³⁸
District probate registrar
Judge Advocate General
Vice Judge Advocate General
Assistant [. . .]²³⁹ Judge Advocate General
[District Judge (Magistrates' Courts)]²⁴⁰
Social Security Commissioner
[. . .]²⁴¹
[President of social security appeal tribunals, medical appeal tribunals and disability appeal tribunals or regional or other full-time chairman of such tribunals]²⁴²
[President of the Employment Tribunals (England and Wales) or member of a panel of [Employment Judges]²⁴³ established by regulations under section 1(1) of the Employment Tribunals Act 1996 for employment tribunals for England and Wales]²⁴⁴
[. . .]²⁴⁵
[. . .]²⁴⁶
[. . .]²⁴⁷

---

²³⁶ Words substituted by Constitutional Reform Act 2005 c. 4 Sch.17(2) para.24 (October 1, 2009).
²³⁷ Words substituted by Constitutional Reform Act 2005 c. 4 Sch.11(2) para.4(1) (October 1, 2009).
²³⁸ Entry for Senior Judge, President and Vice-President of the Court of Protection substituted for entry for Master of the Court of Protection by Mental Capacity Act 2005 c. 9 Sch.6 para.35(2) (October 1, 2007).
²³⁹ Words repealed by Armed Forces Act 2001 c. 19 Sch.7(3) para.1 (October 1, 2001).
²⁴⁰ Words substituted in table by Access to Justice Act 1999 c. 22 Sch.11 para.37 (August 31, **2000**).
²⁴¹ Words repealed by Social Security (Consequential Provisions) Act 1992 c. 6 Sch.1 para.1 (July 1, 1992).
²⁴² Substituted by Disability Living Allowance and Disability Working Allowance Act 1991 c. 21 Sch.2 para.22 (April 6, 1992 as SI 1991/2617).
²⁴³ Word substituted by Crime and Courts Act 2013 c. 22 Sch.14(7) para.13(1) (October 1, 2013: substitution has effect as SI 2013/2200 subject to savings and transitional provisions as specified in 2013 c.22 s.15 and Sch.8).
²⁴⁴ Entry beginning "President of Industrial Tribunals" substituted by Employment Rights (Dispute Resolution) Act 1998 c. 8 Sch.1 para.6 (August 1, 1998).
²⁴⁵ Entry repealed by Transfer of Functions of the Asylum and Immigration Tribunal Order 2010/21 Sch.1 para.8 (February 15, 2010: repeal has effect subject to savings and transitional provisions specified in SI 2010/21 Sch.4).
²⁴⁶ Words repealed by Transfer of Tribunal Functions (Lands Tribunal and Miscellaneous Amendments) Order 2009/1307 Sch.1 para.214 (June 1, 2009).
²⁴⁷ Entry repealed by Transfer of Tribunal Functions and Revenue and Customs Appeals Order 2009/56 Sch.1 para.168(a) (April 1, 2009).

[. . .]²⁴⁸
[Member of the Charity Commission appointed as provided in Schedule 1 to the Charities Act 2011]²⁴⁹
[Senior coroner appointed under paragraph 1 of Schedule 3 to the Coroners and Justice Act 2009]²⁵⁰
.[Member of a Pensions Appeal Tribunal]²⁵¹
[. . .]²⁵²
[. . .]²⁵³
[Judge or other member of the First-tier Tribunal—

(a) appointed under paragraph 1(1) or 2(1) of Schedule 2 to the Tribunals, Courts and Enforcement Act 2007, or

(b) who is a transferred-in judge, or a transferred-in other member, of the First-tier Tribunal (see section 31(2) of that Act)

Judge or other member of the Upper Tribunal—

(a) appointed under paragraph 1(1) or 2(1) of Schedule 3 to the Tribunals, Courts and Enforcement Act 2007, or

(b) who is a transferred-in judge, or a transferred-in other member, of the Upper Tribunal (see section 31(2) of that Act)

Senior President of Tribunals
Chamber President, or Acting Chamber President or Deputy Chamber President, of a chamber of the First-tier Tribunal or of a chamber of the Upper Tribunal.]²⁵⁴

Cremation Act 1902 c. 8

Regulations as to burning

7. The Secretary of State shall make regulations as to the maintenance and inspection of crematoria, and prescribing in what cases and under what conditions the burning of any human remains may take place, and directing the disposition or interment of the ashes, and prescribing the forms of the notices, certificates and [applications]²⁵⁵ to be given or made before any such burning is permitted to take place [. . .]²⁵⁶ and also regulations as to the registration of such burnings as have taken place. [Each such application shall be verified in such manner as the Secretary of State may by such regulations prescribe]²⁵⁷ [. . .]² All statutory provisions relating to the destruction and falsification of registers of burials, and the admissibility of extracts therefrom as evidence in courts and otherwise, shall apply to the register of burnings directed by such regulations to be kept [. . .]²⁵⁸   **A1–232**

---

²⁴⁸ Entry repealed by Transfer of Tribunal Functions and Revenue and Customs Appeals Order 2009/56 Sch.1 para.168(b) (April 1, 2009).
²⁴⁹ Entry substituted by Charities Act 2011 c. 25 Sch.7(2) para.55 (March 14, 2012: substitution has effect subject to transitional provisions and savings specified in 2011 c.25 Sch.7 para.2 and Sch.8).
²⁵⁰ Entry substituted by Coroners and Justice Act 2009 c. 25 Sch.21(1) para.30 (July 25, 2013).
²⁵¹ Words added by Child Support, Pensions and Social Security Act 2000 c. 19 Pt II c.III s.60(5) (April 9, 2001).
²⁵² Entry repealed by Transfer of Tribunal Functions Order 2010/22 Sch.2 para.10 (January 18, 2010).
²⁵³ Entry repealed by Transfer of Functions of the Charity Tribunal Order 2009/1834 Sch.1 para.3 (September 1, 2009).
²⁵⁴ Entries inserted by Tribunals, Courts and Enforcement Act 2007 c. 15 Sch.8 para.16 (November 3, 2008).
²⁵⁵ Word substituted by Cremation Act 1952 (c. 31),.s. 2(1).
²⁵⁶ Words repealed by Cremation Act 1952 (c. 31), s. 2(1)(2).
²⁵⁷ Words inserted by Cremation Act 1952 (c. 31), s. 2(1).
²⁵⁸ Words repealed by Finance Act 1949 (c. 47), Sch. 11 Pt. V.

Penalties for breach of regulations, & c

A1–233 **8.**—(1) Every person who shall contravene any such regulation as aforesaid, or shall knowingly carry out or procure or take part in the burning of any human remains except in accordance with such regulations and the provisions of this Act, shall (in addition to any liability or penalty which he may otherwise incur) be liable, on summary conviction, to a penalty not exceeding [level 3 on the standard scale][259].

[. . .][260]

(2) Every person who shall wilfully make any false[. . .][261] representation, or sign or utter any false certificate, with a view to procuring the burning of any human remains, shall (in addition to any penalty or liability which he may otherwise incur) be liable to imprisonment,[. . .][262] not exceeding two years.

[. . .][263]

Crime and Courts Act 2013 c. 22

Part 2

Courts And Justice

Administration of justice

Enabling the making, and use, of films and other recordings of proceedings

A1–234 **32.**—(1) The Lord Chancellor may, by order made with the concurrence of the Lord Chief Justice, provide that a section mentioned in subsection (2) or any provision of either of those sections—

(a) does not apply in relation to the making of a recording or the making of a prescribed recording;

(b) does not apply in relation to the making of a recording, or the making of a prescribed recording, if prescribed conditions are met, including conditions as to a court or tribunal or any other person being satisfied as to anything or agreeing;

(c) does not apply in relation to prescribed use of a prescribed recording.

(2) Those sections are—

(a) section 41 of the Criminal Justice Act 1925 (no photography or drawing in court of persons involved in proceedings, and no publication of contravening images);

(b) section 9 of the Contempt of Court Act 1981 (no sound recording in court without permission, and no public playing of recordings).

(3) In the case of any particular proceedings of a court or tribunal, the court or tribunal may in the interests of justice or in order that a person is not unduly prejudiced—

---

[259] Words substituted by virtue of (England, Wales) Criminal Justice Act 1982 (c.48), ss. 38, 46 and (Scotland) Criminal Procedure (Scotland) Act 1975 (c.21), ss. 289F, 289G.

[260] Words repealed by Statute Law (Repeals) Act 1993 c. 50 Sch.1(I) para.1 (November 5, 1993).

[261] Words repealed by Prejury Act 1911 (c. 6) Sch. and False Oaths (Scotland) Act 1933 (c. 20). Sch.

[262] Words omitted by virtue of Criminal Justice Act 1948 (c. 58), s. 1(2) and Criminal Justice (Scotland) Act 1949 (c. 94), s. 16(2).

[263] Repealed by Criminal Law Act 1967 (c. 58), Sch. 3 Pt. III.

(a) direct that a provision disapplied in relation to the proceedings by an order under subsection (1) is, despite the order, to apply in relation to the proceedings, or

(b) direct that a provision disapplied in relation to the proceedings by an order under subsection (1) is, despite the order, disapplied in relation to the proceedings only if conditions specified in the direction are met.

(4) No appeal may be made against—

(a) a direction given under subsection (3), or

(b) a decision not to give a direction under that subsection.

(5) In this section—

"recording" means a visual or sound recording on any medium, including (in particular)—

      (a) films and other video-recordings, with or without sound,
      (b) other photographs, and
      (c) sketches and portraits;

"prescribed" means prescribed by an order under subsection (1).

(6) The preceding provisions of this section do not apply in relation to Supreme Court proceedings.
(7) [Amends section 41 of the Criminal Justice Act 1925]
(8) [Amends section 9 of the Contempt of Court Act 1981]

Criminal Justice Act 1925 c. 86

PART III

AMENDMENTS AS TO OFFENCES

Prohibition on taking photographs, &c., in court

41.—(1) No person shall—　　　　　　　　　　A1–235

(a) take or attempt to take in any court any photograph, or with a view to publication make or attempt to make in any court any portrait or sketch, of any person, being a judge of the court or a juror or a witness in or a party to any proceedings before the court, whether civil or criminal; or

(b) publish any photograph, portrait or sketch taken or made in contravention of the foregoing provisions of this section or any reproduction thereof;

and if any person acts in contravention of this section be shall, on summary conviction, be liable in respect of each offence to a fine not exceeding [level 3 on the standard scale].[264]
[(1A) See section 32 of the Crime and Courts Act 2013 for power to provide for exceptions.][265]
(2) For the purposes of this section—

---

[264] Words substituted by Criminal Justice Act 1982 (c. 48), s. 46 subject to transitional provisions specified in s. 47.
[265] Added by Crime and Courts Act 2013 c. 22 Pt 2 s.32(7) (July 15, 2013: insertion has effect as SI 2013/1725 subject to savings and transitional provisions specified in 2013 c.22 s.15 and Sch.8).

[(a) the expression "court" means any court of justice (including the court of a coroner), apart from the Supreme Court;][266]

(b) the expression "Judge" includes [. . .],[267] registrar, magistrate, justice and coroner:

(c) a photograph, portrait or sketch shall be deemed to be a photograph, portrait or sketch taken or made in court if it is taken or made in the court-room or in the building or in the precincts of the building in which the court is held, or if it is a photograph, portrait or sketch taken or made of the person while he is entering or leaving the court-room or any such building or precincts as aforesaid.

Criminal Justice Act 1982 c. 48

PART III

FINES ETC.

Introduction of standard scale of fines

The standard scale of fines for summary offences

A1–236   37.—(1) There shall be a standard scale of fines for summary offences, which shall be known as "the standard scale".

[(2) The standard scale is shown below—

Level at the scale	Amount of fine
1	£ 200
2	£ 500
3	£1,000
4	£2,500
5	£5,000][268]

(3) Where any enactment (whether contained in an Act passed before or after this Act) provides—

(a) that a person convicted of a summary offence shall be liable on conviction to a fine or a maximum fine by reference to a specified level on the standard scale; or

(b) confers power by subordinate instrument to make a person liable on conviction of a summary offence (whether or not created by the instrument) to a fine or maximum fine by reference to a specified level on the standard scale,

it is to be construed as referring to the standard scale for which this section provides as that standard scale has effect from time to time by virtue either of this section or of an order under section 143 of the Magistrates' Courts Act 1980.

---

[266] Substituted by Constitutional Reform Act 2005 c. 4 Pt 3 s.47(1) (October 1, 2009).
[267] Word repealed by Courts Act 1971 (c. 23), Sch. 11 Pt. IV.
[268] Substituted by Criminal Justice Act 1991 c. 53 Pt I s.17(1) (October 1, 1992: represents law in force as at date shown).

Increase of fines

General increase of fines for summary offences under Acts of Parliament

38.—(1) Subject to subsection (5) below and to section 39(1) below, this section applies   **A1–237** to any enactment contained in an Act passed before this Act (however framed or worded) which, as regards any summary offence created not later than 29th July 1977 (the date of the passing of the Criminal Law Act 1977), makes a person liable on conviction to a fine or maximum fine which—

(a) is less than £1,000; and

(b) was not altered by section 30 or 31 of the Criminal Law Act 1977; and

(c) has not been altered since 29th July 1977 or has only been altered since that date by section 35 above.

(2) Subject to subsection (7) below, where an enactment to which this section applies provides on conviction of a summary offence for a fine or maximum fine in respect of a specified quantity or a specified number of things, that fine or maximum fine shall be treated for the purposes of this section as being the fine or maximum fine for the offence.

(3) Where an enactment to which this section applies provides for different fines or maximum fines in relation to different circumstances or persons of different descriptions, they are to be treated separately for the purposes of this section.

(4) An enactment in which section 31(6) and (7) of the Criminal Law Act 1977 (pre 1949 enactments) produced the same fine or maximum fine for different convictions shall be treated for the purposes of this section as if there were omitted from it so much of it as before 29th July 1977 had the effect that a person guilty of an offence under it was liable on summary conviction to a fine or maximum fine less than the highest fine or maximum fine to which he would have been liable if his conviction had satisfied the conditions required for the imposition of the highest fine or maximum fine.

(5) This section shall not affect so much of any enactment as (in whatever words) makes a person liable on summary conviction to a fine or maximum fine for each period of a specified length during which a continuing offence is continued.

(6) The fine or maximum fine for an offence under an enactment to which this section applies shall be increased to the amount at the appropriate level on the standard scale unless it is an enactment in relation to which section 39(2) below provides for some other increase.

(7) Where an enactment to which this section applies provides on conviction of a summary offence for a fine or maximum fine in respect of a specified quantity or a specified number of things but also specifies an alternative fine or maximum fine, subsection (6) above shall have effect to increase—

(a) the alternative fine; and

(b) any amount that the enactment specifies as the maximum which a fine under it may not exceed,

as well as the fine or maximum fine which it has effect to increase by virtue of subsection (2) above.

(8) Subject to subsection (9) below, the appropriate level on the standard scale for the purpose of subsections (6) and (7) above is the level on that scale next above the amount of the fine or maximum fine that falls to be increased.

(9) If the amount of the fine or maximum fine that falls to be increased is £400 or more but less than £500, the appropriate level is £1,000.

(10) Where section 35 above applies, the amount of the fine or maximum fine that falls to be increased is to be taken to be the fine or maximum fine to which a person is liable by virtue of that section.

Application of standard scale to existing enactments

Conversion of references to amounts to references to levels on scale

A1–238   46.—(1) Where—

(a) either—

(i) a relevant enactment makes a person liable to a fine or maximum fine on conviction of a summary offence; or

(ii) a relevant enactment confers power by sub-ordinate instrument to make a person liable to a fine or maximum fine on conviction of a summary offence (whether or not created by the instrument); and

(b) the amount of the fine or maximum fine for the offence is, whether by virtue of this Part of this Act or not, an amount shown in the second column of the standard scale,

a reference to the level in the first column of the standard scale corresponding to that amount shall be substituted for the reference in the enactment to the amount of the fine or maximum fine.

(2) Where a relevant enactment confers a powers such as is mentioned in subsection (1)(a)(ii) above, the power shall be construed as a power to make a person liable to a fine or, as the case may be, a maximum fine not exceeding the amount corresponding to the level on the standard scale to which the enactment refers by virtue of subsection (1) above or not exceeding a lesser amount.

(3) If an order under section 143 of the Magistrates' Courts Act 1980 alters the sums specified in section 37(2) above, the second reference to the standard scale in subsection (1) above is to be construed as a reference to that scale as it has effect by virtue of the order.

(4) In this section "relevant enactment" means—

(a) any enactment contained in an Act passed before this Act[. . .][269];

(b) any enactment contained in this Act;

(c) any enactment contained in an Act passed on the same day as this Act; and

(d) any enactment contained in an Act passed after this Act but in the same Session as this Act.

(5) This section shall not affect so much of any enactment as (in whatever words) makes a person liable on summary conviction to a maximum fine not exceeding a specified amount for each period of a specified length during which a continuing offence is continued.

Criminal Procedure Act 1853 c. 30

Secretary of State may issue his warrant for bringing up a prisoner (not in custody under civil process) to give evidence

A1–239   9. It shall be lawful for [. . .][270] any judge of the [High Court][271] [. . .][272] in any case where he may see fit to do so, upon application by affidavit, to issue a warrant or order under

---

[269] Words repealed by Companies Consolidation (Consequential Provisions) Act 1985 (c.9), ss. 21, 23, 29, 31(8), Sch. 1.

[270] Words repealed by Prison Act 1898 (c. 41), Sch. 1.

[271] Words substituted by virtue of Supreme Court of Judicature (Consolidation) Act 1925 (c. 49), s. 224(1).

[272] Words repealed by Statute Law Revision Act 1892 (c. 19).

his hand for bringing up any prisoner or person confined in any gaol, prison, or place, under any sentence or under commitment for trial or otherwise, (except under process in any civil action, suit, or proceeding,) before any court, judge, justice, or other judicature, to be examined as a witness in any cause or matter, civil or criminal depending or to be inquired of or determined in or before such court, judge, justice, or judicature; and the person required by any such warrant or order to be so brought before such court, judge, justice, or other judicature, shall be so brought under the same care and custody, and be dealt with in like manner in all respects, as a prisoner required by any writ of habeas corpus awarded by any of her Majesty's Superior Courts of Law at [the Royal Courts of Justice][2] to be brought before such court to be examined as a witness in any cause or matter depending before such court is now by law required to be dealt with.

Criminal Procedure Act 1865 c. 18

Provisions of sect. 2. of this Act to apply to trials commenced on or after July 1, 1865

1. The provisions of section two of this Act shall apply to every trial [. . .][273]; and the **A1–240** provisions of sections from three to eight, inclusive, of this Act shall apply to all courts of judicature, as well criminal as all others, and to all persons having, by law or by consent of parties, authority to hear, receive, and examine evidence.

How far witness may be discredited by the party producing

3. A party producing a witness shall not be allowed to impeach his credit by general **A1–241** evidence of bad character; but he may, in case the witness shall in the opinion of the judge prove adverse, contradict him by other evidence, or, by leave of the judge, prove that he has made at other times a statement inconsistent with his present testimony; but before such last-mentioned proof can be given the circumstances of the supposed statement, sufficient to designate the particular occasion, must be mentioned to the witness, and he must be asked whether or not he has made such statement.

As to proof of contradictory statements of adverse witness

4. If a witness, upon cross-examination as to a former statement made by him relative to **A1–242** the subject matter of the indictment or proceeding, and inconsistent with his present testimony, does not distinctly admit that he has made such statement, proof may be given that he did in fact make it; but before such proof can be given the circumstances of the supposed statement, sufficient to designate the particular occasion, must be mentioned to the witness, and he must be asked whether or not he has made such statement.

Cross-examinations as to previous statements in writing

5. A witness may be cross-examined as to previous statements made by him in writing, **A1–243** or reduced into writing, relative to the subject matter of the indictment or proceeding, without such writing being shown to him; but if it is intended to contradict such witness by the writing, his attention must, before such contradictory proof can be given, be called to those parts of the writing which are to be used for the purpose of so contradicting him:

Provided always, that it shall be competent for the judge, at any time during the trial, to require the production of the writing for his inspection, and he may thereupon make such use of it for the purposes of the trial as he may think fit.

---

[273] Words repealed by Criminal Law Act 1967 (c. 58), Sch. 3 Pt. III and (N.I.) Criminal Law Act (Northern Ireland) 1967 (c. 18), Sch. 2 Pt. II.

Crime and Disorder Act 1998 c. 37

PART II

CRIMINAL LAW

Miscellaneous

Abolition of rebuttable presumption that a child is doli incapax

A1–244   **34.** The rebuttable presumption of criminal law that a child aged 10 or over is incapable of committing an offence is hereby abolished.

PART III

CRIMINAL JUSTICE SYSTEM

Functions Of Courts etc.

Early administrative hearings

A1–245   **50.**—(1) Where a person ("the accused") has been charged with an offence at a police station, the magistrates' court before whom he appears or is brought for the first time in relation to the charge may [. . .]²⁷⁴ consist of a single justice.

[(2) At a hearing conducted by a single justice under this section [—]²⁷⁵

[(a) the accused shall be asked whether he wishes to be provided with representation for the purposes of the proceedings under Part 1 of the Legal Aid, Sentencing and Punishment of Offenders Act 2012, and

(b) if he indicates that he does, the necessary arrangements must be made for him to apply for it and, where appropriate, obtain it.]³
      [. . .]²⁷⁶]²⁷⁷

(3) At such a hearing the single justice—

(a) may exercise, subject to subsection (2) above, such of his powers as a single justice as he thinks fit; and

(b) on adjourning the hearing, may remand the accused in custody or on bail.

(4) This section applies in relation to a justices' clerk as it applies in relation to a single justice; but nothing in subsection (3)(b) above authorises such a clerk to remand the accused

---

²⁷⁴ Words repealed by Criminal Justice Act 2003 c. 44 Sch.37(4) para.1 (June 18, 2012: repeal has effect on June 18, 2012 in relation to the relevant local justice areas specified in SI 2012/1320 art.4(1)(d) and purposes specified in SI 2012/1320 art.4(3) subject to savings specified in SI 2012/1320 art.5; November 5, 2012 in relation to local justice areas specified in SI 2012/2574 art.2(1)(d) and purposes specified in SI 2012/2574 art.2(3) subject to saving provisions specified in SI 2012/2574 arts 3 and 4; May 28, 2013 in relation to the relevant local justice areas and purposes specified in SI 2013/1103 art.2(3) subject to savings specified in SI 2013/1103 arts 3 and 4 otherwise).

²⁷⁵ Existing text renumbered as s.50(2)(a), words substituted and s.50(2)(b) added by Legal Aid, Sentencing and Punishment of Offenders Act 2012 c. 10 Sch.5(1) para.47(2) (April 1, 2013 subject to saving and transitional provisions as specified in SI 2013/534 regs 6–13).

²⁷⁶ Repealed by Legal Aid, Sentencing and Punishment of Offenders Act 2012 c. 10 Sch.5(1) para.47(3) (April 1, 2013 subject to saving and transitional provisions as specified in SI 2013/534 regs 6–13).

²⁷⁷ S.50(2) and (2A) substituted for s.50(2) by Criminal Defence Service (Representation Orders and Consequential Amendments) Regulations 2006/2493 reg.8(2) (October 2, 2006).

in custody or, without the consent of the prosecutor and the accused, to remand the accused on bail on conditions other than those (if any) previously imposed.

[(4A) A hearing conducted by a single justice under this section may be—

(a) adjourned to enable the decision mentioned in subsection (2A) above to be taken, and

(b) subsequently resumed by a single justice.]²⁷⁸

[. . .]²⁷⁹

[Sending cases to the Crown Court: adults

51.—(1) Where an adult appears or is brought before a magistrates' court ("the court") charged with an offence and any of the conditions mentioned in subsection (2) below is satisfied, the court shall send him forthwith to the Crown Court for trial for the offence. **A1–246**

(2) Those conditions are—

(a) that the offence is an offence triable only on indictment other than one in respect of which notice has been given under section 51B or 51C below;

(b) that the offence is an either-way offence and the court is required under section 20(9)(b), 21, 23(4)(b) or (5) or 25(2D) of the Magistrates' Courts Act 1980 to proceed in relation to the offence in accordance with subsection (1) above;

(c) that notice is given to the court under section 51B or 51C below in respect of the offence.

(3) Where the court sends an adult for trial under subsection (1) above, it shall at the same time send him to the Crown Court for trial for any either-way or summary offence with which he is charged and which—

(a) (if it is an either-way offence) appears to the court to be related to the offence mentioned in subsection (1) above; or

(b) (if it is a summary offence) appears to the court to be related to the offence mentioned in subsection (1) above or to the either-way offence, and which fulfils the requisite condition (as defined in subsection (11) below).

(4) Where an adult who has been sent for trial under subsection (1) above subsequently appears or is brought before a magistrates' court charged with an either-way or summary offence which—

(a) appears to the court to be related to the offence mentioned in subsection (1) above; and

(b) (in the case of a summary offence) fulfils the requisite condition,

the court may send him forthwith to the Crown Court for trial for the either-way or summary offence.

(5) Where—

(a) the court sends an adult ("A") for trial under subsection (1) or (3) above;

(b) another adult appears or is brought before the court on the same or a subsequent occasion charged jointly with A with an either-way offence; and

---

²⁷⁸ Added by Criminal Defence Service (Representation Orders and Consequential Amendments) Regulations 2006/2493 reg.8(3) (October 2, 2006).

²⁷⁹ Repealed by Access to Justice Act 1999 c. 22 Sch.15(I) para.1 (April 2, 2001 as SI 2001/916).

(c) that offence appears to the court to be related to an offence for which A was sent for trial under subsection (1) or (3) above,

the court shall where it is the same occasion, and may where it is a subsequent occasion, send the other adult forthwith to the Crown Court for trial for the either-way offence.

(6) Where the court sends an adult for trial under subsection (5) above, it shall at the same time send him to the Crown Court for trial for any either-way or summary offence with which he is charged and which—

(a) (if it is an either-way offence) appears to the court to be related to the offence for which he is sent for trial; and

(b) (if it is a summary offence) appears to the court to be related to the offence for which he is sent for trial or to the either-way offence, and which fulfils the requisite condition.

(7) Where—

(a) the court sends an adult ("A") for trial under subsection (1), (3) or (5) above; and

(b) a child or young person appears or is brought before the court on the same or a subsequent occasion charged jointly with A with an indictable offence for which A is sent for trial under subsection (1), (3) or (5) above, or an indictable offence which appears to the court to be related to that offence,

the court shall, if it considers it necessary in the interests of justice to do so, send the child or young person forthwith to the Crown Court for trial for the indictable offence.

(8) Where the court sends a child or young person for trial under subsection (7) above, it may at the same time send him to the Crown Court for trial for any indictable or summary offence with which he is charged and which—

(a) (if it is an indictable offence) appears to the court to be related to the offence for which he is sent for trial; and

(b) (if it is a summary offence) appears to the court to be related to the offence for which he is sent for trial or to the indictable offence, and which fulfils the requisite condition.

(9) Subsections (7) and (8) above are subject to sections 24A and 24B of the Magistrates' Courts Act 1980 (which provide for certain cases involving children and young persons to be tried summarily).

(10) The trial of the information charging any summary offence for which a person is sent for trial under this section shall be treated as if the court had adjourned it under section 10 of the 1980 Act and had not fixed the time and place for its resumption.

(11) A summary offence fulfils the requisite condition if it is punishable with imprisonment or involves obligatory or discretionary disqualification from driving.

(12) In the case of an adult charged with an offence—

(a) if the offence satisfies paragraph (c) of subsection (2) above, the offence shall be dealt with under subsection (1) above and not under any other provision of this section or section 51A below;

(b) subject to paragraph (a) above, if the offence is one in respect of which the court is required to, or would decide to, send the adult to the Crown Court under—

(i) subsection (5) above; or
(ii) subsection (6) of section 51A below,

the offence shall be dealt with under that subsection and not under any other provision of this section or section 51A below.

(13) The functions of a magistrates' court under this section, and its related functions under section 51D below, may be discharged by a single justice.][280]

Data Protection Act 1998 c. 29

PART I

PRELIMINARY

Basic interpretative provisions

1.—(1) In this Act, unless the context otherwise requires—

"data" means information which—

(a) is being processed by means of equipment operating automatically in response to instructions given for that purpose,

(b) is recorded with the intention that it should be processed by means of such equipment,

(c) is recorded as part of a relevant filing system or with the intention that it should form part of a relevant filing system, [. . .][281]

(d) does not fall within paragraph (a), (b) or (c) but forms part of an accessible record as defined by section 68; [or][282]

[(e) is recorded information held by a public authority and does not fall within any of paragraphs (a) to (d);][282]

"data controller" means , subject to subsection (4), a person who (either alone or jointly or in common with other persons) determines the purposes for which and the manner in which any personal data are, or are to be, processed;

"data processor", in relation to personal data, means any person (other than an employee of the data controller) who processes the data on behalf of the data controller;

"data subject" means an individual who is the subject of personal data;

"personal data" means data which relate to a living individual who can be identified—

(a) from those data, or

(b) from those data and other information which is in the possession of, or is likely to come into the possession of, the data controller,

and includes any expression of opinion about the individual and any indication of the intentions of the data controller or any other person in respect of the individual;

"processing", in relation to information or data, means obtaining, recording or holding the information or data or carrying out any operation or set of operations on the information or data, including—

(a) organisation, adaptation or alteration of the information or data,

(b) retrieval, consultation or use of the information or data,

---

[280] Ss 51-51E substituted for s.51 by Criminal Justice Act 2003 c. 44 Sch.3(1) para.18 (June 18, 2012: substitution has effect on June 18, 2012 in relation to the relevant local justice areas subject to savings as specified in SI 2012/1320 art.5; June 18, 2012 for purposes specified in SI 2012/1320 art.4(3) subject to savings as specified in SI 2012/1320 art.5; November 5, 2012 in relation to the relevant local justice areas subject to saving provisions specified in SI 2012/2574 arts 3 and 4; May 28, 2013 in relation to the relevant local justice areas and purposes specified in SI 2013/1103 art.2(3) subject to savings specified in SI 2013/1103 arts 3 and 4 otherwise).

[281] Words repealed by Freedom of Information Act 2000 c. 36 Sch.8(III) para.1 (January 1, 2005).

[282] Added by Freedom of Information Act 2000 c. 36 Pt VII s.68(2)(a) (January 1, 2005 for purposes specified in SI 2004/1909 art.2(1); January 1, 2005 otherwise).

(c) disclosure of the information or data by transmission, dissemination or otherwise making available, or

(d) alignment, combination, blocking, erasure or destruction of the information or data;

["public authority" means a public authority as defined by the Freedom of Information Act 2000 or a Scottish public authority as defined by the Freedom of Information (Scotland) Act 2002;][283]

"relevant filing system" means any set of information relating to individuals to the extent that, although the information is not processed by means of equipment operating automatically in response to instructions given for that purpose, the set is structured, either by reference to individuals or by reference to criteria relating to individuals, in such a way that specific information relating to a particular individual is readily accessible.

(2) In this Act, unless the context otherwise requires—

(a) "obtaining" or "recording", in relation to personal data, includes obtaining or recording the information to be contained in the data, and

(b) "using" or "disclosing", in relation to personal data, includes using or disclosing the information contained in the data.

(3) In determining for the purposes of this Act whether any information is recorded with the intention—

(a) that it should be processed by means of equipment operating automatically in response to instructions given for that purpose, or

(b) that it should form part of a relevant filing system,

it is immaterial that it is intended to be so processed or to form part of such a system only after being transferred to a country or territory outside the European Economic Area.

(4) Where personal data are processed only for purposes for which they are required by or under any enactment to be processed, the person on whom the obligation to process the data is imposed by or under that enactment is for the purposes of this Act the data controller.

[(5) In paragraph (e) of the definition of "data" in subsection (1), the reference to information "held" by a public authority shall be construed in accordance with section 3(2) of the Freedom of Information Act **2000** [or section 3(2), (4) and (5) of the Freedom of Information (Scotland) Act 2002][284].

[(6) Where

(a) section 7 of the Freedom of Information Act **2000** prevents Parts I to V of that Act or

(b) section 7(1) of the Freedom of Information (Scotland) Act 2002 prevents that Act

---

[283] Definition substituted by Freedom of Information (Scotland) Act 2002 (Consequential Modifications) Order 2004/3089 art.2(2)(a) (January 1, 2005).
[284] Words inserted by Freedom of Information (Scotland) Act 2002 (Consequential Modifications) Order 2004/3089 art.2(2)(b) (January 1, 2005).

from applying to certain information held by a public authority, that information is not to be treated for the purposes of paragraph (e) of the definition of "data" in subsection (1) as held by a public authority.][285]][286]

Sensitive personal data

2. In this Act "sensitive personal data" means personal data consisting of information as to—   A1–248

(a) the racial or ethnic origin of the data subject,

(b) his political opinions,

(c) his religious beliefs or other beliefs of a similar nature,

(d) whether he is a member of a trade union (within the meaning of the Trade Union and Labour Relations (Consolidation) Act 1992),

(e) his physical or mental health or condition,

(f) his sexual life,

(g) the commission or alleged commission by him of any offence, or

(h) any proceedings for any offence committed or alleged to have been committed by him, the disposal of such proceedings or the sentence of any court in such proceedings.

The special purposes

3. In this Act "the special purposes" means any one or more of the following—   A1–249

(a) the purposes of journalism,

(b) artistic purposes, and

(c) literary purposes.

The data protection principles

4.—(1) References in this Act to the data protection principles are to the principles set out in Part I of Schedule 1.   A1–250

(2) Those principles are to be interpreted in accordance with Part II of Schedule 1.

(3) Schedule 2 (which applies to all personal data) and Schedule 3 (which applies only to sensitive personal data) set out conditions applying for the purposes of the first principle; and Schedule 4 sets out cases in which the eighth principle does not apply.

(4) Subject to section 27(1), it shall be the duty of a data controller to comply with the data protection principles in relation to all personal data with respect to which he is the data controller.

Application of Act

5.—(1) Except as otherwise provided by or under section 54, this Act applies to a data controller in respect of any data only if—   A1–251

---

[285] Existing text renumbered as s.1(6)(a) and s.1(6)(b) inserted by Freedom of Information (Scotland) Act 2002 (Consequential Modifications) Order 2004/3089 art.2(2)(c) (January 1, 2005).

[286] Added by Freedom of Information Act 2000 c. 36 Pt VII s.68(3) (January 1, 2005 for purposes specified in SI 2004/1909 art.2(1); January 1, 2005 otherwise).

(a) the data controller is established in the United Kingdom and the data are processed in the context of that establishment, or

(b) the data controller is established neither in the United Kingdom nor in any other EEA State but uses equipment in the United Kingdom for processing the data otherwise than for the purposes of transit through the United Kingdom.

(2) A data controller falling within subsection (1)(b) must nominate for the purposes of this Act a representative established in the United Kingdom.

(3) For the purposes of subsections (1) and (2), each of the following is to be treated as established in the United Kingdom—

(a) an individual who is ordinarily resident in the United Kingdom,

(b) a body incorporated under the law of, or of any part of, the United Kingdom,

(c) a partnership or other unincorporated association formed under the law of any part of the United Kingdom, and

(d) any person who does not fall within paragraph (a), (b) or (c) but maintains in the United Kingdom—

    (i) an office, branch or agency through which he carries on any activity, or

    (ii) a regular practice;

and the reference to establishment in any other EEA State has a corresponding meaning.

The Commissioner [. . .]²⁸⁷

A1–252   **6.**—[(1) For the purposes of this Act and of the Freedom of Information Act 2000 there shall be an officer known as the Information Commissioner (in this Act referred to as "the Commissioner").]²⁸⁸

(2) The Commissioner shall be appointed by Her Majesty by Letters Patent.
[. . .]²⁸⁹

(7) Schedule 5 has effect in relation to the Commissioner [. . .].²⁹⁰

PART II

RIGHTS OF DATA SUBJECTS AND OTHERS

Right of access to personal data

A1–253   **7.**—(1) Subject to the following provisions of this section and to [sections 8, 9 and 9A],²⁹¹ an individual is entitled—

(a) to be informed by any data controller whether personal data of which that individual is the data subject are being processed by or on behalf of that data controller,

(b) if that is the case, to be given by the data controller a description of—

---

²⁸⁷ Words repealed by Transfer of Tribunal Functions Order 2010/22 Sch.2 para.25(a) (January 18, 2010).
²⁸⁸ Substituted by Freedom of Information Act 2000 c. 36 Sch.2(I) para.13(2) (January 30, 2001).
²⁸⁹ Repealed by Transfer of Tribunal Functions Order 2010/22 Sch.2 para.25(b) (January 18, 2010).
²⁹⁰ Words repealed by Transfer of Tribunal Functions Order 2010/22 Sch.2 para.25(c) (January 18, 2010).
²⁹¹ Words substituted by Freedom of Information Act 2000 c. 36 Pt VII s.69(1) (November 30, 2000 for conferring powers to make any order, regulations or code of practice; January 1, 2005 for purposes specified in SI 2004/1909 art.2(1); January 1, 2005 otherwise).

    (i) the personal data of which that individual is the data subject,

    (ii) the purposes for which they are being or are to be processed, and

    (iii) the recipients or classes of recipients to whom they are or may be disclosed,

(c) to have communicated to him in an intelligible form—

    (i) the information constituting any personal data of which that individual is the data subject, and

    (ii) any information available to the data controller as to the source of those data, and

(d) where the processing by automatic means of personal data of which that individual is the data subject for the purpose of evaluating matters relating to him such as, for example, his performance at work, his credit worthiness, his reliability or his conduct, has constituted or is likely to constitute the sole basis for any decision significantly affecting him, to be informed by the data controller of the logic involved in that decision-taking.

(2) A data controller is not obliged to supply any information under subsection (1) unless he has received—

(a) a request in writing, and

(b) except in prescribed cases, such fee (not exceeding the prescribed maximum) as he may require.

[(3) Where a data controller—

(a) reasonably requires further information in order to satisfy himself as to the identity of the person making a request under this section and to locate the information which that person seeks, and

(b) has informed him of that requirement,

the data controller is not obliged to comply with the request unless he is supplied with that further information.][292]

(4) Where a data controller cannot comply with the request without disclosing information relating to another individual who can be identified from that information, he is not obliged to comply with the request unless—

(a) the other individual has consented to the disclosure of the information to the person making the request, or

(b) it is reasonable in all the circumstances to comply with the request without the consent of the other individual.

(5) In subsection (4) the reference to information relating to another individual includes a reference to information identifying that individual as the source of the information sought by the request; and that subsection is not to be construed as excusing a data controller from communicating so much of the information sought by the request as can be communicated without disclosing the identity of the other individual concerned, whether by the omission of names or other identifying particulars or otherwise.

(6) In determining for the purposes of subsection (4)(b) whether it is reasonable in all the circumstances to comply with the request without the consent of the other individual concerned, regard shall be had, in particular, to—

(a) any duty of confidentiality owed to the other individual,

---

[292] Substituted by Freedom of Information Act 2000 c. 36 Sch.6 para.1 (May 14, 2001).

(b) any steps taken by the data controller with a view to seeking the consent of the other individual,

(c) whether the other individual is capable of giving consent, and

(d) any express refusal of consent by the other individual.

(7) An individual making a request under this section may, in such cases as may be prescribed, specify that his request is limited to personal data of any prescribed description.

(8) Subject to subsection (4), a data controller shall comply with a request under this section promptly and in any event before the end of the prescribed period beginning with the relevant day.

(9) If a court is satisfied on the application of any person who has made a request under the foregoing provisions of this section that the data controller in question has failed to comply with the request in contravention of those provisions, the court may order him to comply with the request.

(10) In this section—

"prescribed" means prescribed by the [Secretary of State][293] by regulations;
"the prescribed maximum" means such amount as may be prescribed;
"the prescribed period" means forty days or such other period as may be prescribed;
"the relevant day", in relation to a request under this section, means the day on which the data controller receives the request or, if later, the first day on which the data controller has both the required fee and the information referred to in subsection (3).

(11) Different amounts or periods may be prescribed under this section in relation to different cases.

[(12) A person is a relevant person for the purposes of subsection (4)(c) if he—

(a) is a person referred to in paragraph 4(a) or (b) or paragraph 8(a) or (b) of Schedule 11;

(b) is employed by an education authority (within the meaning of paragraph 6 of Schedule 11) in pursuance of its functions relating to education and the information relates to him, or he supplied the information in his capacity as such an employee; or

(c) is the person making the request.][294]

Provisions supplementary to section 7

A1–254   8.—(1) The [Secretary of State][295] may by regulations provide that, in such cases as may be prescribed, a request for information under any provision of subsection (1) of section 7 is to be treated as extending also to information under other provisions of that subsection.

(2) The obligation imposed by section 7(1)(c)(i) must be complied with by supplying the data subject with a copy of the information in permanent form unless—

(a) the supply of such a copy is not possible or would involve disproportionate effort, or

---

[293] Words substituted by Secretary of State for Constitutional Affairs Order 2003/1887 Sch.2 para.9(1)(a) (August 19, 2003).

[294] Deemed to be inserted in relation to data to which SI 2000/414 applies by Data Protection (Subject Access Modification) (Education) Order 2000/414 art.7(2) (March 1, 2000).

[295] Words substituted by Secretary of State for Constitutional Affairs Order 2003/1887 Sch.2 para.9(1)(a) (August 19, 2003).

(b) the data subject agrees otherwise;

and where any of the information referred to in section 7(1)(c)(i) is expressed in terms which are not intelligible without explanation the copy must be accompanied by an explanation of those terms.

(3) Where a data controller has previously complied with a request made under section 7 by an individual, the data controller is not obliged to comply with a subsequent identical or similar request under that section by that individual unless a reasonable interval has elapsed between compliance with the previous request and the making of the current request.

(4) In determining for the purposes of subsection (3) whether requests under section 7 are made at reasonable intervals, regard shall be had to the nature of the data, the purposes for which the data are processed and the frequency with which the data are altered.

(5) Section 7(1)(d) is not to be regarded as requiring the provision of information as to the logic involved in any decision-taking if, and to the extent that, the information constitutes a trade secret.

(6) The information to be supplied pursuant to a request under section 7 must be supplied by reference to the data in question at the time when the request is received, except that it may take account of any amendment or deletion made between that time and the time when the information is supplied, being an amendment or deletion that would have been made regardless of the receipt of the request.

(7) For the purposes of section 7(4) and (5) another individual can be identified from the information being disclosed if he can be identified from that information, or from that and any other information which, in the reasonable belief of the data controller, is likely to be in, or to come into, the possession of the data subject making the request.

[Unstructured personal data held by public authorities

9A.—(1) In this section "unstructured personal data" means any personal data falling   **A1–255** within paragraph (e) of the definition of "data" in section 1(1), other than information which is recorded as part of, or with the intention that it should form part of, any set of information relating to individuals to the extent that the set is structured by reference to individuals or by reference to criteria relating to individuals.

(2) A public authority is not obliged to comply with subsection (1) of section 7 in relation to any unstructured personal data unless the request under that section contains a description of the data.

(3) Even if the data are described by the data subject in his request, a public authority is not obliged to comply with subsection (1) of section 7 in relation to unstructured personal data if the authority estimates that the cost of complying with the request so far as relating to those data would exceed the appropriate limit.

(4) Subsection (3) does not exempt the public authority from its obligation to comply with paragraph (a) of section 7(1) in relation to the unstructured personal data unless the estimated cost of complying with that paragraph alone in relation to those data would exceed the appropriate limit.

(5) In subsections (3) and (4) "the appropriate limit" means such amount as may be prescribed by the [Secretary of State]²⁹⁶ by regulations, and different amounts may be prescribed in relation to different cases .

(6) Any estimate for the purposes of this section must be made in accordance with regulations under section 12(5) of the Freedom of Information Act 2000.]²⁹⁷

---

²⁹⁶ Words substituted by Freedom of Information Act 2000 c. 36 Pt VII s.69 (August 19, 2003: commenced by an amendment).

²⁹⁷ Added by Freedom of Information Act 2000 c. 36 Pt VII s.69(2) (November 30, 2000 for conferring powers to make any order, regulations or code of practice; January 1, 2005 for purposes specified in SI 2004/1909 art.2(1); January 1, 2005 otherwise).

Right to prevent processing likely to cause damage or distress

A1–256   **10.**—(1) Subject to subsection (2), an individual is entitled at any time by notice in writing to a data controller to require the data controller at the end of such period as is reasonable in the circumstances to cease, or not to begin, processing, or processing for a specified purpose or in a specified manner, any personal data in respect of which he is the data subject, on the ground that, for specified reasons—

   (a) the processing of those data or their processing for that purpose or in that manner is causing or is likely to cause substantial damage or substantial distress to him or to another, and

   (b) that damage or distress is or would be unwarranted.

   (2) Subsection (1) does not apply—

   (a) in a case where any of the conditions in paragraphs 1 to 4 of Schedule 2 is met, or

   (b) in such other cases as may be prescribed by the [Secretary of State][298] by order.

   (3) The data controller must within twenty-one days of receiving a notice under subsection (1) ("the data subject notice") give the individual who gave it a written notice—

   (a) stating that he has complied or intends to comply with the data subject notice, or

   (b) stating his reasons for regarding the data subject notice as to any extent unjustified and the extent (if any) to which he has complied or intends to comply with it.

   (4) If a court is satisfied, on the application of any person who has given a notice under subsection (1) which appears to the court to be justified (or to be justified to any extent), that the data controller in question has failed to comply with the notice, the court may order him to take such steps for complying with the notice (or for complying with it to that extent) as the court thinks fit.

   (5) The failure by a data subject to exercise the right conferred by subsection (1) or section 11(1) does not affect any other right conferred on him by this Part.

Compensation for failure to comply with certain requirements

A1–257   **13.**—(1) An individual who suffers damage by reason of any contravention by a data controller of any of the requirements of this Act is entitled to compensation from the data controller for that damage.

   (2) An individual who suffers distress by reason of any contravention by a data controller of any of the requirements of this Act is entitled to compensation from the data controller for that distress if—

   (a) the individual also suffers damage by reason of the contravention, or

   (b) the contravention relates to the processing of personal data for the special purposes.

---

[298] Words substituted by Secretary of State for Constitutional Affairs Order 2003/1887 Sch.2 para.9(1)(a) (August 19, 2003).

(3) In proceedings brought against a person by virtue of this section it is a defence to prove that he had taken such care as in all the circumstances was reasonably required to comply with the requirement concerned.

Rectification, blocking, erasure and destruction

14.—(1) If a court is satisfied on the application of a data subject that personal data of **A1–258** which the applicant is the subject are inaccurate, the court may order the data controller to rectify, block, erase or destroy those data and any other personal data in respect of which he is the data controller and which contain an expression of opinion which appears to the court to be based on the inaccurate data.

(2) Subsection (1) applies whether or not the data accurately record information received or obtained by the data controller from the data subject or a third party but where the data accurately record such information, then—

(a) if the requirements mentioned in paragraph 7 of Part II of Schedule 1 have been complied with, the court may, instead of making an order under subsection (1), make an order requiring the data to be supplemented by such statement of the true facts relating to the matters dealt with by the data as the court may approve, and

(b) if all or any of those requirements have not been complied with, the court may, instead of making an order under that subsection, make such order as it thinks fit for securing compliance with those requirements with or without a further order requiring the data to be supplemented by such a statement as is mentioned in paragraph (a).

(3) Where the court—

(a) makes an order under subsection (1), or

(b) is satisfied on the application of a data subject that personal data of which he was the data subject and which have been rectified, blocked, erased or destroyed were inaccurate,

it may, where it considers it reasonably practicable, order the data controller to notify third parties to whom the data have been disclosed of the rectification, blocking, erasure or destruction.

(4) If a court is satisfied on the application of a data subject—

(a) that he has suffered damage by reason of any contravention by a data controller of any of the requirements of this Act in respect of any personal data, in circumstances entitling him to compensation under section 13, and

(b) that there is a substantial risk of further contravention in respect of those data in such circumstances,

the court may order the rectification, blocking, erasure or destruction of any of those data.

(5) Where the court makes an order under subsection (4) it may, where it considers it reasonably practicable, order the data controller to notify third parties to whom the data have been disclosed of the rectification, blocking, erasure or destruction.

(6) In determining whether it is reasonably practicable to require such notification as is mentioned in subsection (3) or (5) the court shall have regard, in particular, to the number of persons who would have to be notified.

Jurisdiction and procedure

A1–259   **15.**—(1) The jurisdiction conferred by sections 7 to 14 is exercisable [in England and Wales by the High Court or the county court or, in Northern Ireland,]²⁹⁹ by the High Court or a county court or, in Scotland, by the Court of Session or the sheriff.

(2) For the purpose of determining any question whether an applicant under subsection (9) of section 7 is entitled to the information which he seeks (including any question whether any relevant data are exempt from that section by virtue of Part IV) a court may require the information constituting any data processed by or on behalf of the data controller and any information as to the logic involved in any decision-taking as mentioned in section 7(1)(d) to be made available for its own inspection but shall not, pending the determination of that question in the applicant's favour, require the information sought by the applicant to be disclosed to him or his representatives whether by discovery (or, in Scotland, recovery) or otherwise.

Part III

Notification by data controllers

Preliminary

A1–260   **16.**—(1) In this Part "the registrable particulars", in relation to a data controller, means—

(a) his name and address,

(b) if he has nominated a representative for the purposes of this Act, the name and address of the representative,

(c) a description of the personal data being or to be processed by or on behalf of the data controller and of the category or categories of data subject to which they relate,

(d) a description of the purpose or purposes for which the data are being or are to be processed,

(e) a description of any recipient or recipients to whom the data controller intends or may wish to disclose the data,

(f) the names, or a description of, any countries or territories outside the European Economic Area to which the data controller directly or indirectly transfers, or intends or may wish directly or indirectly to transfer, the data, [. . .]³⁰⁰

[(ff) where the data controller is a public authority, a statement of that fact, [. . .]³⁰¹]³⁰⁰

(g) in any case where—

(i) personal data are being, or are intended to be, processed in circumstances in which the prohibition in subsection (1) of section 17 is excluded by subsection (2) or (3) of that section, and

(ii) the notification does not extend to those data,

---

²⁹⁹ Words inserted by Crime and Courts Act 2013 c. 22 Sch.9(3) para.77 (April 22, 2014: insertion has effect as SI 2014/954 subject to savings and transitional provisions specified in 2013 c.22 s.15 and Sch.8 and transitional provision specified in SI 2014/954 arts 2(c) and 3).

³⁰⁰ Added by Freedom of Information Act 2001 c. 36 Pt VII s.71 (January 1, 2005 for purposes specified in SI 2004/1909 art.2(1); January 1, 2005 otherwise).

³⁰¹ Word repealed by Coroners and Justice Act 2009 c. 25 Sch.20(1) para.1(a) (February 1, 2010: repeal comes into force on February 1, 2010 as SI 2010/145 art.2 and Sch.1 para.24 and is also purportedly brought into force on April 6, 2010 by SI 2010/816 art.2 and Sch.1 para.22(d)).

a statement of that fact [, and]³⁰²

[(h) such information about the data controller as may be prescribed under section 18(5A).]³⁰²

(2) In this Part—

"fees regulations" means regulations made by the [Secretary of State]³⁰³ under section 18(5) or 19(4) or (7);

"notification regulations" means regulations made by the [Secretary of State]³⁰³ under the other provisions of this Part;

"prescribed", except where used in relation to fees regulations, means prescribed by notification regulations.

(3) For the purposes of this Part, so far as it relates to the addresses of data controllers—

(a) the address of a registered company is that of its registered office, and

(b) the address of a person (other than a registered company) carrying on a business is that of his principal place of business in the United Kingdom.

Prohibition on processing without registration

17.—(1) Subject to the following provisions of this section, personal data must not be processed unless an entry in respect of the data controller is included in the register maintained by the Commissioner under section 19 (or is treated by notification regulations made by virtue of section 19(3) as being so included). **A1–261**

(2) Except where the processing is assessable processing for the purposes of section 22, subsection (1) does not apply in relation to personal data consisting of information which falls neither within paragraph (a) of the definition of "data" in section 1(1) nor within paragraph (b) of that definition.

(3) If it appears to the [Secretary of State]³⁰⁴ that processing of a particular description is unlikely to prejudice the rights and freedoms of data subjects, notification regulations may provide that, in such cases as may be prescribed, subsection (1) is not to apply in relation to processing of that description.

(4) Subsection (1) does not apply in relation to any processing whose sole purpose is the maintenance of a public register.

Notification by data controllers

18.—(1) Any data controller who wishes to be included in the register maintained under section 19 shall give a notification to the Commissioner under this section. **A1–262**

(2) A notification under this section must specify in accordance with notification regulations—

(a) the registrable particulars, and

(b) a general description of measures to be taken for the purpose of complying with the seventh data protection principle.

---

³⁰² Added by Coroners and Justice Act 2009 c. 25 Sch.20(1) para.1(b) (February 1, 2010).
³⁰³ Words substituted by Secretary of State for Constitutional Affairs Order 2003/1887 Sch.2 para.9(1)(a) (August 19, 2003).
³⁰⁴ Words substituted by Secretary of State for Constitutional Affairs Order 2003/1887 Sch.2 para.9(1)(a) (August 19, 2003).

(3) Notification regulations made by virtue of subsection (2) may provide for the determination by the Commissioner, in accordance with any requirements of the regulations, of the form in which the registrable particulars and the description mentioned in subsection (2)(b) are to be specified, including in particular the detail required for the purposes of section 16(1)(c), (d), (e) and (f) and subsection (2)(b).

(4) Notification regulations may make provision as to the giving of notification—

(a) by partnerships, or

(b) in other cases where two or more persons are the data controllers in respect of any personal data.

(5) The notification must be accompanied by such fee as may be prescribed by fees regulations.

[(5A) Notification regulations may prescribe the information about the data controller which is required for the purpose of verifying the fee payable under subsection (5).][305]

(6) Notification regulations may provide for any fee paid under subsection (5) or section 19(4) to be refunded in prescribed circumstances.

Register of notifications

A1–263   **19.**—(1) The Commissioner shall—

(a) maintain a register of persons who have given notification under section 18, and

(b) make an entry in the register in pursuance of each notification received by him under that section from a person in respect of whom no entry as data controller was for the time being included in the register.

(2) Each entry in the register shall consist of—

(a) the registrable particulars notified under section 18 or, as the case requires, those particulars as amended in pursuance of section 20(4), and

(b) such other information as the Commissioner may be authorised or required by notification regulations to include in the register.

(3) Notification regulations may make provision as to the time as from which any entry in respect of a data controller is to be treated for the purposes of section 17 as having been made in the register.

(4) No entry shall be retained in the register for more than the relevant time except on payment of such fee as may be prescribed by fees regulations.

(5) In subsection (4) "the relevant time" means twelve months or such other period as may be prescribed by notification regulations; and different periods may be prescribed in relation to different cases.

(6) The Commissioner—

(a) shall provide facilities for making the information contained in the entries in the register available for inspection (in visible and legible form) by members of the public at all reasonable hours and free of charge, and

(b) may provide such other facilities for making the information contained in those entries available to the public free of charge as he considers appropriate.

---

[305] Added by Coroners and Justice Act 2009 c. 25 Sch.20(1) para.2 (February 1, 2010).

(7) The Commissioner shall, on payment of such fee, if any, as may be prescribed by fees regulations, supply any member of the public with a duly certified copy in writing of the particulars contained in any entry made in the register.

[(8) Nothing in subsection (6) or (7) applies to information which is included in an entry in the register only by reason of it falling within section 16(1)(h).][306]

Duty to notify changes

20.—(1) For the purpose specified in subsection (2), notification regulations shall include   **A1–264**
provision imposing on every person in respect of whom an entry as a data controller is for the time being included in the register maintained under section 19 a duty to notify to the Commissioner, in such circumstances and at such time or times and in such form as may be prescribed, such matters relating to the registrable particulars and measures taken as mentioned in section 18(2)(b) as may be prescribed.

(2) The purpose referred to in subsection (1) is that of ensuring, so far as practicable, that at any time—

(a) the entries in the register maintained under section 19 contain current names and addresses and describe the current practice or intentions of the data controller with respect to the processing of personal data, and

(b) the Commissioner is provided with a general description of measures currently being taken as mentioned in section 18(2)(b).

(3) Subsection (3) of section 18 has effect in relation to notification regulations made by virtue of subsection (1) as it has effect in relation to notification regulations made by virtue of subsection (2) of that section.

(4) On receiving any notification under notification regulations made by virtue of subsection (1), the Commissioner shall make such amendments of the relevant entry in the register maintained under section 19 as are necessary to take account of the notification.

Offences

21.—(1) If section 17(1) is contravened, the data controller is guilty of an offence.   **A1–265**
(2) Any person who fails to comply with the duty imposed by notification regulations made by virtue of section 20(1) is guilty of an offence.
(3) It shall be a defence for a person charged with an offence under subsection (2) to show that he exercised all due diligence to comply with the duty.

PART IV

EXEMPTIONS

Preliminary

27.—(1) References in any of the data protection principles or any provision of Parts II   **A1–266**
and III to personal data or to the processing of personal data do not include references to data or processing which by virtue of this Part are exempt from that principle or other provision.

(2) In this Part "the subject information provisions" means—

(a) the first data protection principle to the extent to which it requires compliance with paragraph 2 of Part II of Schedule 1, and

(b) section 7.

---

[306] Added by Coroners and Justice Act 2009 c. 25, Sch.20(1) para.3 (February 1, 2010).

(3) In this Part "the non-disclosure provisions" means the provisions specified in subsection (4) to the extent to which they are inconsistent with the disclosure in question.

(4) The provisions referred to in subsection (3) are—

(a) the first data protection principle, except to the extent to which it requires compliance with the conditions in Schedules 2 and 3,

(b) the second, third, fourth and fifth data protection principles, and

(c) sections 10 and 14(1) to (3).

(5) Except as provided by this Part, the subject information provisions shall have effect notwithstanding any enactment or rule of law prohibiting or restricting the disclosure, or authorising the withholding, of information.

National security

A1–267   28.—(1) Personal data are exempt from any of the provisions of—

(a) the data protection principles,

(b) Parts II, III and V, and

(c) [sections 54A and 55][307],

if the exemption from that provision is required for the purpose of safeguarding national security.

(2) Subject to subsection (4), a certificate signed by a Minister of the Crown certifying that exemption from all or any of the provisions mentioned in subsection (1) is or at any time was required for the purpose there mentioned in respect of any personal data shall be conclusive evidence of that fact.

(3) A certificate under subsection (2) may identify the personal data to which it applies by means of a general description and may be expressed to have prospective effect.

(4) Any person directly affected by the issuing of a certificate under subsection (2) may appeal to the Tribunal against the certificate.

(5) If on an appeal under subsection (4), the Tribunal finds that, applying the principles applied by the court on an application for judicial review, the Minister did not have reasonable grounds for issuing the certificate, the Tribunal may allow the appeal and quash the certificate.

(6) Where in any proceedings under or by virtue of this Act it is claimed by a data controller that a certificate under subsection (2) which identifies the personal data to which it applies by means of a general description applies to any personal data, any other party to the proceedings may appeal to the Tribunal on the ground that the certificate does not apply to the personal data in question and, subject to any determination under subsection (7), the certificate shall be conclusively presumed so to apply.

(7) On any appeal under subsection (6), the Tribunal may determine that the certificate does not so apply.

(8) A document purporting to be a certificate under subsection (2) shall be received in evidence and deemed to be such a certificate unless the contrary is proved.

(9) A document which purports to be certified by or on behalf of a Minister of the Crown as a true copy of a certificate issued by that Minister under subsection (2) shall in any legal proceedings be evidence (or, in Scotland, sufficient evidence) of that certificate.

---

[307] Word substituted by Crime (International Co-operation) Act 2003 c. 32 Sch.5 para.69 (April 26, 2004).

(10) The power conferred by subsection (2) on a Minister of the Crown shall not be exercisable except by a Minister who is a member of the Cabinet or by the Attorney General or the [Advocate General for Scotland].[308]

(11) No power conferred by any provision of Part V may be exercised in relation to personal data which by virtue of this section are exempt from that provision.

(12) Schedule 6 shall have effect in relation to appeals under subsection (4) or (6) and the proceedings of the Tribunal in respect of any such appeal.

Crime and taxation

29.—(1) Personal data processed for any of the following purposes—   A1–268

(a) the prevention or detection of crime,

(b) the apprehension or prosecution of offenders, or

(c) the assessment or collection of any tax or duty or of any imposition of a similar nature,

are exempt from the first data protection principle (except to the extent to which it requires compliance with the conditions in Schedules 2 and 3) and section 7 in any case to the extent to which the application of those provisions to the data would be likely to prejudice any of the matters mentioned in this subsection.

(2) Personal data which—

(a) are processed for the purpose of discharging statutory functions, and

(b) consist of information obtained for such a purpose from a person who had it in his possession for any of the purposes mentioned in subsection (1),

are exempt from the subject information provisions to the same extent as personal data processed for any of the purposes mentioned in that subsection.

(3) Personal data are exempt from the non-disclosure provisions in any case in which—

(a) the disclosure is for any of the purposes mentioned in subsection (1), and

(b) the application of those provisions in relation to the disclosure would be likely to prejudice any of the matters mentioned in that subsection.

(4) Personal data in respect of which the data controller is a relevant authority and which—

(a) consist of a classification applied to the data subject as part of a system of risk assessment which is operated by that authority for either of the following purposes—

  (i) the assessment or collection of any tax or duty or any imposition of a similar nature, or

  (ii) the prevention or detection of crime, or apprehension or prosecution of offenders, where the offence concerned involves any unlawful claim for any payment out of, or any unlawful application of, public funds, and

(b) are processed for either of those purposes,

---

[308] Words substituted by Transfer of Functions (Lord Advocate and Advocate General for Scotland) Order 1999/679 Sch.1 para.1 (March 1, 2000: substitution came into force on May 20, 1999 but could not take effect until the commencement of 1998 c.29 s.28(10) on March 1, 2000).

are exempt from section 7 to the extent to which the exemption is required in the interests of the operation of the system.

(5) In subsection (4)—

"public funds" includes funds provided by any [EU][309] institution;
"relevant authority" means—

    (a) a government department,
    (b) a local authority, or
    (c) any other authority administering housing benefit or council tax benefit.

Research, history and statistics

A1–269   33.—(1) In this section—

"research purposes" includes statistical or historical purposes;
"the relevant conditions", in relation to any processing of personal data, means the conditions—

    (a) that the data are not processed to support measures or decisions with respect to particular individuals, and
    (b) that the data are not processed in such a way that substantial damage or substantial distress is, or is likely to be, caused to any data subject.

(2) For the purposes of the second data protection principle, the further processing of personal data only for research purposes in compliance with the relevant conditions is not to be regarded as incompatible with the purposes for which they were obtained.

(3) Personal data which are processed only for research purposes in compliance with the relevant conditions may, notwithstanding the fifth data protection principle, be kept indefinitely.

(4) Personal data which are processed only for research purposes are exempt from section 7 if—

    (a) they are processed in compliance with the relevant conditions, and

    (b) the results of the research or any resulting statistics are not made available in a form which identifies data subjects or any of them.

(5) For the purposes of subsections (2) to (4) personal data are not to be treated as processed otherwise than for research purposes merely because the data are disclosed—

    (a) to any person, for research purposes only,

    (b) to the data subject or a person acting on his behalf,

    (c) at the request, or with the consent, of the data subject or a person acting on his behalf, or

    (d) in circumstances in which the person making the disclosure has reasonable grounds for believing that the disclosure falls within paragraph (a), (b) or (c).

[Manual data held by public authorities

A1–270   33A.—(1) Personal data falling within paragraph (e) of the definition of "data" in section 1(1) are exempt from—

---

[309] Word substituted by Treaty of Lisbon (Changes in Terminology) Order 2011/1043 Pt 2 art.6(1)(c) (April 22, 2011).

(a) the first, second, third, fifth, seventh and eighth data protection principles,

(b) the sixth data protection principle except so far as it relates to the rights conferred on data subjects by sections 7 and 14,

(c) sections 10 to 12,

(d) section 13, except so far as it relates to damage caused by a contravention of section 7 or of the fourth data protection principle and to any distress which is also suffered by reason of that contravention,

(e) Part III, and

(f) section 55.

(2) Personal data which fall within paragraph (e) of the definition of "data" in section 1(1) and relate to appointments or removals, pay, discipline, superannuation or other personnel matters, in relation to—

(a) service in any of the armed forces of the Crown,

(b) service in any office or employment under the Crown or under any public authority, or

(c) service in any office or employment, or under any contract for services, in respect of which power to take action, or to determine or approve the action taken, in such matters is vested in Her Majesty, any Minister of the Crown, the National Assembly for Wales, any Northern Ireland Minister (within the meaning of the Freedom of Information Act 2000) or any public authority,

are also exempt from the remaining data protection principles and the remaining provisions of Part II.][310]

Information available to the public by or under enactment

34. Personal data are exempt from— **A1–271**

(a) the subject information provisions,

(b) the fourth data protection principle and [section 14(1) to (3)][311], and

(c) the non-disclosure provisions,

if the data consist of information which the data controller is obliged by or under any enactment [other than an enactment contained in the Freedom of Information Act 2000][312] to make available to the public, whether by publishing it, by making it available for inspection, or otherwise and whether gratuitously or on payment of a fee.

Disclosures required by law or made in connection with legal proceedings etc.

35.—(1) Personal data are exempt from the non-disclosure provisions where the disclosure is required by or under any enactment, by any rule of law or by the order of a court. **A1–272**

(2) Personal data are exempt from the non-disclosure provisions where the disclosure is necessary—

---

[310] Added by Freedom of Information Act 2000 c. 36 Pt VII s.70(1) (January 1, 2005 for purposes specified in SI 2004/1909 art.2(1); January 1, 2005 otherwise).

[311] Words substituted by Data Protection Act 1998 c. 29 Sch.13 para.3 (October 23, 2007).

[312] Words inserted by Freedom of Information Act 2000 c. 36 Pt VII s.72 (November 30, 2002).

(a) for the purpose of, or in connection with, any legal proceedings (including prospective legal proceedings), or

(b) for the purpose of obtaining legal advice,

or is otherwise necessary for the purposes of establishing, exercising or defending legal rights.

Miscellaneous exemptions

A1–273   **37.** Schedule 7 (which confers further miscellaneous exemptions) has effect.

SCHEDULE 7

MISCELLANEOUS EXEMPTIONS

Confidential references given by the data controller

A1–274   **1.** Personal data are exempt from section 7 if they consist of a reference given or to be given in confidence by the data controller for the purposes of—
       2.

(a) the education, training or employment, or prospective education, training or employment, of the data subject,

(b) the appointment, or prospective appointment, of the data subject to any office, or

(c) the provision, or prospective provision, by the data subject of any service.

Armed forces

A1–275   **3.** Personal data are exempt from the subject information provisions in any case to the extent to which the application of those provisions would be likely to prejudice the combat effectiveness of any of the armed forces of the Crown.

Judicial appointments and honours

A1–276   **4.** Personal data processed for the purposes of—
       5.

(a) assessing any person's suitability for judicial office or the office of Queen's Counsel, or

(b) the conferring by the Crown of any honour [or dignity][313],

are exempt from the subject information provisions.

Legal professional privilege

A1–277   **10.** Personal data are exempt from the subject information provisions if the data consist of information in respect of which a claim to legal professional privilege [or, in Scotland, to confidentiality of communications][314] could be maintained in legal proceedings.

Self-incrimination

A1–278   **11.**—(1) A person need not comply with any request or order under section 7 to the extent that compliance would, by revealing evidence of the commission of any offence [, other than an offence

---

[313] Words added by Freedom of Information Act 2000 c. 36 Sch.6 para.6 (May 14, 2001).
[314] Words substituted by Freedom of Information Act 2000 c. 36 Sch.6 para.7 (May 14, 2001).

under this Act or an offence within sub-paragraph (1A),][315] expose him to proceedings for that offence.

[(1A) The offences mentioned in sub-paragraph (1) are—

(a) an offence under section 5 of the Perjury Act 1911 (false statements made otherwise than on oath),

(b) an offence under section 44(2) of the Criminal Law (Consolidation) (Scotland) Act 1995 (false statements made otherwise than on oath), or

(c) an offence under Article 10 of the Perjury (Northern Ireland) Order 1979 (false statutory declarations and other false unsworn statements).][316]

(2) Information disclosed by any person in compliance with any request or order under section 7 shall not be admissible against him in proceedings for an offence under this Act.

Domestic Violence, Crime and Victims Act 2004 c. 28

PART 1

DOMESTIC VIOLENCE ETC

Causing or allowing the death of a child or vulnerable adult

[The offence

5.—(1) A person ("D") is guilty of an offence if—   **A1–279**

(a) a child or vulnerable adult ("V") dies or suffers serious physical harm as a result of the unlawful act of a person who—

    (i) was a member of the same household as V, and
    (ii) had frequent contact with him,

(b) D was such a person at the time of that act,

(c) at that time there was a significant risk of serious physical harm being caused to V by the unlawful act of such a person, and

(d) either D was the person whose act caused the death or serious physical harm or—

    (i) D was, or ought to have been, aware of the risk mentioned in paragraph (c),
    (ii) D failed to take such steps as he could reasonably have been expected to take to protect V from the risk, and
    (iii) the act occurred in circumstances of the kind that D foresaw or ought to have foreseen.

(2) The prosecution does not have to prove whether it is the first alternative in subsection (1)(d) or the second (sub-paragraphs (i) to (iii)) that applies.

(3) If D was not the mother or father of V—

(a) D may not be charged with an offence under this section if he was under the age of 16 at the time of the act that caused the death or serious physical harm;

---

[315] Words substituted by Coroners and Justice Act 2009 c. 25 Sch.20(4) para.12(2) (April 6, 2010).
[316] Added by Coroners and Justice Act 2009 c. 25 Sch.20(4) para.12(3) (April 6, 2010).

(b) for the purposes of subsection (1)(d)(ii) D could not have been expected to take any such step as is referred to there before attaining that age.

(4) For the purposes of this section—

(a) a person is to be regarded as a "member" of a particular household, even if he does not live in that household, if he visits it so often and for such periods of time that it is reasonable to regard him as a member of it;

(b) where V lived in different households at different times, "the same household as V" refers to the household in which V was living at the time of the act that caused the death or serious physical harm.

(5) For the purposes of this section an "unlawful" act is one that—

(a) constitutes an offence, or

(b) would constitute an offence but for being the act of—

(i) a person under the age of ten, or
(ii) a person entitled to rely on a defence of insanity.

Paragraph (b) does not apply to an act of D.
(6) In this section—

"act" includes a course of conduct and also includes omission;
"child" means a person under the age of 16;
"serious" harm means harm that amounts to grievous bodily harm for the purposes of the Offences against the Person Act 1861 (c. 100);
"vulnerable adult" means a person aged 16 or over whose ability to protect himself from violence, abuse or neglect is significantly impaired through physical or mental disability or illness, through old age or otherwise.

(7) A person guilty of an offence under this section of causing or allowing a person's death is liable on conviction on indictment to imprisonment for a term not exceeding 14 years or to a fine, or to both.
(8) A person guilty of an offence under this section of causing or allowing a person to suffer serious physical harm is liable on conviction on indictment to imprisonment for a term not exceeding 10 years or to a fine, or to both.][317]

Duchy of Lancaster Act 1920 c. 51

Provisions as to the Duchy solicitor

A1–280   **3.**—(1) The person for the time being holding the office of solicitor for the affairs of the Duchy of Lancaster (in this Act referred to as "the Duchy solicitor") shall be a corporation sole by the name of "The solicitor for the affairs of the Duchy of Lancaster," and by that name shall have perpetual succession with a capacity to acquire and hold in that name real and personal property of every description, to execute deeds, using an official seal, to enter into engagements binding on himself and his successors in office, and to do all other acts necessary or expedient to be done in the execution of the duties of his office.

(2) Any document purporting to be sealed with the said official seal shall be receivable in evidence of the particulars stated in that document.

---

[317] Amended by Domestic Violence, Crime and Victims (Amendment) Act 2012 c. 4 s.1 (July 2, 2012: amendments have effect as SI 2012/1432 subject to transitional provisions specified in 2012 c.4 s.1(8)).

(3) Where, by reason of His Majesty having become entitled in right of the Duchy of Lancaster to the personal estate of an intestate or otherwise, any court has power to grant administration of the personal estate of any deceased person to a nominee of His Majesty, [sections two and seven of the Treasury Solicitor Act 1876][318] shall apply as if herein re-enacted and in terms made applicable to this Act, and to the Duchy solicitor, and to property to which His Majesty is entitled in right of the Duchy of Lancaster.

(4) An assistant solicitor for the affairs of the Duchy of Lancaster may, on behalf of the Duchy solicitor, do all such things as an assistant solicitor for the affairs of His Majesty's Treasury is authorised by section three of the Act aforesaid to do on behalf of the Treasury solicitor, and that section, with the necessary adaptations, shall apply accordingly.

Health and Safety at Work etc. Act 1974 c. 37

PART I

HEALTH, SAFETY AND WELFARE IN CONNECTION WITH WORK, AND CONTROL OF DANGEROUS SUBSTANCES AND CERTAIN EMISSIONS INTO THE ATMOSPHERE

Enforcement

Authorities responsible for enforcement of the relevant statutory provisions

18.—(1) It shall be the duty of the Executive to make adequate arrangements for the   **A1–281** enforcement of the relevant statutory provisions except to the extent that some other authority or class of authorities is by any of those provisions or by regulations under subsection (2) below made responsible for their enforcement.

[(1A) The Office for Nuclear Regulation is responsible for the enforcement of the relevant statutory provisions as they apply in relation to GB nuclear sites (within the meaning given in section 68 of the Energy Act 2013 (nuclear safety purposes)).

(1B) Subsection (1A) is subject to any provision of health and safety regulations making the Office of Rail Regulation responsible for the enforcement of any of the relevant statutory provisions to any extent in relation to such sites.][319]

(2) The Secretary of State may by regulations—

[(za) make the Office for Nuclear Regulation responsible for the enforcement of the relevant statutory provisions to such extent as may be prescribed (and may in particular provide for any site or matter in relation to which the Office for Nuclear Regulation is made so responsible to be determined by the Secretary of State or the Office for Nuclear Regulation under the regulations);][320]

(a) make local authorities responsible for the enforcement of the relevant statutory provisions to such extent as may be prescribed;

(b) make provision for enabling responsibility for enforcing any of the relevant statutory provisions to be, to such extent as may be determined under the regulations—

[(zi) transferred from the Executive or local authorities to the Office for Nuclear Regulation, or from the Office for Nuclear Regulation to the Executive or local authorities;][321]

---

[318] Words substituted by Statute Law (Repeals) Act 1981 (c.16), Sch.1 Pt. I.
[319] Added by Energy Act 2013 c. 32 Sch.12(1) para.6(2) (April 1, 2014).
[320] Added by Energy Act 2013 c. 32 Sch.12(1) para.6(3)(a) (April 1, 2014).
[321] Added by Energy Act 2013 c. 32 Sch.12(1) para.6(3)(b) (April 1, 2014).

(i) transferred from the Executive to local authorities or from local authorities to the Executive; or

(ii) assigned to the Executive [, to the Office for Nuclear Regulation][322] or to local authorities for the purpose of removing any uncertainty as to what are by virtue of [subsection (1A) or][323] this subsection their respective responsibilities for the enforcement of those provisions;

[(iii) assigned to the Office of Rail Regulation or the Office for Nuclear Regulation for the purpose of removing any uncertainty as to what are by virtue of any of the relevant statutory provisions their respective responsibilities for the enforcement of any of those provisions;][324]

and any regulations made in pursuance of paragraph (b) above shall include provision for securing that any transfer or assignment effected under the regulations is brought to the notice of persons affected by it.

(3) Any provision made by regulations under the preceding subsection shall have effect subject to any provision made by health and safety regulations [. . .][325] in pursuance of section 15(3)(c).

[(3A) Regulations under subsection (2)(a) may not make local authorities enforcing authorities in relation to any site in relation to which the Office for Nuclear Regulation is an enforcing authority.

(3B) Where the Office for Nuclear Regulation is, by or under subsection (1A) or (2), made responsible for the enforcement of any of the relevant statutory provisions to any extent, it must make adequate arrangements for the enforcement of those provisions to that extent.][326]

(4) It shall be the duty of every local authority—

(a) to make adequate arrangements for the enforcement within their area of the relevant statutory provisions to the extent that they are by any of those provisions or by regulations under subsection (2) above made responsible for their enforcement; and

(b) to perform the duty imposed on them by the preceding paragraph and any other functions conferred on them by any of the relevant statutory provisions in accordance with such guidance as [the Executive][327] may give them.

[(4A) Before the Executive gives guidance under subsection (4)(b) it shall consult the local authorities.

(4B) It shall be the duty of the Executive and the local authorities—

(a) to work together to establish best practice and consistency in the enforcement of the relevant statutory provisions;

(b) to enter into arrangements with each other for securing cooperation and the exchange of information in connection with the carrying out of their functions with regard to the relevant statutory provisions; and

---

[322] Words inserted by Energy Act 2013 c. 32 Sch.12(1) para.6(3)(c)(i) (April 1, 2014).

[323] Words inserted by Energy Act 2013 c. 32 Sch.12(1) para.6(3)(c)(ii) (April 1, 2014).

[324] Added by Energy Act 2013 c. 32 Sch.12(1) para.6(3)(d) (April 1, 2014).

[325] Words repealed by Employment Protection Act 1975 (c. 71), Sch. 18.

[326] Added by Energy Act 2013 c. 32 Sch.12(1) para.6(4) (April 1, 2014).

[327] Words substituted subject to transitional provisions as specified in SI 2008/960 Sch.2 paras 10 and 11 by Legislative Reform (Health and Safety Executive) Order 2008/960 art.10(2) (April 1, 2008: substitution has effect subject to transitional provisions as specified in SI 2008/960 Sch.2 paras 10 and 11).

(c) from time to time to review those arrangements and to revise them when they consider it appropriate to do so.][328]

(5) Where any authority other than [. . .][328], the Executive [, the Office for Nuclear Regulation][329] or a local authority is by any of the relevant statutory provisions [. . .][330] made responsible for the enforcement of any of those provisions to any extent, it shall be the duty of that authority—

(a) to make adequate arrangements for the enforcement of those provisions to that extent; and

(b) [except where that authority is the Office of Rail Regulation,][331] to perform the duty imposed on the authority by the preceding paragraph and any other functions conferred on the authority by any of the relevant statutory provisions in accordance with such guidance as [the Executive][332] may give to the authority.

(6) Nothing in the provisions of this Act or of any regulations made thereunder charging any person in Scotland with the enforcement of any of the relevant statutory provisions shall be construed as authorising that person to institute proceedings for any offence.

(7) In this Part—

(a) "enforcing authority" means the Executive [or the Office for Nuclear Regulation][333] or any other authority which is by any of the relevant statutory provisions or by regulations under subsection (2) above made responsible for the enforcement of any of those provisions to any extent; and

(b) any reference to an enforcing authority's field of responsibility is a reference to the field over which that authority's responsibility for the enforcement of those provisions extends for the time being;

but where by virtue of [subsection (3) of section 13][334] [of this Act or section 95 of the Energy Act 2013 (power for Office for Nuclear Regulation to arrange for exercise of functions by others)][335] the performance of any function of [. . .][336][. . .] [336] the Executive [or the Office for Nuclear Regulation (as the case may be)][337] is delegated to a government department or person, references to [. . .][336] the Executive (or to an enforcing authority where that authority is the Executive [or the Office for Nuclear Regulation][333]) in any provision of this Part which relates to that function shall, so far as

---

[328] Inserted subject to transitional provisions as specified in SI 2008/960 Sch.2 para.11 by Legislative Reform (Health and Safety Executive) Order 2008/960 art.10(3) (April 1, 2008: insertion has effect subject to transitional provisions as specified in SI 2008/960 Sch.2 para.11).

[329] Words inserted by Energy Act 2013 c. 32 Sch.12(1) para.6(5) (April 1, 2014).

[330] Words repealed by Railways Act 2005 c. 14 Sch.13(1) para.1 (June 8, 2005 as SI 2005/1444).

[331] Words inserted by Railways Act 2005 c. 14 Sch.3 para.10(3) (April 1, 2006).

[332] Words substituted subject to transitional provisions as specified in SI 2008/960 Sch.2 para.11 by Legislative Reform (Health and Safety Executive) Order 2008/960 art.10(4) (April 1, 2008: substitution has effect subject to transitional provisions as specified in SI 2008/960 Sch.2 para.11).

[333] Words inserted by Energy Act 2013 c. 32 Sch.12(1) para.6(6)(b) (April 1, 2014).

[334] Words substituted subject to transitional provisions as specified in SI 2008/960 Sch.2 para.11 by Legislative Reform (Health and Safety Executive) Order 2008/960 art.10(5)(a) (April 1, 2008: substitution has effect subject to transitional provisions as specified in SI 2008/960 Sch.2 para.11).

[335] Words inserted by Energy Act 2013 c. 32 Sch.12(1) para.6(6)(a) (April 1, 2014).

[336] Words repealed subject to transitional provisions as specified in SI 2008/960 Sch.2 para.11 by Legislative Reform (Health and Safety Executive) Order 2008/960 art.10(5)(c) (April 1, 2008: repeal has effect subject to transitional provisions as specified in SI 2008/960 Sch.2 para.11).

[337] Words inserted by Energy Act 2013 c. 32 Sch.12(1) para.6(6)(c) (April 1, 2014).

may be necessary to give effect to any agreement under [that subsection][338] [or arrangements under the provision in question],[339] be construed as references to that department or person; and accordingly any reference to the field of responsibility of an enforcing authority shall be construed as a reference to the field over which that department or person for the time being performs such a function.

Human Rights Act 1998 c. 42

Introduction

The Convention Rights

A1–282   **1.**—(1) In this Act "the Convention rights" means the rights and fundamental freedoms set out in—

(a) Articles 2 to 12 and 14 of the Convention,

(b) Articles 1 to 3 of the First Protocol, and

(c) [Article 1 of the Thirteenth Protocol][340],

as read with Articles 16 to 18 of the Convention.

(2) Those Articles are to have effect for the purposes of this Act subject to any designated derogation or reservation (as to which see sections 14 and 15).

(3) The Articles are set out in Schedule 1.

(4) The [Secretary of State][341] may by order make such amendments to this Act as he considers appropriate to reflect the effect, in relation to the United Kingdom, of a protocol.

(5) In subsection (4) "protocol" means a protocol to the Convention—

(a) which the United Kingdom has ratified; or

(b) which the United Kingdom has signed with a view to ratification.

(6) No amendment may be made by an order under subsection (4) so as to come into force before the protocol concerned is in force in relation to the United Kingdom.

Interpretation of Convention rights

A1–283   **2.**—(1) A court or tribunal determining a question which has arisen in connection with a Convention right must take into account any—

(a) judgment, decision, declaration or advisory opinion of the European Court of Human Rights,

(b) opinion of the Commission given in a report adopted under Article 31 of the Convention,

---

[338] Words substituted subject to transitional provisions as specified in SI 2008/960 Sch.2 para.11 by Legislative Reform (Health and Safety Executive) Order 2008/960 art.10(5)(b) (April 1, 2008: substitution has effect subject to transitional provisions as specified in SI 2008/960 Sch.2 para.11).

[339] Words substituted by Energy Act 2013 c. 32 Sch.12(1) para.6(6)(d) (April 1, 2014).

[340] Words substituted by Human Rights Act 1998 (Amendment) Order 2004/1574 art.2(1) (June 22, 2004).

[341] Words substituted by Secretary of State for Constitutional Affairs Order 2003/1887 Sch.2 para.10(1) (August 19, 2003).

(c) decision of the Commission in connection with Article 26 or 27(2) of the Convention, or

(d) decision of the Committee of Ministers taken under Article 46 of the Convention,

whenever made or given, so far as, in the opinion of the court or tribunal, it is relevant to the proceedings in which that question has arisen.

(2) Evidence of any judgment, decision, declaration or opinion of which account may have to be taken under this section is to be given in proceedings before any court or tribunal in such manner as may be provided by rules.

(3) In this section "rules" means rules of court or, in the case of proceedings before a tribunal, rules made for the purposes of this section—

(a) by [the Lord Chancellor or]³⁴² [. . .]³⁴³ the Secretary of State, in relation to any proceedings outside Scotland;

(b) by the Secretary of State, in relation to proceedings in Scotland; or

(c) by a Northern Ireland department, in relation to proceedings before a tribunal in Northern Ireland—

(i) which deals with transferred matters; and

(ii) for which no rules made under paragraph (a) are in force.

Legislation

Interpretation of legislation

3.—(1) So far as it is possible to do so, primary legislation and subordinate legislation must be read and given effect in a way which is compatible with the Convention rights.   **A1-284**

(2) This section—

(a) applies to primary legislation and subordinate legislation whenever enacted;

(b) does not affect the validity, continuing operation or enforcement of any incompatible primary legislation; and

(c) does not affect the validity, continuing operation or enforcement of any incompatible subordinate legislation if (disregarding any possibility of revocation) primary legislation prevents removal of the incompatibility.

Declaration of incompatibility

4.—(1) Subsection (2) applies in any proceedings in which a court determines whether   **A1-285**
a provision of primary legislation is compatible with a Convention right.

(2) If the court is satisfied that the provision is incompatible with a Convention right, it may make a declaration of that incompatibility.

(3) Subsection (4) applies in any proceedings in which a court determines whether a provision of subordinate legislation, made in the exercise of a power conferred by primary legislation, is compatible with a Convention right.

(4) If the court is satisfied—

(a) that the provision is incompatible with a Convention right, and

---

³⁴² Words inserted by Transfer of Functions (Lord Chancellor and Secretary of State) Order 2005/3429 Sch.1 para.3 (January 12, 2006).
³⁴³ Words repealed by Secretary of State for Constitutional Affairs Order 2003/1887 Sch.2 para.10(2) (August 19, 2003).

(b) that (disregarding any possibility of revocation) the primary legislation concerned prevents removal of the incompatibility,

it may make a declaration of that incompatibility.

(5) In this section "court" means—[

(a) the Supreme Court;][344]

(b) the Judicial Committee of the Privy Council;

(c) the [Court Martial Appeal Court][345];

(d) in Scotland, the High Court of Justiciary sitting otherwise than as a trial court or the Court of Session;

(e) in England and Wales or Northern Ireland, the High Court or the Court of Appeal [;][346]

[(f) the Court of Protection, in any matter being dealt with by the President of the Family Division, the [Chancellor of the High Court][347] or a puisne judge of the High Court.][346]

(6) A declaration under this section ("a declaration of incompatibility")—

(a) does not affect the validity, continuing operation or enforcement of the provision in respect of which it is given; and

(b) is not binding on the parties to the proceedings in which it is made.

Right of Crown to intervene

A1–286   **5.**—(1) Where a court is considering whether to make a declaration of incompatibility, the Crown is entitled to notice in accordance with rules of court.

(2) In any case to which subsection (1) applies—

(a) a Minister of the Crown (or a person nominated by him),

(b) a member of the Scottish Executive,

(c) a Northern Ireland Minister,

(d) a Northern Ireland department,

is entitled, on giving notice in accordance with rules of court, to be joined as a party to the proceedings.

(3) Notice under subsection (2) may be given at any time during the proceedings.

(4) A person who has been made a party to criminal proceedings (other than in Scotland) as the result of a notice under subsection (2) may, with leave, appeal to the [Supreme Court][348] against any declaration of incompatibility made in the proceedings.

(5) In subsection (4)—

---

[344] Substituted by Constitutional Reform Act 2005 c. 4 Sch.9(1) para.66(2) (October 1, 2009).

[345] Words substituted by Armed Forces Act 2006 c. 52 Sch.16 para.156 (October 31, 2009).

[346] Added by Mental Capacity Act 2005 c. 9 Sch.6 para.43 (October 1, 2007).

[347] Word substituted by Crime and Courts Act 2013 c. 22 Sch.14(3) para.5(5) (October 1, 2013: substitution has effect as SI 2013/2200 subject to savings and transitional provisions as specified in 2013 c.22 s.15 and Sch.8).

[348] Words substituted by Constitutional Reform Act 2005 c. 4 Sch.9(1) para.66(3) (October 1, 2009).

"criminal proceedings" includes all proceedings before the [Court Martial Appeal Court][349]; and

"leave" means leave granted by the court making the declaration of incompatibility or by the [Supreme Court][1] .

Public authorities

Acts of public authorities

6.—(1) It is unlawful for a public authority to act in a way which is incompatible with   **A1–287**
a Convention right.

(2) Subsection (1) does not apply to an act if—

  (a) as the result of one or more provisions of primary legislation, the authority could not have acted differently; or

  (b) in the case of one or more provisions of, or made under, primary legislation which cannot be read or given effect in a way which is compatible with the Convention rights, the authority was acting so as to give effect to or enforce those provisions.

(3) In this section "public authority" includes—

  (a) a court or tribunal, and

  (b) any person certain of whose functions are functions of a public nature,

but does not include either House of Parliament or a person exercising functions in connection with proceedings in Parliament.

[. . .][350]

(5) In relation to a particular act, a person is not a public authority by virtue only of subsection (3)(b) if the nature of the act is private.

(6) "An act" includes a failure to act but does not include a failure to—

  (a) introduce in, or lay before, Parliament a proposal for legislation; or

  (b) make any primary legislation or remedial order.

Proceedings

7.—(1) A person who claims that a public authority has acted (or proposes to act) in a way   **A1–288**
which is made unlawful by section 6(1) may—

  (a) bring proceedings against the authority under this Act in the appropriate court or tribunal, or

  (b) rely on the Convention right or rights concerned in any legal proceedings,

but only if he is (or would be) a victim of the unlawful act.

(2) In subsection (1)(a) "appropriate court or tribunal" means such court or tribunal as may be determined in accordance with rules; and proceedings against an authority include a counterclaim or similar proceeding.

(3) If the proceedings are brought on an application for judicial review, the applicant is to be taken to have a sufficient interest in relation to the unlawful act only if he is, or would be, a victim of that act.

---

[349] Words substituted by Armed Forces Act 2006 c. 52 Sch.16 para.157 (October 31, 2009).
[340] Repealed by Constitutional Reform Act 2005 c. 4 Sch.18(5) para.1 (October 1, 2009).

(4) If the proceedings are made by way of a petition for judicial review in Scotland, the applicant shall be taken to have title and interest to sue in relation to the unlawful act only if he is, or would be, a victim of that act.

(5) Proceedings under subsection (1)(a) must be brought before the end of—

(a) the period of one year beginning with the date on which the act complained of took place; or

(b) such longer period as the court or tribunal considers equitable having regard to all the circumstances,

but that is subject to any rule imposing a stricter time limit in relation to the procedure in question.

(6) In subsection (1)(b) "legal proceedings" includes—

(a) proceedings brought by or at the instigation of a public authority; and

(b) an appeal against the decision of a court or tribunal.

(7) For the purposes of this section, a person is a victim of an unlawful act only if he would be a victim for the purposes of Article 34 of the Convention if proceedings were brought in the European Court of Human Rights in respect of that act.

(8) Nothing in this Act creates a criminal offence.

(9) In this section "rules" means—

(a) in relation to proceedings before a court or tribunal outside Scotland, rules made by [the Lord Chancellor or]^{351} [. . .]^{352} the Secretary of State for the purposes of this section or rules of court,

(b) in relation to proceedings before a court or tribunal in Scotland, rules made by the Secretary of State for those purposes,

(c) in relation to proceedings before a tribunal in Northern Ireland—

    (i) which deals with transferred matters; and
    (ii) for which no rules made under paragraph (a) are in force,

rules made by a Northern Ireland department for those purposes,

and includes provision made by order under section 1 of the Courts and Legal Services Act 1990.

(10) In making rules, regard must be had to section 9.

(11) The Minister who has power to make rules in relation to a particular tribunal may, to the extent he considers it necessary to ensure that the tribunal can provide an appropriate remedy in relation to an act (or proposed act) of a public authority which is (or would be) unlawful as a result of section 6(1), by order add to—

(a) the relief or remedies which the tribunal may grant; or

(b) the grounds on which it may grant any of them.

(12) An order made under subsection (11) may contain such incidental, supplemental, consequential or transitional provision as the Minister making it considers appropriate.

(13) "The Minister" includes the Northern Ireland department concerned.

---

[351] Words inserted by Transfer of Functions (Lord Chancellor and Secretary of State) Order 2005/3429 Sch.1 para.3 (January 12, 2006).

[352] Words repealed by Secretary of State for Constitutional Affairs Order 2003/1887 Sch.2 para.10(2) (August 19, 2003).

Judicial remedies

8.—(1) In relation to any act (or proposed act) of a public authority which the court finds   **A1-289**
is (or would be) unlawful, it may grant such relief or remedy, or make such order, within its
powers as it considers just and appropriate.

(2) But damages may be awarded only by a court which has power to award damages, or
to order the payment of compensation, in civil proceedings.

(3) No award of damages is to be made unless, taking account of all the circumstances of
the case, including—

(a) any other relief or remedy granted, or order made, in relation to the act in question
(by that or any other court), and

(b) the consequences of any decision (of that or any other court) in respect of that
act,

the court is satisfied that the award is necessary to afford just satisfaction to the person in
whose favour it is made.

(4) In determining—

(a) whether to award damages, or

(b) the amount of an award,

the court must take into account the principles applied by the European Court of Human
Rights in relation to the award of compensation under Article 41 of the Convention.

(5) A public authority against which damages are awarded is to be treated—

(a) in Scotland, for the purposes of section 3 of the Law Reform (Miscellaneous
Provisions) (Scotland) Act 1940 as if the award were made in an action of damages
in which the authority has been found liable in respect of loss or damage to the
person to whom the award is made;

(b) for the purposes of the Civil Liability (Contribution) Act 1978 as liable in respect
of damage suffered by the person to whom the award is made.

(6) In this section—

"court" includes a tribunal;
"damages" means damages for an unlawful act of a public authority; and
"unlawful" means unlawful under section 6(1).

Judicial acts

9.—(1) Proceedings under section 7(1)(a) in respect of a judicial act may be brought   **A1-290**
only—

(a) by exercising a right of appeal;

(b) on an application (in Scotland a petition) for judicial review; or

(c) in such other forum as may be prescribed by rules.

(2) That does not affect any rule of law which prevents a court from being the subject of
judicial review.

(3) In proceedings under this Act in respect of a judicial act done in good faith, damages
may not be awarded otherwise than to compensate a person to the extent required by Article
5(5) of the Convention.

(4) An award of damages permitted by subsection (3) is to be made against the Crown;
but no award may be made unless the appropriate person, if not a party to the proceedings,
is joined.

(5) In this section—

"appropriate person" means the Minister responsible for the court concerned, or a person or government department nominated by him;
"court" includes a tribunal;
"judge" includes a member of a tribunal, a justice of the peace [(or, in Northern Ireland, a lay magistrate)][353] and a clerk or other officer entitled to exercise the jurisdiction of a court;
"judicial act" means a judicial act of a court and includes an act done on the instructions, or on behalf, of a judge; and
"rules" has the same meaning as in section 7(9).

Remedial action

Power to take remedial action

A1–291   **10.**—(1) This section applies if—

(a) a provision of legislation has been declared under section 4 to be incompatible with a Convention right and, if an appeal lies—

(i) all persons who may appeal have stated in writing that they do not intend to do so;
(ii) the time for bringing an appeal has expired and no appeal has been brought within that time; or
(iii) an appeal brought within that time has been determined or abandoned; or

(b) it appears to a Minister of the Crown or Her Majesty in Council that, having regard to a finding of the European Court of Human Rights made after the coming into force of this section in proceedings against the United Kingdom, a provision of legislation is incompatible with an obligation of the United Kingdom arising from the Convention.

(2) If a Minister of the Crown considers that there are compelling reasons for proceeding under this section, he may by order make such amendments to the legislation as he considers necessary to remove the incompatibility.
(3) If, in the case of subordinate legislation, a Minister of the Crown considers—

(a) that it is necessary to amend the primary legislation under which the subordinate legislation in question was made, in order to enable the incompatibility to be removed, and

(b) that there are compelling reasons for proceeding under this section,

he may by order make such amendments to the primary legislation as he considers necessary.
(4) This section also applies where the provision in question is in subordinate legislation and has been quashed, or declared invalid, by reason of incompatibility with a Convention right and the Minister proposes to proceed under paragraph 2(b) of Schedule 2.
(5) If the legislation is an Order in Council, the power conferred by subsection (2) or (3) is exercisable by Her Majesty in Council.
(6) In this section "legislation" does not include a Measure of the Church Assembly or of the General Synod of the Church of England.
(7) Schedule 2 makes further provision about remedial orders.

---

[353] Words in definition s. 9(5) inserted (N.I.)(1.4.2005) by 2002 c. 26, s. 10(6), Sch. 4 para. 39; S.R. 2005/109, art. 2 Sch.

Supplemental

Interpretation, etc.

21.—(1) In this Act—

"amend" includes repeal and apply (with or without modifications);

"the appropriate Minister" means the Minister of the Crown having charge of the appropriate authorised government department (within the meaning of the Crown Proceedings Act 1947);

"the Commission" means the European Commission of Human Rights;

"the Convention" means the Convention for the Protection of Human Rights and Fundamental Freedoms, agreed by the Council of Europe at Rome on 4th November 1950 as it has effect for the time being in relation to the United Kingdom;

"declaration of incompatibility" means a declaration under section 4;

"Minister of the Crown" has the same meaning as in the Ministers of the Crown Act 1975;

"Northern Ireland Minister" includes the First Minister and the deputy First Minister in Northern Ireland;

"primary legislation" means any—

  (a) public general Act;
  (b) local and personal Act;
  (c) private Act;
  (d) Measure of the Church Assembly;
  (e) Measure of the General Synod of the Church of England;
  (f) Order in Council—

   (i) made in exercise of Her Majesty's Royal Prerogative;
   (ii) made under section 38(1)(a) of the Northern Ireland Constitution Act 1973 or the corresponding provision of the Northern Ireland Act 1998; or
   (iii) amending an Act of a kind mentioned in paragraph (a), (b) or (c);

and includes an order or other instrument made under primary legislation (otherwise than by the [Welsh Ministers, the First Minister for Wales, the Counsel General to the Welsh Assembly Government],[354] a member of the Scottish Executive, a Northern Ireland Minister or a Northern Ireland department) to the extent to which it operates to bring one or more provisions of that legislation into force or amends any primary legislation;

"the First Protocol" means the protocol to the Convention agreed at Paris on 20th March 1952;

[. . .][355]

"the Eleventh Protocol" means the protocol to the Convention (restructuring the control machinery established by the Convention) agreed at Strasbourg on 11th May 1994;

---

[354] Words substituted by Government of Wales Act 2006 c. 32 Sch.10 para.56(2) (May 3, 2007 immediately after the ordinary election as specified in 2006 c.32 s.161(1); May 25, 2007 immediately after the end of the initial period for purposes of functions of the Welsh Ministers, the First Minister, the Counsel General and the Assembly Commission and in relation to the Auditor General and the Comptroller and Auditor General as specified in 2006 c.32 s.161(4)-(5)).

[355] Definition repealed by Human Rights Act 1998 (Amendment) Order 2004/1574 art.2(2) (June 22, 2004).

["the Thirteenth Protocol" means the protocol to the Convention (concerning the abolition of the death penalty in all circumstances) agreed at Vilnius on 3rd May 2002;][356]
"remedial order" means an order under section 10;
"subordinate legislation" means any—

    (a) Order in Council other than one—

        (i) made in exercise of Her Majesty's Royal Prerogative;
        (ii) made under section 38(1)(a) of the Northern Ireland Constitution Act 1973 or the corresponding provision of the Northern Ireland Act 1998; or
        (iii) amending an Act of a kind mentioned in the definition of primary legislation;

    (b) Act of the Scottish Parliament;
    [(ba) Measure of the National Assembly for Wales;
    (bb) Act of the National Assembly for Wales;][357]
    (c) Act of the Parliament of Northern Ireland;
    (d) Measure of the Assembly established under section 1 of the Northern Ireland Assembly Act 1973;
    (e) Act of the Northern Ireland Assembly;
    (f) order, rules, regulations, scheme, warrant, byelaw or other instrument made under primary legislation (except to the extent to which it operates to bring one or more provisions of that legislation into force or amends any primary legislation);
    (g) order, rules, regulations, scheme, warrant, byelaw or other instrument made under legislation mentioned in paragraph (b), (c), (d) or (e) or made under an Order in Council applying only to Northern Ireland;
    (h) order, rules, regulations, scheme, warrant, byelaw or other instrument made by a member of the Scottish Executive [, Welsh Ministers, the First Minister for Wales, the Counsel General to the Welsh Assembly Government][358], a Northern Ireland Minister or a Northern Ireland department in exercise of prerogative or other executive functions of Her Majesty which are exercisable by such a person on behalf of Her Majesty;

"transferred matters" has the same meaning as in the Northern Ireland Act 1998; and
"tribunal" means any tribunal in which legal proceedings may be brought.

(2) The references in paragraphs (b) and (c) of section 2(1) to Articles are to Articles of the Convention as they had effect immediately before the coming into force of the Eleventh Protocol.

(3) The reference in paragraph (d) of section 2(1) to Article 46 includes a reference to Articles 32 and 54 of the Convention as they had effect immediately before the coming into force of the Eleventh Protocol.

---

[356] Definition inserted by Human Rights Act 1998 (Amendment) Order 2004/1574 art.2(2) (June 22, 2004).
[357] Added by Government of Wales Act 2006 c. 32 Sch.10 para.56(3) (May 3, 2007 immediately after the ordinary election as specified in 2006 c.32 s.161(1); May 25, 2007 immediately after the end of the initial period for purposes of functions of the Welsh Ministers, the First Minister, the Counsel General and the Assembly Commission and in relation to the Auditor General and the Comptroller and Auditor General as specified in 2006 c.32 s.161(4)-(5)).
[358] Words inserted by Government of Wales Act 2006 c. 32 Sch.10 para.56(4) (May 3, 2007 immediately after the ordinary election as specified in 2006 c.32 s.161(1); May 25, 2007 immediately after the end of the initial period for purposes of functions of the Welsh Ministers, the First Minister, the Counsel General and the Assembly Commission and in relation to the Auditor General and the Comptroller and Auditor General as specified in 2006 c.32 s.161(4)-(5)).

(4) The references in section 2(1) to a report or decision of the Commission or a decision of the Committee of Ministers include references to a report or decision made as provided by paragraphs 3, 4 and 6 of Article 5 of the Eleventh Protocol (transitional provisions). [. . .]³⁵⁹

SCHEDULE 1

THE ARTICLES

PART I

THE CONVENTION RIGHTS AND FREEDOMS

Right to life

Article 2

1. Everyone's right to life shall be protected by law. No one shall be deprived of his life intentionally   **A1–293** save in the execution of a sentence of a court following his conviction of a crime for which this penalty is provided by law.

2. Deprivation of life shall not be regarded as inflicted in contravention of this Article when it results from the use of force which is no more than absolutely necessary:

(a) in defence of any person from unlawful violence;

(b) in order to effect a lawful arrest or to prevent the escape of a person lawfully detained;

(c) in action lawfully taken for the purpose of quelling a riot or insurrection.

Prohibition of torture

Article 3

No one shall be subjected to torture or to inhuman or degrading treatment or punishment.   **A1–294**

Prohibition of slavery and forced labour

Article 4

1. No one shall be held in slavery or servitude.   **A1–295**
2. No one shall be required to perform forced or compulsory labour.
3. For the purpose of this Article the term "forced or compulsory labour" shall not include:

(a) any work required to be done in the ordinary course of detention imposed according to the provisions of Article 5 of this Convention or during conditional release from such detention;

(b) any service of a military character or, in case of conscientious objectors in countries where they are recognised, service exacted instead of compulsory military service;

(c) any service exacted in case of an emergency or calamity threatening the life or well-being of the community;

(d) any work or service which forms part of normal civic obligations.

---

³⁵⁹ Repealed by Armed Forces Act 2006 c. 52 Sch.17 para.1 (October 31, 2009 as SI 2009/1167).

Right to liberty and security

Article 5

A1–296   1. Everyone has the right to liberty and security of person. No one shall be deprived of his liberty save in the following cases and in accordance with a procedure prescribed by law:

(a) the lawful detention of a person after conviction by a competent court;

(b) the lawful arrest or detention of a person for non-compliance with the lawful order of a court or in order to secure the fulfilment of any obligation prescribed by law;

(c) the lawful arrest or detention of a person effected for the purpose of bringing him before the competent legal authority on reasonable suspicion of having committed an offence or when it is reasonably considered necessary to prevent his committing an offence or fleeing after having done so;

(d) the detention of a minor by lawful order for the purpose of educational supervision or his lawful detention for the purpose of bringing him before the competent legal authority;

(e) the lawful detention of persons for the prevention of the spreading of infectious diseases, of persons of unsound mind, alcoholics or drug addicts or vagrants;

(f) the lawful arrest or detention of a person to prevent his effecting an unauthorised entry into the country or of a person against whom action is being taken with a view to deportation or extradition.

2. Everyone who is arrested shall be informed promptly, in a language which he understands, of the reasons for his arrest and of any charge against him.

3. Everyone arrested or detained in accordance with the provisions of paragraph 1(c) of this Article shall be brought promptly before a judge or other officer authorised by law to exercise judicial power and shall be entitled to trial within a reasonable time or to release pending trial. Release may be conditioned by guarantees to appear for trial.

4. Everyone who is deprived of his liberty by arrest or detention shall be entitled to take proceedings by which the lawfulness of his detention shall be decided speedily by a court and his release ordered if the detention is not lawful.

5. Everyone who has been the victim of arrest or detention in contravention of the provisions of this Article shall have an enforceable right to compensation.

Right to a fair trial

Article 6

A1–297   1. In the determination of his civil rights and obligations or of any criminal charge against him, everyone is entitled to a fair and public hearing within a reasonable time by an independent and impartial tribunal established by law. Judgment shall be pronounced publicly but the press and public may be excluded from all or part of the trial in the interest of morals, public order or national security in a democratic society, where the interests of juveniles or the protection of the private life of the parties so require, or to the extent strictly necessary in the opinion of the court in special circumstances where publicity would prejudice the interests of justice.

2. Everyone charged with a criminal offence shall be presumed innocent until proved guilty according to law.

3. Everyone charged with a criminal offence has the following minimum rights:

(a) to be informed promptly, in a language which he understands and in detail, of the nature and cause of the accusation against him;

(b) to have adequate time and facilities for the preparation of his defence;

(c) to defend himself in person or through legal assistance of his own choosing or, if he has not sufficient means to pay for legal assistance, to be given it free when the interests of justice so require;

(d) to examine or have examined witnesses against him and to obtain the attendance and examination of witnesses on his behalf under the same conditions as witnesses against him;

(e) to have the free assistance of an interpreter if he cannot understand or speak the language used in court.

No punishment without law

Article 7

1. No one shall be held guilty of any criminal offence on account of any act or omission which did **A1–298** not constitute a criminal offence under national or international law at the time when it was committed. Nor shall a heavier penalty be imposed than the one that was applicable at the time the criminal offence was committed.

2. This Article shall not prejudice the trial and punishment of any person for any act or omission which, at the time when it was committed, was criminal according to the general principles of law recognised by civilised nations.

Right to respect for private and family life

Article 8

1. Everyone has the right to respect for his private and family life, his home and his correspon- **A1–299** dence.

2. There shall be no interference by a public authority with the exercise of this right except such as is in accordance with the law and is necessary in a democratic society in the interests of national security, public safety or the economic well-being of the country, for the prevention of disorder or crime, for the protection of health or morals, or for the protection of the rights and freedoms of others.

Freedom of thought, conscience and religion

Article 9

1. Everyone has the right to freedom of thought, conscience and religion; this right includes freedom **A1–300** to change his religion or belief and freedom, either alone or in community with others and in public or private, to manifest his religion or belief, in worship, teaching, practice and observance.

2. Freedom to manifest one's religion or beliefs shall be subject only to such limitations as are prescribed by law and are necessary in a democratic society in the interests of public safety, for the protection of public order, health or morals, or for the protection of the rights and freedoms of others.

Freedom of expression

Article 10

1. Everyone has the right to freedom of expression. This right shall include freedom to hold opinions **A1–301** and to receive and impart information and ideas without interference by public authority and regardless of frontiers. This Article shall not prevent States from requiring the licensing of broadcasting, television or cinema enterprises.

2. The exercise of these freedoms, since it carries with it duties and responsibilities, may be subject to such formalities, conditions, restrictions or penalties as are prescribed by law and are necessary in a democratic society, in the interests of national security, territorial integrity or public safety, for the prevention of disorder or crime, for the protection of health or morals, for the protection of the reputation or rights of others, for preventing the disclosure of information received in confidence, or for maintaining the authority and impartiality of the judiciary.

Freedom of assembly and association

Article 11

1. Everyone has the right to freedom of peaceful assembly and to freedom of association with others, **A1–302** including the right to form and to join trade unions for the protection of his interests.

2. No restrictions shall be placed on the exercise of these rights other than such as are prescribed by law and are necessary in a democratic society in the interests of national security or public safety, for the prevention of disorder or crime, for the protection of health or morals or for the protection of the rights and freedoms of others. This Article shall not prevent the imposition of lawful restrictions on the

exercise of these rights by members of the armed forces, of the police or of the administration of the State.

Right to marry

Article 12

A1–303   Men and women of marriageable age have the right to marry and to found a family, according to the national laws governing the exercise of this right.

Prohibition of discrimination

Article 14

A1–304   The enjoyment of the rights and freedoms set forth in this Convention shall be secured without discrimination on any ground such as sex, race, colour, language, religion, political or other opinion, national or social origin, association with a national minority, property, birth or other status.

Restrictions on political activity of aliens

Article 16

A1–305   Nothing in Articles 10, 11 and 14 shall be regarded as preventing the High Contracting Parties from imposing restrictions on the political activity of aliens.

Prohibition of abuse of rights

Article 17

A1–306   Nothing in this Convention may be interpreted as implying for any State, group or person any right to engage in any activity or perform any act aimed at the destruction of any of the rights and freedoms set forth herein or at their limitation to a greater extent than is provided for in the Convention.

Limitation on use of restrictions on rights

Article 18

A1–307   The restrictions permitted under this Convention to the said rights and freedoms shall not be applied for any purpose other than those for which they have been prescribed.

PART II

THE FIRST PROTOCOL

Protection of property

Article 1

A1–308   Every natural or legal person is entitled to the peaceful enjoyment of his possessions. No one shall be deprived of his possessions except in the public interest and subject to the conditions provided for by law and by the general principles of international law.

    The preceding provisions shall not, however, in any way impair the right of a State to enforce such laws as it deems necessary to control the use of property in accordance with the general interest or to secure the payment of taxes or other contributions or penalties.

Right to education

Article 2

A1–309   No person shall be denied the right to education. In the exercise of any functions which it assumes in relation to education and to teaching, the State shall respect the right of parents to ensure such education and teaching in conformity with their own religious and philosophical convictions.

Right to free elections

Article 3

The High Contracting Parties undertake to hold free elections at reasonable intervals by secret ballot,   **A1–310**
under conditions which will ensure the free expression of the opinion of the people in the choice of
the legislature.

PART III

ARTICLE 1 OF THE THIRTEENTH PROTOCOL

[ABOLITION OF THE DEATH PENALTY

The death penalty shall be abolished. No one shall be condemned to such penalty or exe-   **A1–311**
cuted.]³⁶⁰

Human Tissue Act 2004 c. 30

PART 1

REMOVAL, STORAGE AND USE OF HUMAN ORGANS AND OTHER TISSUE FOR
SCHEDULED PURPOSES

Authorisation of activities for scheduled purposes

1.—(1) The following activities shall be lawful if done with appropriate consent—   **A1–312**

  (a) the storage of the body of a deceased person for use for a purpose specified in
     Schedule 1, other than anatomical examination;

  (b) the use of the body of a deceased person for a purpose so specified, other than
     anatomical examination;

  (c) the removal from the body of a deceased person, for use for a purpose specified in
     Schedule 1, of any relevant material of which the body consists or which it con-
     tains;

  (d) the storage for use for a purpose specified in Part 1 of Schedule 1 of any relevant
     material which has come from a human body;

  (e) the storage for use for a purpose specified in Part 2 of Schedule 1 of any relevant
     material which has come from the body of a deceased person;

  (f) the use for a purpose specified in Part 1 of Schedule 1 of any relevant material which
     has come from a human body;

  (g) the use for a purpose specified in Part 2 of Schedule 1 of any relevant material which
     has come from the body of a deceased person.

(2) The storage of the body of a deceased person for use for the purpose of anatomical
examination shall be lawful if done—

  (a) with appropriate consent, and

  (b) after the signing of a certificate—

---

³⁶⁰ Substituted by Human Rights Act 1998 (Amendment) Order 2004/1574 art.2(3) (June 22,
2004).

> > (i) under section 22(1) of the Births and Deaths Registration Act 1953 (c. 20), or
> >
> > (ii) under Article 25(2) of the Births and Deaths Registration (Northern Ireland) Order 1976 (SI 1976/1041 (N.I. 14)),
>
> of the cause of death of the person.

(3) The use of the body of a deceased person for the purpose of anatomical examination shall be lawful if done—

> (a) with appropriate consent, and
>
> (b) after the death of the person has been registered—
>
> > (i) under section 15 of the Births and Deaths Registration Act 1953, or
> >
> > (ii) under Article 21 of the Births and Deaths Registration (Northern Ireland) Order 1976.

(4) Subsections (1) to (3) do not apply to an activity of a kind mentioned there if it is done in relation to—

> (a) a body to which subsection (5) applies, or
>
> (b) relevant material to which subsection (6) applies.

(5) This subsection applies to a body if—

> (a) it has been imported, or
>
> (b) it is the body of a person who died before the day on which this section comes into force and at least one hundred years have elapsed since the date of the person's death.

(6) This subsection applies to relevant material if—

> (a) it has been imported,
>
> (b) it has come from a body which has been imported, or
>
> (c) it is material which has come from the body of a person who died before the day on which this section comes into force and at least one hundred years have elapsed since the date of the person's death.

(7) Subsection (1)(d) does not apply to the storage of relevant material for use for the purpose of research in connection with disorders, or the functioning, of the human body if—

> (a) the material has come from the body of a living person, and
>
> (b) the research falls within subsection (9).

(8) Subsection (1)(f) does not apply to the use of relevant material for the purpose of research in connection with disorders, or the functioning, of the human body if—

> (a) the material has come from the body of a living person, and
>
> (b) the research falls within subsection (9).

(9) Research falls within this subsection if—

> (a) it is ethically approved in accordance with regulations made by the Secretary of State, and

(b) it is to be, or is, carried out in circumstances such that the person carrying it out is not in possession, and not likely to come into possession, of information from which the person from whose body the material has come can be identified.

[(9A) Subsection (1)(f) does not apply to the use of relevant material for the purpose of research where the use of the material requires consent under paragraph 6(1) or 12(1) of Schedule 3 to the Human Fertilisation and Embryology Act 1990 (use of human cells to create an embryo or a human admixed embryo) or would require such consent but for paragraphs 16 and 20 of that Schedule.][361]

(10) The following activities shall be lawful—

(a) the storage for use for a purpose specified in Part 2 of Schedule 1 of any relevant material which has come from the body of a living person;

(b) the use for such a purpose of any relevant material which has come from the body of a living person;

(c) an activity in relation to which subsection (4), (7) or (8) has effect.

[(10A) In the case of an activity in relation to which subsection (8) has effect, subsection (10)(c) is to be read subject to any requirements imposed by Schedule 3 to the Human Fertilisation and Embryology Act 1990 in relation to the activity.][362]

(11) The Secretary of State may by order—

(a) vary or omit any of the purposes specified in Part 1 or 2 of Schedule 1, or

(b) add to the purposes specified in Part 1 or 2 of that Schedule.

(12) Nothing in this section applies to—

(a) the use of relevant material in connection with a device to which Directive 98/79/EC of the European Parliament and of the Council on in vitro diagnostic medical devices applies, where the use falls within the Directive, or

(b) the storage of relevant material for use falling within paragraph (a).

(13) In this section, the references to a body or material which has been imported do not include a body or material which has been imported after having been exported with a view to its subsequently being re-imported.

"Appropriate consent" : children

2.—(1) This section makes provision for the interpretation of "appropriate consent" in **A1–313** section 1in relation to an activity involving the body, or material from the body, of a person who is a child or has died a child ("the child concerned").

(2) Subject to subsection (3), where the child concerned is alive, "appropriate consent" means his consent.

(3) Where—

(a) the child concerned is alive,

(b) neither a decision of his to consent to the activity, nor a decision of his not to consent to it, is in force, and

---

[361] Added by Human Fertilisation and Embryology Act 2008 c. 22 Sch.7 para.22(a) (October 1, 2009).

[362] Added by Human Fertilisation and Embryology Act 2008 c. 22 Sch.7 para.22(b) (October 1, 2009).

(c) either he is not competent to deal with the issue of consent in relation to the activity or, though he is competent to deal with that issue, he fails to do so,

"appropriate consent" means the consent of a person who has parental responsibility for him.

(4) Where the child concerned has died and the activity is one to which subsection (5) applies, "appropriate consent" means his consent in writing.

(5) This subsection applies to an activity involving storage for use, or use, for the purpose of—

(a) public display, or

(b) where the subject-matter of the activity is not excepted material, anatomical examination.

(6) Consent in writing for the purposes of subsection (4) is only valid if—

(a) it is signed by the child concerned in the presence of at least one witness who attests the signature, or

(b) it is signed at the direction of the child concerned, in his presence and in the presence of at least one witness who attests the signature.

(7) Where the child concerned has died and the activity is not one to which subsection (5) applies, "appropriate consent" means—

(a) if a decision of his to consent to the activity, or a decision of his not to consent to it, was in force immediately before he died, his consent;

(b) if paragraph (a) does not apply—

    (i) the consent of a person who had parental responsibility for him immediately before he died, or

    (ii) where no person had parental responsibility for him immediately before he died, the consent of a person who stood in a qualifying relationship to him at that time.

"Appropriate consent" : adults

A1–314   3.—(1) This section makes provision for the interpretation of "appropriate consent" in section 1in relation to an activity involving the body, or material from the body, of a person who is an adult or has died an adult ("the person concerned").

(2) Where the person concerned is alive, "appropriate consent" means his consent.

(3) Where the person concerned has died and the activity is one to which subsection (4) applies, "appropriate consent" means his consent in writing.

(4) This subsection applies to an activity involving storage for use, or use, for the purpose of—

(a) public display, or

(b) where the subject-matter of the activity is not excepted material, anatomical examination.

(5) Consent in writing for the purposes of subsection (3) is only valid if—

(a) it is signed by the person concerned in the presence of at least one witness who attests the signature,

(b) it is signed at the direction of the person concerned, in his presence and in the presence of at least one witness who attests the signature, or

(c) it is contained in a will of the person concerned made in accordance with the requirements of—

    (i) section 9 of the Wills Act 1837 (c. 26), or

    (ii) Article 5 of the Wills and Administration Proceedings (Northern Ireland) Order 1994 (SI 1994/1899 (N.I. 13)).

(6) Where the person concerned has died and the activity is not one to which subsection (4) applies, "appropriate consent" means—

    (a) if a decision of his to consent to the activity, or a decision of his not to consent to it, was in force immediately before he died, his consent;

    (b) if—

        (i) paragraph (a) does not apply, and

        (ii) he has appointed a person or persons under section 4 to deal after his death with the issue of consent in relation to the activity,

    consent given under the appointment;

    (c) if neither paragraph (a) nor paragraph (b) applies, the consent of a person who stood in a qualifying relationship to him immediately before he died.

(7) Where the person concerned has appointed a person or persons under section 4 to deal after his death with the issue of consent in relation to the activity, the appointment shall be disregarded for the purposes of subsection (6) if no one is able to give consent under it.

(8) If it is not reasonably practicable to communicate with a person appointed under section 4 within the time available if consent in relation to the activity is to be acted on, he shall be treated for the purposes of subsection (7) as not able to give consent under the appointment in relation to it.

Nominated representatives

4—(1) An adult may appoint one or more persons to represent him after his death in **A1–315** relation to consent for the purposes of section 1.

(2) An appointment under this section may be general or limited to consent in relation to such one or more activities as may be specified in the appointment.

(3) An appointment under this section may be made orally or in writing.

(4) An oral appointment under this section is only valid if made in the presence of at least two witnesses present at the same time.

(5) A written appointment under this section is only valid if—

    (a) it is signed by the person making it in the presence of at least one witness who attests the signature,

    (b) it is signed at the direction of the person making it, in his presence and in the presence of at least one witness who attests the signature, or

    (c) it is contained in a will of the person making it, being a will which is made in accordance with the requirements of—

        (i) section 9 of the Wills Act 1837 (c. 26), or

        (ii) Article 5 of the Wills and Administration Proceedings (Northern Ireland) Order 1994 (SI 1994/1899 (N.I. 13)).

(6) Where a person appoints two or more persons under this section in relation to the same activity, they shall be regarded as appointed to act jointly and severally unless the appointment provides that they are appointed to act jointly.

(7) An appointment under this section may be revoked at any time.

(8) Subsections (3) to (5) apply to the revocation of an appointment under this section as they apply to the making of such an appointment.

(9) A person appointed under this section may at any time renounce his appointment.

(10) A person may not act under an appointment under this section if—

(a) he is not an adult, or

(b) he is of a description prescribed for the purposes of this provision by regulations made by the Secretary of State.

Prohibition of activities without consent etc.

A1–316   **5.**—(1) A person commits an offence if, without appropriate consent, he does an activity to which subsection (1), (2) or (3) of section 1 applies, unless he reasonably believes—

(a) that he does the activity with appropriate consent, or

(b) that what he does is not an activity to which the subsection applies.

(2) A person commits an offence if—

(a) he falsely represents to a person whom he knows or believes is going to, or may, do an activity to which subsection (1), (2) or (3) of section 1 applies—

(i) that there is appropriate consent to the doing of the activity, or
(ii) that the activity is not one to which the subsection applies, and

(b) he knows that the representation is false or does not believe it to be true.

(3) Subject to subsection (4), a person commits an offence if, when he does an activity to which section 1(2) applies, neither of the following has been signed in relation to the cause of death of the person concerned—

(a) a certificate under section 22(1) of the Births and Deaths Registration Act 1953 (c. 20), and

(b) a certificate under Article 25(2) of the Births and Deaths Registration (Northern Ireland) Order 1976 (SI 1976/1041 (N.I. 14)).

(4) Subsection (3) does not apply—

(a) where the person reasonably believes—

(i) that a certificate under either of those provisions has been signed in relation to the cause of death of the person concerned, or
(ii) that what he does is not an activity to which section 1(2) applies, or

(b) where the person comes into lawful possession of the body immediately after death and stores it prior to its removal to a place where anatomical examination is to take place.

(5) Subject to subsection (6), a person commits an offence if, when he does an activity to which section 1(3) applies, the death of the person concerned has not been registered under either of the following provisions—

(a) section 15 of the Births and Deaths Registration Act 1953, and

(b) Article 21 of the Births and Deaths Registration (Northern Ireland) Order 1976.

(6) Subsection (5) does not apply where the person reasonably believes—

(a) that the death of the person concerned has been registered under either of those provisions, or

(b) that what he does is not an activity to which section 1(3) applies.

(7) A person guilty of an offence under this section shall be liable—

(a) on summary conviction to a fine not exceeding the statutory maximum;

(b) on conviction on indictment—

    (i) to imprisonment for a term not exceeding 3 years, or
    (ii) to a fine, or
    (iii) to both.

(8) In this section, "appropriate consent" has the same meaning as in section 1.

Activities involving material from adults who lack capacity to consent

6. Where—   **A1-317**

(a) an activity of a kind mentioned in section 1(1)(d) or (f) involves material from the body of a person who—

    (i) is an adult, and
    (ii) lacks capacity to consent to the activity, and

(b) neither a decision of his to consent to the activity, nor a decision of his not to consent to it, is in force,

there shall for the purposes of this Part be deemed to be consent of his to the activity if it is done in circumstances of a kind specified by regulations made by the Secretary of State.

Powers to dispense with need for consent

7.—(1) If the Authority is satisfied—   **A1-318**

(a) that relevant material has come from the body of a living person,

(b) that it is not reasonably possible to trace the person from whose body the material has come ("the donor"),

(c) that it is desirable in the interests of another person (including a future person) that the material be used for the purpose of obtaining scientific or medical information about the donor, and

(d) that there is no reason to believe—

    (i) that the donor has died,
    (ii) that a decision of the donor to refuse to consent to the use of the material for that purpose is in force, or
    (iii) that the donor lacks capacity to consent to the use of the material for that purpose,

it may direct that subsection (3) apply to the material for the benefit of the other person.
(2) If the Authority is satisfied—

(a) that relevant material has come from the body of a living person,

(b) that it is desirable in the interests of another person (including a future person) that the material be used for the purpose of obtaining scientific or medical information about the person from whose body the material has come ("the donor"),

(c) that reasonable efforts have been made to get the donor to decide whether to consent to the use of the material for that purpose,

    (d) that there is no reason to believe—

        (i) that the donor has died,

        (ii) that a decision of the donor to refuse to consent to the use of the material for that purpose is in force, or

        (iii) that the donor lacks capacity to consent to the use of the material for that purpose, and

    (e) that the donor has been given notice of the application for the exercise of the power conferred by this subsection,

it may direct that subsection (3) apply to the material for the benefit of the other person.

(3) Where material is the subject of a direction under subsection (1) or (2), there shall for the purposes of this Part be deemed to be consent of the donor to the use of the material for the purpose of obtaining scientific or medical information about him which may be relevant to the person for whose benefit the direction is given.

(4) The Secretary of State may by regulations enable the High Court, in such circumstances as the regulations may provide, to make an order deeming there for the purposes of this Part to be appropriate consent to an activity consisting of—

    (a) the storage of the body of a deceased person for use for the purpose of research in connection with disorders, or the functioning, of the human body,

    (b) the use of the body of a deceased person for that purpose,

    (c) the removal from the body of a deceased person, for use for that purpose, of any relevant material of which the body consists or which it contains,

    (d) the storage for use for that purpose of any relevant material which has come from a human body, or

    (e) the use for that purpose of any relevant material which has come from a human body.

Restriction of activities in relation to donated material

A1–319   8.—(1) Subject to subsection (2), a person commits an offence if he—

    (a) uses donated material for a purpose which is not a qualifying purpose, or

    (b) stores donated material for use for a purpose which is not a qualifying purpose.

(2) Subsection (1) does not apply where the person reasonably believes that what he uses, or stores, is not donated material.

(3) A person guilty of an offence under this section shall be liable—

    (a) on summary conviction to a fine not exceeding the statutory maximum;

    (b) on conviction on indictment—

        (i) to imprisonment for a term not exceeding 3 years, or

        (ii) to a fine, or

        (iii) to both.

(4) In subsection (1), references to a qualifying purpose are to—

    (a) a purpose specified in Schedule 1,

    (b) the purpose of medical diagnosis or treatment,

    (c) the purpose of decent disposal, or

    (d) a purpose specified in regulations made by the Secretary of State.

(5) In this section, references to donated material are to—

   (a) the body of a deceased person, or

   (b) relevant material which has come from a human body,

which is, or has been, the subject of donation.

(6) For the purposes of subsection (5), a body, or material, is the subject of donation if authority under section 1(1) to (3) exists in relation to it.

Existing holdings

9.—(1) In its application to the following activities, section 1(1) shall have effect with the omission of the words "if done with appropriate consent"—   **A1–320**

   (a) the storage of an existing holding for use for a purpose specified in Schedule 1;

   (b) the use of an existing holding for a purpose so specified.

(2) Subsection (1) does not apply where the existing holding is a body, or separated part of a body, in relation to which section 10(3) or (5) has effect.

(3) Section 5(1) and (2) shall have effect as if the activities mentioned in subsection (1) were not activities to which section 1(1) applies.

(4) In this section, "existing holding" means—

   (a) the body of a deceased person, or

   (b) relevant material which has come from a human body,

held, immediately before the day on which section 1(1) comes into force, for use for a purpose specified in Schedule 1.

Existing anatomical specimens

10.—(1) This section applies where a person dies during the three years immediately preceding the coming into force of section 1.   **A1–321**

(2) Subsection (3) applies where—

   (a) before section 1 comes into force, authority is given under section 4(2) or (3) of the Anatomy Act 1984 (c. 14) for the person's body to be used for anatomical examination, and

   (b) section 1 comes into force before anatomical examination of the person's body is concluded.

(3) During so much of the relevant period as falls after section 1 comes into force, that authority shall be treated for the purposes of section 1 as appropriate consent in relation to—

   (a) the storage of the person's body, or separated parts of his body, for use for the purpose of anatomical examination, and

   (b) the use of his body, or separated parts of his body, for that purpose.

(4) Subsection (5) applies where—

   (a) before section 1 comes into force, authority is given under section 6(2) or (3) of the Anatomy Act 1984 for possession of parts (or any specified parts) of the person's body to be held after anatomical examination of his body is concluded, and

(b) anatomical examination of the person's body is concluded—

    (i) after section 1 comes into force, but

    (ii) before the end of the period of three years beginning with the date of the person's death.

(5) With effect from the conclusion of the anatomical examination of the person's body, that authority shall be treated for the purposes of section 1 as appropriate consent in relation to—

(a) the storage for use for a qualifying purpose of a part of the person's body which—

    (i) is a part to which that authority relates, and

    (ii) is such that the person cannot be recognised simply by examination of the part, and

(b) the use for a qualifying purpose of such a part of the person's body.

(6) Where for the purposes of section 1 there would not be appropriate consent in relation to an activity but for authority given under the Anatomy Act 1984 (c. 14) being treated for those purposes as appropriate consent in relation to the activity, section 1(1) to (3) do not authorise the doing of the activity otherwise than in accordance with that authority.

(7) In subsection (3), "the relevant period", in relation to a person, means whichever is the shorter of—

(a) the period of three years beginning with the date of the person's death, and

(b) the period beginning with that date and ending when anatomical examination of the person's body is concluded.

(8) In subsection (5), "qualifying purpose" means a purpose specified in paragraph 6 or 9 of Schedule 1.

(9) The Secretary of State may by order amend subsection (8).

Coroners

A1–322 **11.**—(1) Nothing in this Part applies to anything done for purposes of functions of a coroner or under the authority of a coroner.

(2) Where a person knows, or has reason to believe, that—

(a) the body of a deceased person, or

(b) relevant material which has come from the body of a deceased person,

is, or may be, required for purposes of functions of a coroner, he shall not act on authority under section 1 in relation to the body, or material, except with the consent of the coroner.

Interpretation of Part 1

A1–323 **12.** In this Part, "excepted material" means material which has—

(a) come from the body of a living person, or

(b) come from the body of a deceased person otherwise than in the course of use of the body for the purpose of anatomical examination.

The Human Tissue Authority

13.—(1) There shall be a body corporate to be known as the Human Tissue Authority   **A1–324**
(referred to in this Act as "the Authority").

(2) Schedule 2 (which makes further provision about the Authority) has effect.

Remit

14.—(1) The following are the activities within the remit of the Authority—   **A1–325**

   (a) the removal from a human body, for use for a scheduled purpose, of any relevant material of which the body consists or which it contains;

   (b) the use, for a scheduled purpose, of—

      (i) the body of a deceased person, or

      (ii) relevant material which has come from a human body;

   (c) the storage of an anatomical specimen or former anatomical specimen;

   (d) the storage (in any case not falling within paragraph (c)) of—

      (i) the body of a deceased person, or

      (ii) relevant material which has come from a human body,

   for use for a scheduled purpose;

   (e) the import or export of—

      (i) the body of a deceased person, or

      (ii) relevant material which has come from a human body,

   for use for a scheduled purpose;

   (f) the disposal of the body of a deceased person which has been—

      (i) imported for use,

      (ii) stored for use, or

      (iii) used,

   for a scheduled purpose;

   (g) the disposal of relevant material which—

      (i) has been removed from a person's body for the purposes of his medical treatment,

      (ii) has been removed from the body of a deceased person for the purposes of an anatomical, or post-mortem, examination,

      (iii) has been removed from a human body (otherwise than as mentioned in sub-paragraph (ii)) for use for a scheduled purpose,

      (iv) has come from a human body and been imported for use for a scheduled purpose, or

      (v) has come from the body of a deceased person which has been imported for use for a scheduled purpose.

   [(h) the procurement, processing, preservation, testing, storage, distribution, import or export of tissue or cells, in so far as those activities are activities to which regulation

7(1) or (2) of the 2007 Regulations applies and are not within the remit of the Authority by virtue of paragraphs (a) to (g) [;][363]][364]

[(i) the donation, testing, characterisation, procurement, preservation, transport, transplantation and disposal of human organs, in so far as those activities are activities to which regulation 5(1) of the 2012 Regulations applies and are not within the remit of the Authority by virtue of paragraphs (a) to (h).][2]

(2) Without prejudice to the generality of subsection (1)(a) and (b), the activities within the remit of the Authority include, in particular—

(a) the carrying-out of an anatomical examination, and

(b) the making of a post-mortem examination.

[(2ZA) The activities within the remit of the Authority do not include the use, for a scheduled purpose, of relevant material where the use of the material requires consent under paragraph 6(1) or 12(1) of Schedule 3 to the Human Fertilisation and Embryology Act 1990 (use of human cells to create an embryo or a human admixed embryo) or would require such consent but for paragraphs 16 and 20 of that Schedule.][365]

[(2A) Expressions used in paragraph (h) of subsection (1) and in the 2007 Regulations have the same meaning in that paragraph as in those Regulations; and the reference to activities to which regulation 7(1) or (2) of those Regulations applies is to be read subject to regulation 2(3) of those Regulations.][366]

[(2B) Expressions used in paragraph (i) of subsection (1) and in the 2012 Regulations have the same meaning in that paragraph as in those Regulations.][367]

(3) An activity is excluded from the remit of the Authority if—

(a) it relates to the body of a person who died before the day on which this section comes into force or to material which has come from the body of such a person, and

(b) at least one hundred years have elapsed since the date of the person's death.

(4) The Secretary of State may by order amend this section for the purpose of adding to the activities within the remit of the Authority.

(5) In this section, "relevant material", in relation to use for the scheduled purpose of transplantation, does not include blood or anything derived from blood.

---

[363] Added by Quality and Safety of Organs Intended for Transplantation Regulations 2012/1501 Pt 6 reg.25(2)(a) (July 12, 2012 for purposes specified in SI 2012/1501 reg.1(3); August 27, 2012 otherwise).

[364] Added by Human Tissue (Quality and Safety for Human Application) Regulations 2007/1523 Pt 6 reg.30(2) (May 25, 2007 for the purposes specified in SI 2007/1523 reg.1(3); July 5, 2007 otherwise).

[365] Added by Human Fertilisation and Embryology Act 2008 c. 22 Sch.7 para.23 (October 1, 2009).

[366] Added by Human Tissue (Quality and Safety for Human Application) Regulations 2007/1523 Pt 6 reg.30(3) (May 25, 2007 for the purposes specified in SI 2007/1523 reg.1(3); July 5, 2007 otherwise).

[367] Added by Quality and Safety of Organs Intended for Transplantation Regulations 2012/1501 Pt 6 reg.25(2)(b) (July 12, 2012 for purposes specified in SI 2012/1501 reg.1(3); August 27, 2012 otherwise).

PART 2

REGULATION OF ACTIVITIES INVOLVING HUMAN TISSUE

The Human Tissue Authority

General functions

15. The Authority shall have the following general functions—   **A1–326**

(a) maintaining a statement of the general principles which it considers should be followed—

  (i) in the carrying-on of activities within its remit, and

  (ii) in the carrying-out of its functions in relation to such activities;

(b) providing in relation to activities within its remit such general oversight and guidance as it considers appropriate;

(c) superintending, in relation to activities within its remit, compliance with—

  (i) requirements imposed by or under Part 1 or this Part, and

  (ii) codes of practice under this Act;

(d) providing to the public, and to persons carrying on activities within its remit, such information and advice as it considers appropriate about the nature and purpose of such activities;

(e) monitoring developments relating to activities within its remit and advising the Secretary of State, the National Assembly for Wales and the relevant Northern Ireland department on issues relating to such developments;

(f) advising the Secretary of State, the National Assembly for Wales or the relevant Northern Ireland department on such other issues relating to activities within its remit as he, the Assembly or the department may require.

Licensing

Licence requirement

16.—(1) No person shall do an activity to which this section applies otherwise than under   **A1–327** the authority of a licence granted for the purposes of this section.

(2) This section applies to the following activities—

(a) the carrying-out of an anatomical examination;

(b) the making of a post-mortem examination;

(c) the removal from the body of a deceased person (otherwise than in the course of an activity mentioned in paragraph (a) or (b)) of relevant material of which the body consists or which it contains, for use for a scheduled purpose other than transplantation;

(d) the storage of an anatomical specimen;

(e) the storage (in any case not falling within paragraph (d)) of—

  (i) the body of a deceased person, or

  (ii) relevant material which has come from a human body,

for use for a scheduled purpose;

(f) the use, for the purpose of public display, of—

  (i) the body of a deceased person, or

(ii) relevant material which has come from the body of a deceased person.

[(2A) This section does not apply to the procurement, testing, processing, preservation, storage, distribution, import or export of tissue and cells intended for human application in so far as those activities are activities to which regulation 7(1) or (2) of the 2007 Regulations applies.

(2B) Expressions used in subsection (2A) and in the 2007 Regulations have the same meaning in that subsection as in those Regulations; and the reference to activities to which regulation 7(1) or (2) of those Regulations applies is to be read subject to regulation 2(3) of those Regulations.][368]

(3) The Secretary of State may by regulations specify circumstances in which storage of relevant material by a person who intends to use it for a scheduled purpose is excepted from subsection (2)(e)(ii).

(4) An activity is excluded from subsection (2) if—

(a) it relates to the body of a person who died before the day on which this section comes into force or to material which has come from the body of such a person, and

(b) at least one hundred years have elapsed since the date of the person's death.

(5) The Secretary of State may by regulations amend this section for the purpose of—

(a) adding to the activities to which this section applies,

(b) removing an activity from the activities to which this section applies, or

(c) altering the description of an activity to which this section applies.

(6) Schedule 3 (which makes provision about licences for the purposes of this section) has effect.

(7) In subsection (2)—

(a) references to storage do not include storage which is incidental to transportation, and

(b) "relevant material", in relation to use for the scheduled purpose of transplantation, does not include blood or anything derived from blood.

Persons to whom licence applies

A1–328   17. The authority conferred by a licence extends to—

(a) the designated individual,

(b) any person who is designated as a person to whom the licence applies by a notice given to the Authority by the designated individual, and

(c) any person acting under the direction of—

(i) the designated individual, or
(ii) a person designated as mentioned in paragraph (b).

---

[368] Added by Human Tissue (Quality and Safety for Human Application) Regulations 2007/1523 Pt 6 reg.31(2) (May 25, 2007 for the purposes specified in SI 2007/1523 reg.1(3); July 5, 2007 otherwise).

Duty of the designated individual

18. It shall be the duty of the individual designated in a licence as the person under whose supervision the licensed activity is authorised to be carried on to secure—   **A1–329**

(a) that the other persons to whom the licence applies are suitable persons to participate in the carrying-on of the licensed activity,

(b) that suitable practices are used in the course of carrying on that activity, and

(c) that the conditions of the licence are complied with.

Conduct of licensed activities

23.—(1) Directions may impose requirements in relation to the conduct of the activity which a licence authorises to be carried on.   **A1–330**

(2) Directions under subsection (1) may be given in relation to licences generally, licences of a particular description or a particular licence.

(3) A person shall comply with a requirement imposed by directions under subsection (1) if it is applicable to him.

Changes of licence circumstance

24.—(1) Directions may make provision for the purpose of dealing with a situation arising in consequence of—   **A1–331**

(a) the variation of a licence, or

(b) a licence ceasing to have effect.

(2) Directions under subsection (1)(a) may impose requirements—

(a) on the holder of the licence;

(b) on a person who is the designated individual immediately before, or immediately after, the variation;

(c) on any other person, if he consents.

(3) Directions under subsection (1)(b) may impose requirements—

(a) on the person who is the holder of the licence immediately before the licence ceases to have effect;

(b) on the person who is the designated individual at that time;

(c) on any other person, if he consents.

(4) Directions under subsection (1) may, in particular, require anything kept, or information held, in pursuance of the licence to be transferred in accordance with the directions.

(5) Where a licence has ceased to have effect by reason of the death or dissolution of its holder, anything subsequently done by a person before directions are given under subsection (1) shall, if the licence would have been authority for doing it, be treated as authorised by a licence.

Breach of licence requirement

25.—(1) A person who contravenes section 16(1) commits an offence, unless he reasonably believes—   **A1–332**

(a) that what he does is not an activity to which section 16 applies, or

(b) that he acts under the authority of a licence.

(2) A person guilty of an offence under subsection (1) shall be liable—

(a) on summary conviction to a fine not exceeding the statutory maximum;

(b) on conviction on indictment—

   (i) to imprisonment for a term not exceeding 3 years, or
   (ii) to a fine, or
   (iii) to both.

Possession of anatomical specimens away from licensed premises

A1–333   **30.**—(1) Subject to subsections (2) to (6), a person commits an offence if—

(a) he has possession of an anatomical specimen, and

(b) the specimen is not on premises in respect of which an anatomy licence is in force.

(2) Subsection (1) does not apply where—

(a) the specimen has come from premises in respect of which a storage licence is in force, and

(b) the person—

   (i) is authorised in writing by the designated individual to have possession of the specimen, and
   (ii) has possession of the specimen only for a purpose for which he is so authorised to have possession of it.

(3) Subsection (1) does not apply where—

(a) the specimen is the body of a deceased person which is to be used for the purpose of anatomical examination,

(b) the person who has possession of the body has come into lawful possession of it immediately after the deceased's death, and

(c) he retains possession of the body prior to its removal to premises in respect of which an anatomy licence is in force.

(4) Subsection (1) does not apply where the person has possession of the specimen only for the purpose of transporting it to premises—

(a) in respect of which an anatomy licence is in force, or

(b) where the specimen is to be used for the purpose of education, training or research.

(5) Subsection (1) does not apply where the person has possession of the specimen for purposes of functions of, or under the authority of, a coroner.

(6) Subsection (1) does not apply where the person reasonably believes—

(a) that what he has possession of is not an anatomical specimen,

(b) that the specimen is on premises in respect of which an anatomy licence is in force, or

(c) that any of subsections (2) to (5) applies.

(7) A person guilty of an offence under subsection (1) shall be liable—

(a) on summary conviction to a fine not exceeding the statutory maximum;

(b) on conviction on indictment—

(i) to imprisonment for a term not exceeding 3 years, or
(ii) to a fine, or
(iii) to both.

(8) In this section—
"anatomy licence" means a licence authorising—

(a) the carrying-out of an anatomical examination, or
(b) the storage of anatomical specimens;

"storage licence" means a licence authorising the storage of anatomical specimens.

Anatomy

Possession of former anatomical specimens away from licensed premises

31.—(1) Subject to subsections (2) to (5), a person commits an offence if—   **A1–334**

(a) he has possession of a former anatomical specimen, and

(b) the specimen is not on premises in respect of which a storage licence is in force.

(2) Subsection (1) does not apply where—

(a) the specimen has come from premises in respect of which a storage licence is in force, and

(b) the person—

(i) is authorised in writing by the designated individual to have possession of the specimen, and
(ii) has possession of the specimen only for a purpose for which he is so authorised to have possession of it.

(3) Subsection (1) does not apply where the person has possession of the specimen only for the purpose of transporting it to premises—

(a) in respect of which a storage licence is in force, or

(b) where the specimen is to be used for the purpose of education, training or research.

(4) Subsection (1) does not apply where the person has possession of the specimen—

(a) only for the purpose of its decent disposal, or

(b) for purposes of functions of, or under the authority of, a coroner.

(5) Subsection (1) does not apply where the person reasonably believes—

(a) that what he has possession of is not a former anatomical specimen,

(b) that the specimen is on premises in respect of which a storage licence is in force, or

(c) that any of subsections (2) to (4) applies.

(6) A person guilty of an offence under subsection (1) shall be liable—

(a) on summary conviction to a fine not exceeding the statutory maximum;

(b) on conviction on indictment—

(i) to imprisonment for a term not exceeding 3 years, or
(ii) to a fine, or
(iii) to both.

(7) In this section, "storage licence" means a licence authorising the storage, for use for a scheduled purpose, of relevant material which has come from a human body.

Trafficking

Prohibition of commercial dealings in human material for transplantation

A1–335   32.—(1) A person commits an offence if he—

(a) gives or receives a reward for the supply of, or for an offer to supply, any controlled material;

(b) seeks to find a person willing to supply any controlled material for reward;

(c) offers to supply any controlled material for reward;

(d) initiates or negotiates any arrangement involving the giving of a reward for the supply of, or for an offer to supply, any controlled material;

(e) takes part in the management or control of a body of persons corporate or unincorporate whose activities consist of or include the initiation or negotiation of such arrangements.

(2) Without prejudice to subsection (1)(b) and (c), a person commits an offence if he causes to be published or distributed, or knowingly publishes or distributes, an advertisement—

(a) inviting persons to supply, or offering to supply, any controlled material for reward, or

(b) indicating that the advertiser is willing to initiate or negotiate any such arrangement as is mentioned in subsection (1)(d).

(3) A person who engages in an activity to which subsection (1) or (2) applies does not commit an offence under that subsection if he is designated by the Authority as a person who may lawfully engage in the activity.

[(3A) The Authority may not designate a person under subsection (3) to engage in any activity relating to an organ (within the meaning given by Directive 2010/53/EU of the European Parliament and of the Council on standards of quality and safety of human organs intended for transplantation) for use for the purpose of transplantation.][369]

(4) A person guilty of an offence under subsection (1) shall be liable—

(a) on summary conviction—

---

[369] Added by Quality and Safety of Organs Intended for Transplantation Regulations 2012/1501 Pt 6 reg.25(3) (July 12, 2012 for purposes specified in SI 2012/1501 reg.1(3); August 27, 2012 otherwise).

      (i) to imprisonment for a term not exceeding 12 months, or

     (ii) to a fine not exceeding the statutory maximum, or

    (iii) to both;

  (b) on conviction on indictment—

      (i) to imprisonment for a term not exceeding 3 years, or

     (ii) to a fine, or

    (iii) to both.

(5) A person guilty of an offence under subsection (2) shall be liable on summary conviction—

  (a) to imprisonment for a term not exceeding 51 weeks, or

  (b) to a fine not exceeding level 5 on the standard scale, or

  (c) to both.

(6) For the purposes of subsections (1) and (2), payment in money or money's worth to the holder of a licence shall be treated as not being a reward where—

  (a) it is in consideration for transporting, removing, preparing, preserving or storing controlled material, and

  (b) its receipt by the holder of the licence is not expressly prohibited by the terms of the licence.

(7) References in subsections (1) and (2) to reward, in relation to the supply of any controlled material, do not include payment in money or money's worth for defraying or reimbursing—

  (a) any expenses incurred in, or in connection with, transporting, removing, preparing, preserving or storing the material,

  (b) any liability incurred in respect of—

      (i) expenses incurred by a third party in, or in connection with, any of the activities mentioned in paragraph (a), or

     (ii) a payment in relation to which subsection (6) has effect, or

  (c) any expenses or loss of earnings incurred by the person from whose body the material comes so far as reasonably and directly attributable to his supplying the material from his body.

(8) For the purposes of this section, controlled material is any material which—

  (a) consists of or includes human cells,

  (b) is, or is intended to be removed, from a human body,

  (c) is intended to be used for the purpose of transplantation, and

  (d) is not of a kind excepted under subsection (9).

(9) The following kinds of material are excepted—

  (a) gametes,

  (b) embryos, and

  (c) material which is the subject of property because of an application of human skill.

(10) Where the body of a deceased person is intended to be used to provide material which—

(a) consists of or includes human cells, and

(b) is not of a kind excepted under subsection (9),

for use for the purpose of transplantation, the body shall be treated as controlled material for the purposes of this section.

(11) In this section—

"advertisement" includes any form of advertising whether to the public generally, to any section of the public or individually to selected persons;

"reward" means any description of financial or other material advantage.

Transplants

Restriction on transplants involving a live donor

A1–336   **33.**—(1) Subject to subsections (3) and (5), a person commits an offence if—

(a) he removes any transplantable material from the body of a living person intending that the material be used for the purpose of transplantation, and

(b) when he removes the material, he knows, or might reasonably be expected to know, that the person from whose body he removes the material is alive.

(2) Subject to subsections (3) and (5), a person commits an offence if—

(a) he uses for the purpose of transplantation any transplantable material which has come from the body of a living person, and

(b) when he does so, he knows, or might reasonably be expected to know, that the transplantable material has come from the body of a living person.

(3) The Secretary of State may by regulations provide that subsection (1) or (2) shall not apply in a case where—

(a) the Authority is satisfied—

(i) that no reward has been or is to be given in contravention of section 32, and

(ii) that such other conditions as are specified in the regulations are satisfied, and

(b) such other requirements as are specified in the regulations are complied with.

(4) Regulations under subsection (3) shall include provision for decisions of the Authority in relation to matters which fall to be decided by it under the regulations to be subject, in such circumstances as the regulations may provide, to reconsideration in accordance with such procedure as the regulations may provide.

(5) Where under subsection (3) an exception from subsection (1) or (2) is in force, a person does not commit an offence under that subsection if he reasonably believes that the exception applies.

(6) A person guilty of an offence under this section is liable on summary conviction—

(a) to imprisonment for a term not exceeding 51 weeks, or

(b) to a fine not exceeding level 5 on the standard scale, or

(c) to both.

(7) In this section—

"reward" has the same meaning as in section 32;
"transplantable material" means material of a description specified by regulations made by the Secretary of State.

Information about transplant operations

34.—(1) The Secretary of State may make regulations requiring such persons as may be   **A1–337**
specified in the regulations to supply to such authority as may be so specified such information as may be so specified with respect to transplants that have been or are proposed to be carried out using transplantable material removed from a human body.

(2) Any such authority shall keep a record of information supplied to it in pursuance of regulations under this section.

(3) A person commits an offence if—

(a) he fails without reasonable excuse to comply with regulations under this section, or

(b) in purported compliance with such regulations, he knowingly or recklessly supplies information which is false or misleading in a material respect.

(4) A person guilty of an offence under subsection (3)(a) is liable on summary conviction to a fine not exceeding level 3 on the standard scale.

(5) A person guilty of an offence under subsection (3)(b) is liable on summary conviction to a fine not exceeding level 5 on the standard scale.

(6) In this section, "transplantable material" has the same meaning as in section 33.

Exceptions

Criminal justice purposes

39.—(1) Subject to subsection (2), nothing in section 14(1) or 16(2) applies to anything   **A1–338**
done for purposes related to—

(a) the prevention or detection of crime, or

(b) the conduct of a prosecution.

(2) Subsection (1) does not except from section 14(1) or 16(2) the carrying-out of a post-mortem examination for purposes of functions of a coroner.

(3) The reference in subsection (2) to the carrying-out of a post-mortem examination does not include the removal of relevant material from the body of a deceased person, or from a part of the body of a deceased person, at the first place where the body or part is situated to be attended by a constable.

(4) For the purposes of subsection (1)(a), detecting crime shall be taken to include—

(a) establishing by whom, for what purpose, by what means and generally in what circumstances any crime was committed, and

(b) the apprehension of the person by whom any crime was committed;

and the reference in subsection (1)(a) to the detection of crime includes any detection outside the United Kingdom of any crime or suspected crime.

(5) In subsection (1)(b), the reference to a prosecution includes a prosecution brought in respect of any crime in a country or territory outside the United Kingdom.

(6) In this section, references to crime include a reference to any conduct which—

(a) constitutes one or more criminal offences (whether under the law of a part of the United Kingdom or of a country or territory outside the United Kingdom),

(b) is, or corresponds to, any conduct which, if it all took place in any one part of the United Kingdom, would constitute one or more criminal offences, or

(c) constitutes one or more [service offences within the meaning of the Armed Forces Act 2006][370].

Religious relics

A1–339   **40.**—(1) This section applies—

(a) to the use of—

(i) the body of a deceased person, or
(ii) relevant material which has come from a human body,

for the purpose of public display at a place of public religious worship or at a place associated with such a place, and

(b) to the storage of—

(i) the body of a deceased person, or
(ii) relevant material which has come from a human body,

for use for the purpose mentioned in paragraph (a).

(2) An activity to which this section applies is excluded from sections 14(1) and 16(2) if there is a connection between—

(a) the body or material to which the activity relates, and

(b) the religious worship which takes place at the place of public religious worship concerned.

(3) For the purposes of this section, a place is associated with a place of public religious worship if it is used for purposes associated with the religious worship which takes place there.

Supplementary

Interpretation of Part 2

A1–340   **41.**—(1) In this Part—

["the 2007 Regulations" means the Human Tissue (Quality and Safety for Human Application) Regulations 2007;][371]
["the 2012 Regulations" means the Quality and Safety of Organs Intended for Transplantation Regulations 2012;][372]
"anatomical specimen" means—

(a) the body of a deceased person to be used for the purpose of anatomical examination, or
(b) the body of a deceased person in the course of being used for the purpose of anatomical examination (including separated parts of such a body);

---

[370] Words substituted by Armed Forces Act 2006 c. 52 Sch.16 para.241 (October 31, 2009).
[371] Definition inserted by Human Tissue (Quality and Safety for Human Application) Regulations 2007/1523 Pt 6 reg.32 (May 25, 2007 for the purposes specified in SI 2007/1523 reg.1(3); July 5, 2007 otherwise).
[372] Definition inserted by Quality and Safety of Organs Intended for Transplantation Regulations 2012/1501 Pt 6 reg.25(4) (July 12, 2012 for purposes specified in SI 2012/1501 reg.1(3); August 27, 2012 otherwise).

"appeals committee" has the meaning given by section 20(2);

"designated individual", in relation to a licence, means the individual designated in the licence as the person under whose supervision the licensed activity is authorised to be carried on;

"export" means export from England, Wales or Northern Ireland to a place outside England, Wales and Northern Ireland;

"import" means import into England, Wales or Northern Ireland from a place outside England, Wales and Northern Ireland;

"scheduled purpose" means a purpose specified in Schedule 1.

(2) In this Part, references to the carrying-out of an anatomical examination are to the carrying-out of a macroscopic examination by dissection for anatomical purposes of the body of a deceased person, and, where parts of the body of a deceased person are separated in the course of such an examination, include the carrying-out of a macroscopic examination by dissection of the parts for those purposes.

(3) In this Part, references to a person to whom a licence applies are to a person to whom the authority conferred by the licence extends (as provided by section 17).

PART 3

MISCELLANEOUS AND GENERAL

Miscellaneous

Power of Human Tissue Authority to assist other public authorities

42.—(1) The Authority may if it thinks it appropriate to do so provide assistance to any   **A1–341** other public authority in the United Kingdom for the purpose of the exercise by that authority of its functions.

(2) Assistance provided by the Authority under this section may be provided on such terms, including terms as to payment, as it thinks fit.

Preservation for transplantation

43.—(1) Where part of a body lying in a hospital, nursing home or other institution is   **A1–342** or may be suitable for use for transplantation, it shall be lawful for the person having the control and management of the institution—

(a) to take steps for the purpose of preserving the part for use for transplantation, and

(b) to retain the body for that purpose.

(2) Authority under subsection (1)(a) shall only extend—

(a) to the taking of the minimum steps necessary for the purpose mentioned in that provision, and

(b) to the use of the least invasive procedure.

(3) Authority under subsection (1) ceases to apply once it has been established that consent making removal of the part for transplantation lawful has not been, and will not be, given.

(4) Authority under subsection (1) shall extend to any person authorised to act under the authority by—

(a) the person on whom the authority is conferred by that subsection, or

(b) a person authorised under this subsection to act under the authority.

(5) An activity done with authority under subsection (1) shall be treated—

(a) for the purposes of Part 1, as not being an activity to which section 1(1) applies;

(b) for the purposes of Part 2, as not being an activity to which section 16 applies.

(6) In this section, "body" means the body of a deceased person.

Surplus tissue

A1–343   **44.**—(1) It shall be lawful for material to which subsection (2) or (3) applies to be dealt with as waste.

(2) This subsection applies to any material which consists of or includes human cells and which has come from a person's body in the course of his—

(a) receiving medical treatment,

(b) undergoing diagnostic testing, or

(c) participating in research.

(3) This subsection applies to any relevant material which—

(a) has come from a human body, and

(b) ceases to be used, or stored for use, for a purpose specified in Schedule 1.

(4) This section shall not be read as making unlawful anything which is lawful apart from this section.

Non-consensual analysis of DNA

A1–344   **45.**—(1) A person commits an offence if—

(a) he has any bodily material intending—

(i) that any human DNA in the material be analysed without qualifying consent, and

(ii) that the results of the analysis be used otherwise than for an excepted purpose,

(b) the material is not of a kind excepted under subsection (2), and

(c) he does not reasonably believe the material to be of a kind so excepted.

(2) Bodily material is excepted if—

(a) it is material which has come from the body of a person who died before the day on which this section comes into force and at least one hundred years have elapsed since the date of the person's death,

(b) it is an existing holding and the person who has it is not in possession, and not likely to come into possession, of information from which the individual from whose body the material has come can be identified, or

(c) it is an embryo outside the human body.

(3) A person guilty of an offence under this section—

(a) is liable on summary conviction to a fine not exceeding the statutory maximum;

(b) is liable on conviction on indictment—

    (i) to imprisonment for a term not exceeding 3 years, or

    (ii) to a fine, or

    (iii) to both.

(4) Schedule 4 (which makes provision for the interpretation of "qualifying consent" and "use for an excepted purpose" in subsection (1)(a)) has effect.

(5) In this section (and Schedule 4)—

"bodily material" means material which—

    (a) has come from a human body, and

    (b) consists of or includes human cells;

"existing holding" means bodily material held immediately before the day on which this section comes into force.

General

"Relevant material"

53.—(1) In this Act, "relevant material" means material, other than gametes, which   **A1–345** consists of or includes human cells.

(2) In this Act, references to relevant material from a human body do not include—

    (a) embryos outside the human body, or

    (b) hair and nail from the body of a living person.

General interpretation

54.—(1) In this Act— **A1–346**

"adult" means a person who has attained the age of 18 years;

"anatomical examination" means macroscopic examination by dissection for anatomical purposes;

"anatomical purposes" means purposes of teaching or studying, or researching into, the gross structure of the human body;

"the Authority" has the meaning given by section 13(1);

"child", except in the context of qualifying relationships, means a person who has not attained the age of 18 years;

"licence" means a licence under paragraph 1 of Schedule 3;

"licensed activity", in relation to a licence, means the activity which the licence authorises to be carried on;

"parental responsibility"—

    (a) in relation to England and Wales, has the same meaning as in the Children Act 1989 (c. 41), and

    (b) in relation to Northern Ireland, has the same meaning as in the Children (Northern Ireland) Order 1995 (SI 1995/755 (N.I. 2));

"relevant Northern Ireland department" means the Department of Health, Social Services and Public Safety.

(2) In this Act—

    (a) references to material from the body of a living person are to material from the body of a person alive at the point of separation, and

(b) references to material from the body of a deceased person are to material from the body of a person not alive at the point of separation.

(3) In this Act, references to transplantation are to transplantation to a human body and include transfusion.

(4) In this Act, references to decent disposal include, in relation to disposal of material which has come from a human body, disposal as waste.

(5) In this Act, references to public display, in relation to the body of a deceased person, do not include—

(a) display for the purpose of enabling people to pay their final respects to the deceased, or

(b) display which is incidental to the deceased's funeral.

[(6) In this Act "embryo" and "gametes" have the same meaning as they have by virtue of section 1(1), (4) and (6) of the Human Fertilisation and Embryology Act 1990 in the other provisions of that Act (apart from section 4A).][373]

(7) For the purposes of this Act, material shall not be regarded as from a human body if it is created outside the human body.

(8) For the purposes of this Act, except section 49, a person is another's partner if the two of them (whether of different sexes or the same sex) live as partners in an enduring family relationship.

(9) The following are qualifying relationships for the purposes of this Act, spouse, [civil partner,][374] partner, parent, child, brother, sister, grandparent, grandchild, child of a brother or sister, stepfather, stepmother, half-brother, half-sister and friend of long standing.

(10) The Secretary of State may by order amend subsection (9).

SCHEDULE 1

SCHEDULED PURPOSES

PART 1

PURPOSES REQUIRING CONSENT: GENERAL

A1–347   1 Anatomical examination.

2 Determining the cause of death.

3 Establishing after a person's death the efficacy of any drug or other treatment administered to him.

4 Obtaining scientific or medical information about a living or deceased person which may be relevant to any other person (including a future person).

5 Public display.

6 Research in connection with disorders, or the functioning, of the human body.

7 Transplantation.

8 Clinical audit.

9 Education or training relating to human health.

---

[373] Substituted by Human Fertilisation and Embryology Act 2008 c. 22 Sch.7 para.24 (October 1, 2009).

[374] Words inserted by Civil Partnership Act 2004 (Overseas Relationships and Consequential, etc. Amendments) Order 2005/3129 Sch.4 para.12(3) (December 5, 2005).

PART 2

PURPOSES REQUIRING CONSENT: DECEASED PERSONS

10 Performance assessment.   A1–348
11 Public health monitoring.
12 Quality assurance.

International Headquarters and Defence Organisations Act 1964 c. 5

International headquarters and defence organisations

1.—(1) Where in pursuance of any arrangements for common defence to which Her   A1–349
Majesty's Government in the United Kingdom are for the time being a party any
international headquarters or defence organisation has been or is about to be set up, Her
Majesty may by Order in Council designate the headquarters or organisation for the
purposes of this Act and confer on it the legal capacity of a body corporate and, to such
extent as may be specified in the Order,—

(a) immunity from suit and legal process;

(b) the like privileges as respects the inviolability of official archives as are accorded to
an envoy of a foreign sovereign power accredited to Her Majesty.

(2) Where any headquarters or organisation is designated by an Order in Council under
this section the Visiting Forces Act 1952 shall have effect with the adaptations set out in the
Schedule to this Act, being adaptations for extending certain provisions of that Act to the
headquarters or organisation and certain persons connected with it.

(3) An Order in Council under this section may be varied or revoked by a subsequent
Order in Council.

(4) No recommendation shall be made to Her Majesty in Council to make an Order
under this section unless a draft thereof has been laid before Parliament and approved by a
resolution of each House of Parliament.

SCHEDULE 1

ADAPTATIONS OF VISITING FORCES ACT 1952

Interpretation

1.—(1) In this Schedule—   A1–350

"civilian member of a headquarters" has the meaning assigned to it by paragraph 2 of this
Schedule;
"headquarters" means a headquarters or organisation designated by an Order in Council under
section 1 of this Act;
"member of a headquarters" means military member or civilian member of a headquarters;
"military member of a headquarters" means a member of any country's forces who is for the time
being appointed to serve in the United Kingdom under the orders of a headquarters, except that
it does not include a member of the home forces.

(2) Any reference in this Schedule to a section is a reference to that section of the Visiting Forces Act
1952, and any expression used in this Schedule and in that Act has the same meaning in this Schedule
as in that Act, except that the expression "dependant" does not include any person who is a citizen of
the United Kingdom and Colonies or is ordinarily resident in the United Kingdom.

(3) References in this Schedule to a member of a headquarters belonging to any country are
references, in the case of a military member, to his being a member of that country's forces and, in the
case of a civilian member, to his being employed by that country's forces.

739

2.—(1) In this Schedule "civilian member of a headquarters" means a person who for the time being holds such a passport as is mentioned in paragraph (a) of subsection (1) of section 10, being a passport containing—

(a) an uncancelled entry made by or on behalf of an authority appointed for the purposes of this paragraph by any country outside the United Kingdom or by the headquarters stating that he is a civilian member of the headquarters; and

(b) an uncancelled mark or indication made on behalf of the Secretary of State signifying that the entry has been noted and approved;

and whose recognition as a civilian member of the headquarters has not been withdrawn by a notice in writing given to the said authority by or on behalf of the Secretary of State.

(2) Subsections (3) and (4) of section 10 (which contain supplementary provisions as to the passports mentioned in that section) shall with the necessary modifications apply for the purposes of this paragraph.

3.—(1) Subject to sub-paragraph (2) of this paragraph, a military member of a headquarters who belongs to a country to which section 2 applies shall be included among the persons who are subject to the jurisdiction of the service courts and service authorities of that country in accordance with that section, and subsection (6) of that section shall apply in relation to him as it applies in relation to members of a visiting force.

(2) Sub-paragraph (1) of this paragraph does not apply to a military member of a headquarters who became (or last became) a member of the forces of the country to which he belongs while he was in the United Kingdom, unless it is shown that he did so with his consent.

4.—(1) Section 3 shall apply in relation to a person charged with an offence who at the time the offence is alleged to have been committed was a member of a headquarters and belonged to a country to which that section applies as it applies to a person who at that time was a member of a visiting force of that country or was a member of a civilian component of such a force, according as the first-mentioned person was then a military or civilian member of the headquarters; and, as so applying, shall be further adapted as follows–

(a) the reference in paragraph (a) of subsection (1) to his duty as a member of that force or component shall be construed as a reference to his duty as a member of the headquarters;

(b) the references in paragraphs (b) and (c) of that subsection to a person having a relevant association with a visiting force of that country shall be construed as including references to any person who at the said time was, or was a dependant of, a member of a headquarters belonging to that country;

(c) the references in the said paragraph (c) to property of the sending country shall be construed as references to property of the country to which the person charged belonged, to property of the headquarters, to such property of any other country to which the section applies as was used or to be used for the purposes of the headquarters, and to such property of any other headquarters as was used or to be used for those purposes;

(d) the references in subsection (2) and in paragraph (a) of subsection (3) to the sending country shall be construed as references to the country to which the person charged belonged.

(2) In relation to a person to whom section 3 applies apart from sub-paragraph (1) of this paragraph, that is to say, a person charged with an offence who at the time the offence is alleged to have been committed was a member of a visiting force of any country or a member of a civilian component of such a force, that section shall have effect subject to the adaption that references in paragraphs (b) and (c) of subsection (1) to a person having a relevant association with a visiting force of the same country shall be construed as including references to any person who at the said time was, or was a dependant of, a member of a headquarters belonging to that country.

5. The references in section 6 to service as a member of a visiting force or as a member of a civilian component of such a force shall include references to service as a member of a headquarters.

6. The references in section 7 to a deceased person who at the time of his death had a relevant association with a visiting force shall include references to a deceased person who at the time of his death was a member of a headquarters and belonged to a country to which that section applies or a dependant of such a member.

7. Sections 8 and 9 shall apply in relation to a headquarters and its members and property and persons connected with it as they apply in relation to a visiting force and its members and property and persons connected with it.

8. For the purposes of the Visiting Forces Act 1952 as adapted by this Schedule—

(a) a certificate issued by or on behalf of an authority appointed by a headquarters for the purposes of paragraph 2 of this Schedule stating that at a time specified in the certificate a person so specified either was or was not a military or civilian member of that headquarters and, if he was, belonged to any country so specified;

(b) a certificate so issued stating that an alleged offence, if committed by a person so specified, arose out of and in the course of his duty as a member of that headquarters;

shall be sufficient evidence of the fact so stated unless the contrary is proved.

9. Subsection (3) of section 16 shall apply in relation to any document purporting to be any such certificate as is mentioned in paragraph 8 of this Schedule, and to the authority issuing such a certificate, as it applies in relation to such a certificate and authority as are mentioned in that section.

Industrial Diseases (Notification) Act 1981 c. 25

Regulations

1. [The Secretary of State][375] or with his approval the Registrar General, may make by statutory instrument regulations concerning the notification and certification of death and for the recording of information relating to industrial diseases and matters related thereto.   **A1–351**

Short title, interpretation and extent

2.—(1) This Act may be cited as the Industrial Diseases (Notification) Act 1981.   **A1–352**
(2) In this Act "Registrar General" means—

(a) in England and Wales, the Registrar General for England and Wales; and

(b) in Scotland, the Registrar General of Births, Deaths and Marriages for Scotland.

(3) This Act does not apply to Northern Ireland.

Law Reform (Year and a Day Rule) Act 1996 c. 19

Abolition of "year and a day rule"

1. The rule known as the "year and a day rule" (that is, the rule that, for the purposes of offences involving death and of suicide, an act or omission is conclusively presumed not to have caused a person's death if more than a year and a day elapsed before he died) is abolished for all purposes.   **A1–353**

[Restriction on institution of proceedings for a fatal offence

2.—(1) Proceedings to which this section applies may only be instituted by or with the consent of the Attorney General.   **A1–354**
(2) This section applies to proceedings against a person for a fatal offence if—

(a) the injury alleged to have caused the death was sustained more than three years before the death occurred, or

(b) the person has previously been convicted of an offence committed in circumstances alleged to be connected with the death.

---

[375] Words substituted by Transfer of Functions (Registration) Order 2008/678 Sch.2 para.10 (April 3, 2008).

(3) In subsection (2)"fatal offence" means—

(a) murder, manslaughter, infanticide or any other offence of which one of the elements is causing a person's death,

(b) an offence under section 2(1) of the Suicide Act 1961 (offence of encouraging or assisting suicide) in connection with the death of a person, or

(c) an offence under section 5 of the Domestic Violence, Crime and Victims Act 2004 of causing or allowing the death of a child or vulnerable adult.

(4) No provision that proceedings may be instituted only by or with the consent of the Director of Public Prosecutions shall apply to proceedings to which this section applies.

(5) In the application of this section to Northern Ireland—

(a) the reference in subsection (1) to the Attorney General is to the Attorney General for Northern Ireland,

(aa) the reference in subsection (3)(b) to section 2(1) of the Suicide Act 1961 is to be read as a reference to section 13(1) of the Criminal Justice Act (Northern Ireland) 1966, and

(b) the reference in subsection (4) to the Director of Public Prosecutions is to the Director of Public Prosecutions for Northern Ireland.][376];

Short title, commencement and extent

A1–355 **3.**—(1) This Act may be cited as the Law Reform (Year and a Day Rule) Act 1996.

(2) Section 1 does not affect the continued application of the rule referred to in that section to a case where the act or omission (or the last of the acts or omissions) which caused the death occurred before the day on which this Act is passed.

(3) Section 2 does not come into force until the end of the period of two months beginning with the day on which this Act is passed; but that section applies to the institution of proceedings after the end of that period in any case where the death occurred during that period (as well as in any case where the death occurred after the end of that period).

(4) This Act extends to England and Wales and Northern Ireland.

Legal Aid, Sentencing and Punishment of Offenders Act 2012 c. 10

PART 1

LEGAL AID

Provision of legal aid

Lord Chancellor's functions

A1–356 **1.**—(1) The Lord Chancellor must secure that legal aid is made available in accordance with this Part.

(2) In this Part "legal aid" means—

(a) civil legal services required to be made available under section 9 or 10 or paragraph 3 of Schedule 3 (civil legal aid), and

---

[376] Words substituted by Domestic Violence, Crime and Victims (Amendment) Act 2012 c. 4 Sch.1 para.3 (July 2, 2012).

(b) services consisting of advice, assistance and representation required to be made available under section 13, 15 or 16 or paragraph 4 or 5 of Schedule 3 (criminal legal aid).

(3) The Lord Chancellor may secure the provision of—

(a) general information about the law and the legal system, and

(b) information about the availability of advice about, and assistance in connection with, the law and the legal system.

(4) The Lord Chancellor may do anything which is calculated to facilitate, or is incidental or conducive to, the carrying out of the Lord Chancellor's functions under this Part.

(5) Nothing in this Part affects the powers that the Lord Chancellor has otherwise than under this Part.

Arrangements

2.—(1) The Lord Chancellor may make such arrangements as the Lord Chancellor **A1–357** considers appropriate for the purposes of carrying out the Lord Chancellor's functions under this Part.

(2) The Lord Chancellor may, in particular, make arrangements by—

(a) making grants or loans to enable persons to provide services or facilitate the provision of services,

(b) making grants or loans to individuals to enable them to obtain services, and

(c) establishing and maintaining a body to provide services or facilitate the provision of services.

(3) The Lord Chancellor may by regulations make provision about the payment of remuneration by the Lord Chancellor to persons who provide services under arrangements made for the purposes of this Part.

(4) If the Lord Chancellor makes arrangements for the purposes of this Part that provide for a court, tribunal or other person to assess remuneration payable by the Lord Chancellor, the court, tribunal or person must assess the remuneration in accordance with the arrangements and, if relevant, with regulations under subsection (3).

(5) The Lord Chancellor may make different arrangements, in particular, in relation to—

(a) different areas in England and Wales,

(b) different descriptions of case, and

(c) different classes of person.

Standards of service

3.—(1) The Lord Chancellor may set and monitor standards in relation to services made **A1–358** available under this Part.

(2) The Lord Chancellor may, in particular, make arrangements for the accreditation of persons providing, or wishing to provide, such services by—

(a) the Lord Chancellor, or

(b) persons authorised by the Lord Chancellor.

(3) Arrangements for accreditation must include—

(a) arrangements for monitoring services provided by accredited persons, and

(b) arrangements for withdrawing accreditation where the services provided are unsatisfactory.

(4) The Lord Chancellor may impose charges in connection with—

(a) accreditation,

(b) monitoring services provided by accredited persons, and

(c) authorising accreditation by others.

(5) Persons authorised by the Lord Chancellor may, in accordance with the terms of their authorisation, impose charges in connection with—

(a) accreditation, and

(b) monitoring services provided by accredited persons.

Director of Legal Aid Casework

A1–359 4.—(1) The Lord Chancellor must designate a civil servant as the Director of Legal Aid Casework ("the Director").

(2) The Lord Chancellor must make arrangements for the provision to the Director by civil servants or other persons (or both) of such assistance as the Lord Chancellor considers appropriate.

(3) The Director must—

(a) comply with directions given by the Lord Chancellor about the carrying out of the Director's functions under this Part, and

(b) have regard to guidance given by the Lord Chancellor about the carrying out of those functions.

(4) But the Lord Chancellor—

(a) must not give a direction or guidance about the carrying out of those functions in relation to an individual case, and

(b) must ensure that the Director acts independently of the Lord Chancellor when applying a direction or guidance under subsection (3) in relation to an individual case.

(5) The Lord Chancellor must publish any directions and guidance given under this section.

(6) Directions and guidance under this section may be revised or withdrawn from time to time.

Civil legal aid

Civil legal services

A1–360 8.—(1) In this Part "legal services" means the following types of services—

(a) providing advice as to how the law applies in particular circumstances,

(b) providing advice and assistance in relation to legal proceedings,

(c) providing other advice and assistance in relation to the prevention of disputes about legal rights or duties ("legal disputes") or the settlement or other resolution of legal disputes, and

(d) providing advice and assistance in relation to the enforcement of decisions in legal proceedings or other decisions by which legal disputes are resolved.

(2) The services described in subsection (1) include, in particular, advice and assistance in the form of—

(a) representation, and

(b) mediation and other forms of dispute resolution.

(3) In this Part "civil legal services" means any legal services other than the types of advice, assistance and representation that are required to be made available under sections 13, 15 and 16 (criminal legal aid).

General cases

9.—(1) Civil legal services are to be available to an individual under this Part if—   **A1–361**

(a) they are civil legal services described in Part 1 of Schedule 1, and

(b) the Director has determined that the individual qualifies for the services in accordance with this Part (and has not withdrawn the determination).

(2) The Lord Chancellor may by order—

(a) add services to Part 1 of Schedule 1, or

(b) vary or omit services described in that Part,

(whether by modifying that Part or Part 2, 3 or 4 of the Schedule).

Exceptional cases

10.—(1) Civil legal services other than services described in Part 1 of Schedule 1 are to   **A1–362**
be available to an individual under this Part if subsection (2) or (4) is satisfied.
(2) This subsection is satisfied where the Director—

(a) has made an exceptional case determination in relation to the individual and the services, and

(b) has determined that the individual qualifies for the services in accordance with this Part,

(and has not withdrawn either determination).
(3) For the purposes of subsection (2), an exceptional case determination is a determination—

(a) that it is necessary to make the services available to the individual under this Part because failure to do so would be a breach of—

   (i) the individual's Convention rights (within the meaning of the Human Rights Act 1998), or

   (ii) any rights of the individual to the provision of legal services that are enforceable EU rights, or

(b) that it is appropriate to do so, in the particular circumstances of the case, having regard to any risk that failure to do so would be such a breach.

(4) This subsection is satisfied where—

(a) the services consist of advocacy in proceedings at an inquest under the Coroners Act 1988 into the death of a member of the individual's family,

(b) the Director has made a wider public interest determination in relation to the individual and the inquest, and

(c) the Director has determined that the individual qualifies for the services in accordance with this Part,

(and neither determination has been withdrawn).

(5) For the purposes of subsection (4), a wider public interest determination is a determination that, in the particular circumstances of the case, the provision of advocacy under this Part for the individual for the purposes of the inquest is likely to produce significant benefits for a class of person, other than the individual and the members of the individual's family.

(6) For the purposes of this section an individual is a member of another individual's family if—

(a) they are relatives (whether of the full blood or half blood or by marriage or civil partnership),

(b) they are cohabitants (as defined in Part 4 of the Family Law Act 1996), or

(c) one has parental responsibility for the other.

Qualifying for civil legal aid

A1–363   11.—(1) The Director must determine whether an individual qualifies under this Part for civil legal services in accordance with—

(a) section 21 (financial resources) and regulations under that section, and

(b) criteria set out in regulations made under this paragraph.

(2) In setting the criteria, the Lord Chancellor—

(a) must consider the circumstances in which it is appropriate to make civil legal services available under this Part, and

(b) must, in particular, consider the extent to which the criteria ought to reflect the factors in subsection (3).

(3) Those factors are—

(a) the likely cost of providing the services and the benefit which may be obtained by the services being provided,

(b) the availability of resources to provide the services,

(c) the appropriateness of applying those resources to provide the services, having regard to present and likely future demands for the provision of civil legal services under this Part,

(d) the importance for the individual of the matters in relation to which the services would be provided,

(e) the nature and seriousness of the act, omission, circumstances or other matter in relation to which the services are sought,

(f) the availability to the individual of services provided other than under this Part and the likelihood of the individual being able to make use of such services,

(g) if the services are sought by the individual in relation to a dispute, the individual's prospects of success in the dispute,

   (h) the conduct of the individual in connection with services made available under this Part or an application for such services,

   (i) the conduct of the individual in connection with any legal proceedings or other proceedings for resolving disputes about legal rights or duties, and

   (j) the public interest.

(4) In setting the criteria, the Lord Chancellor must seek to secure that, in cases in which more than one form of civil legal service could be provided for an individual, the individual qualifies under this Part for the form of service which in all the circumstances is the most appropriate having regard to the criteria.

(5) The criteria must reflect the principle that, in many disputes, mediation and other forms of dispute resolution are more appropriate than legal proceedings.

(6) Regulations under subsection (1)(b) may provide that no criteria apply in relation to a prescribed description of individual or services.

Determinations

12.—(1) A determination by the Director that an individual qualifies under this Part for   **A1–364** civil legal services must specify—

   (a) the type of services, and

   (b) the matters in relation to which the services are to be available.

(2) Regulations may make provision about the making and withdrawal of determinations under sections 9 and 10.

(3) Regulations under subsection (2) may, in particular, include—

   (a) provision about the form and content of determinations and applications for determinations,

   (b) provision permitting or requiring applications and determinations to be made and withdrawn in writing, by telephone or by other prescribed means,

   (c) provision setting time limits for applications and determinations,

   (d) provision for a determination to be disregarded for the purposes of this Part if made in response to an application that is made otherwise than in accordance with the regulations,

   (e) provision about conditions which must be satisfied by an applicant before a determination is made,

   (f) provision about the circumstances in which a determination may or must be withdrawn,

   (g) provision requiring information and documents to be provided,

   (h) provision requiring individuals who are the subject of a determination to be informed of the reasons for making or withdrawing the determination, and

   (i) provision for giving information to individuals who do not qualify for civil legal services under this Part about alternative ways of obtaining or funding civil legal services.

(4) The circumstances prescribed under subsection (3)(f) may, in particular, relate to whether the individual who is the subject of the determination has complied with requirements imposed by or under this Part.

(5) Regulations under subsection (2) must make provision establishing procedures for the review of determinations under sections 9 and 10 and of the withdrawal of such determinations.

(6) Regulations under subsection (2) may make provision for appeals to a court, tribunal or other person against such determinations and against the withdrawal of such determinations.

Financial resources

21.—(1) A person may not make a relevant determination that an individual qualifies under this Part for services unless the person has determined that the individual's financial resources are such that the individual is eligible for the services (and has not withdrawn the determination).

(2) Regulations may—

(a) make provision about when an individual's financial resources are such that the individual is eligible under this Part for services, and

(b) make provision for exceptions from subsection (1).

(3) Regulations may provide that an individual is to be treated, for the purposes of regulations under subsection (2), as having or not having financial resources of a prescribed description.

(4) Regulations under subsection (3) may, in particular, provide that the individual is to be treated as having prescribed financial resources of a person of a prescribed description.

(5) Regulations may make provision about the making and withdrawal of determinations under this section.

(6) Regulations under subsection (5) may, in particular, include—

(a) provision about the form and content of determinations,

(b) provision permitting or requiring determinations to be made and withdrawn in writing, by telephone or by other prescribed means,

(c) provision setting time limits for determinations,

(d) provision about conditions which must be satisfied before a determination is made,

(e) provision about the circumstances in which a determination may or must be withdrawn,

(f) provision requiring information and documents to be provided,

(g) provision requiring individuals who are the subject of a determination to be informed of the reasons for making or withdrawing the determination, and

(h) provision for the review of a determination in respect of an individual's financial resources.

(7) The circumstances prescribed under subsection (6)(e) may, in particular, relate to whether the individual who is the subject of the determination has complied with requirements imposed by or under this Part.

(8) In this section "relevant determination" means a determination that is required to be carried out in accordance with this section by—

(a) section 11 or 17, or

(b) regulations under section 15 or paragraph 4 of Schedule 3.

Schedule 1

Civil Legal Services

Part 1

Services

[Note: only paragraphs within the scope of this work are included here]

Judicial review

19.—(1) Civil legal services provided in relation to judicial review of an enactment, decision, act or omission.　　　**A1–366**

General exclusions

(2) Sub-paragraph (1) is subject to—　　　**A1–367**

(a) the exclusions in Part 2 of this Schedule, with the exception of [paragraphs 1, 2, 3, 4, 5, 6, 8, 12, 15, 16 and 18][377] of that Part, and

(b) the exclusion in Part 3 of this Schedule.

Specific exclusion: benefit to individual

(3) The services described in sub-paragraph (1) do not include services provided to an individual in relation to judicial review that does not have the potential to produce a benefit for the individual, a member of the individual's family or the environment.　　　**A1–368**

(4) Sub-paragraph (3) does not exclude services provided in relation to a judicial review where the judicial review ceases to have the potential to produce such a benefit after civil legal services have been provided in relation to the judicial review under arrangements made for the purposes of this Part of this Act.

Specific exclusions: immigration cases

(5) The services described in sub-paragraph (1) do not include services provided in relation to judicial review in respect of an issue relating to immigration where—　　　**A1–369**

(a) the same issue, or substantially the same issue, was the subject of a previous judicial review or an appeal to a court or tribunal,

(b) on the determination of the previous judicial review or appeal (or, if there was more than one, the latest one), the court, tribunal or other person hearing the case found against the applicant or appellant on that issue, and

(c) the services in relation to the new judicial review are provided before the end of the period of 1 year beginning with the day of that determination.

(6) The services described in sub-paragraph (1) do not include services provided in relation to judicial review of removal directions in respect of an individual where the directions were given not more than 1 year after the latest of the following—

(a) the making of the decision (or, if there was more than one, the latest decision) to remove the individual from the United Kingdom by way of removal directions;

(b) the refusal of leave to appeal against that decision;

(c) the determination or withdrawal of an appeal against that decision.

---

[377] Words substituted by Legal Aid, Sentencing and Punishment of Offenders Act 2012 (Amendment of Schedule 1) Order 2013/748 art.6 (April 1, 2013).

(7) Sub-paragraphs (5) and (6) do not exclude services provided to an individual in relation to—

(a) judicial review of a negative decision in relation to an asylum application (within the meaning of the EU Procedures Directive) where there is no right of appeal to the First-tier Tribunal against the decision;

(b) judicial review of certification under section 94 or 96 of the Nationality, Immigration and Asylum Act 2002 (certificate preventing or restricting appeal of immigration decision).

(8) Sub-paragraphs (5) and (6) do not exclude services provided in relation to judicial review of removal directions in respect of an individual where prescribed conditions relating to either or both of the following are met—

(a) the period between the individual being given notice of the removal directions and the proposed time for his or her removal;

(b) the reasons for proposing that period.

Definitions

A1–370   (9) For the purposes of this paragraph an individual is a member of another individual's family if—

(a) they are relatives (whether of the full blood or half blood or by marriage or civil partnership),

(b) they are cohabitants (as defined in Part 4 of the Family Law Act 1996), or

(c) one has parental responsibility for the other.

(10) In this paragraph—

"EU Procedures Directive" means Council Directive 2005/85/EC of 1 December 2005 on minimum standards on procedures in Member States for granting and withdrawing refugee status;
"an issue relating to immigration" includes an issue relating to rights described in paragraph 30 of this Part of this Schedule;
"judicial review" means—

(a) the procedure on an application for judicial review (see section 31 of the Senior Courts Act 1981), but not including the procedure after the application is treated under rules of court as if it were not such an application, and

(b) any procedure in which a court, tribunal or other person mentioned in Part 3 of this Schedule is required by an enactment to make a decision applying the principles that are applied by the court on an application for judicial review;

"removal directions" means directions under—

(a) paragraphs 8 to 10A of Schedule 2 to the Immigration Act 1971 (removal of persons refused leave to enter and illegal entrants);

(b) paragraphs 12 to 14 of Schedule 2 to that Act (removal of seamen and aircrew);

(c) paragraph 1 of Schedule 3 to that Act (removal of persons liable to deportation);

(d) section 10 of the Immigration and Asylum Act 1999 (removal of certain persons unlawfully in the United Kingdom);

(e) section 47 of the Immigration, Asylum and Nationality Act 2006 (removal of persons with statutorily extended leave).

Inquests

A1–371   41.—(1) Civil legal services provided to an individual in relation to an inquest under the Coroners Act 1988 into the death of a member of the individual's family.

Exclusions

A1–372   (2) Sub-paragraph (1) is subject to—

(a) the exclusions in Part 2 of this Schedule, with the exception of paragraph 1 of that Part, and

(b) the exclusion in Part 3 of this Schedule.

Definitions

(3) For the purposes of this paragraph an individual is a member of another individual's family　**A1–373**
if—

(a) they are relatives (whether of the full blood or half blood or by marriage or civil partnership),

(b) they are cohabitants (as defined in Part 4 of the Family Law Act 1996), or

(c) one has parental responsibility for the other.

Connected matters

46—(1) Prescribed civil legal services provided, in prescribed circumstances, in connection with the　**A1–374**
provision of services described in a preceding paragraph of this Part of this Schedule.

Exclusions

(2) Sub-paragraph (1) is subject to—　**A1–375**

(a) the exclusions in Parts 2 and 3 of this Schedule, except to the extent that regulations under this
paragraph provide otherwise, and

(b) any other prescribed exclusions.

Part 2

Excluded Services

The services described in Part 1 of this Schedule do not include the services listed in this Part of this　**A1–376**
Schedule, except to the extent that Part 1 of this Schedule provides otherwise.
[Note: only paragraphs within the scope of this work are included here]

1 Civil legal services provided in relation to personal injury or death.
2 Civil legal services provided in relation to a claim in tort in respect of negligence.
3 Civil legal services provided in relation to a claim in tort in respect of assault, battery or false
imprisonment.
12 (1) Civil legal services provided in relation to a claim for damages in respect of a breach of
Convention rights by a public authority to the extent that the claim is made in reliance on section 7
of the Human Rights Act 1998.
(2) In this paragraph—

"Convention rights" has the same meaning as in the Human Rights Act 1998;
"public authority" has the same meaning as in section 6 of that Act.

[18.—(1) Civil legal services provided in relation to judicial review of an enactment, decision, act or
omission.
(2) In this paragraph "judicial review" means—

(a) the procedure on an application for judicial review (see section 31 of the Senior Courts Act
1981[378]), but not including the procedure after the application is treated under rules of court as
if it were not such an application, and

---

[378] 1981 c. 54; section 31 was amended by SI 2004/1033 and the Tribunals, Courts and Enforcement
Act 2007 (c. 15), section 141.

(b) any procedure in which a court, tribunal or other person mentioned in Part 3 of this Schedule is required by an enactment to make a decision applying the principles that are applied by the court on an application for judicial review.][379];

PART 3

ADVOCACY: EXCLUSION AND EXCEPTIONS

A1–377   The services described in Part 1 of this Schedule do not include advocacy, except as follows—

(a) those services include the types of advocacy listed in this Part of this Schedule, except to the extent that Part 1 of this Schedule provides otherwise;

(b) those services include other types of advocacy to the extent that Part 1 of this Schedule so provides.

[Note: only paragraphs within the scope of this work are included here]

EXCEPTIONS: COURTS

A1–378   1 Advocacy in proceedings in the Supreme Court.
2 Advocacy in proceedings in the Court of Appeal.
3 Advocacy in proceedings in the High Court.

EXCEPTIONS: TRIBUNALS

A1–379   18 Advocacy in proceedings which are brought before the Upper Tribunal (wholly or primarily) to exercise its judicial review jurisdiction under section 15 of the Tribunals, Courts and Enforcement Act 2007.
19 Advocacy where judicial review applications are transferred to the Upper Tribunal from the High Court under section 31A of the Senior Courts Act 1981.

OTHER EXCEPTIONS

A1–380   23 Advocacy in legal proceedings before any person to whom a case is referred (in whole or in part) in any proceedings within any other paragraph of this Part of this Schedule.
25 Advocacy in proceedings before any person for the enforcement of a decision in proceedings within any other paragraph of this Part of this Schedule.

PART 4

INTERPRETATION

A1–381   1 For the purposes of this Part of this Act, civil legal services are described in Part 1 of this Schedule if they are described in one of the paragraphs of that Part (other than in an exclusion), even if they are (expressly or impliedly) excluded from another paragraph of that Part.
2 References in this Schedule to an Act or instrument, or a provision of an Act or instrument—

(a) are references to the Act, instrument or provision as amended from time to time, and

(b) include the Act, instrument or provision as applied by another Act or instrument (with or without modifications).

3 References in this Schedule to services provided in relation to an act, omission or other matter of a particular description (however expressed) include services provided in relation to an act, omission or other matter alleged to be of that description.
4 References in this Schedule to services provided in relation to proceedings, orders and other matters include services provided when such proceedings, orders and matters are contemplated.

---

[379] Added by Legal Aid, Sentencing and Punishment of Offenders Act 2012 (Amendment of Schedule 1) Order 2013/748 art.7 (April 1, 2013).

5—(1) Where a paragraph of Part 1 or 2 of this Schedule describes services that consist of or include services provided in relation to proceedings, the description is to be treated as including, in particular—

(a) services provided in relation to related bail proceedings,

(b) services provided in relation to preliminary or incidental proceedings,

(c) services provided in relation to a related appeal or reference to a court, tribunal or other person, and

(d) services provided in relation to the enforcement of decisions in the proceedings.

(2) Where a paragraph of Part 3 of this Schedule describes advocacy provided in relation to particular proceedings in or before a court, tribunal or other person, the description is to be treated as including services provided in relation to preliminary or incidental proceedings in or before the same court, tribunal or other person.

(3) Regulations may make provision specifying whether proceedings are or are not to be regarded as preliminary or incidental for the purposes of this paragraph.

6 For the purposes of this Schedule, regulations may make provision about—

(a) when services are provided in relation to a matter;

(b) when matters arise under a particular enactment;

(c) when proceedings are proceedings under a particular enactment;

(d) when proceedings are related to other proceedings.

7 In this Schedule "enactment" includes—

(a) an enactment contained in subordinate legislation (within the meaning of the Interpretation Act 1978), and

(b) an enactment contained in, or in an instrument made under, an Act or Measure of the National Assembly for Wales.

Legal Services Act 2007 c. 29

PART 3

RESERVED LEGAL ACTIVITIES

Reserved legal activities

Meaning of "reserved legal activity" and "legal activity"

12.—(1) In this Act "reserved legal activity" means—   **A1–382**

(a) the exercise of a right of audience;

(b) the conduct of litigation;

(c) reserved instrument activities;

(d) probate activities;

(e) notarial activities;

(f) the administration of oaths.

(2) Schedule 2 makes provision about what constitutes each of those activities.

(3) In this Act "legal activity" means—

(a) an activity which is a reserved legal activity within the meaning of this Act as originally enacted, and

(b) any other activity which consists of one or both of the following—

  (i) the provision of legal advice or assistance in connection with the application of the law or with any form of resolution of legal disputes;

  (ii) the provision of representation in connection with any matter concerning the application of the law or any form of resolution of legal disputes.

(4) But "legal activity" does not include any activity of a judicial or quasi-judicial nature (including acting as a mediator).

(5) For the purposes of subsection (3) "legal dispute" includes a dispute as to any matter of fact the resolution of which is relevant to determining the nature of any person's legal rights or liabilities.

(6) Section 24 makes provision for adding legal activities to the reserved legal activities.

Interpretation

Authorised persons

A1–383   **18.**—(1) For the purposes of this Act "authorised person", in relation to an activity ("the relevant activity") which is a reserved legal activity, means—

(a) a person who is authorised to carry on the relevant activity by a relevant approved regulator in relation to the relevant activity [(other than by virtue of a licence under Part 5), or][380]

(b) a licensable body which, by virtue of such a licence, is authorised to carry on the relevant activity by a licensing authority in relation to the reserved legal activity.

(2) A licensable body may not be authorised to carry on the relevant activity as mentioned in subsection (1)(a).

(3) But where a body ("A") which is authorised as mentioned in subsection (1)(a) becomes a licensable body, the body is deemed by virtue of this subsection to continue to be so authorised from that time until the earliest of the following events—

(a) the end of the period of 90 days beginning with the day on which that time falls;

(b) the time from which the relevant approved regulator determines this subsection is to cease to apply to A;

(c) the time when A ceases to be a licensable body.

(4) Subsection (2) is subject to Part 2 of Schedule 5 (by virtue of which licensable bodies may be deemed to be authorised as mentioned in subsection (1)(a) in relation to certain activities during a transitional period).

(5) A person other than a licensable body may not be authorised to carry on the relevant activity as mentioned in subsection (1)(b).

(6) But where a body ("L") which is authorised as mentioned in subsection (1)(b) ceases to be a licensable body, the body is deemed by virtue of this subsection to continue to be so authorised from that time until the earliest of the following events—

(a) the end of the period of 90 days beginning with the day on which that time falls;

---

[380] Words inserted by Legal Services Act 2007 (Commencement No. 6, Transitory, Transitional and Saving Provisions) Order 2009/3250 art.3(1) (October 1, 2011: insertion has effect upon the commencement of 2007 c.29 s.18(2)).

(b) the time from which the relevant licensing authority determines this subsection is to cease to apply to L;

(c) the time when L becomes a licensable body.

Exempt persons

19. In this Act, "exempt person", in relation to an activity ("the relevant activity") which   **A1–384**
is a reserved legal activity, means a person who, for the purposes of carrying on the relevant activity, is an exempt person by virtue of—

(a) Schedule 3 (exempt persons), or

(b) paragraph 13 or 18 of Schedule 5 (additional categories of exempt persons during transitional period).

SCHEDULE 2

THE RESERVED LEGAL ACTIVITIES

Rights of audience

3.—(1) A "right of audience" means the right to appear before and address a court, including the   **A1–385**
right to call and examine witnesses.

(2) But a "right of audience" does not include a right to appear before or address a court, or to call or examine witnesses, in relation to any particular court or in relation to particular proceedings, if immediately before the appointed day no restriction was placed on the persons entitled to exercise that right.

Medical Act 1983 c. 54

PART VII

MISCELLANEOUS AND GENERAL

Interpretation

55.—[(1) In this Act—   **A1–386**

"acceptable overseas qualification" has the meaning given by [section 21B(2)][381] above;
["acceptable programme for provisionally registered doctors" has the meaning given by section 10A(1) above;][382]
"additional qualification" has the meaning given by section 16(2) above;
["CCT" means a certificate of completion of training awarded under section 34L(1);][383]

---

[381] Words substituted by Medical Act 1983 (Amendment) and Miscellaneous Amendments Order 2006/1914 Pt 4 art.41(a) (October 19, 2007: July 19, 2006 for the purpose of conferring powers enabling orders to be made by the Privy Council, or amendments specified in SI 2006/1914 art.1(2)(b)(ii); October 19, 2007 as specified on page 10493 of the London Gazette dated July 20, 2007 otherwise).

[382] Definition inserted by Medical Act 1983 (Amendment) and Miscellaneous Amendments Order 2006/1914 Pt 3 art.33(a) (August 1, 2007: July 19, 2006 for the purpose of conferring powers enabling orders to be made by the Privy Council, or amendments specified in SI 2006/1914 art.1(2)(b)(ii); August 1, 2007 as specified on page 10493 of the London Gazette dated July 20, 2007 otherwise).

[383] Definition inserted by General and Specialist Medical Practice (Education, Training and Qualifications) Order 2010/234 Sch.1 para.16 (April 1, 2010).

[. . .][384]

["competent authority" means any authority or body of a relevant European State designated by that State for the purposes of the Directive as competent to—

(a) receive or issue evidence of qualifications or other information or documents, or

(b) receive applications and take the decisions referred to in the Directive,

in connection with the practice of medicine;"the Directive" has the meaning given by section 5(4) above;][385]

[. . .][386]

"disqualifying decision" has the meaning given by section 44(2) above;

[. . .][387]

[. . .][388]

["exempt person" has the meaning given in section 19(2) above;][389]

[. . .][390]

["fully registered person" means a person for the time being registered under [section 3, 14A, 18A, 19, 19A, 21B, 27A or 27B][391] above as a fully registered medical practitioner, or under Schedule 2A as a visiting medical practitioner from a relevant European State, and—

(a) so far as mentioned in subsection (3) of section 15 (including that subsection as applied by section 15A(4), 21 or 21C above, but not further, includes a person for the time being provisionally registered;

and "fully registered" shall be construed accordingly;][392]

"the General Council" means the General Medical Council;

["General Practitioner Register" means the register kept by the General Council under section 34C;][383]

["the General Systems Regulations" means the European Communities (Recognition of Professional Qualifications) Regulations 2007 (SI 2007/2781);][393]

["GP Registrar" means a medical practitioner who is being trained in general practice whether as part of training leading to the award of a CCT or otherwise;][383]

---

[384] Definitions repealed by Health Care and Associated Professions (Miscellaneous Amendments) Order 2008/1774 Sch.1 para.20(b) (January 1, 2009).

[385] Definitions inserted by European Qualifications (Health and Social Care Professions) Regulations 2007/3101 Pt 2 reg.29(a)(i) (December 3, 2007).

[386] Definition repealed by European Qualifications (Health and Social Care Professions) Regulations 2007/3101 Pt 2 reg.29(a)(ii) (December 3, 2007).

[387] Definition repealed by European Qualifications (Health and Social Care Professions) Regulations 2007/3101 Pt 2 reg.29(a)(iii) (December 3, 2007).

[388] Definition repealed by Health Care and Associated Professions (Miscellaneous Amendments) Order 2008/1774 Sch.1 para.20(b) (January 1, 2009).

[389] Definition inserted by Medical Act 1983 (Amendment) Order 2002/3135 Pt VII art.15(6)(c) (December 17, 2002 for purposes specified in SI 2002/3135 art.1(2)(h); July 7, 2004 for the purpose specified in the London Gazette dated July 2, 2004; November 1, 2004 for the purpose specified in the London Gazette dated October 8, 2004; September 8, 2009 for the purpose specified on page 14478 and 14479 of the London Gazette dated August 21, 2009; on dates to be notified in London, Edinburgh and Belfast Gazettes otherwise).

[390] Definition repealed by European Primary Medical Qualifications Regulations 1996/1591 Sch.2 para.13(2)(c) (July 10, 1996).

[391] Words inserted by Health Care and Associated Professions (Miscellaneous Amendments) Order 2008/1774 Sch.1 para.20(a) (July 10, 2008).

[392] Words substituted by European Qualifications (Health and Social Care Professions) Regulations 2007/3101 Pt 2 reg.29(a)(iv) (December 3, 2007).

[393] Definition inserted by European Qualifications (Health and Social Care Professions) Regulations 2007/3101 Pt 2 reg.29(a)(v) (December 3, 2007).

["impaired", in relation to a person's fitness to practise, has the meaning given in section 35C(2) above;][394]

["licence to practise" has the meaning given in section 29A above;][395]

[. . .][396]

"national", in relation to a [relevant European State][397], has the same meaning as in the [EU][398], but does not include a person who by virtue of Article 2 of Protocol No. 3 (Channel Islands and Isle of Man) to the Treaty of Accession is not to benefit from [EU][399] provisions relating to the free movement of persons and services;

["the necessary knowledge of English", in relation to a person, means the knowledge of English which, in the interests of himself and his patients, is necessary for the practice of medicine in the United Kingdom;][400]

["NHS consultant" means a consultant other than a locum consultant (but including an honorary consultant) employed for the purposes of providing any service as part of any of the UK health services;][383]

[. . .][389]

[. . .][401]

"the prescribed knowledge and skill" has the meaning given by section 5(4) above;

[. . .][402]

"the prescribed standard of proficiency" has the meaning given by section 5(4) above;

"primary European qualification" shall be construed in accordance with section 17 above;

"primary United Kingdom qualification" has the meaning given by section 4(3) above;

["professional performance" includes a medical practitioner's professional competence;][390]

---

[394] Definition inserted by Medical Act 1983 (Amendment) Order 2002/3135 Pt VII art.15(6)(c) (July 7, 2004: as London Gazette dated July 2, 2004).

[395] Definition inserted by Medical Act 1983 (Amendment) Order 2002/3135 Pt VII art.15(6)(c) (September 8, 2009: as London Gazette dated August 21, 2009 page 14478 and 14479).

[396] Definition repealed by Medical Act 1983 (Amendment) and Miscellaneous Amendments Order 2006/1914 Pt 2 art.15(b) (October 19, 2007: July 19, 2006 for the purpose of conferring powers enabling orders to be made by the Privy Council, or amendments specified in SI 2006/1914 art.1(2)(b)(ii); October 19, 2007 as specified on page 10493 of the London Gazette dated July 20, 2007 otherwise).

[397] Words substituted by European Qualifications (Health and Social Care Professions) Regulations 2007/3101 Pt 2 reg.29(a)(vi) (December 3, 2007).

[398] Words substituted by Treaty of Lisbon (Changes in Terminology) Order 2011/1043 Pt 2 art.6(1)(a) (April 22, 2011).

[399] Word substituted by Treaty of Lisbon (Changes in Terminology) Order 2011/1043 Pt 2 art.6(2)(c) (April 22, 2011).

[400] Definition substituted by Medical Act 1983 (Amendment) (Knowledge of English) Order 2014/1101 Pt 4 art.10(2) (April 29, 2014).

[401] Definition repealed by Medical Act 1983 (Amendment) and Miscellaneous Amendments Order 2006/1914 Pt 2 art.15(c) (October 19, 2007: July 19, 2006 for the purpose of conferring powers enabling orders to be made by the Privy Council, or amendments specified in SI 2006/1914 art.1(2)(b)(ii); October 19, 2007 as specified on page 10493 of the London Gazette dated July 20, 2007 otherwise).

[402] Definition repealed by Medical Act 1983 (Amendment) and Miscellaneous Amendments Order 2006/1914 Pt 3 art.33(b) (August 1, 2007: July 19, 2006 for the purpose of conferring powers enabling orders to be made by the Privy Council, or amendments specified in SI 2006/1914 art.1(2)(b)(ii); August 1, 2007 as specified on page 10493 of the London Gazette dated July 20, 2007 otherwise).

"provisionally registered" means provisionally registered under [section 15, 15A, 21 or 21C][403] above;

"qualification", except where the context otherwise requires, means any diploma, degree, fellowship, membership, licence, authority to practise, letters testimonial, certificate or other status or document granted in respect of any branch or branches of medicine by any university, corporation, college or other body or by any department of, or persons acting under the authority of, the government of any country or place;

[. . .][404]

["recognised specialty" means a specialty which the Privy Council have designated as a recognised specialty by order under section 34D(3);][383]

["the register" means the register of medical practitioners;][405]

"the Registrar" has the meaning given by section 2(1) above but subject to sub-paragraph (3) of paragraph 16 of Schedule 1 to this Act;

["relevant European State" means an EEA State or Switzerland;][406]

["revalidation" has the meaning given in section 29A above;][390]

["Specialist Register" means the register kept by the General Council under section 34D;][383]

[. . .][407]

["the statutory committees" has the meaning given in section 1(3A) above;][408]

["the UK health services" means—

(a) the health service as defined by section 275(1) of the National Health Service Act 2006 or section 206(1) of the National Health Service (Wales) Act 2006;

(b) the health service as defined by section 108(1) of the National Health Service (Scotland) Act 1978[409]; and

(c) any of the health services under any enactment which extends to Northern Ireland and which corresponds to section 1(1) of the National Health Service Act 2006;][383][410]

[(2) In relation to anything done before the adoption by the Council of Directive 93/16/EEC, references in this Act to [the Directive],[411] or to any provision of [the

---

[403] Words substituted by Medical Act 1983 (Amendment) and Miscellaneous Amendments Order 2006/1914 Pt 4 art.41(c) (October 19, 2007: July 19, 2006 for the purpose of conferring powers enabling orders to be made by the Privy Council, or amendments specified in SI 2006/1914 art.1(2)(b)(ii); October 19, 2007 as specified on page 10493 of the London Gazette dated July 20, 2007 otherwise).

[404] Definition repealed by Medical Act 1983 (Amendment) Order 2002/3135 Pt VII art.15(6)(a) (December 17, 2002).

[405] Definition substituted by Medical Act 1983 (Amendment) and Miscellaneous Amendments Order 2006/1914 Pt 2 art.15(d) (October 19, 2007: July 19, 2006 for the purpose of conferring powers enabling orders to be made by the Privy Council, or amendments specified in SI 2006/1914 art.1(2)(b)(ii); October 19, 2007 as specified on page 10493 of the London Gazette dated July 20, 2007 otherwise).

[406] Definition inserted by European Qualifications (Health and Social Care Professions) Regulations 2007/3101 Pt 2 reg.29(a)(vii) (December 3, 2007).

[407] Definition repealed by European Primary Medical Qualifications Regulations 1996/1591 Sch.2 para.13(2)(f) (July 10, 1996).

[408] Possible drafting error, definition purportedly inserted in s.55(1) but the definition already exists, therefore definition is substituted by Medical Act 1983 (Amendment) Order 2002/3135 Pt VII art.15(6)(c) (November 1, 2004: as London Gazette dated October 8, 2004).

[409] 1978 c.29. Section 108(1) is amended but that definition has not been amended.

[410] Renumbering existing s.55 as s.55:(1) by European Primary Medical Qualifications Regulations 1996/1591 Sch.2 para.13(1) (July 10, 1996).

[411] Words substituted by European Qualifications (Health and Social Care Professions) Regulations 2007/3101 Pt 2 reg.29(b) (December 3, 2007).

Directive],⁴¹¹ shall be construed as references to, or to the corresponding provision of, the following Directives as for the time being amended, namely—

(a) Council Directive No. 75/362/EEC concerning the mutual recognition of diplomas, certificates and other evidence of formal qualifications in medicine⁴¹²; and

(b) Council Directive No. 75/363/EEC concerning the coordination of provisions in respect of activities of doctors⁴¹³.]⁴¹⁴

[(3) In relation to anything done—

(a) before the adoption by the Council and the European Parliament of the Directive, but

(b) after the adoption by the Council of Directive 93/16/EEC,

references in this Act to the Directive, or to any provision of the Directive, shall be construed as references to, or to any corresponding provision of, Directive 93/16/EEC as for the time being amended.

(4) In this section, "Directive 93/16/EEC" means Council Directive 93/16/EEC⁴¹⁵ of 5th April 1993 to facilitate the free movement of doctors and the mutual recognition of their diplomas, certificates and other evidence of formal qualifications (OJ No. L165, 7.7.93, p.1).]⁴¹⁶

SCHEDULE 6

TRANSITIONAL AND SAVING PROVISIONS

11.—(1) In any enactment passed before 1st January 1979 the expression "legally qualified medical   **A1–387**
practitioner", or "duly qualified medical practitioner", or any expression importing a person recognised by law as a medical practitioner or member of the medical profession, shall, unless the contrary intention appears, be construed to mean a [registered medical practitioner]⁴¹⁷ [who holds a licence to practise].⁴¹⁸

(2) In any enactment passed before 1st January 1979 references (however expressed) to a person registered under the Medical Acts or as a medical practitioner shall, unless the contrary intention

---

⁴¹² Council Directive No. 75/362/EEC was amended by the Act concerning the Conditions of Accession and Adjustments to the Treaties-Accession of the Hellenic Republic (OJ No L291, 19.11.1979, p. 90); Council Directive No 82/76/EEC of 26 January 1982 (OJ No L43, 15.2.1982, p.21); the Act concerning the Conditions of Accession and Adjustments to the Treaties-Accession of the Kingdom of Spain and the Portuguese Republic (OJ No L302, 15.11.1985, p. 158); Council Directive No 89/594/EEC of 30 October 1989 (OJ No L341, 23.11.1989, p.19); and Council Directive No 90/658/EEC of 4 December 1990 (OJ No L353, 17.12.1990, p.73); and was extended by Council Directive No 81/1057/EEC of 14 December 1981 (OJ No. L385, 31.12.1981, p.25).

⁴¹³ Council Directive No 75/363/EEC was amended by Council Directive No 82/76/EEC of 26 January 1982 (OJ No L43, 15.2.1982, p.21); and Council Directive No 89/594/EEC of 30 October 1989 (OJ No L341, 23.11.1989, p.19).

⁴¹⁴ Added by European Primary Medical Qualifications Regulations 1996/1591 Sch.2 para.13(3) (July 10, 1996).

⁴¹⁵ Directive 93/16/EEC was last amended by the Act annexed to the Treaty relating to the conditions of accession of the Czech Republic, the Republic of Estonia, the Republic of Cyprus, the Republic of Latvia, the Republic of Lithuania, the Republic of Hungary, the Republic of Malta, the Republic of Poland, the Republic of Slovenia and the Slovak Republic signed at Athens on 16th April 2003, and was repealed with effect from 20th October 2007 by Directive 2005/36/EC.

⁴¹⁶ Added by European Qualifications (Health and Social Care Professions) Regulations 2007/3101 Pt 2 reg.29(c) (December 3, 2007).

⁴¹⁷ Words substituted by Medical Act 1983 (Amendment) Order 2002/3135, Art 12(8).

⁴¹⁸ Words inserted by General and Specialist Medical Practice (Education, Training and Qualifications) Order 2010/234 Sch.1 para.16 (April 1, 2010).

appears, be construed as references to a [registered medical practitioner][417] [who holds a licence to practise].[418]

Merchant Shipping Act 1995 c. 21

PART IV

SAFETY

Control of, and returns as to, persons on ships

Returns of births and deaths in ships, etc.

A1–388   **108.**—(1) The Secretary of State may make regulations under the following provisions of this section in relation to births and deaths in the circumstances specified in those provisions.

(2) Regulations under this section may require the master of any United Kingdom ship to make a return to a superintendent or proper officer of—

(a) the birth or death of any person occurring in the ship; and

(b) the death of any person employed in the ship, wherever occurring outside the United Kingdom;

and to notify any such death to such person (if any) as the deceased may have named to him as his next of kin.

(3) Regulations under this section may require the master of any ship not registered in the United Kingdom which calls at a port in the United Kingdom in the course of or at the end of a voyage to make a return to a superintendent of any birth or death of a British citizen, a British Dependent Territories citizen or a British Overseas citizen which has occurred in the ship during the voyage.

(4) The returns referred to in subsections (2) and (3) above shall be for transmission to the Registrar General of Shipping and Seamen.

(5) Regulations under this section may require the Registrar General of Shipping and Seamen to record such information as may be specified in the regulations about such a death as is referred to in subsection (2) above in a case where—

(a) it appears to him that the master of the ship cannot perform his duty under that subsection because he has himself died or is incapacitated or missing; and

(b) any of the circumstances specified in subsection (6) below exist.

(6) Those circumstances are that—

(a) the death in question has been the subject of—

(i) an inquest held by a coroner,

(ii) an inquiry held in pursuance of section 271, or

(iii) an inquiry held in pursuance of the Fatal Accidents and Sudden Deaths Inquiry (Scotland) Act 1976;

and the findings of the inquest or inquiry include a finding that the death occurred;

(b) the deceased's body has been the subject of—

(i) a post-mortem examination in England and Wales, or

(ii) a preliminary investigation in Northern Ireland;

and in consequence the coroner [discontinues an investigation under Part 1 of the Coroners and Justice Act 2009 or, as the case may be, is satisfied that an inquest under the Coroners Act (Northern Ireland) 1959 is unnecessary][419]; or

(c) in Scotland, it does not appear to the Lord Advocate, under section 1(1)(b) of the Fatal Accidents and Sudden Deaths Inquiry (Scotland) Act 1976, to be expedient in the public interest that an inquiry under that Act should be held.

(7) Regulations under this section may require the Registrar General of Shipping and Seamen to send a certified copy of any return or record made thereunder to the Registrar General for England and Wales, the Registrar General of Births, Deaths and Marriages for Scotland or the Registrar General for Northern Ireland, as the case may require.

(8) The Registrar General to whom any such certified copies are sent—

(a) shall record the information contained therein in the marine register; and

(b) may record in the marine register such additional information as appears to him desirable for the purpose of ensuring the completeness and correctness of the register;

and the enactments relating to the registration of births and deaths in England, Scotland and Northern Ireland shall have effect as if the marine register were a register of births (other than stillbirths) or deaths or certified copies of entries in such a register had been transmitted to the Registrar General in accordance with those enactments.

(9) Regulations under this section may make a contravention of any provision thereof an offence punishable on summary conviction with a fine not exceeding level 2 on the standard scale or not exceeding a lesser amount.

(10) Regulations under this section may contain provisions authorising the registration of the following births and deaths occurring outside the United Kingdom in circumstances where no return is required to be made under the preceding provisions of this section—

(a) any birth or death of a British citizen, a British Dependent Territories citizen or a British Overseas citizen which occurs in a ship not registered in the United Kingdom;

(b) any death of any such citizen who has been employed in a ship not registered in the United Kingdom which occurs elsewhere than in the ship; and

(c) any death of a person who has been employed in a United Kingdom ship which occurs elsewhere than in the ship.

(11) References in this section to deaths occurring in a ship include references to deaths occurring in a ship's boat.

PART XI

ACCIDENT INVESTIGATIONS AND INQUIRIES

Inquiries into and reports on deaths and injuries

Transmission of particulars of certain deaths on ships

273.—[(1) Where—   A1–389

(a) an inquest is held into a death or subsection (2) below applies; and

---

[419] Words substituted by Coroners and Justice Act 2009, c. 25, Sch.21(1) para.33 (July 25, 2013).

(b) it appears to the coroner that the death in question is such as is mentioned in section 108(2) or in that subsection as extended (with or without amendments) by virtue of section 307,

it shall be the duty of the coroner to send to the Registrar General of Shipping and Seamen particulars in respect of the deceased of a kind prescribed by regulations made by the Secretary of State.

(2) This subsection applies where—

(a) in England and Wales, an investigation under Part 1 of the Coroners and Justice Act 2009 into a person's death is discontinued under section 4 of that Act (cause of death revealed by post-mortem examination); or

(b) in Northern Ireland, a preliminary investigation is made of a dead body as a result of which the coroner is satisfied that an inquest is unnecessary.][420];

PART XIII

SUPPLEMENTAL

Application of Act to certain descriptions of ships, etc.

Application of Act to non-United Kingdom ships

A1–390   **307.**—(1) The Secretary of State may make regulations specifying any description of non-United Kingdom ships and directing that such of the provisions of this Act and of instruments under this Act as may be specified in the regulations—

(a) shall extend to non-United Kingdom ships of that description and to masters and seamen employed in them, or

(b) shall so extend in such circumstances as may be so specified, with such modifications (if any) as may be so specified.

(2) Regulations under this section may contain such transitional, supplementary and consequential provisions as appear to the Secretary of State to be expedient.

(3) In this section "non-United Kingdom ships" means ships which are not registered in the United Kingdom.

Final provisions

Definitions

A1–391   **313.**—(1) In this Act, unless the context otherwise requires—

"British connection" has the meaning given in section 9(9);
"British citizen", "British Dependent Territories citizen", "British Overseas citizen" and "Commonwealth citizen" have the same meaning as in the British Nationality Act 1981;
"British ship" has the meaning given in section 1(1);
"commissioned military officer" means a commissioned officer in Her Majesty's land forces on full pay;
"commissioned naval officer" means a commissioned officer of Her Majesty's Navy on full pay;

---

[420] Existing s.273(1) renumbered as s.273(1), words are substituted and s.273(2) is added by Coroners and Justice Act 2009 c. 25 Sch.21(1) para.35 (July 25, 2013).

"conservancy authority" includes all persons entrusted with the function of conserving, maintaining or improving the navigation of a tidal water (as defined in section 255);

"consular officer", in relation to a foreign country, means the officer recognised by Her Majesty as a consular officer of that foreign country;

"contravention" includes failure to comply (and "failure" includes refusal);

"Departmental inspector" and "Departmental officer" have the meanings given in section 256(9);

"fishing vessel" means a vessel for the time being used (or, in the context of an application for registration, intended to be used) for, or in connection with fishing for sea fish other than a vessel used (or intended to be used) for fishing otherwise than for profit; and for the purposes of this definition "sea fish" includes shellfish, salmon and migratory trout (as defined by section 44 of the Fisheries Act 1981);

"foreign", in relation to a ship, means that it is neither a United Kingdom ship nor a small ship (as defined in section 1(2)) which is a British ship;

"Government ship" has the meaning given in section 308;

"harbour" includes estuaries, navigable rivers, piers, jetties and other works in or at which ships can obtain shelter or ship and unship goods or passengers;

["harbour authority" means, in relation to a harbour—

    (a) the person who is the statutory harbour authority for the harbour, or

    (b) if there is no statutory harbour authority for the harbour, the person (if any) who is the proprietor of the harbour or who is entrusted with the function of managing, maintaining or improving the harbour][421]

"master" includes every person (except a pilot) having command or charge of a ship and, in relation to a fishing vessel, means the skipper;

["Minister of the Crown" has the same meaning as in the Ministers of the Crown Act 1975;][422]

"port" includes place;

"proper officer" means a consular officer appointed by Her Majesty's Government in the United Kingdom and, in relation to a port in a country outside the United Kingdom which is not a foreign country, also any officer exercising in that port functions similar to those of a superintendent;

["qualifying foreign ship" has the meaning given in section 313A·][423]

"the register" and "registered" have the meaning given in section 23(1);

"the registrar", in relation to the registration of ships, has the meaning given in section 8;

"registration regulations" means regulations under section 10;

"relevant British possession" means—

    (a) the Isle of Man;

    (b) any of the Channel Islands; and

    (c) any colony;

"safety regulations" means regulations under section 85;

"seaman" includes every person (except masters and pilots) employed or engaged in any capacity on board any ship;

"ship" includes every description of vessel used in navigation;

["statutory harbour authority" means—

---

[421] Definition substituted by Merchant Shipping and Maritime Security Act 1997 c. 28 Sch.6 para.19(2)(a) (July 17, 1997).

[422] Definition added by Merchant Shipping and Maritime Security Act 1997 c. 28 Sch.6 para.19(2)(b) (March 23, 1997).

[423] Definition added by Merchant Shipping and Maritime Security Act 1997 c. 28 Sch.6 para.19(2)(c) (March 23, 1997).

(a) in relation to Great Britain, a harbour authority within the meaning of the Harbours Act 1964; and

(b) in relation to Northern Ireland, a harbour authority within the meaning of the Harbours Act (Northern Ireland) 1970.][424]

"superintendent" means a mercantile marine superintendent appointed under section 296;

"surveyor of ships" has the meaning given in section 256(9);

"the tonnage regulations" means regulations under section 19;

"United Kingdom ship" (and in Part V" United Kingdom fishing vessel") has the meaning given in section 1(3) except in the contexts there mentioned; and

"wages" includes emoluments.

(2) In this Act—

(a) "United Kingdom waters" means the sea or other waters within the seaward limits of the territorial sea of the United Kingdom; and

(b) "national waters", in relation to the United Kingdom, means United Kingdom waters landward of the baselines for measuring the breadth of its territorial sea.

[(2A) In this Act "right of innocent passage", "right of transit passage" and "straits used for international navigation" shall be construed in accordance with the United Nations Convention on the Law of the Sea 1982.][425]

(3) A vessel for the time being used (or intended to be used) wholly for the purpose of conveying persons wishing to fish for pleasure is not a fishing vessel.

Nuclear Installations Act 1965 c. 57

Miscellaneous And General

[Reporting of and inquiries into dangerous occurrences

A1–392   22.—(1) The provisions of this section apply where any prescribed occurrence happens—

(a) on a licensed site, or

(b) in the course of the carriage of nuclear matter on behalf of any person where a duty with respect to that carriage is imposed on that person by section 7, 10 or 11 of this Act.

(2) The licensee or other person mentioned in subsection (1) must ensure that the occurrence is reported without delay in the prescribed manner—

(a) to the appropriate national authority, and

(b) to such other persons, if any, as may be prescribed in relation to occurrences of that kind.

(3) A person who is required by virtue of subsection (2) to report an occurrence and who fails to do so is guilty of an offence.

---

[424] Definition added by Merchant Shipping and Maritime Security Act 1997 c. 28 Sch.6 para.19(2)(d) (July 17, 1997).

[425] Added by Merchant Shipping and Maritime Security Act 1997 c. 28 Sch.6 para.19(3) (March 23, 1997).

(4) A person convicted of an offence under subsection (3) in England and Wales or Scotland is liable—

(a) on conviction on indictment to imprisonment for a term not exceeding 2 years, or a fine, or both;

(b) on summary conviction to imprisonment for a term not exceeding 12 months, or a fine (in England and Wales) or a fine not exceeding £20,000 (in Scotland), or both.

(5) A person convicted of an offence under subsection (3) in Northern Ireland is liable on summary conviction to imprisonment for a term not exceeding 3 months, or a fine not exceeding level 3 on the standard scale, or both.

(6) In relation to an offence committed before the commencement of section 154(1) of the Criminal Justice Act 2003 (general limit on magistrates' court's power to imprison), the reference to 12 months in subsection (4)(b), as it has effect in England and Wales, is to be read as a reference to 6 months.

(7) Before exercising any function under subsection (1) or (2) in or as regards Scotland, the Secretary of State must consult the Scottish Ministers.

(8) Subsections (9) to (11) have effect only in relation to a prescribed occurrence which happens in Northern Ireland.

(9) The Secretary of State—

(a) may direct an inspector to make a special report with respect to the occurrence, and

(b) may cause any such report, or so much of it as it is not in the Secretary of State's opinion inconsistent with the interests of national security to disclose, to be made public at such time and in such manner as the Secretary of State considers appropriate.

(10) The Secretary of State may direct an inquiry to be held into the occurrence and its causes, circumstances and effects.

(11) Any such inquiry must be held—

(a) in accordance with the provisions of Schedule 2 to this Act, and

(b) in public, except where or to the extent that it appears to the Secretary of State expedient in the interests of national security to direct otherwise.][426]

Oaths Act 1978 c. 19

PART I

ENGLAND, WALES AND NORTHERN IRELAND

Manner of administration of oaths

1.—(1) Any oath may be administered and taken in England, Wales or Northern Ireland   **A1–393**
in the following form and manner–
The person taking the oath shall hold the New Testament, or, in the case of a Jew, the Old Testament, in his uplifted hand, and shall say or repeat after the officer administering the oath the words "I swear by Almighty God that . . . ", followed by the words of the oath prescribed by law.

---

[426] Substituted by Energy Act 2013 c. 32 Sch.12(2) para.23 (April 1, 2014).

(2) The officer shall (unless the person about to take the oath voluntarily objects thereto, or is physically incapable of so taking the oath) administer the oath in the form and manner aforesaid without question.

(3) In the case of a person who is neither a Christian nor a Jew, the oath shall be administered in any lawful manner.

(4) In this section "officer" means any person duly authorised to administer oaths.

Part II

United Kingdom

Oaths

Swearing with uplifted hand

A1–394   **3.** If any person to whom an oath is administered desires to swear with uplifted hand, in the form and manner in which an oath is usually administered in Scotland, he shall be permitted so to do, and the oath shall be administered to him in such form and manner without further question.

Validity of oaths

A1–395   **4.**—(1) In any case in which an oath may lawfully be and has been administered to any person, if it has been administered in a form and manner other than that prescribed by law, he is bound by it if it has been administered in such form and with such ceremonies as he may have declared to be binding.

(2) Where an oath has been duly administered and taken, the fact that the person to whom it was administered had, at the time of taking it, no religious belief, shall not for any purpose affect the validity of the oath.

Solemn affirmations

Making of solemn affirmations

A1–396   **5.**—(1) Any person who objects to being sworn shall be permitted to make his solemn affirmation instead of taking an oath.

(2) Subsection (1) above shall apply in relation to a person to whom it is not reasonably practicable without inconvenience or delay to administer an oath in the manner appropriate to his religious belief as it applies in relation to a person objecting to be sworn.

(3) A person who may be permitted under subsection (2) above to make his solemn affirmation may also be required to do so.

(4) A solemn affirmation shall be of the same force and effect as an oath.

Form of affirmation

A1–397   **6.**—(1) Subject to subsection (2) below, every affirmation shall be as follows–

"I,   do solemnly, sincerely and truly declare and affirm,"

and then proceed with the words of the oath prescribed by law, omitting any words of imprecation or calling to witness.

(2) Every affirmation in writing shall commence–

"I,   of   do solemnly and sincerely affirm," and the form in lieu of jurat shall be "Affirmed at   this   day of   19   , Before me."

Perjury Act 1911 c. 6

Perjury

1.—(1) If any person lawfully sworn as a witness or as an interpreter in a judicial   **A1–398**
proceedings wilfully makes a statement material in that proceeding, which he knows to be
false or does not believe to be true, he shall be guilty of perjury, and shall, on conviction
thereof on indictment, be liable to penal servitude for a term not exceeding seven years, or
to imprisonment [. . .]427 for a term not exceeding two years, or to a fine or to both such
penal servitude or imprisonment and fine.

(2) The expression "judicial proceeding" includes a proceeding before any court,
tribunal, or person having by law power to hear, receive, and examine evidence on oath.

(3) Where a statement made for the purposes of a judicial proceeding is not made before
the tribunal itself, but is made on oath before a person authorised by law to administer an
oath to the person who makes the statement, and to record or authenticate the statement,
it shall, for the purposes of this section, be treated as having been made in a judicial proceeding.

(4) A statement made by a person lawfully sworn in England for the purposes of a judicial
proceeding—

   (a) in another part of His Majesty's dominions; or

   (b) in a British tribunal lawfully constituted in any place by sea or land outside His
       Majesty's dominions; or

   (c) in a tribunal of any foreign state.

shall, for the purposes of this section, be treated as a statement made in a judicial proceeding
in England.

(5) Where, for the purposes of a judicial proceeding in England, a person is lawfully sworn
under the authority of an Act of Parliament—

   (a) in any other part of His Majesty's dominions; or

   (b) before a British tribunal or a British officer in a foreign country, or within the
       jurisdiction of the Admiralty of England;

a statement made by such person so sworn as aforesaid (unless the Act of Parliament under
which it was made otherwise specifically provides) shall be treated for the purposes of this
section as having been made in the judicial proceedings in England for the purposes whereof
it was made.

(6) The question whether a statement on which perjury is assigned was material is a
question of law to be determined by the court of trial.

---

427 Words omitted by virtue of Criminal Justice Act 1948 (c. 58), s. 1(2).

Police and Criminal Evidence Act 1984 c. 60

Part II

Powers Of Entry, Search And Seizure

Seizure etc.

General power of seizure etc.

A1–399   **19.**—(1) The powers conferred by subsections (2), (3) and (4) below are exercisable by a constable who is lawfully on any premises.

(2) The constable may seize anything which is on the premises if he has reasonable grounds for believing—

(a) that it has been obtained in consequence of the commission of an offence; and

(b) that it is necessary to seize it in order to prevent it being concealed, lost, damaged, altered or destroyed.

(3) The constable may seize anything which is on the premises if he has reasonable grounds for believing—

(a) that it is evidence in relation to an offence which he is investigating or any other offence; and

(b) that it is necessary to seize it in order to prevent the evidence being concealed, lost, altered or destroyed.

(4) The constable may require any information which is [stored in any electronic form][428] and is accessible from the premises to be produced in a form in which it can be taken away and in which it is visible and legible [or from which it can readily be produced in a visible and legible form][429] if he has reasonable grounds for believing—

(a) that—

    (i) it is evidence in relation to an offence which he is investigating or any other offence; or

    (ii) it has been obtained in consequence of the commission of an offence; and

(b) that it is necessary to do so in order to prevent it being concealed, lost, tampered with or destroyed.

(5) The powers conferred by this section are in addition to any power otherwise conferred.

(6) No power of seizure conferred on a constable under any enactment (including an enactment contained in an Act passed after this Act) is to be taken to authorise the seizure of an item which the constable exercising the power has reasonable grounds for believing to be subject to legal privilege.

---

[428] Words substituted by Criminal Justice and Police Act 2001 c. 16 Sch.2(2) para.13(2)(a) (April 1, 2003).

[429] Words inserted by Criminal Justice and Police Act 2001 c. 16 Sch.2(2) para.13(2)(a) (April 1, 2003).

Prison Act 1952 c. 52

Provision, maintenance and closing of prisons

Jurisdiction of sheriff, etc.

34.—(1) The transfer under the Prison Act 1877 of prisons and of the power and   **A1–400**
jurisdiction of prison authorities and of justices in sessions assembled and visiting justices
shall not be deemed to have affected the jurisdiction of any sheriff or coroner or, except to
the extent of that transfer, of any justice of the peace or other officer.

(2) The Secretary of State may by order direct that, for the purpose of any enactment, rule
of law or custom dependent on a prison being the prison of any county or place, any prison
situated in that county or in the county in which that place is situated, or any prison
provided by him in pursuance of this Act, shall be deemed to be the prison of that county
or place.

Public Health Act 1936 c. 49

PART VI

LABORATORIES, AMBULANCES, MORTUARIES, &C.

Provision of mortuaries and post-mortem rooms

198.—(1) A local authority or a parish council may, and if required by the Minister shall,   **A1–401**
provide—

(a) a mortuary for the reception of dead bodies before interment;

(b) a post-mortem room for the reception of dead bodies during the time required to
conduct any post-mortem examination ordered by a coroner or other duly
authorised authority;

and may make byelaws with respect to the management, and charges for the use, of any such
place provided by them.

(2) A local authority or parish council may provide for the interment of any dead body
which may be received into their mortuary.

Public Health (Control of Disease) Act 1984 c. 22

PART III

DISPOSAL OF DEAD BODIES

Burial and cremation

46.—(1) It shall be the duty of a local authority to cause to be buried or cremated the   **A1–402**
body of any person who has died or been found dead in their area, in any case where it
appears to the authority that no suitable arrangements for the disposal of the body have been
or are being made otherwise than by the authority.

(2) Any council which is the local authority for the purposes of the Local Authority
Social Services Act 1970 may cause to be buried or cremated the body of any deceased
person who immediately before his death was being provided with accommodation under
Part III of the National Assistance Act 1948 by, or by arrangement with, the council or was
living in a hostel provided by the council under section 29 of that Act.

(3) An authority shall not cause a body to be cremated under subsection (1) or (2) above where they have reason to believe that cremation would be contrary to the wishes of the deceased.

(4) Subsections (1) and (2) above do not affect any enactment regulating or authorising the burial, cremation or anatomical examination of the body of a deceased person.

(5) An authority may recover from the estate of the deceased person [. . .][430] expenses incurred under subsection (1) or subsection (2) above, [. . .].[431]

(6) Without prejudice to any other method of recovery, a sum due to an authority under subsection (5) above is recoverable summarily as a civil debt by proceedings brought within three years after the sum becomes due.

(7) The Secretary of State may cause such inquiries to be held as he may deem necessary or desirable for the purposes of this section.

(8) The Secretary of State may by order made by statutory instrument direct that this section, in its application to the Isles of Scilly, shall have effect subject to exceptions, adaptations and modifications.

PART III

DISPOSAL OF DEAD BODIES

Regulations about dead bodies

A1–403   **47.**—(1) The Secretary of State may make regulations imposing any conditions and restrictions—

(a) with respect to means of disposal of dead bodies otherwise than by burial or cremation,

(b) as to the period of time a body may be retained after death on any premises, or

(c) with respect to embalming or preservation,

which may appear to be desirable in the interests of public health or public safety.

(2) The power to make regulations under this section shall be exercisable by statutory instrument.

Removal of body to mortuary or for immediate burial

A1–404   **48.**—(1) If a justice of the peace (acting, if he deems it necessary, ex parte) is satisfied, on a certificate of the proper officer of the local authority for the district in which a dead body lies, that the retention of the body [in any place would endanger the health of any person],[432] he may order—

(a) that the body be removed by, and at the cost of, the local authority to a mortuary, and

(b) that the necessary steps be taken to secure that it is buried within a time limited by the order or, if he considers immediate burial necessary, immediately.

(2) Where an order is made under subsection (1) above, relatives or friends of the deceased person shall be deemed to comply with the order if they cause the body to be cremated within the time limited by the order or, as the case may be, immediately.

---

[430] Words repealed by Health and Social Care Act 2008, c. 14, Sch.15(5) para.1 (April 6, 2008).
[431] Words repealed by Social Security Act 1986, c. 50, Sch.11.
[432] Words substituted by Health and Social Care Act 2008 c. 14 Sch.11 para.7 (July 26, 2010 as SI 2010/1547).

(3) An order under this section shall be an authority to any officer named in it to do all acts necessary for giving effect to the order.

Road Traffic Act 1988 c. 52

PART VII

MISCELLANEOUS AND GENERAL

Inquiries

General provisions as to accident inquiries

181.—(1) Where an accident arises out of the presence of a [mechanically propelled vehicle][433] on a road, the Secretary of State may direct inquiry to be made into the cause of the accident.

A1-405

(2) Where any accident arising out of the presence of a [mechanically propelled vehicle][433] on a road has occurred, a person authorised by the Secretary of State in that behalf may, on production if so required of his authority, inspect any vehicle in connection with which the accident arose, and for that purpose may enter at any reasonable time any premises where the vehicle is.

(3) If a person obstructs a person so authorised in the performance of his duty under subsection (2) above, he is guilty of an offence.

(4) If in any case the Secretary of State considers that an inquiry to be made by him under this section should be made by means of the holding of a public inquiry, he may direct a public inquiry to be held.

(5) A report made by or to the Secretary of State as the result of an inquiry under this section shall not be used in evidence by or on behalf of a person by or against whom any legal proceedings are instituted in consequence of the accident to which the inquiry relates.

Special provisions as to accident inquiries in Greater London

182.—(1) Where, owing to the presence of a vehicle on a road, an accident occurs within Greater London and it appears to the Secretary of State that the sole or a contributory cause of the accident was—

A1-406

(a) the nature or character of the road or of the road surface, or

(b) a defect in the design or construction of the vehicle or in the materials used in the construction of the road or vehicle,

he may, if he thinks fit, cause an inquiry to be held into the cause of the accident.

(2) In this section "road" includes a highway and a bridge carrying a highway and any lane, mews, footway, square, court, alley or passage whether a thoroughfare or not.

---

[433] Words substituted by Road Traffic Act 1991 c. 40 Sch.4 para.76 (July 1, 1992).

Senior Courts Act 1981 c. 54

PART II

JURISDICTION

Chapter 2 The High Court

Other particular fields of jurisdiction

[Mandatory, prohibiting and quashing orders.][434]

A1–407   **29.**—[(1) The orders of mandamus, prohibition and certiorari shall be known instead as mandatory, prohibiting and quashing orders respectively.

(1A) The High Court shall have jurisdiction to make mandatory, prohibiting and quashing orders in those classes of case in which, immediately before 1st May 2004, it had jurisdiction to make orders of mandamus, prohibition and certiorari respectively.][435]

(2) Every such order shall be final, subject to any right of appeal therefrom.

(3) In relation to the jurisdiction of the Crown Court, other than its jurisdiction in matters relating to trial on indictment, the High Court shall have all such jurisdiction to make [mandatory, prohibiting or quashing orders][436] as the High Court possesses in relation to the jurisdiction of an inferior court.

[(3A) The High Court shall have no jurisdiction to make mandatory, prohibiting or quashing orders in relation to the jurisdiction of the Court Martial in matters relating to—

(a) trial by the Court Martial for an offence; or

(b) appeals from the Service Civilian Court.][437]

(4) The power of the High Court under any enactment to require justices of the peace or a judge or officer of [the county court][438] to do any act relating to the duties of their respective offices, or to require a magistrates' court to state a case for the opinion of the High Court, in any case where the High Court formerly had by virtue of any enactment jurisdiction to make a rule absolute, or an order, for any of those purposes, shall be exercisable by [mandatory order].[439]

[(5) In any statutory provision—

(a) references to mandamus or to a writ or order of mandamus shall be read as references to a mandatory order;

(b) references to prohibition or to a writ or order of prohibition shall be read as references to a prohibiting order;

---

[434] Words substituted by Civil Procedure (Modification of Supreme Court Act 1981) Order 2004/1033 art.3(e) (May 1, 2004).

[435] S.29(1)–(1A) substituted for s.29(1) by Civil Procedure (Modification of Supreme Court Act 1981) Order 2004/1033 art.3(a) (May 1, 2004).

[436] Words substituted by Civil Procedure (Modification of Supreme Court Act 1981) Order 2004/1033 art.3(b) (May 1, 2004).

[437] Substituted by Armed Forces Act 2006 c. 52 Sch.16 para.93 (October 31, 2009).

[438] Words substituted by Crime and Courts Act 2013 c. 22 Sch.9(3) para.52(1)(b) (April 22, 2014: substitution has effect as SI 2014/954 subject to savings and transitional provisions specified in 2013 c.22 s.15 and Sch.8 and transitional provision specified in SI 2014/954 arts 2(c) and 3).

[439] Words substituted by Civil Procedure (Modification of Supreme Court Act 1981) Order 2004/1033 art.3(c) (May 1, 2004).

(c) references to certiorari or to a writ or order of certiorari shall be read as references to a quashing order; and

(d) references to the issue or award of a writ of mandamus, prohibition or certiorari shall be read as references to the making of the corresponding mandatory, prohibiting or quashing order.][440]

[(6) In subsection (3) the reference to the Crown Court's jurisdiction in matters relating to trial on indictment does not include its jurisdiction relating to [requirements to make payments under regulations under section 23 or 24 of the Legal Aid, Sentencing and Punishment of Offenders Act 2012].[441]][442]

PART II

JURISDICTION

Other particular fields of jurisdiction

Injunctions to restrain persons from acting in offices in which they are not entitled to act

30.—(1) Where a person not entitled to do so acts in an office to which this section applies, the High Court may—   **A1–408**

(a) grant an injunction restraining him from so acting; and

(b) if the case so requires, declare the office to be vacant.

(2) This section applies to any substantive office of a public nature and permanent character which is held under the Crown or which has been created by any statutory provision or royal charter.

Application for judicial review

31.—(1) An application to the High Court for one or more of the following forms of relief, namely—   **A1–409**

[(a) a mandatory, prohibiting or quashing order;][443]

(b) a declaration or injunction under subsection (2); or

(c) an injunction under section 30 restraining a person not entitled to do so from acting in an office to which that section applies,

shall be made in accordance with rules of court by a procedure to be known as an application for judicial review.

(2) A declaration may be made or an injunction granted under this subsection in any case where an application for judicial review, seeking that relief, has been made and the High Court considers that, having regard to—

---

[440] Substituted by Civil Procedure (Modification of Supreme Court Act 1981) Order 2004/1033 art.3(d) (May 1, 2004).

[441] Words substituted by Legal Aid, Sentencing and Punishment of Offenders Act 2012 c. 10 Sch.5(1) para.21 (April 1, 2013 subject to saving and transitional provisions as specified in SI 2013/534 regs 6-13).

[442] Added by Access to Justice Act 1999 c. 22 Sch.4 para.23 (April 2, 2001 subject to transitional provisions specified in SI 2001/916 Sch.2 para.2).

[443] Substituted by Civil Procedure (Modification of Supreme Court Act 1981) Order 2004/1033 art.4(a) (May 1, 2004).

(a) the nature of the matters in respect of which relief may be granted by [mandatory, prohibiting or quashing orders][444];

(b) the nature of the persons and bodies against whom relief may be granted by such orders; and

(c) all the circumstances of the case,

it would be just and convenient for the declaration to be made or the injunction to be granted, as the case may be.

(3) No application for judicial review shall be made unless the leave of the High Court has been obtained in accordance with rules of court; and the court shall not grant leave to make such an application unless it considers that the applicant has a sufficient interest in the matter to which the application relates.

[(4) On an application for judicial review the High Court may award to the applicant damages, restitution or the recovery of a sum due if—

(a) the application includes a claim for such an award arising from any matter to which the application relates; and

(b) the court is satisfied that such an award would have been made if the claim had been made in an action begun by the applicant at the time of making the application.][445]

[(5) If, on an application for judicial review, the High Court quashes the decision to which the application relates, it may in addition—

(a) remit the matter to the court, tribunal or authority which made the decision, with a direction to reconsider the matter and reach a decision in accordance with the findings of the High Court, or

(b) substitute its own decision for the decision in question.

(5A) But the power conferred by subsection (5)(b) is exercisable only if—

(a) the decision in question was made by a court or tribunal,

(b) the decision is quashed on the ground that there has been an error of law, and

(c) without the error, there would have been only one decision which the court or tribunal could have reached.

(5B) Unless the High Court otherwise directs, a decision substituted by it under subsection (5)(b) has effect as if it were a decision of the relevant court or tribunal.][446]

(6) Where the High Court considers that there has been undue delay in making an application for judicial review, the court may refuse to grant—

(a) leave for the making of the application; or

(b) any relief sought on the application,

---

[444] Words substituted by Civil Procedure (Modification of Supreme Court Act 1981) Order 2004/1033 art.4(b) (May 1, 2004).
[445] Substituted by Civil Procedure (Modification of Supreme Court Act 1981) Order 2004/1033 art.4(c) (May 1, 2004).
[446] S.31(5)–(5B) substituted for s.31(5) by Tribunals, Courts and Enforcement Act 2007 c. 15 Pt 7 s.141 (April 6, 2008).

if it considers that the granting of the relief sought would be likely to cause substantial hardship to, or substantially prejudice the rights of, any person or would be detrimental to good administration.

(7) Subsection (6) is without prejudice to any enactment or rule of court which has the effect of limiting the time within which an application for judicial review may be made.

[Transfer of judicial review applications to Upper Tribunal

31A.—(1) This section applies where an application is made to the High Court—   A1–410

(a) for judicial review, or

(b) for permission to apply for judicial review.

(2) If Conditions 1, 2 [and 3][447] are met, the High Court must by order transfer the application to the Upper Tribunal.
[. . .][448]

(3) If Conditions 1 [and 2][449] are met, but Condition 3 is not, the High Court may by order transfer the application to the Upper Tribunal if it appears to the High Court to be just and convenient to do so.

(4) Condition 1 is that the application does not seek anything other than—

(a) relief under section 31(1)(a) and (b);

(b) permission to apply for relief under section 31(1)(a) and (b);

(c) an award under section 31(4);

(d) interest;

(e) costs.

(5) Condition 2 is that the application does not call into question anything done by the Crown Court.

(6) Condition 3 is that the application falls within a class specified under section 18(6) of the Tribunals, Courts and Enforcement Act 2007.
[. . .][450][451]

---

[447] Words substituted by Crime and Courts Act 2013 c. 22 Pt 2 s.22(1)(a) (November 1, 2013: substitution has effect as SI 2013/1725 as amended by SI 2013/2200 subject to savings and transitional provisions specified in 2013 c.22 s.15 and Sch.8).

[448] Repealed by Crime and Courts Act 2013 c. 22 Pt 2 s.22(1)(b) (November 1, 2013: repeal has effect as SI 2013/1725 as amended by SI 2013/2200 subject to savings and transitional provisions specified in 2013 c.22 s.15 and Sch.8).

[449] Words substituted by Crime and Courts Act 2013 c. 22 Pt 2 s.22(1)(c) (November 1, 2013: substitution has effect as SI 2013/1725 as amended by SI 2013/2200 subject to savings and transitional provisions specified in 2013 c.22 s.15 and Sch.8).

[450] Repealed by Crime and Courts Act 2013 c. 22 Pt 2 s.22(1)(d) (November 1, 2013: repeal has effect as SI 2013/1725 as amended by SI 2013/2200 subject to savings and transitional provisions specified in 2013 c.22 s.15 and Sch.8).

[451] Added by Tribunals, Courts and Enforcement Act 2007 c. 15 Pt 1 c.2 s.19(1) (November 3, 2008).

Chapter 4 General Provisions

Costs

[Costs in civil division of Court of Appeal, High Court and county courts

A1–411   **51.**—(1) Subject to the provisions of this or any other enactment and to rules of court, the costs of and incidental to all proceedings in—

(a) the civil division of the Court of Appeal;

(b) the High Court; [. . .][452]

[(ba) the family court; and][2]

(c) [the][453] county court,

shall be in the discretion of the court.

(2) Without prejudice to any general power to make rules of court, such rules may make provision for regulating matters relating to the costs of those proceedings including, in particular, prescribing scales of costs to be paid to legal or other representatives [or for securing that the amount awarded to a party in respect of the costs to be paid by him to such representatives is not limited to what would have been payable by him to them if he had not been awarded costs].[454]

(3) The court shall have full power to determine by whom and to what extent the costs are to be paid.

(4) In subsections (1) and (2) "proceedings" includes the administration of estates and trusts.

(5) Nothing in subsection (1) shall alter the practice in any criminal cause, or in bankruptcy.

(6) In any proceedings mentioned in subsection (1), the court may disallow, or (as the case may be) order the legal or other representative concerned to meet, the whole of any wasted costs or such part of them as may be determined in accordance with rules of court.

(7) In subsection (6), "wasted costs" means any costs incurred by a party—

(a) as a result of any improper, unreasonable or negligent act or omission on the part of any legal or other representative or any employee of such a representative; or

(b) which, in the light of any such act or omission occurring after they were incurred, the court considers it is unreasonable to expect that party to pay.

(8) Where—

(a) a person has commenced proceedings in the High Court; but

---

[452] Added by Crime and Courts Act 2013 c. 22 Sch.10(2) para.61(2) (April 22, 2014: insertion has effect as SI 2014/954 subject to savings and transitional provisions specified in 2013 c.22 s.15 and Sch.8 and transitional provision specified in SI 2014/954 arts 2(d) and 3).

[453] Word substituted by Crime and Courts Act 2013 c. 22 Sch.9(2) para.29(a) (April 22, 2014: substitution has effect as SI 2014/954 subject to savings and transitional provisions specified in 2013 c.22 s.15 and Sch.8 and transitional provision specified in SI 2014/954 arts 2(c) and 3).

[454] Words added by Access to Justice Act 1999 c. 22 Pt II s.31 (June 2, 2003).

(b) those proceedings should, in the opinion of the court, have been commenced in [the county court][455] [or family court][456] in accordance with any provision made under section 1 of the Courts and Legal Services Act 1990 or by or under any other enactment,

the person responsible for determining the amount which is to be awarded to that person by way of costs shall have regard to those circumstances.

(9) Where, in complying with subsection (8), the responsible person reduces the amount which would otherwise be awarded to the person in question—

(a) the amount of that reduction shall not exceed 25 per cent; and

(b) on any taxation of the costs payable by that person to his legal representative, regard shall be had to the amount of the reduction.

(10) The Lord Chancellor may by order amend subsection (9)(a) by substituting, for the percentage for the time being mentioned there, a different percentage.

(11) Any such order shall be made by statutory instrument and may make such transitional or incidental provision as the Lord Chancellor considers expedient.

(12) No such statutory instrument shall be made unless a draft of the instrument has been approved by both Houses of Parliament.

(13) In this section "legal or other representative", in relation to a party to proceedings, means any person exercising a right of audience or right to conduct litigation on his behalf.][457]

Treasure Act 1996 c. 24

Meaning of "treasure"

Meaning of "treasure"

1.—(1) Treasure is—   A1–412

(a) any object at least 300 years old when found which—

    (i) is not a coin but has metallic content of which at least 10 per cent by weight is precious metal;

    (ii) when found, is one of at least two coins in the same find which are at least 300 years old at that time and have that percentage of precious metal; or

    (iii) when found, is one of at least ten coins in the same find which are at least 300 years old at that time;

(b) any object at least 200 years old when found which belongs to a class designated under section 2(1);

(c) any object which would have been treasure trove if found before the commencement of section 4;

(d) any object which, when found, is part of the same find as—

---

[455] Words substituted by Crime and Courts Act 2013 c. 22 Sch.9(2) para.29(b) (April 22, 2014: substitution has effect as SI 2014/954 subject to savings and transitional provisions specified in 2013 c.22 s.15 and Sch.8 and transitional provision specified in SI 2014/954 arts 2(c) and 3).

[456] Words inserted by Crime and Courts Act 2013 c. 22 Sch.10(2) para.61(3) (April 22, 2014: insertion has effect as SI 2014/954 subject to savings and transitional provisions specified in 2013 c.22 s.15 and Sch.8 and transitional provision specified in SI 2014/954 arts 2(d) and 3).

[457] Substituted by Courts and Legal Services Act 1990 c. 41 Pt I s.4(1) (October 1, 1991).

(i) an object within paragraph (a), (b) or (c) found at the same time or earlier; or

(ii) an object found earlier which would be within paragraph (a) or (b) if it had been found at the same time.

(2) Treasure does not include objects which are—

(a) unworked natural objects, or

(b) minerals as extracted from a natural deposit,

or which belong to a class designated under section 2(2).

Power to alter meaning

A1–413   **2.**—(1) The Secretary of State may by order, for the purposes of section 1(1)(b), designate any class of object which he considers to be of outstanding historical, archaeological or cultural importance.

(2) The Secretary of State may by order, for the purposes of section 1(2), designate any class of object which (apart from the order) would be treasure.

(3) An order under this section shall be made by statutory instrument.

(4) No order is to be made under this section unless a draft of the order has been laid before Parliament and approved by a resolution of each House.

Supplementary

A1–414   **3.**—(1) This section supplements section 1.

(2) "Coin" includes any metal token which was, or can reasonably be assumed to have been, used or intended for use as or instead of money.

(3) "Precious metal" means gold or silver.

(4) When an object is found, it is part of the same find as another object if—

(a) they are found together,

(b) the other object was found earlier in the same place where they had been left together,

(c) the other object was found earlier in a different place, but they had been left together and had become separated before being found.

(5) If the circumstances in which objects are found can reasonably be taken to indicate that they were together at some time before being found, the objects are to be presumed to have been left together, unless shown not to have been.

(6) An object which can reasonably be taken to be at least a particular age is to be presumed to be at least that age, unless shown not to be.

(7) An object is not treasure if it is wreck within the meaning of Part IX of the Merchant Shipping Act 1995.

Ownership of treasure which is found

A1–415   **4.**—(1) When treasure is found, it vests, subject to prior interests and rights—

(a) in the franchisee, if there is one;

(b) otherwise, in the Crown.

(2) Prior interests and rights are any which, or which derive from any which—

(a) were held when the treasure was left where it was found, or

(b) if the treasure had been moved before being found, were held when it was left where it was before being moved.

(3) If the treasure would have been treasure trove if found before the commencement of this section, neither the Crown nor any franchisee has any interest in it or right over it except in accordance with this Act.

(4) This section applies—

(a) whatever the nature of the place where the treasure was found, and

(b) whatever the circumstances in which it was left (including being lost or being left with no intention of recovery).

Meaning of "franchisee"

5.—(1) The franchisee for any treasure is the person who—

(a) was, immediately before the commencement of section 4, or

(b) apart from this Act, as successor in title, would have been,

the franchisee of the Crown in right of treasure trove for the place where the treasure was found.

(2) It is as franchisees in right of treasure trove that Her Majesty and the Duke of Cornwall are to be treated as having enjoyed the rights to treasure trove which belonged respectively to the Duchy of Lancaster and the Duchy of Cornwall immediately before the commencement of section 4.

Treasure vesting in the Crown

6.—(1) Treasure vesting in the Crown under this Act is to be treated as part of the hereditary revenues of the Crown to which section 1 of the Civil List Act 1952 applies (surrender of hereditary revenues to the Exchequer).

(2) Any such treasure may be transferred, or otherwise disposed of, in accordance with directions given by the Secretary of State.

(3) The Crown's title to any such treasure may be disclaimed at any time by the Secretary of State.

(4) If the Crown's title is disclaimed, the treasure—

(a) is deemed not to have vested in the Crown under this Act, and

(b) without prejudice to the interests or rights of others, may be delivered to any person in accordance with the code published under section 11.

Coroners' jurisdiction

Jurisdiction of coroners

7.—(1) The jurisdiction of coroners which is referred to in section 30 of the Coroners Act 1988 (treasure) is exercisable in relation to anything which is treasure for the purposes of this Act.

(2) That jurisdiction is not exercisable for the purposes of the law relating to treasure trove in relation to anything found after the commencement of section 4.

(3) The Act of 1988 and anything saved by virtue of section 36(5) of that Act (saving for existing law and practice etc.) has effect subject to this section.

(4) An inquest held by virtue of this section is to be held without a jury, unless the coroner orders otherwise.

Duty of finder to notify coroner

A1–419   8.—(1) A person who finds an object which he believes or has reasonable grounds for believing is treasure must notify the coroner for the district in which the object was found before the end of the notice period.

(2) The notice period is fourteen days beginning with—

(a) the day after the find; or

(b) if later, the day on which the finder first believes or has reason to believe the object is treasure.

(3) Any person who fails to comply with subsection (1) is guilty of an offence and liable on summary conviction to—

(a) imprisonment for a term not exceeding three months;

(b) a fine of an amount not exceeding level 5 on the standard scale; or

(c) both.

(4) In proceedings for an offence under this section, it is a defence for the defendant to show that he had, and has continued to have, a reasonable excuse for failing to notify the coroner.

(5) If the office of coroner for a district is vacant, the person acting as coroner for that district is the coroner for the purposes of subsection (1).

[Duty to notify coroner of acquisition of certain objects

A1–420   8A.—(1) A person who—

(a) acquires property in an object, and

(b) believes or has reasonable grounds for believing—

(i) that the object is treasure, and

(ii) that notification in respect of the object has not been given under section 8(1) or this subsection,

must notify the Coroner for Treasure before the end of the notice period.

(2) The notice period is fourteen days beginning with—

(a) the day after the person acquires property in the object; or

(b) if later, the day on which the person first believes or has reason to believe—

(i) that the object is treasure; and

(ii) that notification in respect of the object has not been given under section 8(1) or subsection (1) of this section.

(3) Any person who fails to comply with subsection (1) is guilty of an offence if—

(a) notification in respect of the object has not been given under section 8(1) or subsection (1) of this section; and

(b) there has been no investigation in relation to the object.

(4) Any person guilty of an offence under this section is liable on summary conviction to—

(a) imprisonment for a term not exceeding 51 weeks;

(b) a fine of an amount not exceeding level 5 on the standard scale; or

(c) both.

(5) In proceedings for an offence under this section, it is a defence for the defendant to show that he had, and has continued to have, a reasonable excuse for failing to notify the Coroner for Treasure.

(6) If the office of Coroner for Treasure is vacant, notification under subsection (1) must be given to an Assistant Coroner for Treasure.

(7) In determining for the purposes of this section whether a person has acquired property in an object, section 4 is to be disregarded.

(8) For the purposes of an investigation in relation to an object in respect of which notification has been given under subsection (1), the object is to be presumed, in the absence of evidence to the contrary, to have been found in England and Wales after the commencement of section 4.

(9) This section has effect subject to section 8B.

(10) In this section "investigation" means an investigation under section 26 of the Coroners and Justice Act 2009.

(11) [Applies to Northern Ireland]][458]

[Notice under section 8 or 8A to designated officer

8B.—(1) A requirement under section 8 or 8A to give a notification to the Coroner for **A1–421** Treasure (or an Assistant Coroner for Treasure) may, if the relevant place falls within an area for which there is a designated officer, be complied with by giving the notification to that officer.

(2) A designated officer must notify the Coroner for Treasure of all notifications given under subsection (1).

(3) If the office of Coroner for Treasure is vacant, notification under subsection (2) must be given to an Assistant Coroner for Treasure.

(4) In this section—

"designated officer" means an officer designated by an order made by statutory instrument by the Secretary of State;
"the relevant place" means—

> (a) in relation to a requirement under section 8, the place where the object in question was found;
> (b) in relation to a requirement under section 8A, the place where the treasure in question is located.

(5) A statutory instrument containing an order under this section shall be subject to annulment in pursuance of a resolution of either House of Parliament.

(6) In its application to Northern Ireland this section has effect as if—

> (a) in subsection (1), for "the Coroner for Treasure (or an Assistant Coroner for Treasure)" there were substituted "a coroner";
> (b) in subsection (2), for "Coroner for Treasure" there were substituted "coroner for the district in which the relevant place falls";
> (c) in subsection (3), for the words from "Coroner for Treasure" to "Assistant Coroner for Treasure" there were substituted "coroner for a district is vacant, the person acting as coroner for that district is the coroner for the purposes of subsection (2)".][459]

---

[458] Added by Coroners and Justice Act 2009 c. 25 Pt 1 c.4 s.30(1) (date to be appointed).
[459] Added by Coroners and Justice Act 2009 c. 25 Sch.21(1) para.40 (date to be appointed).

[Offences under section 8 or 8A: period for bringing proceedings

A1–422   8C.—(1) Proceedings for an offence under section 8 or 8A may be brought within the period of six months from the date on which evidence sufficient in the opinion of the prosecutor to warrant the proceedings came to the prosecutor's knowledge; but no such proceedings may be brought by virtue of this subsection more than three years after the commission of the offence.

(2) For the purposes of subsection (1)—

(a) a certificate signed by or on behalf of the prosecutor and stating the date on which the evidence referred to in that subsection came to the prosecutor's knowledge shall be conclusive evidence to that effect; and

(b) a certificate to that effect and purporting to be so signed shall be deemed to be so signed unless the contrary is proved.][460]

Procedure for inquests

A1–423   9.—(1) In this section, "inquest" means an inquest held under section 7.

(2) A coroner proposing to conduct an inquest must notify—

(a) the British Museum, if his district is in England; or

(b) the National Museum of Wales, if it is in Wales.

(3) Before conducting the inquest, the coroner must take reasonable steps to notify—

(a) any person who it appears to him may have found the treasure; and

(b) any person who, at the time the treasure was found, occupied land which it appears to him may be where it was found.

(4) During the inquest the coroner must take reasonable steps to notify any such person not already notified.

(5) Before or during the inquest, the coroner must take reasonable steps—

(a) to obtain from any person notified under subsection (3) or (4) the names and addresses of interested persons; and

(b) to notify any interested person whose name and address he obtains.

(6) The coroner must take reasonable steps to give any interested person notified under subsection (3), (4) or (5) an opportunity to examine witnesses at the inquest.

(7) In subsections (5) and (6), "interested person" means a person who appears to the coroner to be likely to be concerned with the inquest—

(a) as the finder of the treasure or otherwise involved in the find;

(b) as the occupier, at the time the treasure was found, of the land where it was found, or

(c) as having had an interest in that land at that time or since.

[Procedure for inquests: Northern Ireland

A1–424   9A. [*Applies to Northern Ireland*].][461]

---

[460] Added by Coroners and Justice Act 2009 c. 25 Sch.21(1) para.40 (date to be appointed).
[461] Ss 9 and 9A substituted for s.9 by Coroners and Justice Act 2009 c. 25 Sch.21(1) para.41 (date to be appointed).

Rewards, codes of practice and report

Rewards

10.—(1) This section applies if treasure—   A1–425

    (a) has vested in the Crown under section 4, and

    (b) is to be transferred to a museum.

(2) The Secretary of State must determine whether a reward is to be paid by the museum before the transfer.

(3) If the Secretary of State determines that a reward is to be paid, he must also determine, in whatever way he thinks fit—

    (a) the treasure's market value;

    (b) the amount of the reward;

    (c) to whom the reward is to be payable; and

    (d) if it is to be payable to more than one person, how much each is to receive.

(4) The total reward must not exceed the treasure's market value.

(5) The reward may be payable to—

    (a) the finder or any other person involved in the find;

    (b) the occupier of the land at the time of the find;

    (c) any person who had an interest in the land at that time, or has had such an interest at any time since then.

(6) Payment of the reward is not enforceable against a museum or the Secretary of State.

(7) In a determination under this section, the Secretary of State must take into account anything relevant in the code of practice issued under section 11.

(8) This section also applies in relation to treasure which has vested in a franchisee under section 4, if the franchisee makes a request to the Secretary of State that it should.

Codes of practice

11.—(1) The Secretary of State must—   A1–426

    (a) prepare a code of practice relating to treasure;

    (b) keep the code under review; and

    (c) revise it when appropriate.

(2) The code must, in particular, set out the principles and practice to be followed by the Secretary of State—

    (a) when considering to whom treasure should be offered;

    (b) when making a determination under section 10; and

    (c) where the Crown's title to treasure is disclaimed.

(3) The code may include guidance for—

    (a) those who search for or find treasure; and

(b) museums and others who exercise functions in relation to treasure.

(4) Before preparing the code or revising it, the Secretary of State must consult such persons appearing to him to be interested as he thinks appropriate.

(5) A copy of the code and of any proposed revision of the code shall be laid before Parliament.

(6) Neither the code nor any revision shall come into force until approved by a resolution of each House of Parliament.

(7) The Secretary of State must publish the code in whatever way he considers appropriate for bringing it to the attention of those interested.

(8) If the Secretary of State considers that different provision should be made for—

(a) England and Wales, and

(b) Northern Ireland,

or that different provision should otherwise be made for treasure found in different areas, he may prepare two or more separate codes.

Report on operation of Act

A1–427   12. As soon as reasonably practicable after each anniversary of the coming into force of this section, the Secretary of State shall lay before Parliament a report on the operation of this Act in the preceding year.

Miscellaneous

Application of Act to Northern Ireland

A1–428   13. [*Applies to Northern Ireland*]

Consequential amendments

A1–429   14.—[*Makes various consequential amendments*]

Short title, commencement and extent

A1–430   15.—(1) This Act may be cited as the Treasure Act 1996.

(2) This Act comes into force on such day as the Secretary of State may by order made by statutory instrument appoint; and different days may be appointed for different purposes.

(3) This Act does not extend to Scotland.

Treasury Solicitor Act 1876 c. 18

Grant of administration to Solicitor of Treasury

A1–431   2. Where, by reason of Her Majesty having become entitled in right of Her Crown to the personal estate of an intestate or otherwise, any court has power to grant administration of the personal estate of any deceased person to a nominee of Her Majesty, and Her Majesty, by warrant under Her Royal Sign Manual, is pleased to nominate for that purpose the Treasury Solicitor for the time being, the court may grant such administration for the use of Her Majesty to the Treasury Solicitor (by his official name) and his successors, or, if the warrant so provide, to some person nominated in that behalf by the Treasury Solicitor.

A royal warrant may nominate the Treasury Solicitor for the purposes of this section, either in any particular case or class of cases, or in all cases, and may limit such nomination to be during Her Majesty's pleasure, or during any limited period or otherwise, as to Her

Majesty may seem fit; and may, if to Her Majesty seem fit, authorise the Treasury Solicitor to nominate some other person to take out the administration in any particular case or class of cases.

The administration so granted to the Treasury Solicitor, and the office of administrator under such grant, and all the estate, rights, duties, and liabilities of such administrator, shall notwithstanding any change in the person who is Treasury Solicitor, be vested in and imposed on the Treasury Solicitor for the time being without any further grant of administration.

Provided that nothing in this section shall affect any limitation, in duration or otherwise, contained in the grant, or any right of any court to revoke such grant.

[. . .][462]

Definitions

7. In this Act:—   A1–432
[. . .][463]

The expression "administration" means letters of administration of the personal estate and effects of a deceased person, whether general or limited, or with the will annexed or otherwise, and includes confirmation in Scotland.

Tribunals, Courts and Enforcement Act 2007 c. 15

PART 2

JUDICIAL APPOINTMENTS

Judicial appointments: "judicial-appointment eligibility condition"

50.—(1) Subsection (2) applies for the purposes of any statutory provision that—   A1–433

(a) relates to an office or other position, and

(b) refers to a person who satisfies the judicial-appointment eligibility condition on an N-year basis (where N is the number stated in the provision).

(2) A person satisfies that condition on an N-year basis if—

(a) the person has a relevant qualification, and

(b) the total length of the person's qualifying periods is at least N years.

(3) In subsection (2) "qualifying period", in relation to a person, means a period during which the person—

(a) has a relevant qualification, and

(b) gains experience in law (see section 52).

(4) For the purposes of subsections (2) and (3), a person has a relevant qualification if the person—

(a) is a solicitor or a barrister (but see section 51), or

---

[462] Words repealed by Administration of Estates Act 1971 (c. 25), Sch. 2 Pt. II.
[463] Definition of "the Treasury" repealed by Statute Law Revision Act 1894 (c. 56).

(b) holds a qualification that under section 51(1) is a relevant qualification in relation to the office, or other position, concerned.

(5) In this section—

"barrister" means barrister in England and Wales;
"solicitor" means solicitor of the Senior Courts of England and Wales;
"statutory provision" means—

(a) a provision of an Act, or
(b) a provision of subordinate legislation (within the meaning given by section 21(1) of the Interpretation Act 1978 (c. 30)).

(6) Schedule 10, which makes amendments—
for the purpose of substituting references to satisfying the judicial-appointment eligibility condition in place of references to having a qualification mentioned in section 71 of the Courts and Legal Services Act 1990 (c. 41),
for the purpose of reducing qualifying periods for eligibility for appointment to certain judicial offices from ten and seven years to seven and five years respectively, and
for connected purposes, has effect.

(7) At any time before the coming into force of section 59(1) of the Constitutional Reform Act 2005 (c. 4) (renaming of Supreme Court), the reference to the Senior Courts in subsection (5) is to be read as a reference to the Supreme Court.

"Relevant qualification" in section 50: further provision

A1–434
51.—(1) The Lord Chancellor may by order provide for a qualification specified in the order to be a relevant qualification for the purposes of section 50(2) and (3) in relation to an office or other position specified in the order.

(2) A qualification may be specified under subsection (1) only if it is one [awarded by a body which, for the purposes of the Legal Services Act 2007, is an approved regulator in relation to the exercise of a right of audience or the conduct of litigation (within the meaning of that Act).]⁴⁶⁴
[. . .]⁴⁶⁴

(3) An order under subsection (1) may, in relation to a qualification specified in the order, include provision as to when a person who holds the qualification is, for the purposes of section 50, to be taken first to have held it.

(4) Where—

(a) a qualification is specified under subsection (1),

(b) the qualification is one awarded by a body such as is mentioned in subsection [(2)],⁴⁶⁵ and

(c) after the qualification is specified under subsection (1), it becomes the case that [, for the purposes of the Legal Services Act 2007, the body–]⁴⁶⁶

[(i) is not an approved regulator in relation to the exercise of a right of audience (within the meaning of that Act), and
(ii) is not an approved regulator in relation to the conduct of litigation (within the meaning of that Act).]⁴⁶⁶

the provision under subsection (1) specifying the qualification ceases to have effect, subject to any provision made under [section 46 of the Legal Services Act 2007

---

⁴⁶⁴ Words substituted by Legal Services Act 2007 c. 29 Sch.21 para.162(2) (January 1, 2010).
⁴⁶⁵ Word substituted by Legal Services Act 2007 c. 29 Sch.21 para.162(3)(a) (January 1, 2010).
⁴⁶⁶ Words and s.51(4)(c)(i)-(ii) substituted by Legal Services Act 2007 c. 29 Sch.21 para.162(3)(b) (January 1, 2010).

(transitional etc. provision in consequence of cancellation of designation as approved regulator).].[467]

(5) For the purposes of section 50 and this section, a person shall be taken first to become a solicitor when the person's name is entered on the roll kept under section 6 of the Solicitors Act 1974 (c. 47) (Law Society to keep list of all solicitors) for the first time after the person's admission as a solicitor.

(6) For the purposes of section 50 and this section, a person shall be taken first to become a barrister—

(a) when the person completes pupillage in connection with becoming a barrister, or

(b) in the case of a person not required to undertake pupillage in connection with becoming a barrister, when the person is called to the Bar of England and Wales.

(7) For the purposes of section 50—

(a) a barrister,

(b) a solicitor, or

(c) a person who holds a qualification specified under subsection (1),

shall be taken not to have a relevant qualification at times when, as a result of disciplinary proceedings, he is prevented from practising as a barrister or (as the case may be) as a solicitor or as a holder of the specified qualification.

(8) The Lord Chancellor may by order make provision supplementing or amending subsections (5) to (7).

(9) Before making an order under subsection (1) or (8), the Lord Chancellor must consult—

(a) the Lord Chief Justice of England and Wales, and

(b) the Judicial Appointments Commission.

(10) The Lord Chief Justice of England and Wales may nominate a judicial office holder (as defined in section 109(4) of the Constitutional Reform Act 2005 (c. 4)) to exercise his function under subsection (9)(a).

(11) In this section—

"barrister" means barrister in England and Wales;
"solicitor" means solicitor of the Senior Courts of England and Wales.

(12) Power to make an order under this section is exercisable by statutory instrument.

(13) An order under this section may make different provision for different purposes.

(14) No order may be made under this section unless a draft of the statutory instrument containing it (whether alone or with other provision) has been laid before, and approved by a resolution of, each House of Parliament.

(15) At any time before the coming into force of section 59(1) of the Constitutional Reform Act 2005 (renaming of Supreme Court), the reference to the Senior Courts in subsection (11) is to be read as a reference to the Supreme Court.

---

[467] Words substituted by Legal Services Act 2007 c. 29 Sch.21 para.162(3)(c) (January 1, 2010).

Meaning of "gain experience in law" in section 50

A1–435   **52.**—(1) This section applies for the purposes of section 50.

(2) A person gains experience in law during a period if the period is one during which the person is engaged in law-related activities.

(3) For the purposes of subsection (2), a person's engagement in law-related activities during a period is to be disregarded if the engagement is negligible in terms of the amount of time engaged.

(4) For the purposes of this section, each of the following is a "law-related activity"—

(a) the carrying-out of judicial functions of any court or tribunal;

(b) acting as an arbitrator;

(c) practice or employment as a lawyer;

(d) advising (whether or not in the course of practice or employment as a lawyer) on the application of the law;

(e) assisting (whether or not in the course of such practice) persons involved in proceedings for the resolution of issues arising under the law;

(f) acting (whether or not in the course of such practice) as mediator in connection with attempts to resolve issues that are, or if not resolved could be, the subject of proceedings;

(g) drafting (whether or not in the course of such practice) documents intended to affect persons' rights or obligations;

(h) teaching or researching law;

(i) any activity that, in the relevant decision-maker's opinion, is of a broadly similar nature to an activity within any of paragraphs (a) to (h).

(5) For the purposes of this section, an activity mentioned in subsection (4) is a "law-related activity" whether it—

(a) is done on a full-time or part-time basis;

(b) is or is not done for remuneration;

(c) is done in the United Kingdom or elsewhere.

(6) In subsection (4)(i) "the relevant decision-maker", in relation to determining whether a person satisfies the judicial-appointment eligibility condition on an N-year basis in a particular case, means—

(a) where the condition applies in respect of appointment by Her Majesty to an office or other position, the person whose function it is to recommend the exercise of Her Majesty's function of making appointments to that office or position;

(b) where the condition applies in respect of appointment, by any person other than Her Majesty, to an office or other position, that person.

(7) In subsection (6) "appointment", in relation to an office or position, includes any form of selection for that office or position (whether called appointment or selection, or not).

Visiting Forces Act 1952 c. 67

Part I

Visiting Forces

Countries to which Act applies

1.—(1) References in this Act to a country to which a provision of this Act applies are **A1–436** reference to—

(a) Canada, Australia, New Zealand, [South Africa][468][. . .][469], India, [Pakistan][470] [. . .][471] [Ceylon [Ghana, [. . .][472] Malaysia][473] [474] [the Republic of Cyprus,[. . .][475] [476] [Nigeria,[. . .][477] [478] [Sierra Leone,[. . .][479][480] [Tanganyika or Jamaica][481] [Trinidad and Tobago, or][482] [Uganda, or][483] [Kenya, or][484] [Zanzibar, or][485] [Malawi, or][486] [Zambia, or][487] [Malta, or][488] [The Gambia, or][489] [Guyana, or][490] [Botswana, or][491] [Lesotho, or][492] [Singapore, or][493] [Barbados, or][494] [Mauritius, or][495] [Swaziland, or][496] [Tonga, or][497] [Fiji, or][498] [the Bahamas, or][499] [Bangladesh, or][500] [Solomon Islands or][501] [Tuvalu or][502] [Dominica or][503] [St. Lucia or][504]

---

[468] Words inserted by South Africa Act 1995 c. 3 Sch.1 para.5(1) (March 23, 1995).

[469] Words repealed by South Africa Act 1962 (c. 23), Sch. 5.

[470] Words inserted (retrospectively) by Pakistan Act 1990 (c. 14), s. 1, Sch. para. 5.

[471] Words repealed by Pakistan Act 1973 (c. 43), Sch. 4.

[472] Words repealed by Cyprus Act 1960 (c. 52), s. 3(2), Sch. 1 para. 6.

[473] Words substituted by Federation of Malaya Independence Act 1957 (c. 60), s. 2(1), Sch. 1 para. 4(1) as construed with Malaysia Act 1963 (c. 35), s. 3(2), Sch. 2 para. 1(a).

[474] Words substituted by Ghana Independence Act 1957 (c. 6), s. 4(4), Sch. 2 para. 6.

[475] Words repealed by Nigeria Independence Act 1960 (c. 55), s. 3(4), Sch. 2 para. 6.

[476] Words added by Cyprus Act 1960 (c. 52), s. 3(2), Sch. 1 para. 6.

[477] Words repealed by Sierra Leone Independence Act 1961 (c. 16), s. 3(3), Sch. 3 para. 7.

[478] Words added by Nigeria Independence Act 1960 (c. 55), s. 3(4), Sch. 2 para. 6.

[479] Word repealed by Tanganyika Independence Act 1961 (10 & 11 Eliz. 2 c. 1), s. 3(4), Sch. 2 para. 6.

[480] Words added by Sierra Leone Independence Act 1961 (c. 16), s. 3(3), Sch. 3 para. 7.

[481] Words substituted by Jamaica Independence Act 1962 (c. 40), s. 3(5), (6), Sch. 2 para. 6.

[482] Words added by Trinidad and Tobago Independence Act 1962 (c. 54), s. 3(4), (5), Sch. 2 para. 6.

[483] Words added by Uganda Independence Act 1962 (c. 57), s. 3(4), (5), Sch. 3 para. 6.

[484] Words added by Kenya Independence Act 1963 (c. 54), s. 4(4), (5), Sch. 2 para. 6.

[485] Words added by Zanzibar Act 1963 (c. 55), s. 1(2), Sch. 1 para. 7.

[486] Words added by Malawi Independence Act 1964 (c. 46), s. 4(4), (6), Sch. 2 para. 6.

[487] Words added by Zambia Independence Act 1964 (c. 65), s. 2(2), Sch. 1 para. 7.

[488] Words added by Malta Independence Act 1964 (c. 86), s. 4(4), (7), Sch. 2 para. 6.

[489] Words added by Gambia Independence Act 1964 (c. 93), s. 4(4), (6), Sch. 2 para. 6.

[490] Words added by Guyana Independence Act 1966 (c. 14), s. 5(4), (5), Sch. 2 para. 6.

[491] Words added by Botswana Independence Act 1966 (c. 23), s. 2, Sch. 1 Pt. I para. 7.

[492] Words added by Lesotho Independence Act 1966 (c. 24), s. 2(2), Sch. 1 Pt. I para. 7.

[493] Words added by Singapore Act 1966 (c. 29), s. 1, Sch. 1 para. 4.

[494] Words added by Barbados Independence Act 1966 (c. 37), s. 4(5), (6), Sch. 2 para. 6.

[495] Words added by Mauritius Independence Act 1968 (c. 8), s. 4(3), (4), Sch. 2 para. 6.

[496] Words added by Swaziland Independence Act 1968 (c. 56), s. 2(2) Sch. 1 Pt. I para. 7.

[497] Words added by Tonga Act 1970 (c. 22), s. 1(3), Sch. 1 Pt. I para. 6.

[498] Words added by Fiji Independence Act 1970 (c. 50), s. 4(3), (4), Sch. 2 para. 5.

[499] Words added by Bahamas Independence Act 1973 (c. 27), s. 4(3), (4), Sch. 2 para. 4.

[500] Words added retrospectively by Bangladesh Act 1973 (c. 49), Sch.1 para. 2.

[501] Words inserted by Solomon Islands Act 1978 (c. 15), s. 7(4), Sch. para. 3(a).

[502] Words inserted by Tuvalu Act 1978 (c. 20), s. 4(3), Sch. 2 para. 3(a).

[503] Words inserted by SI 1978/1030, Sch. para. 4.

[504] Words inserted by 1978/1899, Sch. para. 4.

[Kiribati or][505] [St Vincent and the Grenadines or][506] [Papua New Guinea, Western Samoa and Nauru, or][507] [Zimbabwe or][508] [the New Hebrides or][509] [Belize or][510] [Antigua and Barbuda or][511] [Saint Christopher and Nevis][512] [Brunei or Maldives, or][513] [Namibia][514] [or Cameroon or Mozambique][515].

(b) any country designated for the purposes of that provision by Order in Council under the next following subsection.

(2) Where it appears to Her Majesty, as respects any country not mentioned in paragraph (a) of the foregoing subsection, that having regard to [(a)][516] any arrangements for common defence [; or (b) any other arrangements for defence co-operation, to][517] which Her Majesty's Government in the United Kingdom and the Government of that country are for the time being parties it is expedient that the following provisions of this Act, or any of those provisions, should have effect in relation to that country, Her Majesty may by Order in Council designate that country for the purposes of the provisions in question.

(3) Her Majesty may by Order in Council provide that in so far as this Act has effect in relation to any country designated under the last foregoing subsection, it shall have effect subject to such limitations, adaptations or modifications as may be specified in the Order.

(4) No recommendation shall be made to Her Majesty in Council to make an Order under the last foregoing subsection unless a draft thereof has been laid before Parliament and approved by resolution of each House of Parliament.

Exercise of powers by service courts and authorities of countries sending visiting forces

A1–437   **2.**—(1) The service courts and service authorities of a country to which this section applies may within the United Kingdom, or on board any of Her Majesty's ships or aircraft, exercise over persons subject to their jurisdiction in accordance with this section all such powers as are exercisable by them according to the law of that country.

(2) The persons subject to the jurisdiction of the service courts and service authorities of a country in accordance with this section are the following, that is to say—

(a) members of any visiting force of that country; and

(b) all other persons who, being neither citizens of the United Kingdom and Colonies nor ordinarily resident in the United Kingdom, are for the time being subject to the service law of that country otherwise than as members of that country's forces:

Provided that for the purposes of this subsection a person shall not be treated as a member of a visiting force of a country if he became (or last became) a member of that country's forces at a time when he was in the United Kingdom unless it is shown that he then became a member of those forces with his consent.

---

[505] Words inserted by Kiribati Act 1979 (c. 27), s. 3(4), Sch. para. 4(a).
[506] Words inserted by SI 1979/917, Sch. para. 4.
[507] Words inserted by Papua New Guinea, Western Samoa and Nauru (Miscellaneous Provisions) Act 1980 (c. 2), s. 3, Sch. para. 9.
[508] Words inserted by SI 1980/701, Sch. para. 11(2).
[509] Words inserted by New Hebrides Act 1980 (c. 16), s. 4(2), Sch. 1 para. 4.
[510] Words inserted by Belize Act 1981 (c. 52), s. 3(4), Sch. 2 para. 3(a).
[511] SI 1981/1105, Sch. para. 1.
[512] Words inserted by SI 1983/882, Sch. para. 3.
[513] Words inserted by Brunei and Maldives Act 1985 (c. 3), s. 1, Sch. para. 6.
[514] Word inserted (retrospectively) by Namibia Act 1991 (c. 4), s. 1, Sch. para. 4.
[515] Words inserted by Commonwealth Act 2002 c. 39 Sch.2 para.3(1) (January 7, 2003).
[516] Word added after the word "to" in the second place it appears by Armed Forces Act 1996 c. 46 s.33(a) (October 1, 1996).
[517] Words substituted for the word "to" in the third place it appears by Armed Forces Act 1996 c. 46 s.33(b) (October 1, 1996).

(3) Where any sentence has, whether within or outside the United Kingdom, been passed by a service court of a country to which this section applies upon a person who immediately before the sentence was passed was subject to the jurisdiction of that court in accordance with this section, then for the purposes of any proceedings in a United Kingdom court the said service court shall be deemed to have been properly constituted, and the sentence shall be deemed to be within the jurisdiction of that court and in accordance with the law of that country, and if executed according to the tenor of the sentence shall be deemed to have been lawfully executed.

(4) Notwithstanding anything in the foregoing provisions of this section, a sentence of death passed by a service court of a country to which this section applies shall not be carried out in the United Kingdom unless under United Kingdom law a sentence of death could have been passed in a similar case.

(5) Any person who—

(a) is detained in custody in pursuance of a sentence as respects which subsection (3) of this section has effect, or

(b) being subject in accordance with this section to the jurisdiction of the service courts of a country to which this section applies, is detained in custody pending or during the trial by such a court of a charge brought against him,

shall for the purposes of any proceedings in any United Kingdom court be deemed to be in legal custody.

(6) For the purpose of enabling the service courts and service authorities of a country to which this section applies to exercise more effectively the powers referred to in subsection (1) of this section, [the Defence Council][518], if so requested by the appropriate authority of that country, may from time to time by general or special orders direct members of the home forces to arrest any person, being a member of a visiting force of that country, who is alleged to be guilty of an offence punishable under the law of that country and to hand him over to such service authority of that country as may be designated by or under the orders.

Provisions as to coroners' inquests and as to removal of bodies of deceased persons

7.—[(1) Subsections (1A) and (1B) of this section apply if a coroner who has jurisdiction **A1–438** to conduct an investigation under Part 1 of the Coroners and Justice Act 2009 into a person's death is satisfied that the deceased person, at the time of the death, had a relevant association with a visiting force.]

(1A) If no investigation into the person's death has begun, the coroner shall not begin an investigation unless directed to do so by the Lord Chancellor.

(1B) If an investigation into the person's death has begun but has not been completed, the coroner shall suspend the investigation unless directed not to do so by the Lord Chancellor.][519]

(2) Subject to [subsections (1) to (1B) of this section, if in the course of an investigation under Part 1 of the Coroners and Justice Act 2009 into a person's death][520] the coroner is satisfied—

(a) that a person who in accordance with section two of this Act is subject to the jurisdiction of the service courts of a country to which this section applies has been charged before a court of that country with the homicide of the deceased person, whether or not that charge has been dealt with, or

---

[518] Words substituted with saving by SI 1964/488.
[519] S.7(1) to (1B) substituted for s.7(1) by Coroners and Justice Act 2009 c. 25 Sch.21(1) para.5(2) (July 25, 2013).
[520] Words substituted by Coroners and Justice Act 2009 c. 25 Sch.21(1) para.5(3)(a) (July 25, 2013).

(b) that such a person is being detained by an authority of that country with a view to being so charged,

then unless the [Lord Chancellor]521 otherwise directs the coroner shall [suspend the investigation]522 and shall furnish the registrar of deaths with a certificate stating the particulars necessary for the registration of the death so far as they have been ascertained [in the course of the investigation].523

[(2A) A coroner who suspends an investigation under this section shall—

(a) adjourn any inquest being held as part of the investigation, and

(b) discharge any jury that has been summoned.

(2B) The suspension of an investigation under this section does not prevent its suspension under Schedule 1 to the Coroners and Justice Act 2009; and vice versa.]524

[(3) Where an investigation is suspended under this section, the coroner shall not resume it except on the direction of the Lord Chancellor.

(3A) Where the investigation is resumed, the coroner must resume any inquest that was adjourned under subsection (2A).

(3B) A resumed inquest may be held with a jury if the coroner thinks that there is sufficient reason for it to be held with one.]525

(4) Section four of the Births and Deaths Registration Act, 1926 (which restricts the removal out of England of the body of a deceased person) shall not apply to the body of a person who at the time of his death had a relevant association with a visiting force:

Provided that this subsection shall not apply as respects the body of a person concerning whose death, by virtue of a direction of [the Lord Chancellor under subsection (1A) or (3) of this section, an investigation is required to be conducted]526 or, if begun, is required to be resumed.

(5) Notwithstanding [subsection (1) of section 24 of the Births and Deaths Registration Act 1953]527 (which relates to certificates to be given to persons giving information concerning deaths), the registrar shall not give a certificate under that subsection to the person giving information concerning a death if that person informs the registrar that the body is one as respects which the last foregoing subsection has effect and that it is proposed to remove the body out of England.

(6) [In this section the expression "homicide" includes—

(a) murder, manslaughter or infanticide,

(b) any offence under the law of the country in question which is analogous to any of the offences within paragraph (a), and

(c) any offence under the law of the country in question which is analogous to an offence under section 2(1) of the Suicide Act 1961 or section 13(1) of the Criminal Justice Act (Northern Ireland) 1966 (encouraging or assisting suicide).]528

[(7) In the application of this section to Northern Ireland—

---

521 Words substituted by Coroners and Justice Act 2009 c. 25 Sch.21(1) para.5(3)(b) (July 25, 2013).
522 Words substituted by Coroners and Justice Act 2009 c. 25 Sch.21(1) para.5(3)(c) (July 25, 2013).
523 Words substituted by Coroners and Justice Act 2009 c. 25 Sch.21(1) para.5(3)(d) (July 25, 2013).
524 Added by Coroners and Justice Act 2009 c. 25 Sch.21(1) para.5(4) (July 25, 2013).
525 S.7(3) to (3B) substituted for s.7(3) by Coroners and Justice Act 2009 c. 25 Sch.21(1) para.5(5) (July 25, 2013).
526 Words substituted by Coroners and Justice Act 2009 c. 25 Sch.21(1) para.5(6) (July 25, 2013).
527 Words substituted by Coroners and Justice Act 2009 c. 25 Sch.21(1) para.5(7) (July 25, 2013).
528 S.7(6)(a)-(c) substituted for words by Coroners and Justice Act 2009 c. 25 Sch.21(2) para.54(a) (February 1, 2010).

(a) in subsection (1), for "a coroner who has jurisdiction to conduct an investigation under Part 1 of the Coroners and Justice Act 2009 into a person's death" there is substituted "a coroner who has jurisdiction under the Coroners Act (Northern Ireland) 1959 to hold an inquest into a person's death";

(b) in subsection (1A), for "no investigation" there is substituted "no inquest" and for "an investigation" there is substituted "an inquest";

(c) in subsection (1B), for "an investigation" there is substituted "an inquest", and for "suspend the investigation" there is substituted "adjourn the inquest";

(d) in subsection (2)—

(i) for "in the course of an investigation under Part 1 of the Coroners and Justice Act 2009" there is substituted "on an inquest";
(ii) for "suspend the investigation" there is substituted "adjourn the inquest";
(iii) for "in the course of the investigation" there is substituted "at the inquest";

(e) in subsection (2A), for the words from "suspends an investigation" to the end there is substituted "adjourns an inquest under this section shall discharge any jury that has been summoned";

(f) in subsection (3), for "investigation is suspended" there is substituted "inquest is adjourned";

(g) subsection (3A) is omitted;

(h) in subsection (3B), for "A resumed inquest" there is substituted "An inquest resumed under this section";

(i) subsections (4) and (5) are omitted.][529]

Definition of membership of civilian component of visiting force

10.—(1) In this Part of this Act references to a member of a civilian component of a   **A1–439** visiting force are references to a person for the time being fulfilling the following conditions, that is to say—

(a) that he holds a passport issued in respect of him by a Government, not being a passport issued by the passport authorities of the United Kingdom or any colony;

(b) that the passport contains an uncancelled entry made by or on behalf of the appropriate authority of the sending country stating that he is a member of a civilian component of a visiting force of that country; and

(c) that the passport contains a note of recognition of that entry by or on behalf of the Secretary of State which has not been cancelled and as respects which no notification in writing has been given by or on behalf of the Secretary of State to the appropriate authority of the sending country stating that the recognition is withdrawn.

(2) The reference in paragraph (c) of the last foregoing subsection to a note of recognition of an entry in a passport is a reference to any mark or indication made in the passport by or on behalf of the Secretary of State signifying that the entry has been noted and approved.

(3) For the purposes of this section the following provisions shall have effect in any proceedings in any United Kingdom court, that is to say—

(a) a document purporting to be a passport issued by or on behalf of a Government and to be so issued in respect of a person bearing the name in which a person is referred

---

[529] Substituted by Coroners and Justice Act 2009 c. 25 Sch.21(1) para.5(8) (July 25, 2013).

to in the proceedings (whether as a party thereto or otherwise) shall, unless the contrary is proved, be deemed to have been issued by that Government and to relate to the person so referred to;

(b) an entry in a passport containing such a statement as is mentioned in paragraph (b) of subsection (1) of this section and purporting to be made by or on behalf of the appropriate authority of the sending country shall, unless the contrary is proved, be deemed to have been so made; and

(c) a mark or indication in a passport purporting to be made by or on behalf of the Secretary of State shall, unless the contrary is proved, be deemed to have been so made.

(4) In this section the expression "passport" includes any document which, in accordance with the United Kingdom law for the time being in force, would be treated as the equivalent of a passport in the case of a person entering the United Kingdom, being a national of the country by whose Government the document is issued.

Evidence for purposes of Part I

A1–440   **11.**—(1) For the purposes of this Part of this Act a certificate issued by or on behalf of the appropriate authority of a country, stating that at a time specified in the certificate a person so specified either was or was not a member of a visiting force of that country, shall in any proceedings in any United Kingdom court be sufficient evidence of the fact so stated unless the contrary is proved.

(2) For the purposes of this Part of this Act a certificate issued by or on behalf of the appropriate authority of a country, stating, as respects a person specified in the certificate,—

(a) that on a date so specified he was sentenced by a service court of that country to such punishment as is specified in the certificate, or

(b) that he is, or was at a time so specified, detained in custody in pursuance of a sentence passed upon him by a service court of that country or pending or during the trial by such a court of a charge brought against him, or

(c) that he has been tried, at a time and place specified in the certificate, by a service court of that country for a crime so specified,

shall in any proceedings in any United Kingdom court be conclusive evidence of the facts so stated.

(3) For the purposes of subsection (2) of section three of this Act a certificate issued by or on behalf of the appropriate authority of a country, stating in connection with any charge against a person of an offence against United Kingdom law, being a charge specified in the certificate, that his case can be dealt with under the law of that country, shall in any such proceedings as aforesaid be conclusive evidence of the fact so stated.

(4) Where a person is charged with an offence against United Kingdom law and at the time when the offence is alleged to have been committed he was a member of a visiting force or a member of a civilian component of such a force, a certificate issued by or on behalf of the appropriate authority of the sending country, stating that the alleged offence, if committed by him, arose out of and in the course of his duty as a member of that force or component, as the case may be, shall in any such proceedings as aforesaid be sufficient evidence of that fact unless the contrary is proved.

Interpretation of Part I

A1–441   **12.**—(1) In this Part of this Act, unless the context otherwise requires, the following expressions have the meanings hereby assigned to them respectively, that is to say—

"court" includes a service court;

"Her Majesty's ships or aircraft" does not include ships or aircraft belonging to Her Majesty otherwise than in right of Her Majesty's Government in the United Kingdom;

"the home forces" means any of the forces of Her Majesty raised in the United Kingdom and for the time being serving in the United Kingdom;

"member", in relation to a visiting force, means a member of the forces of the sending country, being one of the members thereof for the time being appointed to serve with that visiting force;

"the sending country", in relation to a visiting force, means the country to whose forces the visiting force belongs;

"service authorities" means naval, military or air force authorities;

"service court" means a court established under service law and includes any authority of a country who under the law thereof is empowered to review the proceedings of such a court or to try or investigate charges brought against persons subject to the service law of that country; and references to trial by, or to sentences passed by, service courts of a country shall be construed respectively as including references to trial by, and to punishment imposed by, such an authority in the exercise of such powers;

"service law", in relation to a country, means the law governing all or any of the forces of that country; and

"visiting force", means for the purposes of any provision in this Part of this Act, any body, contingent or detachment of the forces of a country to which that provision applies, being a body, contingent or detachment for the time being present in the United Kingdom [(including United Kingdom territorial waters), or in any place to which subsection (1A) below applies][530] on the invitation of Her Majesty's Government in the United Kingdom.

[(1A) This subsection applies to any place on, under or above an installation in a designated area within the meaning of section 1(7) of the Continental Shelf Act 1964 or any waters within 500 metres of such an installation.][531]

(2) References in this Part of this Act to a person's having at any time a relevant association with a visiting force are references to his being at that time a person of one or other of the following descriptions, that is to say—

    (a) a member of that visiting force or a member of a civilian component of that force;

    (b) a person, not being a citizen of the United Kingdom and Colonies or ordinarily resident in the United Kingdom, but being a dependant of a member of that visiting force or of a civilian component of that force.

(3) In determining for the purposes of any provision in this Part of this Act whether a person is, or was at any time, ordinarily resident in the United Kingdom, no account shall be taken of any period during which he has been or intends to be present in the United Kingdom while being a member of a visiting force or of a civilian component of such a force, or while being a dependant of a member of a visiting force or of such a civilian component.

(4) In this section the expression "dependant", in relation to a person, means any of the following, that is to say—

    (a) the wife or husband of that person; and

---

[530] Words inserted by Criminal Justice Act 1988 (c. 33), s. 170(1), Sch. 15 para. 14(1).
[531] S. 12(1A) inserted by Criminal Justice Act 1988 (c. 33), s. 170(1), Sch. 15 para. 14(2).

(b) any other person wholly or mainly maintained by him or in his custody, charge or care.

PART III

SUPPLEMENTARY PROVISIONS

Provisions as to proof of facts by certificate

A1–442   **16.**—(1) For the purposes of this Act—

(a) a certificate issued by or on behalf of the appropriate authority of a country, stating that a body, contingent or detachment of the forces of that country is, or was at a time specified in the certificate, present in the United Kingdom, shall in any proceedings in any United Kingdom court be conclusive evidence of the fact so stated; and

(b) where in any such proceedings it is admitted or proved (whether by means of a certificate under the foregoing paragraph or otherwise) that a body, contingent or detachment of the forces of a country is or was at any time present in the United Kingdom, it shall be assumed in those proceedings, unless the contrary is shown, that the body, contingent or detachment is or was at that time present in the United Kingdom on the invitation of Her Majesty's Government in the United Kingdom.

(2) Where in any certificate issued for the purposes of this Act reference is made to a person by name, and in any proceedings in a United Kingdom court reference is made to a person by that name (whether as a party to the proceedings or otherwise), the references in the certificate and in the proceedings respectively shall, unless the contrary is proved, be deemed to be references to one and the same person.

(3) Any document purporting to be a certificate issued for the purposes of any provision of this Act, and to be signed by or on behalf of an authority specified therein, shall be received in evidence and shall, unless the contrary is proved, be deemed to be a certificate issued by or on behalf of that authority; and where under the provision in question a certificate is required to be issued by or on behalf of the appropriate authority of a country, and the document purports to be signed by or on behalf of an authority of that country, that authority shall, unless the contrary is proved, be deemed to be the appropriate authority of that country for the purposes of that provision.

Interpretation

A1–443   **17.**—(1) In this Act, unless the context otherwise requires, the expression "forces", in relation to a country, means any of the naval, military or air forces of that country, the expression "United Kingdom court" means a court exercising jurisdiction in the United Kingdom under United Kingdom law otherwise than by virtue of section two of this Act, and the expression "United Kingdom law" means the law of the United Kingdom or of any part thereof.

(2) For the purposes of this Act a member of a force of any country which (by whatever name called) is in the nature of a reserve or auxiliary force shall be deemed to be a member of that country's forces so long as, but only so long as, he is called into actual service (by whatever expression described) or is called out for training; and any reference in this Act to a person's becoming a member of a country's forces shall be construed accordingly.

(3) References in any provision of this Act to the appropriate authority of a country are references to such authority as may be appointed by the Government of that country for the purposes of that provision.

(4) References in this Act to the presence of any forces in the United Kingdom at any time shall be construed as including references to their being at that time in transit to the United Kingdom.

(5) In this Act, unless the context otherwise requires, any reference to an enactment shall be construed as a reference to that enactment as amended by or under any other enactment, and in this subsection the expression "enactment" includes an enactment of the Parliament of Northern Ireland.

(6) Any power conferred by the foregoing provisions of this Act to make an Order in Council or order shall be construed as including a power, exercisable in the like manner, to vary or revoke the Order in Council or order; and an Order in Council varying or revoking an Order under subsection (2) of section one of this Act may contain such transitional provisions as appear to Her Majesty in Council expedient in consequence of the variation or revocation.

Welsh Language Act 1993 c. 38

PART III

MISCELLANEOUS

Welsh in legal proceedings

Use of Welsh in legal proceedings

22.—(1) In any legal proceedings in Wales the Welsh language may be spoken by any   **A1–444**
party, witness or other person who desires to use it, subject in the case of proceedings in a court other than a magistrates' court to such prior notice as may be required by rules of court; and any necessary provision for interpretation shall be made accordingly.

(2) Any power to make rules of court includes power to make provision as to the use, in proceedings in or having a connection with Wales, of documents in the Welsh language.

[Oaths and affirmations

23.—(1) The Lord Chancellor may, after consulting the Lord Chief Justice of England   **A1–445**
and Wales, make rules prescribing a translation in the Welsh language of any form for the time being prescribed by law as the form of any oath or affirmation to be administered and taken or made by any person in any court, and an oath or affirmation administered and taken or made in any court in Wales in the translation prescribed by such rules shall, without interpretation, be of the like effect as if it had been administered and taken or made in the English language.

(2) The Lord Chief Justice may nominate a judicial office holder (as defined in section 109(4) of the Constitutional Reform Act 2005) to exercise his functions under this section.][532]

Provision of interpreters

24.—(1) The Lord Chancellor may make rules as to the provision and employment of   **A1–446**
interpreters of the Welsh and English languages for the purposes of proceedings before courts in Wales.

(2) The interpreters shall be paid, out of the same fund as the expenses of the court are payable, such remuneration in respect of their services as the Lord Chancellor may determine.

(3) The Lord Chancellor's powers under this section shall be exercised with the consent of the Treasury.

---

[532] Existing s.23 renumbered as s.23(1), words are inserted and s.23(2) is added by Constitutional Reform Act 2005 c. 4 Sch.4(1) para.232 (April 3, 2006).

Appendix 2

STATUTORY INSTRUMENTS

Armed Forces (Service Inquiries) Regulations 2008/1651

Citation and commencement

A2–001   **1.** These Regulations may be cited as the Armed Forces (Service Inquiries) Regulations 2008 and shall come into force on 1st October 2008.

Interpretation

A2–002   **2.**—(1) In these Regulations—

"the Act" means the Armed Forces Act 2006;

"convening authority" means a person appointed in accordance with regulation 3 as convening authority in relation to a matter or a category of matters;

"convening order" means an order given by the convening authority to convene a service inquiry panel;

"Crown servant" means a person employed by or in the service of the Government of the United Kingdom;

"document" includes information recorded in any form, and see paragraph (2);

"legal representative" means a person who—

    (a) has a general qualification within the meaning of section 71 of the Courts and Legal Services Act 1990;

    (b) is an advocate or solicitor in Scotland;

    (c) is a member of the Bar of Northern Ireland or a solicitor of the Supreme Court of Northern Ireland; or

    (d) has in any of the Channel Islands, the Isle of Man, a Commonwealth country or a British overseas territory rights and duties similar to those of a barrister or solicitor in England and Wales, and is subject to punishment or disability for breach of professional rules;

"live television link" means arrangement by which a person (when not in the place where the proceedings of a service inquiry panel are being conducted) is able to see and hear, and to be seen and be heard by, the panel (and for this purpose any impairment of eyesight or hearing is to be disregarded;

"president" means, in relation to a service inquiry panel, the president of the panel;

"senior non-commissioned officer" means a non-commissioned officer who is of or above the rate or rank of petty officer, sergeant or equivalent rank;

"service court" means, subject to regulation 20 and paragraph 4 of Schedule 3, any of the Summary Appeal Court, the Court Martial, the Service Civilian Court and the Court Martial Appeal Court;

"service inquiry" means an inquiry referred to in section 343 of the Act;

"service inquiry panel" has the same meaning as in section 343 of the Act, and "panel" shall be construed accordingly;

"summary hearing" means, subject to regulation 20 and paragraph 5 of Schedule 3, a summary hearing under section 131 of the Act;

"terms of reference" means, in relation to a service inquiry, its terms of reference, as provided for it under regulation 7(2) or as subsequently amended under regulation 7(3); and

"witness notice" means a witness notice issued under regulation 13(1).

(2) References in these Regulations to producing or providing a document, in relation to information recorded otherwise than in legible form, are to be read as producing or providing a copy of the information in a legible form.

The convening authority

A2–003   **3.**—(1) Subject to paragraph (2), the convening authority in relation to any matter connected with any of Her Majesty's forces, or any category of such matters stated in the terms of his appointment, shall be the person appointed as such by the Defence Council or by an officer authorised by the Defence Council.

(2) A convening authority must be an officer of or above the rank of naval captain, colonel or group captain subject to service law.

Matters for reference to a service inquiry panel

4.—(1) In the event of the death on or after 1st October 2008 of a person while subject to service law—   **A2-004**

(a) a convening authority must have been appointed, or as soon as reasonably practicable be appointed, in relation to that event or to a category of matters which includes that event; and

(b) the convening authority must cause a service inquiry to be held, if he considers that anything of consequence to any of the regular or reserve forces which is not in his opinion apparent from the death may be learned by any of those forces by means of such an inquiry.

(2) Paragraph (1) shall not apply if a service, UK, British overseas territory or overseas police force is conducting, has conducted, or informs the convening authority that it will conduct, an investigation into the events which caused the death.

(3) Subject to paragraph (1)(b), where a convening authority is appointed in relation to a matter or a category of matters, he may cause a service inquiry to be held in relation to that matter or into any matter within that category.

(4) Notwithstanding anything in paragraphs (1) to (3), the Defence Council may cause a service inquiry to be held in relation to any matter connected with any of Her Majesty's forces, and for that purpose may carry out, or appoint a person to carry out, any of a convening authority's functions under these Regulations.

Convening of a service inquiry panel

5. In order to cause a service inquiry to be held in relation to any matter, the convening authority shall convene a service inquiry panel by order specifying—   **A2-005**

(a) that a service inquiry is to be held;

(b) the president and the other members of the panel; and

(c) the date on which, and the time and place at which, the panel shall first assemble.

Composition of a service inquiry panel

6.—(1) Subject to the following paragraphs of this Regulation, a service inquiry panel must consist of a president and at least two other members.   **A2-006**

(2) If in the opinion of the convening authority the president is unable to continue as president the convening authority must as soon as practicable appoint an existing member or a new member to replace him as president.

(3) Subject to paragraphs (4), if in the opinion of the convening authority any other member is unable to continue as a member, the convening authority may appoint a replacement.

(4) If the membership of a service inquiry panel falls below the requirements of paragraph (1), the convening authority must as soon as practicable appoint one or more new members as necessary to meet those requirements.

(5) Subject to paragraph (6), a member of a service inquiry panel must be—

(a) an officer, warrant officer or senior non-commissioned officer of any of Her Majesty's forces; or

(b) a Crown servant.

(6) A person who is a member of an armed force other than any of Her Majesty's forces may be appointed a member of a service inquiry panel, if—

(a) he is of a rank equivalent to that of a senior non-commissioned officer or above; and

(b) in the opinion of the convening authority the terms of reference under regulation 7 will require the service inquiry panel to investigate a mater which is likely to be connected with that force as well as with any of Her Majesty's forces.

(7) The president must be an officer—

(a) subject to service law; and

(b) of or above the rank of lieutenant commander, major or squadron leader.

(8) Notwithstanding paragraph (1), but subject to any provision of these Regulations expressly requiring any action to be taken by all the members of a service inquiry panel, any function under these Regulations of a service inquiry panel may be performed by such one or more of the members of the panel as the president may decide.

Functions of a service inquiry panel

A2–007   7.—(1) Subject to regulation 19, the functions of a service inquiry panel shall be to investigate and report on the facts relating to the matters specified in its terms of reference provided under paragraph (2) and otherwise to comply with those terms of reference.

(2) The convening authority must provide the panel with terms of reference on or before the date on which the panel is required to assemble.

(3) The convening authority may, by notice in writing to the president amend the terms of reference at any time until it has taken action under regulation 19(4)(a).

(4) The terms of reference of a service inquiry panel must specify—

(a) the matters, the facts relating to which the panel is to investigate and report upon; and

(b) any matter about which the panel is required to make recommendations or on which it is required to express an opinion;

and may include such other terms as the convening authority considers appropriate.

Power to defer or suspend service inquiry

A2–008   8.—(1) The convening authority in relation to a matter may at any time defer the convening of a service inquiry panel, or, at any time after making a convening order, issue a suspension notice to the president to suspend the proceedings of the panel. A deferment or suspension must only be for such period as the convening authority considers necessary to allow for—

(a) the carrying out of any other investigation, whether in the United Kingdom or abroad, relating to any of the matters to which the service inquiry relates or would relate, or

(b) the determination of any—

(i) civil proceedings whether in the United Kingdom or abroad;

(ii) proceedings for any criminal offence in any court whether in the United Kingdom or abroad;

(iii) proceedings in a service court; or

(iv) a summary hearing.

(2) The power conferred by paragraph (1) may be exercised whether or not the investigation or proceedings have begun.

(3) A suspension notice under paragraph (1) may suspend the proceedings of the service inquiry panel until a specified day, until the happening of a specified event or until the giving by the convening authority of a further notice to the president to end the suspension.

(4) A suspension notice under paragraph (1) must state the convening authority's reasons for suspending the proceedings of the service inquiry panel.

Termination of a service inquiry

9.—(1) The convening authority in relation to a service inquiry may at any time issue a notice to the president terminating the inquiry from such date as is specified in the notice. The date specified may be the date of issue of the notice or any later date.   **A2–009**

(2) For the purposes of these Regulations a service inquiry comes to an end on—

(a) the date on which, in accordance with regulation 19, the convening authority declares a provisional report to be the final report; or

(b) any earlier date specified in a notice under paragraph (1) terminating the service inquiry.

(3) A notice given under paragraph (1) must state the convening authority's reasons for terminating the service inquiry.

(4) The termination of a service inquiry by a notice under paragraph (1) shall be—

(a) subject to a duty to complete a service inquiry where there is a duty to hold a service inquiry under regulation 4(1); and

(b) without prejudice to the power of the convening authority under regulation 4(3) and the power of the Defence Council under regulation 4(4) to cause a further service inquiry to be held in relation to the same matter.

Procedure and record of proceedings

10.—(1) Subject to any other provision of these Regulations, the procedure of the panel is to be such as the president may direct.   **A2–010**

(2) The panel shall sit on such occasions and in such places as the president may direct.

(3) The president may adjourn the proceedings of the panel.

(4) The president must ensure that a record of the proceedings of the panel is made.

(5) The president must ensure that the convening order and the terms of reference are entered in the record of the proceedings on the date the panel first assembles.

(6) The record of the proceedings under paragraph (4) shall also include—

(a) a transcript of any oral evidence given to the panel;

(b) a copy of any written evidence given to the panel; and

(c) a copy of any other document which the president decides should form part of the record.

Evidence and witnesses

11.—(1) The president shall decide—   **A2–011**

(a) subject to paragraph (9), the persons from whom written or oral evidence is to be requested; and

(b) whether a person is to be requested to produce any document or other thing,

and the president may so decide at any time before or during the proceedings of the service inquiry panel.

(2) Where the president makes a decision under paragraph (1) that a person be requested to provide written evidence or to produce any document or other thing, the panel must send a written request to the person—

(a) to provide written evidence; or

(b) to produce the document or other thing.

(3) The president may allow a witness to give evidence through a live television link or by other means.

(4) Any document or other thing produced to the panel by a witness for use as evidence shall be made an exhibit.

(5) Each exhibit must be attached to or kept with the record of the proceedings unless the president decides that it is not practicable or convenient to do so.

(6) If in accordance with paragraph (5) an exhibit is not attached to or kept with the record of the proceedings, the president shall ensure that such steps as he considers appropriate are taken for its safekeeping until the service inquiry has come to an end in accordance with regulation 9.

(7) Subject to paragraphs (8) and (9), every witness who gives oral evidence may be required by the president to do so on oath.

(8) Where the president would, apart from this paragraph, require a witness to give oral evidence on oath and—

(a) the witness objects to taking an oath; or

(b) it is not reasonably practicable without inconvenience to, or without delaying the proceedings of, the panel to administer an oath to a witness in the manner appropriate to his religious belief,

he must be required to make a solemn affirmation instead of taking an oath.

(9) A witness under the age of fourteen who does not in the opinion of the president understand the nature of an oath or solemn affirmation—

(a) may give evidence to the panel, if in the opinion of the president he understands that he should tell the truth when giving evidence to them; and

(b) must not give evidence to the panel on oath or having solemnly affirmed.

(10) An oath must be administered, or a solemn affirmation made, before the panel and in the form and manner set out in Schedule 1.

Restrictions on admissibility of evidence

A2–012   **12.**—(1) Subject to paragraph (2), evidence given by a person to a service inquiry panel shall not be admissible against a person at a summary hearing or in proceedings before a civilian court or a service court.

(2) Evidence given before a service inquiry panel may be admissible in proceedings referred to in paragraph (1) for—

(a) an offence against section 42 of the Act where the corresponding offence under the law of England and Wales is an offence mentioned in sub–paragraph (b);

(b) an offence under section 2 or 5 of the Perjury Act 1911.

Issue of witness notice on application to a judge advocate

13.—(1) Subject to paragraph (5), a judge advocate may issue a witness notice if he is   **A2–013**
satisfied that a person—

(a) is likely to be able to give or provide material evidence, or to produce or provide any document or other thing likely to be material evidence, for the purpose of a service inquiry,

(b) will not voluntarily attend the proceedings of the service inquiry panel or voluntarily produce or provide that document or other thing, and

(c) is a civilian subject to service discipline, or a person in the United Kingdom, the Isle of Man or a British overseas territory.

(2) A witness notice must require the person referred to in paragraph (1) to—

(a) attend the proceedings of the panel at a time and place stated in the witness notice, and give the evidence, or produce the document or other thing, or

(b) provide the document or other thing to the panel within a specified period.

(3) A witness notice may only be issued on an application by the president in accordance with paragraph 1 of Schedule 2, and paragraph 2 of that Schedule shall apply to the consideration of such an application.

(4) The judge advocate who decides whether to issue a witness notice may refuse to issue the witness notice if any requirement of paragraph 1 of Schedule 2 relating to the application is not met.

(5) A person may not be required to produce or provide any evidence or document if he could not be required to do so if the proceedings of the service inquiry were civil proceedings in a court in England and Wales.

Service of witness notice

14. Where a judge advocate issues a witness notice, the court administration officer shall   **A2–014**
serve it on the person to whom it is addressed by—

(a) delivering it to him;

(b) leaving it at his usual or last known place of residence;

(c) sending it by post to that address; or

(d) transmitting it to him by fax or other electronic means, but only if he has agreed to accept service by that method.

Application to vary or revoke witness notice

15.—(1) If a witness notice has been issued, and the person to whom it is addressed   **A2–015**
applies in accordance with paragraph 3 of Schedule 2 and satisfies a judge advocate
that—

(a) he is unable to comply with the witness notice; or

(b) it is not reasonable in all the circumstances to require him to comply with it,

the judge advocate must vary or revoke the witness notice.

(2) Where the judge advocate varies or revokes a witness notice, the judge advocate may order that the person to whom the witness notice was addressed shall be paid by the relevant authority the whole or a specified part of his costs of the application under paragraph (1).

(3) In paragraph (2) the "relevant authority" means the convening authority or (where the Defence Council has caused an inquiry to be held under regulation 4(4) the Defence Council or a person appointed by the Defence Council to carry out any function of a convening authority.

Offences

A2–016   **16.**—(1) A person is guilty of an offence if he fails without reasonable excuse to do anything that is required to do by a witness notice served upon him in accordance with regulation 14.

(2) A person is guilty of an offence if, during a service inquiry, he does anything that is intended to have the effect of—

(a) distorting or otherwise altering any evidence, document or other thing that is given, produced or provided to a service inquiry panel, or

(b) preventing any evidence, document or other thing from being given, produced or provided to a service inquiry panel,

or does anything that he knows or believes is likely to have such effect.

(3) A person is guilty of an offence if, during a service inquiry—

(a) he intentionally suppresses or conceals a document that is, and that he knows or believes to be, a relevant document, or

(b) he intentionally alters or destroys any such document.

(4) For the purposes of paragraph (3) a document is a "relevant document" if it is likely that the service inquiry panel would (if aware of its existence) wish to be provided with it.

(5) A person does not commit an offence under paragraph (2) or (3) by doing anything that he is authorised to do by the president or by virtue of regulation 13(5).

(6) An offence under any of paragraphs (1) to (3) is triable summarily by a civilian court in the United Kingdom, the Isle of Man or in a British overseas territory, and shall be punishable by a fine not exceeding level 3 on the standard scale.

Persons who may be permitted to attend

A2–017   **17.**—(1) Subject to regulation 18, the president must obtain the consent of the convening authority before permitting a person to be present at the proceedings of the panel, other than as a witness.

(2) Where the president permits a person to be present at the proceedings of the panel, that permission shall—

(a) apply only to such part, or the whole, of those proceedings as the convening authority has agreed before the permission is given; and

(b) be subject to such conditions as the convening authority may reasonably impose when he gives his consent under paragraph (1).

Persons entitled to attend

A2–018   **18.**—(1) Subject to paragraph (2), a potentially affected person shall be entitled to be present at the proceedings of a service inquiry panel.

(2) A potentially affected person's entitlement under paragraph (1) shall be subject to such conditions and exclusions as the president, after consulting the convening authority, may reasonably impose from time to time. Such exclusions may—

(a) include an exclusion from being present at such part of the proceedings of the panel as the president may specify; and

(b) be imposed before or at any time during the proceedings of the panel.

(3) Where under paragraph (1) a potentially affected person is entitled to be present at any part of the proceedings of the panel—

(a) he may be represented at that part by a legal representative or, with the consent of the president, he may be represented by a person other than a legal representative;

(b) he may give evidence, question witnesses or produce any witness to give evidence, in each case as to any other matter as to which, in the opinion of the president, the potentially affected person may be affected in relation to his character or professional reputation by the findings of the panel;

(c) where he is represented, his representative may question witnesses and may, with the permission of the president, address the panel; and

(d) the president shall provide him with a copy of any part of the record of the proceedings of the panel, if the president considers it appropriate to do so.

(4) In this regulation "potentially affected person" means a person who in the opinion of the president may be affected in relation to his character or professional reputation by the findings of the panel.

Submission of reports

19.—(1) When the president considers that the panel has fulfilled the terms of reference, he shall ensure that a provisional report is prepared, that the report is signed by all the members of the panel and that the report is provided, as soon as practicable, to the convening authority. **A2–019**

(2) The provisional report may also contain anything that the president considers to be relevant to the terms of reference, including any recommendations or the expression of any opinion which the president considers it appropriate to make whether or not required to do so by the terms of reference.

(3) The president shall ensure that the provisional report reflects any points of disagreement between the members of the panel.

(4) After considering the provisional report, the convening authority may—

(a) declare the provisional report as the final report; or

(b) require the panel (whether by amending the terms of reference or otherwise) to undertake such further work as he considers appropriate, having regard to the matters which the panel was to investigate under the terms of reference.

(5) If the convening authority requires the panel to undertake further work in accordance with paragraph (4), the panel shall, on completing that work, submit a revised provisional report. Paragraphs (1) to (4) shall then apply to that provisional report.

Children's Homes Regulations 2001/3967

Part III

Conduct Of Children's Homes

Part 3 Records

Notifiable events

A2–020　　**30.**—(1) If, in relation to a children's home, any of the events listed in column 1 of the table in Schedule 5 takes place, the registered person shall without delay notify the persons indicated in respect of the event in column 2 of the table.

(2) The registered person shall without delay notify the parent of any child accommodated in the home of any significant incident affecting the child's welfare unless to do so is not reasonably practicable or would place the child's welfare at risk.

(3) Any notification made in accordance with this regulation which is given orally shall be confirmed in writing.

Schedule 5

Events and Notifications

A2–021

Column 1	Column 2					
Event:	To be notified:					
	[HMCI][1]	Placing authority	Secretary of State	Local authority for the area in which the children's home is situated, if different from the placing authority][2]	Police	[Clinical commissioning groups and the National Health Service Commissioning Board][3]
Death of a child accommodated in the home	yes	yes	yes	yes		yes

[Note: remaining entries in the Table are outside the scope of this work]

---

[1] Word substituted by Children's Homes (Amendment) Regulations 2011/583 reg.26(a) (April 1, 2011).

[2] Words inserted by Children's Homes and Looked after Children (Miscellaneous Amendments) (England) Regulations 2013/3239 Pt 2 reg.15(b) (January 27, 2014).

[3] Words substituted by National Treatment Agency (Abolition) and the Health and Social Care Act 2012 (Consequential, Transitional and Saving Provisions) Order 2013/235 Sch.2(1) para.49(3)(b) (April 1, 2013).

Children's Homes (Wales) Regulations 2002/327

PART III

CONDUCT OF CHILDREN'S HOMES

Part 3 Records

Notifiable events

29.—(1) If, in relation to a children's home, any of the events listed in column 1 of the   **A2–022**
table in Schedule 5 takes place, the registered person shall without delay notify the persons
indicated in respect of the event in column 2 of the table.

(2) A notification under paragraph (1) shall include a child's name only if that is necessary.

(3) The registered person shall without delay notify the parent of any child accommodated in the home of any significant incident affecting the child's welfare unless to do so is
not reasonably practicable or would place the child's welfare at risk.

(4) Any notification made in accordance with this regulation which is given orally shall
be confirmed in writing.

SCHEDULE 5

EVENTS AND NOTIFICATIONS

A2–023

Column 1	Column 2				
Event:	To be notified to:				
	Appropriate office of the National Assembly	Placing authority	Local authority in whose area the home is situated	Appropriate private police officer	Health authority in whose area the home is situated
Death of a child accommodated in the home	yes	yes	yes		yes

[Note: remaining entries in the Table are outside the scope of this work]

Civil Aviation (Investigation of Air Accidents and Incidents) Regulations 1996/2798

2.—(1) In these Regulations, unless the context otherwise requires—   **A2–024**

"accident" means an occurrence associated with the operation of an aircraft which takes
place between the time any person boards the aircraft with the intention of flight
until such time as all such persons have disembarked, in which—

(a) a person suffers a fatal or serious injury as a result of—

— being in or upon the aircraft,
— direct contact with any part of the aircraft, including parts which have
become detached from the aircraft, or
— direct exposure to jet blast,

except when the injuries are from natural causes, self-inflicted or inflicted by other persons, or when the injuries are to stowaways hiding outside the areas normally available to the passengers and crew, or

(b) the aircraft sustains damage or structural failure which—

— adversely affects the structural strength, performance or flight characteristics of the aircraft, and

— would normally require major repair or replacement of the affected component,

except for engine failure or damage, when the damage is limited to the engine, its cowlings or accessories; or for damage limited to propellers, wing tips, antennas, tyres, brakes, fairings, small dents or puncture holes in the aircraft skin; or

(c) the aircraft is missing or is completely inaccessible;

"aerodrome authority" means, in relation to any aerodrome, the person by whom the aerodrome is managed;

"the Annex" means Annex 13 to the Chicago Convention as amended on 23 March 1994[4];

"Chief Inspector" means the Chief Inspector of Air Accidents appointed under regulation 8 below;

"commander" in relation to an aircraft means the member of the flight crew designated as commander of that aircraft by the operator thereof, or failing such a person, the person who is for the time being the pilot in command of the aircraft;

"Contracting State" means any State (including the United Kingdom) which is party to the Chicago Convention;

"crew" includes every person employed or engaged in an aircraft in flight on the business of the aircraft;

"the Directive" means Council Directive 94/56/EC of 21 November 1994 establishing the fundamental principles governing the investigation of civil aviation accidents and incidents[5];

"fatal injury" means an injury which is sustained by a person in an accident and which results in his death within 30 days of the date of the accident;

"incident" means an occurrence, other than an accident, associated with the operation of an aircraft which affects or would affect the safety of operation;

"Inspector" means a person appointed as an Inspector of Air Accidents under regulation 8 below;

"investigating Inspector" means an Inspector carrying out an investigation pursuant to these Regulations;

"owner" means, where an aircraft is registered, the registered owner;

"pilot in command" in relation to an aircraft means a person who for the time being is in charge of the piloting of the aircraft without being under the direction of any other pilot in the aircraft;

"police officer" means any person who is a member of a police force or of the Royal Ulster Constabulary (including, for the avoidance of doubt, the Royal Ulster Constabulary Reserve), and any special constable;

"serious incident" means an incident involving circumstances indicating that an accident nearly occurred;

"serious injury" means an injury which is sustained by a person in an accident and which—

[4] The eighth edition of Annex 13 to the Chicago Convention dated July 1994 is published by the International Civil Aviation Organisation, Montreal Canada.

[5] OJ No. L 319, 12.2.94, p.14; a correction to Article 12, which incorrectly states that the implementation date is 21st November 1994 (the correct date is 21st November 1996), has been published in OJ No. L 191, 12.8.95, p.39.

(a) requires hospitalisation for more than 48 hours, commencing within seven days from the date the injury was received;

(b) results in a fracture of any bone (except simple fractures of fingers, toes, or nose);

(c) involves lacerations which cause severe haemorrhage, nerve, muscle or tendon damage;

(d) involves injury to any internal organ;

(e) involves second or third degree burns, or any burns affecting more than 5 per cent of the body surface; or

(f) involves verified exposure to infectious substances or harmful radiation; and "seriously injured" shall be construed accordingly;

"causes", "investigation", "flight recorder", "undertaking" and "safety recommendation" have the meanings given by Article 3 of the Directive; and

"established" shall have the same meaning as in the Directive.

(2) Any notice or other document required or authorised by any provision of these Regulations to be served on or given to any person may be served or given—

(a) by delivering it to that person;

(b) by leaving it at his usual or last-known residence or place of business, whether in the United Kingdom or elsewhere;

(c) by sending it to him by post at that address; or

(d) by sending it to him at that address by telex, by facsimile transmission or other similar means which produce a document containing a text of the communication, in which event the document shall be regarded as served when it is received.

3. These Regulations apply only to civil aviation accidents and incidents.

4. The sole objective of the investigation of an accident or incident under these Regulations shall be the prevention of accidents and incidents. It shall not be the purpose of such an investigation to apportion blame or liability.

5.—(1) Where an accident or a serious incident occurs in respect of which, by virtue of regulation 8(3) below the Chief Inspector is required to carry out, or to cause an Inspector to carry out, an investigation, the relevant person and, in the case of an accident or a serious incident occurring on or adjacent to an aerodrome, the aerodrome authority shall forthwith give notice thereof to the Chief Inspector by the quickest means of communication available and, in the case of an accident occurring in or over the United Kingdom, shall also notify forthwith a police officer for the area where the accident occurred of the accident and of the place where it occurred.

(2) In this regulation the expression "relevant person" means—

(a) in the case of an accident or serious incident occurring in or over the United Kingdom or occurring elsewhere to an aircraft registered in the United Kingdom, the commander of the aircraft involved at the time of the accident or serious incident or, if he be killed or incapacitated, the operator of the aircraft; and

(b) in the case of a serious incident occurring in or over any country or territory other than a member State or a Contracting State to an aircraft registered elsewhere than in the United Kingdom but operated by an undertaking established in the United Kingdom, that undertaking.

(3) The notice to the Chief Inspector referred to in paragraph (1) above shall contain as much of the following information as is available—

(a) in the case of an accident, the identifying abbreviation "ACCID" or, in the case of a serious incident, the identifying abbreviation "INCID";

(b) the type, model and the nationality and registration marks of the aircraft;

(c) the name of the owner, operator and hirer (if any) of the aircraft;

(d) the name of the commander of the aircraft;

(e) the date and Co-ordinated Universal Time of the accident or serious incident;

(f) the last point of departure and the next point of intended landing of the aircraft;

(g) the position of the aircraft by reference to some easily defined geographical point and latitude and longitude;

(h) the number of—

    (i) crew on board the aircraft at the time of the accident or serious incident and, in the case of an accident, the number of them killed or seriously injured as a result of the accident;

    (ii) passengers on board the aircraft at the time of the accident or serious incident and, in the case of an accident, the number of them killed or seriously injured as a result of the accident;

    (iii) in the case of an accident, other persons killed or seriously injured as a result of the accident;

(i) the nature of the accident or serious incident and the extent of the damage to the aircraft as far as is known.

(4) Where an incident, other than a serious incident, takes place—

(a) in or over the United Kingdom; or

(b) otherwise than in or over the United Kingdom to an aircraft registered in the United Kingdom;

the owner, operator, commander or hirer of the aircraft shall, if so required by notice given to him by the Chief Inspector, send to the Chief Inspector such information as is in his possession or control with respect to the incident in such form and at such times as may be specified in the notice.

8.—(1) For the purpose of carrying out investigations into accidents and incidents to which these Regulations apply, the Secretary of State shall, subject to paragraph (2) below, appoint persons as Inspectors of Air Accidents, one of whom shall be appointed by the Secretary of State as Chief Inspector of Air Accidents.

(2) The body of Inspectors of Air Accidents shall continue to form that part of the Department of Transport known as the Air Accidents Investigation Branch.

(3) Subject to paragraphs (5) and (6) below, the Chief Inspector shall carry out, or cause an Inspector to carry out, an investigation into—

(a) accidents and serious incidents which occur in or over the United Kingdom;

(b) accidents and serious incidents which occur in or over any country or territory which is neither a member State nor a Contracting State to aircraft registered in the United Kingdom when such an investigation is not carried out by another State;

(c) serious incidents which occur in or over any country or territory which is neither a member State nor a Contracting State to aircraft which are registered elsewhere than in the United Kingdom but which are operated by an undertaking established in the United Kingdom when such an investigation is not carried out by another State; and

(d) accidents and serious incidents to aircraft registered in the United Kingdom in the circumstances described in paragraph 5.3 of the Annex.

(4) Subject to paragraphs (5) and (6) below, the Chief Inspector may, when he expects to draw air safety lessons from it, carry out, or cause an Inspector to carry out, an investigation into an incident, other than a serious incident, which occurs—

(a) in or over the United Kingdom; or

(b) otherwise than in or over the United Kingdom to an aircraft registered in the United Kingdom.

(5) The Chief Inspector may delegate the task of carrying out an investigation into an accident or an incident to another member State [or Switzerland][6] or, in accordance with paragraphs 5.1, 5.1.1 or 5.3 of the Annex, to another Contracting State.

(6) Where the Chief Inspector delegates the task of carrying out an investigation pursuant to paragraph (5) above, he shall so far as he is able facilitate inquiries by the investigator appointed by the relevant State.

(7) The Chief Inspector may carry out, or cause an Inspector to carry out, an investigation into an accident or incident where the task of carrying out the investigation has been delegated to the United Kingdom by another member State [or Switzerland][6] or, in accordance with paragraphs 5.1, 5.1.1 or 5.3 of the Annex, by another Contracting State.

(8) Without prejudice to the power of an Inspector to seek such advice or assistance as he may deem necessary in making an investigation, the Secretary of State may at the request of the Chief Inspector appoint persons to assist an Inspector in a particular investigation and such persons shall for the purpose of so doing have such of the powers of an Inspector under these Regulations as may be specified in their appointment.

(9) The Chief Inspector may arrange for any of his powers and obligations under these regulations to be performed on his behalf by an Inspector designated by him to be his deputy.

(10) In any case where the Chief Inspector causes more than one Inspector to carry out an investigation he shall nominate one of them to be in overall charge of the investigation.

Civil Aviation (Investigation of Military Air Accidents at Civil Aerodromes) Regulations 2005/2693

Citation and commencement

1. These Regulations may be cited as the Civil Aviation (Investigation of Military Air   **A2–025** Accidents at Civil Aerodromes) Regulations 2005 and shall come into force on 1st November 2005.

Interpretation

2.—(1) "accident" means an occurrence associated with the operation of a military   **A2–026** aircraft which takes place between the time any person boards the aircraft with the intention of flight until such time as all such persons have disembarked, in which:

    (a) a person suffers a fatal or serious injury as a result of:

        (i) being in or upon the aircraft,

        (ii) direct contact with any part of the aircraft, including parts which have become detached from the aircraft, or

        (iii) direct exposure to jet blast, except when the injuries are from natural causes, self-inflicted or inflicted by other persons, or when the injuries are to stowaways hiding outside the areas normally available to the passengers and crew, or

    (b) the aircraft sustains damage or structural failure which:

---

[6] Words inserted by EC/Swiss Air Transport Agreement (Consequential Amendments) Regulations 2004/1256 reg.7 (June 1, 2004).

(i)   adversely affects the structural strength, performance or flight characteristics of the aircraft, and

(ii) would normally require major repair or replacement of the affected component, except for engine failure or damage when the damage is limited to the engine, its cowlings or accessories; or for damage limited to propellers, wing tips, antennas, tyres, brakes, fairings, small dents or puncture holes in the aircraft skin.

"aerodrome authority" means, in relation to any civil aerodrome, the person by whom the aerodrome is managed;

"accredited representative" means a person designated by a State on the basis of his qualifications, for the purpose of participating in an investigation conducted by another State;

"the Annex" means Annex 13 to the Chicago Convention as amended[7];

"Chief Inspector" means the Chief Inspector of Air Accidents appointed under regulation 8 of the Civil Regulations;

"civil aerodrome" means an aerodrome used wholly or mainly for the purposes of civil aviation;

"Civil Regulations" means the Civil Aviation (Investigation of Air Accidents and Incidents) Regulations 1996;

"commander" in relation to a military aircraft means the person who is for the time being in command of the aircraft;

"crew" includes every person employed or engaged in a military aircraft in flight on the business of the aircraft;

"the Directive" means Council Directive 94/56/EC of 21st November 1994 establishing the fundamental principles governing the investigation of civil aviation accidents[8];

"fatal injury" means an injury which is sustained by a person in an accident and which results in his death within 30 days of the date of the accident;

"flight recorder" means any type of recorder installed in the aircraft for the purposes of facilitating accident investigation;

"Inspector" means a person appointed as an Inspector of Air Accidents under regulation 8 of the Civil Regulations;

"investigation" means a process conducted for the purposes of accident prevention which includes the gathering and analysis of information, the drawing of conclusions including the determination of the cause or causes and, when appropriate, the making of safety recommendations;

"investigating Inspector" means an Inspector carrying out an investigation pursuant to these Regulations;

"operator" in relation to an aircraft means any person, body or undertaking operating or proposing to operate one or more aircraft;

"owner" means, in relation to an aircraft, the registered owner;

"police officer" means any person who is a member of a police force or of the Police Service of Northern Ireland (including for the avoidance of doubt, the Police Service of Northern Ireland Reserve) and any special constable;

"safety recommendation" means any proposal by an investigating Inspector made with the intention of preventing accidents;

"serious injury" means an injury which is sustained by a person in an accident and which—

(a)   requires hospitalisation for more than 48 hours, commencing within 7 days from the date the injury was received;

---

[7] The ninth edition of Annex 13 to the Convention dated 1st July 2001 is published by the International Civil Aviation Organisation, Montreal, Canada.

[8] OJ No. L319, 12.2.94, p.14; a correction to Article 12 which incorrectly states that the implementation date is 21st November 1994 (the correct date is 21st November 1996), has been published in OJ No. L191, 12.8.95, p.39.

(b) results in the fracture of any bone (except simple fractures of fingers, toes or nose);

(c) involves lacerations which cause severe haemorrhage, nerve, muscle or tendon damage;

(d) involves injury to any internal organ;

(e) involves second or third degree burns, or any burns affecting more than 5 per cent of the body surface; or

(f) involves verified exposure to infectious substances or harmful radiation;

and "seriously injured" shall be construed accordingly;

"State of Design" means the State having jurisdiction over the organisation responsible for the type design of the aircraft;

"State of Manufacture" means the State having jurisdiction over the organisation responsible for the final assembly of the aircraft;

"State of the operator" means the State in which the operator's principal place of business is located, or if there is no such place of business, the operator's permanent residence;

"State of Registry" means the State on whose register the aircraft is entered; and

"undertaking" means any natural person, any legal person, whether profit making or not, or any official body whether having its own legal personality or not.

(2) Any notice or other document required or authorised by any provision of these Regulations to be served on or given to any person may be served or given—

(a) by delivering it to that person;

(b) by leaving it at his usual last-known residence or place of business, whether in the United Kingdom or elsewhere;

(c) by sending it to him by post at that address;

(d) by sending it to him at that address by telex, by facsimile transmission, by electronic communication, or other similar means which produce a document containing a text of the communication, in which event the document shall be regarded as served when it is received.

(3) An aircraft shall be treated for the purpose of these Regulations as being a military aircraft if—

(a) it is an aircraft in the ownership of any of Her Majesty's naval, military or air forces, or

(b) not being such an aircraft in sub-paragraph (a), it is an aircraft in the ownership of any of the naval, military or air forces of any other State, or

(c) the Secretary of State for Defence certifies that by reason of the circumstances affecting the aircraft, it is to be treated for the purposes of these Regulations as being a military aircraft.

(4) References in these Regulations to the Secretaries of State are to the Secretary of State for Transport and the Secretary of State for Defence acting jointly.

Application

3.—(1) Where a military aircraft is involved in an accident arising out of or in the course of air navigation occurring in or over the United Kingdom and the Secretaries of State are of the opinion that the accident occurred or may have occurred—   **A2–027**

(a) while the aircraft was on, or in the course of taking off from or landing on, a civil aerodrome, or

(b) in such circumstances that the Secretaries of State, are or may be concerned or interested in its circumstances or causes,

they may, save where the accident is one to which the Civil Regulations apply, direct that the accident shall be treated as an accident to which these Regulations apply.

(2) Public notice of any direction made under this regulation shall be given in such manner as the Secretaries of State may think fit.

(3) References in these Regulations to an accident to which these Regulations apply are references to an accident in respect of which a direction has been given under this regulation.

Purpose of the investigation of accidents

A2–028   **4.** The sole objective of the investigation of an accident to which these Regulations apply shall be the prevention of accidents. It shall not be the purpose of such an investigation to apportion blame or liability.

Duty to furnish information relating to accidents

A2–029   **5.**—(1) Where a military aircraft is involved in an accident to which these Regulations apply and the accident occurs on or adjacent to a civil aerodrome, the aerodrome authority shall—

(a) give notice as soon as possible to the Chief Inspector by the quickest means of communication available, and

(b) notify forthwith a police officer for the area where the accident occurred of the accident and the place where it occurred.

(2) The notice to the Chief Inspector referred to in paragraph (1) shall contain as much of the following information as is available—

(a) the identifying abbreviation "ACCID";

(b) the type, model, nationality and registration marks of the aircraft;

(c) the name of the owner, operator and hirer (if any) of the aircraft;

(d) the name of the commander of the aircraft;

(e) the date and Co-ordinated Universal Time of the accident;

(f) the last point of departure and the next point of intended landing of the aircraft;

(g) the position of the aircraft by reference to some easily defined geographical point and latitude and longitude;

(h) the number of—

(i) crew on board the aircraft at the time of the accident and the number of them killed or seriously injured as a result of the accident;

(ii) passengers on board the aircraft at the time of the accident and the number of them killed or seriously injured as a result of the accident;

(iii) other persons killed or seriously injured as a result of the accident;

(i) the nature of the accident and the extent of the damage to the aircraft and property as far as is known;

(j) the nature of any air cargo, munitions or other dangerous or potentially hazardous items carried on the aircraft.

Publication

A2–030   **6.** Subject to regulation 12, the Chief Inspector may at any time publish, or cause to be published, information relating to an accident to which these Regulations apply.

Removal of damaged aircraft

7.—(1) Subject to paragraph (2) and regulation 9, where an accident occurs to which   **A2–031**
these Regulations apply—

(a) no person other than an authorised person shall have access to the aircraft involved, and

(b) neither the aircraft nor its contents shall, except under the authority of the Secretary of State for Transport or the Secretary of State for Defence, be removed or otherwise interfered with.

(2) Subject to the provisions of section 21(4), (4A) and (5) of the Customs and Excise Management Act 1979[9]—

(a) the aircraft may be removed or interfered with so far as may be necessary for the purposes of saving human life or for the removal of any immediate hazard to human life;

(b) if the aircraft is wrecked on water, the aircraft or any of its contents may be removed to such extent as may be necessary for bringing it or them to a place of safety.

(3) In this regulation the expression "authorised person" means—

(a) any person authorised by the Secretary of State for Transport or the Secretary of State for Defence either generally or specially to have access to any military aircraft involved in an accident;

(b) any police officer;

(c) any officer of Customs and Excise.

Inspectors of Air Accidents

8.—(1) The Chief Inspector shall determine whether or not an investigation shall be   **A2–032**
carried out into any accident to which these Regulations apply and he himself may carry out or cause an Inspector to carry out an investigation of any such accident.
(2) Without prejudice to the power of an Inspector to seek such advice or assistance as he may deem necessary in making an investigation, the Secretary of State for Transport may at the request of the Chief Inspector—

(a) appoint persons to assist an Inspector in a particular investigation; and

(b) such persons shall for the purpose of so doing have such of the powers of an Inspector under these Regulations as may be specified in their appointment.

(3) The Chief Inspector may authorise that any of his powers and obligations under these Regulations shall be performed on his behalf by an Inspector designated by him to be his deputy.
(4) In any case where the Chief Inspector causes more than one Inspector to carry out an investigation he shall nominate one of them to be in overall charge of the investigation.

[9] Section 21(4A) was inserted by regulation 6(5) of the Customs Control on Importation of Goods Regulations 1991 (S.I. 1991/2724).

Powers of Inspectors

A2–033   9.—(1) For the purposes of enabling him to carry out an investigation into an accident to which these Regulations apply in the most efficient way and within the shortest time, an investigating Inspector is hereby authorised to—

(a) have immediate free access to the site of the accident as well as to the aircraft, its contents or wreckage;

(b) ensure an immediate listing of evidence and controlled removal of debris or components for examination or analysis purposes;

(c) have immediate access to and use of the contents of the flight recorders and any other recordings;

(d) have access to the results of examinations of the bodies of victims or of tests made upon samples taken from the bodies of the victims;

(e) have access to the results of examinations of the people involved in the operation of the aircraft or of the tests made on samples taken from such people;

(f) examine witnesses; and

(g) have free access to any relevant information or records held by the owner, the operator or the manufacturer of the aircraft and by the authorities responsible for civil and military aviation or aerodrome operation.

(2) For the purposes of paragraph (1) above an inspecting Investigator shall have power—

(a) by summons under his hand—

(i) to call before him and examine all such persons as he thinks fit;

(ii) to require such persons to answer any question or furnish any information or produce any books, papers, documents and articles which he may consider relevant; and

(iii) to retain any such books, papers, documents and articles until the completion of the investigation;

(b) to take such statements from all such persons as he thinks fit and to require any such person to make and sign a declaration of the truth of the statement made by him;

(c) on production if required of his credentials, to enter and inspect any place, building or aircraft if it appears to him to be necessary for the purposes of the investigation;

(d) on production if required of his credentials, to remove, test, take measures for the preservation of or otherwise deal with any aircraft or any part of such aircraft or anything carried thereon other than an aircraft involved in the accident where it appears to him necessary for the purposes of the investigation; and

(e) to take such measures for the preservation of evidence as he considers appropriate.

(3) Every person summoned by an investigating Inspector under paragraph 2(a) shall be allowed such expenses as the Secretaries of State may determine.

Form and conduct of investigations

A2–034   10.—(1) The extent of investigations and the procedure to be followed in carrying out investigations authorised under these Regulations shall be determined by the Chief

Inspector taking account of the purpose described in regulation 4 and the lessons he expects to draw from the accident for the improvement of safety.

(2) The Chief Inspector shall notify the Secretaries of State in writing of his decision to proceed or not proceed with an investigation into an air accident to which these Regulations apply.

Inspector's report

11.—(1) On completion of an investigation into an accident to which these Regulations **A2–035** apply, the investigating Inspector shall prepare a report of the investigation in a form appropriate to the type and seriousness of the accident.

(2) If it appears to the investigating Inspector that the investigation of an accident to which these Regulations apply has been completed but for the investigation of matters affecting the discipline or internal administration of—

(a) Her Majesty's naval, military or air forces; or

(b) the naval, military or air forces of any other State

which are more appropriate for the investigation by some other person or body, the investigation may be treated for the purposes of paragraph (1) as if it had been completed without such matters being investigated under these Regulations.

(3) In a case covered by paragraph (2) the report of the investigation into the accident shall state those matters to which the investigation has not extended by reason of that paragraph.

(4) The report of an investigation into an accident to which these Regulations apply shall state the sole objective of the investigation as described in regulation 4 and contain, where appropriate, safety recommendations.

(5) A safety recommendation shall in no case create a presumption of blame or liability for an accident.

(6) The Chief Inspector shall submit a copy of every report prepared pursuant to paragraph (1) to the Secretaries of State without delay.

(7) In this regulation and regulation 12, the expression "investigating Inspector" in a case where more than one Inspector is carrying out the task of investigation means the Inspector nominated by the Chief Inspector to be in overall charge of the investigation, and that person shall not be the Chief Inspector.

Notice of Inspector's report and representations thereon

12.—(1) No report which is required by regulation 13 to be published shall be published **A2–036** if, in the investigating Inspector's opinion, it is likely to adversely affect the reputation of any person, until he has—

(a) where it appears to him to be practicable so to do, served a notice under this regulation upon that person, or if that person is a deceased individual, upon the person who appears to him, at the time he proposes to serve the notice pursuant to this paragraph, to represent best the interest of the deceased in the matter, and

(b) made such changes to the report as he thinks fit following his consideration of any representations made to him in accordance with paragraph (3) by or on behalf of the person served with such notice.

(2) The notice referred to in paragraph (1)(a) shall include particulars of any proposed analysis of facts and conclusions as to the cause or causes of the accident which may affect the person on whom or in respect of whom the notice is served.

(3) Any representations made pursuant to paragraph (1)(b) shall be in writing and shall, subject to paragraph (6), be served on the investigating Inspector within 28 days of service of the notice referred to in paragraph (1)(a).

(4) A copy of the report submitted to the Secretaries of State under regulation 11(6) shall be served by the investigating Inspector on any person who has been served with a notice pursuant to paragraph (1).

(5) No person shall disclose or permit to be disclosed any information contained in a notice or report served on him pursuant to paragraphs (1) or (4) to any other person without the prior consent in writing of the Chief Inspector.

(6) The Chief Inspector shall have power to extend the period of 28 days prescribed in paragraph (3) and this power shall be exercisable notwithstanding that that period has expired.

Publication of reports

A2–037   **13.** Subject to regulation 12(1), the Chief Inspector shall cause the report of an investigation to be made public in the shortest time possible (and, if possible, within 12 months of the date of the accident) and in such manner as he thinks fit.

Safety recommendations

A2–038   **14.**—(1) The Chief Inspector shall cause the report referred to in regulation 13, including the safety recommendations contained therein, to be communicated to the undertakings or national aviation authorities concerned in the accident.

(2) Any undertaking or authority to which a safety recommendation is communicated pursuant to paragraph (1) shall, without delay—

    (a) take that recommendation into consideration and, where appropriate, act upon it;

    (b) send to the Secretaries of State—

        (i) full details of the measures, if any, it has taken to or proposes to take to implement the recommendation and, in the case where it proposes to implement measures, the timetable for securing that implementation; or

        (ii) a full explanation as to why the recommendation is not to be the subject of the measures taken to implement it; and

    (c) give notice to the Secretaries of State if at any time any information provided to the Secretaries of State in accordance with paragraph (2)(b)(i) concerning the measures it proposes to take or the timetable for securing their implementation is rendered inaccurate by any change of circumstances.

Reopening of investigation

A2–039   **15.**—(1) The Chief Inspector may cause the investigation of any accident to which these Regulations apply to be re-opened and shall do so—

    (a) if, after the completion of the investigation, evidence has been disclosed which is in his opinion both new and important; or

    (b) if for any other reason there is in his opinion ground for suspecting that the reputation of any person has been unfairly and adversely affected.

(2) Without prejudice to regulation 19(3) any investigation re-opened shall be subject to and conducted in accordance with the provisions of these regulations.

Accredited representatives

A2–040   **16.**—(1) Where an investigation of an accident is being carried out by an investigating Inspector pursuant to regulation 8, an accredited representative appointed by—

    (a) the State of Registry;

(b) the State of Design;

(c) the State of Manufacture;

(d) the State of the operator;

(e) any other State which has, on request, furnished information, facilities or experts to the investigating Inspector in connection with the accident;

may take part in the investigation.

(2) For the purposes of paragraph (1) an accredited representative shall be permitted to—

(a) visit the scene of the accident;

(b) examine the wreckage;

(c) question witnesses;

(d) receive copies of all pertinent documents (saving all just exceptions as may be determined by the investigating Inspector);

(e) have access to all relevant evidence and make submissions; and

(f) be accompanied by such technical and other advisers as may be considered necessary by the authorities of the State by which he is appointed.

(3) In this regulation the expression "investigating Inspector" in a case where more than one Inspector is carrying out the task of investigation means the Inspector nominated under regulation 8(4).

Obstruction of investigation

17.—(1) No person shall obstruct or impede any investigating Inspector or any person   **A2–041** acting under the authority of the Secretaries of State in the exercise of any powers under these Regulations.

(2) No person shall without reasonable excuse fail, after having had the expenses (if any) to which he is entitled under these Regulations tendered to him, to comply with any summons of an investigating Inspector.

Disclosure of relevant records

18.—(1) Subject to paragraphs (2) and (4) to (6) no relevant record shall be made available   **A2–042** by the Secretaries of State to any person for purposes other than accident investigation.

(2) Nothing in paragraph (1) shall preclude a person making a relevant record available to any other person where—

(a) in a case where the other person is a party to or otherwise entitled to appear at judicial proceedings, the relevant court has ordered that the relevant record shall be made available to him for the purposes of those proceedings, or

(b) in any other circumstances, the relevant court has ordered that the relevant record shall be made available to him for the purposes of those circumstances.

(3) In this regulation—

"judicial proceedings" includes any proceedings before any court, tribunal or person having by law the power to hear, receive and examine evidence on oath:
"relevant court" in the case of judicial proceedings or an application for disclosure, made in—

(a) England, Wales or Northern Ireland means the High Court, and

(b) In the case of Scotland means the Court of Session.

"relevant record" means any item in the possession, custody or power of the Secretaries of State which is of a kind referred to in sub-paragraphs (a) to (e) of paragraph 5.12 of the Annex; and

"Secretaries of State" includes any officer of theirs.

(4) Subject to paragraph (6) no order shall be made under paragraph (2) unless the relevant court is satisfied that the interests of justice in the circumstances in question outweigh the adverse domestic and international impact which disclosure may have—

(a) on the investigation into the accident to which the record relates; or

(b) on any future accident investigation undertaken in the United Kingdom.

(5) A relevant record or part thereof shall not be treated as having been made available under paragraph (1) in any case where that record or part is included in the final report (or the appendices to the final report) of the accident.

(6) The provisions of this regulation shall be without prejudice to any rule of law which authorises or requires the withholding of any relevant record or part thereof on the ground that the disclosure of it would be injurious to the public interest.

Community Legal Service (Cost Protection) Regulations 2000/824

Costs order against Commission

A2–043   **5.**—(1) The following paragraphs of this regulation apply where:

(a) funded services are provided to a client in relation to proceedings;

(b) those proceedings are finally decided in favour of a non-funded party; and

(c) cost protection applies.

(2) The court may, subject to the following paragraphs of this regulation, make an order for the payment by the Commission to the non-funded party of the whole or any part of the costs incurred by him in the proceedings (other than any costs that the client is required to pay under a section 11(1) costs order).

(3) An order under paragraph (2) may only be made if all the conditions set out in sub-paragraphs (a), (b), (c) and (d) are satisfied:

(a) a section 11(1) costs order is made against the client in the proceedings, and the amount (if any) which the client is required to pay under that costs order is less than the amount of the full costs;

(b) [unless there is a good reason for the delay,][10] the non-funded party makes a request under regulation 10(2) of the Community Legal Service (Costs) Regulations 2000 within three months of the making of the section 11(1) costs order;

(c) as regards costs incurred in a court of first instance, the proceedings were instituted by the client [, the non-funded party is an individual,][11] and the court is satisfied that

---

[10] Words inserted by Community Legal Service (Cost Protection) (Amendment No. 2) Regulations 2001/3812 reg.4(1) (December 3, 2001).

[11] Words inserted by Community Legal Service (Cost Protection) (Amendment No. 2) Regulations 2001/3812 reg.4(2)(a) (December 3, 2001).

the non-funded party will suffer [. . .]¹² financial hardship unless the order is made; and

(d) in any case, the court is satisfied that it is just and equitable in the circumstances that provision for the costs should be made out of public funds.

[(3A) An order under paragraph (2) may be made—

(a) [in relation to proceedings in the Supreme Court, by such officers as may be appointed by the President]¹³;

(b) in relation to proceedings in the Court of Appeal, High Court [, family court]¹⁴ or a county court, by a costs judge or a district judge;

(c) in relation to proceedings in a magistrates' court, by a single justice or by the justices' clerk;

(d) in relation to proceedings in the Employment Appeal Tribunal, by the Registrar of that tribunal.]¹⁵

(4) Where the client receives funded services in connection with part only of the proceedings, the reference in paragraph (2) to the costs incurred by the non-funded party in the relevant proceedings shall be construed as a reference to so much of those costs as is attributable to the part of the proceedings which are funded proceedings.

(5) Where a court decides any proceedings in favour of the non-funded party and an appeal lies (with or without permission) against that decision, any order made under this regulation shall not take effect:

(a) where permission to appeal is required, unless the time limit for applications for permission to appeal expires without permission being granted;

(b) where permission to appeal is granted or is not required, unless the time limit for appeal expires without an appeal being brought.

(6) Subject to paragraph (7), in determining whether the conditions in paragraph (3)(c) and (d) are satisfied, the court shall have regard to the resources of the non-funded party and of his partner.

(7) The court shall not have regard to the resources of the partner of the non-funded party if the partner has a contrary interest in the funded proceedings.

(8) Where the non-funded party is acting in a representative, fiduciary or official capacity and is entitled to be indemnified in respect of his costs from any property, estate or fund, the court shall, for the purposes of paragraph (3), have regard to the value of the property, estate or fund and the resources of the persons, if any, including that party where appropriate, who are beneficially interested in that property, estate or fund.

---

¹² Word repealed by Community Legal Service (Cost Protection) (Amendment No. 2) Regulations 2001/3812 reg.4(2)(b) (December 3, 2001).

¹³ Words substituted by Constitutional Reform Act 2005 (Consequential Amendments) Order 2009/2468 art.3 (October 1, 2009).

¹⁴ Words inserted by Crime and Courts Act 2013 (Family Court: Consequential Provision) (No.2) Order 2014/879 Pt 2 art.78 (April 22, 2014).

¹⁵ Added by Community Legal Service (Cost Protection) (Amendment) Regulations 2001/823 reg.3 (April 2, 2001).

Coroners and Justice Act 2009 (Alteration of Coroner Areas) Order 2013/1626

A2–044   **1.**—(1) This Order may be cited as the Coroners and Justice Act 2009 (Alteration of Coroner Areas) Order 2013.

2. This Order comes into force on the 26th July 2013.

3. In this Order—

"coroner area" means a coroner area constituted by the Coroners and Justice Act 2009 (Coroner Areas and Assistant Coroners) Transitional Order 2013;

"altered coroner area" means a new coroner area resulting from the amalgamation of coroner areas as set out in this Order.

4. Coroner areas listed in the first column of the table in the Schedule to this Order shall be amalgamated into the single coroner area listed in the corresponding entry in the second column.

SCHEDULE 1

A2–045

Coroner areas to be amalgamated	Altered coroner area
1. Carmarthenshire/Sir Gaerfyrddin	Carmarthenshire and Pembrokeshire/Sir Gaerfyrddin a Sir Benfro
2. Pembrokeshire/Sir Benfro	
1. Darlington and South Durham	County Durham and Darlington
2. North Durham	
1. Derby and South Derbyshire	Derby and Derbyshire
2. North Derbyshire	
1. Bournemouth, Poole and Eastern Dorset	Dorset
2. Western Dorset	
1. Essex and Thurrock	Essex
2. Southend and South East Essex	
1. Plymouth and South West Devon	Plymouth, Torbay and South Devon
2. Torbay and South Devon	
1. Bridgend and Glamorgan Valleys/Pen-y-bont ar Ogwr a Chymoedd Morgannwg	Powys, Bridgend and Glamorgan Valleys/Powys, Pen-y-bont ar Ogwr a Chymoedd Morgannwg
2. Powys	
1. Mid and North West Shropshire	Shropshire, Telford and Wrekin
2. South Shropshire	
3. Wrekin	
1. Neath Port Talbot/Castell-nedd Port Talbot	Swansea and Neath Port Talbot/Abertawe a Chastell-nedd Port Talbot
2. Swansea/Abertawe	

Coroners and Justice Act 2009 (Commencement No. 3 and Transitional Provision) Order 2010/145

Citation and interpretation

1.—(1) This Order may be cited as the Coroners and Justice Act 2009 (Commencement No. 3 and Transitional Provision) Order 2010.   **A2–046**

(2) In this Order, "the 2009 Act" means the Coroners and Justice Act 2009.

Appointed days

2.—(1) [Outside the scope of this work]   **A2–047**

(2) The provisions of the 2009 Act specified in the Schedule shall come into force on 1st February 2010.

SCHEDULE 1

PROVISIONS WHICH COME INTO FORCE ON 1ST FEBRUARY 2010

1. Section 35 (Chief Coroner and Deputy Chief Coroners).   **A2–048**
21. Schedule 8 (Chief Coroner and Deputy Chief Coroners).

Coroners and Justice Act 2009 (Commencement No. 10) Order 2012/2374

Citation and interpretation

1.—(1) This Order may be cited as the Coroners and Justice Act 2009 (Commencement No. 10) Order 2012.   **A2–049**

(2) In this Order, "the 2009 Act" means the Coroners and Justice Act 2009.

Appointed days

2. The following provisions of the 2009 Act shall come into force on 24th September 2012—   **A2–050**

(a) section 12 (death of service personnel abroad, investigation in Scotland); and

(b) [*Outside the scope of this work*].

Coroners and Justice Act 2009 (Commencement No. 11) Order 2013/250

Citation

1. This Order may be cited as the Coroners and Justice Act 2009 (Commencement No. 11) Order 2013.   **A2–051**

Appointed day

2. The following provisions of the Coroners and Justice Act 2009 shall come into force on 12th February 2013—   **A2–052**

(a) section 178 (repeals), in so far as it relates to the provision specified in sub–paragraph (b); and

(b) in Part 1 (coroners etc) of Schedule 23 (repeals), the entry relating to the Coroners Act 1988 in so far as it relates to section 5(2) of that Act.

Coroners and Justice Act 2009 (Commencement No. 14) Order 2013/1628

Citation

A2–053   1. This Order may be cited as the Coroners and Justice Act 2009 (Commencement No. 14) Order 2013.

Commencement

A2–054   2. The following provisions of the Coroners and Justice Act 2009 come into force on the day after the date on which this Order is made—

(a) section 43 (coroners regulations); and

(b) section 45 (coroners rules).

Coroners and Justice Act 2009 (Commencement No. 15, Consequential and Transitory Provisions) Order 2013/1869

Citation

A2–055   1. This Order may be cited as the Coroners and Justice Act 2009 (Commencement No. 15, Consequential and Transitory Provisions) Order 2013.

Commencement of provisions of the Coroners and Justice Act 2009

A2–056   2. The following provisions of the Coroners and Justice Act 2009 are commenced on 25th July 2013—

(a) sections 1 to 11 and sections 13 to 17 (investigations into deaths);

(b) sections 22 to 24 (coroner areas, appointments etc.);

(c) section 32 only in so far as it relates to paragraphs 1, 2, 6 and 7 of Schedule 5 and sections 33 to 34 (further provision to do with investigations and deaths);

(d) section 36 with the exclusion of subsection (4)(c), section 37, section 41 only in so far as it relates to paragraphs 1, 3 and 5 of Schedule 10 and section 42 (governance etc.);

(e) section 46 (coroner of the Queen's household);

(f) section 177(1) (consequential etc. amendments, and transitional and saving provisions) to the extent that it relates to the provisions specified in sub-paragraph (o);

(g) section 178 (repeals) only to the extent that it relates to the provisions specified in sub-paragraph (p);

(h) Schedule 1 (duty or power to suspend or resume investigations);

(i)   Schedule 2 (coroner areas);

(j)   Schedule 3 (appointment etc. of senior coroners, area coroners and assistant coroners);

(k)   paragraphs 1, 2, 6 and 7 of Schedule 5 (powers of coroners);

(l)   Schedule 6 (offences);

(m)   Schedule 7 (allowances, fees and expenses);

(n)   paragraphs 1, 3 and 5 of Schedule 10 (investigation by Chief Coroner or Coroner for Treasure or by judge, former judge or former coroner);

(o)   in Part 1 of Schedule 21 (minor and consequential amendments)—

   (i)   paragraphs 1 to 7;
   (ii)   paragraph 8(4);
   (iii) paragraph 9(3)(d);
   (iv)   paragraph 11(3);
   (v)   paragraph 15(1), (3), and (4);
   (vi)   paragraph 15(2) but only in so far as substituting subsection (2) of section 23 of the Births and Deaths Registration Act 1953 with a new subsection (2) and not subsection (2ZA);
   (vii) paragraph 18(1) and (2) to the extent that those provisions introduce a new subsection (3B) only into section 29 of the Births and Deaths Registration Act 1953;
   (viii) paragraph 18(3) and (4) (and paragraph 18(1) in so far as relating to those provisions);
   (ix)   paragraph 21(1) but only in relation to the definition of "the 2009 Act";
   (x)   paragraph 21(2) but only in so far as inserting a new subsection (3) into section 41 of the Birth and Deaths Registration Act 1953 and not a new subsection (2);
   (xi)   paragraphs 22 to 25;
   (xii) paragraph 26 with the exception of the words "Coroner for Treasure";
   (xiii) paragraph 28;
   (xiv) paragraph 30;
   (xv)   paragraphs 32 to 36;
   (xvi) paragraphs 44 and 45; and
   (xvii) paragraph 51 to the extent that it relates to the Deputy Chief Coroner only; and

(p)   Part 1 of Schedule 23 (repeals: coroners etc.) to the extent that it relates to the entry for the Coroners Act 1988 except for sections 4A(8) and 13(1) and (2) of that Act.

Transitory modification provision in relation to treasure inquests

3. From the time when the provision in article 2(p) of this Order is commenced until   **A2–057** such time as sections 25 to 31 (investigations concerning treasure) of, and Schedule 4 to, the Coroners and Justice Act 2009 come into force—

(a)   the Coroners Act 1988 is to be treated as not repealed, in so far as it relates to the exercise of a coroner's jurisdiction in relation to treasure inquests as provided by section 30 of that Act;

(b) any reference to a coroner in the Coroners Act 1988 is to be treated as a reference to a coroner appointed under section 23 of, and Schedule 3 to, the Coroners and Justice Act 2009; and

(c) any reference to a coroner district in the Coroners Act 1988 is to be treated as a reference to a coroner area constituted under section 22 of, and Schedule 2 to, the Coroners and Justice Act 2009.

Consequential amendments

A2–058   4. The amendments made in the Schedule shall have effect on 25th July 2013.

SCHEDULE 1

CONSEQUENTIAL AMENDMENTS

A2–059   *[Makes consequential amendments]*

Coroners and Justice Act 2009 (Consequential Provisions) Order 2013/1874

Citation, commencement and extent

A2–060   1.—(1) This Order may be cited as the Coroners and Justice Act 2009 (Consequential Provisions) Order 2013, and comes into force on the day after the day on which it is made.

(2) The amendments made by Article 2 have the same extent as the enactments to which they each relate.

Amendment of the Coroners Act 1988

A2–061   2.—*[Amends the Coroners Act 1988]*

Coroners and Justice Act 2009 (Coroner Areas and Assistant Coroners) Transitional Order 2013/1625

A2–062   1.—(1) This Order may be cited as the Coroners and Justice Act 2009 (Coroner Areas and Assistant Coroners) Transitional Order 2013.

2. This Order comes into force on the 25th July 2013.

3. In this Order—

"coroner's district" means a coroner's district constituted under the Coroners Act 1988, as it exists immediately before the day on which this Order comes into force;
"coroner area" means a coroner area specified by this Order.

4. Each coroner's district listed in the table in the Schedule to this Order is specified as a coroner area with the same name (but ending with "coroner area" instead of "coroner' district").

5. At least one assistant coroner must be appointed for each coroner area specified by this Order.

SCHEDULE 1

Coroner's district to be specified as a corresponding coroner area
Avon
Bedfordshire and Luton
Berkshire
Birmingham and Solihull
Black Country
Blackburn, Hyndburn and Ribbl Valley
Blackpool and Fylde
Bournemouth, Poole and Eastern Dorset
Bridgend and Glamorgan Valleys/Pen-y-bont ar Ogwr a Chymoedd Morgannwg
Brighton and Hove
Buckinghamshire
Cardiff and Vale of Glamorgan
Carmarthenshire/Sir Gaerfyrddin
Central and South East Kent
Central Hampshire
Central Lincolnshire
Ceredigion
Cheshire
City of London
Cornwall
Coventry
Darlington and South Durham
Derby and South Derbyshire
East Lancashire
East London
East Riding and Hull
East Sussex
Essex and Thurrock
Exeter and Greater Devon
Gateshead and South Tyneside
Gloucestershire
Gwent
Hartlepool
Herefordshire

Coroner's district to be specified as a corresponding coroner area—*continued*
Hertfordshire
Inner North London
Inner South London
Inner West London
Isle of Wright
Isles of Scilly
Leicester City and South Leicestershire
Liverpool
Manchester (City)
Manchester North
Manchester South
Manchester West
Mid and North West Shropshire
Mid Kent and Medway
Milton Keynes
Neath Port Talbot/Castell-nedd Port Talbot
Newcastle-upon-Tyne
Norfolk
Northamptonshire
North and East Cambridgeshire
North and West Cumbria
North Derbyshire
North Durham
North East Hampshire
North East Kent
North Lincolnshire and Grimsby
North London
North Northumberland
North Tyneside
North Wales (East and Central)/Gogledd Cymru (Dwyrain a Chanol
North West Kent
North West Wales/Gogledd Orllewin Cymru
North Yorkshire (Eastern)
North Yorkshire (Western)
Nottinghamshire and Nottingham
Oxfordshire

Coroner's district to be specified as a corresponding coroner area—*continued*
Pembrokeshire/Sir Benfro
Peterborough
Plymouth and South West Devon
Portsmouth and South East Hampshire
Powys
Preston and West Lancashire
Rutland and North Leicestershire
Sefton, St Helens and Knowsley
Somerset (Eastern)
Somerset (Western)
South and East Cumbria
South and West Cambridgeshire
South Lincolnshire
South London
South Northumberland
South Shropshire
South Staffordshire
South Yorkshire (East)
South Yorkshire (West)
Southampton and New Forest
Southend and South East Essex
Stoke on Trent and North Staffordshire
Suffolk
Sunderland
Surrey
Swansea/Abertawe
Teesside
The Wrekin
Torbay and South Devon
Warwickshire
Western Dorset
West London
West Sussex
West Yorkshire (Eastern)
West Yorkshire (Western)
Wiltshire and Swindon

Coroner's district to be specified as a corresponding coroner area—*continued*
Wirral
Worcestershire
York

Coroners Allowances, Fees and Expenses Regulations

PART 1

INTRODUCTION

Citation and commencement

A2–064   **1.** These Regulations may be cited as the Coroners Allowances, Fees and Expenses Regulations 2013 and shall come into force on 25th July 2013.

Interpretation

A2–065   **2.** In these Regulations—

"copy" means in relation to a document, anything on which information recorded in a document has been copied, by whatever means and whether directly or indirectly;

"coroner" means:

    (a) a senior coroner, area coroner or assistant coroner;

    (b) the Chief Coroner when conducting an investigation under paragraph 1 of Schedule 10 to the Coroners and Justice Act 2009; and

    (c) a judge, former judge or former coroner conducting an investigation under paragraph 3 of Schedule 10 to the Coroners and Justice Act 2009,

unless a provision of these Regulations specifically provides otherwise;

"document" means any medium in which information of any description is recorded or stored;

"expert witness" means a person of any calling, profession or trade who gives evidence at an inquest because of his or her expertise, other than a professional witness;

"ordinary witness" means any person who gives evidence at an inquest and is not an expert or professional witness;

"professional witness" means any person who is practising as a member of the medical profession or as a dentist who gives medical evidence at an inquest;

"relevant authority" means the local authority designated as such in accordance with the Coroners and Justice Act 2009 for a particular coroner area; and

"witness" means an expert witness, ordinary witness or professional witness.

Delegation of administrative functions

A2–066   **3.** A coroner may delegate administrative functions to coroner's officers and other staff.

PART 2

CALCULATION, DETERMINATION AND PAYMENT OF ALLOWANCES, FEES AND EXPENSES

Calculation and payment by the coroner

A2–067   **4.** Any allowance, fee or expense payable to a person under these Regulations is to be calculated by the coroner or the coroner's relevant authority, and paid by the coroner or the coroner's relevant authority.

Determination by the coroner

5. A coroner may require a person claiming an expense under these Regulations to provide receipts, invoices or other documents proving the expense incurred before determining and making any payment under these Regulations.

A2–068

Explanation by the coroner

6. A coroner must, if requested to do so by a person claiming an allowance, fee or expense under these Regulations, provide that person with information on how his or her particular allowance, fee or expense has been calculated.

A2–069

Unusual allowance, fee or expense

7.—(1) A coroner must report any unusual allowance, fee or expense likely to be incurred in relation to an investigation to his or her relevant authority before it is incurred.

(2) Where it is not possible to report the unusual allowance, fee or expense before it is incurred under paragraph (1), the coroner must—

(a) report the unusual allowance, fee or expense on the date it is incurred; or

(b) as soon as reasonably practicable after that date.

A2–070

Provision of allowances, fees and expenses

8. The Schedule to these Regulations provides for the allowances, fees and expenses that are payable by or on behalf of a coroner.

A2–071

Expert witness fee for preparatory work

9. A coroner may pay an expert witness who has carried out preparatory work directly related to the giving of evidence at an inquest a fee that the coroner considers reasonable having regard to the nature and complexity of the preparatory work carried out.

A2–072

Expert witness fee for attending an inquest

10.—(1) A coroner may pay an expert witness a fee that the coroner considers reasonable for attending and giving expert evidence at an inquest.

(2) When considering a fee which is reasonable under paragraph (1) the coroner shall have regard to the nature and complexity of the evidence provided by the expert witness.

A2–073

Additional expenses

11. A coroner may reimburse a suitable practitioner, juror or witness for any additional expenses, other than those prescribed by these Regulations, which the coroner believes have been reasonably incurred.

A2–074

Fee for disclosure after an inquest

12.—(1) This regulation applies where a coroner discloses a document to an interested person after an inquest.

(2) No fee shall be payable where a document is disclosed by email by a coroner to an interested person.

(3) Where a document is disclosed by a coroner as a paper copy, a fee of £5 for a document of 10 pages or less shall be payable, with an additional 50p payable for each subsequent page.

(4) A fee of £5 per document shall be payable where a document is disclosed in any other medium, other than by email or as a paper copy.

A2–075

(5) The fee for a transcription of an inquest hearing shall be as follows—

(a) for a copy consisting of 360 words or less, £6.20;

(b) for a copy consisting of between 361 words and up to an including 1439 words, £13.10; and

(c) for a copy consisting of 1440 words or more, £13.10 for the first 1440 words and 70p for each additional 72 words or part thereof.

13.—(1) A coroner must provide his or her relevant authority with an account of all allowances, fees and expenses paid under these Regulations at time intervals agreed with that relevant authority.

(2) An account provided to the relevant authority under paragraph (1) shall include any receipt, invoice or other document that proves the sum incurred.

(3) A relevant authority shall, on being satisfied that an account submitted under paragraph (1) is correct, reimburse the coroner in respect of the payments to which the account relates.

14.—(1) A coroner and his or her relevant authority must each keep a record of all allowances, fees and expenses paid under these Regulations for 3 years.

(2) A coroner and his or her relevant authority must, if so requested by the Chief Coroner, provide the Chief Coroner with a copy of any records held under this Part.

PART 4

RECORD KEEPING AND INDEMNITIES

Record of allowances, fees and expenses

A2–076   **15.** A coroner and his or her relevant authority must, if so requested by a person, return any receipts, invoices or other documents submitted by that person.

16. A coroner must retain all receipts, invoices or other documents (or copies of such if the original documents are to be returned to a person under regulation 15) submitted under these Regulations, in a format and for a period agreed by that coroner's relevant authority.

Indemnity

A2–077   **17.**—(1) A coroner shall be indemnified by his or her relevant authority in respect of—

(a) any costs which the coroner reasonably incurs in or in connection with proceedings in respect of anything done or omitted in the exercise (or purported exercise) of the coroner's duty;

(b) any costs which the coroner reasonably incurs in taking steps to dispute any claim which might have been made in such proceedings;

(c) any damages awarded against or ordered to be paid by the coroner in any such proceedings;

(d) any sums payable by the coroner in connection with any reasonable settlement of any such proceedings or claim.

(2) Paragraph (1) applies in relation to proceedings brought by a coroner only if and to the extent that the relevant authority for that coroner area agrees in advance to indemnify the coroner.

(3) A coroner may appeal to the Lord Chancellor or any person appointed by the Lord Chancellor for the purpose, from any decision of the relevant authority made under paragraph (2).

SCHEDULE 1

TABLES OF ALLOWANCES, FEES AND EXPENSES

Overnight allowance

1. A suitable practitioner, juror, or witness who is necessarily absent from his or her place of residence overnight for the purposes of serving at or attending an inquest hearing shall be paid up to a maximum allowance per night of—

Within a 5 mile radius of Charing Cross	£100.70
Elsewhere in England and Wales	£69.20

Travel expenses

2.—(1) A suitable practitioner, juror or witness shall have his or her travel expenses reimbursed as follows—

(a) where travel is by public transport the coroner may reimburse the actual fare paid (in the case of railway or air, the economy fare only, unless the coroner otherwise directs);

(b) where travel is by taxi or other privately hired vehicle, such costs may only be reimbursed where the coroner believes that such transport was reasonable;

(c) where travel is by private transport an allowance per mile each way may be paid as follows—

Car/motorcycle public transport rate	25p
Car/motorcycle standard rate	45p
Bicycle rate	20p

(2) Public transport rate must be paid unless the coroner is satisfied that no adequate public transport was available on the date on which the journey was made.

(3) Any parking fees reasonably incurred may be reimbursed.

(4) The allowances set out in paragraph (1) for car travel may be increased by 2p per mile each way if a passenger is carried to whom an allowance would otherwise have been payable for travel to and from an inquest, and by an additional 1p per mile for any further additional passenger so carried.

Subsistence allowance

3.—(1) A juror who is necessarily absent from his or her place of residence or work for the purpose of serving at an inquest hearing, may be paid a daily subsistence up to a maximum of—

Attendance of up to and including 10 hours	£5.71
Attendance of more than 10 hours	£12.17

(2) An ordinary witness who is necessarily absent from his or her place of residence or work for the purpose of providing evidence at an inquest hearing, may be paid a daily subsistence allowance up to a maximum of—

Attendance of up to and including 5 hours	£2.25
Attendance of more than 5 hours up to and including 10 hours	£4.50
Attendance of more than 10 hours	£9.75

Financial loss allowance

A2–081   **4.** A juror or ordinary witness who loses earnings or benefits or incurs expenses as a direct result of serving at or attending an inquest hearing, may be paid a maximum allowance of—

Length of attendance at the inquest hearing	Time spent each day	Maximum daily allowance
Up to and including 10 days	Up to and including 4 hours	£32.47
Up to and including 10 days	More than 4 hours	£64.95
On the 11th and all subsequent days	Up to and including 4 hours	£64.95
On the 11th and all subsequent days	More than 4 hours	£129.91

Professional witness allowance

A2–082   **5.** A professional witness who attends an inquest hearing to give evidence, shall be paid a maximum daily fee of—

If the professional witness does not employ a person to take care of his or her practice during his or her absence:	
Up to and including 2 hours	£83.50
More than 2 hours up to and including 4 hours	£117.00
More than 4 hours up to and including 6 hours	£174.00
More than 6 hours	£234.00
Or: If the professional witness necessarily incurs expense in the provision of a person to take care of his or her practice during his or her absence:	
Up to and including 2 hours	£89.00
More than 2 hours up to and including 4 hours	£125.00
More than 4 hours	£250.00

Fee for making a post-mortem examination

A2–083   **6.** A suitable practitioner is to be paid a fee of—

For making a post-mortem examination and reporting the result to the coroner	£96.80
For making a post-mortem examination involving additional skills and reporting the result to the coroner	£276.90

Coroners (Inquests) Rules 2013/1616

PART 1

INTRODUCTION

Citation and commencement

A2–084   **1.** These Rules may be cited as the Coroners (Inquests) Rules 2013 and shall come into force on 25th July 2013.

Interpretation

2.—(1) In these Rules—   **A2–085**

"the 2009 Act" means the Coroners and Justice Act 2009;
"bank holiday" means a day designated as a bank holiday in England and Wales under the
  Banking and Financial Dealings Act 1971;
"copy" means in relation to a document, anything on to which information recorded in
  the document has been copied, by whatever means and whether directly or indirectly;
"coroner" means—

(a) a senior coroner, area coroner or assistant coroner;
(b) the Chief Coroner when conducting an inquest; or
(c) a judge, former judge or former coroner conducting an inquest in
    accordance with Schedule 10 to the 2009 Act;

"document" means any medium in which information of any description is recorded or
  stored;
"working day" means a day that is not a Saturday, a Sunday, a bank holiday, Christmas Day
  or Good Friday.

(2) All references to section and schedule provisions in these Rules are references to
provisions in the 2009 Act, unless a rule specifically states otherwise.
(3) Any reference to a Form in these Rules is a reference to a Form in the Schedule to
these Rules.

Application to existing inquests

3.—(1) These Rules apply to any inquest which has not been completed before 25th July   **A2–086**
2013.
(2) Any direction, time limit, adjournment or other decision made by the coroner in
relation to an inquest made before 25th July 2013 shall stand.
4. This Part applies where a coroner is under a duty to hold an inquest under section
6.

PART 2

FORMALITIES

Opening of an inquest

5.—(1) An inquest must be opened as soon as reasonably practicable after the date on   **A2–087**
which the coroner considers that the duty under section 6 applies.
(2) At the opening of the inquest, the coroner must, where possible, set the dates on
which any subsequent hearings are scheduled to take place.

Pre-inquest review hearing

6. A coroner may at any time during the course of an investigation and before an inquest   **A2–088**
hearing hold a pre-inquest review hearing.

Days on which an inquest may be held

7. An inquest must be held on a working day, unless the coroner considers that there is   **A2–089**
an urgent reason for holding it on some other day.

Timing of an inquest

A2–090   **8.** A coroner must complete an inquest within six months of the date on which the coroner is made aware of the death, or as soon as is reasonably practicable after that date.

Notification of inquest hearing arrangements

A2–091   **9.**—(1) A coroner must notify the next of kin or personal representative of the deceased of the date, time and place of the inquest hearing within one week of setting the date of the inquest hearing.

(2) A coroner must notify any other interested persons who have made themselves known to the coroner of the date, time and place of the inquest hearing within one week of setting the date of the inquest hearing.

(3) Where an inquest hearing is to be held, the coroner must make details of the date, time and place of the inquest hearing publicly available before the inquest hearing commences.

Coroner to notify interested persons of any alteration of arrangements for an inquest hearing

A2–092   **10.**—(1) Where the date, time or place of the inquest hearing is altered the coroner must notify the next of kin or personal representative of the deceased, and any other interested persons who have made themselves known to the coroner, of the alteration within one week of the decision to alter.

(2) The coroner must make the details of any alteration made under paragraph (1) publicly available within one week of the decision to alter.

Inquest hearings to be held in public

A2–093   **11.**—(1) A coroner must open an inquest in public.

(2) Where the coroner does not have immediate access to a court room or other appropriate premises, the coroner may open the inquest privately and then announce that the inquest has been opened at the next inquest hearing held in public.

(3) An inquest hearing and any pre-inquest hearing must be held in public unless paragraph (4) or (5) applies.

(4) A coroner may direct that the public be excluded from an inquest hearing, or any part of an inquest hearing if the coroner considers it would be in the interests of national security to do so.

(5) A coroner may direct that the public be excluded from a pre-inquest review hearing if the coroner considers it would be in the interests of justice or national security to do so.

PART 3

DISCLOSURE

A2–094   **12.** This Part applies to the disclosure of documents by the coroner during or after the course of an investigation, pre-inquest review or inquest.

Disclosure of documents at the request of an interested person

A2–095   **13.**—(1) Subject to rule 15, where an interested person asks for disclosure of a document held by the coroner, the coroner must provide that document or a copy of that document, or make the document available for inspection by that person as soon as is reasonably practicable.

(2) Documents to which this rule applies include—

(a) any post-mortem examination report;

(b) any other report that has been provided to the coroner during the course of the investigation;

(c) where available, the recording of any inquest hearing held in public, but not in relation to any part of the hearing from which the public was excluded under rule 11(4) or (5);

(d) any other document which the coroner considers relevant to the inquest.

Managing disclosure

14. A coroner may— **A2–096**

(a) disclose an electronic copy of a document instead of, or in addition to, a paper copy;

(b) disclose a redacted version of all or part of a document; or

(c) make a document available for inspection at a particular time and place.

Restrictions on disclosure

15. A coroner may refuse to provide a document or a copy of a document requested **A2–097** under rule 13 where—

(a) there is a statutory or legal prohibition on disclosure;

(b) the consent of any author or copyright owner cannot reasonably be obtained;

(c) the request is unreasonable;

(d) the document relates to contemplated or commenced criminal proceedings; or

(e) the coroner considers the document irrelevant to the investigation.

Costs of disclosure

16. A coroner may not charge a fee for any document or copy of any document, disclosed **A2–098** to an interested person before or during an inquest.

PART 4

MANAGEMENT OF THE INQUEST HEARING

Evidence by video link

17.—(1) A coroner may direct that a witness may give evidence at an inquest hearing **A2–099** through a live video link.

(2) A direction may not be given under paragraph (1) unless the coroner determines that giving evidence in the way proposed would improve the quality of the evidence given by the witness or allow the inquest to proceed more expediently.

(3) Before giving a direction under paragraph (1), the coroner must consider all the circumstances of the case, including in particular—

(a) any views expressed by the witness or any interested person;

(b) whether it would be in the interests of justice or national security to give evidence by video link; and

(c) whether in the opinion of the coroner, giving evidence by video link would impede the effectiveness of the questioning of the witness.

(4) A direction may be given under paragraph (1)—

(a) on an application by the witness, or in the case of a child witness the parent or legal guardian of that witness;

(b) on an application by an interested person; or

(c) on the coroner's own initiative.

Evidence given from behind a screen

A2–100   **18.**—(1) A coroner may direct that a witness may give evidence at an inquest hearing from behind a screen.

(2) A direction may not be given under paragraph (1) unless the coroner determines that giving evidence in the way proposed would be likely to improve the quality of the evidence given by the witness or allow the inquest to proceed more expediently.

(3) In making that determination, the coroner must consider all the circumstances of the case, including in particular—

(a) any views expressed by the witness or an interested person;

(b) whether it would be in the interests of justice or national security to allow evidence to be given from behind a screen; and

(c) whether giving evidence from behind a screen would impede the effectiveness of the questioning of the witness by an interested person or a representative of the interested person.

(4) A direction may be given under paragraph (1)—

(a) on the application by the witness, or in the case of a child witness the parent or legal guardian of that witness;

(b) on an application of an interested person; or

(c) on the coroner's own initiative.

Entitlement to examine witnesses

A2–101   **19.**—(1) A coroner must allow any interested person who so requests, to examine any witness either in person or by the interested person's representative.

(2) A coroner must disallow any question put to the witness which the coroner considers irrelevant.

Evidence given on oath or affirmation

A2–102   **20.**—(1) A witness providing evidence at an inquest hearing shall be examined by the coroner on oath or affirmation subject to paragraph (2).

(2) A child under the age of 14, or a child aged 14 or over who is considered by the coroner to be unable to understand the nature of an oath or affirmation, may, on promising to tell the truth, be permitted to give unsworn evidence.

Examination of witnesses

A2–103   **21.** Unless the coroner otherwise determines, a witness at an inquest hearing must be examined in the following order—

(a) first by the coroner;

(b) then by any interested person who has asked to examine the witness; and

(c) if the witness is represented at the inquest, lastly by the witness's representative.

Self incrimination

22.—(1) No witness at an inquest is obliged to answer any question tending to incriminate him or her.

(2) Where it appears to the coroner that a witness has been asked such a question, the coroner must inform the witness that he or she may refuse to answer it.

Written evidence

23.—(1) Written evidence as to who the deceased was and how, when and where the deceased came by his or her death is not admissible unless the coroner is satisfied that—

   (a) it is not possible for the maker of the written evidence to give evidence at the inquest hearing at all, or within a reasonable time;

   (b) there is a good and sufficient reason why the maker of the written evidence should not attend the inquest hearing;

   (c) there is a good and sufficient reason to believe that the maker of the written evidence will not attend the inquest hearing; or

   (d) the written evidence (including evidence in admission form) is unlikely to be disputed.

(2) Before admitting such written evidence the coroner must announce at the inquest hearing—

   (a) what the nature of the written evidence to be admitted is;

   (b) the full name of the maker of the written evidence to be admitted in evidence;

   (c) that any interested person may object to the admission of any such written evidence; and

   (d) that any interested person is entitled to see a copy of any written evidence if he or she so wishes.

(3) A coroner must admit as evidence at an inquest hearing any document made by a deceased person if the coroner is of the opinion that the contents of the document are relevant to the purposes of the inquest.

(4) A coroner may direct that all or parts only of any written evidence submitted under this rule may be read aloud at the inquest hearing.

Inquiry findings

24.—(1) A coroner may admit the findings of an inquiry, including any inquiry under the Inquiries Act 2005, if the coroner considers them relevant to the purposes of the inquest.

(2) Before admitting such inquiry findings as evidence, the coroner must announce publicly that—

   (a) the findings of the inquiry may be admitted as evidence;

   (b) the title of the inquiry, date of publication and a brief account of the findings; and

   (c) that any interested person is entitled to see a copy of the inquiry findings if he or she so wishes.

Adjournment and resumption of an inquest

A2–107   **25.**—(1) A coroner may adjourn an inquest if the coroner is of the view that it is reasonable to do so.

(2) The coroner must inform the next of kin or personal representative of the deceased and any other interested persons who have made themselves known to the coroner as soon as reasonably practicable of the decision to adjourn, the date of the decision to adjourn and the reason for the adjournment.

(3) The coroner must inform the next of kin or personal representative of the deceased and any other interested persons who have made themselves known to the coroner as soon as reasonably practicable of the date, time and place at which an adjourned inquest is to be resumed.

(4) A coroner must adjourn an inquest and notify the Director of Public Prosecutions, if during the course of the inquest, it appears to the coroner that the death of the deceased is likely to have been due to a homicide offence and that a person may be charged in relation to the offence.

Recording inquest hearings

A2–108   **26.** A coroner must keep a recording of every inquest hearing, including any pre-inquest review hearing.

No address as to facts

A2–109   **27.** No person may address the coroner or the jury as to the facts of who the deceased was and how, when and where the deceased came by his or her death.

PART 5

JURY INQUESTS

A2–110   **28.** This Part applies to inquests heard or to be heard with a jury.

Method of summoning jurors

A2–111   **29.**—(1) A juror must be summoned using Form 1.

(2) Form 1 must be sent by post with a return envelope, to the juror or delivered by hand at his or her address as shown in the electoral register.

Summoning in exceptional circumstances

A2–112   **30.** If it appears to the coroner that a jury will be, or probably will be, incomplete, the coroner may require any persons up to the number needed who are in, or in the vicinity of, the place of the inquest hearing to be summoned (without any written notice) for jury service.

Certificate of attendance

A2–113   **31.** A person duly attending an inquest hearing to serve on a jury in compliance with a summons issued under rule 29 or rule 30 is entitled on request to the coroner to a certificate recording that fact.

Validity of proceedings where jury not present

A2–114   **32.** Where an inquest hearing begins without a jury but a jury is subsequently summoned, the validity of anything done by the coroner before the jury was summoned is still effective.

Summing up and directions to the jury

33. Where the coroner sits with a jury, the coroner must direct the jury as to the law and   **A2–115**
provide the jury with a summary of the evidence.

PART 6

RECORD

Record of the inquest

34. A coroner or in the case of an inquest heard with a jury, the jury, must make a   **A2–116**
determination and any findings required under section 10 using Form 2.

SCHEDULE

Form 1   **A2–117**
Juror Summons

Coroner (insert name) summons—
(insert juror name) of (insert juror address)
You are hereby summoned to appear before him or her as a juror on (insert date, time and place) until
you are no longer needed.
You must attend at the date, time and place specified above unless you are told by an officer authorised
by the coroner that you do not need to do so.
Date:
Coroner:
Coroner signature:
YOU MUST COMPLETE THE ATTACHED FORM AND RETURN IT TO (Insert name of the
officer authorised by the coroner) IN THE ENVELOPE PROVIDED WITHIN THREE DAYS OF
THE RECEIPT OF THIS SUMMONS
WARNING: IT IS AN OFFENCE TO SERVE ON A JURY AT AN INQUEST IF YOU ARE
DISQUALIFIED FROM JURY SERVICE (SEE DETACHABLE FORM BELOW) AND KNOW
THAT YOU ARE DISQUALIFIED FROM JURY SERVICE.
A person guilty of such an offence is liable on summary conviction to a fine not exceeding level 5 on
the standard scale.
IT IS AN OFFENCE TO REFUSE WITHOUT REASONABLE EXCUSE TO ANSWER THE
QUESTIONS IN THE DETACHABLE FORM AS TO WHETHER YOU ARE QUALIFIED TO
SERVE AS A JUROR AT THE INQUEST, TO GIVE AN ANSWER TO SUCH A QUESTION
KNOWING THE ANSWER. TO BE FALSE IN A MATERIAL PARTICULAR, OR RECK-
LESSLY TO GIVE AN ANSWER TO SUCH A QUESTION THAT IS FALSE IN A MATERIAL
PARTICULAR.
A person guilty of such an offence is liable on summary conviction to a fine not exceeding level 3 on
the standard scale.
IT IS AN OFFENCE FOR A PERSON WHO IS DULY SUMMONED AS A JUROR. AT AN
INQUEST TO MAKE ANY FALSE REPRESENTATION, OR TO CAUSE OR PERMIT TO BE
MADE ANY FALSE REPRESENTATION ON YOUR BEHALF WITH THE INTENTION OF
EVADING SERVICE AS A JUROR AT AN INQUEST.
A person guilty of such an offence is liable on summary conviction to a fine not exceeding level 3 on
the standard scale.
IT IS AN OFFENCE FOR A PERSON TO MAKE OR CAUSE TO BE MADE, ON BEHALF OF
A PERSON WHO HAS BEEN DULY SUMMONED AS A JUROR AT AN INQUEST, ANY
FALSE REPRESENTATION WITH THE INTENTION OF ENABLING THE OTHER
PERSON TO EVADE SERVICE AS A JUROR AT AN INQUEST.
A person guilty of such an offence is liable on summary conviction to a fine not exceeding level 3 on
the standard scale.
A coroner may impose a fine not exceeding £1000 on you if you fail without reasonable excuse to
attend in accordance with the summons, or attend in accordance with the summons but refuse without
reasonable excuse to serve as a juror. A fine may not be imposed under this paragraph. unless the
summons was served on you not later than 14 days before the day on which you were/are required to
attend.

<DETACHABLE FORM>

This form should be returned in the envelope provided within three days of receiving it. Jurors details—
This form should be returned in the envelope provided within three days of receiving it. Jurors details—
Surname ....
Forename(s) ....Date of Birth ....
Address ....
........................Telephone number ....
Or possible please provide a telephone number where you can be contacted between 9a.m. and 5p.m.)
INFORMATION GIVEN WILL BE TREATED IN THE STRICTEST CONFIDENCE
YOU ARE QUALIFIED for jury service if you—
(a) are not less that eighteen not more than seventy years of age;
(if you will be under eighteen on or have reached your seventieth birthday by the date on which your appearance is required you will NOT be eligible to serve as a juror)
(b) are registered as a parliamentary or local government elector;
(c) have lived in the United Kingdom, the Channel Islands or the Isle of Man for a period of at least five years since attaining the age of thirteen; and
(d) are not one of the persons described in Parts I and II of Schedule 1 to the Juries Act 1974.

1. Are you QUALIFIED to serve as a juror? Please tick the appropriate:
YES NO
If you have answered NO to question 1, please answer question 2 and sign the form at the end.

If you have answered YES and wish to be excused from jury service on this occasion, please go to question 3 below and then sign the form at the end.
2. I AM NOT QUALIFIED to serve on a jury because—

3. YOU ARE ENTITLED TO BE EXCUSED if you—
(a) are a full time serving member of Her Majesty's navy, military or air forces and your commanding officer certifies that it would be prejudicial to the efficiency of the service if you were required to be absent from duty;
(b) are a coroner within the same coroner area in which you have been summoned to attend as a juror; or
(c) are otherwise excused from attending by the coroner before whom you are summoned.
YOU MAY BE EXCUSED at the discretion of the Coroner or of the officer authorised by the Coroner on the grounds of poor health, illness, physical disability, insufficient understanding of English, holiday arrangements or any other good reason.
I WISH TO BE EXCLUDED from jury service on this occasion because--
(if you have any doubts as to whether you may be excused from jury service please write to the officer authorised by the Coroner at the address on the front of the summons.)
When you attend as a juror you may be discharged if there is doubt as to your capacity to serve on a jury because of physical disability or insufficient understanding of English.
I HAVE READ THE WARNING IN THE SUMMONS AND THE INFORMATION I HAVE GIVEN IS TRUE.

Signed ....Dated ....

Form 2
RECORD OF INQUEST

The following is the record of the inquest (including the statutory determination and, where required, findings)—

1. Name of deceased:
2. Medical cause of death:
3. How, when and where, and for investigations where section 5(2) of the Coroners and Justice Act 2009 applies, in what circumstances the deceased came by his death:
4. Conclusion of the coroner/jury as to the death (see notes (i) and (ii)):
5. Further particulars required by the Births and Deaths Registration Act 1953 to be registered concerning the death:

(1)	(2)	(3)	(4)	(5)	(6)
Date and place of death	Name and surname of deceased	Sex	Maiden surname of woman who has married	Date and place of birth	Occupation and usual address

Signature of coroner (and jurors):

NOTES:

(i) One of the following short-form conclusions may be adopted:—
I. accident or misadventure
II. alcohol / drug related
III. industrial disease
IV. lawful/ unlawful killing
V. natural causes
VI. open
VII. road traffic collision
VIII. stillbirth
IX. suicide
(ii) As an alternative, or in addition to one of the short-form conclusions listed under NOTE (i), the coroner or where applicable the jury, may make a brief narrative conclusion.
(iii) The standard of proof required for the short form conclusions of "unlawful killing" and "suicide" is the criminal standard of proof. For all other short-form conclusions and a narrative statement the standard of proof is the civil standard of proof.

Coroners (Investigations) Regulations 2013/1629

PART 1

INTRODUCTION

Citation and commencement

1. These Regulations may be cited as the Coroners (Investigations) Regulations 2013 and shall come into force on 25th July 2013. **A2–118**

Interpretation

2.—(1) In these Regulations— **A2–119**

"2009 Act" means the Coroners and Justice Act 2009;
"bank holiday" means a day designated as a bank holiday in England and Wales under the Banking and Financial Dealings Act 1971;
"coroner" means—

    (a) a senior coroner, area coroner or assistant coroner;
    (b) the Chief Coroner when conducting an investigation under paragraph 1 of Schedule 10 to the 2009 Act; or
    (c) a judge, former judge or former coroner conducting an investigation under paragraph 3 of Schedule 10 to the 2009 Act;

"document" means any medium in which information of any description is recorded or stored;
"enforcing authority" has the same meaning as in section 18(7) of the Health and Safety at Work etc. Act 1974;

"investigation" means an investigation into a death conducted under Part 1 of the 2009 Act;

"working day" means a day that is not a Saturday, a Sunday, a bank holiday, Christmas Day or Good Friday.

(2) All references to sections and schedule provisions in these Regulations are references to provisions in the 2009 Act, unless a regulation specifically states otherwise.

(3) A reference to a Form in these Regulations is a reference to a Form in the Schedule to these Regulations.

Application

A2–120   **3.**—(1) These Regulations shall have effect in relation to any investigation (including any inquest) which has not been completed before 25th July 2013.

(2) Any decision of the coroner made in relation to an investigation, or inquest as the case may be, including any decision relating to a post-mortem examination before 25th July 2013 shall stand.

PART 2

GENERAL

Coroner availability for urgent matters

A2–121   **4.** A coroner must be available at all times to address matters relating to an investigation into a death which must be dealt with immediately and cannot wait until the next working day.

Register of reported deaths

A2–122   **5.**—(1) The senior coroner must keep a register of all deaths reported in his or her coroner area.

(2) The senior coroner must record in the register, the following information, when known—

(a) the date on which a death was reported under section 1;

(b) the deceased's full name, gender, age and full address;

(c) any other information that aids the identification of the deceased; and

(d) the place of death or, if that is unknown, the place where the body was found.

Informing the deceased's next of kin or personal representative

A2–123   **6.** A coroner who is under a duty to investigate a death under section 1, must attempt to identify the deceased's next of kin or personal representative and inform that person, if identified, of the coroner's decision to begin an investigation.

Delegation of administrative functions

A2–124   **7.** A coroner may delegate administrative, but not judicial functions, to coroner's officers and other support staff.

Providing information to the registrar of births and deaths

A2–125   **8.** Where a coroner suspends an investigation under paragraph 1, 2, 3 or 5 of Schedule 1 the coroner must provide the registrar of births and deaths with the particulars required to register the death under the Births and Deaths Registration Act 1953.

Interim certificate of fact of death

9.—(1) Where a coroner has begun but not yet completed or discontinued an investigation, he or she may, if requested to do so by the next of kin or personal representative of the deceased, provide that person with a certificate of the fact of death.   **A2–126**

(2) A coroner must use Form 1 when issuing a certificate of the fact of death.

Resumption of investigation

10. Where a coroner resumes a suspended investigation in accordance with paragraph 7 of Schedule 1, the coroner must notify—   **A2–127**

(a) The next of kin or personal representative of the deceased; and

(b) any other interested persons who have made themselves known to the coroner,

of the resumption and the reason for the resumption of the investigation.

Part 3

Post-mortem examinations

Delay in post-mortem examination to be avoided

11. A coroner who considers that a post-mortem examination should be made under section 14, shall request a suitable practitioner to make that post-mortem examination as soon as reasonably practicable.   **A2–128**

Post-mortem examination where homicide offence is suspected

12. Where a coroner is informed by a chief officer of police that a homicide offence is suspected in connection with the death of the deceased, the coroner must consult that chief officer of police about who should make the post-mortem examination.   **A2–129**

Notification of post-mortem examination

13.—(1) Where a coroner has requested a suitable practitioner to make a post-mortem examination, the coroner must notify the persons or bodies listed in paragraph (3) of the date, time and place at which that post-mortem examination is to be made.   **A2–130**

(2) A coroner need not give such notification, where it is impracticable or where to do so would cause the post-mortem examination to be unreasonably delayed.

(3) The persons to be notified are—

(a) the next of kin or the personal representative of the deceased or any other interested person who has notified the coroner in advance of his or her desire to be represented at the post-mortem examination;

(b) the deceased's regular medical practitioner, if he or she has notified the coroner of his or her desire to be represented at the post-mortem examination;

(c) if the deceased died in hospital, that hospital;

(d) if the death of the deceased may have been caused by an accident or disease which must be reported to an enforcing authority, to that enforcing authority or the appropriate inspector or representative of that authority;

(e) a Government department which has notified the coroner of its desire to be represented at the examination; and

(f) if the chief officer of police has notified the coroner of his or her desire to be represented at the examination, the chief officer of police.

(4) Any of the persons or bodies listed in paragraph (3) are entitled to be represented at a post-mortem examination by a medical practitioner, or if they are a medical practitioner, may attend themselves.

(5) The following persons may attend a post-mortem examination—

(a) A representative of the chief officer of police from the police force of which he or she is chief officer; and

(b) any other person including a trainee doctor, medical student or other medical practitioner but only with the consent of the coroner.

Preservation or retention of material from a post-mortem examination

14.—(1) Where a suitable practitioner conducts a post-mortem examination under section 14 and preserves or retains material which in his or her opinion relates to the cause of death or identity of the deceased, he or she must provide the coroner with written notification of that fact.

(2) A suitable practitioner who preserves or retains material under paragraph (1) must provide the coroner with a written notification that—

(a) identifies the material being preserved or retained; and

(b) explains why that practitioner is of the opinion set out in paragraph (1).

(3) A written notification under paragraph (2) may—

(a) specify the period of time for which the suitable practitioner believes the material should be preserved or retained; and

(b) specify different periods of time in relation to different preserved or retained material.

(4) On receiving a notification under paragraph (1), the coroner must notify the suitable practitioner of the period of time for which he or she requires the material to be preserved or retained for the purposes of fulfilling his or her functions under the 2009 Act.

(5) On making the notification under paragraph (4) the coroner must also notify, where known—

(a) the next of kin or personal representative of the deceased; and

(b) any other relative of the deceased who has notified the coroner of his or her desire to be represented at the post-mortem examination,

that material is being preserved or retained, the period or periods for which it is required to be preserved or retained and the options for dealing with the material under paragraph (6) once the period or periods of preservation or retention has or have expired.

(6) The options for dealing with material are—

(a) disposal of the material by burial, cremation or other lawful disposal by the suitable practitioner;

(b) return of the material to a person listed in sub-paragraph (a) or (b) of paragraph (5); or

(c) retention of the material with the consent of a person listed in sub-paragraph (a) or (b) of paragraph (5) for medical research or other purposes in accordance with the Human Tissue Act 2004.

Further provisions relating to preservation or retention of material from post-mortem examinations

15.—(1) A coroner who—   A2–132

(a) receives a request from a prosecuting authority, Provost Marshal or the Director of Service Prosecutions under paragraph 1 of Schedule 1 to suspend an investigation because a person may be charged with an offence in relation to the death of the deceased; or

(b) becomes aware or is informed under paragraph 2 of Schedule 1 that a person has been charged with an offence in relation to, or connected with, the death of the deceased,

must notify the chief officer of police or prosecuting authority, of any period for which the coroner requires material to be preserved or retained under regulation 14(4).

(2) Where the coroner is informed that a public inquiry is to be held instead of an inquest, the coroner must notify the chairman of that inquiry of any period for which the coroner requires material to be preserved or retained under regulation 14(4).

(3) A coroner may from time to time vary a period notified under regulation 14(4) and must notify both the suitable practitioner and any person notified under regulation 14(5), 15(1) and 15(2) of the variation.

(4) Where a suitable practitioner has received a notification from a coroner under regulation 14(4) and the suitable practitioner believes that the material should be preserved or retained for a different period, the suitable practitioner may request that the coroner vary the time by providing a notification in accordance with regulation 14(2).

(5) Where a suitable practitioner has retained material in accordance with regulation 14 and the period notified under regulation 14(4) has expired, that suitable practitioner must record the fact that—

(a) the material has been disposed by the suitable practitioner or on behalf of the suitable practitioner;

(b) the material has been delivered into the possession of a specified person; or

(c) the material has been dealt with in accordance with regulation 14(6).

(6) Any record made by a suitable practitioner under paragraph (5) must be retained by him or her.

Post-mortem examination report

16.—(1) A suitable practitioner, on completion of a post-mortem examination, must   A2–133
report to the coroner as soon as practicable after the examination has been made.

(2) Unless authorised in writing by the coroner, the suitable practitioner who made the post-mortem examination may not supply any other person with the post-mortem examination report or any copy of that report.

Discontinuance of investigation where cause of death is revealed by post-mortem examination

17. Where a coroner discontinues an investigation in accordance with section 4(1)   A2–134
because the post-mortem examination reveals the cause of death, the coroner must record the cause of death and notify the next of kin or personal representative of the deceased using Form 2.

PART 4

TRANSFER OF INVESTIGATIONS

Transfer of investigations

A2–135   18.—(1) Where Coroner A and Coroner B agree to transfer an investigation under section 2, or the Chief Coroner directs Coroner B to conduct an investigation under section 3—

(a) Coroner A must provide Coroner B with all relevant evidence, documents and information;

(b) Coroner B must notify the next of kin or personal representative of the deceased of the transfer; and

(c) Coroner B must notify any other interested persons who have made themselves known to the coroner of the transfer.

(2) A coroner must fulfil their obligations under this regulation within 5 working days of the date the transfer is either agreed or directed, unless there are exceptional circumstances.

Costs of a transferred investigation

A2–136   19.—(1) Where Coroner A and Coroner B agree to transfer an investigation in accordance with section 2, the relevant authority for Coroner B's coroner area will be responsible for all costs related to the transferred investigation and any associated inquest from the date the transfer is made.

(2) Where the Chief Coroner directs Coroner B to conduct an investigation in accordance with section 3, the relevant authority for Coroner A's coroner area shall be responsible for all costs related to the transferred investigation and any associated inquest from the date the transfer is made, unless the Chief Coroner otherwise directs.

PART 5

POWERS IN RELATION TO BODIES

Release of bodies

A2–137   20.—(1) A coroner must release the body for burial or cremation as soon as is reasonably practicable.

(2) Where a coroner cannot release the body within 28 days of being made aware that the body is within his or her area, the coroner must notify the next of kin or personal representative of the deceased of the reason for the delay.

Burial or cremation order

A2–138   21.—(1) A coroner may only issue an order authorising the burial or cremation of a body where the coroner no longer needs to retain the body for the purposes of the investigation.

(2) A coroner must use Form 3 when issuing an order to bury a body.

Exhumation

A2–139   22.—(1) A coroner may issue a direction to exhume a body lying within England and Wales.

(2) Where such a direction is made the coroner must use Form 4.

Part 6

Disclosure and provision of information

23. Part 3 of the Coroners (Inquests) Rules 2013 applies to the disclosure of documents **A2–140** to an interested person made by the coroner at any time during the course of an investigation.

Providing information to a Local Safeguarding Children Board

24.—(1) Where a coroner decides to conduct an investigation into a death under section **A2–141** 1 or directs that a post-mortem examination should be made under section 14, and the coroner believes the deceased was under the age of 18, the coroner must notify the appropriate Local Safeguarding Children Board within 3 days of making the decision or direction.

(2) A coroner must provide all information to the appropriate Local Safeguarding Children Board.

(3) In this regulation—

"the appropriate Local Safeguarding Children Board" means the Board established under section 13(1) or 31(1) of the Children Act 2004 within whose area the deceased died or within whose area the body was found; and

"information" means any information that is—

(a) held by the coroner for the purposes of an investigation under Part 1 of the 2009 Act; and

(b) relates to the death of a person who was or may have been under the age of 18 at the time of death.

Power of the Chief Coroner to require information

25.—(1) The Chief Coroner may at any time require information from a coroner in **A2–142** relation to a particular investigation or investigations that have or are being conducted by that coroner.

(2) A coroner must provide the Chief Coroner with the information requested under paragraph (1).

Investigations lasting more than a year

26.—(1) Where an investigation has not been completed or discontinued within a year **A2–143** of the date that the death was reported, the coroner must notify the Chief Coroner of that fact as soon as is reasonably practicable from the date that the investigation becomes a year old and explain why the investigation has not been completed or discontinued.

(2) A coroner who completes or discontinues an investigation that the coroner has previously notified to the Chief Coroner under paragraph (1), must notify the Chief Coroner of the date the investigation is completed or discontinued and provide a reason for any further delay in completing or discontinuing the investigation.

Retention and release of documents

27.—(1) Any document in the possession of a coroner in connection with an **A2–144** investigation or post-mortem examination must, unless a court or the Chief Coroner otherwise directs, be retained by or on behalf of the coroner for at least 15 years from the date that the investigation is completed.

(2) The coroner may provide any document or copy of any document to any person who in the opinion of the coroner is a proper person to have possession of it.

(3) A coroner may charge for the provision of any document or copy of any document in accordance with any regulations made under Schedule 7.

PART 7

ACTION TO PREVENT OTHER DEATHS

Report on action to prevent other deaths

A2–145   **28.**—(1) This regulation applies where a coroner is under a duty under paragraph 7(1) of Schedule 5 to make a report to prevent other deaths.

(2) In this regulation, a reference to "a report" means a report to prevent other deaths made by the coroner.

(3) A report may not be made until the coroner has considered all the documents, evidence and information that in the opinion of the coroner are relevant to the investigation.

(4) The coroner—

(a) must send a copy of the report to the Chief Coroner and every interested person who in the coroner's opinion should receive it;

(b) must send a copy of the report to the appropriate Local Safeguarding Children Board (which has the same meaning as in regulation 24(3)) where the coroner believes the deceased was under the age of 18; and

(c) may send a copy of the report to any other person who the coroner believes may find it useful or of interest.

(5) On receipt of a report the Chief Coroner may—

(a) publish a copy of the report, or a summary of it, in such manner as the Chief Coroner thinks fit; and

(b) send a copy of the report to any person who the Chief Coroner believes may find it useful or of interest.

Response to a report on action to prevent other deaths

A2–146   **29.**—(1) This regulation applies where a person is under a duty to give a response to a report to prevent other deaths made in accordance with paragraph 7(1) of Schedule 5.

(2) In this regulation, a reference to "a report" means a report to prevent other deaths made by the coroner.

(3) The response to a report must contain—

(a) details of any action that has been taken or which it is proposed will be taken by the person giving the response or any other person whether in response to the report or otherwise and set out a timetable of the action taken or proposed to be taken; or

(b) an explanation as to why no action is proposed.

(4) The response must be provided to the coroner who made the report within 56 days of the date on which the report is sent.

(5) The coroner who made the report may extend the period referred to in paragraph (4) (even if an application for extension is made after the time for compliance has expired).

(6) On receipt of a response to a report the coroner—

(a) must send a copy of the response to the report to the Chief Coroner;

(b) must send a copy to any interested persons who in the coroner's opinion should receive it; and

(c) may send a copy of the response to any other person who the coroner believes may find it useful or of interest.

(7) On receipt of a copy under paragraph (6)(a) the Chief Coroner may—

(a) publish a copy of the response, or a summary of it, in such manner as the Chief Coroner thinks fit; and

(b) send a copy of the response to any person who the Chief Coroner believes may find it useful or of interest (other than a person who has been sent a copy of the response under paragraph (6)(b) or (c)).

(8) A person giving a response to a report may make written representations to the coroner about—

(a) the release of the response; or

(b) the publication of the response.

(9) Representations under paragraph (8) must be made to the coroner no later than the time when the response to the report to prevent other deaths is provided to the coroner under paragraph (4).

(10) The coroner must pass any representations made under paragraph (8) to the Chief Coroner who may then consider those representations and decide whether there should be any restrictions on the release or publication of the response.

SCHEDULE 1

FORMS

Form 1
Coroner's certificate of fact of death

A2–147

To whom it may concern,

C.D. (insert name): ....
of (insert address): ....
died on (insert date): ....
The precise cause of death, *was as follows/*has yet to be established
*Delete as appropriate

Date: ....
Signature: ....
Coroner: ....

Form 2
Notice of Discontinuance

To (insert name): ....

The investigation into the death of C.D. has been discontinued under section 4 of the Coroners and Justice Act 2009.
The investigation was discontinued for the following reason(s):

Date: ....
Signature: ....
Coroner: ....

Form 3
Order for burial

I authorise the burial of C.D. (insert, name)
aged, (insert age)
who died at, (insert time and place)
on, (insert date)

Date: ....
Signature: ....
Coroner: ....

Form 4
Direction to exhume

To

(insert the names of the Minister and churchwardens or other persons having control over the churchyard, cemetery, or other place where the body is buried).
I have been informed that the body of C.D., has been buried in
(insert the name of the churchyard, cemetery or other place where the body is buried), and it appears to me that it is necessary for the body to be exhumed and examined for the purposes of:
1. conducting an investigation into the death of the deceased under Part I of the Coroners and Justice Act 2009; or
2. discharging a coroner's function in relation to the body or death of the deceased, namely:
(insert function)
I direct that you allow the body of C.D. to be exhumed.

Date: ....
Signature: ....
Coroner: ....

Cremation (England and Wales) Regulations 2008/2841

PART 1

PRELIMINARY

Citation, commencement and extent

A2–148   **1.**—(1) These Regulations may be cited as the Cremation (England and Wales) Regulations 2008 and come into force on 1st January 2009.
(2) These Regulations extend to England and Wales only.

Interpretation

A2–149   **2.**—(1) In these Regulations—

"the 1953 Act" means the Births and Deaths Registration Act 1953;
[. . .]¹⁶
"the 2004 Act" means the Human Tissue Act 2004;
["the 2009 Act" means the Coroners and Justice Act 2009;]¹⁷

---

¹⁶ Definition repealed by Coroners and Justice Act 2009 (Commencement No. 15, Consequential and Transitory Provisions) Order 2013/1869 Sch.1 para.4(2)(a) (July 25, 2013 as SI 2013/1869 art.4).
¹⁷ Definition inserted by Coroners and Justice Act 2009 (Commencement No. 15, Consequential and Transitory Provisions) Order 2013/1869 Sch.1 para.4(2)(b) (July 25, 2013 as SI 2013/1869 art.4).

"applicant" means the person making an application for cremation in accordance with regulation 15;

"body parts" means material which consists of, or includes, human cells from—

(a) a deceased person, whether or not separation from the body occurred before or after death; or

(b) a stillborn child;

"cremation" means the burning of human remains;

"cremation authority" means any burial authority or any person who has opened a crematorium and, in article 3(a), includes any burial authority or person who intends to open a crematorium;

"deputy medical referee" means a person appointed under regulation 6(2);

"five years' standing", in relation to a registered medical practitioner, means that the medical practitioner—

(a) has been a fully registered person within the meaning of section 55 of the Medical Act 1983 for at least five years; and

(b) if paragraph 10 of Schedule 1 to the Medical Act 1983 (Amendment) Order 2002 has come into force, has held a licence to practise under the 1983 Act—

(i) for at least five years; or

(ii) since the coming into force of that paragraph;

["investigation" means an investigation into the death of a deceased person under Part 1 of the 2009 Act;][18]

"medical certificate" and "confirmatory medical certificate" are references to the certificates so named given in accordance with regulation 17(1) and (2) respectively;

"medical referee" means a person appointed under regulation 6(1);

"registrar" means a person appointed under regulation 31;

"stillborn" and "stillbirth" apply to any child born after the twenty-fourth week of pregnancy and which did not at any time after birth, breathe or show any other signs of life.

(2) In calculating the time periods referred to in regulations 22(3), 23(1)(d) and (2) and 32(2), any period must be disregarded if it falls on—

(a) a Saturday or a Sunday;

(b) Christmas Day or Good Friday; or

(c) a day which is a bank holiday under the Banking and Financial Dealings Act 1971 in England and Wales.

PART 2

MAINTENANCE AND INSPECTION OF CREMATORIUM

[Outside the scope of this work]

---

[18] Definition substituted by Coroners and Justice Act 2009 (Commencement No. 15, Consequential and Transitory Provisions) Order 2013/1869 Sch.1 para.4(2)(c) (July 25, 2013 as SI 2013/1869 art.4).

Appointment of medical referee and deputy medical referee

A2–150   6.—(1) The Secretary of State must appoint a medical referee for each cremation authority.

(2) The Secretary of State must appoint as many deputy medical referees for each cremation authority as the Secretary of State thinks appropriate.

Qualifications of medical referee and deputy medical referee

A2–151   7.—(1) To be eligible for appointment as a medical referee or a deputy medical referee, a person must be a registered medical practitioner of at least five years' standing.

(2) The Secretary of State must appoint as medical referee and deputy medical referee such persons as may be nominated by the cremation authority who have the character, experience and qualifications to discharge the duties required by these Regulations.

Guidance by the Secretary of State

A2–152   8.   The Secretary of State may issue guidance about the character, experience and qualifications that a person appointed as a medical referee or a deputy medical referee is expected to have.

Termination of office

A2–153   9. The Secretary of State may remove a medical referee or a deputy medical referee from office for incapacity or misbehaviour.

Functions of deputy medical referee

A2–154   10.—(1) The functions of the medical referee for a cremation authority may—

(a) be performed by a deputy medical referee for the cremation authority—

    (i) during any period when the medical referee is absent or unavailable;

    (ii) in any case in which the medical referee has been the usual medical attendant of the deceased person in relation to whom an application for cremation has been made;

    (iii) during any vacancy in the office of medical referee; or

    (iv) in any other case, with the consent of the medical referee; and

(b) be performed by a medical referee or a deputy medical referee for any other cremation authority in an emergency.

(2) Accordingly, a reference in these Regulations to a medical referee is to be read, where relevant, as including a deputy medical referee.

Report to the Secretary of State

A2–155   11. A medical referee must give such reports to the Secretary of State as the Secretary of State may from time to time require.

Supplementary powers of medical referee

A2–156   12. A medical referee—

(a) who has investigated the cause of death of a deceased person, may issue a confirmatory medical certificate in an emergency;

(b) who has made a post-mortem examination of the body of the deceased person under regulation 24(2), may issue a certificate under regulation 24(3); and

(c) who is a coroner, may issue a certificate under regulation 16(1)(c)(ii).

PART 4

CONDITIONS FOR CREMATION

Place where cremation may take place

13. No cremation may take place except in a crematorium the opening of which has been notified to the Secretary of State.   **A2–157**

Forms

14.—(1) Subject to regulation 37(3) and this regulation, the forms set out in Schedule 1   **A2–158**
must be used in the cases to which they apply.

(2) In the case of an application for cremation of the remains of a deceased person—

(a) if the death of the deceased person occurred in any place outside the British Islands an application for cremation which contains all the particulars required by the application for cremation set out in Schedule 1 may be used instead of the application set out in Schedule 1; and

(b) if the death of the deceased person occurred in Scotland, Northern Ireland, the Isle of Man or the Channel Islands, an application for cremation and certificates—

(i) which contain all the particulars required by the application for cremation and, as the case may be, by the medical certificate, the confirmatory medical certificate, the certificate of coroner or the certificate following anatomical examination set out in Schedule 1; and

(ii) which are used in accordance with the law relating to cremation for the time being in force in Scotland, Northern Ireland, the Isle of Man, the Bailiwick of Jersey or the Bailiwick of Guernsey,

may be used instead of the application or certificates set out in Schedule 1.

(3) In the case of an application for cremation of body parts, if the death of the deceased person, the stillbirth or the post-mortem examination occurred in any place outside England and Wales, certificates which contain all the particulars given in the certificate or certified copy referred to in regulation 19(b) or in the certificate releasing body parts for cremation set out in Schedule 1 may be given instead of those certificates or that certified copy.

(4) In the case of an application for cremation of a stillborn child, if the stillbirth occurred outside England and Wales, a certificate which contains all the particulars given in the certificate of stillbirth set out in Schedule 1 may be given by a person entitled to practise as a medical practitioner or midwife in the place where the stillbirth occurred instead of the certificate set out in Schedule 1.

Application for cremation

15.—(1) Subject to paragraph (2), an application for cremation must be made to the   **A2–159**
cremation authority by—

(a) an executor of the deceased person; or

(b) a near relative who has attained the age of 16.

(2) An application for cremation may be made by any other person if the medical referee is satisfied—

(a) that the person is a proper person to make the application; and

(b) as to the reason why the application is not made by an executor or a near relative who has attained the age of 16.

(3) In this regulation, "near relative" means the widow, widower or surviving civil partner of the deceased person, or a parent or child of the deceased person, or any other relative usually residing with the deceased person, or a parent of a stillborn child.

Cremation of the remains of a deceased person

A2–160   **16.**—(1) No cremation of the remains of a deceased person may take place unless—

(a) an application for cremation is made in accordance with regulation 15;

(b) except where regulation 18 applies,—

   (i) a certificate is given under section 24(1), (2) or (4) of the 1953 Act (certificates as to registration of death) in relation to the death of the deceased person; or

   (ii) a certified copy of the entry in the relevant register is issued under sections 30 to 32 of the 1953 Act in relation to the death of the deceased person;

(c) (i) a medical certificate and, subject to regulation 17(3), a confirmatory medical certificate are given in accordance with regulation 17(1) and (2) respectively;

   (ii) where regulation 18 applies, a certificate is given by a coroner; or

   (iii) a certificate is given that the body of the deceased person has undergone an anatomical examination under the authority of a licence granted under the 2004 Act for that purpose; and

(d) written authority is given by a medical referee in accordance with regulation 23.

(2) This regulation does not apply to the cremation of the exhumed remains of a deceased person who has already been buried for a period of one year or more.

Medical certificate and confirmatory medical certificate

A2–161   **17.**—(1) A medical certificate giving the cause of death of the deceased person may be given by a registered medical practitioner.

(2) A confirmatory medical certificate giving the cause of death of the deceased person may be given by a registered medical practitioner of at least five years' standing who is not—

(a) a relative of the deceased person;

(b) the medical practitioner who issued the medical certificate; or

(c) a relative, or partner or colleague in the same practice or clinical team, of the medical practitioner who issued the medical certificate.

(3) A confirmatory medical certificate is not required where—

(a) the death of the deceased person occurred in a hospital in which the deceased person was an in-patient; and

(b) a medical practitioner mentioned in paragraph (2) has made or supervised a post-mortem examination of the body of the deceased person and the medical practitioner giving the medical certificate (in accordance with paragraph (1)) knows the result of that examination before giving that certificate.

(4) In this regulation, "hospital" means any institution for the reception and treatment of persons suffering from illness or mental disorder, any maternity home, and any institution for the reception and treatment of persons during convalescence.

Certificate of coroner

18. This regulation applies if—   A2–162

(a) a post-mortem examination has been made under [section 14 of the 2009 Act][19] and the cause of death of the deceased person has been certified by the coroner under [a post-mortem examination made under section 14 of the 2009 Act has revealed the cause of death of the deceased and the coroner does not think it necessary to continue the investigation][1];

(b) an [investigation has begun][20]; or

(c) the death of the deceased person occurred outside the British Islands and no post-mortem examination or [investigation][21] is necessary.

Cremation of body parts

19. No cremation of body parts may take place unless—   A2–163

(a) an application for cremation is made in accordance with regulation 15;

(b) (i) a certificate is given under section 24(1), (2) or (4) of the 1953 Act (certificates as to registration of death) or under section 11(2) or (3) of the 1953 Act (certificates as to registration of stillbirth) in relation to the death of the deceased person or to the stillborn child to whom the body parts belonged; or

   (ii) a certified copy of the entry in the relevant register is issued under sections 30 to 32 of the 1953 Act in relation to the death of the deceased person or to the stillborn child to whom the body parts belonged;

(c) (i) a certificate is given on behalf of the hospital trust or other authority holding the body parts that there is no reason for further inquiry or examination of the body parts and that they are released for cremation; or

   (ii) evidence is produced that the body parts were removed in the course of a post-mortem examination made of the body of the deceased person; and

(d) written authority is given by a medical referee in accordance with regulation 25.

---

[19] Words substituted by Coroners and Justice Act 2009 (Commencement No. 15, Consequential and Transitory Provisions) Order 2013/1869 Sch.1 para.4(3)(a) (July 25, 2013 as SI 2013/1869 art.4).
[20] Words substituted by Coroners and Justice Act 2009 (Commencement No. 15, Consequential and Transitory Provisions) Order 2013/1869 Sch.1 para.4(3)(b) (July 25, 2013 as SI 2013/1869 art.4).
[21] Word substituted by Coroners and Justice Act 2009 (Commencement No. 15, Consequential and Transitory Provisions) Order 2013/1869 Sch.1 para.4(3)(c) (July 25, 2013 as SI 2013/1869 art.4).

Cremation of a stillborn child

A2–164   **20.**—(1) No cremation of a stillborn child may take place unless—

(a) an application for cremation is made in accordance with regulation 15;

(b) a certificate is given under section 11(2) or (3) of the 1953 Act (certificates as to registration of stillbirth);

(c) (i) a certificate is given by a registered medical practitioner or a registered midwife who has examined the body and who can certify that the child was stillborn; or

  (ii) where paragraph (2) applies, a declaration is given by a person who is qualified to give information concerning the birth; and

(d) written authority is given by a medical referee in accordance with regulation 26.

(2) This paragraph applies where the child was stillborn and either—

(a) no registered medical practitioner or registered midwife was present at the birth or has examined the body; or

(b) a certificate under paragraph (1)(c)(i) cannot be obtained from a registered medical practitioner or a registered midwife who was present at the birth.

Cremation of exhumed remains of deceased person who has already been buried for one year or more

A2–165   **21.** The cremation of the exhumed remains of a deceased person who has already been buried for a period of one year or more may take place subject to such conditions as may be imposed by—

(a) the Secretary of State in an exhumation licence granted under section 25 of the Burial Act 1857; or

(b) a faculty granted by the ordinary.

Right to inspect medical certificate and confirmatory medical certificate and to make representations to medical referee

A2–166   **22.**—(1) Paragraph (2) applies where the applicant for cremation of the remains of a deceased person—

(a) (i) has informed the cremation authority to which the application for cremation was made that they would like to inspect the medical certificate and confirmatory medical certificate; or

  (ii) has nominated another person to inspect those certificates; and

(b) has given one or more telephone numbers to the cremation authority at which the applicant, or the person nominated by the applicant, may be contacted.

(2) As soon as the cremation authority receives the medical certificate and confirmatory medical certificate it must make all reasonable efforts to notify the applicant for cremation or any person nominated by that person, by telephone on the number (or one of the numbers) provided, of the receipt of those certificates.

(3) Within 48 hours, beginning with the time at which the cremation authority notifies the person under paragraph (2), that person may—

(a) at a time and place agreed with the cremation authority, inspect the medical certificate and confirmatory medical certificate; and

(b) make representations to the medical referee about any matter contained in such a certificate or the inquiry made by the person who gave the certificate.

Authorisation of cremation of the remains of a deceased person by medical referee

23.—(1) A medical referee may not authorise a cremation under regulation 16(1)(d) unless the medical referee is satisfied— **A2–167**

(a) that the requirements of regulation 16(1)(a), (b) and (c) have been complied with;

(b) that the inquiry made by a person giving a certificate under regulation 16(1)(c) has been adequate;

(c) that the fact and cause of death of the deceased person have been definitely ascertained; and

(d) subject to paragraph (2), in any case where notification has been given under regulation 22(2),—

    (i) at least 48 hours have passed since that notification was given; and

    (ii) where certificates have been inspected under regulation 22(3)(a), at least 24 hours have passed since the time of the inspection.

(2) Where the medical referee is satisfied that a cremation authority has made all reasonable efforts to comply with regulation 22(2) but has been unable to do so within 48 hours, beginning with the time at which the cremation authority received the medical certificate and confirmatory medical certificate, the medical referee may authorise cremation of the remains of a deceased person.

(3) If a coroner has decided to hold an inquest, a medical referee may not authorise cremation of the remains of the deceased person until the inquest has been opened.

Medical referee not satisfied about the cause of death of the deceased person

24.—(1) Paragraph (2) applies if— **A2–168**

(a) the medical referee is not satisfied that the fact and cause of death of the deceased person have been definitely ascertained; or

(b) the death of the deceased person may have been violent or unnatural.

(2) The medical referee may make a post-mortem examination of the body of the deceased person or request any person to do so if—

(a) the medical referee, or the person so requested by the medical referee, is entitled to make a post-mortem examination under the authority of a licence granted under section 16 of the 2004 Act (licence requirement) for that purpose; and

(b) the medical referee has obtained the appropriate consent for a post-mortem examination in accordance with the provisions of that Act.

(3) If a certificate is given by the person who has made the post-mortem examination stating the cause of death to the satisfaction of the medical referee, the medical referee may authorise cremation of the remains of the deceased person.

(4) Paragraph (5) applies if—

(a) a post-mortem examination fails to satisfy the medical referee that the fact and cause of death have been definitely ascertained; or

(b) it appears to the medical referee that the cause of death is violent or unnatural, or there are other suspicious circumstances connected with the death of the deceased person, whether revealed in the medical certificate or confirmatory medical certificate or otherwise.

(5) The medical referee may not authorise cremation of the remains of the deceased person unless an inquest is opened and a certificate is given under regulation 16(1)(c)(ii).

Authorisation of cremation of body parts by medical referee

A2–169   **25.** A medical referee may not authorise a cremation under regulation 19(d) unless the medical referee is satisfied that the requirements of regulation 19(a), (b) and (c) have been complied with.

Authorisation of cremation of a stillborn child by medical referee

A2–170   **26.** A medical referee may not authorise a cremation under regulation 20(1)(d) unless the medical referee is satisfied—

(a) that the requirements of regulation 20(1)(a), (b) and (c) have been complied with;

(b) that the examination made by the person giving the certificate under regulation 20(1)(c)(i) has been adequate; and

(c) that there is no reason for further examination.

Authorisation of cremation by medical referee—inquiries by medical referee

A2–171   **27.**—(1) Before authorising a cremation, a medical referee may make such inquiry as the medical referee thinks appropriate with regard to—

(a) an application for cremation;

(b) a certificate referred to in regulation 16(1)(c), 19(c)(i) or 20(1)(c)(i); or

(c) a declaration given under regulation 20(1)(c)(ii).

(2) Inquiries under paragraph (1) may be made on the medical referee's own initiative or, in relation to a certificate given in accordance with regulation 17(1) and (2), as a result of representations made under regulation 22(3)(b).

(3) If inquiries are made as a result of representations made under regulation 22(3)(b), the medical referee must inform the person who made the representations of the result of the inquiries made.

Refusal to authorise cremation

28. A medical referee who refuses to authorise a cremation must give written reasons to the applicant. **A2–172**

Incineration of body parts

29.—(1) Body parts which are not cremated under regulation 19 may be incinerated in accordance with a permit which authorises the disposal of a matter listed in code 18 01 02 or 18 01 03 of Schedule 1 to the List of Wastes Regulations. **A2–173**

(2) In this regulation—

"incinerated" means burnt in an incinerator as part of one of the following activities in section 5.1 of Part 2 of Schedule 1 to the Environmental Permitting (England and Wales) Regulations 2007—

    (a) activities in Part A(1)(a), (c), (d) and (e);
    (b) activities in Part A(2)(a); and
    (c) activities in Part B(a);

"List of Wastes Regulations" means—

    (a) in relation to England, the List of Wastes (England) Regulations 2005; and
    (b) in relation to Wales, the List of Wastes (Wales) Regulations 2005; and

"permit" means a permit granted under regulation 13 of the Environmental Permitting (England and Wales) Regulations 2007.

PART 6

DISPOSAL OF ASHES

Disposal of ashes

30.—(1) Subject to paragraph (2), after a cremation the cremation authority must give the ashes to the applicant or a person nominated for that purpose by the applicant. **A2–174**

(2) If the applicant does not want to be given the ashes and has not nominated any person for that purpose, the cremation authority must retain the ashes.

(3) Subject to any special arrangement for the burial or preservation of ashes, any ashes retained by a cremation authority must be decently interred in a burial ground or in part of a crematorium reserved for the burial of ashes, or scattered there.

(4) In relation to ashes left temporarily in the care of a cremation authority, the authority may not inter or scatter the ashes unless 14 days notice of their intention to do so has been given to the applicant.

PART 7

REGISTRATION OF CREMATIONS

Appointment of registrar

31. A cremation authority must appoint a registrar. **A2–175**

SCHEDULE 1

FORMS

Application for cremation of the body of a person who has died

A2–176

Application for cremation of the body of a person who has died

Cremation 1
replacing Form A

01.09

This form can only be completed by a person who is at least 16 years of age.
Please complete this form in full, if a part does not apply enter 'N/A'.

Part 1 Details of the crematorium

Name of crematorium where cremation will take place

Name of funeral director

Telephone number

Part 2 Your details (the applicant)

Your full name

Address

Telephone number

Part 3 Details of the person who has died

Full name

Address

Occupation or last occupation if retired or not in work at date of death

continued over the page ⇨

Regulation 16(1)(a) of the Cremation (England and Wales) Regulations 2008

Part 3 continued

Age at date of death

Sex
☐ Male ☐ Female

Status
☐ married/civil partnership ☐ widow/widower/surviving civil partner ☐ Single

Part 4 The application

1. Are you a near relative or an executor of the person who has died? ☐ Yes ☐ No

Near relative means the widow, widower or surviving civil partner of the person
who has died, or a parent or child of the person who has died, or any other relative
usually residing with the person who has died.

If No, please give the nature of your relationship and explain why you are
making the application rather than a near relative or an executor.

2. Is there any near relative(s) or executor(s) who has not been informed of the
proposed cremation? ☐ Yes ☐ No

If Yes, please give the name(s) and the reason(s) why they have not been contacted.

3. Has any near relative or executor expressed any objection to the
proposed cremation? ☐ Yes ☐ No

If Yes, please give details.

4. What was the date and time of death of the person who has died?

Date ☐☐/☐☐/☐☐☐☐

Time

continued over the page ⇨

2

865

Part 4 continued

5. Please give the address where the person died.

Address

☐☐☐☐ ☐☐☐

Please state whether it was the residence of the person who has died or a hotel, hospital, or nursing home etc.

☐ Their home   ☐ Hospital   ☐ Other (please specify)

☐ Hotel   ☐ Nursing home

6. Do you know or suspect that the death of the person who has died was violent or unnatural?   ☐ Yes   ☐ No

7. Do you consider that there should be any further examination of the remains of the person who has died?   ☐ Yes   ☐ No

If you have answered Yes to questions **6** or **7**, please give reasons below.

8. What is the name, address and telephone number of the usual doctor of the person who has died?

Doctor's name

Address   Telephone number

☐☐☐☐ ☐☐☐

continued over the page ▷

866

Part 4 continued

9. Please give the name, address and telephone number of the doctor(s) who attended the person who has died during their last illness.

Doctor's name

Address

Telephone number

Doctor's name

Address

Telephone number

10. Was any implant placed in the body which may become hazardous when the body is cremated (e.g. a pacemaker, radioactive device or "Fixion" intramedullary nailing system)?

☐ Yes ☐ No

☐ I don't know

Implants may damage cremation equipment if not removed from the body of the deceased before cremation and some radioactive treatments may endanger the health of crematorium staff.

If Yes, please give details and state whether it has been removed.

Part 5 Inspection of certificates

You are entitled to inspect the certificates (if any) given by doctors under regulation 16(c)(i) of the Cremation Regulations 2008 (forms Cremation 4 and Cremation 5). If you do not wish to inspect any such certificates yourself you may nominate another person to inspect them instead of you.

Such certificates will only be available for inspection at the offices of the cremation authority for **48 hours** from the time that the cremation authority notifies you, or the person you have nominated, that the certificates are available to be inspected. You may take someone with you when you attend to inspect the certificates. If you, or the person nominated by you, do not attend to inspect the certificates at the time agreed with the cremation authority, the cremation may then proceed.

Please state if you would like to inspect the certificates given by the doctors or whether you would like to nominate someone else to do so instead and give a contact telephone number.

If certificates are given by medical practitioners:-

☐ I would like to inspect the certificates and

   my contact telephone number is

☐ I nominate

   to inspect the certificates and their
   contact telephone number is

Part 6 Statement of truth

I apply for the body of the person who has died to be cremated and I certify that I am at least 16 years of age.

I believe that the facts given in this application are true. I am aware that it is an offence to wilfully make a false statement with a view to obtaining the cremation of any human remains.

Print your full name

Signed   Dated ☐☐/☐☐/☐☐☐☐

Cremation 1   5

868

Application for cremation of body parts

Cremation 2
replacing Form AA

01.09

Body parts means material consisting of, or including, human cells from a deceased person or stillborn baby.

This form can only be completed by a person who is at least 16 years of age.
Please complete this form in full, if a part does not apply enter 'N/A'.

If your application is about a stillborn baby, replace the words 'person who has died' throughout this form with the words 'stillborn baby'.

Part 1 Details of the crematorium

Name of crematorium where cremation will take place

Name of funeral director

Telephone number

Part 2 Your details (the applicant)

Your full name

Address

Telephone number

Part 3 Details of the person who has died

In the case of a stillborn baby who has not been given a name, in place of the name and address insert a description sufficient to identify the baby.

Full name

Address

continued over the page ⇨

Regulation 19(a) of the Cremation (England and Wales) Regulations 2008

Part 3 continued

Age at date of death

Sex

☐ Male ☐ Female

Status

☐ married/civil partnership ☐ widow/widower/surviving civil partner ☐ Single

Part 4 The application

1. Are you a near relative or an executor of the person who has died? ☐ Yes ☐ No

   Near relative means the widow, widower or surviving civil partner of the person who has died, or a parent or child of the person who has died, or any other relative usually residing with the person who has died, or a parent of a stillborn baby.

   If No, please give the nature of your relationship and explain why you are making the application rather than a near relative or an executor.

2. Is there any near relative(s) or executor(s) who has not been informed of the proposed cremation? ☐ Yes ☐ No

   If Yes, please give the name(s) and the reason(s) why they have not been contacted.

3. Has any near relative or executor expressed any objection to the proposed cremation? ☐ Yes ☐ No

   If Yes, please give details.

continued over the page ⇨

Cremation 2

Part 4 continued

4. What was the date and place of the death or stillbirth?

Date

☐☐ / ☐☐ / ☐☐☐☐

Address

☐☐☐☐ ☐☐☐☐

5. Please give the name and address of the cemetery, churchyard or crematorium where the body of the person who has died was buried or cremated.

Name of cemetery, churchyard or crematorium

Address

☐☐☐☐ ☐☐☐☐

6. Please give the date that the burial or cremation took place.

Date

☐☐ / ☐☐ / ☐☐☐☐

7. Please state whether the body parts were removed from the body of the person who has died at a:

☐ Coroner's post-mortem examination   ☐ Hospital post-mortem examination

☐ Other (please specify)

continued over the page ⇨

871

Part 4 continued

8. Do you consider that there should be any further examination of the remains of the person who has died?   ☐ Yes   ☐ No

If Yes, please give reasons below.

Part 5 Statement of truth

I apply for the following body parts of the person who has died to be cremated and I certify that I am at least 16 years of age.

Specify body parts to be cremated.

I believe that the facts given in this application are true. I am aware that it is an offence to wilfully make a false statement with a view to obtaining the cremation of any human remains.

Print your full name

Signed   Dated
                                          ☐☐ / ☐☐ / ☐☐☐☐

Application for cremation of stillborn baby

Cremation 3
introduced in 2009 | 01.09

This form can only be completed by a person who is at least 16 years of age.
Please complete this form in full, if a part does not apply enter 'N/A'.

Part 1 Details of the crematorium

Name of crematorium where cremation will take place

Name of funeral director

Telephone number

Part 2 Your details (the applicant)

Your full name

Address

Telephone number

Part 3 Details of the stillborn baby

In the case of a stillborn baby who has not been given a name, in place of the name insert a description sufficient to identify the baby.

Full name of baby

Sex
☐ Male ☐ Female

Date of stillbirth
☐☐ / ☐☐ / ☐☐☐☐

continued over the page ⇒

Regulation 20(1)(a) of the Cremation (England and Wales) Regulations 2008

Part 4 The application

1. Are you a parent of the stillborn baby?   ☐ Yes   ☐ No

    If No, please give the nature of your relationship and explain why you are
    making the application.

2. Have both parents been informed of the proposed cremation?   ☐ Yes   ☐ No

    If No, please give the name of the parent and the reason(s) why they have not been contacted.

3. Has a parent of the stillborn baby expressed any objection to the   ☐ Yes   ☐ No
    proposed cremation?

    If Yes, please give details.

4. Please give the address where the baby was stillborn.

    Address

    Please state whether it was the applicant's own home, hospital etc.

continued over the page ➪

Part 4 continued

5. Do you know or suspect that the baby was not stillborn? ☐ Yes ☐ No

6. Do you consider that there should be any further examination of the stillborn baby's remains? ☐ Yes ☐ No

If you have answered Yes to questions **5** or **6**, please give reasons below.

Part 5 Statement of truth

I apply for the stillborn baby to be cremated and I certify that I am at least 16 years of age.

I believe that the facts given in this application are true. I am aware that it is an offence to wilfully make a false statement with a view to obtaining the cremation of any human remains.

Print your full name

Signed   Dated
                                               ☐☐ / ☐☐ / ☐☐☐☐

Medical certificate

Medical certificate

| Cremation 4 |
| replacing Form B |

01.09

This form can only be completed by a registered medical practitioner.
Please complete this form in full, if a part does not apply enter 'N/A'.

Part 1 Details of the deceased

Full name

Address

Occupation or last occupation if retired or not in work at the date of death

Where a past occupation of the deceased person may suggest that the death was due to industrial disease, you should consider whether to refer the death to a coroner.

Part 2 The report on the deceased

1. What was the date and time of death of the deceased?

Date ☐☐ / ☐☐ / ☐☐☐☐   Time

2. Please give the address where the deceased died.

Address

Please state whether it was the residence of the deceased or a hotel, hospital, or nursing home etc.

☐ Their home   ☐ Hospital   ☐ Other (please specify)

☐ Hotel   ☐ Nursing home

continued over the page ➪

Regulation 16(c)(i) of the Cremation (England and Wales) Regulations 2008

Part 2 continued

3. Are you a relative of the deceased? ☐ Yes ☐ No

    If Yes, please give the nature of your relationship.

4. Have you, so far as you are aware, any pecuniary interest in the death of the deceased? ☐ Yes ☐ No

    If Yes, please give details.

5. Were you the deceased's usual medical practitioner? ☐ Yes ☐ No

    If Yes, please state for how long.

    If No, please give details of your medical role in relation to the deceased.

6. Please state for how long you attended the deceased during their last illness?

7. Please state the number of days and hours before the deceased's death that you last saw them alive?

    Days   Hours

8. Please state the date and time that you saw the body of the deceased and the examination that you made of the body.

    Date   □□ / □□ / □□□□   Time

    Examination

continued over the page ☞

Part 2 continued

9. From your medical notes, and the observations of yourself and others immediately before and at the time of the deceased's death, please describe the symptoms and other conditions which led to your conclusions about the cause of death.

10. If the deceased died in a hospital at which they were an in-patient, has a hospital post-mortem examination been made or supervised by a registered medical practitioner of at least five years' standing who is neither a relative of the deceased nor a relative of yours or a partner or colleague in the same practice or clinical team as you?

☐ Yes ☐ No

If Yes, are the results of that examination known to you?

☐ Yes ☐ No

Note: 'Five years' standing' means a medical practitioner who has been a fully registered person within the meaning of the Medical Act 1983 for at least five years and, if paragraph 10 of Schedule 1 to the Medical Act 1983 (Amendment) Order 2002 (S.I. 2002/3135) has come into force, has held a licence to practice for at least five years or since the coming into force of that paragraph.

continued over the page ⇨

Part 2 continued

11. Please give the cause of death

1. (a) Disease or condition directly leading to death (this does not mean the mode of dying, such as heart failure, asphyxia, asthenia, etc: it means the disease, injury, or complication which caused death)

(b) Other disease or condition, if any, leading to (a)

(c) Other disease or condition, if any, leading to (b)

2. Other significant conditions contributing to the death but not related to the disease or condition causing it.

12. Did the deceased undergo any operation in the year before their death?   ☐ Yes   ☐ No

If Yes, what was the date and nature of the operation and who performed it.

Date of operation

☐☐ / ☐☐ / ☐☐☐☐

Who performed it

Nature of operation

13. Do you have any reason to believe that the operation(s) shortened the life of the deceased?   ☐ Yes   ☐ No

If Yes, please give details.

continued over the page ➧

Part 2 continued

14. Please give the full name and address details of any person who nursed the deceased during their last illness (Say whether professional nurse, relative, etc. If the illness was a long one, this question should be answered with reference to the period of four weeks before the death.)

15. Were there any persons present at the moment of death? ☐ Yes ☐ No

    If Yes, please give the full name and address details of those persons and whether you have spoken to them about the death.

16. If there were persons present at the moment of death, did those persons have any concerns regarding the cause of death? ☐ Yes ☐ No

    If Yes, please give details

17. In view of your knowledge of the deceased's habits and constitution do you have any doubts whatever about the character of the disease or condition which led to the death? ☐ Yes ☐ No

18. Have you any reason to suspect that the death of the deceased was

    Violent ☐ Yes ☐ No
    Unnatural ☐ Yes ☐ No

19. Have you any reason at all to suppose a further examination of the body is desirable? ☐ Yes ☐ No

    If you have answered Yes to questions **17**, **18** or **19** please give details below:

continued over the page ⇨

Part 2 continued

20. Has a coroner been informed about the death? ☐ Yes ☐ No

If Yes, please state the outcome.

```
```

21. Has there been any discussion with a coroner's office about the death of the deceased? ☐ Yes ☐ No

If Yes, please state the coroner's office that was contacted and the outcome of the discussions.

```
```

22. Have you given the certificate required for registration of death? ☐ Yes ☐ No

If No, please give the full name and contact details of the medical practitioner who has

Full name

```
```

Address   Telephone number

```
```

23. Was any hazardous implant placed in the body (e.g. a pacemaker, radioactive device or 'Fixion' intramedullary nailing system)? ☐ Yes ☐ No

Implants may damage cremation equipment if not removed from the body of the deceased before cremation and some radioactive treatments may endanger the health of crematorium staff.

If Yes, has it been removed? ☐ Yes ☐ No

continued over the page ▷

Cremation 4   6

Part 3 Statement of truth

I certify that I am a registered medical practitioner.

I certify that the information I have given above is true and accurate to the best of my knowledge and belief and that I know of no reasonable cause to suspect that the deceased died either a violent or unnatural death or a sudden death of which the cause is unknown or in a place or circumstance which requires an inquest in pursuance of any Act.

I am aware that it is an offence to wilfully make a false statement with a view to procuring the cremation of any human remains.

Your full name

Address   Telephone number

Registered qualifications

GMC Reference number

Signed   Dated □□ / □□ / □□□□

Once completed, this certificate must be handed or sent in a closed envelope by, or on behalf of, the medical practitioner who signs it to the medical practitioner who is to give the confirmatory medical certificate except in a case where question 10 is answered in the affirmative, in which case the certificate must be so handed or sent to the medical referee at the cremation authority at which the cremation is to take place.

Cremation 4   7

Confirmatory medical certificate

Confirmatory medical certificate

| Cremation 5
replacing Form C | 01.09 |

This form may only be completed by a registered medical practitioner of at least five years' standing who is not either a relative of the deceased, the medical practitioner who issued the medical certificate (form Cremation 4) or a relative or a partner or colleague in the same practice or clinical team as the medical practitioner who issued that certificate.

'Five years' standing' means a medical practitioner who has been a fully registered person within the meaning of the Medical Act 1983 for at least five years and, if paragraph 10 of Schedule 1 to the Medical Act 1983 (Amendment) Order 2002 (S.I. 2002/3135) has come into force, has held a licence to practice for at least five years or since the coming into force of that paragraph.

Please complete this form in full, if a part does not apply enter 'N/A'.

Part 1 Details of the deceased

Full name

Address

Occupation or last occupation if retired or not in work at the date of death

Part 2 The report on the deceased

1. Have you questioned the medical practitioner who gave the Medical Certificate (form Cremation 4)?   ☐ Yes   ☐ No

If No, please give reasons.

continued over the page ⇨

Regulation 16(c)(i) of the Cremation (England and Wales) Regulations 2008

883

Part 2 continued

In answer to questions 2, 3, 4, and 5, please give names and addresses of persons questioned and say whether you spoke to them in person or by telephone. Any failure to answer one of these questions in the affirmative may be treated as inadequate enquiry.

2. Have you questioned any other medical practitioner who attended the deceased?   ☐ Yes   ☐ No

If Yes, please give the full name and address details of the medical practitioner(s).

3. Have you questioned any person who nursed the deceased during their last illness, or who was present at the death?   ☐ Yes   ☐ No

If Yes, please give the full name and address details.

4. Have you questioned any of the relatives of the deceased?   ☐ Yes   ☐ No

If Yes, please give the full name and address details.

5. Have you questioned any other person?   ☐ Yes   ☐ No

If Yes, please give the full name and address details.

continued over the page ⇨

Part 2 continued

6. Please state the date and time that you saw the body of the deceased and the examination that you made of the body.

Date

☐☐ / ☐☐ / ☐☐☐☐

Time

Examination

7. Do you agree with the cause of death given in question 11 of Part 2 of the Medical Certificate (form Cremation 4)?

☐ Yes ☐ No

If No, please give reasons and give the cause of death.

Reason(s) for disagreeing

1. (a) Disease or condition directly leading to death (this does not mean the mode of dying, such as heart failure, asphyxia, asthenia, etc: it means the disease, injury, or complication which caused death)

(b) Other disease or condition, if any, leading to (a)

(c) Other disease or condition, if any, leading to (b)

2. Other significant conditions contributing to the death but not related to the disease or condition causing it.

continued over the page ⇨

Cremation 5   3

Part 3 Statement of truth

I certify that I am a registered medical practitioner of at least five years' standing and I am not a relative of the deceased, or a relative or a partner or colleague in the same practice or clinical team as the medical practitioner who has given the Medical Certificate (form Cremation 4).

I certify that the information I have given above is true and accurate to the best of my knowledge and belief and that I know of no reasonable cause to suspect that the deceased died either a violent or unnatural death or a sudden death of which the cause is unknown or in a place or circumstance which requires an inquest in pursuance of any Act.

I am aware that it is an offence to wilfully make a false statement with a view to procuring the cremation of any human remains.

Your full name

Address   Telephone number

Registered qualifications

GMC reference number

Signed   Dated

Once completed, this certificate and the Medical Certificate (form Cremation 4) must be handed or sent in a closed envelope by one of the medical practitioners giving the certificates to the medical referee at the cremation authority at which the cremation is to take place.

Cremation 5   4

Certificate of coroner [ORIGINAL IMAGE: See footnotes for amendments[22]] [23]

A2–181

Certificate of coroner

| Cremation 6
replacing Form E

09
01.09

Please complete this form in full, if a part does not apply enter 'N/A'.

Part 1 Details of the deceased

Full name

Age at date of death

Sex
☐ Male ☐ Female

Date of death

☐☐/☐☐/☐☐☐☐

Place of death or where body found

Registration district and sub-district in which the death is to be registered

Cause of death or insert unascertained

1. (a) Disease or condition directly leading to death (this does not mean mode of dying, such as heart failure, asphyxia, asthenia, etc: it means the disease, injury, or complication which caused death)

   (b) Other disease or condition, if any, leading to (a)

   (c) Other disease or condition, if any, leading to (b)

2. Other significant conditions contributing to the death but not related to the disease or condition causing it.

continued over the page ⇨

Regulation 16(c)(ii) of the Cremation (England and Wales) Regulations 2008

---

[22] Amendments made by SI 2013/1869 Sch.1 para.4(4)(a).
[23] Words substituted by Coroners and Justice Act 2009 (Commencement No. 15, Consequential and Transitory Provisions) Order 2013/1869 Sch.1 para.4(4)(a) (July 25, 2013 as SI 2013/1869 art.4).

Part 2 Certification of coroner

I certify that:

☐ a post-mortem examination of the body of the deceased has been made by my direction or at my request and as a result I am satisfied that an inquest is unnecessary.

☐ I have opened an inquest on the body of the deceased.

☐ the death occurred outside the British Islands and no post-mortem examination or inquest is necessary.

In my opinion there is no need for any further examination of the body.

Print your full name

Signed   District

Dated

☐☐/☐☐/☐☐☐☐

Part 3 Notification by Registrar of Cremation

(Section 3(1) of the Births and Deaths Registration Act 1926)

Name of deceased

Date of death

☐☐/☐☐/☐☐☐☐

Place of death

was cremated on

☐☐/☐☐/☐☐☐☐

Name of crematorium

Print your full name

Signed

Dated

☐☐/☐☐/☐☐☐☐

A2–182

Certificate following anatomical examination

| Cremation 7
| replacing Form H   01.00

Please complete this form in full, if a part does not apply enter 'N/A'.

Part 1 Details of the deceased

Full name

Age at date of death   Sex
                              ☐ Male ☐ Female   Date of death
                                                        ☐☐ / ☐☐ / ☐☐☐☐

Part 2 Certification of anatomical examination

I certify that the body of the deceased has undergone an anatomical examination under the authority of a licence granted under the Human Tissue Act 2004[1] for that purpose.

The examination took place at

Your full name

Address

☐☐☐☐ ☐☐☐☐

Registered qualifications

Signed   Dated
                                              ☐☐ / ☐☐ / ☐☐☐☐

[1] If the anatomical examination took place before the implementation of the Human Tissue Act 2004 on 1 September 2006, for the words 'Human Tissue Act 2004' substitute a reference to the relevant Anatomy Act under which the examination was authorised.

Regulation 16(c)(ii) of the Cremation (England and Wales) Regulations 2008

Certificate releasing body parts for cremation [ORIGINAL IMAGE: See footnotes for amendments[24]][25]

Certificate releasing body parts for cremation

| Cremation 8 |
| replacing Form DD |

01.09

Please complete this form in full, if a part does not apply enter 'N/A'.

Part 1 Details of the deceased

Full name

Address

Age at date of death

Sex

☐ Male   ☐ Female

Date of death

☐☐ / ☐☐ / ☐☐☐☐

Place of death

Part 2 Body parts for release

I confirm on behalf of (insert name and address of hospital trust or other authority lawfully holding the body parts)

that the following body parts are held in respect of the deceased—

☐ Heart   ☐ Brain   ☐ Chest   ☐ Abdominal

(please specify)

☐ other Organs

continued over the page ➪

Regulation 19(c)(i) of the Cremation (England and Wales) Regulations 2008

---

[24] Amendments made by SI 2013/1869 Sch.1 para.4(4)(b).
[25] Word substituted by Coroners and Justice Act 2009 (Commencement No. 15, Consequential and Transitory Provisions) Order 2013/1869 Sch.1 para.4(4)(b) (July 25, 2013 as SI 2013/1869 art.4).

Part 2 continued

'delete if not applicable

I certify that there is no reason for any further inquiry or examination concerning the above body parts and that they are [with the consent of the coroner for the following district]¹ now released for cremation in a suitably safe and prepared condition. I am aware that it is an offence to wilfully make a false statement with a view to procuring the cremation of any human remains .

Name of coroner's district (if applicable)

Your full name

Address

Registered qualifications

GMC reference number

Signed

Dated

□□ / □□ / □□□□

Certificate of stillbirth

| **Cremation 9**
introduced in 2009 | 09
01.09 |

Please complete this form in full, if a part does not apply enter 'N/A'.

Part 1 The stillborn child

Full name of child or description

Sex
☐ Male ☐ Female

Date of stillbirth
☐☐ / ☐☐ / ☐☐☐☐

Part 2 Certificate of stillbirth

I am a registered
☐ medical practitioner
☐ midwife

I certify that I have examined the body of the stillborn child and can certify that the child was stillborn.

I certify that the information I have given above is true and accurate to the best of my knowledge and belief. I am aware that it is an offence to wilfully make a false statement with a view to procuring a cremation.

Your full name

Address

Registered qualifications

GMC reference number / Nursing and Midwifery Council Personal Indentification number (PIN)

Signed

Dated
☐☐ / ☐☐ / ☐☐☐☐

Regulation 20(1)(c)(i) of the Cremation (England and Wales) Regulations 2008

Authorisation of cremation of deceased person by medical referee

A2–185

Authorisation of cremation of deceased person by medical referee

Cremation 10
replacing Form F
01.09

Please complete this form in full, if a part does not apply enter 'N/A'.

Part 1 Details of the deceased

Full name

Address

Occupation or last occupation if retired or not in work at date of death

Part 2 Authorisation by medical referee

An application has been made for the cremation of the remains of the deceased.

I am satisfied that—

(a) the requirements of the Cremation (England and Wales) Regulations 2008 have been complied with;

(b) the inquiry/examination made by the persons who gave the relevant certificates has been adequate; and

(c) the fact and cause of death have been definitely ascertained or, if not ascertained, a coroner has opened an inquest.

Accordingly, I authorise the Registrar of the following crematorium to cremate the remains of the deceased within that crematorium—

Name of crematorium

Print your full name

Cremation authority

Signed

Dated ☐☐/☐☐/☐☐☐☐

Regulation 23(1) of the Cremation (England and Wales) Regulations 2008

Certificate after post-mortem examination

Certificate after post-mortem examination

Cremation 11
replacing Form D

01.09

Please complete this form in full, if a part does not apply enter 'N/A'.

Part 1 Details of the deceased

Full name

Address

Occupation or last occupation if retired or not in work at date of death

Part 2 Certification of person making post-mortem examination

I certify that I have made a post-mortem examination of the remains of the deceased under the authority of a licence granted under the Human Tissue Act 2004 for that purpose and the appropriate consents required by that Act having been obtained.

I am satisfied that the cause of death was

1. (a) Disease or condition directly leading to death (this does not mean the mode of dying, such as heart failure, asphyxia, asthenia, etc: it means the disease, injury, or complication which caused death)

(b) Other disease or condition, if any, leading to (a)

(c) Other disease or condition, if any, leading to (b)

continued over the page ⇨

Regulation 24(3) of the Cremation (England and Wales) Regulations 2008

Part 2 continued

2. Other significant conditions contributing to the death but not related to the disease or condition causing it.

☐ I am satisfied that there is no reason for making any toxicological analysis.

If a toxicology analysis has been made have the results been stated in this certificate or are they attached?   ☐ stated in this certificate   ☐ attached to this certificate

☐ I am satisfied that there is no reason for the holding of an inquest.

If the cause of death is such as to require that an inquest be held, the coroner should issue a certificate and meet the costs of the post-mortem examination by paying the fee prescribed by the Secretary of State.

I am aware that it is an offence to wilfully make a false statement with a view to obtaining the cremation of any human remains.

Your full name

Address

Registered qualifications

GMC reference number

Signed   Dated ☐☐ / ☐☐ / ☐☐☐☐

Cremation 11   2

Authorisation of cremation of body parts by medical referee

Authorisation of cremation of body parts by medical referee

Cremation 12
replacing Form FF

01.09

Please complete this form in full, if a part does not apply enter 'N/A'.

Part 1 The deceased/stillborn child

In the case of a stillborn child who has not been given a name, insert a description sufficient to identify the body.

Full name

Address

Part 2 Authorisation by medical referee

An application has been made for the cremation of the body parts of the deceased/stillborn child.

I am satisfied that the requirements of the Cremation (England and Wales) Regulations 2008 have been complied with.

Accordingly, I authorise the Registrar of the following crematorium to cremate the remains of the deceased within that crematorium—

Name of crematorium

Print your full name

Cremation authority

Signed

Dated ☐☐/☐☐/☐☐☐☐

Regulation 25 of the Cremation (England and Wales) Regulations 2008

A2–188

Authorisation of cremation of stillborn child by medical referee

Cremation 13
introduced in 2009

01.09

Please complete this form in full, if a part does not apply enter 'N/A'.

Part 1 The stillborn child

Full name of child or description

Sex

☐ Male   ☐ Female

Part 2 Authorisation by medical referee

An application has been made for the cremation of the stillborn child.

I am satisfied that—

(a) the requirements of the Cremation (England and Wales) Regulations 2008 have been complied with;

(b) the examination made by the person who gave the relevant certificate has been adequate; and

(c) there is no reason for further examination.

Accordingly, I authorise the Registrar of the following crematorium to cremate the stillborn child within that crematorium—

Name of crematorium

Print your full name

Cremation authority

Signed

Dated ☐☐/☐☐/☐☐☐☐

Regulation 26 of the Cremation (England and Wales) Regulations 2008

Detention Centre Rules 2001/238

Part II

Detained Persons

Health Care

Notification of illness or death

36.—(1) If a detained person dies, becomes seriously ill, sustains any severe injury or is   A2–189
removed to hospital on account of mental disorder, the manager shall inform the Secretary
of State without delay and the Secretary of State shall at once inform—

(a) the detained person's spouse or next of kin (if he knows of their contact details);
and

(b) any other person who the detained person may reasonably have asked should be
informed.

(2) In any case in which the Secretary of State is under a duty to inform the detained
person's spouse or next of kin under paragraph (1), this shall be done in person by the
appropriate officer wherever it is reasonably practicable to do so.

(3) Without prejudice to paragraph (1), if a detained person dies, the manager shall give
notice immediately to the police, to the coroner or procurator fiscal having jurisdiction, to
the visiting committee and to the Secretary of State.

Electricity Safety, Quality and Continuity Regulations 2002/2665

Part I

Introductory

Citation, commencement and interpretation

1.—(1) These Regulations may be cited as the Electricity Safety, Quality and Continuity   A2–190
Regulations 2002 and shall come into force on 31st January 2003.

(2) Any requirement in these Regulations for goods or materials to comply with a
specified standard shall be satisfied by compliance with an equivalent standard or code of
practice of a national standards or equivalent body of any EEA State, in so far as the standard
or code of practice in question enables electricity safety, quality or continuity considerations
to be met in an equivalent manner.

(3) In paragraph (2) the expression "EEA State" means a State which is a Contracting
Party to the Agreement on the European Economic Area signed at Oporto on 2nd May
1992 as adjusted by the Protocol signed at Brussels on 17th March 1993.

(4) Unless the context otherwise requires, any reference in these Regulations to the
provision of information "in writing" shall include the provision of such information by
electronic mail, facsimile or similar means which are capable of producing a document
containing the text of any communication.

(5) In these Regulations, unless the context otherwise requires—

"British Standard Requirements" means the British Standard Requirements for Electrical
   Installations BS 7671: [2008 IEE Wiring Regulations 17th Edition (ISBN
   978-0-86341-844-0)][26] 16th Edition ISBN 0 85296 988 0, 2001 (as amended by

---

[26] Words substituted by Electricity Safety, Quality and Continuity (Amendment) Regulations 2009/639
reg.2(2) (April 6, 2009).

Amendment No. 1 (AMD 13628) February 2002 [and as further amended by Amendment No. 2 (AMD 14905) March 2004][27]);

"conductor" means an electrical conductor arranged to be electrically connected to a network but does not include conductors used or intended to be used solely for the purposes of control, protection or regulation of supply or for communication;

"connected with earth" means connected with earth in such manner as will at all times provide a rapid and safe discharge of energy, and cognate expressions shall be construed accordingly;

"consumer" means any person supplied or entitled to be supplied by a supplier but in regulations 24, 25 and 26 shall not include, in respect of any supply to meet haulage or traction requirements, any person who is an operator of a network within the meaning of Part I of the Railways Act 1993[28] [or an operator of a tramway, a trolley vehicle system or guided transport][29];

"consumer's installation" means the electric lines situated upon the consumer's side of the supply terminals together with any equipment permanently connected or intended to be permanently connected thereto on that side;

"danger" includes danger to health or danger to life or limb from electric shock, burn, injury or mechanical movement to persons, livestock or domestic animals, or from fire or explosion, attendant upon the generation, transmission, transformation, distribution or use of energy;

"distributing main" means a low voltage electric line which connects a distributor's source of voltage to one or more service lines or directly to a single consumer's installation;

"distributor" means a person who owns or operates a network, except for a network where that person is an operator of a network within the meaning of Part I of the Railways Act 1993 [or an operator of a tramway, a trolley vehicle system or guided transport][4];

"earth" means the general mass of the earth;

"earth electrode" means a conductor or group of conductors in intimate contact with, and providing a connection with, earth;

"electric line" means any line which is used or intended to be used for carrying electricity for any purpose and includes, unless the context otherwise requires—

(a) any equipment connected to any such line for the purpose of carrying electricity; and

(b) any wire, cable, tube, pipe, insulator or other similar thing (including its casing or coating) which surrounds or supports, or is associated with, any such line;

"energy" means electrical energy;

"equipment" includes plant, meters, lines, supports, appliances and associated items used or intended to be used for carrying electricity for the purposes of generating, transmitting or distributing energy, or for using or measuring energy;

"generating station" means those parts of any premises which are principally used for the purpose of generating energy;

"generator" means a person who generates electricity at high voltage for the purpose of supplying consumer's installations via a network;

"high voltage" means any voltage exceeding low voltage;

"insulation" means non-conducting material enclosing or surrounding a conductor or any part thereof and of such quality and thickness as to withstand the operating voltage of the equipment;

---

[27] Words inserted by Electricity Safety, Quality and Continuity (Amendment) Regulations 2006/1521 reg.2 (October 1, 2006).

[28] See sections 6(2) and 83.

[29] Words inserted by Electricity Safety, Quality and Continuity (Amendment) Regulations 2006/1521 reg.3(a) (October 1, 2006).

"insulator" means a device which supports a live conductor or which electrically separates the upper and lower parts of a stay wire;

"low voltage" means—

(a) in relation to alternating current, a voltage exceeding 50 volts measured between phase conductors (or between phase conductors and earth), but not exceeding 1000 volts measured between phase conductors (or 600 volts if measured between phase conductors and earth), calculated by taking the square root of the mean of the squares of the instantaneous values of a voltage during a complete cycle; and

(b) in relation to direct current, a voltage exceeding 120 volts measured between live conductors (or between live conductors and earth), but not exceeding 1500 volts measured between live conductors (or 900 volts if measured between live conductors and earth),

with any variations of voltage allowed by these Regulations;

"metalwork" does not include any electric line or conductor used for earthing purposes;

"meter operator" means a person who installs, maintains or removes metering equipment used for measuring the flow of energy to or from a network at or near the supply terminals;

"network" means an electrical system supplied by one or more sources of voltage and comprising all the conductors and other equipment used to conduct electricity for the purposes of conveying energy from the source or sources of voltage to one or more consumer's installations, street electrical fixtures, or other networks, but does not include an electrical system which is situated entirely on an offshore installation;

"neutral conductor" means a conductor which is, or is intended to be, connected to the neutral point of an electrical system and intended to contribute to the carrying of energy;

"overhead line" means any electric line which is placed above ground and in the open air;

"phase conductor" means a conductor for the carrying of energy other than a neutral conductor or a protective conductor or a conductor used for earthing purposes;

"protective conductor" means a conductor which is used for protection against electric shock and which connects the exposed conductive parts of equipment with earth;

"service line" means an electric line which connects either a street electrical fixture, or no more than four consumer's installations in adjacent buildings, to a distributing main;

["smart meter communication provider" means a person who holds a licence under section 6(1)(f) of the Electricity Act 1989;][30]

"street electrical fixture" means a permanent fixture which is or is intended to be connected to a supply of electricity and which is in, on, or is associated with a highway;

"substation" means any premises or part thereof which contain equipment for either transforming or converting energy to or from high voltage (other than transforming or converting solely for the operation of switching devices or instruments) or for switching, controlling or regulating energy at high voltage, but does not include equipment mounted on a support to any overhead line;

"supplier" means a person who contracts to supply electricity to consumers;

"supply" means the supply of electricity;

---

[30] Definition inserted by Electricity and Gas (Smart Meters Licensable Activity) Order 2012/2400 Pt 5 art.35(2) (September 19, 2012).

"supply neutral conductor" means the neutral conductor of a low voltage network which is or is intended to be connected with earth, but does not include any part of the neutral conductor on the consumer's side of the supply terminals;

"supply terminals" means the ends of the electric lines at which the supply is delivered to a consumer's installation;

"support" means any structure, pole or other device, in, on, by or from which any electric line is or may be supported, carried or suspended and includes stays and struts, but does not include insulators, their fittings or any building or structure the principal purpose of which is not the support of electric lines or equipment;

"switching device" includes any device which can either make or break a current, or both; [. . .]³¹

["tramway", "trolley vehicle system" and "guided transport" have the same meanings as in section 67(1) of the Transport and Works Act 1992; and]⁶

"underground cable" means any conductor surrounded by insulation which is placed below ground.

(6) In relation to a distributor, generator or meter operator a reference in these Regulations to his network, his overhead line, his substation or his equipment is a reference to a network, an overhead line, a substation or equipment (as the case may be) owned or operated by him.

(7) Words and expressions to which meanings are assigned by these Regulations shall (unless the contrary intention appears) have the same meanings in any document issued by the Secretary of State under these Regulations.

PART VIII

MISCELLANEOUS

Notification of specified events

A2–191   31.—(1) Notice shall be given to the Secretary of State in accordance with this regulation by the distributor in respect of any event which is of a type specified in paragraph (2)(b) where the event involves a consumer's installation which is connected to the distributor's network and by the generator, distributor or meter operator, as the case may be, in respect of any event which is an event of a type otherwise specified in paragraph (2) and involves a network or equipment which is in the ownership of, under the control of, or used by, the generator, distributor or meter operator, as the case may be.

(2) The events referred to in paragraph (1) are—

(a) any event attributable in whole or in part to the generating, transforming, control or carrying of energy up to and including the supply terminals, which has given rise to—

   (i) the death of any person other than a person engaged by the generator, distributor or meter operator for the purposes of his business; or

   (ii) an injury (including any electric shock) to any person other than a person engaged by the generator, distributor or meter operator for the purposes of his business; or

   (iii) any fire; or

   (iv) any explosion or implosion;

(b) any event attributable in whole or in part to the presence of energy on the consumer's side of the supply terminals on any non-industrial and non-commercial premises resulting in the death of any person;

³¹ Definitions inserted by Electricity Safety, Quality and Continuity (Amendment) Regulations 2006/1521 reg.3(b) (October 1, 2006).

(c) any event, whether or not accompanied by an event specified in sub-paragraph (a), which caused an overhead line to be at a height less than that required by regulation 17(2);

(d) the occurrence of any damage to any underground cable resulting from an event not specified in sub-paragraphs (a) and (b); and

(e) any event other than those listed in sub-paragraph (a), (c) or (d) which, taking into account the circumstances of that event, was likely to cause any of the events listed in sub-paragraph (a).

(3) In respect of any event specified in paragraph (2)(a)—

(a) the requirement to give notice in accordance with paragraph (4) (so far as applicable) applies in addition to the requirement to give notice in accordance with paragraph (5) unless the notice given satisfies the requirements of both paragraphs; and

(b) the requirement to give notice in accordance with paragraphs (4) and (5) applies in addition to the requirement to give notice in accordance with paragraph (6).

(4) In respect of any event specified in paragraph (2)(a)(i) or (in the case of a serious injury) in paragraph (2)(a)(ii), notice of the event shall be given to the Secretary of State by telephone or other immediate means of communication immediately after the event becomes known to the generator, distributor or meter operator, as the case may be.

(5) In respect of any event specified in paragraph (2)(a) or (2)(b), notice containing the relevant particulars shall, subject to paragraph (8), as soon as possible after the event becomes known to the generator, distributor or meter operator, as the case may be, be given to the Secretary of State in writing by the quickest practicable means.

(6) In respect of any event notifiable under paragraph (2)(a), (2)(c) or (2)(e), notice shall be given to the Secretary of State by post within 15 days of the end of the month in which the event becomes known to the generator, distributor or meter operator as the case may be, in the form of a computer disc which—

(a) conforms to the description specified in the Department's publication; and

(b) subject to paragraph (8), contains the information comprising the relevant particulars, arranged in a form which complies with the technical requirements specified in that publication.

(7) In respect of any event specified in paragraph (2)(d), notice containing the relevant particulars shall be sent to the Secretary of State by means of a return in writing to be submitted within one month of the end of the period of 3 months ending on 31st March, 30th June, 30th September or 31st December (as the case may be) in which the event became known to the generator, distributor or meter operator as the case may be.

(8) The notices required by paragraphs (5) and (6) shall, where the giver of the notice is unable to provide full particulars, contain such of the relevant particulars as are available to the giver of the notice at the time of giving it, and the remaining particulars shall be supplied to the Secretary of State in writing by the quickest practicable means immediately after they have become known.

(9) In this regulation—

"the Department's publication" means the publication entitled (under the heading "ELECTRICITY SAFETY, QUALITY AND CONTINUITY REGULATIONS 2002") "COMPUTERISATION OF THE NOTIFICATION OF CERTAIN SPECIFIED EVENTS UNDER REGULATION 31", subtitled "SPECIFICA-TION OF THE DATA FILES", and published in September 2002 by the Department of Trade and Industry, a copy of which was certified as such by the signature of the Minister of State for Energy and Construction, Department of Trade and Industry;

"event" means any event of the kind specified irrespective of whether it was accidental;

"relevant particulars" means—

(i) in respect of an event specified in paragraph (2)(a), (2)(b) or (2)(d), the particulars specified in Parts I, II and IV, respectively, of Schedule 3; and

(ii) in respect of an event specified in paragraph (2)(c) or (2)(e), the particulars specified in Part III of Schedule 3; and

"serious injury" means any injury which results in the person injured being admitted into hospital as an in-patient.

European Communities (Lawyer's Practice) Regulations 2000/1119

PART II

PRACTICE OF PROFESSIONAL ACTIVITIES BY A REGISTERED EUROPEAN LAWYER

Representation in legal proceedings

A2–192   11.—(1) Subject to paragraph (2), no enactment or rule of law or practice shall prevent a registered European lawyer from pursuing professional activities relating to the representation of a client in any proceedings before any court, tribunal or public authority (including addressing the court, tribunal or public authority) only because he is not a solicitor or barrister.

(2) In proceedings referred to in paragraph (1), where the professional activities in question may (but for these Regulations) be lawfully provided only by a solicitor, barrister or other qualified person, a registered European lawyer shall act in conjunction with a solicitor or barrister who is entitled to practise before the court, tribunal or public authority concerned and who could lawfully provide those professional activities.

(3) The solicitor or barrister referred to in paragraph (2) shall, where necessary, be answerable to the court, tribunal or public authority concerned.

[(4) Paragraph (2) does not apply to professional activities relating to the representation of a client in proceedings before the Asylum and Immigration Tribunal or the Asylum Support Tribunal, or any tribunal hearing an appeal from those tribunals.][32]

Health Protection (Notification) Regulations 2010/659

Citation, commencement and application

A2–193   1.—(1) These Regulations may be cited as the Health Protection (Notification) Regulations 2010 and shall come into force—

(a) for the purposes of all regulations except regulation 4 on 6th April 2010; and

(b) for the purposes of regulation 4 on 1st October 2010.

(2) These Regulations apply in relation to England only.

---

[32] Added by Legal Services Act 2007 (Registered European Lawyers) Order 2009/1587 art.2(3) (July 1, 2009).

[(3) In these Regulations, "Public Health England" means the executive agency of the Department of Health known as Public Health England.][33]

Duty to notify suspected disease, infection or contamination in patients

2.—(1) A registered medical practitioner (R) must notify the proper officer[34] of the   **A2–194**
relevant local authority where R has reasonable grounds for suspecting that a patient (P) whom R is attending—

    (a) has a notifiable disease;

    (b) has an infection[35] which, in the view of R, presents or could present significant harm to human health; or

    (c) is contaminated[36] in a manner which, in the view of R, presents or could present significant harm to human health.

(2) The notification must include the following information insofar as it is known to R—

    (a) P's name, date of birth and sex;

    (b) P's home address including postcode;

    (c) P's current residence (if not home address);

    (d) P's telephone number;

    (e) P's NHS number;

    (f) P's occupation (if R considers it relevant);

    (g) the name, address and postcode of P's place of work or education (if R considers it relevant);

    (h) P's relevant overseas travel history;

    (i) P's ethnicity;

    (j) contact details for a parent of P (where P is a child);

    (k) the disease or infection which P has or is suspected of having or the nature of P's contamination or suspected contamination;

    (l) the date of onset of P's symptoms;

    (m) the date of R's diagnosis; and

    (n) R's name, address and telephone number.

(3) The notification must be provided in writing within 3 days beginning with the day on which R forms a suspicion under paragraph (1).

(4) Without prejudice to paragraph (3), if R considers that the case is urgent, notification must be provided orally as soon as reasonably practicable.

(5) In determining whether the case is urgent, R must have regard to—

---

[33] Added by National Treatment Agency (Abolition) and the Health and Social Care Act 2012 (Consequential, Transitional and Saving Provisions) Order 2013/235 Sch.2(1) para.148(2) (April 1, 2013).

[34] See section 74 of the Public Health (Control of Disease) Act 1984 (c.22) ("the 1984 Act") for the definition of "proper officer".

[35] See section 45A of the 1984 Act for the interpretation of "infection".

[36] See section 45A of the 1984 Act for the interpretation of "contamination" and related expressions.

(a) the nature of the suspected disease, infection or contamination;

(b) the ease of spread of that disease, infection or contamination;

(c) the ways in which the spread of the disease, infection or contamination can be prevented or controlled; and

(d) P's circumstances (including age, sex and occupation).

(6) This regulation does not apply where R reasonably believes that the proper officer of the relevant local authority has already been notified with regard to P and the suspected disease, infection or contamination by another registered medical practitioner in accordance with this regulation.

(7) In this regulation—

"child" means a person under the age of 18 years;
"notifiable disease" means a disease listed in Schedule 1;
"parent" has the meaning given to it by section 576 of the Education Act 1996; and
"relevant local authority" means the local authority within whose area R attended P on the occasion of forming a suspicion under paragraph (1).

Duty to notify suspected disease, infection or contamination in dead persons

A2–195   3.—(1) A registered medical practitioner (R) must notify the proper officer of the relevant local authority where R has reasonable grounds for suspecting that a person (P) whom R is attending has died whilst—

(a) infected with a notifiable disease;

(b) infected with a disease which, in the view of R, presents or could present, or presented or could have presented (whilst P was alive), significant harm to human health; or

(c) contaminated in a manner which, in the view of R, presents or could present, or presented or could have presented (whilst P was alive), significant harm to human health.

(2) The notification must include the following information insofar as it is known to R—

(a) P's name, date of birth and sex;

(b) P's date of death;

(c) P's home address including postcode;

(d) P's place of residence at time of death (if different from home address);

(e) P's NHS number;

(f) P's occupation at time of death (if R considers it relevant);

(g) the name, address and postcode of P's place of work or education at the time of death (if R considers it relevant);

(h) P's relevant overseas travel history;

(i) P's ethnicity;

(j) the disease or infection which P had or is suspected of having had or the nature of P's contamination or suspected contamination;

(k) the date of onset of P's symptoms;

(l) the date of R's diagnosis; and

(m) R's name, address and telephone number.

(3) The notification must be provided in writing within 3 days beginning with the day on which R forms a suspicion under paragraph (1).

(4) Without prejudice to paragraph (3), if R considers that the case is urgent, notification must be provided orally as soon as reasonably practicable.

(5) In determining whether the case is urgent, R must have regard to—

(a) the nature of the suspected disease, infection or contamination;

(b) the ease of spread of that disease, infection or contamination;

(c) the ways in which the spread of the disease, infection or contamination can be prevented or controlled; and

(d) P's circumstances (including age, sex and occupation).

(6) This regulation does not apply where R reasonably believes that the proper officer of the relevant local authority has already been notified with regard to P and the suspected disease, infection or contamination by another registered medical practitioner in accordance with this regulation or regulation 2(1).

(7) In this regulation—

"notifiable disease" has the same meaning it has in regulation 2; and
"relevant local authority" means the local authority within whose area R attended P on the occasion of forming a suspicion under paragraph (1).

Duty to notify causative agents found in human samples

4.—(1) The operator of a diagnostic laboratory must notify [Public Health England][37] in accordance with this regulation where the diagnostic laboratory identifies a causative agent in a human sample.   **A2–196**

(2) The notification must include the following information insofar as it is known to the operator of the diagnostic laboratory—

(a) name and address of the diagnostic laboratory;

(b) details of the causative agent identified;

(c) date of the sample;

(d) nature of the sample;

(e) name of person (P) from whom the sample was taken;

(f) P's date of birth and sex;

(g) P's current home address including postcode;

(h) P's current residence (if not home address);

(i) P's ethnicity;

(j) P's NHS number; and

(k) the name, address and organisation of the person who solicited the test which identified the causative agent.

---

[37] Words substituted by National Treatment Agency (Abolition) and the Health and Social Care Act 2012 (Consequential, Transitional and Saving Provisions) Order 2013/235 Sch.2(1) para.148(3)(a) (April 1, 2013).

(3) The notification must be provided in writing within 7 days beginning with the day on which the causative agent is identified.

(4) Without prejudice to paragraph (3), if the operator of the diagnostic laboratory considers that the case is urgent, the notification must be provided orally as soon as reasonably practicable.

(5) In determining whether the case is urgent, the operator of the diagnostic laboratory must have regard to—

(a) the nature of the causative agent;

(b) the nature of the disease which the causative agent causes;

(c) the ease of spread of the causative agent;

(d) the ways in which the spread of the causative agent can be prevented or controlled; and

(e) where known, P's circumstances (including age, sex and occupation).

(6) This regulation does not apply where the operator of the diagnostic laboratory reasonably believes that [Public Health England][38] has already been notified in accordance with this regulation by the operator of another diagnostic laboratory in relation to the same causative agent being found in a sample from the same person.

(7) For the purposes of paragraph (1), a diagnostic laboratory identifies a causative agent where—

(a) the diagnostic laboratory identifies the causative agent; or

(b) the causative agent is identified by another laboratory under an arrangement made with that diagnostic laboratory.

(8) Where paragraph (7)(b) applies, the day on which the causative agent is identified for the purposes of paragraph (3), is the day on which the diagnostic laboratory became aware of the identification by the other laboratory.

(9) It is an offence for the operator of a diagnostic laboratory to fail without reasonable excuse to comply with this regulation.

(10) Any person who commits an offence under this regulation is liable on summary conviction to a fine not exceeding level 5 on the standard scale.

(11) In this regulation—

"causative agent" means—

(a) a causative agent listed in Schedule 2, or
(b) evidence of an infection caused by such an agent;

"diagnostic laboratory" means an institution (or facility within an institution) which is equipped with apparatus and reagents for the performance of diagnostic tests for human infections;

"director of a diagnostic laboratory" means—

(a) the clinical microbiologist, consultant pathologist or other registered medical practitioner or other person in charge of a diagnostic laboratory, or

(b) any other person working in the diagnostic laboratory to whom the function of making a notification under this regulation has been delegated by the person mentioned in paragraph (a); and

---

[38] Words substituted by National Treatment Agency (Abolition) and the Health and Social Care Act 2012 (Consequential, Transitional and Saving Provisions) Order 2013/235 Sch.2(1) para.148(3)(b) (April 1, 2013).

"operator of a diagnostic laboratory" means the corporate body that operates the diagnostic laboratory or, if there is no such body, the director of the diagnostic laboratory.

Duty to provide information to [Public Health England][39]

5.—(1) This regulation applies where a notification has been made by the operator of a diagnostic laboratory to [Public Health England][40] under regulation 4.

    A2–197

(2) [Public Health England][41] may request that the person (R) who solicited the laboratory test which identified the causative agent to which the notification relates, provide to it the information listed at regulation 4(2) insofar as that information was not included in the notification.

(3) R must provide the information requested under paragraph (2) insofar as it is known to R.

(4) The information must be provided in writing within 3 days beginning with the day on which the request is made.

(5) Without prejudice to paragraph (4), if [Public Health England][42] considers the case to be urgent and informs R of this fact when making the request, the information must be provided orally as soon as reasonably practicable.

(6) In determining whether the case is urgent, [Public Health England][43] must have regard to—

    (a) the nature of the causative agent to which the notification relates;

    (b) the nature of the disease which the causative agent causes;

    (c) the ease of spread of the causative agent;

    (d) the ways in which the spread of the causative agent can be prevented or controlled; and

    (e) where known, the circumstances of the person from whom the sample was taken (including age, sex and occupation).

Duty on the relevant local authority to disclose notification to others

6.—(1) This regulation applies where the proper officer of a local authority has received a notification under regulation 2 or 3.

    A2–198

(2) The proper officer of the local authority must disclose the fact of the notification and its contents to—

---

[39] Words substituted by National Treatment Agency (Abolition) and the Health and Social Care Act 2012 (Consequential, Transitional and Saving Provisions) Order 2013/235 Sch.2(1) para.148(4)(a) (April 1, 2013).

[40] Words substituted by National Treatment Agency (Abolition) and the Health and Social Care Act 2012 (Consequential, Transitional and Saving Provisions) Order 2013/235 Sch.2(1) para.148(4)(b) (April 1, 2013).

[41] Words substituted by National Treatment Agency (Abolition) and the Health and Social Care Act 2012 (Consequential, Transitional and Saving Provisions) Order 2013/235 Sch.2(1) para.148(4)(c) (April 1, 2013).

[42] Words substituted by National Treatment Agency (Abolition) and the Health and Social Care Act 2012 (Consequential, Transitional and Saving Provisions) Order 2013/235 Sch.2(1) para.148(4)(d) (April 1, 2013).

[43] Words substituted by National Treatment Agency (Abolition) and the Health and Social Care Act 2012 (Consequential, Transitional and Saving Provisions) Order 2013/235 Sch.2(1) para.148(4)(e) (April 1, 2013).

[(a) Public Health England;]⁴⁴

(b) the proper officer of the local authority in whose area P usually resides (if different); and

(c) the proper officer of the port health authority or local authority in whose district or area a ship, hovercraft, aircraft or international train is or was situated from which P has disembarked (if known to the disclosing proper officer and if that officer considers disclosure appropriate).

(3) The disclosure must be made in writing within 3 days beginning with the day that the proper officer receives the notification.

(4) Without prejudice to paragraph (3), if the disclosing proper officer considers that the case is urgent, disclosure must be made orally as soon as reasonably practicable.

(5) In determining whether a case is urgent, the disclosing proper officer must have regard to—

(a) the nature of the disease, infection or contamination or the suspected disease, infection or contamination notified;

(b) the ease of spread of the disease, infection or contamination;

(c) the ways in which the spread of the disease, infection or contamination can be prevented or controlled; and

(d) where known, the patient's circumstances (including age, sex and occupation).

Electronic communications

A2–199   **7.**—(1) This regulation applies to—

(a) notifications provided under regulation 2(1), 3(1) and 4(1);

(b) information provided under regulation 5(3);

(c) disclosures made under regulation 6(2);

(d) lists provided under regulation 3 of the Health Protection (Local Authority Powers) Regulations 2010 (requirement to provide details of children attending school); and

(e) reports provided under regulations 10(1) (duty to report Part 2A applications) and 11(1) (duty to report variations or revocations of Part 2A orders) of the Health Protection (Part 2A Orders) Regulations 2010.

(2) Notifications, information, disclosures, lists and reports, which are required to be in writing, may be communicated electronically if—

(a) the recipient has consented in writing to receiving the notification, information, disclosure list or report (as the case may be) by an electronic communication; and

(b) the communication is sent to the number or address specified by the recipient when giving that consent.

---

⁴⁴ Substituted by National Treatment Agency (Abolition) and the Health and Social Care Act 2012 (Consequential, Transitional and Saving Provisions) Order 2013/235 Sch.2(1) para.148(5) (April 1, 2013).

SCHEDULE 1

NOTIFIABLE DISEASES

Acute encephalitis
Acute meningitis
Acute poliomyelitis
Acute infectious hepatitis
Anthrax
Botulism
Brucellosis
Cholera
Diphtheria
Enteric fever (typhoid or paratyphoid fever)
Food poisoning
Haemolytic uraemic syndrome (HUS)
Infectious bloody diarrhoea
Invasive group A streptococcal disease and scarlet fever
Legionnaires' Disease
Leprosy
Malaria
Measles
Meningococcal septicaemia
Mumps
Plague
Rabies
Rubella
SARS
Smallpox
Tetanus
Tuberculosis
Typhus
Viral haemorrhagic fever (VHF)
Whooping cough
Yellow fever

A2–200

SCHEDULE 2

CAUSATIVE AGENTS

Bacillus anthracis
Bacillus cereus (only if associated with food poisoning)
Bordetella pertussis
Borrelia spp
Brucella spp
Burkholderia mallei
Burkholderia pseudomallei
Campylobacter spp
Chikungunya virus
Chlamydophila psittaci
Clostridium botulinum
Clostridium perfringens (only if associated with food poisoning)
Clostridium tetani
Corynebacterium diphtheriae
Corynebacterium ulcerans
Coxiella burnetii
Crimean-Congo haemorrhagic fever virus
Cryptosporidium spp
Dengue virus
Ebola virus
Entamoeba histolytica
Francisella tularensis

A2–201

Giardia lamblia
Guanarito virus
Haemophilus influenzae (invasive)
Hanta virus
Hepatitis A, B, C, delta, and E viruses
Influenza virus
Junin virus
Kyasanur Forest disease virus
Lassa virus
Legionella spp
Leptospira interrogans
Listeria monocytogenes
Machupo virus
Marburg virus
Measles virus
Mumps virus
Mycobacterium tuberculosis complex
Neisseria meningitidis
Omsk haemorrhagic fever virus
Plasmodium falciparum, vivax, ovale, malariae, knowlesi
Polio virus (wild or vaccine types)
Rabies virus (classical rabies and rabies-related lyssaviruses)
Rickettsia spp
Rift Valley fever virus
Rubella virus
Sabia virus
Salmonella spp
SARS coronavirus
Shigella spp
Streptococcus pneumoniae (invasive)
Streptococcus pyogenes (invasive)
Varicella zoster virus
Variola virus
Verocytotoxigenic Escherichia coli (including E.coli O157)
Vibrio cholerae
West Nile Virus
Yellow fever virus
Yersinia pestis

Health Protection (Notification) (Wales) Regulations 2010/1546

Title, commencement and application

A2–202   1.—(1) The title of these Regulations is the Health Protection (Notification) (Wales) Regulations 2010 and they come into force—

(a) for the purposes of all regulations except regulation 4 on 26 July 2010; and

(b) for the purposes of regulation 4 on 1 October 2010.

(2) These Regulations apply in relation to Wales.

Duty to notify suspected disease, infection or contamination in patients

A2–203   2.—(1) A registered medical practitioner (R) must notify the proper officer[45] of the relevant local authority where R has reasonable grounds for suspecting that a patient (P) whom R is attending—

---

[45] See section 74 of the Public Health (Control of Disease) Act 1984 (c. 22) ("the 1984 Act") for the definition of "proper officer".

(a) has a notifiable disease;

(b) has an infection[46] which, in the view of R, presents or could present significant harm to human health; or

(c) is contaminated[47] in a manner which, in the view of R, presents or could present significant harm to human health.

(2) The notification must include the following information insofar as it is known to R—

(a) P's name, date of birth and sex;

(b) P's home address including postcode;

(c) P's current residence (if not home address);

(d) P's telephone number;

(e) P's NHS number;

(f) P's occupation;

(g) the name, address and postcode of P's place of work or education (if R considers it relevant);

(h) P's relevant overseas travel history;

(i) P's ethnicity;

(j) contact details for a parent of P (where P is a child);

(k) the disease or infection which P has or is suspected of having or the nature of P's contamination or suspected contamination;

(l) the date of onset of P's symptoms;

(m) the date of R's diagnosis; and

(n) R's name, address and telephone number.

(3) The notification must be provided in writing within 3 days beginning with the day on which R forms a suspicion under paragraph (1).

(4) Without prejudice to paragraph (3), if R considers that the case is urgent, notification must be provided orally as soon as reasonably practicable.

(5) In determining whether the case is urgent, R must have regard to—

(a) the nature of the suspected disease, infection or contamination;

(b) the ease of spread of that disease, infection or contamination;

(c) the ways in which the spread of the disease, infection or contamination can be prevented or controlled; and

(d) P's circumstances (including age, sex and occupation).

(6) This regulation does not apply where R reasonably believes that the proper officer of the relevant local authority has already been notified with regard to P and the suspected disease, infection or contamination by another registered medical practitioner in accordance with this regulation.

(7) In this regulation—

---

[46] See section 45A of the 1984 Act for the interpretation of "infection".

[47] See section 45A of the 1984 Act for the interpretation of "contamination" and related expressions.

"child" ("plentyn") means a person under the age of 18 years;

"notifiable disease" ("clefyd hysbysadwy") means a disease or syndrome listed in Schedule 1;

"parent" ("rhiant") has the meaning given to it by section 576 of the Education Act 1996; and

"relevant local authority" ("awdurdod lleol perthnasol") means the local authority within whose area R attended P on the occasion of forming a suspicion under paragraph (1).

Duty to notify suspected disease, infection or contamination in dead persons

A2–204   **3.**—(1) A registered medical practitioner (R) must notify the proper officer of the relevant local authority where R has reasonable grounds for suspecting that a person (P) whom R is attending has died whilst—

(a) infected with a notifiable disease;

(b) infected with a disease which, in the view of R, presents or could present, or presented or could have presented (whilst P was alive), significant harm to human health; or

(c) contaminated in a manner which, in the view of R, presents or could present, or presented or could have presented (when P was alive), significant harm to human health.

(2) The notification must include the following information insofar as it is known to R—

(a) P's name, date of birth and sex;

(b) P's date of death;

(c) P's home address including postcode;

(d) P's place of residence at time of death (if different from home address);

(e) P's NHS number;

(f) P's occupation at time of death (if R considers it relevant);

(g) the name, address and postcode of P's place of work or education at time of death (if R considers it relevant);

(h) P's relevant overseas travel history;

(i) P's ethnicity;

(j) the disease or infection which P had or is suspected of having had or the nature of P's contamination or suspected contamination;

(k) the date of onset of P's symptoms;

(l) the date of R's diagnosis; and

(m) R's name, address and telephone number.

(3) The notification must be provided in writing within 3 days beginning with the day on which R forms a suspicion under paragraph (1).

(4) Without prejudice to paragraph (3), if R considers that the case is urgent, notification must be provided orally as soon as reasonably practicable.

(5) In determining whether the case is urgent, R must have regard to—

(a) the nature of the suspected disease, infection or contamination;

(b) the ease of spread of that disease, infection or contamination;

(c) the ways in which the spread of the disease, infection or contamination can be prevented or controlled; and

(d) P's circumstances (including age, sex and occupation).

(6) This regulation does not apply where R reasonably believes that the proper officer of the relevant local authority has already been notified with regard to P and the suspected disease, infection or contamination by another registered medical practitioner in accordance with this regulation or regulation 2(1).

(7) In this regulation—

"notifiable disease" ("clefyd hysbysadwy") has the same meaning it has in regulation 2; and

"relevant local authority" ("awdurdod lleol perthnasol") means the local authority within whose area R attended P on the occasion of forming a suspicion under paragraph (1).

Duty to notify causative agents found in human samples

4.—(1) The operator of a diagnostic laboratory must notify the proper officer of the relevant local authority in accordance with this regulation where the diagnostic laboratory identifies a causative agent in a human sample.   **A2–205**

(2) The notification must include the following information insofar as it is known to the operator of the diagnostic laboratory—

(a) name and address of the diagnostic laboratory;

(b) details of the causative agent identified;

(c) date of the sample;

(d) nature of the sample;

(e) name of person (P) from whom the sample was taken;

(f) P's date of birth and sex;

(g) P's current home address including postcode;

(h) P's current residence (if not home address);

(i) P's ethnicity;

(j) P's NHS number; and

(k) the name, address and organisation of the person who solicited the test which identified the causative agent.

(3) The notification must be provided in writing within 7 days beginning with the day on which the causative agent is identified.

(4) Without prejudice to paragraph (3), if the operator of the diagnostic laboratory considers that the case is urgent, the notification must be provided orally as soon as reasonably practicable.

(5) In determining whether the case is urgent, the operator of the diagnostic laboratory must have regard to—

(a) the nature of the causative agent;

(b) the nature of the disease which the causative agent causes;

(c) the ease of spread of the causative agent;

(d) the ways in which the spread of the causative agent can be prevented or controlled; and

(e)   where known, P's circumstances (including age, sex and occupation).

(6) This regulation does not apply where the operator of the diagnostic laboratory reasonably believes that the proper officer of the relevant local authority has already been notified in accordance with this regulation by the operator of another diagnostic laboratory in relation to the same causative agent being found in a sample from the same person.

(7) For the purposes of paragraph (1), a diagnostic laboratory identifies a causative agent where—

(a)   the diagnostic laboratory identifies the causative agent; or

(b)   the causative agent is identified by another laboratory under an arrangement made with that diagnostic laboratory.

(8) Where paragraph (7)(b) applies, the day on which the causative agent is identified for the purposes of paragraph (3), is the day on which the diagnostic laboratory became aware of the identification by the other laboratory.

(9) It is an offence for the operator of a diagnostic laboratory to fail without reasonable excuse to comply with this regulation.

(10) Any person who commits an offence under this regulation is liable on summary conviction to a fine not exceeding level 5 on the standard scale.

(11) In this regulation—

"causative agent" ("cyfrwng achosol") means—

(a)   a causative agent listed in Schedule 2, or

(b)   evidence of an infection caused by such an agent;

"diagnostic laboratory" ("labordy diagnostig") means an institution (or facility within an institution) which is equipped with apparatus and reagents for the performance of diagnostic tests for human infections;

"director of a diagnostic laboratory" ("cyfarwyddwr labordy diagnostig") means—

(a)   the clinical microbiologist, consultant pathologist or other registered medical practitioner or other person in charge of a diagnostic laboratory; or

(b)   any other person working in the diagnostic laboratory to whom the function of making a notification under this regulation has been delegated by the person mentioned in sub-paragraph (a);

"operator of a diagnostic laboratory" ("gweithredwr labordy diagnostig") means the corporate body that operates the diagnostic laboratory or, if there is no such body, the director of the diagnostic laboratory; and

"relevant local authority" ("awdurdod lleol perthnasol") means the local authority within whose area the organisation of the person who solicited the test which identified the causative agent is situated.

Duty to provide information to the proper officer

A2–206   5.—(1) This regulation applies where a notification has been made by the operator of a diagnostic laboratory to the proper officer under regulation 4.

(2) The proper officer may request that the person (R) who solicited the laboratory test which identified the causative agent to which the notification relates, provide to him or her the information listed at regulation 4(2) insofar as that information was not included in the notification.

(3) R must provide the information requested under paragraph (2) insofar as it is known to R.

(4) The information must be provided in writing within 3 days beginning with the day on which the request is made.

(5) Without prejudice to paragraph (4), if the proper officer considers the case to be urgent and informs R of this fact when making the request, the information must be provided orally as soon as reasonably practicable.

(6) In determining whether the case is urgent, the proper officer must have regard to—

(a) the nature of the causative agent to which the notification relates;

(b) the nature of the disease which the causative agent causes;

(c) the ease of spread of the causative agent;

(d) the ways in which the spread of the causative agent can be prevented or controlled; and

(e) where known, the circumstances of the person from whom the sample was taken (including age, sex and occupation).

(7) In this regulation, "causative agent" ("cyfrwng achosol") has the same meaning it has in regulation 4(11).

Duty on the proper officer to disclose notifications to others

6.—(1) This regulation applies where the proper officer has received a notification under regulation 2, 3 or 4. **A2–207**

(2) The proper officer must disclose the fact of the notification and its contents to—

(a) the Public Health Wales National Health Service Trust[48];

(b) the proper officer of the local authority in whose area P usually resides (if different); and

(c) the proper officer of the port health authority or local authority in whose district or area a ship, hovercraft, aircraft or international train is or was situated from which P has disembarked (if known to the disclosing proper officer and if that officer considers disclosure appropriate).

(3) The disclosure must be made in writing within 3 days beginning with the day that the proper officer receives the notification.

(4) Without prejudice to paragraph (3), if the disclosing proper officer considers that the case is urgent, disclosure must be made orally as soon as reasonably practicable.

(5) In determining whether a case is urgent, the disclosing proper officer must have regard to—

(a) the nature of the disease, infection or contamination or the suspected disease, infection or contamination notified;

(b) the ease of spread of the disease, infection or contamination;

(c) the ways in which the spread of the disease, infection or contamination can be prevented or controlled; and

(d) where known, P's circumstances (including age, sex and occupation).

Electronic communications

7.—(1) This regulation applies to— **A2–208**

(a) notifications provided under regulations 2(1), 3(1) and 4(1);

(b) information provided under regulation 5(3);

---

[48] ???

(c) disclosures made under regulation 6(2);

(d) lists provided under regulation 3 (requirement to provide details of children attending school) of the Health Protection (Local Authority Powers) (Wales) Regulations 2010; and

(e) reports provided under regulations 10(1) (duty to report Part 2A applications) and 11(1) (duty to report variations or revocations of Part 2A orders) of the Health Protection (Part 2A Orders) (Wales) Regulations 2010.

(2) Notifications, information, disclosures, lists and reports, which are required to be in writing, may be communicated electronically if—

(a) the recipient has consented in writing to receiving the notification, information, disclosure, list or report (as the case may be) by an electronic communication; and

(b) the communication is sent to the number or address specified by the recipient when giving that consent.

Schedule 1

Notifiable Diseases And Syndromes

A2–209 Anthrax
Botulism
Brucellosis
Cholera
Diphtheria
Encephalitis (acute)
Enteric fever (typhoid or paratyphoid fever)
Food poisoning
Haemolytic uraemic syndrome (HUS)
Infectious bloody diarrhoea
Infectious hepatitis (acute)
Invasive group A streptococcal disease and scarlet fever
Legionnaires' Disease
Leprosy
Malaria
Measles
Meningitis (acute)
Meningococcal septicaemia
Mumps
Plague
Poliomyelitis (acute)
Rabies
Rubella
SARS
Smallpox
Tetanus
Tuberculosis
Typhus
Viral haemorrhagic fever (VHF)
Whooping cough
Yellow fever

Schedule 2

Causative Agents

A2–210 Bacillus anthracis
Bacillus cereus (only if associated with food poisoning)

Bordetella pertussis
Borrelia spp
Brucella spp
Burkholderia mallei
Burkholderia pseudomallei
Campylobacter spp
Chikungunya virus
Chlamydophila psittaci
Clostridium botulinum
Clostridium perfringens (only if associated with food poisoning)
Clostridium tetani
Corynebacterium diphtheriae
Corynebacterium ulcerans
Coxiella burnetii
Crimean-Congo haemorrhagic fever virus
Cryptosporidium spp
Dengue virus
Ebola virus
Entamoeba histolytica
Francisella tularensis
Giardia lamblia
Guanarito virus
Haemophilus influenzae (invasive)
Hanta virus
Hepatitis A, B, C, delta, and E viruses
Influenza virus
Junin virus
Kyasanur Forest disease virus
Lassa virus
Legionella spp
Leptospira interrogans
Listeria monocytogenes
Machupo virus
Marburg virus
Measles virus
Mumps virus
Mycobacterium tuberculosis complex
Neisseria meningitidis
Omsk haemorrhagic fever virus
Plasmodium falciparum, vivax, ovale, malariae, knowlesi
Polio virus (wild or vaccine types)
Rabies virus (classical rabies) and rabies-related lyssaviruses
Rickettsia spp
Rift Valley fever virus
Rubella virus
Sabia virus
Salmonella spp
SARS coronavirus
Shigella spp
Streptococcus pneumoniae (invasive)
Streptococcus pyogenes (invasive)
Varicella zoster virus
Variola virus
Verocytotoxigenic Escherichia coli (including E.coli O157)
Vibrio cholerae
West Nile Virus
Yellow fever virus
Yersinia pestis

Ionising Radiations Regulations 1999/3232

PART I

INTERPRETATION AND GENERAL

Interpretation

A2–211   **2.**—(1) In these Regulations, unless the context otherwise requires—

"accelerator" means an apparatus or installation in which particles are accelerated and which emits ionising radiation with an energy higher than 1MeV;

"appointed doctor" means, subject to regulation 39(5) (which relates to transitional provisions), a registered medical practitioner who is for the time being appointed in writing by the Executive for the purposes of these Regulations;

"approved" means approved for the time being in writing for the purposes of these Regulations by the Health and Safety Commission or the Executive, as the case may be, and published in such form as the Health and Safety Commission or the Executive respectively considers appropriate;

"approved dosimetry service" means, subject to regulation 39(3) (which relates to transitional provisions), a dosimetry service approved in accordance with regulation 35;

"calendar year" means a period of 12 calendar months beginning with the 1st January;

"classified person" means—

(a) a person designated as such pursuant to regulation 20(1); and

(b) in the case of an outside worker employed by an undertaking in Northern Ireland or in another member State, a person who has been designated as a Category A exposed worker within the meaning of Article 21 of the Directive;

"comforter and carer" means an individual who (other than as part of his occupation) knowingly and willingly incurs an exposure to ionising radiation resulting from the support and comfort of another person who is undergoing or who has undergone any medical exposure;

"contamination" means the contamination by any radioactive substance of any surface (including any surface of the body or clothing) or any part of absorbent objects or materials or the contamination of liquids or gases by any radioactive substance;

"controlled area" means—

(a) in the case of an area situated in Great Britain, an area which has been so designated in accordance with regulation 16(1); and

(b) in the case of an area situated in Northern Ireland or in another member State, an area subject to special rules for the purposes of protection against ionising radiation and to which access is controlled as specified in Article 19 of the Directive;

"the Directive" means Council Directive 96/29/Euratom laying down basic safety standards for the protection of the health of workers and the general public against the dangers arising from ionising radiation;

"dose" means, in relation to ionising radiation, any dose quantity or sum of dose quantities mentioned in Schedule 4;

"dose assessment" means the dose assessment made and recorded by an approved dosimetry service in accordance with regulation 21;

"dose constraint" means a restriction on the prospective doses to individuals which may result from a defined source;

"dose limit" means, in relation to persons of a specified class, the limit on effective dose or equivalent dose specified in Schedule 4 in relation to a person of that class;

"dose rate" means, in relation to a place, the rate at which a person or part of a person would receive a dose of ionising radiation from external radiation if he were at that place being a dose rate at that place averaged over one minute;

"dose record" means, in relation to a person, the record of the doses received by that person as a result of his exposure to ionising radiation, being the record made and maintained on behalf of the employer by the approved dosimetry service in accordance with regulation 21;

"employment medical adviser" means an employment medical adviser appointed under section 56 of the Health and Safety at Work etc. Act 1974;

"the Executive" means the Health and Safety Executive;

"external radiation" means, in relation to a person, ionising radiation coming from outside the body of that person;

"health record" means, subject to regulation 39(7) (which relates to transitional provisions), in relation to an employee, the record of medical surveillance of that employee maintained by the employer in accordance with regulation 24(3);

"internal radiation" means, in relation to a person, ionising radiation coming from inside the body of that person;

"ionising radiation" means the transfer of energy in the form of particles or electro-magnetic waves of a wavelength of 100 nanometres or less or a frequency of $3 \times 10 > 15 >$ hertz or more capable of producing ions directly or indirectly;

"licensee" has the meaning assigned to it by section 26(1) of the Nuclear Installations Act 1965[49];

"local rules" means rules made in accordance with regulation 17;

"maintained", where the reference is to maintaining plant, apparatus, equipment or facilities, means maintained in an efficient state, in efficient working order and good repair;

"medical exposure" means exposure of a person to ionising radiation for the purpose of his medical or dental examination or treatment which is conducted under the direction of a suitably qualified person and includes any such examination for legal purposes and any such examination or treatment conducted for the purposes of research;

"member State" means a member State of the Communities;

"outside worker" means a classified person who carries out services in the controlled area of any employer (other than the controlled area of his own employer);

"overexposure" means any exposure of a person to ionising radiation to the extent that the dose received by that person causes a dose limit relevant to that person to be exceeded or, in relation to regulation 26(2), causes a proportion of a dose limit relevant to any employee to be exceeded;

"practice" means work involving—

(a) the production, processing, handling, use, holding, storage, transport or disposal of radioactive substances; or

(b) the operation of any electrical equipment emitting ionising radiation and containing components operating at a potential difference of more than 5kV,

which can increase the exposure of individuals to radiation from an artificial source, or from a radioactive substance containing naturally occurring radionuclides which are processed for their radioactive, fissile or fertile properties;

"radiation accident" means an accident where immediate action would be required to prevent or reduce the exposure to ionising radiation of employees or any other persons;

"radiation employer" means an employer who in the course of a trade, business or other undertaking carries out work with ionising radiation and, for the purposes of regulations 5, 6 and 7, includes an employer who intends to carry out such work;

---

[49] Relevant amending instruments are SI 1974/2056 and SI 1990/1918.

"radiation passbook" means—

    (a) in the case of an outside worker employed by an employer in Great Britain—

        (i) a passbook approved by the Executive for the purpose of these Regulations; or

        (ii) a passbook to which regulation 39(4) (transitional provisions) applies; and

    (b) in the case of an outside worker employed by an employer in Northern Ireland or in another member State, a passbook authorised by the competent authority for Northern Ireland or that member State, as the case may be;

"radiation protection adviser" means, subject to regulation 39(6) (which relates to transitional provisions), an individual who, or a body which, meets such criteria of competence as may from time to time be specified in writing by the Executive;

"radioactive substance" means any substance which contains one or more radionuclides whose activity cannot be disregarded for the purposes of radiation protection;

["relevant authority" means—

    (a) in so far as these Regulations apply in relation to, or in relation to any activity carried out on, any nuclear premises, the Office for Nuclear Regulation;

    (b) otherwise, the Executive;

"nuclear premises" means premises which are or are on—

    (a) a GB nuclear site (within the meaning given in section 68 of the Energy Act 2013);

    (b) an authorised defence site (within the meaning given in regulation 2(1) of the Health and Safety (Enforcing Authority) Regulations 1998);

    (c) a new nuclear build site (within the meaning given in regulation 2A of those Regulations); or

    (d) a nuclear warship site (within the meaning given in regulation 2B of those Regulations).][50]

"sealed source" means a source containing any radioactive substance whose structure is such as to prevent, under normal conditions of use, any dispersion of radioactive substances into the environment, but it does not include any radioactive substance inside a nuclear reactor or any nuclear fuel element;

"short-lived daughters of radon 222" means polonium 218, lead 214, bismuth 214 and polonium 214;

"supervised area" means an area which has been so designated by the employer in accordance with regulation 16(3);

"trainee" means a person aged 16 years or over (including a student) who is undergoing instruction or training which involves operations which would, in the case of an employee, be work with ionising radiation;

"transport" means, in relation to a radioactive substance, carriage of that substance on a road within the meaning of, in relation to England and Wales, section 192 of the Road Traffic Act 1988 and, in relation to Scotland, the Roads (Scotland) Act 1984 or through another public place (whether on a conveyance or not), or by rail, inland waterway, sea or air and, in the case of transport on a conveyance, a substance shall be deemed as being transported from the time that it is loaded onto the conveyance for the purpose of transporting it until it is unloaded from that conveyance, but a substance shall not be considered as being transported if—

---

[50] Definitions inserted by Energy Act 2013 (Office for Nuclear Regulation) (Consequential Amendments, Transitional Provisions and Savings) Order 2014/469 Sch.3(3) para.99 (April 1, 2014).

    (a) it is transported by means of a pipeline or similar means; or

    (b) it forms an integral part of a conveyance and is used in connection with the operation of that conveyance;

"woman of reproductive capacity" means a woman who is made subject to the additional dose limit for a woman of reproductive capacity specified in paragraphs 5 and 11 of Schedule 4 by an entry in her health record made by an appointed doctor or employment medical adviser;

"work with ionising radiation" means work to which these Regulations apply by virtue of regulation 3(1).

(2) In these Regulations, unless the context otherwise requires, any reference to—

    (a) an employer includes a reference to a self-employed person and any duty imposed by these Regulations on an employer in respect of his employee shall extend to a self-employed person in respect of himself;

    (b) an employee includes a reference to—

        (i) a self-employed person, and

        (ii) a trainee who but for the operation of this sub-paragraph and paragraph (3) would not be classed as an employee;

    (c) exposure to ionising radiation is a reference to exposure to ionising radiation arising from work with ionising radiation;

    (d) a person entering, remaining in or working in a controlled or supervised area includes a reference to any part of a person entering, remaining in or working in any such area.

(3) For the purposes of these Regulations and Part I of the Health and Safety at Work etc. Act 1974—

    (a) the word "work" shall be extended to include any instruction or training which a person undergoes as a trainee and the meaning of "at work" shall be extended accordingly; and

    (b) a trainee shall, while he is undergoing instruction or training in respect of work with ionising radiation, be treated as the employee of the person whose undertaking (whether for profit or not) is providing that instruction or training and that person shall be treated as the employer of that trainee except that the duties to the trainee imposed upon the person providing instruction or training shall only extend to matters under the control of that person.

(4) In these Regulations, where reference is made to a quantity specified in Schedule 8, that quantity shall be treated as being exceeded if—

    (a) where only one radionuclide is involved, the quantity of that radionuclide exceeds the quantity specified in the appropriate entry in Schedule 8; or

    (b) where more than one radionuclide is involved, the quantity ratio calculated in accordance with Part II of Schedule 8 exceeds one.

(5) Nothing in these Regulations shall be construed as preventing a person from entering or remaining in a controlled area or a supervised area where that person enters or remains in any such area—

    (a) in the due exercise of a power of entry conferred on him by or under any enactment; or

    (b) for the purpose of undergoing a medical exposure.

(6) In these Regulations—

(a) any reference to an effective dose means the sum of the effective dose to the whole body from external radiation and the committed effective dose from internal radiation; and

(b) any reference to equivalent dose to a human tissue or organ includes the committed equivalent dose to that tissue or organ from internal radiation.

(7) In these Regulations—

(a) a numbered Regulation or Schedule is a reference to the Regulation or Schedule in these Regulations so numbered;

(b) a numbered paragraph is a reference to the paragraph so numbered in the Regulation or Schedule in which that reference appears.

PART VI

ARRANGEMENTS FOR THE CONTROL OF RADIOACTIVE SUBSTANCES, ARTICLES AND EQUIPMENT

[Notification of certain occurrences

A2–212   **30.**—(1) Every radiation employer shall forthwith notify the Executive in any case where a quantity of a radioactive substance which was under his control and which exceeds the quantity specified for that substance in column 4 of Schedule 8—

(a) has been released or is likely to have been released into the atmosphere as a gas, aerosol or dust; or

(b) has been spilled or otherwise released in such a manner as to give rise to significant contamination.

(2) Paragraph (1) shall not apply where such release—

(a) was in accordance with an environmental permit under the Environmental Permitting (England and Wales) Regulations 2010 in respect of mobile radioactive apparatus within the meaning of those Regulations;

(b) was in a manner specified in such an environmental permit in respect of radioactive waste within the meaning of those Regulations; or

(c) did not, under regulation 12 of those Regulations, require an environmental permit.

(3) Where a radiation employer has reasonable cause to believe that a quantity of a radioactive substance which exceeds the quantity for that substance specified in column 5 of Schedule 8 and which was under his control is lost or has been stolen, the employer shall forthwith notify the Executive of that loss or theft, as the case may be.

(4) Where a radiation employer suspects or has been informed that an occurrence notifiable under paragraph (1) or (3) may have occurred, he shall make an immediate investigation and, unless that investigation shows that no such occurrence has occurred, he shall forthwith make a notification in accordance with the relevant paragraph.

(5) A radiation employer who makes any investigation in accordance with paragraph (4) shall make a report of that investigation and shall, unless the investigation showed that no such occurrence occurred, keep that report or a copy thereof for at least 50 years from the date on which it was made or, in any other case, for at least 2 years from the date on which it was made.][51]

---

[51] Amended by SI 1999/983.

Judicial Appointments Order 2008/2995

1.—(1) This Order may be cited as the Judicial Appointments Order 2008.   **A2–213**
(2) This Order shall come into force—

(a) for the purposes of article 7(b), on 30th November 2010; and

(b) for all other purposes five days after the day on which it is made.

Interpretation

[**2.** In this Order—   **A2–214**

"the 1998 Act" means the Social Security Act 1998;
"the 2007 Act" means the Tribunals, Courts and Enforcement Act 2007;
"registered patent attorney" has the meaning assigned to it by section 275 of the
     Copyright, Designs and Patents Act 1988;
"registered trade mark attorney" has the meaning assigned to it by section 83 of the Trade
     Marks Act 1994;][52]

Specified qualifications under the 1998 Act

3. [*Outside the scope of this work*]   **A2–215**

Specified and relevant qualifications under the 2007 Act

4. Articles 5 and 6 are subject to articles 7 and 8.   **A2–216**
[**5.** For the purposes of section 50(2) and (3) of the 2007 Act, a person holds a relevant
qualification if the person is—

(a) a Fellow of the Institute of Legal Executives;

(b) a registered patent attorney; or

(c) a registered trade mark attorney.][53]

[**6.** For the purposes of section 50 of the 2007 Act, a person shall be taken first to
become—

(a) a Fellow of the Institute of Legal Executives when the person is admitted or enrolled
as a Fellow of the Institute of Legal Executives;

(b) a registered patent attorney when the person's name is entered on the register of
patent attorneys in accordance with section 275 of the Copyright, Designs and
Patents Act 1988; or

(c) a registered trade mark attorney when the person's name is entered on the register
of trade mark attorneys in accordance with section 83 of the Trade Marks Act
1994.][54]

---

[52] Amended by Legal Services Act 2007 (Consequential Amendments) Order 2009/3348 art.21(2)
(January 1, 2010 being the day on which 2007 c.29 s.13 comes into force).
[53] Amended by Legal Services Act 2007 (Consequential Amendments) Order 2009/3348 art.21(3)
(January 1, 2010 being the day on which 2007 c.29 s.13 comes into force).
[54] Amended by Legal Services Act 2007 (Consequential Amendments) Order 2009/3348 art.21(4)
(January 1, 2010 being the day on which 2007 c.29 s.13 comes into force).

Specified offices under the 2007 Act

A2–217   **7.** A person who is a Fellow of the Institute of Legal Executives holds a relevant qualification for the purposes of section 50(2) and (3) of the 2007 Act in relation to the offices specified in—

(a) Part 1 of Schedule 1 to this Order; and

(b) Part 2 of Schedule 1 to this Order.

[*Outside the scope of this work.*]

SCHEDULE 1

OFFICES FOR WHICH A FELLOW OF THE INSTITUTE OF LEGAL EXECUTIVES HOLDS A
RELEVANT QUALIFICATION

PART 1

[*Outside the scope of this work*]

PART 2

A2–218   [District Judge appointed under section 6(1) of the County Courts Act 1984[55],
District Judge (Magistrates' Courts) appointed under section 22(1) of the Courts Act 2003[56].
Senior coroners, area coroners and assistant coroners appointed under section 23 of, and Part 1 of Schedule 3 to, the Coroners and Justice Act 2009.][57]

Judicial Discipline (Prescribed Procedures) Regulations 2013/1674

PART 1

INTRODUCTION

Citation and commencement

A2–219   **1.** These Regulations may be cited as the Judicial Discipline (Prescribed Procedures) Regulations 2013 and shall come into force on 1st October 2013.

Interpretation

A2–220   **2.**—(1) In these Regulations—

"the Act" means the Constitutional Reform Act 2005;
"advisory committee" means one of the Lord Chancellor's advisory committees on justices of the peace;
"area coroner" means a person appointed as such under paragraph 2 of Schedule 3 to the Coroners and Justice Act 2009;
"assistant coroner" means a person appointed as such under paragraph 2 of Schedule 3 to the Coroners and Justice Act 2009;

---

[55] Section 6(1) was amended by the Constitutional Reform Act 2005, Schedule 3, paragraph 1(1).
[56] Section 22(1) was amended by the Tribunals, Courts and Enforcement Act 2007, Schedule 10, paragraph 38(1) and (2).
[57] Words inserted by Judicial Appointments (Amendment) Order 2013/3022 art.3 (December 3, 2013).

"bank holiday" means a bank holiday under the Banking and Financial Dealings Act 1971 in the part of the United Kingdom where service is to take place;

"business day" means any day other than a Saturday, Sunday, Christmas Day, Good Friday or a day which is a bank holiday in any part of the United Kingdom;

"case" means a complaint or issue of misconduct being considered under these Regulations;

"complaint" means a complaint containing an allegation of misconduct by a person holding judicial office or other office;

"disciplinary action" means—

    (a) the exercise by the Lord Chancellor of the Lord Chancellor's power to remove a person from office;

    (b) the exercise by the Lord Chief Justice of any of the Lord Chief Justice's powers under section 108(3), (4)(b) and (c) and (5) of the Act[58]; or

    (c) a decision that the Lord Chancellor will move an Address for the removal of a senior judge by both Houses of Parliament;

"disciplinary panel" has the meaning given by regulation 11;

"investigating judge" has the meaning given by regulation 10;

"justice of the peace" means a justice of the peace who is not a District Judge (Magistrates' Courts);

"nominated judge" has the meaning given by regulation 9;

"office" means an office listed in regulation 3;

"office holder concerned" means the holder of an office whose conduct is being considered in accordance with these Regulations;

"relevant President" in relation to a tribunal means a President or other office holder with disciplinary responsibility for tribunal members and includes any office holder designated to exercise such disciplinary responsibility under rules made under regulation 7;

"senior coroner" means a person appointed as such under paragraph 1 of Schedule 3 to the Coroners and Justice Act 2009;

"tribunal member" has the meaning given by regulation 8.

(2) In these Regulations, unless the contrary intention appears, a reference to the Lord Chief Justice is to be read—

    (a) in relation to an office holder who exercises functions wholly or mainly in Scotland, as a reference to the Lord President of the Court of Session;

    (b) in relation to an office holder who exercises functions wholly or mainly in Northern Ireland, as a reference to the Lord Chief Justice of Northern Ireland;

    (c) otherwise, as a reference to the Lord Chief Justice of England and Wales.

Application

3. These Regulations apply to—   **A2–221**

    (a) a judicial office;

---

[58] 2005 c.4; section 108 was extended by the Coroners and Justice Act 2009 (c.25), Schedule 3, paragraph 14.

(b) the offices of senior coroner, area coroner or assistant coroner;

(c) an office that has been designated by an order under section 118 of the Act.

The Judicial Conduct Investigations Office

A2–222   4.—(1) The Lord Chancellor must, with the agreement of the Lord Chief Justice, the Lord President of the Court of Session and the Lord Chief Justice of Northern Ireland, designate officials for the purpose of performing functions under these Regulations.

(2) Officials designated by the Lord Chancellor under paragraph (1) are known collectively as the Judicial Conduct Investigations Office.

(3) The Judicial Conduct Investigations Office may undertake such enquiries as are necessary for it to perform its functions under these Regulations or under any rules made under these Regulations.

(4) The Judicial Conduct Investigations Office may provide advice to any person regarding the application and interpretation of these Regulations and any rules made under these Regulations.

(5) For the purpose of paragraph (4) advice may include advice regarding any proposed disciplinary action.

(6) The Judicial Conduct Investigations Office may provide administrative assistance to a nominated judge, a relevant President, an investigating judge or a disciplinary panel in relation to the exercise of their functions under these Regulations or rules made under these Regulations.

Measurement of time for doing an act

A2–223   5. In these Regulations the time for doing any act in response to a notification, invitation or request ("the document") starts on the day that corresponds to the method of delivery used in relation to the notification, invitation or request shown in the table below—

Method of delivery	Starting day
First class post (or other method which provides for delivery on the next business day).	The second business day after the day on which the document was posted.
Second class post.	The third business day after the day on which the document was posted.
Delivering the document to or leaving it at a permitted address.	If it is delivered to or left at the permitted address on a business day before 4.30pm, that day; or if delivered at, or after, 4.30pm, the next business day.
Fax.	If the transmission of the fax is completed on a business day before 4.30pm, that day; or if transmitted at, or after, 4.30pm, the next business day.
Other electronic method.	If an e-mail or other electronic transmission is sent on a business day before 4.30pm, that day; or if an e-mail or other electronic transmission is sent at, or after, 4.30pm, the next business day.

Part 2

Complaints and investigation of complaints

Complaint of misconduct

6.—(1) Subject to paragraphs (2) and (3), a complaint about an office holder must be **A2–224**
made to the Judicial Conduct Investigations Office.

(2) A complaint about a justice of the peace must be made to the advisory committee for
the local justice area to which the justice of the peace is assigned under section 10(2) of the
Courts Act 2003.[59]

(3) A complaint about a tribunal member, other than a President, must be made to the
relevant President of the tribunal concerned.

Investigation process

7.—(1) The Lord Chief Justice, with the agreement of the Lord Chancellor, may make **A2–225**
rules about the process to be applied when a complaint is made under regulation 6.[60]

(2) Rules under paragraph (1) shall not apply in relation to an office holder who exercises
functions wholly or mainly in Scotland, unless they are made with the agreement of the
Lord President of the Court of Session.

(3) Rules under paragraph (1) shall not apply in relation to an office holder who exercises
functions wholly or mainly in Northern Ireland, unless they are made with the agreement
of the Lord Chief Justice of Northern Ireland.

(4) The rules may include provision as to any of the following—

(a) the form of a complaint;

(b) the information to be contained in a complaint;

(c) time limits for taking any step and procedures for extending or shortening time
limits;

(d) the circumstances in which a complaint or a part of a complaint may be dismissed;

(e) the circumstances in which an investigation may be undertaken (on the making of
a complaint or otherwise);

(f) the conduct of an investigation, including steps to be taken by the office holder
concerned, by a complainant or any other person;

(g) the circumstances in which an investigation may be conducted by the Judicial
Conduct Investigations Office, a nominated judge, an investigating judge, a
disciplinary panel, a relevant President or a person delegated by a relevant President;

(h) the circumstances in which a complaint may be dealt with under a summary
procedure;

---

[59] Section 10(2) was amended by the Constitutional Reform Act 2005 (c.4), Schedule 4, paragraphs 308
and 313.

[60] Section 117 of the Constitutional Reform Act 2005 (c.4) provides the Lord Chief Justice with a
power to make rules under the Regulations.

    (i) the steps to be taken by a person investigating a complaint where they wish to recommend that the Lord Chief Justice should exercise the power to suspend an office holder under section 108(7) of the Act;

    (j) the circumstances in which a complaint or part of a complaint which has initially been dismissed may be reconsidered.

Tribunal member

A2–226   **8.** A tribunal member for the purposes of these Regulations is a person specified as such under rules made under regulation 7.

Nominated judge

A2–227   **9.**—(1) A nominated judge means an office holder who is nominated by the Lord Chief Justice to deal with a case in accordance with rules made under regulation 7.

    (2) The Lord Chief Justice may nominate different office holders to deal with different cases or to deal with different aspects of the same case.

    (3) In a particular case, a nominated judge must be of at least the same rank as the office holder concerned.

Investigating judge

A2–228   **10.**—(1) An investigating judge means an office holder or a former office holder who is nominated by the Lord Chief Justice to investigate a case in accordance with rules made under regulation 7.

    (2) The Lord Chief Justice may nominate different office holders to investigate different cases or to investigate different aspects of the same case.

    (3) An investigating judge must be of a higher rank than the office holder concerned.

    (4) In relation to a former office holder reference to their rank means the rank they held immediately before they ceased to hold office.

Disciplinary panel

A2–229   **11.**—(1) A disciplinary panel is a panel consisting of—

    (a) either an office holder or former office holder who is of a higher rank than the office holder concerned;

    (b) either an office holder or former office holder who is of the same rank as the office holder concerned; and

    (c) two other members, neither of whom has been—

        (i) an office holder, or
        (ii) a practising or employed lawyer.

    (2) In relation to a former office holder, reference to their rank means the rank they held immediately before they ceased to hold office.

    (3) The Lord Chief Justice must nominate the members of a disciplinary panel under paragraph (1)(a) and (b).

    (4) The Lord Chancellor must nominate with the agreement of the Lord Chief Justice the other members in paragraph (1)(c).

(5) A person is ineligible for membership of a disciplinary panel if that person has had any previous involvement in the disciplinary process relating to the case that is being referred to the disciplinary panel.

(6) The office holder nominated under paragraph (1)(a) must chair the disciplinary panel and must exercise a casting vote if necessary.

Part 3

Decisions

Consideration of advice

12. Before making a decision under regulation 15 in relation to a case, the Lord Chancellor and the Lord Chief Justice must consider any advice provided by a person who or a body that has conducted an investigation into a complaint in accordance with rules made under regulation 6. **A2–230**

Further investigation

13.—(1) This regulation applies where the Lord Chancellor and the Lord Chief Justice have considered advice in accordance with regulation 12 and they require further investigation before making a decision under regulation 15. **A2–231**

(2) If the Lord Chancellor and the Lord Chief Justice agree, they may refer a complaint to a person or body listed in paragraph (3) to investigate further that complaint.

(3) The persons and bodies are—

(a) a nominated judge;

(b) in relation to a tribunal member, a relevant President or their designate;

(c) in relation to a magistrate, an advisory committee;

(d) an investigating judge; or

(e) a disciplinary panel.

(4) Any further investigation must be carried out in accordance with rules made under regulation 7.

Removal when other disciplinary power is recommended

14.—(1) This regulation applies where— **A2–232**

(a) advice has been provided to the Lord Chief Justice and the Lord Chancellor by a person who or a body that has conducted an investigation into a complaint in accordance with rules made under regulation 7; and

(b) that advice does not recommend the removal or suspension of an office holder from office but the Lord Chancellor and the Lord Chief Justice consider removal or suspension to be the appropriate disciplinary action.

(2) The Lord Chancellor and the Lord Chief Justice must constitute a disciplinary panel and refer the complaint to it.

(3) The disciplinary panel must—

(a) investigate the complaint in accordance with rules made under regulation 7; and

(b) advise the Lord Chancellor and the Lord Chief Justice whether disciplinary action should be taken, and if so, what disciplinary action should be taken.

(4) The Lord Chancellor and the Lord Chief Justice must consider the advice provided by the disciplinary panel before making a decision in accordance with regulation 15.

Decision

A2–233 **15.**—(1) This regulation applies where the Lord Chancellor and the Lord Chief Justice have considered advice in accordance with regulation 12 and determine not to exercise, or exercise further, their powers in regulation 13 and regulation 14 does not apply.

(2) The Lord Chancellor and the Lord Chief Justice may agree—

(a) to dismiss a complaint; or

(b) to take a particular disciplinary action.

(3) Where a complaint is dismissed, the Lord Chancellor and the Lord Chief Justice may agree that—

(a) the alleged conduct referred to in a complaint took place but did not constitute misconduct; and

(b) the Lord Chief Justice may deal with the matter informally.

Notification of final decision

A2–234 **16.**—(1) The Judicial Conduct Investigations Office must inform the persons listed in paragraph (2) of the decision made by the Lord Chancellor and Lord Chief Justice under regulation 15.

(2) The persons referred to in paragraph (1) are—

(a) the office holder concerned;

(b) the complainant;

(c) if the complaint is about a tribunal member, the relevant President;

(d) if the complaint is about a justice of the peace, the chairman of the advisory committee and the bench chairman.

Interim suspension

A2–235 **17.**—(1) If the Lord Chief Justice decides to suspend an office holder from their office under section 108(4)(a), (6) or (7) of the Act, the Lord Chief Justice must—

(a) notify the office holder of the proposed suspension, the reasons for it and the time when it is proposed that it will come into effect;

(b) notify the office holder of the factors that will be taken into account in determining when the suspension will end; and

(c) invite the office holder to make representations.

(2) The office holder must make any representations within ten business days of the notification under paragraph (1).

(3) Where, after a suspension comes into effect, any of the factors which the Lord Chief Justice has indicated would be taken into account in accordance with paragraph (1)(b) become operative, or any other matter which the Lord Chief Justice and the Lord Chancellor consider relevant arises, the Lord Chief Justice and the Lord Chancellor must—

(a) decide whether continuation of the suspension is appropriate;

(b) notify the office holder of their decision under sub-paragraph (a) and of the reasons for that decision; and

(c) invite the office holder to make representations.

(4) The office holder must make any representations within ten business days of a notification under paragraph (3).

Publication of decision

18.—(1) The Lord Chancellor and the Lord Chief Justice may agree to the publication of information about disciplinary proceedings or the taking of disciplinary action.   **A2–236**
(2) Publication for this purpose means any form of communication which is addressed to an individual, a section of the public or the public at large.

PART 4

MISCELLANEOUS

Requirements in relation to reviews by the Ombudsman

19.—(1) If the Ombudsman requests from any person information for the purposes of a review carried out under section 111 of the Act[61], and such information is not provided within ten business days of the notification of the request, or within such other period as the Ombudsman indicates, they may—   **A2–237**

(a) prepare their review without regard to that information, and

(b) may disregard any representations made out of time by the person concerned.

(2) The Lord Chancellor, the Lord Chief Justice or any person or body conducting an investigation in accordance with rules made under regulation 6 must provide the Ombudsman with such information as the Ombudsman may reasonably require for the purposes of a review carried out under section 111 or section 113 of the Act[62].
(3) Where the Ombudsman directs under section 111(7)(b) of the Act that an investigation should be undertaken or undertaken again, the case must be investigated in accordance with the rules made under regulation 7.

Delegation

20. The Lord Chief Justice may delegate any functions under these Regulations other than those under regulation 7(1).   **A2–238**

Scotland and Northern Ireland: eligibility to exercise functions

21. [*Applies to Scotland and Northern Ireland*]   **A2–239**

Scotland and Northern Ireland: Judicial Appointments and Conduct Ombudsman

22. [*Applies to Scotland and Northern Ireland*]   **A2–240**

---

[61] 2005 c.4; section 111 was extended by the Coroners and Justice Act 2009 (c.25), Schedule 3, paragraph 14.
[62] 2005 c4; sections 111 and 113 were extended by the Coroners and Justice Act 2009 (c.25), Schedule 3, paragraph 14.

Ceasing to hold office

A2–241   **23.**—(1) Subject to paragraphs (2) and (4), where the office holder concerned ceases to hold their office, consideration of the complaint under these Regulations or rules made under regulation 7 must cease.

(2) The Lord Chancellor and the Lord Chief Justice may continue to deal with the case and then make a finding of misconduct in relation to the office holder concerned where the circumstances in paragraph (3) apply.

(3) The circumstances are—

(a) the office holder concerned ceases to hold their office;

(b) a disciplinary panel or an investigating judge proposes to advise, or has advised, the Lord Chief Justice and the Lord Chancellor that the office holder concerned should be removed from holding their office; and

(c) no decision has been made under regulation 15.

(4) Paragraph (1) does not apply where—

(a) the office holder concerned has ceased to hold their office; but

(b) the Ombudsman directs under section 111(7)(b) of the Act that an investigation should be undertaken or undertaken again.

Transitional provision

A2–242   **24.**—(1) Subject to paragraph (2), these Regulations apply to any complaint made before these Regulations come into force which has not been withdrawn, dismissed or determined.

(2) Where the circumstances in paragraph (3) apply a complaint is to be considered as though these Regulations had not come into force and the Judicial Discipline (Prescribed Procedures) Regulations 2006[63] had not been revoked.

(3) The circumstances are—

(a) a complaint has been made before these Regulations come into force and the complaint has not been dismissed or withdrawn; and

(b) a notification has been made by the Lord Chancellor or the Lord Chief Justice under regulation 27(1)(a) of the Judicial Discipline (Prescribed Procedures) Regulations 2006.

Revocations

A2–243   **25.** The following Regulations are revoked—

(a) the Judicial Discipline (Prescribed Procedures) Regulations 2006; and

(b) the Judicial Discipline (Prescribed Procedures) (Amendment) Regulations 2008.

---

[63] amended by SI 2008/2098.

Magistrates' Courts Rules 1981/552

Satisfaction, Enforcement And Application Of Payments

Notice to defendant of fine or forfeited recognizance

46.—(1) Where under [section 140(1) of the Act of 2000],[64] section 49 of the Criminal   **A2–244**
Justice Act 1967 or section 19(5) of the Coroners Act 1887 a magistrates' court is required
to enforce payment of a fine imposed or recognizance forfeited by the Crown Court or by
a coroner or where a magistrates' court allows time for payment of a sum adjudged to be
paid by a summary conviction, or directs that the sum be paid by instalments, or where the
offender is absent when a sum is adjudged to be paid by a summary conviction, the
[[designated officer][65] for][66] the court shall serve on the offender notice in writing stating
the amount of the sum and, if it is to be paid by instalments, the amount of the instalments,
the date on which the sum, or each of the instalments, is to be paid and the places and times
at which payment may be made; and a warrant of [control][67] or commitment shall not be
issued until the preceding provisions of this rule have been complied with.

(2) A notice under this rule shall be served by delivering it to the offender or by sending
it to him by post in a letter addressed to him at his last known or usual place of
abode.[[68]][69]

Merchant Shipping Act 1970 (Unregistered Ships) Regulations 1991/1366

Extension to ships entitled to be registered of 24 metres or more in length

2. It is hereby directed that—   **A2–245**

(a) the provisions of the Merchant Shipping Act 1970 specified in column 1 of Part I
of Schedule 1 to these Regulations; and

(b) the provisions of the Regulations made under that Act specified in column 1 of Part
II of that Schedule;

shall extend to ships (other than fishing vessels) of the following description, that is to say,
sea-going ships—

(i) which are wholly owned by a person resident in, or by a body corporate (not being
a general lighthouse authority) having a principal place of business in, the United
Kingdom;

(ii) which are entitled to be registered in the United Kingdom under the Merchant
Shipping Act 1894 but are not registered, whether in the United Kingdom or
elsewhere; and

---

[64] Words substituted by Magistrates' Courts (Miscellaneous Amendments) Rules 2003/1236 rule 29
(June 20, 2003).

[65] Words substituted by Courts Act 2003 (Consequential Provisions) (No. 2) Order 2005/617 Sch.1
para.85 (April 1, 2005).

[66] Words substituted by Magistrates' Courts (Amendment No. 2) Rules 2001/610 rule 3. (April 1,
2001).

[67] Word substituted by Tribunals, Courts and Enforcement Act 2007 (Consequential, Transitional and
Saving Provision) Order 2014/600 Sch.1(1) para.1(b) (April 6, 2014).

[68] In relation to criminal matters: SI 1981/552 rule 46 is substantively re-enacted by SI 2005/384 rule
52.1.

[69] Superseded in relation to criminal matters as authorised by Criminal Procedure Rules 2005/384 Pt
2 rule 2.1 (April 4, 2005).

(iii) which are 24 metres or more in length;

and to masters and seamen employed in them, with such exceptions, adaptations or modifications (if any) as are specified in column 2 of that Schedule.

3. It is hereby directed that—

(a) the provisions of the Merchant Shipping Act 1970 specified in column 1 of Part I of Schedule 2 to these Regulations; and

(b) the provisions of the Regulations made under that Act specified in column 1 of Part II of that Schedule;

shall extend to ships (other than fishing vessels) of the following description, that is to say, sea-going ships

(i) which are wholly owned by a person resident in, or a body corporate (not being a general lighthouse authority) having a principal place of business in, the United Kingdom; and

(ii) which are entitled to be registered in the United Kingdom under the Merchant Shipping Act 1894 but are not registered, whether in the United Kingdom or elsewhere; and

(iii) which are less than 24 metres in length;

and to masters and seamen employed in them, with such exceptions, adaptations and modifications (if any) as are specified in column 2 of that Schedule.

SCHEDULE 1

EXTENSION TO UNREGISTERED SHIPS OF THE DESCRIPTION CONTAINED IN REGULATION 2

PART I

A2–246

Column 1	Column 2
Provision of the Merchant Shipping Act 1970	*Exception, adaptation or modification to which extension is subject*
Sections 1 to 4.	
Section 5.	Subject to the modification that, for the reference to a ship ceasing to be registered in the United Kingdom, there shall be substituted a reference to its ceasing to be entitled to be registered under the Merchant Shipping Act 1894.
Sections 7 to 14.	
Section 22.	
Sections 25 and 26.	
Section 28.	
Section 30.	
Section 33.	
Sections 39 to 42.	
Sections 43, 44, 45 and 47.	

Column 1	Column 2
Provision of the Merchant Shipping Act 1970	*Exception, adaptation or modification to which extension is subject*
Section 48.	
Sections 61 to 64.	
Sections 67 to 69.	
Section 74.	
Sections 76 to 79.	

PART II

A2–247

Column 1	Column 2
Regulations made under the Merchant Shipping Act 1970	*Exception, adaptation or modification to which extension is subject*
The Merchant Shipping (Crew Agreements, Lists of Crew and Discharge of Seamen) Regulations 1972.	
The Merchant Shipping (Seamen's Wages and Accounts) Regulations 1972.	
The Merchant Shipping (Seamen's Wages) (Contributions) Regulations 1972.	
The Merchant Shipping (Seamen's Allotments) Regulations 1972.	
The Merchant Shipping (Repatriation) Regulations 1979.	
The Merchant Shipping (Official Log Books) Regulations 1981.	

Merchant Shipping (Returns of Births and Deaths) Regulations 1979/1577

Death in ship registered in the United Kingdom and death of person employed in such a ship

3. Where—

A2–248

(a) any person dies in a ship registered in the United Kingdom; or

(b) any person employed in any such ship dies outside the United Kingdom the master of the ship shall—

    (i) make a return of the death in accordance with regulations 5 and 6; and

    (ii) as soon as practicable but not more than 3 days after the death, notify the death to such person (if any) as the deceased may have named to him as his next of kin.

Birth and death in ship not registered in the United Kingdom

4. Where—

A2–249

(a) a citizen of the United Kingdom and Colonies is born or dies in a ship not registered in the United Kingdom; and

(b) the ship thereafter calls at a port in the United Kingdom in the course of or at the end of the voyage during which the birth or death occurs

the master of the ship shall make a return of the birth or of the death in accordance with regulations 5 and 6.

Returns of births and deaths

A2-250   **5.**—(1) Any return of a birth or of a death required to be made under regulation 2 or 3 shall be made by the master of the ship as soon as practicable after (but within 6 months after) the birth or death to which it relates and—

(a) in the case of a birth or of a death which occurs in the ship, shall be made to a superintendent or proper officer for the place where the ship is at the time of the birth or of the death, as the case may be, or at which it next calls thereafter; and

(b) in the case of a death which occurs elsewhere than in the ship, shall be made to a superintendent or proper officer for the place where the ship is when the master first becomes aware of the death or at which it next calls thereafter.

(2) Any return of a birth or of a death required to be made under regulation 4 shall be made by the master of the ship to a superintendent for the port referred to in paragraph (b) of that regulation before the ship leaves that port.

(3) Without prejudice to the preceding provisions of this regulation and to the provisions of regulation 13, a return of a birth or of a death required to be made under regulation 2, 3 or 4 which is not made within the period prescribed for the making thereof or is made to a superintendent or proper officer other than that specified by the preceding provisions of this regulation, shall not be invalid by reason only that it is not made within that period or to such specified person.

Contents of returns

A2-251   **6.** A return of a birth or of a death required to be made under these Regulations—

(a) shall be in writing;

(b) shall be signed by the master of the ship as informant; and

(c) shall contain—

(i) (in the case of a birth) the particulars specified in Schedule 1 to these Regulations; or

(ii) (in the case of a death) the particulars specified in Schedule 2 to these Regulations;

or so many of those particulars as the master may reasonably be able to obtain, having regard to the circumstances of the birth or of the death.

Records of deaths where master unable to act

A2-252   **7.** Where it appears to the Registrar General of Shipping and Seamen that the master of the ship cannot perform the duty imposed on him by virtue of regulation 3 of these Regulations in respect of the death because he has himself died or is incapacitated or missing and either—

(1) the death in question has been the subject of an inquest held by the coroner or an inquiry held in pursuance of section 61 of the Merchant Shipping Act 1970 or in pursuance of the Fatal Accidents and Sudden Deaths Inquiry (Scotland) Act 1976

and the findings of the inquest or inquiry include a finding that the death occurred, or

(2) a post-mortem examination, or a preliminary investigation in Northern Ireland, has been made of the deceased's body and in consequence the coroner is satisfied that an inquest is unnecessary, or

(3) in Scotland, it does not appear to the Lord Advocate, under section 1(1)(b) of the said Act of 1976, to be expedient in the public interest that an inquiry under that Act should be held

then the Registrar General of Shipping and Seamen shall record such of the information specified in Schedule 2 to these Regulations as he may be able to obtain in the circumstances of the death.

Particulars of deaths to be supplied by coroners

8. Where—   **A2–253**

(1) an inquest is held on a dead body or touching a death or a post-mortem examination, or a preliminary investigation in Northern Ireland, is made of a dead body as a result of which the coroner is satisfied that an inquest is unnecessary; and

(2) it appears to the coroner that the death in question is such as is mentioned in paragraph (a) or (b) of regulation 3, as extended by regulation 12(1) of these Regulations

it shall be the duty of the coroner to send to the Registrar General of Shipping and Seamen particulars in respect of the deceased of the kind specified in Schedule 3 to these Regulations.

Certified copies of returns or records to be sent to the Registrar General

9. When a return made in accordance with regulations 5 and 6 has been transmitted to   **A2–254**
him, or a record in accordance with regulation 7 has been made by him, the Registrar
General of Shipping and Seamen shall send a copy, certified by him or by a person
authorised by him for that purpose to be a true copy of that return or record, to the
appropriate Registrar General ascertained under the provisions of regulation 11.

Other births and deaths outside the United Kingdom

10.—(1) This regulation applies to the following births and deaths occurring outside the   **A2–255**
United Kingdom in circumstances where no return or record is required to be made under
the preceding provisions of these Regulations—

(a) any birth or death of a citizen of the United Kingdom and Colonies which occurs in a ship not registered in the United Kingdom;

(b) any death of a citizen of the United Kingdom and Colonies who has been employed in such a ship which occurs elsewhere than in the ship; and

(c) any death of a person who has been employed in a ship registered in the United Kingdom which occurs elsewhere than in the ship.

(2) If he is satisfied that a birth or a death to which this regulation applies has occurred, the appropriate Registrar General ascertained under the provisions of regulation 11 may record in the marine register—

(a) (in the case of a birth) such of the particulars specified in Schedule 1 to these Regulations; or

(b) (in the case of a death) such of the particulars specified in Schedule 2 to these Regulations

as he thinks fit.

[Rules for ascertaining appropriate Registrar General

A2–256   **11.** (1) The appropriate Registrar General for the purposes of regulations 9 and 10 is—

(a)   (i) in the case of the birth of a child the father or second female parent of whom or, if the child is illegitimate, the mother of whom was at the time of the birth usually resident in Scotland or Northern Ireland; or

(ii) in the case of the death of a person who at the date of his death was usually resident in Scotland or in Northern Ireland

the Registrar General of Births, Deaths and Marriages for Scotland or the Registrar General for Northern Ireland, as the case may require; and

(b) in any other case, the Registrar General for England and Wales.

(2) In paragraph (1), "second female parent" means the woman who is a parent of the child by virtue of—

(a) section 42 of the Human Fertilisation and Embryology Act 2008 (which relates to treatment provided to a woman who at the time of treatment is married to another woman, or in certain circumstances is a party to a void marriage with another woman, or party to a civil partnership or in certain circumstances a void civil partnership); or

[(b)   section 43 of that Act (which relates to treatment provided to a woman where she agrees a second woman is to be the parent of the child) where the woman—

(i) is married to, or the civil partner of, the child's mother at the time of the child's birth, or

(ii) was married to, or the civil partner of, the child's mother at any time during the period beginning with the time mentioned in section 43(b) of that Act[70] and ending with the child's birth.][71]][72]

Extensions to unregistered British ships

A2–257   **12.**—(1) It is hereby directed that the provisions of section 72 of the Merchant Shipping Act 1970 and of these Regulations (except regulations 4 and 10(1)(a) and (b)) shall extend to British ships (which are not registered in the United Kingdom or elsewhere) of the following description, that is to say, sea-going ships which are owned by a person resident in, or by a body corporate having a principal place of business in the United Kingdom, and to masters and seamen employed in them.

---

[70] Existing reg.11 renumbered as reg.11(1) and reg.11(2) inserted by Human Fertilisation and Embryology (Consequential Amendments and Transitional and Saving Provisions) Order 2009/1892 Sch.1(2) para.8(3) (September 1, 2009).

[71] Substituted by Marriage (Same Sex Couples) Act 2013 (Consequential Provisions) Order 2014/107 Sch.1 para.7(b) (March 13, 2014).

[72] Words substituted by Marriage (Same Sex Couples) Act 2013 (Consequential Provisions) Order 2014/107 Sch.1 para.7(a) (March 13, 2014).

(2) Paragraph 1 of Schedule 1 and paragraph 1 of Schedule 2 to these Regulations as extended by paragraph (1) of this regulation shall have effect with the modification that for sub-paragraphs (a) and (b) of each of those regulations there shall be substituted—

"(a) name of the ship and sufficient description to identify the ship;

(b) the name of the owner; and

(c) the address of his residence in the United Kingdom, or, if the owner is a body corporate having a principal place of business in the United Kingdom, the address of that place of business."

Offences

13. (1) The master of a ship who fails to comply with any provision of regulation 2, 3,   **A2–258**
4, 5, or 6 or of regulation 2, 3, 5 or 6 as extended by regulation 12 shall be guilty of an offence.

(2) Any offence under these Regulations shall be punishable on summary conviction with a fine not exceeding [level 3 on the standard scale].[73]

SCHEDULE 2

PARTICULARS REQUIRED TO BE CONTAINED IN RETURNS OR RECORDS OF DEATHS UNDER REGULATION 3, 4, 5, 6 AND 7 OR AUTHORISED TO BE RECORDED IN THE MARINE REGISTER UNDER REGULATION 10

1. Ship in which death occurred or in which the deceased was employed

(a) name of ship;   **A2–259**

(b)(i) wherever it is registered, its port of registry and official number or, in the case of a fishing vessel, letters and number; and

(ii) if it is not registered in the United Kingdom, the name of its owner and his address.

2. The deceased

(a) date of death or loss;   **A2–260**

(b)(i) if the death took place in the ship or in a ship's boat or if the deceased was lost from the ship or a ship's boat, the place of death or, if at sea, the position of the ship or ship's boat by latitude and longitude at the time of the death or loss (as the case may require); and

(ii) in any other case, the place of death;

(c) name and surname;

(d) sex;

(e) date of birth (if known) or age;

(f) (if known) maiden surname of woman who has been married (being the name under which she contracted her marriage or, where she has been married more than once, her first marriage);

(g) occupation, rank or profession;

(h) usual residence at time of death or loss;

(i) nationality; and

(j) cause of death or loss (certified if possible by ship's doctor or other medical practitioner).

---

[73] Word substituted by Criminal Justice Act 1988 c. 33 Pt V s.55 (October 12, 1988 as SI 1988/1676).

3. Informant

A2–261
    (a) name and surname of master; or

    (b) in the case of a death authorised to be recorded in the marine register under regulation 10—

        (i) name and surname;
        (ii) usual address; and
        (iii) qualification; or

    (c) in the case of a death authorised to be recorded under regulation 7 and where no informant is notified the name and office of the proper officer or superintendent who conducted the inquiry or of the coroner who held the inquest or was satisfied that no inquest was necessary.

SCHEDULE 3

PARTICULARS REQUIRED TO BE SENT BY CORONERS IN RESPECT OF DEATHS UNDER REGULATION 8

1. Ship in which death occurred or in which the deceased was employed

A2–262
    (a) name of ship;

    (b)(i) where it is registered, its port of registry and official number or, in the case of a fishing vessel, letters and number; and

    (ii) where it is unregistered, its type and the name of its owner and his address.

2. The deceased

A2–263
    (a) date of death or loss;

    (b)(i) if the death took place in the ship or in a ship's boat or if the deceased was lost from the ship or a ship's boat, the place of death or, if at sea, the position of the ship or ship's boat by latitude and longitude at the time of the death or loss (as the case may require); and

    (ii) in any other case, the place of death;

    (c) name and surname;

    (d) sex;

    (e) date of birth (if known) or age;

    (f) (if known) maiden surname of woman who has been married (being the name under which she contracted her marriage or, where she has been married more than once, her first marriage);

    (g) occupation, rank or profession;

    (h) usual residence at time of death or loss;

    (i) nationality.

3. Coroner's certificate

A2–264 Certification by the coroner that:

    (a) an inquest was held or

    (b) a post-mortem examination/preliminary investigation was held; and

    (c) the cause of death.

Non-Contentious Probate Rules 1987/2024

Order of priority for grant in case of intestacy

A2–265
    22.—(1) Where the deceased died on or after 1st January 1926, wholly intestate, the person or persons having a beneficial interest in the estate shall be entitled to a grant of administration in the following classes in order of priority, namely—

(a) the surviving [spouse or civil partner][74];

(b) the children of the deceased and the issue of any deceased child who died before the deceased;

(c) the father and mother of the deceased;

(d) brothers and sisters of the whole blood and the issue of any deceased brother or sister of the whole blood who died before the deceased;

(e) brothers and sisters of the half blood and the issue of any deceased brother or sister of the half blood who died before the deceased;

(f) grandparents;

(g) uncles and aunts of the whole blood and the issue of any deceased uncle or aunt of the whole blood who died before the deceased;

(h) uncles and aunts of the half blood and the issue of any deceased uncle or aunt of the half blood who died before the deceased.

(2) In default of any person having a beneficial interest in the estate, the Treasury Solicitor shall be entitled to a grant if he claims bona vacantia on behalf of the Crown.

(3) If all persons entitled to a grant under the foregoing provisions of this rule have been cleared off, a grant may be made to a creditor of the deceased or to any person who, notwithstanding that he has no immediate beneficial interest in the estate, may have a beneficial interest in the event of an accretion thereto.

(4) Subject to paragraph (5) of rule 27, the personal representative of a person in any of the classes mentioned in paragraph (1) of this rule or the personal representative of a creditor of the deceased shall have the same right to a grant as the person whom he represents provided that the persons mentioned in sub-paragraphs (b) to (h) of paragraph (1) above shall be preferred to the personal representative of a spouse [or a civil partner][75] who has died without taking a beneficial interest in the whole estate of the deceased as ascertained at the time of the application for the grant.

Order of priority for grant in pre-1926 cases

23. Where the deceased died before 1st January 1926, the person or persons entitled to a grant shall, subject to the provisions of any enactment, be determined in accordance with the principles and rules under which the court would have acted at the date of death.

A2–266

Right of assignee to a grant

24.—(1) Where all the persons entitled to the estate of the deceased (whether under a will or on intestacy) have assigned their whole interest in the estate to one or more persons, the assignee or assignees shall replace, in the order of priority for a grant of administration, the assignor or, if there are two or more assignors, the assignor with the highest priority.

A2–267

(2) Where there are two or more assignees, administration may be granted with the consent of the others to any one or more (not exceeding four) of them.

(3) In any case where administration is applied for by an assignee the original instrument of assignment shall be produced and a copy of the same lodged in the registry.

---

[74] Words substituted by Civil Partnership Act 2004 (Amendments to Subordinate Legislation) Order 2005/2114 Sch.6 para.2(2) (December 5, 2005).

[75] Words inserted by Civil Partnership Act 2004 (Amendments to Subordinate Legislation) Order 2005/2114 Sch.6 para.2(3) (December 5, 2005).

Exceptions to rules as to priority

A2–268   **28.**—(1) Any person to whom a grant may or is required to be made under any enactment shall not be prevented from obtaining such a grant notwithstanding the operation of rules 20, 22, 25 or 27.

(2) Where the deceased died domiciled outside England and Wales rules 20, 22, 25 or 27 shall not apply except in a case to which paragraph (3) of rule 30 applies.

Nuclear Installations (Dangerous Occurrences) Regulations 1965/1824

Dangerous occurrences

A2–269   **3.**—(1) The Minister of Power and the Secretary of State hereby prescribe for the purposes of section 22(1) of the Act occurrences of each of the following classes or descriptions, that is to say—

  (a) any occurrence on a licensed site involving the emission of ionising radiations or the release of radioactive or toxic substances in such circumstances as to cause or be likely to cause—

   (i) the death of, or serious injury to the health of, persons outside the site at the time of the occurrence, whether or not persons on the site are also affected thereby; or

   (ii) the death of, or serious injury to the health of, persons on the site at the time of the occurrence;

  (b) any occurrence in the course of carriage of nuclear matter (not being excepted matter) on behalf of any person other than the Authority or a government department, being—

   (i) an occurrence which that person has reason to believe has caused or may be likely to cause the death of, or serious injury to the health of, any person by reason of the radioactive properties of such nuclear matter; or

   (ii) an occurrence involving the breaking open of any outside container in which such nuclear matter is being carried;

  (c) any explosion or outbreak of fire on a licensed site, being an explosion or outbreak affecting or likely to affect the safe working or safe condition of the nuclear installation;

  (d) any uncontrolled criticality excursion.

(2) The requirements of sub-paragraphs (b), (c) and (d) of the last preceding paragraph shall be without prejudice to the generality of the requirements of sub-paragraph (a) thereof.

[Manner in which occurrences are to be reported to the appropriate national authority

A2–270   **4.**—(1) A report required to be made under section 22(2) of the Act to the appropriate national authority must be made in the manner prescribed in paragraph (2).

(2) The report must—

  (a) be made by the quickest means available; and

  (b) be subsequently confirmed in writing.

(3) Where a report is confirmed in writing, it must contain the information (or such part of that information as may be applicable to the occurrence concerned) specified in the Schedule.][76]

Prison Rules 1999/728

PART II

PRISONERS

Medical Attention

Notification of illness or death

22.—(1) If a prisoner dies, becomes seriously ill, sustains any severe injury or is removed to hospital on account of mental disorder, the governor shall, if he knows his or her address, at once inform the prisoner's spouse or next of kin, and also any person who the prisoner may reasonably have asked should be informed.

A2–271

(2) If a prisoner dies, the governor shall give notice immediately to the coroner having jurisdiction, to the [independent monitoring board][77] and to the Secretary of State.

Railways and Other Guided Transport Systems (Safety) Regulations 2006/599

PART 1

INTRODUCTION

Interpretation and application

2.—(1) In these Regulations—

A2–272

"building operation" means the—

    (a) construction, structural alteration, repair or maintenance of a building and "maintenance" shall include repointing, redecoration and external cleaning of the structure;

    (b) demolition of a building; or

    (c) preparation for and laying the foundation of an intended building,

but does not include any operation which is a work of engineering construction;
"bus" means a motor vehicle which is designed or adapted to travel along roads and to carry more than eight passengers but which is not a tramcar;
"cableway installation" means an installation made up of several components that—

    (a) is used or intended to be used for the purpose of providing an operational system for carrying persons in vehicles, on chairs or by towing devices;

    (b) uses cables positioned along the line of travel to provide suspension or traction or both; and

    (c) is one of the following—

---

[76] Regs 4 and 4A substituted for reg.4 by Energy Act 2013 (Office for Nuclear Regulation) (Consequential Amendments, Transitional Provisions and Savings) Order 2014/469 Sch.3(3) para.29 (April 1, 2014).

[77] Words substituted by Prison (Amendment) Rules 2008/597 rule 4(a) (April 1, 2008).

> > (i) cable car (including a gondola and chair lift) where the cabins or chairs are lifted or displaced by one or more carrier cables;
> > (ii) drag lift, where users with appropriate equipment are dragged by means of a cable; or
> > (iii) funicular railway or other installation with vehicles mounted on wheels or on other suspension devices where traction is provided by one or more cables;

> but does not include cable operated tramways, rack railways or lifts;

"carriageway" has the same meaning as in the Highways Act 1980[78], or in Scotland the Roads (Scotland) Act 1984[78];

["certification body" has the same meaning as in the ECM Regulation;][79]

"common safety methods" ("CSMs") means the methods, developed pursuant to article 6 of the Directive, to describe how—

> (a) safety levels;
> (b) achievement of safety targets; and
> (c) compliance with other safety requirements,

> are assessed, as revised and reissued from time to time;

"common safety targets" ("CSTs") means the safety levels, developed pursuant to article 7 of the Directive, that must be reached by—

> (a) different parts of the mainline railway system; and
> (b) that system as a whole,

> expressed in risk acceptance criteria, as revised and reissued from time to time;

"competent person" means, except for the purposes of Part 4, a person who—

> (a) has sufficient skills, knowledge, experience and resources to undertake the safety verification in relation to which he is appointed;
> (b) has not borne such responsibility in relation to any of the matters he has to consider in undertaking that safety verification that might compromise his objectivity; and
> (c) is sufficiently independent of a management system, or a part thereof, which has borne responsibility for any of the matters he has to consider in undertaking the safety verification, to ensure that he will be objective in carrying out the safety verification for which he is appointed;

"conventional Directive" means Council Directive 2001/16 of the European Parliament and of the Council on the interoperability of the conventional rail system[80];

[. . .][81]

["the Directive" means Directive 2004/49/EC[82] of the European Parliament and of the Council on safety on the Community's railways as amended by the Interoperability Directive, Directive 2008/110/EC[83] of the European Parliament and of the Council on safety on the Community's railways and Commission Directive 2009/149/EC[84] on Common Safety Indicators and common methods to calculate accident costs;][85]

---

[78] To which there are amendments not relevant to these Regulations.

[79] Definition inserted by Railways and Other Guided Transport Systems (Miscellaneous Amendments) Regulations 2013/950 reg.3(2)(a) (May 21, 2013).

[80] O.J. No. L110, 20.04.2001, p1, as amended by Directive 2004/50/EC of the European Parliament and the Council of 29th April 2004 (O.J. No. L164, 30.04.2004, p114).

[81] Definitions repealed by Railways and Other Guided Transport Systems (Miscellaneous Amendments) Regulations 2013/950 reg.3(2)(b) (May 21, 2013).

[82] O.J. No. L164, 30.4.2004, p44.

[83] O.J. No. L345, 23.12.2008, p62.

[84] O.J. No. L313, 28.11.2009, p65.

[85] Definition substituted by Railways and Other Guided Transport Systems (Safety) (Amendment) Regulations 2011/1860 reg.2(2)(a) (August 26, 2011).

["ECM certificate" means a certificate issued in accordance with the ECM Regulation to an entity in charge of maintenance for the purposes of Article 14a(4) of the Directive or a certificate or self-declaration recognised as being equivalent for those purposes in accordance with Article 12(3) to (7) of the ECM Regulation;"ECM Regulation" means Commission Regulation (EU) No 445/2011 on a system of certification of entities in charge of maintenance for freight wagons and amending Regulation (EC) No 653/2007[86];] [87]

"engineering possession" means a section of track which is closed to normal traffic and where the closure is for the purpose of carrying out maintenance which shall include any repair alteration, reconditioning, examination or testing of infrastructure;

["entity in charge of maintenance" means an entity in charge of maintenance of a vehicle, and includes a transport undertaking, an infrastructure manager or a keeper;][88]

"European Railway Agency" means the Community agency for railway safety and interoperability established by Regulation (EC) No. 881/2004 of the European Parliament and of the Council establishing a European Railway Agency;

"factory" means a factory within the meaning of section 175 of the Factories Act 1961[89] and premises to which section 123(1) or (2) or 125(1) of that Act applies;

["freight wagon" means a non-self-propelled-vehicle designed for the purpose of transporting freight or other materials to be used for activities such as construction or infrastructure maintenance;][90]

"guided bus system" means a system of transport, used wholly or mainly for the carriage of passengers, that employs buses which for some or all of the time when they are in operation—

    (a) travel along roads; and

    (b) are guided (whether while on the road or at other times) by means of—

        (i) apparatus, a structure or other device which is fixed and not part of the bus; or

        (ii) a guidance system which is automatic;

"guided transport" means a system of transport, used wholly or mainly for the carriage of passengers, employing vehicles which for some or all of the time when they are in operation are guided by means of—

    (a) rails, beams, slots, guides or other apparatus, structures or devices which are fixed and not part of the vehicle; or

    (b) a guidance system which is automatic;

"harbour" and "harbour area" have the meanings assigned to them by regulation 2(1) of the Dangerous Substances in Harbour Areas Regulations 1987[79];

[. . .][91]

---

[86] O.J. No. L122, 11.05.2011, p22.

[87] Definitions inserted by Railways and Other Guided Transport Systems (Miscellaneous Amendments) Regulations 2013/950 reg.3(2)(c) (May 21, 2013).

[88] Definition inserted by Railways and Other Guided Transport Systems (Safety) (Amendment) Regulations 2011/1860 reg.2(2)(b) (August 26, 2011).

[89] Subsection (2)(n) of section 175 was amended by the Factories Act 1961 etc. (the Metrication Regulations 1983 (S.I. 1983/978), regulation 3(1) and Schedule 1; section 123(2) was amended by SI 1974/1941, regulation 2(a) and Schedule 1 ; there are amendments to the Act not relevant to these Regulations.

[99] Definition inserted by Railways and Other Guided Transport Systems (Miscellaneous Amendments) Regulations 2013/950 reg.3(2)(d) (May 21, 2013).

[91] Definition repealed by Railways and Other Guided Transport Systems (Miscellaneous Amendments) Regulations 2013/950 reg.3(2)(e) (May 21, 2013).

"high-speed Directive" means Council Directive 96/48/EC on the interoperability of the trans-European high-speed rail system[92];

"infrastructure" means fixed assets used for the operation of a transport system which shall include, without prejudice to the generality of the foregoing—

    (a) its permanent way or other means of guiding or supporting vehicles;

    (b) any station; and

    (c) plant used for signalling or exclusively for supplying electricity for operational purposes to the transport system;

"infrastructure manager" means the person who—

    (a) in relation to infrastructure other than a station, is responsible for developing and maintaining that infrastructure or, in relation to a station, the person who is responsible for managing and operating that station, except that it shall not include any person solely on the basis that he carries out the construction of that infrastructure or station or its maintenance, repair or alteration; and

    (b) manages and uses that infrastructure or station, or permits it to be used, for the operation of a vehicle;

["Interoperability Directive" means Directive 2008/57/EC of the European Parliament and of the Council of 17th June 2008 on the interoperability of the rail system within the Community (Recast)[93];][94]

"Interoperability Regulations" means the [Railways (Interoperability) Regulations 2011][95];

["keeper" means the person who, being the owner of a vehicle or having the right to use it, exploits the vehicle as a means of transport and is registered as being the keeper in the National Vehicle Register;][96]

"mainline application" means an application for—

    (a) a safety certificate or an amended safety certificate; or

    (b) a safety authorisation or an amended safety authorisation,

made in relation to an operation on the mainline railway;

["mainline railway" means any railway except for any railway or part of a railway—

    (a) that the Office of Rail Regulation determines in accordance with regulation 2A (determination of exclusion from the mainline railway) falls within one of the categories listed in paragraph (1) of that regulation; or

    (b) which is privately owned infrastructure that exists solely for use by the infrastructure owner for its own freight operations;][97]

"mainline railway system" means the mainline railway and the management and operation of the mainline railway as a whole;

---

[92] O.J. No. L235, 17.09.97, p6, corrected by O.J. L262, 16.10.96, p8 and as amended by Directive 2004/50/EC of the European Parliament and the Council of 29th April 2004 (O.J. No. L164, 30.04.2004, p114).

[93] O.J. No. L191, 18.7.2008, p1, as amended by Commission Directive 2009/131/EC (O.J. No. L273, 17.10.2009, p12).

[94] Definition inserted by Railways and Other Guided Transport Systems (Safety) (Amendment) Regulations 2011/1860 reg.2(2)(c) (August 26, 2011).

[95] Word substituted by Railways (Interoperability) Regulations 2011/3066 Sch.1 para.3(a)(i) (January 16, 2012).

[96] Definition inserted by Railways and Other Guided Transport Systems (Safety) (Amendment) Regulations 2011/1860 reg.2(2)(d) (August 26, 2011).

[97] Definition substituted by Railways and Other Guided Transport Systems (Miscellaneous Amendments) Regulations 2013/950 reg.3(2)(f) (May 21, 2013).

["maintenance file" means the written file that contains all the technical and management information that is necessary to carry out the maintenance of a vehicle;"maintenance rules" means any rules, applicable [in][98] Great Britain, which set out requirements relating to the maintenance of vehicles;][99]

"material" includes plant;

"military establishment" means an establishment intended for use for naval, military or air force purposes or for the purposes of the Department of the Secretary of State responsible for defence;

"mine" has the meaning assigned to it by section 180 of the Mines and Quarries Act 1954[100];

"national safety rules" means any legislation and other requirements—

    (a) applicable [in][101] Great Britain; and

    [(b) which contain requirements (including common operating rules) relating to railway safety which are imposed on more than one transport undertaking operating on the mainline railway;][102]

except that where the requirements in sub-paragraph (b) consist of common operating rules of the mainline railway it shall not include such rules which regulate matters which are covered by a TSI;

["National Vehicle Register" means the register of vehicles authorised in Great Britain, required by [regulation 36][103] of the Interoperability Regulations[104];][105]

"new" in relation to regulations 5 and 6 means new to the transport system in question;

"non-mainline application" means an application for—

    (a) a safety certificate or an amended safety certificate; or

    (b) a safety authorisation or an amended safety authorisation,

made in relation to an operation on a transport system other than the mainline railway;

"operator of last resort" means a transport operator appointed by the Secretary of State to provide transport services in accordance with section 30 of the Railways Act 1993;

["owner", in relation to a vehicle, means any person who has an estate or interest in, or a right over, that vehicle, and whose permission is needed before another may use it;][106]

---

[98] Words substituted by Railways and Other Guided Transport Systems (Miscellaneous Amendments) Regulations 2013/950 reg.3(2)(g) (May 21, 2013).

[99] Definitions inserted by Railways and Other Guided Transport Systems (Safety) (Amendment) Regulations 2011/1860 reg.2(2)(e) (August 26, 2011).

[100] Section 180(1) was substituted by SI 1993/1897, regulation 41(2) and Schedule 3, Part II; section 180(2) was repealed by SI 1999/2024, regulation 47(1) and Schedule 2, Part I; section 180(3)(b) was repealed by SI 1999/2024regulation 47(1) and Schedule 2, Part 1 and amended by SI 1999/2024, regulation 47(2) and Schedule 2, Part II; section 180(4) was amended by SI 1999/2024, regulation 47(2) and Schedule 2, Part II and SI 1974/2013, regulation 2(1)(b) and Schedule 2, paragraph 3; section 180(5) was amended by SI 1999/2024, regulation 47(2) and Schedule 2, Part II and by SI 1974/2013, regulation 2(1)(b) and Schedule 2, paragraph 3.

[101] Words substituted by Railways and Other Guided Transport Systems (Miscellaneous Amendments) Regulations 2013/950 reg.3(2)(h)(i) (May 21, 2013).

[102] Substituted by Railways and Other Guided Transport Systems (Miscellaneous Amendments) Regulations 2013/950 reg.3(2)(h)(ii) (May 21, 2013).

[103] Word substituted by Railways (Interoperability) Regulations 2011/3066 Sch.1 para.3(a)(ii) (January 16, 2012).

[104] S.I. 2006/397, to which there are amendments not relevant to these Regulations.

[105] Definition inserted by Railways and Other Guided Transport Systems (Safety) (Amendment) Regulations 2011/1860 reg.2(2)(f) (August 26, 2011).

[106] Definition inserted by Railways and Other Guided Transport Systems (Safety) (Amendment) Regulations 2011/1860 reg.2(2)(g) (August 26, 2011).

"Part A of a safety certificate" means that part of a safety certificate certifying the matters set out in regulation 7(4)(b)(i) and related expressions shall be construed accordingly;

"Part B of a safety certificate" means that part of a safety certificate certifying the matters set out in regulation 7(4)(b)(ii) and related expressions shall be construed accordingly;

["placed in service" means when a vehicle or infrastructure, having been constructed, upgraded or renewed, is first operated in the provision of a transport service, and in ascertaining when this takes place no regard shall be had to any trials or testing that take place to the vehicle or infrastructure, and cognate expressions shall be construed accordingly;][107]

"quarry" has the meaning assigned to it by regulation 3 of the Quarries Regulations 1999[79];

"railway" means a system of transport employing parallel rails which—

(a) provide support and guidance for vehicles carried on flanged wheels; and

(b) form a track which either is of a gauge of at least 350 millimetres or crosses a carriageway (whether or not on the same level),

but does not include a tramway;

"relevant infrastructure manager" means the infrastructure manager for any infrastructure used in relation to the operation in question;

"relevant infrastructure or vehicle" means any new or altered—

(a) infrastructure; or

(b) vehicle,

falling within regulation 5(4) or 6(4) and related expressions shall be construed accordingly;

"responsible person" means in relation to any relevant infrastructure or vehicle, any person who—

(a) has contracted with another person for the manufacture or construction by that other person of that infrastructure or vehicle; or

(b) manufactures or constructs that infrastructure or vehicle for his own use, or for sale to, or use by, another person but not where he is contracted to do so by a person falling under sub-paragraph (a),

and includes an authorised representative established in Great Britain of such a person.

"risk" means in Parts 1 and 2 a risk to the safety of a person;

"road" means in the definition of "guided bus system" and "tramway"—

(a) in England and Wales, any length of highway or of any other road to which the public has access, and includes bridges over which a road passes; and

(b) in Scotland, has the same meaning as in the Roads (Scotland) Act 1984;

"rolling stock" has the meaning in section 83(1) of the Railways Act 1993[79];

"ROTS" means the Railways and Other Transport Systems (Approval of Works, Plant and Equipment) Regulations 1994[108];

"safety authorisation" means a safety authorisation issued by the Office of Rail Regulation in accordance with regulation 10 or 12;

"safety authority" means—

(a) as regards a member State other than the United Kingdom, the authority established in that State in accordance with article 16.1 of the Directive;

---

[107] Definition substituted by Railways and Other Guided Transport Systems (Miscellaneous Amendments) Regulations 2013/950 reg.3(2)(i) (May 21, 2013).

[108] As amended by SIs 1997/553, 2002/1166 and SI 2004/129.

(b) as regards Great Britain, the Office of Rail Regulation; or

(c) as regards Northern Ireland, the Department for Regional Development established by article 3(1) of the Departments (Northern Ireland) Order 1999[109];

"safety certificate" means a safety certificate issued by the Office of Rail Regulation in accordance with regulation 7 or 9;

"safety management system" means the organisation and arrangements established by a transport operator to ensure the safe management of its operation;

"significant safety risk" means, in relation to new or altered infrastructure or a new or altered vehicle the design or construction of which incorporates significant changes compared to any infrastructure or vehicle already in use on the transport system, the capability of significantly increasing an existing safety risk or creating a significant safety risk to—

(a) passengers on the transport system in question; or

(b) members of the public on roads and any other location where the transport system in question operates and to which the public have access (including a place to which the public has access only on making a payment), except a location which is a crossing subject to an Order made under section 1 of the Level Crossings Act 1983[110];

"station" means a passenger stop, station or terminal on a transport system but does not include any permanent way or other means of guiding or supporting vehicles or plant used for signalling or exclusively for supplying electricity for operational purposes to a transport system;

["subsystem" has the same meaning as in the Interoperability Directive;][111]

"technical specifications for interoperability" ("TSIs") means technical specifications for interoperability which are published in the Official Journal of the European Communities pursuant to—

(a) Article 6.1 of the high-speed Directive; [. . .][112]

(b) Article 6.1 of the conventional Directive [; or][113]

[(c) Article 6.1 of the Interoperability Directive,][114]

and in force;

"train" includes any rolling stock;

"tramway" means a system of transport used wholly or mainly for the carriage of passengers—

(a) which employs parallel rails which—

(i) provide support and guidance for vehicles carried on flanged wheels;

---

[109] S.I. 1999/283 (N.I. 1) as amended by the Industrial Development (Northern Ireland) Act 2002, c. 1 (N.I.), section 5(4) and Schedule 4.

[110] Sections 1(1A), (4A), (10A) and (10B) were inserted, section 1(3) was repealed and sections 1(6) and (6A) were substituted for section 1(6) as originally enacted by SI 1997/487, regulations 3(6), 4(2) to (4) and (7) and section 1(7) and (9) were substituted by SI 1997/487, regulation 4(5) and (6), section 1(11) was amended by the Local Government (Wales) Act 1994 (c. 19), sections 22(1), 66(8) and Schedule 7, paragraph 31 and Schedule 18, the Local Government Act 1985 (c.51), section 102 and Schedule 17, the Local Government etc. (Scotland) Act 1994 (c. 39), section 180(1), Schedule 13, paragraph 131, the Transport and Works Act 1992, section 51 (c.42), SI 1997/487, regulation 4(8), and the Road Traffic Regulation Act 1984 (c. 27), section 146 and Schedule 13.

[111] Definition inserted by Railways and Other Guided Transport Systems (Safety) (Amendment) Regulations 2011/1860 reg.2(2)(i) (August 26, 2011).

[112] Word repealed by Railways and Other Guided Transport Systems (Safety) (Amendment) Regulations 2011/1860 reg.2(2)(j)(i) (August 26, 2011).

[113] Added by Railways and Other Guided Transport Systems (Safety) (Amendment) Regulations 2011/1860 reg.2(2)(j)(ii) (August 26, 2011).

      (ii) are laid wholly or partly along a road or in any other place to which the public has access (including a place to which the public has access only on making a payment); and

    (b) on any part of which the permitted maximum speed is such as to enable the driver to stop a vehicle in the distance he can see to be clear ahead;

"transport operator" means any transport undertaking or infrastructure manager;

"transport system" means a railway, a tramway, or any other system using guided transport where that other system is used wholly or mainly for the carriage of passengers but a transport system does not include—

    (a) a guided bus system;
    (b) a trolley vehicle system;
    (c) any part of a transport system—

      (i) within a harbour or harbour area or which is part of a factory, mine or quarry;
      (ii) used solely for the purpose of carrying out a building operation or work of engineering construction;
      (iii) within a maintenance or goods depot;
      (iv) within a siding except where Part 4 applies; or
      (v) which is within a military establishment;

    (d) any fairground equipment;
    (e) any cableway installation; or
    (f) any transport system where the track forms a gauge of less than 350mm except where such a track crosses a carriageway (whether or not on the same level),

except where the transport system in question forms part of the mainline railway;

"transport undertaking" means any person who operates a vehicle in relation to any infrastructure but shall not include a person who operates a vehicle solely within an engineering possession;

"trolley vehicle system" means a system of transport by vehicles constructed or adapted for use on roads without rails under electric power transmitted to them by overhead wires (whether or not there is in addition a source of power on board the vehicles);

["vehicle"—

    (a) includes a mobile traction unit; and
    (b) in respect of the mainline railway, means a vehicle that runs on its own wheels on railway lines of a gauge of at least 350 millimetres, with or without traction, and is composed of one or more structural and functional subsystems or parts of such subsystems;][114]

"work of engineering construction" means the—

    (a) construction of any line or siding otherwise than on an existing transport system; and
    (b) construction, structural alteration, repair (including repointing and repainting) or demolition of any tunnel, bridge or viaduct except where carried on upon a transport system; and

"writing" apart from its usual meaning includes any text transmitted using electronic communications that is received, or accessible by the person to whom it is sent, in legible form.

---

[114] Definition substituted by Railways and Other Guided Transport Systems (Safety) (Amendment) Regulations 2011/1860 reg.2(2)(k) (August 26, 2011).

(2) Any reference in these Regulations to a person who operates a train or a vehicle is a reference to the person operating the train or vehicle for the time being in the course of a business or other undertaking carried on by him, whether for profit or not, but it does not include a self-employed person by reason only that he drives or otherwise controls the movement of a train or vehicle.

(3) Parts 2 and 3 of these Regulations shall not apply to or in relation to the operation of a train or the management or use of infrastructure in the tunnel system within the meaning of section 1(7) of the Channel Tunnel Act 1987.[79]

Registration of Births and Deaths Regulations 1987/2088

PART I

PRELIMINARY

Interpretation

2.—(1) In these Regulations, unless the context otherwise requires—   **A2–273**

["the 2009 Act" means the Coroners and Justice Act 2009;][115]
"the Act" means the Births and Deaths Registration Act 1953;
"approved form" means a form approved by the Registrar General for the purpose for which it is used;
"certificate of cause of death" means a certificate required to be signed by a medical practitioner pursuant to section 22(1) of the Act;
["coroner" includes—

    (a) a senior coroner, area coroner and assistant coroner;
    (b) the Chief Coroner when conducting an investigation under paragraph 1 of Schedule 10 to the 2009 Act; and
    (c) a judge, former judge, or former coroner conducting an investigation under paragraph 3 of Schedule 10 to the 2009 Act;][116]

"description", in relation to a coroner, means his official designation and the area of his jurisdiction;
"entry" means a record of the particulars relating to a live-birth, still-birth or death completed by the registrar in the appropriate spaces in form 1, 9 or 13;
"inquest" includes an inquest which [is conducted as part of an investigation under Part 1 of the Coroners and Justice Act 2009 (including any inquest which has been adjourned)][117];
[["maiden surname" means the surname with which a woman entered into her first marriage or civil partnership, and, where a woman has entered into a civil partnership and marriage, it means the surname with which she entered the first of these ceremonies;][118]] [119]
"name", in relation to a person, excludes surname;

---

[115] Definition inserted by Coroners and Justice Act 2009 (Commencement No. 15, Consequential and Transitory Provisions) Order 2013/1869 Sch.1 para.2(2)(a) (July 25, 2013 as SI 2013/1869 art.4).
[116] Definition substituted by Coroners and Justice Act 2009 (Commencement No. 15, Consequential and Transitory Provisions) Order 2013/1869 Sch.1 para.2(2)(b) (July 25, 2013 as SI 2013/1869 art.4).
[117] Words substituted by Coroners and Justice Act 2009 (Commencement No. 15, Consequential and Transitory Provisions) Order 2013/1869 Sch.1 para.2(2)(c) (July 25, 2013 as SI 2013/1869 art.4).
[118] Definition substituted by Registration of Births and Deaths (Amendment) (England and Wales) Regulations 2009/2165 reg.2(2) (September 1, 2009).
[119] Substituted by Registration of Births and Deaths (Amendment) Regulations 1994/1948 reg.2 (April 1, 1995).

"name, surname and qualification", in relation to a registered medical practitioner who has issued a certificate of cause of death, means his name and surname as stated on the certificate and his registered professional qualification;

["other parent" means a woman who is a parent by virtue of section 42 or 43 of the Human Fertilisation and Embryology Act 2008;][120]

["relevant registrar", in relation to the registration of a birth or death, means (subject to paragraph (3)(b) below) the registrar of the sub-district in which the birth or death occurred.][121]

(2) In these Regulations, unless the context otherwise requires—

(a) any reference to a numbered regulation is to the regulation in these Regulations bearing that number and any reference in a regulation to a numbered paragraph is to the paragraph of that Regulation bearing that number;

(b) any reference to a numbered form is to the form bearing that number in Schedule 2 to these Regulations and any reference to a numbered space in a form is to the space bearing that number in that form.

(3) Where a still-born child is found exposed or a dead body is found, any reference in these Regulations to—

(a) the date of the still-birth or of the death of the deceased person, is to be construed as a reference to the date on which the still-born child or the deceased was found;

(b) the place where the still-birth or death occurred is, if the place is unknown, to be construed as a reference to the place where the still-born child or the deceased was found.

PART II

GENERAL PROVISIONS AS TO REGISTRATION

[Preparation of draft particulars

A2–274   3.—(1) Before commencing registration of a birth or death whether or not in the presence of a qualified informant, the registrar shall, except where paragraph (2) applies, prepare a draft of the particulars to be entered in the register, either–

(a) on an approved form; or

(b) if he has a computer, on that computer.

(2) Before a qualified informant makes a declaration under [[Regulation 13, 34A, or 42A][122],][123] or a statement under [Regulation 17(7)(a)][124] the officer before whom the declaration or statement is to be made shall prepare a draft of the particulars to be entered in the register, either–

(a) on an approved form; or

---

[120] Definition inserted by Registration of Births and Deaths (Amendment) (England and Wales) Regulations 2009/2165 reg.2(3) (September 1, 2009).

[121] Definition substituted by Registration of Births and Deaths Regulations 1987 (Amendment) Regulations 2012/1203 reg.2 (May 28, 2012).

[122] Words substituted by Registration of Births and Deaths Regulations 1987 (Amendment) Regulations 2012/1203 reg.3 (May 28, 2012).

[123] Words substituted by Registration of Births and Deaths (Amendment) Regulations 1997/844 reg.4(2) (April 1, 1997).

[124] Words substituted by Registration of Births and Deaths (Amendment) (England and Wales) Regulations 2009/2165 reg.3 (September 1, 2009).

(b) if he has a computer, on that computer.

(3) Having prepared a draft of the particulars in accordance with paragraph (1) or (2), where the informant is present the officer shall show or read them to him and shall correct any error or omission.][125]

Absence of particulars

4. Where during the registration of a birth or death it appears to the registrar that he **A2–275** cannot enter the particulars required in any space on the appropriate form, other than space 17 on form 1, he shall, subject to any other provision of these Regulations, [enter a line through that space][126] before the informant is called upon to certify the entry.

Signature by mark or in foreign characters

5. Where— **A2–276**

(a) under any provision of these Regulations a person is required to sign a register, declaration or statement in the presence of [. . .][127] a registrar;

(b) that person makes a mark or signs in characters other than those used in the English or Welsh language,

the [. . .][128] registrar concerned shall write against the mark or signature the words "The mark [or signature] of . . . ", inserting the name and surname of the person.

Registration in more than one place

6.—(1) A registrar shall not register a birth or death which has already been registered **A2–277** except—

(a) in accordance with Regulation 36, 45 or 47(4); or

(b) where the Registrar General gives his authority.

(2) Where it appears to a registrar that a birth or death has nevertheless been registered more than once—

(a) if there is no material difference in the particulars recorded, he shall write in the margin of every entry but the original the words "Inadvertently re-registered. For correct entry see No . . . Register No . . . ", inserting the number of the original entry and the number of the register in which it is recorded;

(b) if there is any material difference, he shall report the matter to the Registrar General and shall make such note in the margins of all or any of the entries as the Registrar General may authorise.

(3) Where a birth or death is re-registered on the authority of the Registrar General, the registrar making the new entry and the registrar or superintendent registrar having custody

---

[125] Substituted by Registration of Births and Deaths (Amendment) Regulations 1992/2753 reg.3 (January 1, 1993).
[126] Words substituted by Registration of Births and Deaths (Amendment) Regulations 2006/2827 reg.2 (November 13, 2006).
[127] Words repealed by Registration of Births and Deaths Regulations 1987 (Amendment) Regulations 2012/1203 reg.4(2) (May 28, 2012).
[128] Words repealed by Registration of Births and Deaths Regulations 1987 (Amendment) Regulations 2012/1203 reg.4(3) (May 28, 2012).

of the register in which the original entry was made shall make such notes, if any, in the margin of the respective entries as the Registrar General may authorise.

PART VIII

REGISTRATION OF STILL-BIRTHS

Particulars to be registered and form of register

A2–278   **31.** The particulars concerning a still-birth required to be registered pursuant to section 1(1) of the Act[129] shall, subject to the provisions of this Part of these Regulations, be those required in spaces 1 to 13 in form 9 and that form shall be the prescribed form for registration of still-births for the purposes of section 5 of the Act (which provides for registration of births free of charge).

Certificate and declaration in connection with registration

A2–279   **32.**—(1) The form of the certificate to be signed, pursuant to section 11(1)(a) of the Act,[130] by a registered medical practitioner or a registered midwife for delivery by the qualified informant to the registrar shall be form 10.

(2) The form of the declaration to be made by a qualified informant, pursuant to section 11(1)(b) of the Act,[131] where no certificate is obtained shall be form 11.

Reference to coroner

A2–280   **33.**—(1) Where [the relevant registrar][132] is given information of an alleged still-birth and he has reason to believe that the child was born alive he shall report the matter to the coroner on an approved form.

(2) The registrar shall not register a still-birth which to his knowledge has been reported to the coroner until he has received either a coroner's certificate after inquest or a notification from the coroner that he does not intend to hold an inquest.

[Report to the Registrar General

A2–281   **33A.**—(1) Where a relevant registrar is informed that a still-birth which occurred more than twelve months previously has not been registered, he shall make a report to the Registrar General stating, to the best of his knowledge and belief—

(a) the particulars required to be registered concerning the birth;

(b) the source of his information; and

(c) the name, surname and address of any qualified information available to give information for the registration.

(2) Where a report has been, or is required to be, made to the coroner in accordance with regulation 33, the relevant registrar shall also inform the Registrar General of this fact and, upon receiving a coroner's certificate after inquest or being informed that the coroner does not intend to hold an inquest, notify the Registrar General accordingly.

---

[129] Section 1(1) was amended by paragraph 13(1) of Schedule 3 to the Children Act 1975 (c.72).

[130] Section 11(1)(a) was substituted by section 2(1) of the Population (Statistics) Act 1960 (c.32) and amended by paragraph 7 of Schedule 7 to the Nurses, Midwives and Health Visitors Act 1979 (c.36).

[131] Section 11(1)(b) was amended by paragraph 7 of Schedule 7 to the Nurses, Midwives and Health Visitors Act 1979 (c.36).

[132] Words substituted by Registration of Births and Deaths (Amendment) Regulations 1997/844 reg.2(3) (April 1, 1997).

(3) On being satisfied that the Registrar General has issued his written authority to the relevant registrar for the registration of the still-birth, that registrar, on registering the birth, shall enter in space 15 the words "on the authority of the Registrar General".][133]

Registration where no reference to coroner

34.—(1) In the case of a still-birth in respect of which—   A2–282

(a) a certificate in form 10 or a declaration in form 11 has been delivered to the relevant registrar;

(b) a report has not been, and is not required to be, made to the coroner; and

(c) [. . .][134] the relevant registrar receives personally from a qualified informant information of the particulars required to be registered concerning the birth,

the relevant registrar shall forthwith register the birth and the particulars, if not previously registered, in the presence of the informant on form 9, entering the particulars required in spaces 1 to 13.

(2) Regulations 7(2), 9 and 10 shall apply to the completion of form 9 as they apply to the completion of form 1 but with any necessary modifications, in particular the following—

(a) in space 1 [a][135]—

(i) where a still-born child is found exposed and the date and place of the still-birth are unknown the registrar shall enter the words "Found . . . on . . . ", inserting the relevant place and date,
[. . .][136]

[(aa) in space 1(b) (name and surname) any name and surname given by the informant in respect of the child;][137]

(b) in space 2—

(i) where a certificate in form 10 has been produced, the registrar shall enter the cause of death precisely as stated in the certificate, followed by the words "Certified by . . . " and the name, surname and qualification of the registered medical practitioner or, as the case may be, the name and surname of the midwife and the words "Registered Midwife",

(ii) where a declaration in form 11 has been produced, the registrar shall enter the words "Declaration by informant",

and, except where head (ii) applies, the informant shall not be required to verify the particulars entered in space 2.

---

[133] Added by Registration of Births and Deaths Regulations 1987 (Amendment) Regulations 2012/1203 reg.13 (May 28, 2012).
[134] Words repealed by Registration of Births and Deaths Regulations 1987 (Amendment) Regulations 2012/1203 reg.14 (May 28, 2012).
[135] Word added by Registration of Births and Deaths (Amendment) Regulations 1994/1948 reg.5 (April 1, 1995).
[136] Revoked by Registration of Births and Deaths (Amendment) Regulations 1994/1948 reg.5 (April 1, 1995).
[137] Added by Registration of Births and Deaths (Amendment) Regulations 1994/1948 reg.5 (April 1, 1995).

[Declaration and registration of a still-birth under section 9 of the Act

A2–283   **34A.**—(1) In relation to a still-birth, the officer before whom a declaration for the purposes of section 9(1) of the Act (giving of information to a person other than the registrar) may be made shall be any registrar other than the relevant registrar.

(2) The officer before whom the declaration is to be made shall—

(a) enter in the declaration the particulars required to be registered concerning the still-birth, using an approved form for the purpose;

(b) [show or read the declaration to the informant and correct any error or omission, requiring the informant to initial any amendment if the declaration is prepared in manuscript, and then to sign the declaration][138];

(c) attest the declaration himself; and

(d) send the declaration and either the certificate in form 10 or the declaration in form 11 to the relevant registrar in accordance with section 11(1B)(b) of the Act.

(3) Except in a case to which regulation 33 applies, where it appears to the relevant registrar that the particulars contained in the declaration are in any material respect not proper to be registered, he shall return the declaration to the officer before whom it was attested together with a note of the matters in which it appears to need amendment, and—

(a) that officer shall then in the presence of the declarant amend any error by striking out any incorrect particulars and inserting the correct particulars;

(b) any amendment so made shall be initialled by the declarant and the declaration shall be returned to the relevant registrar.

(4) On receiving the declaration and either the certificate in form 10 or the declaration in form 11 the registrar shall, subject to paragraph (3), enter the particulars of the birth in the register in the following manner—

(a) in spaces 1 and 3 to 13 of form 9, he shall enter the particulars as appearing in the corresponding spaces of the declaration, except that where any particulars have been corrected in pursuance of paragraph (3) he shall enter in the register only the particulars as corrected, omitting any incorrect particular which has been struck out and the initials of the declarant;

(b) in space 2 of form 9, he shall enter the cause of death and nature of the evidence that the child was still-born—

(i) if he has received a certificate in form 10, as they appear in that certificate; or

(ii) if he has received a declaration in form 11, as they appear in the corresponding spaces of the declaration for the purposes of section 9(1) of the Act, except that where those particulars have been corrected in pursuance of paragraph (3) he shall enter in the register only the particulars as corrected, omitting any incorrect particular which has been struck out and the initials of the declarant.

(c) in space 14 of form 9—

---

[138] Words substituted by Registration of Births and Deaths (Amendment) Regulations 2006/2827 reg.8 (November 13, 2006).

    (i) he shall enter the name of the declarant in the form in which he signed the declaration and shall add the words "by declaration dated . . . ", inserting the date on which the declaration was made and signed;

    (ii) if, pursuant to section 9(4) of the Act, a request made under paragraph (b) or (c) of section 10(1) [, or paragraphs (b) or (c) of section 10(1B)][139] of the Act was included in the declaration, he shall after the words required by head (i) make the same addition as, on completion of registration under regulation 10, would be required under (as the case may be) head (ii) or (iii) of paragraph (1)(b) [or (ii) or (iii) of paragraph (1)(c)][140] of that regulation;

    [(iii) if, pursuant to section 9(4A) of the Act, a request made under section 10ZA of the Act was included in the declaration, he shall after the words required by head (i) make the same addition as, on completion of registration under regulation 10, would be required under [paragraph 1(d) of regulation 10][141];][142]

    (d) in space 15 of form 9 he shall enter the date on which the entry is made; and

    (e) in space 16 of form 9 he shall sign the entry, adding his official description.][143]

Registration on coroner's notification where no inquest is held

35.—(1) Where, [in relation to][144] a still-birth which has not already been registered, the relevant registrar receives from a coroner notification that he does not intend to hold an inquest, the registrar shall, subject to [paragraph (2)],[145] take such action as may be required to register the still-birth and the particulars on form 9 in the presence of a qualified informant, entering the particulars required in spaces 1 to 13 in accordance with Regulation 34(2) [or, if a declaration is made for the purposes of section 9(1) of the Act, in accordance with regulation 34A(4)].[146]

    (2) Where the coroner—

    (a) certifies in his notification that an examination made by his direction has disclosed that the child was still-born or that there was not sufficient evidence to show that the child was born alive; and

    (b) delivers to the registrar a certificate showing the result of the examination,

the registrar shall enter in space 2 of form 9 the cause of death precisely as stated in the certificate, followed by the words "Certified by . . . after post-mortem held by direction of . . . ", inserting respectively the name, surname and qualification of the registered medical

A2–284

---

[139] Words inserted by Registration of Births and Deaths (Amendment) (England and Wales) Regulations 2009/2165 reg.19(1) (September 1, 2009).

[140] Words inserted by Registration of Births and Deaths (Amendment) (England and Wales) Regulations 2009/2165 reg.19(2) (September 1, 2009).

[141] Words substituted by Registration of Births and Deaths (Amendment) (England and Wales) Regulations 2009/2165 reg.19(3) (September 1, 2009).

[142] Added by Registration of Births and Deaths (Amendment) Regulations 2003/3048 reg.6 (December 1, 2003).

[143] Added by Registration of Births and Deaths (Amendment) Regulations 1997/844 reg.2(4) (April 1, 1997).

[144] Words substituted by Registration of Births and Deaths Regulations 1987 (Amendment) Regulations 2012/1203 reg.15(2)(a) (May 28, 2012).

[145] Words substituted by Registration of Births and Deaths Regulations 1987 (Amendment) Regulations 2012/1203 reg.15(2)(b) (May 28, 2012).

[146] Words inserted by Registration of Births and Deaths (Amendment) Regulations 1997/844 reg.2(5) (April 1, 1997).

practitioner who made the examination and the name, surname and description of the coroner.

[. . .]¹⁴⁷

Registration on coroner's certificate after inquest

A2–285   **36.**—(1) Where [. . .]¹⁴⁸ the relevant registrar receives a coroner's certificate after inquest from which it appears that the child was still-born or that there was not sufficient evidence to show that the child was born alive, the registrar shall forthwith register the still-birth and the particulars (whether or not already registered) on form 9 as follows—

   (a) in spaces 1 [a, 1b]¹⁴⁹ and 3 to 10, he shall enter, precisely as stated in the coroner's certificate, the particulars contained in the certificate as the particulars to be entered in the respective spaces;

   (b) in space 2, he shall enter the cause of death precisely as stated in the coroner's certificate followed by the words "Certificate after inquest held on . . . ", inserting the date of the inquest as stated in the certificate;

   (c) in spaces 11 and 12 together, he shall enter the name, surname and description of the coroner;

   (d) he shall draw a line through spaces 13 and 14;

   (e) in space 15, he shall enter the date on which the entry is made;

   (f) in space 16 he shall sign the entry and add his official description.

   [(2) If the still-birth has already been registered, the relevant registrar shall register the still-birth and the particulars in accordance with paragraph (1) without making any alteration of the original entry.]¹⁵⁰

Noting of previous entry after coroner's certificate after inquest

A2–286   **37.** Where, in any case to which Regulation 36 applies, the registrar ascertains that an entry in respect of the child has previously been made in any register of live-births, still-births or deaths he shall, after registering the still-birth in accordance with that Regulation—

   (a) if the previous entry is in a still-birth register in his custody, write in the margin of the previous entry the words "Re-registered on coroner's certificate at entry No . . . ", inserting the number of the new entry;

   (b) if the previous entry is in a live-birth or death register in his custody, write in the margin of the previous entry the words "This entry relates to a still-birth and is registered at entry No. . . . in the still-birth register No. . . . ", inserting the numbers of the new entry and of the register;

   (c) if the previous entry is in a live-birth or death register in the custody of a superintendent registrar, give him a copy of the new entry together with particulars of the previous entry whereupon the superintendent registrar shall write in the

---

¹⁴⁷ Revoked by Registration of Births and Deaths Regulations 1987 (Amendment) Regulations 2012/1203 reg.15(3) (May 28, 2012).

¹⁴⁸ Words repealed by Registration of Births and Deaths Regulations 1987 (Amendment) Regulations 2012/1203 reg.16(2) (May 28, 2012).

¹⁴⁹ Words added by Registration of Births and Deaths (Amendment) Regulations 1994/1948 reg.6 (April 1, 1995).

¹⁵⁰ Substituted by Registration of Births and Deaths Regulations 1987 (Amendment) Regulations 2012/1203 reg.16(3) (May 28, 2012).

margin of the previous entry the words "This entry relates to a still-birth and is registered at entry No. . . . . in the still-birth register No. . . . . ", inserting the numbers of the new entry and of the register;

(d) if the previous entry is in a still-birth register in the custody of the Registrar General, send to the Registrar General a copy of the new entry together with particulars of the previous entry.

PART IX

DISPOSAL OF BODIES OF STILL-BORN CHILDREN

Certificates for disposal

38.—(1) The form of the certificate of a registrar to be given under section 11(2) of the Act[151] (preliminaries to disposal of body) that he has registered a still-birth shall be form 12.   **A2–287**

(2) The certificate of a registrar under section 11(2) of the Act that he has received notice of a still-birth shall be given on an approved form but a certificate shall not be given except for the purpose of burial in a burial ground in England or Wales, and then only—

(a) where the case is one which is not required to be reported to the coroner; or

(b) where the case has been reported to the coroner and the registrar has been informed by the coroner that he has completed any investigation which he intends to make and has not issued any order authorising the disposal of the body.

PART X

REGISTRATION OF DEATHS

Particulars to be registered

39. The particulars concerning a death required to be registered pursuant to section 15 of the Act shall, subject to the provisions of this Part of these Regulations, be those required in spaces [1 to 7 and 9][152] in form 13 and that form shall be the prescribed form for registration of deaths for the purpose of section 20 of the Act (which provides for registration of deaths free of charge).   **A2–288**

Certificate of cause of death

40.—(1) Subject to paragraph (2)—   **A2–289**

(a) the form of a certificate of cause of death required to be signed by a registered medical practitioner pursuant to section 22(1) of the Act shall be—

　(i) except in the case of a child who dies within 28 days of birth, form 14,

　(ii) in the case of such a child, form 15;

(b) the form of notice of signing of the certificate of cause of death required by section 22(2) of the Act to be given by the medical practitioner to a qualified informant shall be form 16.

---

[151] Section 11(2) was amended by section 3(3) of the Population (Statistics) Act 1960 (c.32).
[152] Words substituted by Registration of Births and Deaths (Amendment) Regulations 2006/2827 reg.9 (November 13, 2006).

(2) Where the place of death is in England but the certificate of cause of death is issued in Wales—

(a) the form of the certificate or notice may instead be the corresponding form (11, 12 or 13 as the case may be) prescribed by Regulation 2(a) of the Registration of Births and Deaths (Welsh Language) Regulations 1987;

(b) where the corresponding form 11 or 12 is used under sub-paragraph (a) above the version in Welsh shall be disregarded for any other purpose of these Regulations.

Reference to coroner

A2–290   **41.**—(1) Where the relevant registrar is informed of the death of any person he shall, subject to paragraph (2), report the death to the coroner on an approved form if the death is one—

(a) in respect of which the deceased was not attended during his last illness by a registered medical practitioner; or

(b) in respect of which the registrar—

  (i) has been unable to obtain a duly completed certificate of cause of death, or
  (ii) has received such a certificate with respect to which it appears to him, from the particulars contained in the certificate or otherwise, that the deceased was not seen by the certifying medical practitioner either after death or within 14 days before death; or

(c) the cause of which appears to be unknown; or

(d) which the registrar has reason to believe to have been unnatural or to have been caused by violence or neglect or by abortion or to have been attended by suspicious circumstances; or

(e) which appears to the registrar to have occurred during an operation or before recovery from the effect of an anaesthetic; or

(f) which appears to the registrar from the contents of any medical certificate of cause of death to have been due to industrial disease or industrial poisoning.

(2) Where the registrar has reason to believe, with respect to any death of which he is informed or in respect of which a certificate of cause of death has been delivered to him, that the circumstances of the death were such that it is the duty of some person or authority other than himself to report the death to the coroner, he shall either satisfy himself that it has been reported or report it himself.

(3) The registrar shall not register any death—

(a) which he has himself reported to the coroner;

(b) which to his knowledge it is the duty of any other person or authority to report to the coroner; or

(c) which to his knowledge has been reported to the coroner,

until he has received either a coroner's certificate after inquest or a notification from the coroner that he does not intend to hold an inquest.

Registration within twelve months from date of death where no report to coroner

A2–291   **42.**—(1) Where—

(a) a certificate of cause of death has been delivered to the relevant registrar;

(b) the death is not one which has been, or is required to be, reported to the coroner; and

(c) before the expiration of 12 months from the date of death the relevant registrar receives personally from any qualified informant information of the particulars required to be registered concerning the person's death,

the relevant registrar shall forthwith register the death and the particulars, if not previously registered, in the presence of the informant on form 13, entering the particulars required in spaces [1 to 7 and 9][153] in accordance, where applicable, with the following provisions of this Regulation.

(2) In space 1 (date and place of death)—

(a) where a child lived for less than 24 hours, the registrar shall enter after the date of the child's death the word "Aged . . . ", inserting the age in completed hours or, if less than one hour, in minutes;

(b) where the date, but not the place, of death is known, the registrar shall enter the date of death followed by the words "Found dead . . . ", inserting the place where the body was found;

(c) where the place, but not the date, of death is known the registrar shall enter the words "On or about . . . ", inserting the date on which the body was found followed by the place of death;

(d) where both the date and place of death are unknown, the registrar shall enter the words "Deceased found on . . . ", inserting the date on which the body was found followed by the place where it was found.

(3) In space 6 (occupation and usual address of deceased person)—

(a) where the deceased was a child under the age of 16 years, the registrar shall enter the words "son [or daughter] of . . . ", inserting the name, surname and occupation of the father [or other parent][154], if that information is given, and the name, surname and occupation of the mother preceded where appropriate by the word "and" so however that if—

[(i) the names and surnames of the mother, father and other parent are to be entered, whichever is appropriate, and the surname of the mother if it is different from the surname of the father or other parent; and][155]

[(ii) it is within the knowledge of the informant that the mother was known by the surname of the father or the surname of the other parent at any time during the lifetime of the child,][156]

the registrar shall enter in respect of the mother that surname followed by her name and surname as at the death of the child preceded by the word "now" or, if the mother is deceased, the name and surname as at her death preceded by the word "afterwards";

---

[153] Words substituted by Registration of Births and Deaths (Amendment) Regulations 2006/2827 reg.10(1) (November 13, 2006).

[154] Words inserted by Registration of Births and Deaths (Amendment) (England and Wales) Regulations 2009/2165 reg.20(1) (September 1, 2009).

[155] Substituted by Registration of Births and Deaths (Amendment) (England and Wales) Regulations 2009/2165 reg.20(2) (September 1, 2009).

[156] Substituted by Registration of Births and Deaths (Amendment) (England and Wales) Regulations 2009/2165 reg.20(3) (September 1, 2009).

(b) where the deceased was a married woman or widow, the registrar shall, after her occupation enter the words "Wife [or Widow] of . . . ", inserting the name, surname and occupation of her [spouse][157] or deceased [spouse][158] [;][158]

[(ba) where the deceased was a married man or widower, the registrar shall, after his occupation enter the words "Husband [or Widower] of . . . ", inserting the name, surname and occupation of his [spouse][159] or deceased [spouse][160];

(bb) where the deceased was a civil partner or surviving civil partner, the registrar shall, after his occupation enter the words "Civil partner [or Surviving civil partner] of . . . ", inserting the name, surname and occupation of his civil partner or deceased civil partner [;] [160][159]

[(bc) the name, surname and occupation of adoptive parent(s) shall also be entered in space 6.][161]

(4) In space [9][161] (cause of death), the registrar shall enter the cause of death precisely as stated in the certificate of cause of death, followed by the words "Certified by . . . ", inserting the name, surname and qualification of the registered medical practitioner who signed the certificate.

(5) After entering the required particulars in spaces [1 to 7 and 9],[162] the registrar shall call upon the informant to verify the particulars in spaces 1 to 7.

(6) If any error has been made in those particulars, the registrar shall, in the presence of the informant, make the necessary correction as provided in Regulation 54 [when the entry is being prepared in manuscript].[163]

(7) The registrar shall then—

(a) call upon the informant to sign the entry in space [8][164];

(b) enter in space 10 the date on which the entry is made; and

(c) sign the entry in space 11, adding his official description.

[Declaration and registration under section 23A of the Act

A2–292   **42A.**—(1) The officer before whom a declaration for the purposes of section 23A of the Act (giving of information concerning a death to a person other than the registrar) may be made shall be any registrar other than the relevant registrar.

(2) The officer before whom a declaration is to be made shall—

(a) enter in the declaration the particulars required to be registered concerning the death, using an approved form for the purpose;

---

[157] Word substituted by Marriage (Same Sex Couples) Act 2013 (Consequential Provisions) Order 2014/107 Sch.1 para.11(4)(a) (March 13, 2014).

[158] Added by Registration of Births, Deaths and Marriages (Amendment) Regulations 2005/3177 reg.6(2) (December 5, 2005).

[159] Word substituted by Marriage (Same Sex Couples) Act 2013 (Consequential Provisions) Order 2014/107 Sch.1 para.11(4)(b) (March 13, 2014).

[160] Added by Registration of Births and Deaths (Amendment) (England and Wales) Regulations 2009/2165 reg.20(4) (September 1, 2009).

[161] Word substituted by Registration of Births and Deaths (Amendment) Regulations 2006/2827 reg.10(2) (November 13, 2006).

[162] Words substituted by Registration of Births and Deaths (Amendment) Regulations 2006/2827 reg.10(3) (November 13, 2006).

[163] Words inserted by Registration of Births and Deaths (Amendment) Regulations 2006/2827 reg.10(4) (November 13, 2006).

[164] Word substituted by Registration of Births and Deaths (Amendment) Regulations 2006/2827 reg.10(5) (November 13, 2006).

(b) show or read the particulars entered on the form to the informant and correct any error or omission, [where the declaration is being prepared in manuscript][165] requiring the informant to initial any amendment and then to sign the declaration;

(c) attest the declaration himself; and

(d) send the declaration to the relevant registrar in accordance with section 23A(3) of the Act.

(3) Except in a case to which regulation 41 applies, where it appears to the relevant registrar that the particulars contained in the declaration are in any material respect not proper to be registered, he shall return the declaration to the officer before whom it was attested together with a note of the matters in which it appears to need amendment, and—

(a) that officer shall then in the presence of the declarant amend any error by striking out any incorrect particulars and inserting the correct particulars;

(b) any amendment so made shall be initialled by the declarant and the declaration shall be returned to the relevant registrar.

(4) On receiving the declaration the registrar shall subject to paragraph (3), enter the particulars of the death in the register in the following manner—

(a) in spaces 1 to 7 of form 13, he shall enter the particulars as appearing in the corresponding spaces of the declaration, except that where any particulars have been corrected in pursuance of paragraph (3) he shall enter in the register only the particulars as corrected, omitting any incorrect particular which has been struck out and the initials of the declarant;

(b) in space [9][166] of form 13 he shall enter the cause of death as it appears in the certificate of cause of death delivered to the registrar under section 22(1) of the Act;

(c) in space [8][167] of form 13 he shall enter the name of the declarant in the form in which he signed the declaration and shall add the words "by declaration dated . . . ", inserting the date on which the declaration was made and signed;

(d) in space 10 of form 13 he shall enter the date on which the entry is made; and

(e) in space 11 of form 13 he shall sign the entry, adding his official description.][167]

Registration where inquest is not held

43.—(1) Where, before the expiration of 12 months from the date of a death which has   **A2–293** not been registered, the relevant registrar is notified by the coroner that he does not intend to hold an inquest, the registrar shall, subject to paragraph (4), take such action as may be required to register the death and the particulars on form 13 in the presence of a qualified informant, entering the particulars required in spaces [1 to 7 and 9, in accordance with regulation 42(2) to (7) or, if a declaration is made for the purposes of section 23A of the Act,

---

[165] Words inserted by Registration of Births and Deaths (Amendment) Regulations 2006/2827 reg.11(1) (November 13, 2006).

[166] Word substituted by Registration of Births and Deaths (Amendment) Regulations 2006/2827 reg.11(2) (November 13, 2006).

[167] Added by Registration of Births and Deaths (Amendment) Regulations 1997/844 reg.3(2) (April 1, 1997).

in accordance with regulation 42A(4) but subject, in relation to space 9 of form 13 (cause of death), to paragraphs (2) and (3) below][168].

(2) Where the coroner in his notification certifies the cause of death disclosed by any report on a post-mortem examination of the body made [upon a request under section 14 of the 2009 Act][169], the registrar shall enter in space [9][170] of form 13 the cause of death precisely as stated in the notification followed by the words "Certified by . . . ", inserting the name, surname and description of the coroner followed by the words "after post-mortem without inquest".

(3) Where the coroner's notification shows that no post-mortem examination was held by his direction, and the registrar is unable to obtain delivery of a certificate of cause of death, he shall enter in space [9][171] of form 13 the cause of death—

   (a) if the cause is stated in the coroner's notification, precisely as so stated;

   (b) in any other case, as stated by the informant who shall then also verify space [9][172] (as well as spaces 1 to 7).

(4) After the expiration of 12 months from its date a death shall not be registered under this Regulation.

Noting of existing entry on coroner's notification of cause of death

A2–294   **44.** Where the registrar receives a notification as mentioned in Regulation 43(2) in respect of a death which he has already registered on the information of a qualified informant—

   (a) if the register containing the entry is in his custody, he shall, without altering the entry in space [9][172] of form 13, enter in its margin the words "Post-mortem without inquest held by the direction of . . . ", inserting the name, surname and description of the coroner, followed by the words "and cause of death disclosed as . . . ", inserting the cause of death as certified by the coroner;

   (b) if the register containing the entry is in the custody of the superintendent registrar, he shall deliver the notification to the superintendent registrar who shall, without altering the entry of the death, enter in its margin the particulars required by paragraph (a).

[Registration after receipt of declaration and coroner's notification of cause of death

A2–295   **44A.** Where the registrar receives a cation as mentioned in regulation 43(2) in respect of a death in respect of which a declaration has been made for the purposes of section 23A of the Act, but that death has not yet been registered, he shall register that death in accordance with regulation 42A and shall enter in the margin of the entry the particulars required by regulation 44(a).][173]

---

[168] Words substituted by Registration of Births and Deaths (Amendment) Regulations 2006/2827 reg.12(1) (November 13, 2006).

[169] Words substituted by Coroners and Justice Act 2009 (Commencement No. 15, Consequential and Transitory Provisions) Order 2013/1869 Sch.1 para.2(3) (July 25, 2013 as SI 2013/1869 art.4).

[170] Word substituted by Registration of Births and Deaths (Amendment) Regulations 2006/2827 reg.12(2) (November 13, 2006).

[171] Word substituted by Registration of Births and Deaths (Amendment) Regulations 2006/2827 reg.12(3) (November 13, 2006).

[172] Word substituted by Registration of Births and Deaths (Amendment) Regulations 2006/2827 reg.13 (November 13, 2006).

[173] Added by Registration of Births and Deaths (Amendment) Regulations 1997/844 reg.3(4) (April 1, 1997).

Registration after inquest

45. Where, before the expiration of 12 months from the date of a death, the relevant **A2–296** registrar receives with reference to that death a coroner's certificate after an inquest he shall register the death (whether or not it has already been registered) as follows—

(a) in spaces 1 to 6 and [9][174] in form 13, he shall enter the particulars contained in the certificate, precisely as stated in the certificate, except that if any person is named in the certificate as having caused the death his name and surname shall be omitted;

(b) in space 7—

    (i) subject to head (ii) below, he shall enter the words "Certificate received from . . .", inserting the name, surname and description of the coroner followed by the words "Inquest held on . . . ", inserting the date of inquest as stated in the certificate,

    (ii) if the inquest was adjourned, instead of the words "Certificate received from" he shall enter the words "Certificate on inquest adjourned received from",

(c) he shall draw a line through space [8][175];

(d) in space 10, he shall enter the date on which the entry is made;

(e) in space 11, he shall sign the entry and add his official description.

Noting of previous entry on registration after inquest

46. Where under regulation 45 or 47(4) the registrar registers a death which has already **A2–297** been registered on the information of a qualified informant—

(a) if the registrar has custody of the register containing the previous entry, he shall, without altering that entry, write in its margin the words "Re-registered on coroner's certificate at entry No . . . ", inserting the number of the new entry;

(b) where the previous entry is in a register in the custody of a superintendent registrar, he shall give him a copy of the new entry together with particulars of the previous entry whereupon the superintendent registrar shall, without altering the previous entry, write in its margin the words "Re-registered on coroner's certificate at entry No . . . in register No . . . ", inserting the number of the new entry and of the register.

Registration after twelve months

47.—(1) Where in respect of a death which occurred more than 12 months previously **A2–298** a relevant registrar—

(a) is informed that the death has not been registered; or

(b) whether or not it has already been registered on the information of a qualified informant, receives a coroner's certificate upon an inquest with respect to the death,

he shall make a report to the Registrar General enclosing any certificate of the cause of death and any coroner's notification that he does not intend to hold an inquest or coroner's certificate after an inquest.

---

[174] Word substituted by Registration of Births and Deaths (Amendment) Regulations 2006/2827 reg.14(1) (November 13, 2006).
[175] Word substituted by Registration of Births and Deaths (Amendment) Regulations 2006/2827 reg.14(2) (November 13, 2006).

(2) Except in a case to which paragraph (1)(b) applies, the registrar shall, in his report to the Registrar General, state—

(a) to the best of his knowledge and belief, the particulars required to be registered concerning the death;

(b) the source of his information; and

(c) the name, surname and address of any qualified informant available to give information for the registration.

(3) On receiving the Registrar General's written authority to register the death on the information of a qualified informant, the registrar shall arrange for that informant to attend at his office and shall register the death in his presence [or shall enter in the register the particulars of death given in a declaration made for the purposes of section 23A of the Act, in accordance with regulation 42A][176].

(4) On receiving the Registrar General's written authority to register a death in respect of which the registrar has received a coroner's certificate after an inquest the registrar shall proceed to register the death.

(5) Subject to paragraph (6), the provisions of Regulations 42, 43 (other than paragraph (4)) or 45 (as the case may be) shall apply to registration under paragraph (3) or (4) as they apply on a registration within 12 months.

(6) In space 10, after entering the date on which the entry is made, the registrar shall enter the words "On the authority of the Registrar General".

PART XI

DISPOSAL OF BODIES OF DECEASED PERSONS

Interpretation of Part XI

A2–299   **48.** In this Part of these Regulations—

"the 1926 Act" means the Births and Deaths Registration Act 1926;

"certificate for disposal" means any certificate under subsection (1) of section 24 of the Act (certificates as to receipt of notice of and as to registration of death) and "certificate for disposal before registration" means a certificate of a registrar under that subsection that he has received written notice of a death;

"notification of disposal" means a notification as to the date, place and means of disposal of the body of a deceased person which a person effecting the disposal is required by section 3(1) of the 1926 Act to deliver to the relevant registrar.

Certificates and declaration for disposal

A2–300   **49.**—(1) A certificate for disposal shall be given by the relevant registrar on an approved form which, for the use of the person effecting the disposal, shall embody a form of notification of disposal in form 17.

(2) [A registrar may give a certificate for disposal before registration for the purpose of burial or cremation, in England and Wales, but only][177]—

(a) if the death is one which is not required to be reported to the coroner; or

---

[176] Words inserted by Registration of Births and Deaths (Amendment) Regulations 1997/844 reg.3(5) (April 1, 1997).
[177] Words substituted by Registration of Births and Deaths (Amendment) Regulations 2006/2827 reg.15 (November 13, 2006).

(b) if the death has been reported, unless the registrar has received a coroner's certificate after inquest or a notification from a coroner that he does not intend to hold an inquest and the registrar is satisfied that a coroner's order has not been issued authorising the disposal of the body.

(3) The form of a declaration for the purpose of the proviso to section 1(1) of the 1926 Act (disposal by burial on declaration that certificate of registrar or order of coroner has been issued) shall be form 18.

Notification of disposal

50. The person effecting the disposal of the body of a deceased person shall—   **A2–301**

(a) except where paragraph (b) applies—

    (i) write, sign and date the notification of disposal embodied in form 17 or in the coroner's order with regard to the deceased, and

    (ii) detach the notification and deliver it to the relevant registrar;

(b) where a declaration has been made as mentioned in regulation 49(3), notify the relevant registrar in writing in the terms used in form 17.

Enquiry in default of notification of disposal

51.—(1) The period after the issue of a certificate for disposal, or a coroner's order   **A2–302** authorising the disposal of the body, on the expiration of which the registrar (if he has not previously received a notification for disposal) is required to make enquiry under section 24(5) of the Act shall be a period of 14 days after the date of the issue of the certificate of order.

(2) Where in response to such an enquiry the registrar is informed that the body of the deceased person has not been disposed of, he shall, unless he is informed that the body is being held for the purposes of the Anatomy Acts 1832 and 1871 or the Human Tissue Act 1961, report the matter to the officer responsible for matters of environmental health for the district in which the body is lying.

(3) Where after such an enquiry it appears to the registrar that the body has been disposed of and notification of disposal has not been made to him within the time required by section 3(1) of the 1926 Act—

(a) he shall immediately ask the person effecting the disposal of the body to deliver the notification to him; and

(b) if the notification is not received within three days he shall report the matter to the Registrar General.

Certificate that death is not required to be registered

52. The form of a certificate of a registrar for the purposes of section 24(2) of the Act that   **A2–303** a death is not required to be registered in England or Wales shall be form 19.

Time when entry is complete

53. An entry of a birth or death made by a registrar shall for the purposes of these   **A2–304** Regulations be deemed to have been completed when the registrar has signed the entry and added his official description.

PART XII

CORRECTION OF ERRORS

Correction of entry before completion

A2–305   **54.**—(1) Where under these Regulations a registrar is required to correct an error in an entry [, which he is preparing in manuscript]^{178} of a birth or death before the completion of the entry, he shall, subject to paragraph (2), make the correction in the following manner—

(a) if a word is incorrect, he shall strike it out by a line drawn through it, but so that the word remains legible, and shall write the correct word above it;

(b) if in any group of figures one or more is incorrect, he shall strike out all the figures by a line drawn through them, but so that they remain legible, and shall write the correct figures above them;

(c) if a word has been omitted, he shall place a caret where the omission occurs and above the caret he shall write the omitted word, except that if there is sufficient space he shall write the word where the omission occurs and underline it;

[. . .]^{179}

(e) if the particulars required to be entered in any two spaces have been inadvertently transposed, the registrar shall, without any other correction, write in the margin of the entry a note of the error in the following form: "The particulars in . . . and . . . inadvertently transposed", inserting the numbers of the spaces and adding his initials.

(2) If it appears that an error has been made in his signature, the informant shall make the correction [. . .].^{180}

Correction of minor clerical errors after completion

A2–306   **55.**—(1) Where it appears or is represented to the superintendent registrar or the registrar that in any completed entry made [. . .]^{181} in a register of live-births, still-births or deaths in his custody there is any clerical error to which this Regulation applies he shall [correct the error as provided in regulation 55(3)].^{182}

(2) The clerical errors to which this Regulation applies are—

(a) any error—

(i) in spelling any word which is not the name or surname of any person, or

(ii) consisting of the misplacement or incorrect repetition of any such word,

made on entering the particulars other than by copying from a document specified in sub-paragraph (f);

---

^{178} Words inserted by Registration of Births and Deaths (Amendment) Regulations 2006/2827 reg.16(1) (November 13, 2006).

^{179} Revoked by Registration of Births and Deaths (Amendment) Regulations 2006/2827 reg.16(2) (November 13, 2006).

^{180} Words repealed by Registration of Births and Deaths (Amendment) Regulations 2006/2827 reg.16(3) (November 13, 2006).

^{181} Words repealed by Registration of Births and Deaths (Amendment) Regulations 2006/2827 reg.17(1)(a) (November 13, 2006).

^{182} Words substituted by Registration of Births and Deaths (Amendment) Regulations 2006/2827 reg.17(1)(b) (November 13, 2006).

(b) the incorrect statement or omission—

    (i) in the date of registration, of the day or the month (but not both) provided it is evident from the preceding and succeeding entries which day or month should have been inserted,

    (ii) of the year of the birth or death to which an entry relates or of the year of registration (but not of both);

(c) the omission of all the words required to be added, in space 14 of a birth entry, [under these Regulations][183];

[(cc) omission of the words required to be added in space 15 of a birth entry [under these Regulations][184];][185]

(d) the omission of any of the words (including the date) required to be added, following the entry of a name in space 17 of a birth entry, by Regulation 14(2)(a) or (b);

[(e) the omission of—

    (i) any of the words (including the name, surname and qualification of the registered medical practitioner) "Certified by . . . " required to be entered, in space [9][186] of a death entry, by Regulation 42(4),

    (ii) any of the words (including the name, surname and description of the coroner) "Certified by . . . after post-mortem without inquest" required to be entered, in space [9][7] of a death entry by Regulation 43(2),

    (iii) any of the words (including the name, surname and description of the coroner and the date of inquest) "Certificate received from . . . Inquest held on . . . " required to be entered, in space 7 of a death entry, by Regulation 45(b)(i),

    (iv) any of the words (including the name, surname and description of the coroner) "Certificate on inquest adjourned received from . . . " required to be entered in space 7 of a death entry, by Regulation 45(b)(ii);][187]

(f) any error in copying any particulars required to be copied from—

    (i) a declaration made in accordance with Regulation 13 [, 34A or 42A],[188]

    (ii) a certificate of name given in baptism, or a certificate of name given other than in baptism, delivered in pursuance of section 13(1) of the Act,[189]

    (iii) a certificate of cause of death,

    (iv) a doctor's or midwife's certificate of still-birth,

    (v) a coroner's notification after post-mortem without inquest; or

    (vi) a coroner's certificate after inquest;

---

[183] Words substituted by Registration of Births and Deaths (Amendment) Regulations 2006/2827 reg.17(2) (November 13, 2006).

[184] Words substituted by Registration of Births and Deaths (Amendment) Regulations 2006/2827 reg.17(3) (November 13, 2006).

[185] Added by Registration of Births and Deaths (Amendment No. 2) Regulations 1997/1533 reg.2(5)(a) (July 1, 1997).

[186] Word substituted by Registration of Births and Deaths (Amendment) Regulations 2006/2827 reg.17(4) (November 13, 2006).

[187] Substituted by Registration of Births and Deaths (Amendment) Regulations 1989/497 reg.9(2) (April 1, 1989).

[188] Words inserted by Registration of Births and Deaths (Amendment) Regulations 1997/844 reg.4(3)(b) (April 1, 1997).

[189] Section 13(1) was amended by Schedule 2 to the Registration of Births, Deaths and Marriages (Fees) Order 1968 (S.I. 1968/1242).

(g) [any error, in space 14 of a birth entry, in copying the date of a statutory declaration as required by regulations 10(1)(b)(ii) or (iii), or 10(1)(c)(ii) or (iii) or 17(2)(b)(i) or (ii), or 17(4)(i)or(ii)],[190]

and the references in this paragraph to provisions of these Regulations include any corresponding provision of regulations revoked by these Regulations.

[(3) Where any correction is made under paragraph (1), the superintendent registrar or registrar concerned shall enter a marginal note providing details of the correction and where an error has occurred the following wording shall apply—

"In space [or column] . . . corrected to . . . on . . . by me . . . registrar [or superintendent registrar]"

and the registrar or superintendent registrar shall complete and sign the note in the places provided;
where an omission has occurred the following wording shall apply—

"In space [or column] . . . for . . . read . . . corrected on . . . by me . . . registrar [or superintendent registrar]"

and the registrar or superintendent registrar shall complete and sign the note in the places provided; and
where particulars have been transposed the following wording shall apply—

"The particulars in . . . and . . . inadvertently transposed",

and the registrar or superintendent registrar shall complete and sign the marginal note.][191]
[. . .][192]

Correction of other minor clerical errors after completion

56.—[(1) Where it appears or is represented to the superintendent registrar or the registrar that there is any clerical error to which this regulation applies in a completed entry made on the information of a qualified informant in a register of live-births in his custody, he shall correct the error in the presence of an informant.][193]

[(2) Where an error is corrected in accordance with paragraph (1) the following wording shall apply—

"In space [or column] . . . corrected to . . . on . . . by me . . . registrar [or superintendent registrar] in the presence of . . . ",

and where an omission is corrected in accordance with paragraph (1) the following wording shall apply—

"In space [or column] . . . for . . . read . . . corrected on . . . by me . . . registrar [or superintendent registrar] in the presence of . . . "

---

[190] Substituted by Registration of Births and Deaths (Amendment) (England and Wales) Regulations 2009/2165 reg.21 (September 1, 2009).
[191] Substituted by Registration of Births and Deaths (Amendment) Regulations 2006/2827 reg.17(5) (November 13, 2006).
[192] Revoked by Registration of Births and Deaths (Amendment) Regulations 2006/2827 reg.17(6) (November 13, 2006).
[193] Substituted by Registration of Births and Deaths (Amendment) Regulations 2006/2827 reg.18(1) (November 13, 2006).

and the registrar or superintendent registrar shall complete and sign the note in the places provided.][194]

(3) [This][195] Regulation applies to the following clerical errors—

(a) in a live-birth entry (form 1)—

    (i) in space 1, in the date or place of birth, but not both, provided the correct place of birth is within the sub-district where the birth was registered and the correct date of birth is within 3 months of the date of registration,

    (ii) in space 5, in the father's [or other parent's][196] place of birth,

    (iii) in space 6, in the father's [or other parent's][197] occupation,

    [(iv) in space 8a, in the mother's place of birth and in space 8b in the mother's occupation,][198]

    (v) in space 10, in the mother's usual address,

    (vi) in space 12, in the qualification of the informant, unless neither the father nor the mother [nor the other parent][199], provided the identity of the informant is clear from the signature in space 14 and this is consistent with the information in space 4 or 7,

    (vii) in space 13, in the usual address of informant,

(b) in a death entry (form 13)—

    (i) in space 1, in the date or place of death, but not both, provided the corrected place of death is within the sub-district in which the death was registered and the corrected date of death is within 12 months of the date of registration,

    (ii) in space 3, consisting of the omission of the sex of the deceased provided the sex as corrected is consistent with the name of the deceased in space 2,

    (iii) in space 4, in the deceased's maiden surname,

    (iv) in space 5, consisting of the incorrect statement or omission of one, but not both, of the date or place of birth but, in the case of an incorrect statement of the [former][200] only if the date is not corrected by more than one year,

    (v) in space 6, consisting of the incorrect statement or omission of the occupation of the deceased or of the deceased's husband [or wife or civil partner][201] or parents or of the usual address of the deceased or of the omission of the words "son [or daughter] of . . . " and of the names and surnames of the deceased's parents,

    (vi) in space 7(a), in the informant's name or surname provided this is consistent with the signature in space 9,

    (vii) in space 7(c), in the informant's usual address.

    [. . .][202]

---

[194] Substituted by Registration of Births and Deaths (Amendment) Regulations 2006/2827 reg.18(2) (November 13, 2006).

[195] Words substituted by Registration of Births and Deaths (Amendment) Regulations 2006/2827 reg.18(3) (November 13, 2006).

[196] Words inserted by Registration of Births and Deaths (Amendment) (England and Wales) Regulations 2009/2165 reg.22(1) (September 1, 2009).

[197] Words inserted by Registration of Births and Deaths (Amendment) (England and Wales) Regulations 2009/2165 reg.22(2) (September 1, 2009).

[198] Para.(iv) substituted for paras.(iiia) and (iv) subject to savings by Registration of Births and Deaths (Amendment) Regulations 1994/1948 reg.7 (April 1, 1995).

[199] Words inserted by Registration of Births and Deaths (Amendment) (England and Wales) Regulations 2009/2165 reg.22(3) (September 1, 2009).

[200] Word substituted by Registration of Births and Deaths (Amendment) Regulations 1989/497 reg.10(b) (April 1, 1989).

[201] Words inserted by Registration of Births, Deaths and Marriages (Amendment) Regulations 2005/3177 reg.6(3) (December 5, 2005).

[202] Revoked by Registration of Births and Deaths (Amendment) Regulations 2006/2827 reg.18(4) (November 13, 2006).

Correction of other clerical after completion

A2–308   **57.**—(1) Where it appears or is represented to a superintendent registrar or a registrar that in a completed entry made [. . .]²⁰³, on the information of a qualified informant, in a register of live-births, still-births, or deaths in his custody, there is a clerical error other than one to which [Regulation 55, 56 or 59(2)]²⁰⁴ applies, he shall send a report to the Registrar General and shall include with his report—

    (a) such evidence as the Registrar General may require for the purpose of verifying the facts;

    (b) the name and surname of the qualified informant (if any) who will be available to witness correction of the error; and

    (c) a copy of the entry.

(2) On receiving the authority of the Registrar General the superintendent registrar or the registrar concerned shall correct the error [. . .]²⁰⁵ in the presence of the qualified informant specified in the authority of the Registrar General.

[(3) Where any correction is made under paragraph (2) the registrar or the superintendent registrar concerned shall enter a marginal note in the following form—

"In space [or column] . . . corrected to . . . on . . . by me . . . [registrar or superintendent registrar] in the presence of . . . on the authority of the Registrar General"

and he shall complete and sign the note in the places provided, whereupon—

    (a) the informant shall sign the note in the place provided; and

    (b) the superintendent registrar or the registrar concerned shall after the signature of the informant add the informant's qualification for giving information concerning the correction.

(4) Where no qualified informant is available to witness the correction, the superintendent registrar or the registrar concerned shall write a marginal note in the following form—

"In space [or column] . . . corrected to . . . on . . . by me . . . registrar [or superintendent registrar] on the authority of the Registrar General"

and he shall complete and sign the note in the places provided.]²⁰⁶

Correction of errors of fact or substance

A2–309   **58.**—(1) Where it appears or is represented to a superintendent registrar or a registrar that there is an error of fact or substance in a completed entry in a register of live-births, still-births or deaths in his custody, other than an entry to which Regulation 59 applies, he shall—

---

²⁰³ Words repealed by Registration of Births and Deaths (Amendment) Regulations 2006/2827 reg.19(1) (November 13, 2006).

²⁰⁴ Figure substituted by Registration of Births and Deaths (Amendment) Regulations 1988/638 reg.5 (April 4, 1988).

²⁰⁵ Words repealed by Registration of Births and Deaths (Amendment) Regulations 2006/2827 reg.19(2) (November 13, 2006).

²⁰⁶ Substituted by Registration of Births and Deaths (Amendment) Regulations 2006/2827 reg.19(3) (November 13, 2006).

(a) send a report to the Registrar General giving such information as the Registrar General may require and enclosing a copy of the entry; and

(b) comply with any instructions which the Registrar General may give for the purpose of verifying the facts of the case and ascertaining whether there are available two persons qualified to make a statutory declaration required by section 29(3) of the Act[207].

(2) On being informed by the Registrar General that the error may be corrected on production of such a statutory declaration, the superintendent registrar or the registrar concerned shall on production to him of the statutory declaration correct the error in the following manner—

[. . .][208]

(b) he shall write in the margin of the entry a note in the following form (or such other form as the Registrar General may authorise in any particular case)—

"In No . . . . in . . . . for . . . . read . . . . Corrected on . . . . by me . . . . Superintendent Registrar (or Registrar) on production of a statutory declaration made by . . . . and . . . .",

and he shall enter the particulars of the correction and of the declarants and complete and sign the note in the places provided.

Correction of error on coroner's certificate

59.—(1) Where the superintendent registrar or the registrar having the custody of a register containing an entry made in pursuance of a coroner's certificate after inquest receives— **A2–310**

(a) notification from the coroner of a clerical error in the certificate [. . .][209]; or

(b) a certificate relating to that entry given by the coroner pursuant to section 29(4)(a) or (b) of the Act[210], as to an error of fact or substance in the certificate after inquest and as to the true facts of the case,

he shall send a report to the Registrar General, enclosing a copy of the entry and (as the case may be) of the coroner's certificate and notification, or of the coroner's certificates, relating to the entry.

[(2) Where the error is a clerical error, the superintendent registrar or the registrar shall correct the error by entering a marginal note in the following form—

"Clerical error in space [or column] . . . corrected to . . . on . . . by me . . . registrar [or superintendent registrar] on receipt of notification from the Coroner",

and he shall complete and sign the note in the places provided.][211]

---

[207] Section 29(3) was amended by Schedule 2 to the Registration of Births, Deaths and Marriages (Fees) Order 1968 (S.I. 1968/1242).

[208] Revoked by Registration of Births and Deaths (Amendment) Regulations 2006/2827 reg.20 (November 13, 2006).

[209] Words repealed by Registration of Births and Deaths (Amendment) Regulations 2006/2827 reg.21(1) (November 13, 2006).

[210] Section 29(4) was amended by Schedule 12 to the Criminal Law Act 1977 (c.45) and by Schedule 2 to the Coroners Act 1980 (c.38).

[211] Substituted by Registration of Births and Deaths (Amendment) Regulations 2006/2827 reg.21(2) (November 13, 2006).

(3) Where the error is one of fact or substance the superintendent registrar or the registrar shall correct the error by—

[. . .]²¹²

[(b) entering a marginal note in the following form—

"In space [or column] . . . corrected to . . . on . . . by me . . . registrar [or superintendent registrar] on the authority of a certificate from the Coroner",]²¹³

and he shall complete and sign the note in the places provided.

Copy of corrected or annotated entry to be sent to Registrar General

A2–311   **61.**—(1) Where a superintendent registrar or a registrar makes any correction or annotation to a completed entry in a register of live-births, still-births or deaths, whether by marginal note or otherwise, he shall, subject to paragraph (2), within seven days make and send to the Registrar General a copy of the entry as corrected or annotated (or both), including a copy of any marginal note, certified by—

(a) the registrar, if the register containing the entry is in his custody [. . .]²¹⁴; or

[. . .]¹

(c) the superintendent registrar, where the register containing that entry is in his custody,

together, in any case where a birth is re-registered under section 10A of the Act,²¹⁵ with a copy of the new entry, certified by the registrar who made that entry.

(2) Paragraph (1) shall apply in relation to a correction or annotation made by a registrar under Regulations 55 and 56 only if the correction or annotation is made after the registrar has certified a true copy of the original entry pursuant to section 26(1)(a) of the Act (quarterly returns).

(3) Where a registrar has re-registered a birth under either [section 10A, 14(1) or 14A]²¹⁶ of the Act²¹⁷ and the previous entry is in a register in the custody of a superintendent registrar the registrar shall within seven days of the re-registration provide the superintendent registrar with a certified copy of the new entry.

[(4) Where the information in a completed entry in a register of live-births, still-births or deaths exists in an electronic form approved by the Registrar General under the Act, then the information in a correction or annotation made under paragraph (1) must be incorporated into the information in that electronic form after the correction or annotation has been made.]²¹⁸

---

²¹² Revoked by Registration of Births and Deaths (Amendment) Regulations 2006/2827 reg.21(3) (November 13, 2006).

²¹³ Substituted by Registration of Births and Deaths (Amendment) Regulations 2006/2827 reg.21(4) (November 13, 2006).

²¹⁴ Words repealed by Registration of Births and Deaths (Amendment) Regulations 2006/2827 reg.23(1) (November 13, 2006).

²¹⁵ Section 10A was inserted by section 93(2) of the Children Act 1975 (c.72).

²¹⁶ Words substitued by Registration of Births and Deaths (Amendment) Regulations 1988/638 reg.6 (April 4, 1988).

²¹⁷ Section 14(1) was amended by paragraph 13(3) of Schedule 3 to the Children Act 1975 (c.72) and by paragraph 1(b) of Schedule 1 to the Matrimonial Causes Act 1973 (c.18).

²¹⁸ Added by Registration of Births and Deaths (Amendment) Regulations 2006/2827 reg.23(2) (November 13, 2006).

SCHEDULE 2

PRESCRIBED FORMS

Contents

Form	Relevant Regulation	Description	Statutory purpose
9	31	Particulars of still-birth	The Act, sections 1(1) and 5
10	32(1)	Medical certificate of still-birth	The Act, section 11(1)(a)
11	32(2)	Declaration as to still-birth	The Act, section 11(1)(b)
12	38(1)	Certificate that registrar has registered still-birth	The Act, section 11(2)
13	39	Particulars of death	The Act, sections 15 and 20
14	40(1)(a)(i)	Medical certificate of cause of death except for child dying within 28 days of birth	The Act, section 22(1)
15	40(1)(a)(ii)	Medical certificate of cause of death for child dying within 28 days of birth	The Act, section 22(1)
16	40(1)(b)	Medical practitioner's notice to informant of death	The Act, section 22(2)
17	49(1)	Notification	Births and Deaths Registration Act 1926, section 3(1)
18	49(3)	Declaration that certificate or order has been issued	Births and Deaths Registration Act 1926, section 1(1)
19	52	Certificate that death is not required to be registered	The Act, section 24(2)

[FORM 9

A2–313

Stillbirth

	STILL- BIRTH	Entry No.
Registration district		Administrative area
Sub-district		
1.(a) Date and place of birth	**CHILD**	
1.(b) Name and surname		
2. Cause of death and nature of evidence that child was still-born		**3. Sex**
4. Name and surname	**FATHER/PARENT**	
5. Place of birth	**6.** Occupation	
7. Name and surname	**MOTHER**	
8.(a) Place of birth	**8.(b)** Occupation	
9.(a) Maiden surname	**9.(b)** Surname at marriage/civil partnership if different from maiden surname	
10. Usual address (if different from place of child's birth)		
11. Name and surname (if not the mother or father/parent) **INFORMANT** **12.** Qualification		
13. Usual address (if different from that in 10 above)		
14. I certify that the particulars entered above are true to the best of my knowledge and belief		Signature of informant
15. Date of registration	**16.** Signature of registrar	

][219]

---

[219] Forms substituted by Registration of Births and Deaths (Amendment) (England and Wales) Regulations 2009/2165 Sch.1 para.1 (September 1, 2009).

FORM 10

MEDICAL CERTIFICATE OF STILL-BIRTH

Regulation 32(1)   Births and Deaths Registration Act 1953, s.11(1)(*a*)   **A2–314**

★ I was present at the still-birth of a $\dfrac{\text{male}★}{\text{female}★}$ child born

I have examined the body of a $\dfrac{\text{male}★}{\text{female}★}$ child which I am informed and believed was born

on .... day of .... to ....

(name of mother)

at ....

(place of birth)

† 1. The certified cause of death has been confirmed by post-mortem.

2. Information from post-mortem may be available later.

3. Post-mortem not being held.

Weight of fetus .... grams

Estimated duration of pregnancy
State (a) the number of weeks at delivery ....
(b) when the child died
   (i) before labour★
   (ii) during labour★
   (iii) not known★

† Please ring appropriate digit
★ Strike out the words that do not apply

CAUSE OF DEATH

a. Main diseases or conditions in fetus

b. Other diseases or conditions in fetus

c. Main maternal diseases or conditions affecting fetus

d. Other maternal diseases or conditions affecting fetus

e. Other relevant causes

I hereby certify that (i) the child was not born alive, and
                    (ii) to the best of my knowledge and belief the cause of death and the estimated duration of pregnancy of the mother were as stated above.

Signature .... Date ....

Qualifications as registered by General
Medical Council, or Registered no. as
Registered Midwife   ....

Address ....

For still-births in hospital:
Please give the name of the consultant responsible for the care of the mother.

....

[FORM 11

DECLARATION AS TO STILL-BIRTH

A2–315

DECLARATION AS TO STILL-BIRTH

Date of still-birth ....

Place of still-birth ....

Name and surname of mother of
still-born child ....

Usual address of mother of child ....

Reason why a certificate that the child was not born alive cannot be obtained from a registered medical practitioner or registered midwife

....

....

....

I, declare that the particulars stated above are true to the best of my knowledge and belief, and that the child mentioned above was not born alive.

Signature ....   Date ....

State whether "Mother", "Father", of the
child or in what other capacity liable to
give information concerning the still-
birth ....

][220]

FORM 12

A2–316   CERTIFICATE THAT REGISTRAR HAS REGISTERED STILL-BIRTH

Regulation 38(1)   Births and Deaths Registration Act 1953, s.11(2)

I, the undersigned registrar, do hereby certify that I have this day registered the birth of the still-born

child of ....

....

which took place on .... at ....

Entry No. .... Signature of registrar ....

Date ....

Registration District .... Sub-District ....

---

[220] Forms substituted by Registration of Births and Deaths (Amendment) Regulations 1994/1948 Sch.1 para.1 (April 1, 1995).

[FORM 13

PARTICULARS OF DEATH

PARTICULARS OF DEATH

DEATH	Entry No.	
Registration district Sub-district	Administrative area	
1. Date and place of death		
2. Name and surname	3. Sex	
	4. Maiden surname of woman who has married	
5. Date and place of birth		
6. Occupation and usual address		
7.(a) Name and surname of informant	(b) Qualification	
(c) Usual address		
8. I certify that the particulars given by me above are true to the best of my knowledge and belief	Signature of informant	
9. Cause of death		
10. Date of registration	11. Signature of registrar	

]221

---

221 Form substituted by Registration of Births and Deaths (Amendment) Regulations 2006/2827 Sch.1 para.1 (November 13, 2006).

FORM 14

MEDICAL CERTIFICATE OF CAUSE OF DEATH EXCEPT FOR CHILD DYING WITHIN 28 DAYS OF BIRTH

A2–318   Regulation 40(1)(*a*)(i)   Births and Deaths Registration Act 1953, s.22(1)

Name of deceased ....

Date of death as stated to me .... day of .... Age as stated to me ....

Place of death ....

Last seen alive by me .... day of ....

1. The certified cause of death takes account of information obtained from post-mortem.
2. Information from post-mortem may be available later.
3. Post-mortem not being held.
4. I have reported this death to the Coroner for further action.

Please ring appropriate digit(s) and letter.

a. Seen after death by me.
b. Seen after death by another medical practitioner but not by me.
c. Not seen after death by a medical practitioner.

CAUSE OF DEATH	
The condition thought to be the 'Underlying Cause of Death' should appear in the lowest completed line of Part I.	These particulars not to be entered in death registered
	Approximate interval between onset and death
I(a) Disease or condition directly leading to death†	....
(b) Other disease or condition, if any, leading to I(a)	....
(c) Other disease or condition, if any, leading to I(b)	....
II Other significant condition CONTRIBUTING TO THE DEATH but not related to the disease or condition causing it.	....

The death might have been due to or contributed to by the employment followed ☐ Please tick where at some time by the deceased.   applicable.

† This does not mean the mode of dying, such as heart failure, asphyxia, asthenia, etc: it means the disease, injury, or complication which caused death.

I hereby certify that I was in medical attendance during the above named deceased's last illness, and that the particulars and cause of death above written are true to the best of my knowledge and belief.

Signature ....

Residence ....

Qualifications as registered by General Medical Council

Date ....

For deaths in hospital: Please give the name of the consultant responsible for the above named as a patient ....

FORM 15

MEDICAL CERTIFICATE OF CAUSE OF DEATH FOR CHILD DYING WITHIN 28 DAYS OF BIRTH

Regulation 40(1)(*a*)(ii)   Births and Deaths Registration Act 1953, s.22   **A2–319**

Name of child ....   Sex ....

Date of death ....   day of ....

Age at death .... days (complete period of 24 hrs) .... hours

Place of death ....

Place of birth ....

Last seen alive by me .... day of ....

1. The certified cause of death has been confirmed by post-mortem.

   a. Seen after death by me.
   b. Seen after death by another medical practitioner but not by me.
   c. Not seen after death by a medical practitioner.

2. Information from post-mortem may be available later.

3. Post-mortem not being held.

4. I have reported this death to the Coroner for further action.

† Please ring appropriate digit(s) and letter

CAUSE OF DEATH

a.   Main diseases or conditions in infant

b.   Other diseases or conditions in infant

c.   Main maternal diseases or conditions affecting infant

d.   Other maternal diseases or conditions affecting infant

e.   Other relevant causes

I hereby certify that I was in medical attendance durng the above-named deceased's last illness and that the particulars and cause of death above written are true to the best of my knowledge and belief.

Signature .... Date ....

Qualifications as registered by General Medical Council ....

Address ....

For deaths in hospital:

Please give the name of the consultant responsible for the above-named as a patient.

....

FORM 16

MEDICAL PRACTITIONER'S NOTICE TO INFORMANT OF DEATH

A2–320   Regulation 40(1)(*b*)   Births and Deaths Registration Act 1953, s.22(2)

I hereby give notice that I have this day signed a medical certificate of cause of death of ....

....

Signature ....   Date ....

This notice is to be delivered by the informant to the registrar of births and deaths for the sub-district in which the death occurred.

FORM 17

NOTIFICATION

A2–321   Regulation 49(1)   Births and Deaths Registration Act 1926, s.3(1)

This is to notify that the body of .... deceased,

who died on .... at ....

was buried/cremated★ on .... at ....

Signature ....

on behalf of ....

Date ....

★ Strike out whichever does not apply

FORM 18

DECLARATION THAT CERTIFICATE OR ORDER HAS BEEN ISSUED

A2–322   Regulation 49(3)   Births and Deaths Registration Act 1926, s.1(1)

I, ... of ....

in pursuance of the Births and Deaths Registration Act 1926, declare:—

(1) That I am the person procuring the burial of the body of ....

who died at .... on the ....

(2) that a $\frac{\text{registrar's certificate}★}{\text{coroner's order}}$ authorising burial was issued by the

$\frac{\text{registrar}★}{\text{coroner}}$ .... at ....

to .... living at ....

on ....; and,

(3) that the reason why the said document cannot be delivered before burial is that

....

....

....

....

I make this declaration believing the same to be true.

Signature of declarant ....

Date ....

* Strike out whichever does not apply

FORM 19

CERTIFICATE THAT DEATH IS NOT REQUIRED TO BE REGISTERED   **A2–323**

Regulation 52   Births and Deaths Registration Act 1953, s.24(2)

I, the undersigned registrar, hereby certify that, on the information declared before me, it appears that the death of ....
is not required by law to be registered in England or Wales.

Date .... Signature ....
Registrar of Births and Deaths

Registration District .... Sub-District ....

Registration of Births and Deaths (Welsh Language) Regulations 1987/2089

Citation, commencement and interpretation

1.—(1) These Regulations may be cited as the Registration of Births and Deaths (Welsh   **A2–324** Language) Regulations 1987 and shall come into force on 1st January 1988.

(2) In these Regulations, unless the context otherwise requires—

(a) "the Act" means the Births and Deaths Registration Act 1953;

(b) "the principal Regulations" means the Registration of Births and Deaths Regulations 1987 and any expression used in these Regulations which is also used in the principal Regulations has the same meaning as in those Regulations;

(c) any reference in a regulation to a numbered paragraph is to the paragraph of that regulation bearing that number;

(d) any reference to a numbered form is to the form bearing that number in Schedule 2 to these Regulations.

(3) Where a still-born child is found exposed or a dead body is found, any reference in these Regulations to the place where the still-birth or death occurred is, if the place is unknown, to be construed as a reference to the place where the still-born child or the deceased was found.

Prescribed forms for registration of births and deaths

2. Subject to the provisions of regulation 6(2) of these Regulations, in relation to births   **A2–325** and deaths occurring in Wales—

(a) forms 1 to 16 in Schedule 2 to these Regulations shall be the prescribed forms in place of the corresponding forms ("the English forms"), [that is to say forms 1 to 6B, 9 to 11, 13 to 18 and 20, in Schedule 2][222] to the principal Regulations;

---

[222] Words substituted by Registration of Births and Deaths (Welsh Language) (Amendment) Regulations 1992/1504 reg.2 (August 1, 1992).

(b) references to any of the English forms in the principal Regulations shall have effect as referring instead to the corresponding form in Schedule 2 to these Regulations.

Prescribed words

A2–326   **3.** Where a regulation in the principal Regulations specified in column (1) of Schedule 3 to these Regulations requires the use of a form of words set out in column (2), the form of words set out opposite thereto in column (3) shall be used in any Welsh version.

Registration of still-births occurring in Wales

A2–327   **5.**—(1) Forms 8 and 9 may be completed in English only or in both English and Welsh.

[(2) Subject to paragraph (2A), where a qualified informant, giving information relating to the registration of a still-birth which occurred in Wales, elects for the particulars required by Part VIIIof the principal Regulations to be entered in Welsh as well as in English, the registrar shall enter those particulars accordingly.

(2A) Paragraph (2) of this regulation shall apply only where—

(a) the informant gives the requisite information either—

(i) personally to the relevant registrar; or
(ii) by declaration under section 9 of the Act, before a registrar in Wales; and

(b) the informant gives such information in Welsh and the officer to or before whom he gives it can understand and write Welsh.][223]

(3) When completing space 2 of the entry (other than in a case in which paragraph (4) applies)—

(a) if the still-birth is registered on production of a form 8 or of a notification from the coroner that he does not intend to hold an inquest, the registrar shall enter the cause of death, in accordance with regulation 34(2)(b) or 35 of the principal Regulations, precisely as stated on the form or the notification except that any particulars recorded in Welsh shall, if the informant so requests, be excluded from the entry if the still-birth is to be registered in English only;

(b) if the still-birth is registered on production of a form 9, the registrar shall enter the words prescribed by regulation 34(2)(b)(ii) in English only if the form was completed in English only and he shall enter also the Welsh version of those words if the form was completed in Welsh as well as in English,

and where the particulars in space 2 are entered in Welsh as well as in English the registrar shall also enter the Welsh version of any words prescribed by regulation 34(2)(b)(i) or 35(2).

(4) Where a still-birth is registered on production of a coroner's certificate after inquest—

(a) the registrar shall enter the particulars precisely as stated in the certificate in accordance with regulation 36(1) of the principal Regulations; and

(b) if the certificate is completed by the coroner in Welsh as well as in English, the registrar shall also enter the Welsh version of the words prescribed by sub-paragraph

---

[223] Reg.5(2) and (2A) substituted for reg.5(2) by Registration of Births and Deaths (Amendment) Regulations 1997/844 reg.5(2) (April 1, 1997).

(b), and of the particulars prescribed by sub-paragraphs (c), (e) and (f), of regulation 36(1).

Registration of deaths occurring in Wales

6.—(1) Forms 11 to 15 may be completed in English only or in both English and   **A2–328**
Welsh.

(2) Instead of forms 11 to 13, the corresponding forms (that is to say forms 14 to 16) in Schedule 2 to the principal Regulations may be used where the place of death is in Wales but the certificate of cause of death is issued in England.

[(3) Subject to paragraphs (3A) and (4) where a qualified informant giving information relating to the registration of a death which occurred in Wales, elects for the particulars required by Part X of the principal Regulations to be entered in Welsh as well as in English, the registrar shall enter those particulars accordingly.

(3A) Paragraph (3) shall apply only where—

(a) the informant gives the requisite information either—

(i) personally, to the relevant registrar; or
(ii) by declaration under section 23A of the Act, before a registrar in Wales; and

(b) the informant gives the requisite information in Welsh and the officer to or before whom he gives it can understand and write Welsh.][224]

---

[224] Reg.6(3) and (3A) substituted for reg.6(3) by Registration of Births and Deaths (Amendment) Regulations 1997/844 reg.5(3) (April 1, 1997).

(4) When completing space [9]²²⁵ of the entry (other than in a case in which paragraph (5) applies)—

    (a) if the death is registered on production of a certificate of cause of death or of a notification from the coroner that he does not intend to hold an inquest the registrar shall enter the cause of death in accordance with regulation 42(4), 43(2) or (3) or 47(5) of the principal Regulations and precisely as stated on the certificate or notification or (as the case may be) as stated by the informant except that any particulars recorded in Welsh shall, if the informant so requests, be excluded from the entry if the death is to be registered in English only;

    (b) where the particulars in space [9]² are entered in Welsh as well as in English the registrar shall also enter the Welsh version of any words prescribed by regulation 42(4) or 43(2).

(5) Where a death is registered on production of a coroner's certificate after inquest—

    (a) the registrar shall enter the particulars precisely as stated in the certificate in accordance with regulation 45(a) of the principal Regulations; and

    (b) if the certificate is completed by the coroner in Welsh as well as in English, the registrar shall also enter the Welsh version of the words prescribed by sub-paragraph (b), and of the particulars prescribed by sub-paragraphs (d) and (e), of regulation 45.

Correction of errors in birth and death entries

A2-329   7. Where an error requires to be corrected in an entry in a register of births or deaths kept in Wales, the marginal note specified by regulation 54(1)(e), 55(3), 56(2), 57(3) or (4),

---

²²⁵ Word substituted by Registration of Births and Deaths (Amendment) Regulations 2006/2827 reg.27(2) (November 13, 2006).

58(2)(b) or 59(2) or (3)(b) (as the case may be) of the principal Regulations shall be entered in English if the error occurs in particulars entered in English and in Welsh if the error occurs in particulars entered in Welsh.

Certified copies

10. Where a certified copy of an entry in a register of live-births, still-births or deaths   **A2–330**
containing English only, or in a certified copy of such a register, is made on a form
containing both English and Welsh but the particulars in the original entry and those
entered in the certified copy of that entry do not differ in any other respect the certified
copy shall be treated as a true copy of the original entry.

Schedule 2

Prescribed Forms

Contents

A2–331

Form	Description	Statutory purpose	Corresponding form in principal regulations
9	31	Particulars of still-birth	The Act, sections 1(1) and 5
10	32(1)	Medical certificate of still-birth	The Act, section 11(1)(a)
11	32(2)	Declaration as to still-birth	The Act, section 11(1)(b)
12	38(1)	Certificate that registrar has registered still-birth	The Act, section 11(2)
13	39	Particulars of death	The Act, sections 15 and 20
14	40(1)(a)(i)	Medical certificate of cause of death except for child dying within 28 days of birth	The Act, section 22(1)
15	40(1)(a)(ii)	Medical certificate of cause of death for child dying within 28 days of birth	The Act, section 22(1)
16	40(1)(b)	Medical practitioner's notice to informant of death	The Act, section 22(2)
17	49(1)	Notification	Births and Deaths Registration Act 1926, section 3(1)
18	49(3)	Declaration that certificate or order has been issued	Births and Deaths Registration Act 1926, section 1(1)
19	52	Certificate that death is not required to be registered	The Act, section 24(2)

[*FORM 7*

A2–332

STILL-BIRTH – MARW-ANEDIG	Entry No. Cofaed Rhif

Registration district
Dosbarth cofrestra

Administrative area
....

Sub-district
Is-ddosbarth

Rhanbarth gweinyddol

1.(a) Date and place of birth   **CHILD – Y PLENTYN**

....

    Dyddiad a lle y ganwyd

1.(b) Name and surname
    Enw a chyfenw

---

2. Cause of death and nature of evidence that child was still-born
    Achos marwolaeth a natur y dystiolaeth fod y plentyn wedi ei eni 'm farw

3. Sex
....
Rhyw

---

4. Name and surname   **FATHER – TAD/PARENT – RHIANT**
    Enw a chyfenw

---

5. Place of birth

....

    Lley ganwyd

6. Occupation

....

    Gwaith

---

7. Name and surname   **MOTHER – MAM**
    Enw a chyfenw

8.(a) Place of birth

....

    Lley ganwyd

8.(b) Occupation

....

    Gwaith

9.(a) Maiden surname
    Cyfenw morwynol

9.(b) Surname at marriage/civil partnership
    if different from maiden surname
    Cyfenw adeg priodi/partneriaeth sifil
    os ya wabamol i'r cyfenw morwynol

---

10. Usual address (if different from place of
    child's birth

Cyfeiriad arferol (os ya wahanol i le geni'r
    plentyn)

INFORMANT – HYSBYSYDD

11. Name and surname (if not the mother or father/parent Enw a chyfenw (os nad y tad/rhiant mea'r fam)	12. Qualification .... Cymhwyster
13. Usual address (if different from that in 10 above)	Cyfeiriad arferol (os yn wahanol i'r hyn sydd yn 10 uchod)
14. I certify that the particulars entered above are true to the best of my knowledge and belief Tystiaf fod y manylion a gofnodir uchod yn gywir hyd y gwn ac y credaf i	Signature of informant Llofnod yr hysybsydd
15. Date of registration .... Dyddiad cofrestru	16. Signature of registrar Llofnod y cofrestrydd

]226

226 Form substituted by Registration of Births and Deaths (Amendment) (England and Wales) Regulations 2009/2165 Sch.2 para.1 (September 1, 2009).

FORM 8

MEDICAL CERTIFICATE OF STILL-BIRTH

A2–333

Regulation 2(a)   Births and Deaths Registration Act 1953, s.11(1)(a)

★
$\Big\{$
I was present at the still-birth of a $\frac{male★}{female★}$ child born

Yr oeddwn yn bresennol yn ystod marw-enedigaeth plentn $\frac{gwryw★}{benyw★}$ a anwyd

★
$\Big\{$
I have examined the body of the $\frac{male★}{female★}$ child which I am informed and believe was born

Yr wyf wedi archwilio corff plentyn $\frac{gwryw★}{benyw★}$ y dywedir wrthyf ac y credaf iddo gael ei eni

on .... day of .... 19 .... to ....
ar   dydd o fis   i (name of mother)
                                                          (enw'r fam)

at ....
yn   (place of birth)   (lle y ganwyd)

†
$\Big\{$
1. The certified cause of death has been confirmed by post-mortem.
Cadarnhawyd a post-mortem achos ardystiedig y farwolaeth.

2. Information from post-mortem may be available later.
Dichon y bydd gwybodaeth a gafwyd o'r post-mortem ar gael yn ddiweddarach.

3. Post-mortem not being held.
Ni chynhelir post-mortem.

Weight of fetus .... grams
Pwysau'r ffetws   gram
Estimated duration of pregnancy
Amcangyfrif o barhad y beichiogiad
State (a) the number of weeks at delivery ....
Nodwch (a) nifer yr wythnosau adeg y marw-eni.

            (b) when the child died
                 pryd y bu'r plentyn farw
                 (i) before labour★
                     cyn yr esgor★
                 (ii) during labour★
                     yn ystod yr esgor★
                 (iii) not known★
                     nid yw'n hysbys★

† Please ring appropriate digit
   Rhowch gylch am y ffigur cymwys.
★ Strike out the words that do not apply.
   Dylid dileu y geiriau anghymwys.

CAUSE OF DEATH
ACHOS Y FARWOLAETH

---

a. Main diseases or conditions in fetus.
   Prif glefydau neu gyflyrau a berthynai i'r ffetws.

b. Other diseases or conditions in fetus.
   Clefydau eraill neu gyflyrau a berthynai i'r ffetws.

c. Main maternal diseases or conditions affecting fetus.
   Prif glefydau mamol neu gyflyrau a effeithiai ar y ffetws.

d. Other maternal diseases or conditions affecting fetus.
   Clefydau mamol eraill ne gyflyrau a effeithiai ar y ffetws.

e. Other relevant causes.
   Achosion perthnasol eraill.

I hereby certify that   (i) the child was not born alive, and
                               (ii) to the best of my knowledge and belief the cause of death and the estimated duration of pregnancy of the mother were as stated above.

Tystiaf drwy hyn

    (i) na anwyd y plentyn yn fyw, a

    (ii) hyd y gwn ac y credaf i fod achos y farwolaeth ac amcangyfrif o barhad beichiogiad y fam fel a fynegir uchod.

Signature .... Date ....
Llofnod   Dyddiad

Qualifications as registered by General Medical Council, or Registered no. as Registered Midwife ....
Cymwysterau fel y cofrestrwyd hwy gan y Cyngor Meddygol Cyffredinol neu Rhif Cofrestru fel Bydwraig Gofrestredig.

Address ....
Cyfeiriad

For still-births in hospital:
Please give the name of the consultant responsible for the care of the mother.
Yn achos marw-eni mewn ysbyty:
Rhowch enw'r ymgynghorydd oedd yn gyfrifol am edrych ar ol y fam.

[FORM 9

DECLARATION AS TO STILL-BIRTH

FORMW09   **A2–334**

Regulation 2(*a*)   Births and Deaths Registration Act 1953, s.11(1)(*b*)

Date of still-birth ....

Dyddiad y marw-eni ....

Place of still birth ....

lle'r marw-eni ....

Name and surname of mother of the still-born child.

Enw a chyfenw mam y plentyn marw-anedig.   }

Usual address of mother of child ....

Cyfeiriad arferol mam y plentyn ....

Reason why a certificate that the child was not born alive cannot be obtained from a registered medical practitioner or registered midwife:
....

....

Rheswm pam na ellir cael tystysgrif oddi wrth feddyg cofrestredig neu fydwraig gofrestredig yn tystio na chafodd y plentyn ei eni'n fyw:
....

....

I declare that the particulars stated above are true to the best of my knowledge and belief, and that the child mentioned above was not born alive.

Yr wyf yn datgan fod y manylion a roddwyd uchod yn wir hyd eithaf fy ngwybodaeth a'm cred ac na chafodd y plentyn y cyfeirir ato uchod ei eni'n fyw.

Signature
Llofnod
} ....

State whether "Mother", "Father" of the child or
in what other capacity liable to give information
concerning the still-birth
}
....

Dywedwch ai "Mam", "Tad", y plentyn, neu
ynteu mewn safle arall sy'n rhwym o roi gwybodaeth ynghylch y marw-eni
}
....

Date ....

Dyddiad ....]²²⁷

FORM 10

PARTICULARS OF DEATH

A2–335

FORM 10

PARTICULARS OF DEATH

Regulation 2(a)   Births and Deaths Registration Act 1953, ss.15 and 20

DEATH – MARWOLAETH	Entry No. Cofnod Rhif

Registration district Dosbarth cofrestru	Administrative area

Sub-district   Rhanbarth gweinyddol
Is-ddosbarth

1. Date and place of death

....

Dyddiad a lle y bu farw

2. Name and Surname Enw a chyfenw	3. Sex .... Rhyw
	4. Maiden surname of woman who has married Cyfenw morwynol y wraig sydd wedi priodi

5. Date and Place of birth

....

Dyddiad a lle y ganwyd

6. Occupation and usual address

....

Gwaith a chyfeiriad arferol

---

²²⁷ Form substituted by Registration of Births and Deaths (Welsh Language) (Amendment) Regulations
1995/818 Sch.1 para.1 (April 1, 1995).

7. (a) Name and surname of informant Enw a chyfenw'r hysbysydd	(b) Qualification .... Cymhwyster
(c) Usual address .... Cyfeiriad arferol	
8. Cause of death Achos marwolaeth	
9. I certify that the particulars given by me above are true to the best of my knowledge and belief Tystiaf fod y manylion a roddwyd gennyf uchod yn gywir y hyd gwn ac y credaf i	Signature of informant Llofnod yr hysbysydd
10. Date of registration .... Dyddiad cofrestru	11. Signature of registrar Llofnod y cofrestrydd

FORM 11

MEDICAL CERTIFICATE OF CAUSE OF DEATH EXCEPT FOR CHILD DYING WITH 28 DAYS OF BIRTH

Regulation 2(a)   Births and Deaths Registration Act 1953, s.22(1)   **A2–336**

Name of deceased ....
Enw'r madawedig

Date of death as stated to me .... day of .... 19 ....
Dyddiad y bu farw yn ôl a ddywedwyd wrthyf   dydd o fis

Age as stated to me ....
Oedran yn ôl a ddywedwyd wrthyf

Place of death ....
Man y farwolaeth

Last seen alive by me .... day of .... 19 ....
Gwelwyd yn fyw am y tro diwethaf gennyf ar   dydd o fis

1. The certified cause of death takes account of information obtained from post-mortem.
   Y mae achos ardystiedig y farwolaeth yn cymryd i ystyriaeth wybodaeth a gafwyd o'r post-mortem
2. Information from post-mortem may be available later.
   Dichon y bydd gwybodaeth a gafwyd o'r post-mortem ar gael yn ddiweddarach.
3. Post-mortem not being held.
   Ni chynhelir post-mortem.
4. I have reported this death to the Coroner for further action.
   Yr wyf wedi hysbysu'r Crwner am y farwolaeth hon iddo weithredu ymhellach.

Please ring appropriate digits(s) and letter.
Rhowch gylch o gwmpas y ffigur (au) a'r llythyren gymwys.

a. seen after death by me.
   Gwelwyd ar ôl marw gennyf i.
b. See after death by another medical practitioner but not by me.
   Gwelwyd ar ôl marw gan feddyg arall ond nid gennyf i.
c. Not seen after death by a medical practitioner.
   Nis gwelwyd ar ôl marw gan feddyg.

CAUSE OF DEATH ACHOS Y FARWOLAETH The condition thought to be the 'Underlying Cause of Death' shoud appear in the lowest completed line of Part I Dylid cynnwys y cyflwr a ystyriwyd fel 'Achos Sylfaenol y Farwolaeth' yn y llinell olaf a lanwyd yn Rhan I	These particulars not to be entered in death register Ni ddylid cofnodi'r manylion hyn ar gofrestr marwolaeth
	Approximate interval between onset and death Amcangyfrif o'r amser rhwng yr ymosodiad a'r farwolaeth

I(a) Disease or condition directly leading to death†
Afiechyd neu gyflwr yn arwain i farwolaeth yn uniongyrchol†
 	
  (b) Other disease or condition, if any, leading to I(a)
Afiechyd neu gyflwr arall, os oedd un yn arwain i I(a)
 	
  (c) Other disease or condition, if any, leading to I(b)
Afiechyd neu gyflwr arall, os oedd un, yn arwain i I(b)
 	
II   Other significant conditions CONTRIBUTING TO THE DEATH but not related to the disease or condition causing it
Cyflyrau arwyddocaol eraill, YN CYFRANNU AT Y FARWOLAETH ond heb fod â pherthynas â'r clefyd neu â'r cyflwr a achosodd y farwolaeth
	....
	
	....
	
	....
	
	....
	 ....
	
	....
	
	....
	
	....

The death might have been due to or contributed to by the employment followed at some time by the deceased. Dichon fod y farwolaeth wedi deillio neu ei bod yn gysylltiedig â'r gyflogaeth a ddilynid rywbryd gan yr ymadawedig.	Please tick where ☐ applicable Rhowch ✓ yn ôl y galw

† This does not mean the mode of dying, such as heart failure, asphyxia, asthenia, etc: it means the disease, injury or complication which caused death.
Nid yw hyn yn golygu y modd y bu farw, fel y galon yn methu tagfa, asthenia, etc: y mae'n golygu y clefyd, y niwed neu'r cymhlethdod a achosodd y farwolaeth.

I hereby certify that I was in medical attendance during the above named deceased's last illness, and that the particulars and cause of death above written are true to the best of my knowledge and belief.
Tystiaf drwy hyn i mi weini'n feddygol ar yr ymadawedig a enwyd uchod yn ystod ei salwch olaf a bod y manylion ac achos y farwolaeth a ysgrifennwyd uchod yn gywir hyd y gwn ac y credaf i.
For deaths in hospital: Please give the name of the consultant responsible for the above named as a patient

Yn achos marwolathau mewn ysbytai: Rhowch enw'r ymgynghorydd a oedd yn gyfrifol am y person uchod pan oedd yn glaf

Qualifications as
registered by General
Signature .... Medical Council ....
Llofnod   Cymwysterau fel y
cofrestrwyd hwy gan y
Cyngor Meddygol
Cyffredinol

Residence .... Date ....
Preswylfa   Dyddiad

....

FORM 12

MEDICAL CERTIFICATE OF CAUSE OF DEATH FOR CHILD DYING WITH 28 DAYS OF BIRTH

Regulation 2(*a*)   Births and Deaths Registration Act 1953, s.22(1)   **A2–337**

Name of child .... Sex ....
Enw'r plentyn   Rhyw

Date of death .... day of ....
Dyddiad y farwolaeth   dydd o fis

Age at death .... days (complete period of 24 hrs).....hours
Ei oed pan fu farw   diwrnod (24 awr cyflawn)   awr

Place of death ....
Man y farwolaeth

Place of birth ....
Lle y ganwyd

Last seen alive by me .... day of ....
Gwelwyd yn fyw am y tro diwethaf gennyfar   dydd o fis

1. The certified cause of death has been confirmed by post-mortem.
   Cadarnhawyd a post-mortem achos ardystiedig y farwolaeth.

2. Information from post-mortem may be available later.
   Dichon y bydd gwybodaeth a gafwyd o'r post-mortem ar gael yn ddiweddarach.

3. Post-mortem not being held.
   Ni chynhelir post-mortem.

4. I have reported this death to the Coroner for further action.
   Yr wyf wedi hysbysu'r Crwner am y farwolaeth hon iddo weithredu ymhellach.

Please ring appropriate digits(s) and letter.
Rhowch gylch o gwmpas y ffigur (au) a'r llythyren gymwys.

a. seen after death by me.
   Gwelwyd ar ôl marw gennyf i.

b. See after death by another medical practitioner but not by me.
   Gwelwyd ar ôl marw gan feddyg arall ond nid gennyfi.

c. Not seen after death by a medical practitioner.
   Nis gwelwyd ar ôl marw gan feddyg.

CAUSE OF DEATH
ACHOS Y FARWOLAETH

a. Main diseases or conditions in infant
   Prif glefydau neu gyflyrau a berthynai i'r baban

b. Other disease or conditions in infant
   Clefydau eraill neu gyflyrau a berthynai i'r baban

---

c. Main maternal diseases or conditions affecting infant
   Prif glefydau mamol neu gyflyrau a effeithiai ar y baban

d. Other maternal diseases or conditions affecting infant
   Clefydau mamoll erail neu gyflyrau a effeithiai ar y baban

---

e. Other relevant causes
   Achosion perthnasol eraill

I hereby certify that I was in medical attendance during the above-named deceased's last illness, and that the particulars and cause of death above written are true to the best of my knowledge and belief.	Signature .... Llofnod	Qualifications as registered by General Medical Council .... Cymwysterau fel y cofrestrwyd hwy gan y Cyngor Meddygo Cyffredinol
Tystiaf drwy hyn i mi weini'n feddygol ar yr ymadawedig a enwyd uchod yn ystod ei salwch olaf a bod y manylion ac achos y farwolaeth a ysgrifennwyd uchod yn gywir hyd y gwn ac y credaf i.	Address .... Cyfeiriad	Date .... Dyddiad

For deaths in hospital: Please give the name of the consultant responsible for the above-named as a patient

....

Yn achos marwolaethau mewn ysbyty: Rhowch enw'r mgynghorydd a oedd yn gyfrifol am y person uchod pan oedd yn glaf.

FORM 13

MEDICAL PRACTITIONER'S NOTICE TO INFORMANT OF DEATH

A2–338   Regulation 2(a)   Births and Deaths Registration Act 1953, s.22(2)

————————

I hereby give notice that I have this day signed a medical certificate of cause of death

Hysbysaf drwy hyn i mi heddiw lofnodi tystysgrif feddygol a rydd achos marwolaeth

of   } ....

Signature   }
Llofnod   } ....   Date   ....
                                                                Dyddiad ....

This notice is to be delivered by the informant to the registrar of births and deaths for the sub-district in which the death occurred.

Y mae'n ofynnol i'r hysbysydd drosglwyddo'r hysbysiad hwn i gofrestrydd genedigaethau a marwolaethau yr isddosbarth lle digwyddodd y farwolaeth

FORM 14

NOTIFICATION

A2–339   Regulation 2(a)   Births and Deaths Registration Act 1926, s.3(1)

This is to notify that the body of   }
                                       } ....   deceased.
Hyn sydd i hysbysu bod corff   }
                                       } ....   yr ymadawedig.

who died at .... at ....

a fu farw ar .... yn ....

was buried/cremated* on .... at ....

wedi ei gladdu/gorfflosgi* ar .... yn ....

Signature
Llofnod   } ....

on behalf of
ar ran   } ....

Date   ....
Dyddiad

★ } Strike out whichever does not apply.
  ∫ Dylid dileu fel y bo'r achos.

FORM 15

DECLARATION THAT CERTIFICATE OR ORDER HAS BEEN ISSUED

Regulation 2(a)   Births and Deaths Registration Act 1926, s.1(1)   **A2–340**

———————

I
Yr wyfi } .... of ....
                                                           o ....

in pursuance of the Births and Deaths Registration Act 1926, declare:–
yn ôl Births and Deaths Registration Act 1926, yn datgan:–

(1) That I am the person procuring the burial
     of the body of
     Mai myfi yw'r person sy'n cael gofal claddu   } ....
     corff

     who died at .... on the ....

     a fu farw yn .... ar ....

                  registrar's certificate★
(2) that a ————————————————— authorising burial was issued by the
                  coroner's order

         tystysgrif cofrestrydd★
     fod ————————————————— yn awdurdodi claddu wedi ei rhoi gan y
         gorchymyn crwner

     registrar★   at ....
     cofrestrydd ....

     coroner★
     crwner★   yn ....

     to }
         } ....   living at ....
     i   }
                                         sy'n byw yn ....

     on ....; and

     ar ....; ac

(3) that the reason why the said document cannot be delivered before burial is that ....

....

....

mai'r rheswm pam na ellir trosglwyddo'r ddogfen a enwyd cyn y gladdedigaeth yw.........................

....

....

I make this declaration believing the same to be true.
Gwnaf y datganiad hwn gan gredu ei fod yn gywir.

Signature of declarant ⎱
Llofnod y datganwr ⎰ ....

Date ....
Dyddiad ....

★ ⎱ Strike out whichever does not apply.
  ⎰ Dylid dileu fel y bo'r achos.

SCHEDULE 3

SCHEDULE 3

[

Regulations	Form of words required	Welsh version
Reg. 5	The mark (or signature) of	No (neu Llofnod)
9(4)(a)	now	naw
	afterwards	wedyn
9(5)(b)	deceased	ymadawedig
9(5)(c)	now	nawr
9(6)(a)	now	nawr
	afterwards	wedyn
10(1)(b)(ii) and (iii)	Statutory declaration made by ... on ...	Datganiad statudol a wnaethpwyd gan ... ar y ...
10(1)(b)(iv)	Pursuant to section 10(d) of the Births and Deaths Registration Act 1953	Yn unol ag adran 10(d)Births and Deaths Registration Act 1953
10(1)(b)(v)	Pursuant to section 10(e) of the Births and Deaths Registration Act 1953	Yn unol ag adran 10(e)Births and Deaths Registration Act 1953
10(1)(b)(vi)	Pursuant to section 10(f) of the Births and Deaths Registration Act 1953	Yn unol ag adran 10(f)Births and Deaths Registration Act 1953
10(1)(b)(vii)	Pursuant to section 10(g) of the Births and Deaths Registration Act 1953	Yn unol ag adran 10(g)Births and Deaths Registration Act 1953
10(1)(c)(ii)	Statutory declaration made by ... on ...	Datganiad statudol a wnaethpwyd gan ... ar y ...

Regulations	Form of words required	Welsh version
10(1)(c)(iii)	Statutory declaration made by … on …	Datganiad statudol a wnaethpwyd gan … ar y …
10(1)(c)(iv)	Pursuant to section 10(1B)(d) of the Births and Deaths Registration Act 1953	Yn unol ag adran 10(1B)(d)Births and Deaths Registration Act 1953
10(1)(c)(v)	Pursuant to section 10(1B)(e) of the Births and Deaths Registration Act 1953	Yn unol ag adran 10(1B)(e)Births and Deaths Registration Act 1953
10(1)(c)(vi)	Pursuant to section 10(1B)(f) of the Births and Deaths Registration Act 1953	Yn unol ag adran 10(1B)(f)Births and Deaths Registration Act 1953
10(1)(d)	Pursuant to section 10ZA of the Births and Deaths Registration Act 1953	Yn unol ag adran 10ZABirths and Deaths Registration Act 1953
12(3)	On the authority of the Registrar General	Dan awdurdod y Cofrestrydd Cyffredinol
13(4)(b)(i)	by declaration dated …	trwy ddatganiad dyddiedig y …
13(4)(b)(iii)	Pursuant to section 10ZA of the Births and Deaths Registration Act 1953	Yn unol ag adran 10ZABirths and Deaths Registration Act 1953
13(5)(c)(iii)	On the authority of the Registrar General	Dan awdurdod y Cofrestrydd Cyffredinol
14(2)(a)	by baptism on …	trwy fedydd ar y …
14(2)(b)	on certificate of naming dated …	ar dystysgrif enwi dyddiedig y …
17(2)(b)(i)	Statutory declaration made by … on …	Datganiad statudol a wnaethpwyd gan … ar y …
17(2)(b)(ii)	Statutory declaration made by … on …	Datganiad statudol a wnaethpwyd gan … ar y …
17(2)(b)(iii)	Pursuant to section 10A(1)(d) of the Births and Deaths Registration Act 1953	Yn unol ag adran 10A(1)(d)Births and Deaths Registration Act 1953
17(2)(b)(iv)	Pursuant to section 10A(1)(e) of the Births and Deaths Registration Act 1953	Yn unol ag adran 10A(1)(e)Births and Deaths Registration Act 1953
17(2)(b)(v)	Pursuant to section 10A(1)(f) of the Births and Deaths Registration Act 1953	Yn unol ag adran 10A(1)(f)Births and Deaths Registration Act 1953
17(2)(b)(vi)	Pursuant to section 10A(1)(ff) of the Births and Deaths Registration Act 1953	Yn unol ag adran 10A(1)(ff)Births and Deaths Registration Act 1953
17(2)(b)(vii)	Pursuant to section 10A(1)(g) of the Births and Deaths Registration Act 1953	Yn unol ag adran 10A(1)(g)Births and Deaths Registration Act 1953
17(4)(i)	Statutory declaration made by … on …	Datganiad statudol a wnaethpwyd gan … ar y …
17(4)(ii)	Statutory declaration made by … on …	Datganiad statudol a wnaethpwyd gan … ar y …
17(4)(iii)	Pursuant to section 10A(1B)(d) of the Births and Deaths Registration Act 1953	Yn unol ag adran 10A(1B)(d)Births and Deaths Registration Act 1953

Regulations	Form of words required	Welsh version
17(4)(iv)	Pursuant to section 10A(1B)(e) of the Births and Deaths Registration Act 1953	Yn unol ag adran 10A(1B)(e)Births and Deaths Registration Act 1953
17(4)(v)	Pursuant to section 10A(1B)(f) of the Births and Deaths Registration Act 1953	Yn unol ag adran 10A(1B)(f)Births and Deaths Registration Act 1953
17(4)(vi)	Pursuant to section 10A(1B)(g) of the Births and Deaths Registration Act 1953	Yn unol ag adran 10A(1B)(g)Births and Deaths Registration Act 1953
17(5)	On the authority of the Registrar General	Dan awdurdod y Cofrestrydd Cyffredinol
17(9)(b)(i)	by declaration dated ...	trwy ddatganiad dyddiedig y ...
18(i)	Re-registered under section 10A of the Births and Deaths Registration Act 1953 on ...	Ail-gofrestrwyd dan adran 10ABirths and Deaths Registration Act 1953 ar y
18(ii)	Re-registered under section 10A(1B) of the Births and Deaths Registration Act 1953 on ...	Ail-gofrestrwyd dan adran 10A(1(B)Births and Deaths Registration Act 1953 ar y
20(1)(c)	On the authority of the Registrar General	Dan awdurdod y Cofrestrydd Cyffredinol
22(b)	Father	Tad
	Mother	Mam
	Parent	Rhiant
23(b)	On the authority of the Registrar General	Dan awdurdod y Cofrestrydd Cyffredinal
24	Re-registered under section 14 of the Births and Deaths Registration Act 1953 on	Ail-gofrestrwyd dan adran 14Births and Deaths Registration Act 1953 ar y
26(2)(b)	Re-registered under section 14 of the Births and Deaths Registration Act 1953 on	Ail-gofrestrwyd dan adran 14Births and Deaths Registration Act 1953 ar y
26A(b)(i)	Pursuant to section 14A of the Births and Deaths Registration Act 1953 on the authority of the Registrar General	Yn unol ag adran 14ABirths and Deaths Registration Act 1953 dan awdurdod y Cofrestrydd Cyffredinol
26A(b)(ii)	On the authority of the Registrar General	Dan awdurdod y Cofrestrydd Cyffredinol
26B	Re-registered under section 14A of the Births and Deaths Registration Act 1953 on	Ail-gofrestrwyd dan adran 14ABirths and Deaths Registration Act 1953 ar y
26C(b)	Re-registered under section 14 of the Births and Deaths Registration Act 1953 on	Ail-gofrestrwyd dan adran 14Births and Deaths Registration Act 1953 ar y
30	Re-registered under section 3A(5)of the Births and Deaths Registration Act 1953 on	Ail-gofrestrwyd dan adran 3A(5)Births and Deaths Registration Act 1953 ar y
Reg. 34(2)(a)(i)	Found at .. .. on ..	Daethpwyd o hyd i'r corff .. .. ar .. ..
Reg. 34(2)(b)(i)	Certified by .. .. Registered Midwife	Tystiwyd gan .. .. Bydwraig Gofrestredig
Reg. 34(2)(b)(2)	Declaration by informant	Datganiad gan hysbysydd

Regulations	Form of words required	Welsh version
Reg. 35	Certified by .. .. after post-mortem held by direction of	Tystiwyd gan .. .. ar ôl post-mortem a gynhaliwyd yn ôl cyfarwyddyd .. ..
Reg. 36(1)(b)	Certificate after inquest held on	Tystysgrif ar ôl cwest a gynhaliwyd ar .. ..
Reg. 42(2)(a)	Aged	Oed .. ..
Reg. 42(2)(b)	Found dead	Cafwyd yn farw .. ..
Reg. 42(2)(c)	On or about	Ar neu oddeutu .. ..
Reg. 42(2)(d)	Deceased found on ..	Daethpwyd o hyd i'r ymadawedlg ar .. ..
Reg. 42(3)(a)	Son (or daughter) of .. and, now, afterwards	mab (neu merch) .. . a, nawr, wedyn
Reg. 42(3)(b)	wife (or widow) of ..	gwraig (neu gweddw) ..
Reg. 42(4)	Certified by	Tystiwyd gan .. ..
Reg. 43(2)	Certified by .. .. after post-mortem without inquest	Tystiwyd gan .. .. ar ôl post-mortem heb gwest
Reg. 44(a)	Post-mortem without inquest held by the direction of .. .. and cause of death disclosed as	Post-mortem heb gwest a gynhaliwyd yn ôl cyfarwyddyd .. .. a datgelwyd mai achos y farwolaeth oedd .. ..
Reg. 45(b)(i)	Certificate received from .. .. Inquest held	Tystysgrif a dderbyniwyd oddi wrth Cynhaliwyd cwest ar .. ..
Reg. 45(b)(ii)	Certificate on inquest adjourned received from	Tystysgrif ar gwest a ohiriwyd a dderbyniwyd oddi wrth .. ..
Reg. 47(6)	On the authority of the Registrar General	Dan awdurdod y Cofrestrydd Cyffredinol
Reg. 54(1)(d)	one	un
Reg. 54(1)(e)	The particulars in .. .. and .. .. inadvertently transposed	Trawsddodwyd y manylion yn .. .. a .. .. yn ddamweiniol
Reg. 55(3)	Error in .. corrected on .. .. by me .. .. Registrar	Camgymeriad yn .. .. a gywirwyd ar .. .. gennyf i .. Cofrestrydd
Reg. 55(4)	Error in .. .. corrected on .. .. by me .. .. Superintendent Registrar	Camgymeriad yn .. .. a gywirwyd ar .. .. gennyfi .. .. Cofrestrydd Arolygol
Reg. 56(2)	Error in .. .. corrected on .. .. by me .. .. Registrar, in the presence of .. and Superintendent Registrar Error in .. .. corrected on .. .. by me .. .. Superintendent Registrar, in the presence of	Camgymeriad yn .. .. a gywirwyd ar .. .. gennyfi .. .. Cofrestrydd, yng ngwydd .. .. a .. .. Cofrestrydd Arolygol Camgymeriad yn .. .. a gywirwyd ar .. .. gennyfi .. .. Cofrestrydd Arolygol, yng ngwydd ..
Reg. 57(3)	Error in .. .. corrected on .. .. by me .. .. Superintendent Registrar (or Registrar) in the presence of .. .. on the authority of the Registrar General	Camgymeriad yn .. .. a gywirwyd ar .. .. gennyfi .. Cofrestrydd Arolygol (neu Cofrestrydd) yng ngwydd .. .. dan awdurdod Cofrestrydd Cyffredinol
Reg. 57(4)	Error .. .. corrected on .. .. by me .. .. Superintendent Registrar (or Registrar) on the authority of the Registrar General	Camgymeriad yn .. .. a gywirwyd ar .. .. gennyfi .. .. Cofrestrydd (neu Cofrestrydd Arolygol) dan awdurdod y Cofrestrydd Cyffredinol

Regulations	Form of words required	Welsh version
Reg. 58(2)(b)	In No .. .. in .. .. for .. .. read .. .. Corrected on .. .. by me .. .. Superintendent Registrar (or Registrar) on production of a statutory declaration made by .. .. and	Yn Rhif .. .. yn .. .. yn lle .. .. darllener .. .. Cywirwyd ar .. .. gennyfi .. .. Cofrestrydd Arolygol (neu Cofrestrydd) ar ôl i mi weld datganiad cyfreithiol a wnaethpwyd gan .. .. a .. ..
Reg. 59(2)	Error in .. .. corrected on .. .. by me .. .. Superintendent Registrar (or Registrar) on receipt of notification from the Coroner	Camgymeriad yn .. .. a gywirwyd ar y .. .. gennyfi .. .. Cofrestrydd Arolygol (neu Cofrestrydd) ar ôl cael hysbysiad oddi wrth y Crwner
Reg. 59(3)(b)	In No .. .. in .. .. for .. .. read .. .. Corrected on .. .. by me .. .. Superintendent Registrar (or Registrar) on the authority of a certificate from a Coroner	Yn Rhif .. .. yn .. .. yn lle .. .. darllener .. .. Cywirwyd ar y .. .. gennyfi .. .. Cofrestrydd Arolygol (neu Cofrestrydd) dan awdurdod tystysgrif oddi wrth y Crwner

]²²⁸

Removal of Bodies Regulations 1954/448

A2–342   **1.** These regulations may be cited as the Removal of Bodies Regulations, 1954, and shall come into operation on the first day of May, 1954.

2. The Interpretation Act, 1889, applies to the interpretation of these regulations as it applies to the interpretation of an Act of Parliament.

4. Every person intending to remove the body of a deceased person out of England shall give notice of his intention in the form set forth in the first schedule to these regulations, or in a form substantially to the like effect, to the coroner within whose jurisdiction the body is lying, and when the deceased person died in England and a certificate has been given by a registrar under section 24 of the Births and Deaths Registration Act, 1953, or a coroner's order for burial or certificate for cremation has been issued, the certificate or order shall be delivered to the coroner with the notice.

5.—(1) Upon receiving any such notice the coroner shall forthwith send or deliver—

    (a) to the person who gave the notice, or the undertaker or other person designated by that person for the purpose, an acknowledgment of the receipt of the notice in the form set forth in the second schedule to these regulations or in a form substantially to the like effect, and

    (b) to the registrar for the sub-district in which the death occurred, or in which the dead body was found, a notification that a notice of intention to remove the body out of England has been received, and, if a certificate given by that registrar under section 24 of the Births and Deaths Registration Act, 1953, was sent to the coroner under regulation 4 of these regulations, the certificate so sent.

[(2) Any coroner's order for burial or certificate for cremation sent to the coroner under regulation 4 of these regulations shall be retained by him unless he is notified in writing by the person wishing to remove the body out of England that it is intended that the body shall be cremated in Scotland, Northern Ireland, the Channel Islands or the Isle of Man, in which case the coroner shall endorse the certificate with words to the effect that it shall henceforth be valid only for cremation in Scotland, Northern Ireland, the Channel Islands ot the Isle

---

²²⁸ Entries substituted by Registration of Births and Deaths (Amendment) (England and Wales) Regulations 2009/2165 Sch.3 para.1 (September 1, 2009).

of Man, as the case may be, and return it to the person receiving the acknowledgment of the receipt of notice under sub-paragraph (a) of paragraph (1) of this regulation.][229]

6. The body shall not be removed out of England before the expiration of a period of four clear days after the day on which notice of intention to remove the body was received by the coroner:

Provided that, where the coroner states in his acknowledgment of receipt of the notice that after making due enquiry he is satisfied that no further enquiries by him are necessary concerning the death, the body may be removed out of England at any time after the acknowledgment has been received by the person to whom it is addressed, notwithstanding that the said period of four days has not expired.

7. Any notice, acknowledgment or notification required by these regulations to be given, sent or delivered may be sent by post.

[SCHEDULE 1

FORM OF NOTICE TO A CORONER OF INTENTION TO REMOVE A BODY OUT OF ENGLAND

To the Coroner for   **A2–343**

I/We
of (full postal address)

in pursuance of section 4 of the Births and Deaths Registration Act 1926, hereby give you notice that I/we intend to remove out of England the body, now lying within your jurisdiction at
(Here state address or place where body is lying)
     of   deceased, who
died at (or whose body was found at)
on
—and I/we deliver herewith the certificate for disposal given by the registrar of births and deaths*
—and I/we deliver herewith the coroner's order for burial or certificate for cremation of the deceased.*
—and I/we declare that it is intended to remove the body to Scotland/Northern Ireland/the Channel Islands/the Isle of Man and to cremate it there.*
—and I/we declare that to the best of my/our knowledge and belief no certificate for disposal has been given by a registrar of births and deaths in England and Wales and no coroner's order for burial or certificate for cremation has been issued.*
—and I/we declare that the death took place out of England and Wales.*

     † You are requested to send any communication regarding this notice to–
     (Name)
     Full postal address
     Signature of person giving notice
     Date

* Delete where applicable
† This paragraph is for use only where the person giving notice desires the coroner's acknowledgement to be sent to some other person.][230]

---

[229] Substituted by Removal of Bodies (Amendment) Regulations 1971/1354 reg.3 (October 1, 1971).
[230] Substituted by Removal of Bodies (Amendment) Regulations 1971/1354 reg.3 (October 1, 1971).

SCHEDULE 2

FORM OF ACKNOWLEDGMENT BY A CORONER OF RECEIPT OF NOTICE OF INTENTION
TO REMOVE A BODY OUT OF ENGLAND

Regulation 5

A2–344   To........ (Here state the name of the person by whom notice was given, or of such other person as may have been designated in the notice to receive the coroner's acknowledgment)

Address........

1. I hereby acknowledge that I have this.... day of........ 20.... received the notice given by........ for the purpose of section 4 of the Births and Deaths Registration Act 1926 that it is intended to remove out of England the body, now lying within my jurisdiction, of........ deceased.

2. (a) I am satisfied that there is no necessity for me to make further enquiries concerning the death and the body may be removed out of England upon receipt of this acknowledgment.

   (b) The body may be removed out of England on or after the fifth day after the date aforesaid unless any lawful direction to the contrary has been given in the meanwhile.

Signature........
Coroner. Deputy Coroner, Assistant Deputy Coroner.
for........

Strike out (a) or (b).

Reporting of Injuries, Diseases and Dangerous Occurrences Regulations 2013/1471

Citation and commencement

A2–345   1.—(1) These Regulations may be cited as the Reporting of Injuries, Diseases and Dangerous Occurrences Regulations 2013.
(2) Subject to paragraph (3), these Regulations come into force on 1st October 2013.
(3) Regulation 18(2) comes into force immediately after the coming into force of the other regulations.

Interpretation

A2–346   2.—(1) In these Regulations—

"the 1954 Act" means the Mines and Quarries Act 1954[231];
"the 1969 Act" means the Mines and Quarries (Tips) Act 1969[232];
"the 1974 Act" means the Health and Safety at Work etc. Act 1974;
"the 1999 Regulations" means the Quarries Regulations 1999[233];

---

[231] Section 180 was amended by SI 1974/2013, SI 1993/1897 and SI 1999/2024; section 123 was amended by SI 1985/2023 and SI 1999/2024; there are other amending instruments but none is relevant.
[232] Section 2(2) was amended by SI 1999/2024; there are other amending instruments but none is relevant.
[233] To which there are amendments not relevant to these Regulations.

"the 2002 Regulations" means the Control of Substances Hazardous to Health Regulations 2002[234];

"the 2006 Regulations" means the Railways and Other Guided Transport Systems (Safety) Regulations 2006[235];

"the 2013 Order" means the Health and Safety at Work etc. Act 1974 (Application Outside Great Britain) Order 2013;

"accident" includes an act of non-consensual physical violence done to a person at work;

"approved manner" means published in a form considered appropriate and approved for the time being for the purposes of these Regulations—

(a) by the Executive; or

(b) in relation to activities covered by regulation 3 of the Health and Safety (Enforcing Authority for Railways and Other Guided Transport Systems) Regulations 2006, by the ORR;

"biological agent" has the meaning given by regulation 2(1) of the 2002 Regulations;

"carcinogen" has the meaning given by regulation 2(1) of the 2002 Regulations;

"consecutive days" includes any days which are not or would not have been working days;

"construction site" has the meaning given by regulation 2(1) of the Construction (Design and Management) Regulations 2007;

"dangerous occurrence" means an occurrence which arises out of or in connection with work and is of a class specified in—

(a) Part 1 of Schedule 2;

(b) Part 2 of Schedule 2 and takes place anywhere except an offshore workplace;

(c) Part 3 of Schedule 2 and takes place at a mine;

(d) Part 4 of Schedule 2 and takes place at a quarry;

(e) Part 5 of Schedule 2 and takes place where a relevant transport system is operated; or

(f) Part 6 of Schedule 2 and takes place at an offshore workplace;

"disease" includes a medical condition;

"diagnosis" means a registered medical practitioner's identification (in writing, where it pertains to an employee) of—

(a) new symptoms; or

(b) symptoms which have significantly worsened;

"diving contractor" and "diving project" have the meanings they are given by regulation 2(1) of the Diving at Work Regulations 1997;

"dock" means any place to which section 125(1) of the Factories Act 1961[236] applies;

"the Executive" means the Health and Safety Executive;

"explosives" has the meaning given by regulation 2(1) of the Manufacture and Storage of Explosives Regulations 2005;

"factory" has the meaning given by section 175 of the Factories Act 1961;

"flammable gas" and "flammable liquid" have the meanings associated with those hazard classes in Part 2 of Annex I of Regulation (EC) No 1272/2008 (the CLP Regulation)[237];

---

[234] Regulation 2(1) was amended by SI 2003/978; there are other amending instruments but none is relevant.

[235] To which there are amendments not relevant to these Regulations.

[236] Section 175 was amended by SI 1983/978; there are other amending instruments but none is relevant.

[237] OJ No L 353, 31.12.2008, p1. Annex I is amended from time to time.

"mine" has the meaning given by section 180 of the 1954 Act and for the purposes of these Regulations includes a closed tip within the meaning of section 2(2)(b) of the 1969 Act which is associated with such a mine;

"mutagen" has the meaning given by regulation 2(1) of the 2002 Regulations;

"nominated person" means, in relation to a mine or quarry, the person (if any) who is for the time being nominated—

    (a) in a case where there is an association or body representative of a majority of the total number of persons employed at a mine or quarry, by that association or body; or

    (b) in any other case, jointly by associations or bodies which are together representative of such a majority,

to receive notices under paragraph 4 of Part 1 of Schedule 1 on behalf of the persons employed at that mine or quarry;

"non-passenger train" means any train except a passenger train;

"offshore installation" has the meaning given by article 4(2) of the 2013 Order;

"offshore workplace" means any place where activities are carried on, or any premises, such that prescribed provisions of the 1974 Act are applied to those activities or premises by article 4, 5 or 6 of the 2013 Order (which for this purpose are deemed to apply to activities or premises within Great Britain which are in tidal waters or on the foreshore or other land intermittently covered by such waters as they apply to activities or premises within territorial waters or a designated area within the meaning of article 2(1) of that Order);

"operator" means—

    (a) in relation to a pipeline, the person identified as such by regulation 2(1) of the Pipelines Safety Regulations 1996; and

    (b) in relation to a quarry, the person in overall control of the working of the quarry;

"the ORR" means the Office of Rail Regulation;

"owner" in relation to a mine means the person who is for the time being entitled to work it;

"passenger train" means a train carrying passengers or made available for that purpose;

"pipeline" and "pipeline works" have the meanings given by article 6(2) of the 2013 Order;

"quarry" means a quarry to which the 1999 Regulations apply;

"railway" has the meaning given by regulation 2(1) of the 2006 Regulations;

"relevant transport system" means—

    (a) a railway;

    (b) a tramway as defined by regulation 2(1) of the 2006 Regulations;

    (c) a trolley vehicle system as defined by section 67 of the Transport and Works Act 1992, except when it operates on a road; or

    (d) any other system using guided transport as defined by regulation 2(1) of the 2006 Regulations,

except at a factory, dock, construction site, mine or quarry, and does not include a guided bus system as defined by regulation 2(1) of the 2006 Regulations;

"reportable incident" means an incident giving rise to a notification or reporting requirement under these Regulations;

"reporting procedure" means, in relation to—

    (a) an injury, death or dangerous occurrence (except at a mine or quarry), the procedure described in paragraph 1 of Part 1 of Schedule 1;

    (b) an occupational disease or a disease offshore, the procedure described in paragraph 2 of Part 1 of Schedule 1;

    (c) exposure to a carcinogen, mutagen or biological agent, the procedure described in paragraph 3 of Part 1 of Schedule 1; or

(d) an injury, death or dangerous occurrence at a mine or quarry, the procedure described in paragraph 4 of Part 1 of Schedule 1;

"responsible person" means the person identified in accordance with regulation 3;

"road" includes bridges over which a road passes, and—

(a) in relation to England and Wales, means any highway and any other road to which the public has access;

(b) in relation to Scotland, means any road within the meaning of the Roads (Scotland) Act 1984[238] and any other way to which the public has access;

"road vehicle" means any vehicle on a road, other than a train;

"routine work" means work which a person might reasonably be expected to do, either under that person's contract of employment, or, if there is no such contract, in the normal course of that person's work;

"running line" means any line ordinarily used for the passage of trains which is not a siding;

"specified injury" means any injury or condition specified in regulation 4(1)(a) to (h);

"train" includes a locomotive, tramcar or other power unit, and any vehicle used on a relevant transport system;

"well" includes any structures and devices on top of a well;

"workmen's inspectors" means workmen's inspectors exercising the powers conferred on them by either section 123 of the 1954 Act or regulation 40 of the 1999 Regulations;

"work-related accident" means an accident arising out of or in connection with work.

(2) In these Regulations, any reference to a work-related accident or dangerous occurrence includes an accident or dangerous occurrence attributable to—

(a) the manner of conducting an undertaking;

(b) the plant or substances used for the purposes of an undertaking; or

(c) the condition of the premises used for the purposes of an undertaking or any part of them.

(3) For the purposes of these Regulations, a person at an offshore workplace is deemed to be at work at all times when that person is at that workplace in connection with that person's work.

Responsible person

3.—(1) In these Regulations, the "responsible person" is—   **A2–347**

(a) in relation to an injury, death or dangerous occurrence reportable under regulation 4, 5, 6 or 7 or recordable under regulation 12(1)(b) involving—

(i) an employee, that employee's employer; or

(ii) a person not at work or a self-employed person, or in relation to any other dangerous occurrence, the person who by means of their carrying on any undertaking was in control of the premises where the reportable or recordable incident happened, at the time it happened; or

(b) in relation to a diagnosis reportable under regulation 8, 9 or 10 in respect of—

---

[238] The definition of "road" in section 151 was amended by paragraph 94 of Schedule 8 to the New Roads and Street Works Act 1991 (c.22); there are other amending instruments but none is relevant.

(i) an employee, that employee's employer; or

(ii) a self-employed person, that self-employed person.

(2) Despite paragraph (1), in these Regulations the "responsible person" is—

(a) in relation to a mine, the manager of that mine;

(b) in relation to a closed tip, the owner of the mine with which that tip is associated;

(c) in relation to a quarry, the operator of that quarry;

(d) in relation to a dangerous occurrence—

(i) at a pipeline, the operator of that pipeline; or

(ii) at a well, the person appointed to organise and supervise the drilling of, and operations using, that well by any person granted a licence under section 3 of the Petroleum Act 1998, or where no such person is appointed, that licensee; or

(e) except in relation to a diagnosis reportable under regulation 8, 9 or 10—

(i) at an offshore installation, the duty holder for the purposes of the Offshore Installations and Pipeline Works (Management and Administration) Regulations 1995[239] (provided that for the purposes of this provision regulation 3(2)(c) of those Regulations is deemed not to apply); or

(ii) in relation to a diving project, the diving contractor.

Work-related fatalities

A2–348   6.—(1) Where any person dies as a result of a work-related accident, the responsible person must follow the reporting procedure.

(2) Where any person dies as a result of occupational exposure to a biological agent, the responsible person must follow the reporting procedure.

(3) Where an employee has suffered an injury reportable under regulation 4 which is a cause of his death within one year of the date of the accident, the employer must notify the relevant enforcing authority of the death in an approved manner without delay, whether or not the injury has been reported under regulation 4.

(4) This regulation is subject to regulations 14 and 15, and does not apply to a self-employed person who suffers a fatal accident or fatal exposure on premises controlled by that self-employed person.

Dangerous occurrences

A2–349   7. Where there is a dangerous occurrence, the responsible person must follow the reporting procedure, subject to regulations 14 and 15.

Occupational diseases

A2–350   8. Where, in relation to a person at work, the responsible person receives a diagnosis of—

(a) Carpal Tunnel Syndrome, where the person's work involves regular use of percussive or vibrating tools;

(b) cramp in the hand or forearm, where the person's work involves prolonged periods of repetitive movement of the fingers, hand or arm;

---

[239] To which there are amendments not relevant to these Regulations.

(c) occupational dermatitis, where the person's work involves significant or regular exposure to a known skin sensitizer or irritant;

(d) Hand Arm Vibration Syndrome, where the person's work involves regular use of percussive or vibrating tools, or the holding of materials which are subject to percussive processes, or processes causing vibration;

(e) occupational asthma, where the person's work involves significant or regular exposure to a known respiratory sensitizer; or

(f) tendonitis or tenosynovitis in the hand or forearm, where the person's work is physically demanding and involves frequent, repetitive movements,

the responsible person must follow the reporting procedure, subject to regulations 14 and 15.

Gas-related injuries and hazards

11.—(1) Where a conveyor of flammable gas through a fixed pipe distribution system, or **A2–351** a filler, importer or supplier (except by retail) of a refillable container containing liquefied petroleum gas, receives notification of the death, loss of consciousness or taking to hospital of a person because of an injury arising in connection with that gas, that person must—

(a) notify the Executive of the incident without delay; and

(b) send a report of the incident to the Executive in an approved manner within 14 days of the incident.

(2) Where an approved person has sufficient information to decide that the design, construction, manner of installation, modification or servicing of a gas fitting is or could have been likely to cause the death, loss of consciousness or taking to hospital of a person because of—

(a) the accidental leakage of gas;

(b) the incomplete combustion of gas; or

(c) the inadequate removal of the products of combustion of gas,

the approved person must send a report of that information to the Executive in an approved manner within 14 days of acquiring that information.
(3) Nothing is reportable—

(a) under this regulation, if it is notifiable or reportable elsewhere in these Regulations;

(b) under paragraph (2), in relation to any gas fitting undergoing testing or examination at a place set aside for that purpose; or

(c) under paragraph (2), if the approved person has previously reported that information.

(4) In this regulation—

"approved person" means an employer or self-employed person who is a member of a class of persons approved by the Executive for the purposes of regulation 3(3) of the Gas Safety (Installation and Use) Regulations 1998;

"gas fitting" means a gas fitting defined in those Regulations or any flue or ventilation used in connection with that fitting; and

"liquefied petroleum gas" means commercial butane (that is, a hydrocarbon mixture consisting predominantly of butane, butylene or any mixture of them) or commercial propane (that is, a hydrocarbon mixture consisting predominantly of propane, propylene or any mixture of them) or any mixture of commercial butane and commercial propane.

Recording and record-keeping

A2–352   **12.**—(1) The responsible person must keep a record of any—

(a) reportable incident under regulation 4, 5, 6 or 7, which contains the particulars specified in paragraphs 5 to 11 of Part 2 of Schedule 1;

(b) diagnosis reportable under regulation 8, 9 or 10, which contains the particulars specified in paragraphs 12 to 17 of Part 2 of Schedule 1;

(c) injury to a person at work resulting from an accident arising out of or in connection with that work, incapacitating that person for routine work for more than three consecutive days (excluding the day of the accident), which contains the particulars specified in paragraphs 18 to 21 of Part 2 of Schedule 1; and

(d) other particulars approved by the Executive or the ORR for demonstrating compliance with the approved manner of reporting under Part 1 of Schedule 1.

(2) An entry in the record referred to in paragraph (1) must be kept for at least three years from the date on which it was made, and the record must be—

(a) kept at the place where the work to which it relates is carried on, or at the usual place of business of the responsible person; and

(b) in the case of a mine or quarry, available for inspection by any nominated person and workmen's inspectors (excluding any health record of an identifiable individual).

(3) The responsible person must send to the relevant enforcing authority such extracts from the record required to be kept under paragraph (1) as that enforcing authority may require.

(4) Any record of injuries, deaths, dangerous occurrences or diseases which the responsible person keeps for any other purpose satisfies the requirements of paragraph (1) if it covers the injuries recordable under these Regulations and includes the particulars specified in Part 2 of Schedule 1.

Mines, quarries and offshore site disturbance

A2–353   **13.**—(1) Where there is a reportable incident under regulation 4, 5 or 6 at a mine, quarry or offshore workplace, or where there is a dangerous occurrence at a mine or quarry, then the place where it happened must not be disturbed, or anything at that place tampered with before—

(a) the expiration of three clear days after the matter has been notified in accordance with these Regulations; or

(b) the place has been visited by an inspector and, in the case of a mine or quarry, by workmen's inspectors, if that is sooner.

(2) Nothing in this regulation prohibits any person doing anything by or with the consent of an inspector, or which was necessary—

(a) in the case of a mine or quarry, to secure the safety of the mine or quarry, or of any person; or

(b) in the case of an offshore workplace, to secure the safety or integrity of the workplace or of any person, plant, vessel or well.

(3) In relation to a mine or quarry, this regulation does not apply if an appropriate person—

(a) has taken adequate steps to ascertain that disturbing the site—

    (i) is unlikely to prejudice any investigation by an inspector into the circumstances of the reportable incident; and

    (ii) is necessary to secure the safety of any person at the mine or quarry or to avoid disrupting the normal working of the mine or quarry;

(b) has notified any nominated person, or any person designated in writing by a nominated person to receive any such notification, of the proposed disturbance, and gives such a person a reasonable opportunity to visit the site before it is disturbed (except in the case of a non-fatal accident or dangerous occurrence where any nominated person or person designated by them cannot be contacted within a reasonable time);

(c) has taken adequate steps to ensure that such information is obtained as will enable the preparation, without delay, of a full and accurate plan showing the position of any equipment or item relevant to the reportable incident immediately after it happened;

(d) ensures that that plan is signed by the person who prepared it and bears the date on which it was prepared, and that a copy of that plan is supplied on request to any nominated person or any inspector; and

(e) ensures that any equipment or item relevant to the reportable incident is kept as it was immediately after the incident, until an inspector agrees that it may be disposed of.

(4) In paragraph (3), "appropriate person" means the responsible person or—

(a) in the case of a coal mine, a person appointed in the management structure of that mine established pursuant to regulation 10(1) of the Management and Administration of Safety and Health at Mines Regulations 1993; or

(b) in the case of a quarry, a person appointed in the management structure of that quarry established pursuant to regulation 8(1) of the 1999 Regulations.

Restrictions on the application of regulations 4 to 10

14.—(1) Where the injury or death of a person arises out of the conduct of any operation **A2–354** on, or any examination or other medical treatment of, that person (such operation, examination or other treatment being conducted by or under the supervision of a registered medical practitioner or a registered dentist), the requirements of regulations 4, 5, 6(1) and 12(1)(b) do not apply.

(2) In paragraph (1), "registered dentist" has the meaning given by section 53(1) of the Dentists Act 1984.

(3) Where the injury or death of a person arises out of or in connection with the movement of a vehicle on a road, the requirements of regulations 4, 5, 6 and 12(1)(b) do not apply, unless that person—

(a) was injured or killed by an accident involving a train;

(b) was injured or killed by exposure to a substance being conveyed by the vehicle;

(c) was engaged in work connected with the loading or unloading of any article or substance onto or off the vehicle at the time of the accident, or was injured or killed by the activities of another person who was so engaged; or

(d) was engaged in, or was injured or killed by the activities of another person who was at the time of the accident engaged in, work on or alongside a road.

(4) In paragraph (3)(d), "work on or alongside a road" means work concerned with the construction, demolition, alteration, repair or maintenance of—

(a) the road or the markings or equipment on the road;

(b) the verges, fences, hedges or other boundaries of the road;

(c) pipes or cables on, under, over or adjacent to the road; or

(d) buildings or structures adjacent to or over the road.

(5) The injury, death or diagnosis of a member of the armed forces of the Crown or of a visiting force, on duty at the time, is not subject to the requirements of regulation 4, 6, 8, 9, 10 or 12(1)(b) (and for the purposes of this paragraph a visiting force has the meaning given by section 12(1) of the Visiting Forces Act 1952[240]).

(6) Except in relation to an offshore workplace, regulations 4 to 9 do not apply to anything which must be notified under—

(a) the Nuclear Installations Act 1965;

(b) the Merchant Shipping Act 1988;

(c) Orders and Regulations made or to be made under the enactments in (a) and (b);

(d) the Civil Aviation (Investigation of Air Accidents and Incidents) Regulations 1996[241];

(e) the Ionising Radiations Regulations 1999[2];

(f) the Electricity Safety, Quality and Continuity Regulations 2002[2]; or

(g) the Civil Aviation (Investigation of Military Air Accidents at Civil Aerodromes) Regulations 2005.

Restriction on parallel requirements

A2–355   15.—(1) Where the responsible person is under more than one requirement to make a notification under these Regulations, only one notification is required if the conditions in paragraph (3) are met.

(2) Where the responsible person is under more than one requirement to make a report under these Regulations, only one report is required if the conditions in paragraph (3) are met.

(3) The conditions referred to in paragraphs (1) and (2) are—

(a) the facts giving rise to each requirement are identical;

(b) the information required to be provided by each requirement is provided;

(c) where the requirements have different time limits, the shortest time limit is complied with; and

(d) in the case of a mine or quarry, all steps referred to in paragraph 4 of Part 1 of Schedule 1 are complied with.

(4) Where the responsible person is under more than one requirement to keep a record under these Regulations, only one record is required if the facts giving rise to each

---

[240] The definition of "visiting force" was amended by paragraph 14(1) of Schedule 15 to the Criminal Justice Act 1988 (c.33).
[241] To which there are amendments not relevant to these Regulations.

requirement are identical and the particulars required by each requirement are contained in the record.

SCHEDULE 1

REPORTING AND RECORDING PROCEDURES

PART 1 REPORTING PROCEDURE

Injuries, fatalities and dangerous occurrences

1.—(1) Where required to follow the reporting procedure by regulation 4, 5, 6 or 7 (except in relation to a mine or quarry), the responsible person must—   **A2–356**

(a) notify the relevant enforcing authority of the reportable incident by the quickest practicable means without delay; and

(b) send a report of that incident in an approved manner to the relevant enforcing authority within 10 days of the incident.

(2) Sub-paragraph (1)(a) does not apply to a self-employed person who is injured at premises owned or occupied by that self-employed person, and it is sufficient compliance with sub-paragraph (1)(b) for a self-employed person to make arrangements for the report to be sent to the relevant enforcing authority by some other person.

Diseases

2.—(1) Where required to follow the reporting procedure by regulation 8 or 10, the responsible person must send a report of the diagnosis in an approved manner to the relevant enforcing authority without delay.   **A2–357**

(2) It is sufficient compliance with sub-paragraph (1) for a self-employed person to make arrangements for the report to be sent to the relevant enforcing authority by some other person.

Carcinogens, mutagens and biological agents

3. Where required to follow the reporting procedure by regulation 9 the responsible person must notify the relevant enforcing authority in an approved manner.   **A2–358**

Mines and quarries

4.—(1) Where required to follow the reporting procedure by regulation 4, 5, 6 or 7 in the case of a mine or quarry, the responsible person must—   **A2–359**

(a) notify the relevant enforcing authority and any nominated person of the reportable incident by the quickest practicable means without delay; and

(b) send a report of that incident in an approved manner—

    (i) to any nominated person within seven days of the incident; and
    (ii) to the relevant enforcing authority within 10 days of the incident.

(2) Where the responsible person becomes aware of a person subsequently dying as the result of an accident which gave rise to an injury reported in accordance with sub-paragraph (1), the responsible person must notify any nominated person of the death.

SCHEDULE 2

DANGEROUS OCCURRENCES

PART 1 GENERAL

Lifting equipment

1. The collapse, overturning or failure of any load-bearing part of any lifting equipment, other than an accessory for lifting.   **A2–360**

2. The failure of any closed vessel or of any associated pipework (other than a pipeline) forming part of a pressure system as defined by regulation 2(1) of the Pressure Systems Safety Regulations 2000, where that failure could cause the death of any person.

Overhead electric lines

A2–361　　**3.** Any plant or equipment unintentionally coming into—

(a) contact with an uninsulated overhead electric line in which the voltage exceeds 200 volts; or

(b) close proximity with such an electric line, such that it causes an electrical discharge.

Electrical incidents causing explosion or fire

A2–362　　**4.** Any explosion or fire caused by an electrical short circuit or overload (including those resulting from accidental damage to the electrical plant) which either—

(a) results in the stoppage of the plant involved for more than 24 hours; or

(b) causes a significant risk of death.

Explosives

A2–363　　**5.** Any unintentional—

(a) fire, explosion or ignition at a site where the manufacture or storage of explosives requires a licence or registration, as the case may be, under regulation 9, 10 or 11 of the Manufacture and Storage of Explosives Regulations 2005; or

(b) explosion or ignition of explosives (unless caused by the unintentional discharge of a weapon, where, apart from that unintentional discharge, the weapon and explosives functioned as they were designed to),

except where a fail-safe device or safe system of work prevented any person being endangered as a result of the fire, explosion or ignition.

6. The misfire of explosives (other than at a mine or quarry, inside a well or involving a weapon) except where a fail-safe device or safe system of work prevented any person being endangered as a result of the misfire.

7. Any explosion, discharge or intentional fire or ignition which causes any injury to a person requiring first-aid or medical treatment, other than at a mine or quarry.

8.—(1) The projection of material beyond the boundary of the site on which the explosives are being used, or beyond the danger zone of the site, which caused or might have caused injury, except at a quarry.

(2) In this paragraph, "danger zone" means the area from which persons have been excluded or forbidden to enter to avoid being endangered by any explosion or ignition of explosives.

9. The failure of shots to cause the intended extent of collapse or direction of fall of a structure in any demolition operation.

Biological agents

A2–364　　**10.** Any accident or incident which results or could have resulted in the release or escape of a biological agent likely to cause severe human infection or illness.

Radiation generators and radiography

A2–365　　**11.**—(1) The malfunction of—

(a) a radiation generator or its ancillary equipment used in fixed or mobile industrial radiography, the irradiation of food or the processing of products by irradiation, which causes it to fail to de-energise at the end of the intended exposure period; or

(b) equipment used in fixed or mobile industrial radiography or gamma irradiation, which causes a radioactive source to fail to return to its safe position by the normal means at the end of the intended exposure period.

(2) In this paragraph, "radiation generator" means any electrical equipment emitting ionising radiation and containing components operating at a potential difference of more than 5kV.

Breathing apparatus

12. The malfunction of breathing apparatus—   **A2–366**

(a) where the malfunction causes a significant risk of personal injury to the user; or

(b) during testing immediately prior to use, where the malfunction would have caused a significant risk to the health and safety of the user had it occurred during use,

other than at a mine.

Diving operations

13. The failure, damaging or endangering of—   **A2–367**

(a) any life support equipment, including control panels, hoses and breathing apparatus; or

(b) the dive platform, or any failure of the dive platform to remain on station,

which causes a significant risk of personal injury to a diver.
14. The failure or endangering of any lifting equipment associated with a diving operation.
15. The trapping of a diver.
16. Any explosion in the vicinity of a diver.
17. Any uncontrolled ascent or any omitted decompression which causes a significant risk of personal injury to a diver.

Collapse of scaffolding

18. The complete or partial collapse (including falling, buckling or overturning) of—   **A2–368**

(a) a substantial part of any scaffold more than 5 metres in height;

(b) any supporting part of any slung or suspended scaffold which causes a working platform to fall (whether or not in use); or

(c) any part of any scaffold in circumstances such that there would be a significant risk of drowning to a person falling from the scaffold.

Train collisions

19. The collision of a train with any other train or vehicle, other than a collision reportable under   **A2–369**
Part 5 of this Schedule, which could have caused the death, or specified injury, of any person.

Wells

20. In relation to a well (other than a well sunk for the purpose of the abstraction of water)—   **A2–370**

(a) a blow-out (which includes any uncontrolled flow of well-fluids from a well);

(b) the coming into operation of a blow-out prevention or diversion system to control flow of well-fluids where normal control procedures fail;

(c) the detection of hydrogen sulphide at a well or in samples of well-fluids where the responsible person did not anticipate its presence in the reservoir drawn on by the well;

(d) the taking of precautionary measures additional to any contained in the original drilling programme where a planned minimum separation distance between adjacent wells was not maintained; or

(e) the mechanical failure of any part of a well whose purpose is to prevent or limit the effect of the unintentional release of fluids from a well or a reservoir being drawn on by a well, or whose failure would cause or contribute to such a release.

Pipelines or pipeline works

A2–371   **21.** In relation to a pipeline or pipeline works—

(a) any damage to, accidental or uncontrolled release from or inrush of anything into a pipeline;

(b) the failure of any pipeline isolation device, associated equipment or system; or

(c) the failure of equipment involved with pipeline works,

which could cause personal injury to any person, or which results in the pipeline being shut down for more than 24 hours.

22. The unintentional change in position of a pipeline, or in the subsoil or seabed in the vicinity, which requires immediate attention to safeguard the pipeline's integrity or safety.

SCHEDULE 2

DANGEROUS OCCURRENCES

PART 2 DANGEROUS OCCURENCES REPORTABLE EXCEPT IN RELATION TO AN OFFSHORE WORKPLACE

Structural collapse

A2–372   **23.** The unintentional collapse or partial collapse of—

(a) any structure, which involves a fall of more than 5 tonnes of material; or

(b) any floor or wall of any place of work,

arising from, or in connection with, ongoing construction work (including demolition, refurbishment and maintenance), whether above or below ground.

24. The unintentional collapse or partial collapse of any falsework.

Explosion or fire

A2–373   **25.** Any unintentional explosion or fire in any plant or premises which results in the stoppage of that plant, or the suspension of normal work in those premises, for more than 24 hours.

Release of flammable liquids and gases

A2–374   **26.** The sudden, unintentional and uncontrolled release—

(a) inside a building—

    (i) of 100 kilograms or more of a flammable liquid;

    (ii) of 10 kilograms or more of a flammable liquid at a temperature above its normal boiling point;

    (iii) of 10 kilograms or more of a flammable gas; or

(b) in the open air, of 500 kilograms or more of a flammable liquid or gas.

Hazardous escapes of substances

A2–375   **27.** The unintentional release or escape of any substance which could cause personal injury to any person other than through the combustion of flammable liquids or gases.

PART 3 DANGEROUS OCCURRENCES REPORTABLE IN RELATION TO A MINE

Fires or ignition of gas

A2–376   **28.** Any outbreak of fire below ground.

Fires or ignition of gas

A2–377   **29.** Any person being caused to leave any place pursuant to regulation 11(1) of the Coal and Other Mines (Fire and Rescue) Regulations 1956 or section 79 of the 1954 Act, as a result of smoke or other indication that a fire may have broken out below ground.

30. Any fire on the surface which endangers the operation of any winding or haulage apparatus installed at a shaft or unwalkable outlet or of any mechanically operated apparatus for producing ventilation below ground.

31. The ignition of any gas (other than in a safety lamp) or dust below ground.

32. The unintentional ignition of any gas in part of a firedamp drainage system on the surface or in an exhauster house.

Escapes of gas with solid matter

33. The violent unintentional escape of gas together with coal or other solid matter into the mine workings.

A2–378

Failures of plant or equipment

34. The breakage or unintentional uncoupling of any belt, rope, chain, coupling, balance rope, guide rope, rope tensioning system, suspension gear or other gear used for or in connection with—

A2–379

(a) carrying persons through any shaft or staple shaft;

(b) transporting persons below ground; or

(c) a belt conveyor designated by the mine manager as a man-riding conveyor.

35. The overwinding of—

(a) any conveyance being used for the carriage of persons; or

(b) any other conveyance, which becomes detached from its winding rope.

36. The bringing to rest of any conveyance operated using the friction of a rope on a winding sheave by the apparatus provided—

(a) in the headframe of the shaft; or

(b) in the part of the shaft below the lowest landing for the time being in use,

for the purpose of bringing the conveyance to rest in the event of it being overwound.

37. The stoppage of any ventilating apparatus (other than an auxiliary fan) for over 30 minutes, except for planned maintenance, which causes a reduction in mine ventilation resulting in dangerous levels of noxious or flammable gases.

38. The collapse of any headframe, winding engine house, fan house or storage bunker.

Breathing apparatus

39. The malfunction of, or development of a defect in, breathing apparatus or a smoke helmet or other apparatus serving the same purpose or a self-rescuer where—

A2–380

(a) the malfunction or defect causes, or is likely to cause, a significant risk of personal injury to the user; or

(b) immediately after use and as a result of its use any person receives first-aid or medical treatment because of that person's unfitness or suspected unfitness.

Emergency escape apparatus

40. The use of any apparatus—

A2–381

(a) provided at a mine in accordance with regulation 4 of the Mines (Safety of Exit) Regulations 1988; or

(b) used to leave a mine when apparatus and equipment normally so used is unavailable,

other than for the purpose of training and practice.

Inrushes of gas or flowing material

41. The inrush of noxious or flammable gas from old workings.

A2–382

42. The inrush of water or material which flows when wet from any source.

Insecure tips

A2–383   **43.** Any event (including any movement of material or any fire) which indicates that a tip to which Part 1 of the 1969 Act applies is or is likely to become insecure.

Locomotives

A2–384   **44.** The bringing to rest of an underground locomotive by means other than its safety circuit protective devices or normal service brakes, when not used for testing purposes.

Falls of ground

A2–385   **45.** Any fall of ground which—

(a) results from a failure of an underground support system; and

(b) prevents persons travelling through the area affected by the fall, or otherwise exposes them to danger,

other than one which is part of the normal operations at a mine.

Accidents causing specified injuries

A2–386   **46.** Any accident in which any person suffers a specified injury.

PART 4 DANGEROUS OCCURENCES WHICH ARE REPORTABLE IN RELATION TO A QUARRY

Collapse of storage bunkers

A2–387   **47.** The collapse of any storage bunker.

Sinking of craft

A2–388   **48.** The sinking of any water-borne craft or hovercraft.

Projection of substances outside quarry

A2–389   **49.**—(1) Following a blasting operation, the projection of any material beyond the designated danger zone or the projection of any material which caused or might have caused injury.

(2) In this paragraph, "danger zone" means the area determined for each blast under the shotfiring rules required by regulation 25(2)(a)(i) and (b) of the 1999 Regulations.

Misfires

A2–390   **50.** Any misfire, as defined by regulation 2(1) of the 1999 Regulations.

Insecure tips

A2–391   **51.** Any event (including any movement of material or any fire) which indicates that a tip to which the 1999 Regulations apply is or is likely to become insecure.

Movement of slopes or faces

A2–392   **52.** Any movement or failure of an excavated slope or face which—

(a) could cause the death of any person; or

(b) adversely affects any building, contiguous land, transport system, footpath, public utility or service, watercourse, reservoir or area of public access.

Explosion or fire in vehicles or mobile plant

A2–393   **53.** Any explosion or fire in—

(a) a dump truck with a load capacity of at least 50 tonnes; or

(b) an excavator with a bucket capacity of at least 5 cubic metres,

which results in the stoppage of that vehicle or plant for more than 24 hours, and which affects—

     (i) any place where persons normally work; or
     (ii) the route of egress from such a place.

PART 5 DANGEROUS OCCURRENCES WHICH ARE REPORTABLE IN RESPECT OF A RELEVANT TRANSPORT SYSTEM

Collision or derailment of passenger trains

54. Any collision between a passenger train and another train.   **A2–394**
55. The derailment of the whole or part of a passenger train.

Collision or derailment not involving passenger trains

56. Any collision between non-passenger trains—   **A2–395**

(a) on a running line, which causes damage to a train; or

(b) in a siding, which causes damage to a train and an obstruction to a running line.

57. The derailment of a non-passenger train—

(a) on a running line, except a derailment during shunting operations which does not obstruct any other running line; or

(b) in a siding, which causes an obstruction to a running line.

Accidents involving any train

58. Any collision between a train and a buffer stop which causes damage to the train, except a   **A2–396** collision in a siding.
59. A train striking any cattle or horse, whether or not damage is caused to the train, or striking any other animal which causes damage necessitating immediate temporary or permanent repair (including damage to the windows of the driver's cab but excluding other damage consisting solely in the breakage of glass).
60. A train on a running line striking or being struck by any object which causes damage necessitating immediate temporary or permanent repair (including damage to the windows of the driver's cab but excluding other damage consisting solely in the breakage of glass) or which might have been liable to derail the train.
61. A train, other than one on a railway, striking or being struck by a road vehicle.
62. A passenger train, or a non-passenger train not fitted with continuous self-applying brakes, becoming unintentionally divided.

Failure of train parts

63. The failure of—   **A2–397**

(a) an axle;

(b) a wheel or tyre, including a tyre loose on its wheel;

(c) a rope or the rope's fastenings;

(d) a winding plant or equipment involved in working an incline; or

(e) any part of a train which is likely to cause an accident to that or any other train, or to cause personal injury to any person,

which occurs or is discovered whilst the train is on a running line.

Fire

64. Any fire—   **A2–398**

(a) in or on any part of a passenger train or a train carrying dangerous goods within the meaning of the Carriage of Dangerous Goods and Use of Transportable Pressure Equipment Regulations 2009;

(b) in or on any part of a non-passenger train which was extinguished by a fire-fighting service;

(c) seriously affecting the functioning of signalling equipment;

(d) affecting the permanent way or works of a relevant transport system which necessitates the suspension of services over any line, or the closure of any part of a station or signal box or other premises, for a period—

    (i) of more than 30 minutes in the case of any part of a relevant transport system below ground; and

    (ii) in any other case, of more than 1 hour; or

(e) causing damage which could affect the running of a relevant transport system.

Severe electrical arcing or fusing

A2–399   **65.** Severe electrical arcing or fusing—

(a) in or on any part of any train; or

(b) which seriously affects the functioning of signalling equipment.

Level crossings

A2–400   **66.** Any train striking a road vehicle or gate at a level crossing.
67. Any train running onto a level crossing when not authorised to do so.
68. The failure of equipment at a level crossing which could cause a significant risk of personal injury to users of the road or path crossing the railway.

The permanent way and other works

A2–401   **69.** The failure of a rail in a running line or of a rack rail, which results in—

(a) a complete fracture of the rail through its cross-section; or

(b) in a piece becoming detached from the rail which requires the immediate stoppage of traffic or the immediate imposition of a lower speed restriction.

The permanent way and other works

A2–402   **70.** The buckle of a running line which requires the immediate stoppage of traffic or the immediate imposition of a lower speed restriction.
71. An aircraft or vehicle of any kind either landing on, running onto or coming to rest across the line, or damaging the line, so as to cause damage—

(a) which obstructs the line; or

(b) to any railway equipment at a level crossing.

72. The runaway of an escalator, lift or passenger conveyor.
73. The following classes of accident where they are likely to cause an accident to a train or a significant risk of personal injury to any person—

(a) the failure of a tunnel, bridge, viaduct, culvert, station or other structure or any part of it including the fixed electrical equipment of an electrified relevant transport system;

(b) any failure in the signalling system which could cause a significant risk to the safe passage of trains other than a failure of a traffic light controlling the movement of vehicles on a road;

(c) a slip of a cutting or of an embankment;

(d) flooding of the permanent way;

(e) the striking of a bridge by a vessel or by a road vehicle or its load; or

(f) the failure of any other portion of the permanent way or works.

Incidents of signals passed without authority

A2–403   **74.** Any train, travelling on a running line or entering a running line from a siding, passing a signal displaying a stop aspect without authority, unless the stop aspect was not displayed in sufficient time for the driver to stop safely at the signal.

Part 6 Dangerous Occurrences Which Are Reportable In Respect Of An Offshore Workplace

Release of petroleum hydrocarbon

75. The unintentional release of petroleum hydrocarbon on or from an offshore installation **A2–404**
which—

(a) results in—

    (i) a fire or explosion; or
    (ii) the taking of action to prevent or limit the consequences of a potential fire or explosion; or

(b) could cause a specified injury to, or the death of, any person.

76. Any fire or explosion at an offshore installation, other than one caused by the release of petroleum hydrocarbon, which results in the stoppage of plant or the suspension of normal work.
77. The unintentional or uncontrolled release or escape of any substance (other than petroleum hydrocarbon) on or from an offshore installation which could cause a significant risk of personal injury to any person.
78. Any unintentional collapse or partial collapse of any offshore installation or of any plant on an offshore installation which jeopardises the overall structural integrity of the installation.

Equipment

79. The failure of equipment required to maintain a floating offshore installation on station which **A2–405**
could cause a specified injury to, or the death of, any person.

Dropping objects

80. The dropping of any object on an offshore installation or on an attendant vessel or into the water **A2–406**
adjacent to an installation or vessel which could cause a specified injury to, or the death of, any person.

Weather damage

81. Any damage to or on an offshore installation caused by adverse weather conditions and which **A2–407**
could cause a specified injury to, or the death of, any person.

Collisions

82. Any collision between a vessel or aircraft and an offshore installation which causes damage to the **A2–408**
installation, the vessel or the aircraft.
83. Any occurrence with the potential for a collision between a vessel and an offshore installation where, had a collision occurred, it might have jeopardised the overall structural integrity of the installation.

Subsidence or collapse of seabed

84. Any subsidence or collapse of the seabed likely to affect the foundations or the overall structural **A2–409**
integrity of an offshore installation.

Loss of stability or buoyancy

85. Any incident which causes the loss of stability or buoyancy of a floating offshore installation. **A2–410**

Evacuation

86. The partial or complete evacuation of an offshore installation in the interests of safety. **A2–411**

Falls into water

87. Any fall of a person into water from more than 2 metres. **A2–412**

Service Custody and Service of Relevant Sentences Rules 2009/1096

PART 3

TREATMENT, EMPLOYMENT AND DISCIPLINE OF DETAINEES

Deaths in service custody premises

A2–413   39.—(1) If a detainee dies, the commandant shall—

(a) if the death occurs in England, Wales or Northern Ireland, immediately report the fact to the coroner having jurisdiction in the place where the service custody premises is situated;

(b) if the death occurs in Scotland, immediately report the fact to the procurator fiscal having jurisdiction in the place where the service custody premises is situated;

(c) if the death occurs outside the United Kingdom, report the fact to any local civil authority which is authorised or required to inquire into the cause of death.

(2) Nothing in this rule shall affect the duty of the commandant to record or report the death to meet the requirements of any other rules, regulations or instructions.

Treasure (Designation) Order 2002/2666

Citation, commencement and application

A2–414   1.—(1) This Order may be cited as the Treasure (Designation) Order 2002 and shall come into force on 1st January 2003.

(2) This Order applies only in relation to objects found on or after the date when it comes into force.

Interpretation

A2–415   2. In this Order—

"the Act" means the Treasure Act 1996;
"base metal" means any metal other than gold or silver; and
"of prehistoric date" means dating from the Iron Age or any earlier period.

Designation of classes of objects of outstanding historical, archaeological or cultural importance

A2–416   3. The following classes of objects are designated pursuant to section 2(1) of the Act.

(a) any object (other than a coin), any part of which is base metal, which, when found is one of at least two base metal objects in the same find which are of prehistoric date;

(b) any object, (other than a coin) which is of prehistoric date, and any part of which is gold or silver.

Young Offender Institution Rules 2000/3371

PART II

INMATES

Medical Attention

Notification of illness or death

29.—(1) If an inmate dies, or becomes seriously ill, sustains any severe injury or is   **A2–417**
removed to hospital on account of mental disorder, the governor shall, if he knows his or
her address, at once inform the inmate's spouse or next of kin, and also any person who the
inmate may reasonably have asked should be informed.

(2) If an inmate dies, the governor shall give notice immediately to the coroner having
jurisdiction, to the [independent monitoring board]²⁴² and to the Secretary of State.

---

²⁴² Words substituted by Young Offender Institution (Amendment) Rules 2008/599 rule 4(a) (April 1,
2008).

Appendix 3

FORMS

A3–01 This Appendix contains suggested forms (as set out above) for use where none has been prescribed or is provided by the appropriate government department or body. For the sake of completeness another list (below) is given of forms which are prescribed or otherwise provided, together with their source. Forms for judicial review and similar court proceedings are set out in Appendix 4.

A3–02 A number of forms were prescribed by the Coroners Rules 1984 (now repealed), but have not been prescribed under the new Coroners (Inquests) Rules 2013 or the Coroners (Investigations) Regulations 2013. In practice, these forms have continued to be used, though now without statutory authority, and sometimes with necessary modifications. These forms are also referred to in the following list.

A3–03 The following abbreviations are used:

CR	Coroners Rules 1984 (as amended, and now repealed)
Inq Rules	Coroners (Inquests) Rules 2013
Inv Regs	Coroners (Investigations) Regulations 2013
RBR	Removal of Bodies Regulations 1954 (as amended)
RBD Regs	Registration of Births and Deaths Regulations 1987 (as amended)
RBDW Regs	Registration of Births and Deaths (Welsh Language) Regulations 1987 (as amended)
C Regs	Cremation (England and Wales) Regulations 2008 (as amended)
R–G	Registrar General of England and Wales

H.S.E.   Health and Safety Executive

Description of Form	Prescribed/ provided by	Para. in this work (if applicable)
Direction to Exhume	Inv Regs, Form 4	A2–147
Coroner's Certificate of the Fact of Death	Inv Regs, Form 1	A2–147
Coroner's Order for Burial	Inv Regs, Form 3	A2–147
Notice of Discontinuance	Inv Regs, Form 2	A2–147
Summons to Juror	Inq Rules, Form 1	A2–117
Record of Inquest	Inq Rules, Form 2	A2–117
Post-Mortem Examination Report	CR, r. 10, Sched. 2	Not applicable
Coroner's Register of Deaths	*ibid.* r. 54, Sched. 3	Not applicable
Form of Declaration of Office of Coroner	*ibid.* r. 60, Sched. 4, Form 1	Not applicable
Warrant to Summon Jury	*ibid.* Form 3	Not applicable
Notice to Accompany Summons and Reply Thereto	*ibid.* Form 5	Not applicable
Certificate of Attendance	*ibid.* Form 6	Not applicable
Form of Oath of Juror	*ibid.* Form 7	Not applicable
Summons to Witness	*ibid.* Form 8	Not applicable
Oath of Witness	*ibid.* Form 9	Not applicable
Direction to Medical Practitioner to make a Post-Mortem Examination	*ibid.* Form 10	Not applicable
Certificate of Fine	*ibid.* Form 11	Not applicable
Form of Recognizance	*ibid.* Form 12	Not applicable
Notice of Inquest Arrangements	*ibid.* Form 13	Not applicable
Coroner's Interim Certificate of the Fact of Death	*ibid.* Form 14	Not applicable
Notice of Non-Resumption of an Adjourned Inquest	*ibid.* Form 15	Not applicable
Notice of Resumption of an Adjourned Inquest	*ibid.*, Form 16	Not applicable
Notice of Discharging Witness from Attendance at Resumed Inquest	*ibid.* Form 17	Not applicable
Notice of Alteration of Time or Place for Resumption of Inquest	*ibid.* Form 18	Not applicable
Certificate of Forfeiture of Recognizance	*ibid.* Form 19	Not applicable
Order to Remove Body for Inquest or Post-Mortem Examination	*ibid.* Form 20	Not applicable
Notice of Intention to Remove Body out of England and Wales	RBR, Sched. 1 (R–G Form 104, REV)	A2–343
Acknowledgement of Notice of Intention to Remove Body	*ibid.* Sched. 2 (R–G Form 103, Part B)	A2–344
Coroner's Notice of Registrar of Body's Impending Removal	R–G Form 103, Part C	[See Note 1]
Application for Cremation of Body	C Regs, Sched., Form 1	A2–176
Application for Cremation of Body Parts	*ibid.* Sched., Form 2	A2–177
Application for Cremation of Stillborn Baby	*ibid.* Sched., Form 3	A2–178
Medical Certificate for Cremation	*ibid.* Sched., Form 4	A2–179
Confirmatory Medical Certificate for Cremation	*ibid.* Sched., Form 5	A2–180
Coroner's Certificate for Cremation	*ibid.* Sched., Form 6	A2–181
Certificate of Anatomical Examination	*ibid.* Sched., Form 7	A2–182
Certificate Releasing Body Parts for Cremation	*ibid.* Sched., Form 8	A2–183

Description of Form	Prescribed/ provided by	Para. in this work (if applicable)
Certificate of Still-birth	*ibid*. Sched., Form 9	A2–184
Medical Referee's Certificate for Cremation	*ibid*. Sched., Form 10	A2–185
Certificate of Post-Mortem Examiner for Cremation	*ibid*. Sched., Form 11	A2–186
Authority to Cremate Body Parts	*ibid*. Sched., Form 12	A2–187
Authority to Cremate Stillborn Baby	*ibid*. Sched., Form 13	A2–188
Particulars of Still-birth	RBD Regs, Schd. 2 Form 9	A2–313
	RBSW Regs, Sched. 2, Form 7;	A2–332
Certificate of Still-birth	RBD Regs, Sched. 2, Form 10	A2–314
	RBDW Regs, Sched. 2, Form 8;	A2–333
Declaration as to Still-birth	RBD Regs, Sched. 2, Form 11	A2–315
	RBDW Regs, Sched. 2, Form 9	A2–334
Certificate of Registration of Still-birth	RBD Regs, Sched. 2, Form 12;	A2–316
Particulars of Death	RBD Regs, Sched. 2, Form 13	A2–317
	RBDW Regs, Sched. 2, Form 10	A2–335
Death Certificate	RBD Regs, Sched. 2, Form 14 (R–G Form 66)	A2–318
	RBDW Regs, Sched. 2, Form 11;	A2–336
Death Certificate for Child less than 28 days old	RBD Regs, Sched. 2, Form 15	A2–319
	RBDW Regs, Sched. 2, Form 12;	A2–337
Notice to Informant of Death	RBD Regs, Sched. 2, Form 16	A2–320
	RBDW Regs, Sched. 2, Form 13;	A2–338
Notification of Disposal	RBD Regs, Sched. 2, Form 17	A2–321
	RBDW Regs, Sched. 2, Form 14;	A2–339
Declaration that Certificate or Order Issued	RBD Regs, Sched. 2, Form 18	A2–322
	RBDW Regs, Sched. 2, Form 15	A2–340
Certificate that Death not Required to be Registered	RBD Regs, Sched 2, Form 19	A2–323
Certificate relating to Visiting Forces	R–G Form 90	[See Note 1]
Certificate after Inquest	*ibid*. Form 99 REV	[See Note 1]
Certificate of Still-birth	*ibid*. Form 99A	[See Note 1]
Certificate After Inquest Adjourned	*ibid*. Form 120	[See Note 1]
Certificate After Resumed Inquest	*ibid*. Form 121	[See Note 1]
Annual Return	Ministry of Justice	[See Note 2]
Merchant Shipping Death Return	Registrar General of Shipping and Seamen, Form RBD 13	[See Note 3]

Note 1: The Registrar General for England and Wales is based at the General Register Office (now part of Hm Passport Office), PO Box2, Southport, PR8 2JD; tel no. 0300 123 1837; *www.gro.gov.uk*.

Note 2: The Ministry of Justice sends the form of Annual return to coroners each year.

Note 3: The Registry of Shipping is part of the Maritime and Coastguard Agency (Spring Place, 105 Commercial Road, Southampton, SO15 1EG; tel no. 023 8032 9365; *www.dft.gov.uk/mca/mcga07-home/*).

A3–04 1. *Appointment of Senior Coroner*

Pursuant to paragraph 1 of Schedule 3 to the Coroners and Justice Act 2014, [*name*] the relevant authority for [*name of coroner area*], [do hereby appoint [*name*] now of [*address*] to be the senior coroner for that area. [This appointment does not constitute a contract of employment.]

Dated this   day   20

       [*Signed*]
       On behalf of [*name of relevant authority*]

Approved by me this   day of   20

       [*Signed*]
       Lord Chancellor

Approved by me this   day of   20

       [*Signed*]
       Chief Coroner

A3–05 2. *Appointment of Area or Assistant Coroner*

Pursuant to paragraph 2 of Schedule 3 to the Coroners and Justice Act 2014, [*name*] the relevant authority for [*name of coroner area*], [do hereby appoint [*name*] now of [*address*] to be an [Area *or* Assistant] Coroner for that area. [This appointment does not constitute a contract of employment.]

Dated this   day   20

       [*Signed*]
       On behalf of [*name of relevant authority*]

Approved by me this   day of   20

       [*Signed*]
       Lord Chancellor

Approved by me this   day of   20

       [*Signed*]
       Chief Coroner

A3–06 3. *Notice to Witness under Schedule 5 para 1(2)*

To [*name of witness*], of [*address*].

By virtue of the power contained in the Coroners and Justice Act 2009, s 32 and Sch 5 paragraph 1(2), I hereby require you by [*date and time*]

[to provide to me evidence in the form of a written statement about the matters listed in the [Second] Schedule to this notice, being matters relevant to the investigation into the death of [*name of deceased*]] [to produce the documents listed in the First Schedule to this notice, and any other document in your custody or under your control which relate to the matters set out in the Second Schedule, being matters relevant to the investigation into the death of [*name of deceased*]]

[to produce for inspection, examination or testing the thing(s) listed in the First Schedule or any other thing in your custody or under your control which relate(s) to the matters set out in the Second Schedule, being matters relevant to the investigation into the death of [*name of deceased*]].

The possible consequences of not complying with this notice include a fine in a sum not exceeding £1,000 under paragraph 6 of Schedule 6 of the Coroners and Justice Act 2009. In addition there are various offences connected with distorting or altering any evidence, document or other thing given, produced or provided for the purposes of a coroner's investigation (which includes an inquest), and with suppressing or concealing, or altering or destroying such documents, under paragraph 7 of Schedule 6 of the same Act.

If you wish to make a claim that you are unable to comply with this notice, or that it is not reasonable in all the circumstances to require you to comply with this notice, then you must apply to me for that purpose, either in person or in writing and I will determine your application. However, it may be necessary for me to give an opportunity to others affected by your application before determining it, and for that purpose I may need to hold a hearing at which you and such others may be heard. If so, I will appoint a time and place for such hearing, and give you notice of it.

[First Schedule

[*List of documents or things for production*]]

[[Second] Schedule

[*List of matters relevant to the investigation*]]

[*name*]

HM [Senior/Area/Assistant] Coroner for [*coroner area*]

4. *Notice to Witness under Schedule 5 para 1(1)*   **A3–07**

To [*name of witness*], of [*address*].

By virtue of the power contained in the Coroners and Justice Act 2009, s 32 and Sch 5 paragraph 1(1), I hereby require you to attend at [*address*], at [*time*] on [*date*] [*for attendance to give evidence, add*: and for so long thereafter as may be necessary]

[to give evidence at the inquest into the death of [*name of deceased*]]

[to produce the documents listed in the First Schedule to this notice, and any other document in your custody or under your control which relate to the matters set out in the Second Schedule, being matters relevant to the inquest into the death of [*name of deceased*]]

[to produce for inspection, examination or testing the thing(s) listed in the First Schedule or any other thing in your custody or under your control which relate(s) to the matters set out in the Second Schedule, being matters relevant to the inquest into the death of [*name of deceased*]].

The possible consequences of not complying with this notice include a fine in a sum not exceeding £1,000 under paragraph 6 of Schedule 6 of the Coroners and Justice Act 2009.

In addition there are various offences connected with distorting or altering any evidence, document or other thing given, produced or provided for the purposes of a coroner's investigation (which includes an inquest), and with suppressing or concealing, or altering or destroying such documents, under paragraph 7 of Schedule 6 of the same Act.

If you wish to make a claim that you are unable to comply with this notice, or that it is not reasonable in all the circumstances to require you to comply with this notice, then you must apply to me for that purpose, either in person or in writing and I will determine your application. However, it may be necessary for me to give an opportunity to others affected by your application before determining it, and for that purpose I may need to hold a hearing at which you and such others may be heard. If so, I will appoint a time and place for such hearing, and give you notice of it.

[First Schedule

[*List of documents or things for production*]]

[Second Schedule

[*List of matters relevant to the inquest*]]

[*name*]

HM [Senior/Area/Assistant] Coroner for [*coroner area*]

A3–08   5. *Formal Proclamation of Opening Court without Jury*

Oyez oyez oyez.

All manner of persons who have anything to do at this Court before The Queen's Coroner for this coroner area touching the death of [*name*], draw near and give your attendance, and if anyone can give evidence, on behalf of our Sovereign Lady the Queen, when, how, and by what means [*name*] came to his death, let him come forth, and he shall be heard.

A3–09   6. *Formal Proclamation for Opening of Court with Jury*

[*As in Form 5*] and you good men of this coroner area summoned to appear here this day, to enquire for our Sovereign, when, how by what means [*name*] came to his death, answer to your names as you shall be called, each at the first call, upon the pains and perils that shall fall thereon.

A3–10   7. *Formal Proclamation for Adjourning Court*

All manner of persons who have anything more to do at this court before The Queen's Coroner for this coroner area may depart home at this time, and give their attendance [here again *or at* [*the adjourned place*]] on [*name of day*] next, being the [*date*] day of [*month*] at [*time*] precisely—God Save the Queen.

A3–11   8. *Formal Proclamation for Resuming an Adjourned Inquest*

All manner of persons who have anything more to do at this court, before The Queen's Coroner for this coroner area, on this inquest now to be taken, and adjourned over to this time and place, draw near and give your attendance; and you members of the jury who have been impanelled and sworn upon this inquest to inquire touching the death of [*name*], answer severally to your names and save your recognizances.

A3–12   9. *Formal Proclamation for Default of Jurors*

You good men and women who have been already severally called, and have made default, answer to your names and save your fines.

10. *Oath on Voir Dire*   **A3–13**

You shall true answer make to all such questions as the court shall demand of you. So help you God.

11. *Bench Warrant*   **A3–14**

The [*name of coroner area*], *to wit.*

WHEREAS I, [*name*], Her Majesty's [Senior/Area/Assistant] Coroner for the coroner area of [*name*], have received credible information that [*name*] of [*address*], [*occupation*], can give evidence on behalf of our Sovereign Lady The Queen, touching the death of [*name*]; and whereas the said [*name*] (having been duly summoned by notice under paragraph 1 of Schedule 5 to the Coroners and Justice Act 2009 to appear and give evidence before me and my inquest, touching the premises, at the time and place specified in the said notice, of which oath hath been duly made before me) has refused and neglected so to do, to the great hindrance and delay of justice:

THESE ARE THEREFORE, by virtue of my office, in Her Majesty's name, to charge and command you, or one of you, without delay, to apprehend and bring before me, [*name*], HM [Senior/Area/Assistant] Coroner for the coroner area of [*name*], now sitting at [*place*], by virtue of my said office, the body of the said [*name*], that he may be dealt with according to law:

AND FOR SO DOING this shall be your warrant.

Given under my hand this [   ] day of [   ] 20[ ].

HM [Senior/Area/Assistant] Coroner for the coroner area of [*name*].

TO all constables and others Her Majesty's officers of the peace, and also to [*name*], my special officer

12. *Warrant Against Juror or Witness for Contempt of Summons*   **A3–15**

TO the Coroner's officer(s) and to each and all the constables and others Her Majesty's officers of the peace in and for the coroner area of [*name*]:

WHEREAS I, [*name*], Her Majesty's [Senior/Area/Assistant] Coroner for the coroner area of [*name*], have received credible information that [*name*], of [*address*] [is duly qualified for being a juror of the inquest now to be held before me] [can give evidence on behalf of our Sovereign Lady the Queen], touching the death of [*name of deceased*], and WHEREAS the said [*name*], having been duly summoned to [attend as a juror] [appear and give evidence] before me and my inquest, touching the premises, at the time and place in the said summons specified, of which oath has been duly made before me, has refused and neglected so to do, to the great hindrance and delay of justice:

THESE ARE THEREFORE, by virtue of my office, in Her Majesty's name, to charge and command you, or any of you, without delay, to apprehend and bring before me the said [*name of juror or witness*], that he may be dealt with according to law.

AND FOR SO DOING this is your warrant;

GIVEN UNDER MY HAND this   day of   20

                         [*Signed*]
                         Her Majesty's [Senior/Area/Assistant] Coroner, coroner area of [*name*]

A3–16   13. *Oath of Jury in Treasure Inquest*

I swear by Almighty God that I will diligently inquire on behalf of our Sovereign Lady the Queen into certain treasure lately found and to be here produced, and give a true verdict according to the evidence.

A3–17   14. *Oath in the Scottish Form (with uplifted hand)*

I swear by Almighty God, as I shall answer to God at the Great Day of Judgment, that I will tell the truth, the whole truth, and nothing but the truth.

A3–18   15. *Affirmation*

I, [*name*], do solemnly, sincerely and truly declare and affirm that the evidence that I shall give shall be the truth, the whole truth and nothing but the truth.

A3–19   16. *Oath of Interpreter*

I swear by Almighty God that I will well and truly interpret unto the witness(es) here produced on behalf of our Sovereign Lady The Queen, touching the death of [*name*], the oath that shall be administered unto [him/her/them], and also the questions and demands which shall be made to the witness(es) by the Court [or the jury] concerning the matters of this inquiry, and I will well and truly interpret the answers which the witness(es) shall thereunto give, according to the best of my skill and ability.

A3–20   17. *Warrant to Commit Witness for Refusing to Give Evidence*

TO the constables and others Her Majesty's officers of the peace in and for the coroner area of [*name*], AND ALSO TO the Governor of H.M. Prison at [*place*]:

WHEREAS [*name*] of [*address*], having appeared before me, Her Majesty's [Senior/Area/Assistant] Coroner for the coroner area of [*name*], [and a jury] sitting at [*place*] and having been duly required to give evidence and be examined before me and my inquest, on Her Majesty's behalf, touching the death of [*name*], the said [*name*] has wilfully and absolutely refused, and still does wilfully and absolutely refuse to [take an oath] [give evidence and be examined touching the premises], or to give any just or sufficient reason for this refusal, in wilful and open violation and delay of justice:

THESE ARE THEREFORE, by virtue of my office, in Her Majesty's name, to charge and command you, or one of you, the said constables, and others Her Majesty's officers of the peace in and for the said coroner area, forthwith to convey the said [*name*] to her Majesty's prison aforesaid, and safely to deliver to the Governor of the said prison there; AND THESE ARE, LIKEWISE, to will and require you the said Governor to receive the said [*name*] into your custody, and him safely to keep in the prison for the period of [*period not exceeding 1 month*] or until he shall be discharged from thence by due course of law;

AND FOR SO DOING this is your warrant.

GIVEN UNDER MY HAND this   day of   20

[*Signed*]
Her Majesty's [Senior/Area/Assistant] Coroner, coroner area of [*name*]

A3–21   18. *Warrant to Commit for Contempt of Court*

[*Begin as in Form 17*]

WHEREAS at an inquest held this day before me [*name*], Her Majesty's [Senior/Area/Assistant] Coroner for the coroner area of [*name*], [and a jury] sitting at [*place*], touching the death of [*name*], [*name*] [*here set out the action or actions amounting to a contempt*] in wilful and open violation of justice:

THESE ARE, THEREFORE, . . .

[*Conclude as in Form 17*].

19. Oath of Officer in Charge of Jury
A3–22

I swear by Almighty God that I shall well and truly keep the jury upon this inquiry, that I shall not suffer any person to speak to them, nor shall I speak to them myself, unless it be to ask them if they have agreed upon their verdicts, until they shall be so agreed.

20. Treasure Inquisition
A3–23

AN INQUISITION taken for our Sovereign Lady The Queen at [*place*], in the coroner area of [*name*], on the day of 20 [and by adjournment on the day of 20], before me [*name*], Her Majesty's [Senior/Area/Assistant] Coroner for the coroner area of [*name*], [upon the oath of the under-mentioned jurors, good and lawful men (and women), duly sworn and charged to inquire for our said Lady The Queen] of and concerning certain chattels, lately found [and now here produced], when, where, how and by what means and by whom the said chattels were found and whether they were or not treasure, and having heard evidence upon oath, [do upon their oath] [I] say as follows:

1) that the said find, consisting of [*set out what the treasure consisted of*], was, on the day of 20 , found by [*name of finder*] at [*place*] [*set out the circumstances of the find, including whether it was part of another find*];
2) that the said chattels [are][are not] treasure;
3) that [no-one] [*name*] has a prior interest in them [that is, [*describe prior interest*]].

I, the said coroner, have [taken and seized the said treasure trove into Her Majesty's hands] [released the said chattels into the hands of [*name*]].

[*Signed*]
Her Majesty's [Senior/Area/Assistant] Coroner, coroner area of [*name*]

[*Signatures of Jurors*]

21. Formal Proclamation for Closing Court without Jury
A3–24

Oyez oyez oyez.

All manner of persons who have had anything to do at this court before The Queen's Coroner for this coroner area touching the death of [*name*], having discharged your duty may depart hence and take your ease.

22. Formal Proclamation for Closing Court with Jury
A3–25

Oyez oyez oyez.

All manner of persons who have had anything to do at this Court before The Queen's Coroner for this coroner area touching the death of [*name*], having discharged your duty, and you good men [and women] of the jury having returned your verdict, may depart hence and take your ease.

23. Coroner's Certificate to Correct Errors of Substance in Certificate after Inquest
A3–26

WHEREAS on the day of 20 at [*place*] an inquest was held touching the death of [*name*], before me, [*name*], Her Majesty's [Senior/Area/Assistant] Coroner for the coroner area of [*name*], and a jury];

AND WHEREAS I, the said coroner, on the day of 20 transmitted to the Registrar of Births and Deaths for [*name of district or sub-district*] my certificate after inquest held:

NOW I DO CERTIFY that I am satisfied by evidence given upon [oath *or* statutory declaration] that an error of fact or substance occurred in the said certificate after inquest, in that [*state the error and the necessary correction*], and I therefore give this certificate that the error in the register of deaths may be corrected.

DATED this day of 20

> [*Signed*]
> Her Majesty's [Senior/Area/Assistant] Coroner, coroner area of [*name*]

A3–27 24. *Coroner's Certificate to Correct Clerical Errors in Certificate after Inquest*]

[*Begin as in form 23*]

NOW I DO CERTIFY that the said certificate after inquest contains a clerical error in [*state part of certificate*] thereof, namely that [*state clerical error and correction*], and I give this certificate that the error in the register of deaths may be corrected.

DATED this day of 20

> [*Signed*]
> Her Majesty's [Senior/Area/Assistant] Coroner, coroner area of [*name*]

A3–28 25. *Statutory Declaration to Support Certificate to Correct Errors*

IN THE MATTER OF THE CORONERS AND JUSTICE ACT 2009 AND IN THE MATTER OF AN INQUEST INTO THE DEATH OF [*NAME*]

I, [*name*], of [*address*], do solemnly and sincerely declare as follows:

1) That at an inquest held at [*place*] on the day of 20 I received evidence [*state the evidence which was in error*].
2) That since the said inquest I have discovered that there was an error in that evidence, in that [*set out error and means of discovery*].
3) I therefore believe that [*set out correct facts*].
4) That [save as above stated] I declare to the above facts from my own personal knowledge and make this declaration conscientiously believing it to be true and by virtue of the Statutory Declarations Act 1835.

> Declared at [*place*]
> this day of 20
> before me

A Commissioner for Oaths/Solicitor/Justice of the Peace for [*place*]

A3–29 *Form 26: Draft letter of request to foreign judicial authority*

[*Name and address of competent judicial authority*]

I, [*name*], HM [Senior Coroner/Area Coroner/Assistant Coroner] for the area of [*name*], present my compliments to the competent judicial authority for [*name of foreign country*], and have the honour to inform [him/her] of the following:

I have to conduct an investigation and hold an inquest on behalf of Her Britannic Majesty into the death of [*name*], who died on [*date*] in [*place of death*].
In accordance with [*title of relevant legislation*]:

[*Here set out text of primary and secondary legislation relevant to the case giving jurisdiction to the coroner and also setting out the functions to be performed by the investigation/inquest; in most cases this will be CJA 2009 ss 1(1),(2), 5(1), 6, 10(1).*]

Reason for the request:

[*Here explain the reason for the request, e.g. that documents exist in the hands of a particular person in that country which are relevant to the purposes of the inquest, or that a particular witness is believed to have relevant information, but despite requests, the document holder or witness has declined to assist the investigation so far, or that a particular thing or place needs to be examined for the purposes of the inquest.*]

Assistance requested:

[*Here explain the assistance requested, e.g. that the persons having relevant documents (identifying them so far as possible) disclose them to the coroner, or that the coroner or someone on his/her behalf interview the witness(es), explaining the subject matter of the questions to be put, or that that the coroner or someone on his/her behalf examine a particular place or thing, and take photographs or videos of that place or thing.*]

In thanking the competent judicial authority of [*name*] in advance for their co-operation and assistance in this case, HM [Senior Coroner/Area Coroner/Assistant Coroner] for the area of [*name*] avails [himself/herself] of this opportunity to renew to them the assurance of [his/her] highest esteem.

[*Signature and name of coroner*]

Appendix 4

PRECEDENTS FOR JUDICIAL REVIEW

1. Memorial to the Attorney-General for his/her fiat

IN THE MATTER OF THE CORONERS ACT 1988 **A4–01**

-and-

IN THE MATTER OF THE DEATH OF [*name of deceased*]

To Her Majesty's Attorney-General

THE HUMBLE MEMORIAL OF [*name of applicant*]

SHEWETH:

1) Your Memorialist is [*here give particulars of applicant's occupation, address and relationship to deceased*].
2) On the   day of   20   at the Coroner's Court   [*address*], an inquest was held before [*name*], Her Majesty's [Senior/Area/Assistant] Coroner for [*name of area*], [and a jury,] as part of an investigation into the death of [*name of deceased*], who died on the   day of   20 .
3) At the said inquest [the jury returned and] the coroner recorded a determination [and findings] that [*name*] had died [*here give particulars of determination and findings*].
4) [*Here set out allegations in numbered paragraphs which give rise to grounds for quashing the determination and findings specified in Section 13 of the Coroners Act 1988.*]

Your Memorialist therefore humbly prays that you will be pleased to grant your authority under Section 13 of the Coroners Act 1988 to enable [him/her] to make application to the High Court of Justice for an Order [to cause an investigation to be conducted and an inquest to be held into the death of [*name of deceased*] *or* quashing the said determination [and findings] on the grounds of [*here set out such of the grounds specified in Section 13 of the 1988 Act as are applicable to the particular case*] and directing another investigation to be conducted and inquest to be held into the death of the said [*name of deceased*]].

[*signature of applicant*]

2. Statutory Declaration verifying Memorial to Attorney-General

IN THE MATTER OF THE CORONERS ACT 1988 **A4–02**

-and-

IN THE MATTER OF AN INQUEST INTO THE DEATH OF [*name of deceased*]

I [*name*], of [*address*], do solemnly and sincerely declare that the Memorial now produced and shown to me and marked "A" is as to its contents true to the best of my knowledge and belief. And I the said [*name of applicant*]. do make this solemn declaration, conscientiously believing the same to be true and by virtue of the Statutory Declarations Act 1835.

Declared at [*name of place*]
this   day of   20 .

Before me

A Commissioner for Oaths/A Solicitor/
A Justice of the Peace for [*place*]

A4–03   3. *CPR Part 8 Claim Form*

		In the HIGH COURT OF JUSTICE ADMINISTRATIVE COURT
	Claim Form (CPR Part 8)	
		Claim No

Claimant

[*name*]

SEAL

Defendant(s)

HM [Senior/Area/Assistant] Coroner for [*name of area*]

Does your claim include any issues under the Human Rights Act 1998?   ☐ Yes   ☐ No

Details of claim (*see also overleaf*)

1.   This claim is brought under section 13 of the Coroners Act 1988, with the authority of the Attorney General dated [*date*], for an order [that the Defendant conduct an investigation and hold an inquest into the death of [*name of deceased*]] [that the determination [and findings] of the investigation and inquest held by the Defendant [with a jury] into the death of [*name of deceased*] be quashed [and that the Defendant conduct a fresh investigation and hold a fresh inquest into the death]].

Defendant's name and address

Court fee	£
Solicitor's costs	£
Issue date	

The court office at

is open between 10 am and 4 pm Monday to Friday. When corresponding with the court, please address forms or letters to the Court Manager and quote the claim number.

N208 Claim form (CPR Part 8) (October 2000)   © Crown Copyright.

Claim No	

Details of claim (continued)

2. [The Defendant's decision not to hold an inquest into the death of [*name of deceased*] is set out in his letter to [me/*other name*] dated [*date*], a copy of which] [A copy of the inquisition on the inquest] is exhibited to [my witness statement] [the witness statement of [*name*]], together with a copy of the said authority of the Attorney General.

3. [*State Claimant's relationship to deceased, and also whether acting in representative capacity, e.g. personal representative.*]

4. The legal basis for the claim is as follows:

[*Set out concisely and in logical order the various allegations constituting the legal basis for the claim, in particular taking account, if it is a case of refusal, why the coroner was obliged to hold an investigation or an inquest, and if it is a case of quashing the determination and/or findings, the defect(s) under section 13(1)(b) that render(s) it "necessary or desirable in the interest of justice that another inquest or ... investigation should be held".*]

Statement of Truth

* (I believe) (The Claimant believes) that the facts stated in these particulars of claim are true.
* I am duly authorised by the Claimant to sign this statement.

Full name _____

Name of Claimant's solicitor's firm _____

Signed _____ position or office held
_____

* (Claimant) (Litigation friend) (Claimant's solicitor) (if signing on behalf of firm or company)
* delete as appropriate

Claimant's or Claimant's solicitor's address to which documents should be sent if different from overleaf. If you are prepared to accept service by DX, fax or e-mail, please add details.

N208 Claim form (CPR Part 8) (October 2000)   © Crown Copyright.

A4–04   4. *Witness statement in support of Part 8 claim*

Filed on behalf of the
Claimant
[*name of witness*]
[1st] witness statement
[*date made*]
Exhibit(s) [*nos*]

Claim No.

IN THE HIGH COURT OF JUSTICE
QUEEN'S BENCH DIVISION
ADMINISTRATIVE COURT [IN WALES]

[*name*]   Claimant

H.M. Coroner for [*name of district*]   Defendant

I, [*name*] of [*address*] say as follows—

1) I am the Claimant herein, and all facts and matters which I state are within my own knowledge and are true [*or as the case may be, giving the source of any matters of belief*].

2) I am the [*state relationship*] of the late [*name of deceased*] ("the deceased"), who died on the day of   20   at [*place*].

3) [*Set out the circumstances in which the inquest was held, where one was held.*]

4) [*Where an inquest has been held*] There are now produced and shown to be marked "★1", true copies of a bundle of relevant documents. At pages   to   are copies of the record of the said inquest [and at pages   to   are [*state other documents produced, or recording the evidence, at the inquest*]].

5) [I *or* My solicitors, [*name*] on my behalf] applied to Her Majesty's Attorney-General for [his/her] authority pursuant to section 13 of the Coroners Act 1988. A copy of the said authority, dated the   day of 20   , is at pages   to   of "★1".

6) [*Where an inquest has been held, set out criticisms of inquest, being factual allegations falling within the grounds set out in Section 13 of the 1988 Act*].

7) [*Where the coroner has refused to conduct an investigation or hold an inquest, set out circumstances giving the coroner jurisdiction to conduct or hold one, e.g. within Section 1 of the 2009 Act*].

8) [*Where the coroner has refused to conduct an investigation or hold an inquest, set out the circumstances in which he or she so refused, exhibiting any correspondence between the Claimant (or his or her solicitors) and the coroner*].

9) In these circumstances, I respectfully submit that [a miscarriage of justice has occurred and that it is necessary and desirable in the interests of justice that the determination [and findings] should be quashed and that a fresh investigation and inquest should be conducted and held *or* the coroner has wrongfully refused to conduct an investigation and hold an inquest], and I respectfully ask this Honourable Court to make an Order in the terms set out in the [Claim Form].

10) I believe that the facts stated in this witness statement are true.

Dated the   day of   20   .

[Signature]

[*Initials of Claimant to be inserted here.*]

5. *Part 8 Acknowledgment of Service form by Coroner* **A4–05**

Acknowledgment of Service
(Part 8 claim)

You should read the "Notes for Defendant" attached
to the claim form which will tell you how to complete
this form, and when and where to send it.

In the HIGH COURT OF JUSTICE ADMINISTRATIVE COURT	
Claim No.	
Claimant (including ref)	
Defendant	HM [Senior/Area/Assistant] Coroner for [*name of area*]

Tick and complete sections A – E as appropriate
In all cases you must complete sections F and G

Section A

☐ **I do not** intend to contest this claim
  Give details of any order, direction, etc you are seeking from the court.

Section B

☐ I intend to contest this claim
  Give brief details of any different remedy you are seeking.

Section C

☐ I intend to dispute the court's jurisdiction
  (Please note, any application must be filed within 14 days of the date on which you file this acknowledgment of service)

The court office at

is open between 10 am and 4 pm Monday to Friday. When corresponding with the court, please address forms or letters to the
Court Manager and quote the claim number

Claim No.	

Section D

☐ I object to the claimant issuing under this procedure
My reasons for objecting are:

Section E

☐ I intend to rely on written evidence

My written evidence:
☐ is filed with this form
☐ will be filed within 14 days as agreed with the other party(ies). A copy of the written agreement is attached to this form

Section F

Full name of defendant filing this acknowledgment   **HM [Senior/Area/Assistant] Coroner for**
[*name of area*]

Section G

Signed (To be signed by you or by your solicitor or litigation friend)	*(I believe)(The defendant believes) that the facts stated in this form are true. *I am duly authorised by the defendant to sign this statement *delete as appropriate	**Position or office held** (if signing on behalf of firm or company)	

Date | |

Give an address to which notices about this case can be sent to you			if applicable	
		Ref no	
		Fax no	
	Post code	DX no	
	Tel no	e-mail	

6. *Witness statement of coroner in Reply*   **A4–06**

Filed on behalf of the
Claimant
[*name of witness*]
[1st] witness statement
[*date made*]
Exhibit(s) [*nos*]

Claim No.

IN THE HIGH COURT OF JUSTICE
QUEEN'S BENCH DIVISION
ADMINISTRATIVE COURT [IN WALES]

[Headings as in Form 4]

I, [*name*] of [*address*] say as follows—

1) I am the Defendant herein, and all the facts and matters which I state are within my own knowledge and are true [*or as the case may be, giving the source of any matters of belief*].

2) I am a [barrister/Solicitor of the Senior Courts/fully registered medical practitioner] and since [*date*] I have been Her Majesty's [Senior/Area/Assistant] Coroner for the [*name*] area. [*Mention any other relevant background information.*] [*If the coroner is seeking merely to assist the court, and not to descend into the arena, add:* I have no personal interest in the outcome of these proceedings, and do not seek to play an adversarial role in them, but adopt a neutral position, and take part merely to assist the Court in providing such information and other help as I can in relation to the facts and to the specialist coroners' law involved.]

3) I have read what purports to be a true copy of the witness statement made on [*date*] by [*name*], the Claimant herein.

4) [*Where an investigation and inquest have been held, but the Claimant has not exhibited the record of the inquest or any other relevant document to his or her own statement, this should now be exhibited by the coroner*].

5) [*If it is a case of refusal to conduct an investigation or hold an inquest, set out the circumstances of such refusal to the extent that they are not accurately stated in the Claimant's statement, together with any additional or justifying facts and matters. Where an investigation has been conducted and/or inquest has been held, similarly state the circumstances in which this took place, so far as this is not accurately stated in the Claimant's statement, again with any further relevant facts and matters.*]

6) [*If the coroner is taking a full part in the proceedings*] In these circumstances I respectfully submit that [I was right to decline to take jurisdiction in this case] [there is no necessity to quash the determination [and findings] on the inquest already held, not to conduct a fresh investigation/hold a fresh inquest], and I respectfully ask this Honourable Court to decline to grant the relief sought.
or

7) [*If the coroner is seeking merely to assist the court, add suitable information on relevant coroners' law, and conclude:*] As a neutral judicial officer, I do not seek to make substantive submissions on the merits of the claim made by the Claimant, and so, subject to any further assistance which I may be able to provide, I leave it up to the Court as to whether the relief sought by the Claimant should be granted, in whole or in part.

[*Continue as in Form 4*]

Judicial Review
Claim Form

Notes for guidance are available which explain how to complete the judicial review claim form. Please read them carefully before you complete the form.

For Court use only	
Administrative Court Reference No.	
Date filed	

In the High Court of Justice
Administrative Court

(Seal)

name

SECTION 1   Details of the claimant(s) and defendant(s)

Claimant(s) name and address(es)

┌ name ┐

┌ address ┐

┌ Telephone no. ┐   ┌ Fax no. ┐

┌ E-mail address ┐

Claimant's or Claimant's solicitors' address to which documents should be sent.

┌ address ┐

┌ Telephone no. ┐   ┌ Fax no. ┐

┌ E-mail address ┐

Claimant's counsel's details

┌ address ┐

┌ Telephone no. ┐   ┌ Fax no. ┐

┌ E-mail address ┐

1st Defendant

┌ HM [Senior/Area/Assistant] Coroner for [*name of area*] ┐

Defendant's or (where known) Defendant's solicitors' address to which documents should be sent.

┌ address ┐

┌ Telephone no. ┐   ┌ Fax no. ┐

┌ E-mail address ┐

2nd Defendant

┌ name ┐

Defendant's or (where known) Defendant's solicitors' address to which documents should be sent.

┌ name ┐

┌ address ┐

┌ Telephone no. ┐   ┌ Fax no. ┐

┌ E-mail address ┐

SECTION 2   Details of other interested parties

Include name and address and, if appropriate, details of DX, telephone or fax numbers and e-mail

name

name

address

address

Telephone no.   Fax no.

Telephone no.   Fax no.

E-mail address

E-mail address

SECTION 3   Details of the decision to be judicially reviewed

Decision:

[The record of the inquest into the death of [*name*], *or* The decision of the Defendant not to call [*name*] to give evidence at the inquest into the death of [*name*], *or as the case may be.*]

Date of decision:

Name and address of the court, tribunal, person or body who made the decision to be reviewed.

name

HM [Senior/Area/Assistant] Coroner for [*name of area*]

address

SECTION 4   Permission to proceed with a claim for judicial review

I am seeking permission to proceed with my claim for Judicial Review.

Is this application being made under the terms of Section 18 Practice Direction 54 (Challenging removal)? ☐ Yes ☐ No

Are you making any other applications? If Yes, complete Section 7. ☐ Yes ☐ No

Is the claimant in receipt of a Community Legal Service Fund (CLSF) certificate? ☐ Yes ☐ No

Are you claiming exceptional urgency, or do you need this application determined within a certain time scale? If Yes, complete Form N463 and file this with your application. ☐ Yes ☐ No

Have you complied with the pre-action protocol? If No, give reasons for non-compliance in the space below. ☐ Yes ☐ No

Have you issued this claim in the region with which you have the closest connection? (Give any additional reasons for wanting it to be dealt with in this region in the box below). If No, give reasons in the box below. ☐ Yes ☐ No

Does the claim include any issues arising from the Human Rights Act 1998?
If Yes, state the articles which you contend have been breached in the space below. ☐ Yes   ☐ No

SECTION 5   Detailed statement of grounds

☐ set out below   ☐ attached

1. This claim is for the relief in section 7 below, in relation to the Defendant's decision [*describe including date and form taken, e.g. by letter, or orally*].

  2. [*State Claimant's relationship to deceased, and also whether acting in representative capacity, e.g. personal representative.*]

  3. The legal basis for the claim is as follows:
  4. [*Set out concisely and logically the various allegations constituting the grounds for the claim.*]

SECTION 6   Aarhus Convention claim

I contend that this claim is an Aarhus Convention claim.   ☐ Yes ☐ No
If Yes, indicate in the following box if you do not with the costs limits under CPR 45.43 to apply.

SECTION 7   Details of remedy (including any interim remedy) being sought

[*E.g.* An order quashing the refusal of the Defendant to conduct an investigation or hold an inquest into the death of [*name*], and an order requiring him/her to conduct auch an investigation and hold such an inquest, *or* An order quashing the decision of the Defendant not to call [*name*] to give evidence at the inquest into the death of [*name*], and an order requiring him/her to call [*name*] to give such evidence, *or as the case may be.*]

SECTION 8   Other applications

I wish to make an application for:

[*E.g.* An order extending the time limit for filing the claim form, *or* An order for directions.]

SECTION 9   Statement of facts relied on

1. All the facts and matters stated are within my own knowledge [except for *state*] which I derive from [*name source*]].

2. I am the [*state relationship*] of the late [*name*] ("the deceased"), who died on the   day of   20 .

3. On the   day of   20   , the Defendant, H.M. Senior/Area/Assistant Coroner for the [*name of area*] decided [*state decision, or describe other action complained of*].

4. [*Set out facts in chronological order on which reliance is placed*].

Statement of Truth

I believe (The Claimant believes) that the facts stated in this claim form are true.

Full name   _____

Name of Claimant's solicitor's firm   _____

Position or office
Signed   _____   held   _____

       Claimant ('s solicitor)   (if signing on behalf of firm or company)

SECTION 10 Supporting documents

If you do not have a document that you intend to use to support your claim, identify it, give the date when you expect it to be available and give reasons why it is not currently available in the box below.

Please tick the papers you are filing with this claim form and any you will be filing later.

☐ Statement of grounds   ☐ included   ☐ attached

☐ Statement of the facts relied on   ☐ included   ☐ attached

☐ Application to extend the time limit for filing the claim form   ☐ included   ☐ attached

☐ Application for directions   ☐ included   ☐ attached

☐ Any written evidence in support of the claim or application to extend time

☐ Where the claim for judicial review relates to a decision of a court or tribunal, an approved copy of the reasons for reaching that decision

☐ Copies of any documents on which the claimant proposes to rely

☐ A copy of the legal aid or CSLF certificate *(if legally represented)*

☐ Copies of any relevant statutory material

☐ A list of essential documents for advance reading by the court *(with page references to the passages relied upon)*

If Section 18 Practice Direction 54 applies, please tick the relevant box(es) below to indicate which papers you are filing with this claim form:

☐ a copy of the removal directions and the decision to which the application relates   ☐ included   ☐ attached

☐ a copy of the documents served with the removal directions including any documents which contains the Immigration and Nationality Directorate's factual summary of the case   ☐ included   ☐ attached

☐ a detailed statement of the grounds   ☐ included   ☐ attached

Reasons why you have not supplied a document and date when you expect it to be available:

Signed _____ Claimant ('s Solicitor) _____

Judicial Review

Application for urgent consideration

This form must be completed by the Claimant or the Claimant's Advocate if exceptional urgency is being claimed and the application needs to be determined within a certain time scale.

The Claimant, or the Claimant's solicitors must serve this form on the defendant(s) and any Interested Parties with the N461 Judicial review claim form.

To the Defendant(s) and Interested Party(ies) Representations as to the urgency of the claim may be made by defendants or interested parties to the relevant Administrative Court Office by fax or email:

For cases proceeding in

In the High Court of Justice Administrative Court	
Claim No.	
Claimant(s) *(including ref.)*	
Defendant(s)	
Interested Party(ies)	

London
Fax: 020 7947 6802 **email:** administrativecourtoffice.generaloffice@hmcts.x.gsi.gov.uk

Birmingham
Fax: 0121 250 6730 **email:** administrativecourtoffice.birmingham@hmcts.x.gsi.gov.uk

Cardiff
Fax: 02920 376461 **email:** administrativecourtoffice.cardiff@hmcts.x.gsi.gov.uk

Leeds
Fax: 0113 306 2581 **email:** administrativecourtoffice.leeds@hmcts.x.gsi.gov.uk

Manchester
Fax: 0161 240 5315 **email:** administrativecourtoffice.manchester@hmcts.x.gsi.gov.uk

SECTION 1 Reasons for urgency

[E.g. The Defendant proposes [tomorrow *[date]*] to release the body of the late *[name]* to the [First] Interested Party, who proposes to remove it out of the jurisdiction of this Honourable Court so soon thereafter as possible, thus defeating the claim of the Claimant to be entitled to possession of the said body for the purposes of a funeral.]

SECTION 2 Proposed timetable *(tick the boxes and complete the following statements that apply)*

☐ a) The N461 application for permission should be considered within _____ hours/days

  If consideration is sought within 48 hours, you must complete Section 3 below

☐ b) Abridgement of time is sought for the lodging of acknowledgments of service

☐ c) If permission for judicial review is granted, a substantive hearing is sought by _____ (date)

SECTION 3 Justification for request for immediate consideration

If it is decided that your application will be dealt with as an immediate application, we will notify you of the outcome by email as soon as the judge has reached a determination. You will subsequently be sent a hard copy of the judge's order in the post. Please provide an email address to which you would like notification sent.

Email address:

Please note: if you do not provide a valid email address, you will only be notified of the outcome by post, which will take at least 2–3 days to be processed and delivered.

Date and time when it was first appreciated that an immediate application might be necessary.

Date

Time

Please provide reasons for any delay in making the application

What efforts have been made to put the Defendant and any Interested Party on notice of the application?

SECTION 4 Interim relief (*state what interim relief is sought and why in the box below*)

A draft order must be attached.

[*E.g.* An injunction to restrain the Defendant, until the hearing of this application for judicial review or further order, from releasing or delivering up the body of the late [*name*] to anyone, whether the [First] Interested Party or otherwise, other than the Claimant.]

SECTION 5 Service

A copy of this form of application was served on the defendant(s) and interested parties as follows:

Defendant

☐ by fax machine to   time sent
    Fax no.   time

☐ by handing it to or leaving it with
    name

☐ by email to
    email address

Date served
Date

Interested Party

☐ by fax machine to   time sent
    Fax no.   time

☐ by handing it to or leaving it with
    name

☐ by email to
    email address

Date served
Date

I confirm that all relevant facts have been disclosed in this application.

Name of Claimant's Advocate

Name

Claimant (Claimant's Advocate)

Signed

A4–09   9. *Acknowledgment of Service by Coroner*

Judicial Review **Acknowledgment of Service**	**In the High Court of Justice** **Administrative Court**	
	Claim No.	
Name and address of person to be served	**Claimant(s)** *(including ref.)*	
name		
address	**Defendant(s)**	HM [Senior/Area/Assistant] Coroner for [*name of area*]
	Interested Parties	

SECTION A

Tick the appropriate box

1. I intend to contest all of the claim	☐	
2. I intend to contest part of the claim	☐	} complete sections B, C, D and F
3. I do not intend to contest the claim	☐	complete section F
4. The defendant (interested party) is a court or tribunal and **intends** to make a submission.	☐	complete sections B, C and F
5. The defendant (interested party) is a court or tribunal and **does not intend** to make a submission.	☐	complete sections B and F
6. The applicant has indicated that this a claim to which the Aarhus Convention applies.	☐	complete sections E and F

Note: If the application seeks to judicially review the decision of a court or tribunal, the court or tribunal need only
provide the Administrative Court with as much evidence as it can about the decision to help the Administrative
Court perform its judicial function.

SECTION B

Insert the name and address of any person you consider should be added as an interested party.

name	name
address	address
Telephone no.	Fax no.	Telephone no.	Fax no.
E-mail address	E-mail address

SECTION C

Summary of grounds for contesting the claim. If you are contesting only part of the claim, set out which part before you give your grounds for contesting it. If you are a court or tribunal filing a submission, please indicate that this is the case.

1. I am HM [Senior/Area/Assistant] Coroner for [*name of area*] and this claim is brought against me in that capacity, in respect of my decision [*state or describe*].

2. I make this summary of grounds for contesting the claim in the same capacity.

3. The Claimant is not entitled to the remedy sought [or any remedy] because:

[*state grounds, e.g.* S/he has no sufficient standing,

or This claim was made out of time and/or there has been inordinate delay on the Claimant's part

or The decision complained of was not wrong in law/procedurally flawed [*etc*], as alleged by the Claimant or at all.]

or as the case may be.

4. [*Set out relevant facts so far as not accurately set out in claim.*]

5. [*Set out relevant law so far as not set out accurately in claim.*]

SECTION D

Give details of any directions you will be asking the court to make, or tick the box to indicate that a separate application notice is attached.

If you are seeking a direction that this matter be heard at an Administrative Court venue other than that at which this claim was issued, you should complete, lodge and serve on all other parties Form N464 with this acknowledgment of service.

SECTION E

Response to the claimant's contention that the claim is an Aarhus claim

Do you deny that the claim is an Aarhus Convention claim?   ☐ Yes ☐ No

If Yes, please set out your grounds for denial in the box below.

SECTION F

*delete as appropriate

*(I believe)(The Defendant believes) that the facts stated in this form are true.
*I am duly authorised by the defendant to sign this statement.

(if signing on behalf of firm or company, court or tribunal)

Position or office held

(To be signed by you or by your solicitor or litigation friend)

Signed

Date

Give an address to which notices about this case can be sent to you

name

address

Telephone no.

Fax no.

E-mail address

If you have instructed counsel, please give their name address and contact details below.

name

address

Telephone no.

Fax no.

E-mail address

Completed forms, together with a copy, should be lodged with the Administrative Court Office (court address, over the page), at which this claim was issued within 21 days of service of the claim upon you, and further copies should be served on the Claimant(s), any other Defendant(s) and any interested parties within 7 days of lodgement with the Court.

Administrative Court addresses

- Administrative Court in **London**

  Administrative Court Office, Room C315, Royal Courts of Justice, Strand, London, WC2A 2LL.

- Administrative Court in **Birmingham**

  Administrative Court Office, Birmingham Civil Justice Centre, Priory Courts, 33 Bull Street, Birmingham,B4 6DS.

- Administrative Court in **Wales**

  Administrative Court Office, Cardiff Civil Justice Centre, 2 Park Street, Cardiff, CF10 1ET.

- Administrative Court in **Leeds**

  Administrative Court Office, Leeds Combined Court Centre, 1 Oxford Row, Leeds, LS1 3BG.

- Administrative Court in **Manchester**

  Administrative Court Office, Manchester Civil Justice Centre, 1 Bridge Street West, Manchester, M3 3FX.

10. *Witness Statement of coroner in reply* **A4–10**

> Filed on behalf of the
> Claimant
> [*name of witness*]
> [1st] witness statement
> [*date made*]
> Exhibit(s) [*nos*]
>
> Claim No.

IN THE HIGH COURT OF JUSTICE
QUEEN'S BENCH DIVISION
ADMINISTRATIVE COURT [IN WALES]

The Queen on the application of [*name*]   Claimant

– and –

H.M. Coroner for [*name of district*]   Defendant

[*Continue as in Form 6, amending as appropriate*]
to suit the facts of the particular case].

A4–11   11. *Application for directions as to venue*

Application for directions as to venue for administration and determination

Name and address of party making application

name ————————————————————

address ————————————————————

In the High Court of Justice Administrative Court	
Claim No.	
Claimant(s)/ Appellant(s)	
Defendant(s)/ Respondent(s)	HM [Senior/Area/Assistant] Coroner for [*name of area*]
Interested Party(ies)	

I/We apply to the court for a direction that this matter be administered and determined at the:

☐ Royal Courts of Justice in **London**

☐ District Registry of the High Court at **Birmingham**

☐ District Registry of the High Court at **Cardiff**

☐ District Registry of the High Court at **Leeds**

☐ District Registry of the High Court at **Manchester**

for the following reason(s): *(please refer to paragraph 5.2 of PD54D set out overleaf)*

[*Here set out reasons for changing venue, e.g.convenience of the parties, etc*]

(To be signed by you or by your solicitor or litigation friend)   Signed ————————————————   Date ————————

Name ————————————————   Position or office held ————

(if signing on behalf of firm or company, court)

Please send your completed form to the Administrative Court Office which is currently administering this matter, within 21 days of service of the proceedings upon you. You must also serve copies of your completed application on all other parties.

Practice Direction 54D 5.2

5.2 The general expectation is that proceedings will be administered and determined in the region with which the claimant/appellant has the closest connection, subject to the following considerations as applicable—

1) any reason expressed by any party for preferring a particular venue;

2) the region in which the defendant/respondent or any relevant office or department of the defendant/respondent is based;

3) the region in which the claimant's/appellant's legal representatives are based;

4) the ease and cost of travel to a hearing;

5) the availability and suitability of alternative means of attending a hearing (for example, by videolink);

6) the extent and nature of media interest in the proceedings in any particular locality;

7) the time within which it is appropriate for the proceedings to be determined;

8) whether it is desirable to administer or determine the claim in another region in the light of the volume of claims issued at, and the capacity, resources and workload of, the court at which it is issued;

9) whether the claim raises issues sufficiently similar to those in another outstanding claim to make it desirable that it should be determined together with, or immediately following, that other claim; and

10) whether the claim raises devolution issues and for that reason whether it should more appropriately be determined in London or Cardiff.

Response to application for directions as to venue for administration and determination

In the High Court of Justice Administrative Court	
Claim No.	
Claimant(s)/ Appellant(s)	
Defendant(s)/ Respondent(s)	HM [Senior/Area/Assistant] Coroner for [*name of area*]
Interested Party(ies)	

You must serve this form **within 7 days** of receiving form *N464 Application for directions as to venue for administration and determination*.

Name and address of party responding to application

name

address

I/We oppose the application for directions as to the venue for administration and determination, for the following reason(s):

(To be signed by you or by your solicitor or litigation friend)   **Signed**

Date

Name

(if signing on behalf of firm or company, court)

Position or office held

Please send your completed form to the Administrative Court Office which is currently administering this matter, **within 7 days** of receiving form N464 Application for directions as to venue from administration and determination. You must also serve copies of your completed form on all other parties.

N465 Response to application as to venue for administration and determination (04.09)   © Crown copyright 2009

Appendix 5

DEATH

Definition and Diagnosis

Introduction

The jurisdiction of the coroner can only arise where someone has died.[1] But in English law there is no specific test laid down by statute to determine that death has occurred. Moreover, a registered medical practitioner who has attended a patient in the last illness can give a medical certificate of the cause of death (MCCD) without seeing the patient after death.[2] In the majority of cases, it is obvious that the person is no longer alive. The classical medical basis for determining death was the irreversible cessation of respiration and circulation. Modern advances in resuscitation and the need to remove organs and tissue for transplantation have modified the position. Some surgical techniques require the use of artificial circulation for long periods. **A5–01**

The various organs and tissues of the body can resist anoxia (lack of oxygen) for differing times. The cells of the central nervous system in particular are highly susceptible to anoxia and will be irreversibly damaged within minutes at normal temperatures.[3] This has led to the concepts of "brain death" and "brain stem death" being equated for English legal purposes with death.[4] If the criteria are met, the patient is dead and the life support apparatus may be disconnected, or left to oxygenate the dead body while organs and tissues that are more resistant to anoxia, and are still alive, can then be taken for transplantation. **A5–02**

The problem of the definition of death has arisen mainly in the context of the removal of organs from the dead with the aim of transplanting them into the living.[5] There are two major criteria which must be satisfied before transplantation can proceed. The paramount criterion is that the donor must be dead before organs are removed. The other criterion is that the time interval between cessation of circulation and removal of the donor organs must be kept to the absolute minimum (a matter of minutes). Otherwise the donor organ will begin to degenerate and will be of no value to the recipient. **A5–03**

These considerations carry the implication that it must be possible to define death in a precise way so that there is no doubt about it, and to do so in a way which does not depend on the functions of circulation and respiration, since these may be maintained by artificial means so that the organs can be kept oxygenated and removed under surgical conditions. **A5–04**

The matter is of some complexity, and not easily summarised. The criteria for the recognition and confirmation of death are kept under review. The reader is referred to the detailed guidance of the Academy of Medical Royal Colleges (AoMRC)[6] and its publication, *A Code of Practice for the Diagnosis and Conformation of Death*, published in **A5–05**

---

[1] See 5-01.
[2] See 5-28.
[3] However, an individual may sometimes survive for a prolonged period without any form of circulation in some circumstances, such as when the body temperature is extremely low, provided that the oxygenation of organs and tissues is sustained sufficiently to prevent irreversible damage.
[4] See 5-14.
[5] See 8-78ff.
[6] See http://www.aomrc.org.uk for further details.

October 2008. They are too long and complex to set out here, but are available online, where they may be consulted in their most up to date version.[7]

A5–06   The AoMRC code of practice explains that the diagnosis and confirmation of death is required in a number of different situations. The code is intended as a working document aimed primarily at doctors and other healthcare workers rather than the lay public. The code deals with the diagnosis and confirmation of death whatever the cause, irrespective of any surrounding issues, such as organ donation and transplantation.

A5–07   Death entails the irreversible loss of those essential characteristics which are necessary to the existence of a living human person. Thus the code states[8] that the definition of death should be regarded as the irreversible loss of the capacity for consciousness, combined with the irreversible loss of the capacity to breathe.

A5–08   The code goes on to provide *general* guidance about

- Death following the irreversible cessation of brain-stem function (para 2.1);
- Death following cessation of cardiorespiratory function (para 2.2).

A5–09   It then provides *detailed* guidance about

- Diagnosing and confirming death after cardiorespiratory arrest (para 3);
- Diagnosis and confirmation of death in a patient in coma (para 4);
- Conditions necessary for the diagnosis and confirmation of death (para 5);
- The diagnosis of death following irreversible cessation of brain-stem function (para 6).

---

[7] http://www.aomrc.org.uk/doc_view/42-a-code-of-practice-for-the-diagnosis-and-confirmation-of-death. For another perspective on the diagnosis of brain death, the reader may also wish to refer to Calixto Machado, "Diagnosis of brain death" (June 21, 2010), Neurology International, http://www.ncbi.nlm.nih.gov/pmc/articles/PMC3093212 [Accessed July 9, 2014].

[8] At para 2.

Appendix 6

FORENSIC MEDICINE AND PATHOLOGY

In earlier editions of this work there was a specific chapter on this subject. This could never **A6–01** be more than the barest outline of a technical subject which coroners in fact did not need to master because they would invariably retain expert pathologists to examine and report on dead bodies. Moreover, since the subject is constantly changing as science evolves, any treatment soon becomes out of date. In order to free space in this edition for matters more relevant to the coroner's work, the former chapter has been dropped. The aim of this Appendix is therefore much more modest. It is to give the reader some references to those aspects of medicine, particularly pathology, which relate to an inquiry into the cause of death. The first part consists of a short introduction to pathology pertinent to coroners' investigations. There is also a short bibliography of useful works. Finally, there are some internet sites that may prove helpful.

Introduction

The majority of coroners' autopsies[1] (also called 'post-mortem examinations' or 'nec- **A6–02** ropsies') in England and Wales are performed by NHS-consultant histopathologists. Relatively few are performed by forensic pathologists registered on a list of forensic pathologists maintained by The Home Office. The primary difference, insofar as coroners are concerned, is that NHS histopathologists are not trained in forensic issues in the same way that registered forensic pathologists are.[2] Few NHS histopathologists hold specialist forensic academic qualifications such as the DMJ(Path) and The Royal College of Pathologists provides a code of practice for pathologists performing autopsies on non-suspicious deaths.[3]

Where deaths are of unknown cause but not obviously suspicious, an autopsy performed **A6–03** by a histopathologist presents no particular difficulties. However, if there is anything suspicious about the circumstances of the death, or if it is violent or unnatural, consideration should be given to requesting a registered forensic pathologist to perform the autopsy. The Register of Forensic Pathologists[4] is regularly updated by staff in the Pathology Delivery Board of the Home Office. Entry to the list is strictly regulated and registered members are required to comply with a code of practice.[5] The Forensic Science Regulator[6] has oversight of all forensic services, including pathology.

---

[1] See also paras 8–39 to 8–69, above.

[2] See *R v Clarke and Morabir* [2013] EWCA Crim. 162.

[3] Royal College of Pathologists, *Standards for Coroners' pathologists in post-mortem examinations of deaths that appear not to be suspicious*, February 2014: *http://www.rcpath.org/Resources/RCPath/Migrated%20-Resources/Documents/G/G136_CoronersPMsPerfStands_Feb14.pdf* [Accessed July 11, 2014].

[4] Home Office Register of Registered Forensic Pathologists: *https://www.gov.uk/government/uploads/system/uploads/attachment_data/file/303730/RegisterForensicPathologists.pdf* [Accessed July 11, 2014].

[5] Pathology Delivery Board, Code of practice and performance standards for forensic pathology in England, Wales and Northern Ireland: *https://www.gov.uk/government/uploads/system/uploads/attach-ment_data/file/115698/code-practice-forensic-pathology.pdf* [Accessed July 11, 2014]. See para.8–48 above.

[6] Forensic Science Regulator: *https://www.gov.uk/government/organisations/forensic-science-regulator* [Accessed July 11, 2014].

A6–04   A naked eye or macroscopic autopsy may not reveal a cause of death and additional investigations may be necessary, such as histological examination of tissues and organs, toxicological testing, etc. The pathologist will usually advise on such matters. Toxicology results require considerable care in their interpretation and a coroner may require the attendance of a toxicologist as well as a pathologist at the inquest. Radiology and radiologists are now also increasingly used.[7]

A6–05   Histopathology is subdivided into many sub-specialties. These include neuropathology, cardiac pathology (of especial importance in unexplained sudden deaths in young persons, especially where there is a family history) paediatric pathology, lung pathology and pathologists who have a particular interest, such as in the investigation of maternal deaths.

A6–06   All pathologists must not only be registered with the General Medical Council[8] (GMC) but must also undergo regular accreditation and must have a current licence to practise.[9] Autopsies must be conducted on premises that are licensed by the Human Tissue Authority (HTA),[10] and this includes emergency mortuaries. The HTA regulates and inspects mortuaries and also publishes a number of codes of practice, including one for post-mortem examinations. All are available on its website.[11]

Bibliography

A6–07   Burton, J.L. and Rutty, G.N. (eds) *The Hospital Autopsy*, 3rd edn (London: Hodder Arnold, 2010).

Byard, R.W., *Sudden Death in the Young*, 3rd edn (Cambridge: Cambridge University Press, 2010).

Byard, R., Corey, T., Henderson, C. and Payne-James, J., *Encyclopedia of Forensic and Legal Medicine* (London: Academic Press, 2005).

Cowan, S. and Hunt, A.C., *Mason's Forensic Medicine for Lawyers*, 5th edn (Haywards Heath: Tottel Publishing, 2008).

Di Maio, V.J.M. and Di Maio, D.J., *Forensic Pathology*, 2nd edn (Boca Raton, CRC Press, 2001).

Dolinak, D., Matshes E.W. and Lew, E.O., *Forensic Pathology: Principles and Practice* (London: Academic Press, 2005).

Kumar, P. and Clark, M. (eds) *Kumar and Clark's Clinical Medicine*, 7th edn (Edinburgh: Saunders Elsevier, 2009).

Kumar, V., Abbas, A.K., Fausto, N. and Aster, J.C., *Robbins and Cotran Pathologic Basis of Disease*, 8th edn (Oxford: Elsevier Health Sciences, 2010).

Longmore, M., Wilkinson, I., Davidson, E., Foulkes, A. and Mafi, A., *Oxford Handbook of Clinical Medicine*, 8th edn (Oxford: Oxford University Press, 2010).

Mason, J.K. and Purdue, B.N., *The Pathology of Trauma*, 3rd edn (London: Arnold, 2000).

Payne-James, J., Busuttil S., and Smock, W., *Forensic Medicine Clinical and Pathological Aspects* (Cambridge: Cambridge University Press, 2003).

Prahlow, J.A. and Byard, R.W., *Atlas of Forensic Pathology* (New York: Springer, 2012).

Royal Institute of Public Health and Hygiene, *A Handbook of Mortuary Practice and Safety for Anatomical Pathology Technicians* (London: RIBHH, 1991).

Saukko, P.J. and Knight, B., *Knight's Forensic Pathology*, 3rd edn (London: Arnold, 2004).

Shkrum, M. and Ramsay, D., *Forensic Pathology of Trauma, Common Problems for the Pathologist* (New York: Humana Press, 2006).

---

[7] See paras 8–67 to 8–68, above.
[8] General Medical Council: *http://www.gmc-uk.org/* [Accessed July 11, 2014].
[9] *Chief Coroner's Guide to the Coroners and Justice Act 2009*, para.75.
[10] See para.8–58 above.
[11] Human Tissue Authority: *http://www.hta.gov.uk/* [Accessed July 11, 2014].

Spitz, W.U., *Spitz and Fisher's Medicolegal Investigation of Death: Guidelines for the Application of Pathology to Crime Investigation* (Springfield: Charles C Thomas Publishing, 2005).
Tsokos, M., *Forensic Pathology Review* (New York: Humana Press, 2006).

Internet links

ACPO, *Forensic Pathology Practice Advice For Police, http://library.college.police.uk/docs/ACPO/* **A6–08**
ACPO-Forensic-Pathology-Practice-Advice-2013.pdf [Accessed July 11, 2014].
ACPO, *Murder Investigation Manual* (2006), *http://www.acpo.police.uk/documents/crime/2006/2006CBAMIM.pdf* [Accessed July 11, 2014].
deaths that appear not to be suspicious, (February 2014), *http://www.rcpath.org/Resources/RCPath/Migrated%20Resources/Documents/G/G136_CoronersPMsPerfStands_Feb14.pdf* [Accessed July 11, 2014].
Dundee University Department of Forensic Medicine, LLB Forensic Medicine Course Lecture Notes, *http://www.dundee.ac.uk/forensicmedicine/notes/notes.html* [Accessed July 11, 2014].
Forensic Pathology—role within the Home Office: *https://www.gov.uk/forensic-pathology-role-within-the-home-office* [Accessed July 11, 2014].
Forensic Science Regulator, *Guidance on legal issues in Forensic Pathology and Tissue Retention,* 2nd edn (2014), *https://www.gov.uk/government/uploads/system/uploads/attachment_data/file/314874/Legal_Issues_in_Forensic_Pathology_and_Tissue_Retention_Issue_3.pdf* [Accessed July 11, 2014].
http://www.rcpath.org/Resources/RCPath/Migrated%20Resources/Documents/G/G129_PMImaging_Oct12_BS.pdf [Accessed July 11, 2014].
http://www2.le.ac.uk/departments/emfpu/Can%20Cross-Sectional%20Imaging%20as%2-0an%20Adjunct%20and-or%20Alternative%20to%20the%20Invasive%20Autopsy%20-be%20Implemented%20within%20the%20NHS%20-%20FINAL.pdf [Accessed July 11, 2014].
ICRC and others, *Management of dead bodies after disasters: a field manual for first responders,* 3rd edn (2009), *http://www.icrc.org/eng/assets/files/other/icrc-002-0880.pdf* [Accessed July 11, 2014].
Pathology Delivery Board, Code of Practice and performance standards for Forensic Pathology in England, Wales and Northern Ireland, *https://www.gov.uk/government/uploads/system/uploads/attachment_data/file/115698/code-practice-forensic-pathology.pdf* [Accessed July 11, 2014].
Pathology Delivery Board: *https://www.gov.uk/forensic-pathology-role-within-the-home-office-£pathology-delivery-board* [Accessed July 11, 2014].
Protocol For Membership Of The Home Office Register Of Forensic Pathologists, *https://www.gov.uk/government/uploads/system/uploads/attachment_data/file/115693/ho-reg-forensic-pathologist.pdf* [Accessed July 11, 2014].
R. v Clarke and Morabir [2013] EWCA Crim. 162 (when is a pathologist qualified to give an opinion on the cause of death?): *http://www.bailii.org/ew/cases/EWCA/Crim/2013/162.html* [Accessed July 11, 2014].
Report from the NHS Implementation Sub-Group of the Department of Health Post Mortem, Forensic and Disaster Imaging Group (PMFDI) (October 2012), Royal College of Pathologists, *Standards for Coroners' pathologists in post-mortem examinations of* Royal College of Radiologists and the Royal College of Pathologists, Standards for medico-legal post-mortem cross-sectional imaging in adults (October 2012), The list of Home Office approved forensic pathologists and their practice areas: *https://www.gov.uk/government/publications/home-office-register-of-forensic-pathologists-february-2013* [Accessed July 11, 2014].

Appendix 7

USEFUL WEBSITES

(Please note that these are under the control of third parties and are subject to change or deletion without notice)

CORONERS

Office of the Chief Coroner:
http://www.judiciary.gov.uk/about-the-judiciary/office-chief-coroner

Coroners' Society of England and Wales:
http://www.coronersociety.org.uk/

Coroner statistics:
https://www.gov.uk/government/collections/coroners-and-burials-statistics

Coroners Officers and Staff Association:
http://www.coasa.org.uk

Coroners' Courts Support Service:
http://www.coronerscourtssupportservice.org.uk/

Judicial Conduct Investigations Office:
http://judicialconduct.judiciary.gov.uk/index.htm

INQUIRIES AND INQUESTS

The Shipman Inquiry:
http://webarchive.nationalarchives.gov.uk/20090808154959/http:/www.the-shipman-inquiry.org.uk/reports.asp

The Francis Inquiry:
http://www.midstaffspublicinquiry.com/

The Bristol Royal Infirmary Inquiry:
http://webarchive.nationalarchives.gov.uk/+/www.dh.gov.uk/en/Publicationsandstatis
tics/Publications/PublicationsPolicyAndGuidance/DH_4005620

The Royal Liverpool Children's Inquiry Report (Alder Hey):
https://www.gov.uk/government/publications/the-royal-liverpool-childrens-inquiry-report

The Thames Safety Inquiry (Lord Justice Clarke):
http://www.epcollege.com/EPC/media/MediaLibrary/Knowledge%20Hub%20Docu
ments/F%20Inquiry%20Reports/Marchionness-Clarke-(2000).pdf?ext=.pdf

Marchioness-Bowbelle Formal Investigation:
http://webarchive.nationalarchives.gov.uk/20101013092119/http:/www.marchioness-bowbelle.org.uk/

Marchioness MAIB Reports:
http://www.maib.gov.uk/publications/investigation_reports/1990_to_1998/marchio
ness.cfm

The Hutton Inquiry:
http://webarchive.nationalarchives.gov.uk/20090128221546/http://www.the-hutton-inquiry.org.uk/
also
http://hutton.dracos.co.uk/
and
http://www.hutton.softblade.com/

Inquests into the deaths of Diana, Princess of Wales, and Dodi Fayed:
http://webarchive.nationalarchives.gov.uk/20090607230252/http://www.scottbaker-inquests.gov.uk/

Inquests into the deaths following the London 7/7 bombings:
http://webarchive.nationalarchives.gov.uk/20120216072438/http:/7julyinquests.indepen dent.gov.uk/

Inquest into the death of Ian Tomlinson:
http://www.tomlinsoninquest.org.uk/tomlinson/

REPORTS

Coroner reform: The Government's Draft Bill, 2006:
https://www.gov.uk/government/publications/coroner-reform-improving-death-investi gation-in-england-and-wales

House of Commons Constitutional Affairs Committee, Report on Reform of the Coro ners'
System and Death Certification, 2006:
http://www.publications.parliament.uk/pa/cm200506/cmselect/cmconst/902/902i.pdf

Government Response to the Constitutional Affairs Select Committee's Report:
https://www.gov.uk/government/publications/reform-of-the-coroners-system-and-death-certification

LAW

British and Irish Legal Information Institute :
http://www.bailii.org/

ECHR decisions:
http://hudoc.echr.coe.int/sites/eng/Pages/search.aspx#

POLICE AND PROSECUTION SERVICES

National Police Website:
http://www.police.uk/

Association of Chief Police Officers:
http://www.acpo.police.uk/Home.aspx

British Transport Police:
http://www.btp.police.uk

Royal Military Police:
http://www.army.mod.uk/agc/provost/23207.aspx

Crown Prosecution Service:
http://www.cps.gov.uk

FORENSIC PATHOLOGY

Royal College of Pathologists:
http://www.rcpath.org/home

Home Office Forensic Pathology – including current list of Registered Forensic Pathologists:
https://www.gov.uk/forensic-pathology-role-within-the-home-office

Home Office Register of Forensic Pathologists:
https://www.gov.uk/government/publications/home-office-register-of-forensic-pathologists-february-2013

British Academy of Forensic Sciences:
http://bafs.org.uk

Expert Witness Institute:
http://www.ewi.org.uk

The Faculty of Forensic & Legal Medicine:
http://fflm.ac.uk

The Forensic Science Society:
http://www.forensic-science-society.org.uk/Home

Code of Practice for the Diagnosis and Confirmation of Death (Academy of Medical Royal Colleges):
http://www.aomrc.org.uk/doc_view/42-a-code-of-practice-for-the-diagnosis-and-confirmation-of-death

Report from the NHS Implementation Sub-Group of the Department of Health Post Mortem, Forensic and Disaster Imaging Group (PMFDI), October 2012:
http://www2.le.ac.uk/departments/emfpu/Can%20Cross-Sectional%20Imaging%20as%20an%20Adjunct%20and-or%20Alternative%20to%20the%20Invasive%20Autopsy%20be%20Implemented%20within%20the%20NHS%20-%20FINAL.pdf

Standards for medico-legal post-mortem cross-sectional imaging in adults from the Royal College of Radiologists and the Royal College of Pathologists, October 2012:
http://www.rcpath.org/Resources/RCPath/Migrated%20Resources/Documents/G/G129_PMImaging_Oct12_BS.pdf

GOVERNMENT AND GOVERNMENT AGENCIES

What to do after someone dies:
https://www.gov.uk/after-a-death/overview

Ministry of Justice, Coroners Team:
http://www.justice.gov.uk/coroners-burial-cremation

Ministry of Justice, Coroners' Guides
https://www.gov.uk/government/publications/guide-to-coroner-services-and-coroner-investigations-a-short-guide (general guide)
also
http://www.justice.gov.uk/coroners-burial-cremation/coroners/rule-43 (prevention of future death reports)

Other Ministry of Justice guidance:
http://www.justice.gov.uk/coroners-burial-cremation/burials
http://www.justice.gov.uk/coroners-burial-cremation/cremation
http://www.justice.gov.uk/coroners-burial-cremation/flu-pandemic
http://www.justice.gov.uk/coroners-burial-cremation/richard-III

Coroner statistics
https://www.gov.uk/government/collections/coroners-and-burials-statistics

Department of Health
https://www.gov.uk/government/organisations/department-of-health

Public Health England
https://www.gov.uk/government/organisations/public-health-england

Human Tissue Authority
http://www.hta.gov.uk/

Maritime and Coastguard Agency
https://www.gov.uk/government/organisations/maritime-and-coastguard-agency

Deaths abroad:
https://www.gov.uk/government/uploads/system/uploads/attachment_data/file/193657/Death_Overseas_web_13.pdf

Public Record Office (The National Archives)
http://www.nationalarchives.gov.uk/

AMBULANCE SERVICES

London Ambulance Service:
http://www.londonambulance.nhs.uk/

Scottish Ambulance Service:
http://www.scottishambulance.com/

Welsh Ambulance Service:
http://www.ambulance.wales.nhs.uk/

West Midlands Ambulance Service:
http://www.wmas.nhs.uk/Pages/default.aspx

East Midlands Ambulance Service:
http://www.emas.nhs.uk/

North West Ambulance Service:
http://www.nwas.nhs.uk/

North East Ambulance Service:
http://www.neas.nhs.uk/

South Central Ambulance Service:
http://www.southcentralambulance.nhs.uk/

South East Coast Ambulance Service:
http://www.southcentralambulance.nhs.uk/

East of England Ambulance Service:
http://www.eastamb.nhs.uk/

South West Ambulance Service:
http://www.swast.nhs.uk/

Yorkshire Ambulance Service:
http://www.yas.nhs.uk/

Northern Ireland Ambulance Service:
http://www.niamb.co.uk/

LAWYERS

INQUEST Lawyers Group:
http://www.inquest.org.uk/ilg/home

Bar Pro Bono Unit:
http://www.barprobono.org.uk/

PRISONS

National Offender Management Service:
https://www.gov.uk/government/organisations/national-offender-management-service

National Probation Service:
http://www.justice.gov.uk/offenders/probationservice

Prisons and Probation Ombudsman:
http://www.ppo.gov.uk

Independent Advisory Panel on Deaths in Custody:
http://iapdeathsincustody.independent.gov.uk/

TREASURE

Portable Antiquities Scheme:
http://finds.org.uk/

Treasure:
http://finds.org.uk/treasure/advice/summary

Code of Practice:
http://finds.org.uk/documents/treasure_act.pdf

National Council for Metal Detecting:
http://www.ncmd.co.uk/

OTHER INVESTIGATIVE BODIES

Independent Police Complaints Commission:
http://www.ipcc.gov.uk

Health and Safety Executive:
http://www.hse.gov.uk/index.htm

Prisons and Probation Ombudsman:
http://www.ppo.gov.uk

Care Quality Commission:
http://www.cqc.org.uk

Air Accidents Investigation Branch:
http://www.aaib.gov.uk/home/index.cfm

Marine Accident Investigation Branch:
http://www.maib.gov.uk/home/index.cfm

Rail Accident Investigation Branch:
http://www.raib.gov.uk/home/index.cfm

Medicines and Healthcare Products Regulatory Authority (Regulating Medicines and Medical Devices):
http://www.mhra.gov.uk

RELEVANT CHARITIES

INQUEST (a charity providing free advice to people bereaved by a death in custody):
http://www.inquest.org.uk

Cardiac Risk in the Young:
http://www.c-r-y.org.uk

Child Bereavement UK:
http://www.childbereavementuk.org

Foundation for Study into Infant Deaths (FSID) since rebranded as the Lullaby Trust:
http://www.lullabytrust.org.uk

MIND:
http://www.mind.org.uk/

COURTS AND TRIBUNALS

HM Courts and Tribunals Service:
http://www.justice.gov.uk/about/hmcts/

Mental Health Review Tribunals:
http://www.justice.gov.uk/tribunals/mental-health

HEALTH PROFESSIONALS

General Medical Council:
http://www.gmc-uk.org

The Nursing and Midwifery Council:
http://www.nmc-uk.org

Academy of Medical Royal Colleges:
http://www.aomrc.org.uk

Health and Care Professions Council:
http://www.hpc-uk.org

OTHER HEALTH ORGANISATIONS

National Institute for Health and Care Excellence:
http://www.nice.org.uk

National Treatment Agency for Substance Misuse (part of Public Health England):
http://www.nta.nhs.uk

National Confidential Enquiry into Patient Outcome and Deaths:
http://www.ncepod.org.uk

Healthcare Quality Improvement Partnership:
http://www.hqip.org.uk

MBRRACE-UK – UK Mothers and Babies – Confidential Enquiries Reports:
https://www.npeu.ox.ac.uk/mbrrace-uk

DEATHS ABROAD

General:
https://www.gov.uk/government/uploads/system/uploads/attachment_data/file/
193657/Death_Overseas_web_13.pdf

Memorandum of Understanding between the Foreign Office, ACPO and Coroners' Society
regarding homicide abroad:
https://www.gov.uk/government/uploads/system/uploads/attachment_data/file/
141958/mou-fco-acpo-coroners.pdf

INDEX

INDEX

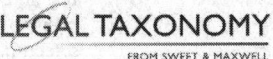

This index has been prepared using Sweet and Maxwell's Legal Taxonomy. Main index entries conform to keywords provided by the Legal Taxonomy except where references to specific documents or non-standard terms (denoted by quotation marks) have been included. These keywords provide a means of identifying similar concepts in other Sweet & Maxwell publications and online services to which keywords from the Legal Taxonomy have been applied. Readers may find some minor differences between terms used in the text and those which appear in the index. Suggestions to *sweet-andmaxwell.taxonomy@thomson.com*.

(All references are to paragraph number)